LEARNSMART® >

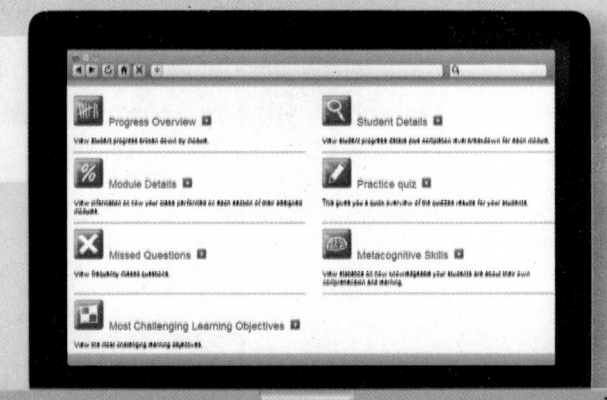

The market-leading **adaptive study tool** proven to strengthen memory recall, increase class retention, and boost grades.

> Moves students beyond memorizing

> Allows instructors to align content with their goals

> Allows instructors to spend more time teaching higher-level concepts

SMARTBOOK® >

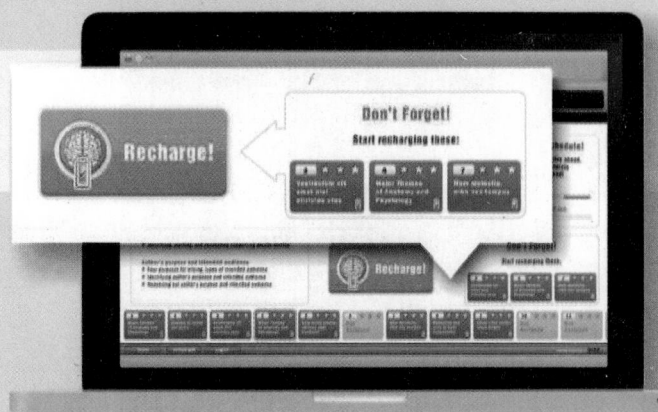

The first—and only—adaptive reading experience designed to transform the way students read.

> Engages students with a personalized reading experience

> Ensures students retain knowledge

LEARNSMART
PREP®

An adaptive course preparation tool that quickly and efficiently helps students prepare for college-level work.

> Levels out student knowledge

> Keeps students on track

LEARNSMART
ACHIEVE®

A learning system that continually adapts and provides learning tools to teach students the concepts they don't know.

> Adaptively provides learning resources

> A time management feature ensures students master course material to complete their assignments by the due date

Human Nutrition:
Science for Healthy Living Updated with 2015-2020 *Dietary Guidelines for Americans*

Tammy J. Stephenson PhD
University of Kentucky

Wendy J. Schiff MS, RDN

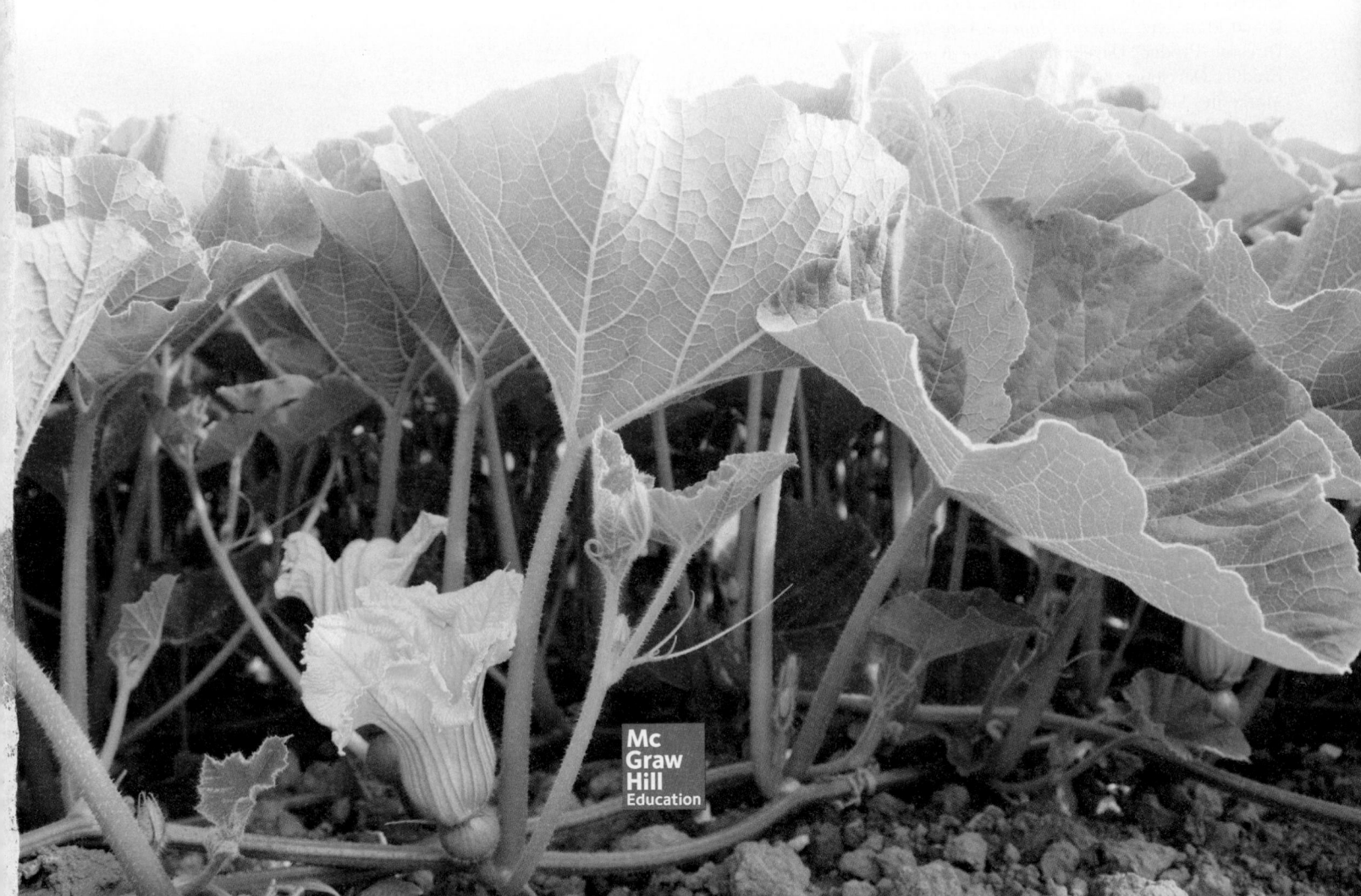

McGraw Hill Education

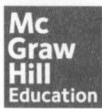

HUMAN NUTRITION: SCIENCE FOR HEALTHY LIVING Updated with *2015–2020 Dietary Guidelines for Americans*

Published by McGraw–Hill Education, 2 Penn Plaza, New York, NY 10121. Copyright © 2016 by McGraw–Hill Education. All rights reserved. Printed in the United States of America. No part of this publication may be reproduced or distributed in any form or by any means, or stored in a database or retrieval system, without the prior written consent of McGraw–Hill Education, including, but not limited to, in any network or other electronic storage or transmission, or broadcast for distance learning.

Some ancillaries, including electronic and print components, may not be available to customers outside the United States.

This book is printed on acid–free paper.

1 2 3 4 5 6 7 8 9 DOW 21 20 19 18 17 16

ISBN 978–1–259–91683–0
MHID 1–259–91683–9

Senior Vice President, Products & Markets: *Kurt L. Strand*
Vice President, General Manager, Products & Markets: *Marty Lange*
Vice President, Content Design & Delivery: *Kimberly Meriwether David*
Managing Director: *Michael S. Hackett*
Director of Digital Content: *Michael G. Koot, PhD*
Brand Managers: *Marija Magner/Amy Reed*
Director, Product Development: *Rose Koos*
Product Developer: *Darlene Schueller*
Marketing Manager: *Kristine Rellihan*
Digital Product Analyst: *Christine Carlson*
Director, Content Design & Delivery: *Linda Avenarius*
Program Manager: *Angela R. FitzPatrick*
Content Project Managers: *Mary Jane Lampe/Brent Dela Cruz*
Buyer: *Jennifer Pickel*
Designers: *Michelle D. Whitaker/Matt Backhaus*
Content Licensing Specialists: *Lori Hancock (images)/Lorraine Buczek (text)*
Cover Image: *©237/Anthony Lee/Ocean/Corbis/RF*
Compositor: *SPi Global*
Printer: *R. R. Donnelley*

All credits appearing on page or at the end of the book are considered to be an extension of the copyright page.

Library of Congress Cataloging–in–Publication Data

Names: Stephenson, Tammy J. | Schiff, Wendy.
Title: Human nutrition: science for healthy living / Tammy J. Stephenson, Ph.D.,
   Wendy J. Schiff, M.S., R.D.FPO.
Description: Updated with 2015–2020 dietary guidelines for Americans. | New York, NY:
   McGraw–Hill Education, c2016. | Includes index.
Identifiers: LCCN 2016008800 | ISBN 9781259916830 (alk. paper)
Subjects: LCSH: Human nutrition—Textbooks.
Classification: LCC QP141 .S647 2016b | DDC 612.3—dc23
LC record available at https://lccn.loc.gov/2016008800

The Internet addresses listed in the text were accurate at the time of publication. The inclusion of a website or photo or mention of a specific product does not indicate an endorsement by the authors or McGraw–Hill Education, and McGraw–Hill Education does not guarantee the accuracy of the information presented at these sites.

www.mhhe.com

About the Authors

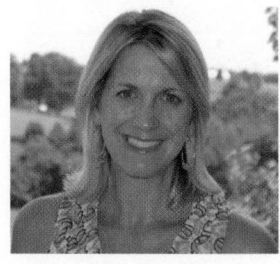

Tammy J. Stephenson, PhD, received her BS in Food Science and Human Nutrition and PhD in Nutritional Sciences from the University of Kentucky. She has taught a wide variety of food, nutrition, and wellness courses, including introductory nutrition, to majors and nonmajors in the Department of Dietetics and Human Nutrition at the University of Kentucky for the past 15 years. Dr. Stephenson is an active member of the Academy of Nutrition and Dietetics, serving as Chair of the Nutrition Educators of Health Professionals practice group. She has published and presented on service learning, technology in teaching, student–centered learning, and other related topics. Dr. Stephenson has a passion for teaching engaging, interesting, and relevant nutrition courses that has been recognized through multiple teaching and mentoring awards at the university, state, and national levels. Outside of the classroom, she enjoys running, yoga, coaching youth soccer, gardening, cooking, and spending time with her family.

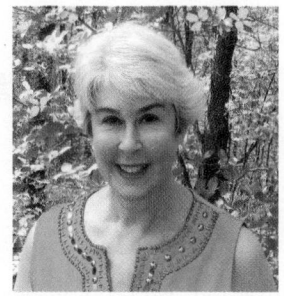

Wendy J. Schiff, MS, RDN, received her BS in Biological Health/Medical Dietetics and MS in Human Nutrition from The Pennsylvania State University. She has taught introductory food and nutrition courses at the University of Missouri–Columbia as well as nutrition, biology, and personal health courses at St. Louis Community College–Meramec. She has worked as a public health nutritionist at the Allegheny County Health Department (Pittsburgh, Pennsylvania) and State Food and Nutrition Specialist for Missouri Extension at Lincoln University in Jefferson City, Missouri. In addition to coauthoring *Human Nutrition: Science for Healthy Living*, Wendy has authored *Nutrition for Healthy Living* and *Nutrition Essentials: A Personal Approach*. She is a registered dietitian nutritionist and member of the Academy of Nutrition and Dietetics.

Welcome to Human Nutrition: Science for Healthy Living Updated with the 2015-2020 *Dietary Guidelines for Americans*

Dear Students,

Welcome to the study of human nutrition! Before you begin your studies, it is important to understand that nutrition is a science that draws upon knowledge from other sciences, particularly biology, human anatomy and physiology, general chemistry, and biological chemistry. The science of human nutrition also involves learning scientific information about foods and nutrition, and how this information is used to develop dietary recommendations for healthy people and nutritional therapies for those who are not healthy. By understanding the contents of this introductory nutrition textbook, you will recognize the effects that peoples' food choices can have on their health. In addition, you will appreciate the valuable role that registered dietitian nutritionists (RDNs) play as members of the health care team and be well prepared to take more advanced human nutrition courses, if you decide to become a dietitian.

Human Nutrition: Science for Healthy Living has been developed by a team of nutrition educators who have extensive college teaching experience and a passion for teaching relevant, student—centered nutrition, foods, health, and wellness courses. Our overall goal is to prepare you for your career in a health care discipline, and we want you to enjoy your introductory study of human nutrition. Learning about any science can be challenging if the information is not presented in an appealing, interesting manner. We've made a distinct effort to write the content of this book in an understandable way and to provide clear descriptions of concepts that can be difficult to convey, such as the processes of digestion, absorption, and energy metabolism. To enhance your learning, numerous meaningful illustrations and photographs accompany the narrative. Such graphics facilitate learning for all students, but especially for those who are "visual learners." By reviewing pages xv—xxiv of this Preface, you will learn about the features of this book and how to use them to facilitate your study of human nutrition.

We hope you will enjoy using this textbook!

Tammy J. Stephenson

Wendy J. Schiff

Brief Contents

Contents

Preface

Tammy Stephenson and Wendy Schiff had a vision of writing an interesting, engaging, and evidence–based introductory nutrition textbook that has a wide variety of pedagogical features to promote active learning. To that end, this updated edition of *Human Nutrition: Science for Healthy Living* is learner–centered, easy to read, and richly illustrated with figures that clearly show physiological processes. Furthermore, the author team felt students and faculty would appreciate a textbook that was clinically oriented and provided ample opportunities for students to practice using their nutrition knowledge and critical thinking skills. *Human Nutrition: Science for Healthy Living* is the result of Tammy and Wendy's efforts.

The clinical emphasis of the textbook is of particular relevance to those studying nutrition, dietetics, or other health science professions, including nursing. Specific real–life examples, current statistics, and scientific evidence from professional resources are provided to support nutrition concepts. Features designed to attract students' interest, such as *Did You Know?* and *Fresh Tips* boxes, provide up–to–date information on current and sometimes controversial topics, as well as practical recommendations for everyday healthy living.

Human Nutrition: Science for Healthy Living provides the framework for students to *learn* how nutrition information is often interrelated and to *apply* the science of nutrition to clinical situations. Furthermore, students can use their foods and nutrition knowledge throughout their lives.

Features Designed Around Student-Centered Learning

Human Nutrition: Science for Healthy Living was written by authors who have extensive experience teaching introductory nutrition classes to both majors and nonmajors. The authors recognize the diverse learning needs of today's students and how the modern learning environment in higher education—large lecture classes, online classes, and flipped/hybrid classrooms—often challenge even the most experienced nutrition educators. The textbook and its supportive interactive materials are designed to help instructors create a learner–centered teaching environment that maximizes student engagement and knowledge acquisition. This current, evidence–based introductory textbook has a wide variety of pedagogical features to promote active learning among students.

What's New in This Updated Edition?

This version of *Human Nutrition: Science for Healthy Living* has incorporated information from the *2015–2020 Dietary Guidelines for Americans*.

Chapter 3, Section 3.4:

- Highlights the five overarching guidelines that recommend basic food– and nutrition–related practices for consumers, such as "Focus on variety, nutrient density, and amount of food" and "Shift to healthier food and beverage choices."
- Presents the components of a healthy eating pattern, according to the new Dietary Guidelines.
- Identifies "nutrients of public health concern," according to the 2015–2020 edition of the Dietary Guidelines.
- Includes some practical recommendations of the new guidelines, such as: "Choose a variety of protein foods, including dried beans and peas." and "Caffeine consumption should be limited to less than 400 mg/day..."
- Suggests limits for alcohol consumption among adults who drink alcohol–containing beverages.
- Provides recommendations for fish consumption, including for women who are pregnant or breastfeeding.
- Has a revised Table 3.10, which helps support the updated narrative by listing the overarching guidelines.
- Includes a new "Did You Know?" box, which briefly explains the process that led to the publication of the 8th edition of the Dietary Guidelines.

Chapter 3, Section 3.5:

- Provides information concerning changes the USDA made to ChooseMyPlate.gov that reflect the new Dietary Guidelines.
- Lists leading sources of empty calories in American diets.

Additionally, specific information from the *2015–2020 Dietary Guidelines for Americans* has been woven into other chapters to update them. For example:

- Chapter 5 mentions the importance of consuming foods that supply dietary fiber (a nutrient of public health concern) and the need to limit intakes of foods and beverages that contain added sugars.
- Chapter 6 presents the new recommendation for dietary cholesterol intake ("as low as possible").
- Chapter 9 identifies vitamin D as a nutrient of public health concern.
- Chapter 11 states the maximum daily limit for sodium intake and identifies calcium and potassium as nutrients of public health concern.
- Chapter 12 identifies iron as a nutrient of public health concern for pregnant women.

Features

Case Study—Each chapter begins with a case study addressing a realistic scenario. These high–interest scenarios engage the student by showing how the chapter's content is relevant to their future professions and can be utilized in a practical or clinical situation. Students are encouraged to consider the case study as they study the chapter. A suggested **Case Study Response** is provided at the end of the chapter to allow students to self–assess their understanding of the material and its applications.

5 Carbohydrates:
Sugars, Starches, and Fiber

CASE STUDY
Carbohydrates for breakfast?

JERRY IS A GRADUATE STUDENT WORKING on his doctorate. Two months ago, Jerry read an article posted on an Internet website about the importance of limiting intakes of carbohydrates, particularly at breakfast. Since reading the article, Jerry has consumed only a fried egg, three pieces of bacon, and a glass of water for breakfast. He also avoids eating carbohydrate-containing foods at other meals. Although Jerry does not need to lose weight, he does have a family history of type 2 diabetes.

- Describe to Jerry the different categories of carbohydrates and how each of these classes may influence his health.
- Provide Jerry with two examples of breakfasts that incorporate healthy, nutrient-dense carbohydrates.
- Explain to Jerry why eating carbohydrates does not necessarily cause diabetes.

The suggested Case Study Response can be found on page 142.

connect | NUTRITION   Check out the Connect site at www.mcgrawhillconnect.com to further explore this case study.

QUIZ Yourself

Would sweetening cereal with honey be a healthier choice than using table sugar? Is fiber good for one's health? Check your knowledge of carbohydrates by taking the following quiz. The answers are found on page 146.

1. The carbohydrate found in milk is called lactose. _T _F
2. Ounce per ounce, sugar provides more energy than starch. _T _F
3. Digestion of starch begins in the mouth. _T _F
4. Eating a high-fiber diet can improve the functioning of the large intestine and reduce blood cholesterol levels. _T _F
5. Individuals with diabetes should follow a carbohydrate-free diet. _T _F

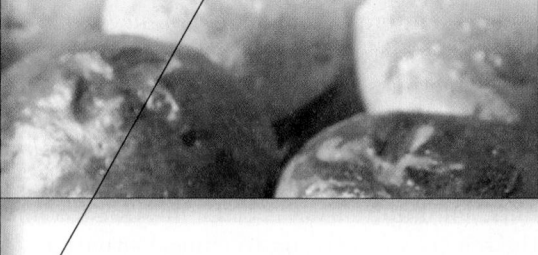

CASE STUDY RESPONSE

CARBOHYDRATES FOR BREAKFAST?

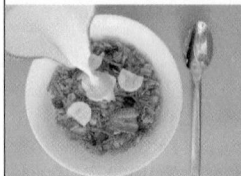

MANY AMERICANS CONSUME EXCESSIVE AMOUNTS of sucrose. Eating sugary foods can cause one's blood glucose concentration to rise rapidly and then drop quickly. By replacing simple sugars with oligosaccharides and polysaccharides, a person may reduce his or her risk of developing serious chronic diseases, particularly obesity and type 2 diabetes.

Jerry should focus on eating foods that are rich sources of complex carbohydrates, particularly dietary fiber. Nutrient-dense, carbohydrate-rich breakfast options include:

- Low-fat yogurt mixed with fresh berries, granola, and nuts
- "Quick-cooking" oatmeal mixed with berries, raisins, and nuts
- Whole-grain, ready-to-eat cereal with fresh fruit and low-fat milk
- Whole-grain waffles or pancakes sprinkled with wheat germ and topped with fresh fruit

Results of scientific studies indicate that carbohydrates as a nutrient category are not a direct cause of diabetes. Consuming too much of any digestible macronutrient and excessive weight gain can contribute to one's risk of developing type 2 diabetes.

Quiz Yourself—This pretest, which is next to the Case Study, stimulates interest in reading the chapter. By taking the quiz, students may be surprised to learn how little or how much they know about the chapter's contents.

Learning Outcomes—Each major section of a chapter opens with a list of learning outcomes. The Learning Outcomes help students prepare for reading the section and also clarify major concepts they are expected to learn. These measurable outcomes are further supported by assessment methods and study aids found within the chapters and within McGraw–Hill Education's Connect®.

3.5 Food Guides for Dietary Planning

LEARNING OUTCOMES

1. *Explain how to use MyPlate to develop nutritionally adequate daily menus for healthy adults and children.*
2. *Describe educational resources available at www.choosemyplate.gov.*
3. *Identify tools people with diabetes can use for diet planning.*

Assess Your Progress—These review questions, which appear at the end of each major section within a chapter, apply to the section's learning outcomes and often involve critical thinking skills. Such questions enable students to test their knowledge and understanding of information provided within that section.

Fresh Tips—These practical suggestions help students apply the chapter's content to their current situations. The *Fresh Tips* are also valuable for future health care professionals who want to provide useful health, food, and nutrition advice to their clients. Such features include tips for including more seafood in diets, maintaining a healthy body weight, preventing choking in children, and keeping foods safe to eat.

FRESH TIPS

- Eat seafood, especially fatty fish, two times a week. Before cooking, marinate fresh fish in olive or canola oil that has been seasoned with a small amount of garlic, pepper, and lemon juice. The light coating of oil on fish can help keep the fish from drying out during cooking.
- Bake, grill, or broil fish.
- Add drained, water-packed tuna to salads, or mix the tuna with a little olive oil and pickle relish, and spread on whole-wheat toast.
- When olive oil is not desired, use canola oil, soybean oil, or soft margarines made from these oils for frying or sautéing.
- Sprinkle chopped walnuts on salads, yogurt, or cereal, or eat the nuts as a snack.

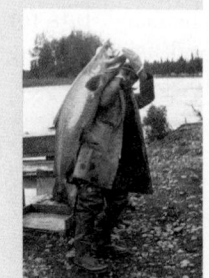

A fisherman in Kenai, Alaska, carrying a king salmon. Alaskans consume significantly more omega-3 fatty acids than the general U.S. population.

DID **YOU** KNOW?

Medical researchers have limited animal models to use for studying the disease *diabetes mellitus* ("diabetes"). Scientists at the National Marine Mammal Foundation in San Diego are investigating the bottlenose dolphin as an animal model for diabetes research. These dolphins can develop diabetes. Rather than conduct research on dolphins in a laboratory setting, researchers perform tests on the animals' blood and urine samples to determine possible links with the human form of the disease.[3] Chapter 5 provides more information about diabetes.

Did You Know?—This feature presents bits of information concerning topics that support the chapter's content and are of interest to introductory nutrition students. Some of these features dispel beliefs about food and nutrition that are commonly held but inaccurate, such as "stick" margarine being more fattening than butter. Other "Did You Know" features report results of current and unusual areas of research, such as how certain dolphins are used to study diabetes in humans.

Real People, Real Stories—This unique feature provides information about real people, many of whom are college students who have recovered from or are currently living with nutrition—related conditions. Such conditions include PKU, celiac disease, type 1 diabetes, eating disorders, smell disorders, and hypertension. This feature is designed to help students recognize the daily challenges faced by people with such conditions and the roles that diet and physical activity play in managing one's health.

REAL People, **REAL** Stories

Dallas Clasen

Dallas Clasen is majoring in engineering at the University of Wisconsin–Platteville. In addition to keeping up with his coursework, he runs cross country at school and participates in triathlons. Like most college students, Dallas is very busy, but unlike most students, he has to pay very close attention to his diet. Dallas was born with a rare inherited metabolic disorder called phenylketonuria (PKU).

A few days after birth, Dallas underwent standard newborn blood testing. The results of the test indicated that the level of phenylalanine in his blood was about 40 times higher than the normal amount, a sign of PKU. To avoid developing severe brain damage and

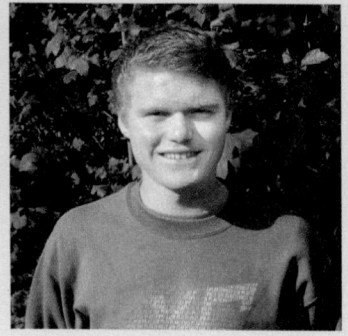

Test Kitchen: Modifying Recipes for Healthy Living—This unique feature provides students with the opportunity to apply nutrition and food information to situations that commonly arise in clinical settings. Students modify an existing recipe to make it healthier, using information they have learned in each chapter. This feature allows students to experiment with recipe modifications, such as substituting "healthy" fats for "unhealthy" ones and using less sugar and salt in recipes.

TEST KITCHEN

Modifying Recipes for Healthy Living

For this activity, compare the ingredients in a serving of a commercial energy drink to a serving of a smoothie that you can make at home. Then, answer the following questions.

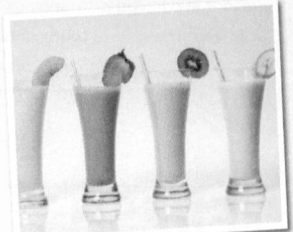

Commercial Energy Drink			High-Caliber Smoothie†		
Ingredients		kcal	Ingredients		kcal
Water	12 oz	0	Nonfat milk	1 cup (8 oz)	80
Sucrose	1 Tbsp	120	Nonfat plain yogurt	¼ cup	35
Glucose	1 tsp	40	Frozen raspberries, unsweetened	¼ cup	30
Caffeine	100 mg		Frozen blueberries, unsweetened	¼ cup	20
B vitamins*			Banana	1 medium	100
Niacin	20 mg				
B-6	1.5 mg				
B-12	2.5 µg				
Pantothenic acid	10 mg				
Total kcal:		160	Total kcal:		265

*All amounts at least 100% of RDA
†To make the smoothie, combine all ingredients and blend until smooth.

1. What are the sources of energy in the two drinks?
2. Not long after the drinks are consumed, blood sugar levels begin to rise. which stimulates the pancreas to release insulin. Assume the person consuming the commercial energy drink does not need the calories from the beverage for energy. In this situation, what effect would the insulin have on the body?
3. Which drink is a healthier source of energy? Explain your choice of drinks.

PERSONAL Dietary Analysis

1. Refer to your 3-day food log from the "Personal Dietary Analysis" feature in Chapter 5.

    a. Find the RDA/AI values for minerals under your life stage/sex group category in the DRI tables (see the last pages of this book). Write those values under the "My RDA/AI" column in the table below.

    b. Review your personal dietary assessment. Find your 3-day average intakes of iron, iodine, zinc, selenium, fluoride, and chromium. Write those values under the "My Average Intake" column of the table.

    c. Calculate the percentage of the RDA/AI you consumed for each mineral by dividing your intake by the RDA/AI amount and multiplying the figure you obtain by 100. For example, if your average intake of iron was 9 mg/day and your RDA for the mineral is 18 mg, you would divide 18 mg by 9 mg to obtain .50. To multiply this figure by 100, simply move the decimal point two places to the right, and replace the decimal point with a percentage sign (50%). Thus, your average daily intake of iron was 50% of the RDA. Place the percentages for each mineral under the "% of My RDA/AI" column.

    d. Under the ">, <, or =" column, indicate whether your average daily intake was greater than (>), less than (<), or equal to (=) the RDA/AI.

2. Use the information you calculated in the first part of this activity to answer the following questions:

    a. Which of your average trace mineral intakes equaled or exceeded the RDA/AI? If one or more were above the RDA/AI, what is a possible consequence of the overconsumption? _____

    b. Which of your average trace mineral intakes was below the RDA/AI? _____

    c. What foods would you eat to increase your intake of the minerals that was less than the RDA/AI levels? (Review sources of the minerals in this chapter.) _____

Personal Dietary Analysis: Trace Minerals

Mineral	My RDA/AI	My Average Intake	% of My RDA/AI	>, <, or =
Iron				
Iodine				
Zinc				
Selenium				
Fluoride				
Chromium				

connect
|NUTRITION

Complete the Personal Dietary Analysis activity online at www.mcgrawhillconnect.com, where you will also find McGraw-Hill LearnSmart®, SmartBook®, NutritionCalc Plus, and many other dynamic learning tools.

Personal Dietary Analysis—Students can gain insight into their eating habits by completing this activity. Many of these activities can be completed with the use of a dietary analysis software program, such as McGraw—Hill's NutritionCalc Plus.

End of Chapter—Each chapter ends with:

- a bulleted chapter Summary;
- Critical Thinking questions that involve higher–level cognition skills, including applying, analyzing, synthesizing, and evaluating information;
- a series of multiple–choice Practice Test questions that assess students' comprehension and recall of information presented in the chapter; and
- References.

SUMMARY

SECTION 12.1 What Is a Trace Mineral?

- Trace minerals are essential nutrients required in very small amounts, generally less than 100 mg/day. Trace minerals include iron, iodine, zinc, selenium, fluoride, chromium, copper, manganese, molybdenum and possibly, some other minerals.

SECTION 12.2 Iron

- Iron plays a critical role in oxygen delivery for energy metabolism as part of hemoglobin and myoglobin.
- Dietary iron can be found in two forms, heme and nonheme. The intestinal tract absorbs more of the heme iron than nonheme iron in foods. Naturally occurring components of plant foods, such as phytates and polyphenols, reduce iron absorption.
- Serum ferritin concentrations are the most common method of assessing iron status. Total body iron can be measured by calculating the ratio of blood transferrin receptor to ferritin.
- Iron deficiency occurs in three stages. Iron deficiency anemia has widespread negative effects on the body. Excess iron in the blood acts as an oxidant and causes damage to cell membranes, proteins, and DNA. Iron overload occurs when toxic amounts of iron supplements are ingested, but the condition also results from certain genetic conditions.

SECTION 12.3 Iodine (Iodide)

- Adequate iodine is essential to form thyroid hormone. Major dietary sources of iodine include saltwater fish, seafood, seaweed, and iodized salt.
- Most Americans have adequate iodine intakes. Needs for iodine increase for pregnant and lactating women. Both deficiency and toxicity in iodine causes goiter and hypothyroidism. Infants of iodine-deficient women are likely to be born with cretinism.

SECTION 12.4

- Zinc is importa
  healing, the se

Critical Thinking

1. Identify at least six factors that influence your food and beverage selections. Which of these factors is the most important? Explain why.
2. Analyze your current eating habits. Based on your analysis, is your diet nutritionally adequate? Explain why your diet is or is not nutritionally adequate.
3. "Everything in moderation." Explain what this statement means in terms of your diet.
4. Consider your parents' and grandparents' health (or causes of death). Based on your family history, which chronic health conditions do you have a higher than average risk of developing? If you were at risk of developing a chronic health condition that could be prevented by changing your diet, would you make the necessary changes at this stage of your life? Explain why or why not.
5. Eric spends about $100 each month on purchases of dietary supplements, including protein powders, vitamin pills, and herbal extracts. He thinks it is necessary to take the products to achieve optimal health and prevent chronic illnesses. Based on the information in this chapter, what would you tell Eric about his use of the supplements?

Practice Test

Select the best answer.

1. Diet is a
   a. practice of restricting energy intake.
   b. usual pattern of food choices.
   c. method of reducing portion sizes.
   d. technique to reduce carbohydrate intake.

8. Which of the following conditions is a chronic disease?
   a. heart disease   c. scurvy
   b. common cold   d. influenza

9. In the United States, the primary cause of preventable cancer deaths is
   a. physical inactivity.   c. high-fat diet.

References

1. Linus Pauling Institute Micronutrient Information Center: *Iron.* Last modified April 2009. http://lpi.oregonstate.edu/infocenter/minerals/iron/ Accessed: February 12, 2014.
2. Office of Dietary Supplements, National Institutes of Health: *Dietary supplement fact sheet: Iron.* Updated August 2007. http://ods.od.nih.gov/factsheets/Iron-HealthProfessional/ Accessed: February 12, 2014.
3. Food and Nutrition Board: *Dietary Reference Intakes for vitamin A, vitamin K, arsenic, boron, chromium, copper, iodine, iron, manganese, molybdenum, nickel, silicon, vanadium, and zinc.* Washington, DC: National Academy Press, 2000.
4. Korus A and others: Effect of different technological and culinary treatments on iron retention, nutritional density and recommended dietary intake in fourteen vegetable species. *International Journal of Food Science and Technology* 47:1882, 2012
5. Collings R and others: The absorption of iron from whole diets: A systematic review. *American Journal of Clinical Nutrition* 98:65, 2013.
6. U.S. Department of Agriculture, Agricultural Research Service: Nutrient intakes from food and beverages: Mean amounts consumed per individual, by gender and age, in the United States, 2011-2012, 2014. http://www.ars.usda.gov/Services/docs.htm?docid=18349. Accessed: November 4, 2014.

21. Evans JR, Lawrenson JG: Antioxidant vitamin and mineral supplements for preventing age-related macular degeneration. *Cochrane Database System Reviews* 6:1, 2012.
22. Office of Dietary Supplements, National Institutes of Health: *Selenium.* Updated July 2013. http://ods.od.nih.gov/factsheets/Selenium-HealthProfessional/ Accessed: February 12, 2014.
23. Linus Pauling Institute Micronutrient Information Center: *Selenium.* Last updated January 2009. http://lpi.oregonstate.edu/infocenter/minerals/selenium/ Accessed: February 12, 2014.
24. Berr C and others: Selenium and cognitive impairment: A brief review based on results from the EVA study. *Biofactors* 38(2):139, 2012.
25. Linus Pauling Institute Micronutrient Information Center: *Fluoride.* Last reviewed January 2014. http://lpi.oregonstate.edu/infocenter/minerals/fluoride/ Accessed: February 12, 2014.
26. Centers for Disease Control and Prevention: *2012 water fluoridation statistics.* 2013. http://www.cdc.gov/fluoridation/statistics/2012stats.htm Accessed: April 20, 2014.
27. U.S. Department of Health and Human Services: *Healthy people 2020: Nutrition and weight status.* Last updated 2013. http://www.healthypeople.gov/2020/

Artwork That Enhances Learning

Dimensional, full–color illustrations, some with numbered labels and explanatory text, help teach and/or show the progression of a complicated concept.

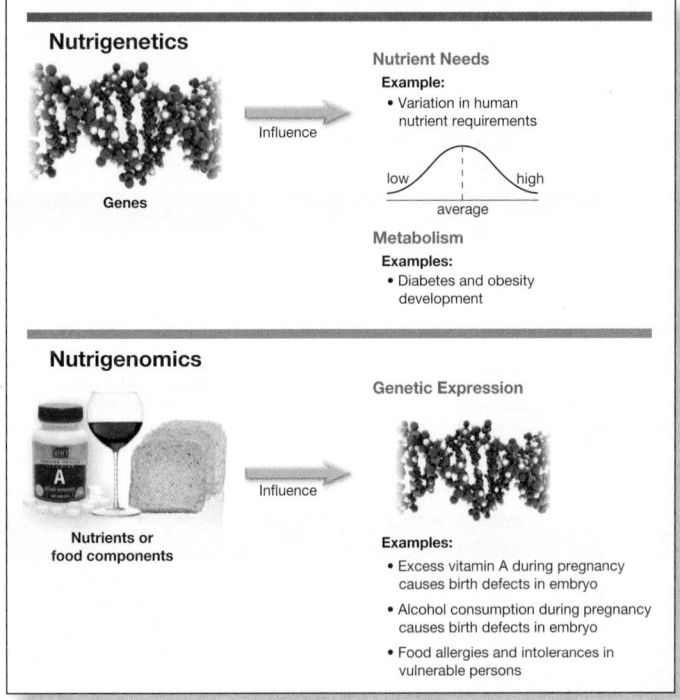

FIGURE 7.22 Nutritional genomics.

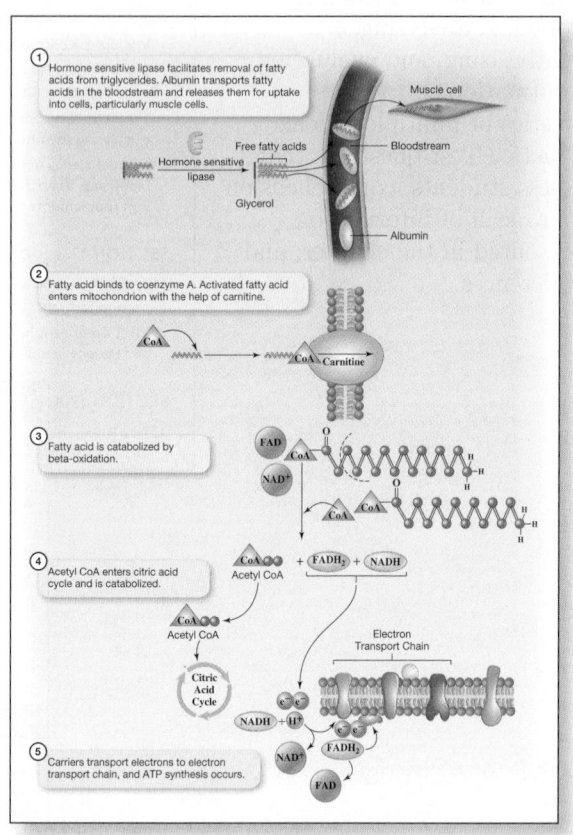

FIGURE 8.27 Summary of fat catabolism.

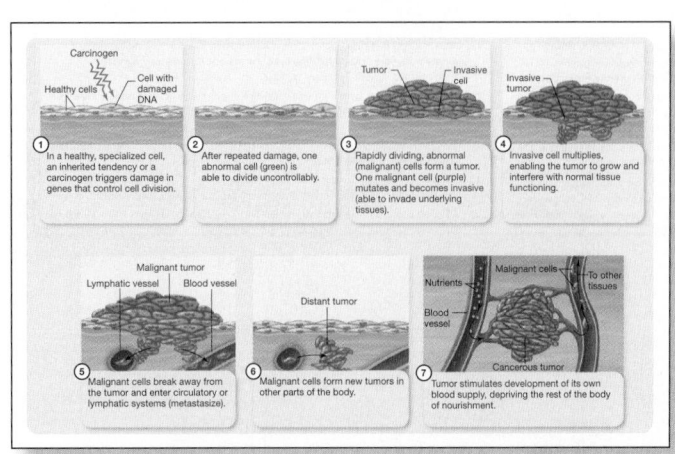

FIGURE 10.15 Cancer development and progression. Several steps are involved as a normal cell progresses into a cancer cell that multiplies out of control.

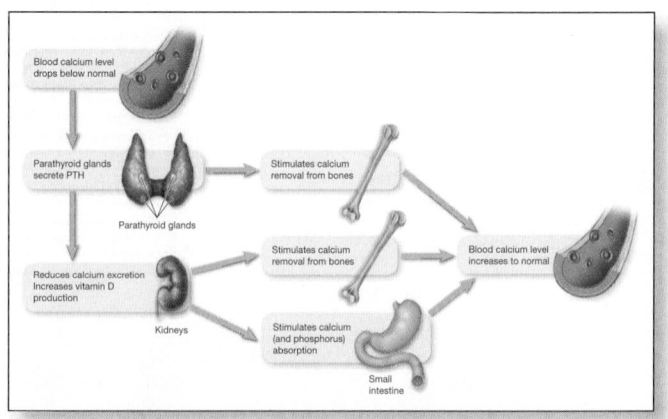

FIGURE 9.16 Maintaining normal blood calcium levels. When the level of calcium in blood drops below normal, a variety of complex physiological responses help raise the level to normal.

Numerous high—quality photos support the text and provide examples of nutrition—related medical conditions as well as microscopic views of clinical cases from the human body.

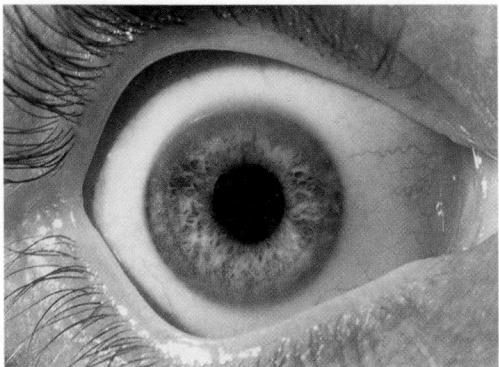

FIGURE 12.11 Kayser-Fleischer ring.

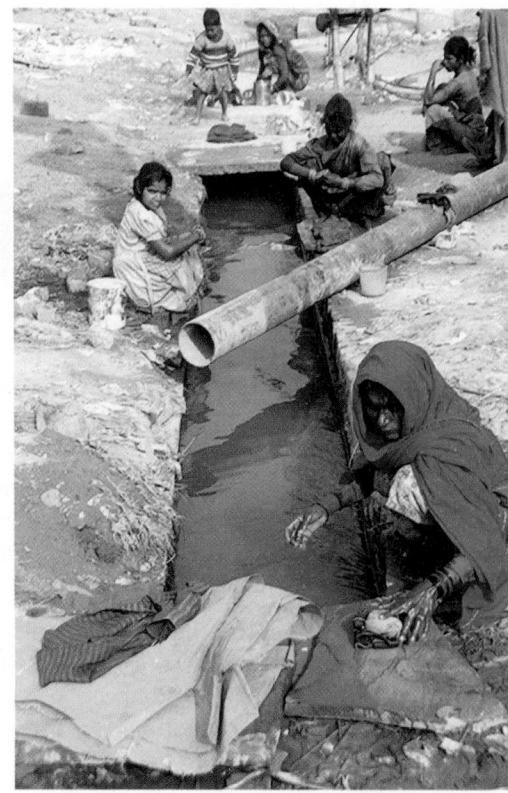

In developing countries, poor sanitation practices and lack of clean cooking and drinking water contribute to the spread of diseases.

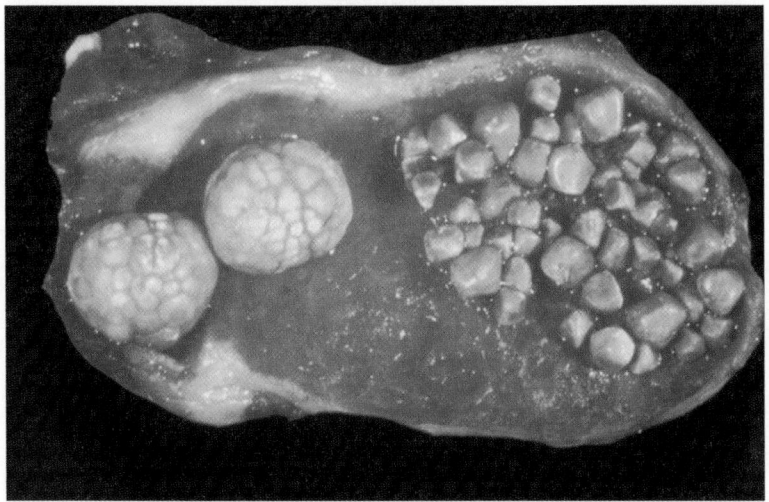

FIGURE 6.16 Gallstones. Gallstones can form in the gallbladder. The stones usually consist of cholesterol.

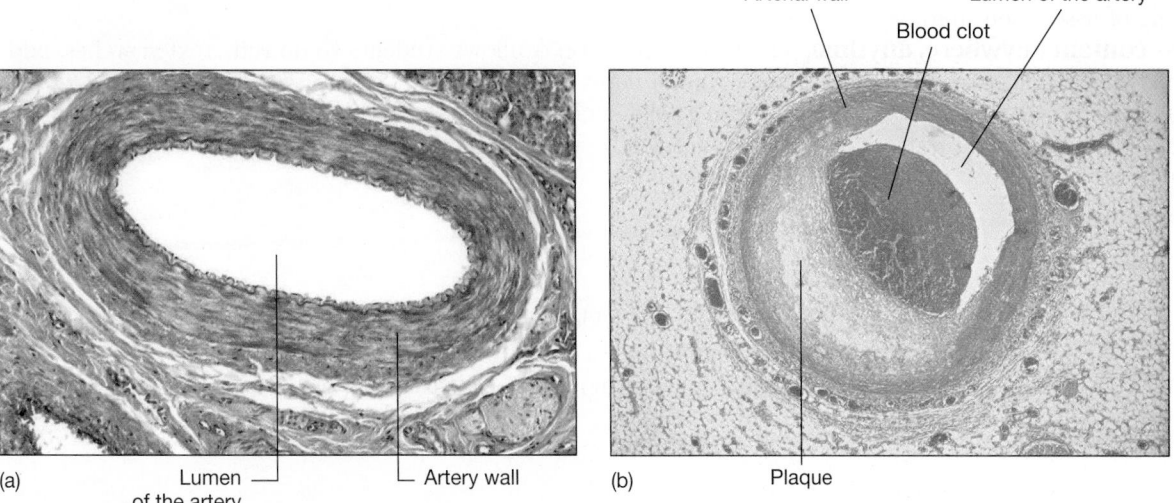

FIGURE 6.18 Healthy and atherosclerotic arteries. Note the differences between the cross section of a healthy artery (a) and that of an artery nearly completely blocked by atherosclerosis (b).

Personalized Teaching and Learning Environment

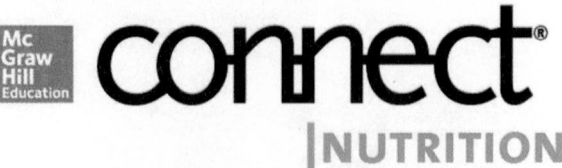

McGraw–Hill Education Connect® Nutrition is a digital teaching and learning environment that saves students and instructors time, while improving performance over a variety of critical outcomes. From in–site tutorials, to tips and best practices, to live help from colleagues and specialists, instructors are never left alone to maximize Connect's potential.

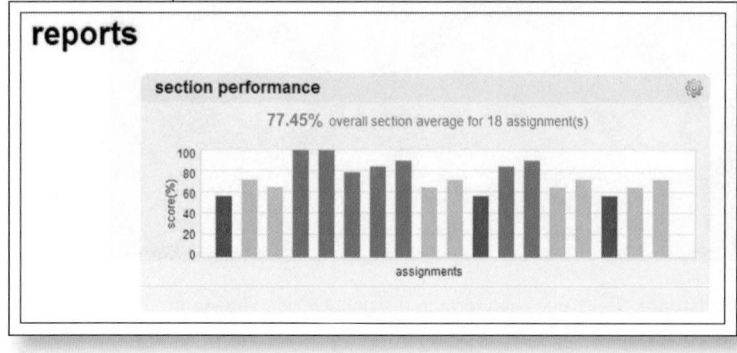

- **Auto–grade assessments and tutorials.** Instructors can easily create customized assessments that will be automatically graded. All Connect content is created by nutrition instructors so it is pedagogical, instructional, and at the appropriate level. Interactive questions using high–quality art from the textbook and animations and videos from a variety of sources take students way beyond multiple choice.
- **Gather assessment information.** All Connect questions are tagged to a learning outcome, specific section and topic, and Bloom's level for easy tracking of assessment data.
- **Access content anywhere, anytime.** The media–rich eBook allows students to do full–text searches, add notes and highlights, and access their instructor's shared notes and highlights.
- **Streamline lecture creation.** Presentation tools, such as PowerPoint® lecture outlines including art, photos, tables, and animations, allow instructors to customize their lectures.

LEARNSMART PREP®

Fueled by LearnSmart—the most widely used and intelligent adaptive learning resource— **LearnSmart Prep®** is designed to get students ready for a forthcoming course by quickly and effectively addressing prerequisite knowledge gaps that may cause problems down the road.

▦LEARNSMART®

Learn faster, study more efficiently. McGraw–Hill LearnSmart® is a diagnostic, adaptive learning system proven to help students get better grades. LearnSmart effectively assesses students' skill levels to determine which topics students have mastered and which require further practice. With over 1 billion questions answered, LearnSmart is the leading adaptive learning tool that focuses students' study where it is needed the most. Experience success with LearnSmart.

Digital Efficacy Study Shows LearnSmart Results!

Digital efficacy study final analysis shows students experience higher success rates when they are required to use LearnSmart.

- Passing rates increased by an average of 11.5% across the schools and by a weighted average of 7% across all students.
- Retention rates increased an average of 10% across the schools and by a weighted average of 8% across all students.

Study details:

- The study included two state universities and four community colleges.

- Control sections assigned chapter assignments consisting of test bank questions, and the experimental sections assigned LearnSmart; both were assigned through Connect.
- Both types of assignments were counted as a portion of the grade, and all other course materials and assessments were consistent.
- 358 students opted into the LearnSmart sections and 332 students opted into the sections where test bank questions were assigned.

▦SMARTBOOK®

Transform the way students read. SmartBook® is the first and only adaptive reading experience available for the higher education market. Powered by LearnSmart, SmartBook facilitates the reading process by identifying what content a student knows and doesn't know through adaptive assessments. As the student reads, the reading material constantly adapts to ensure the student is focused on the content needed the most to close any knowledge gaps.

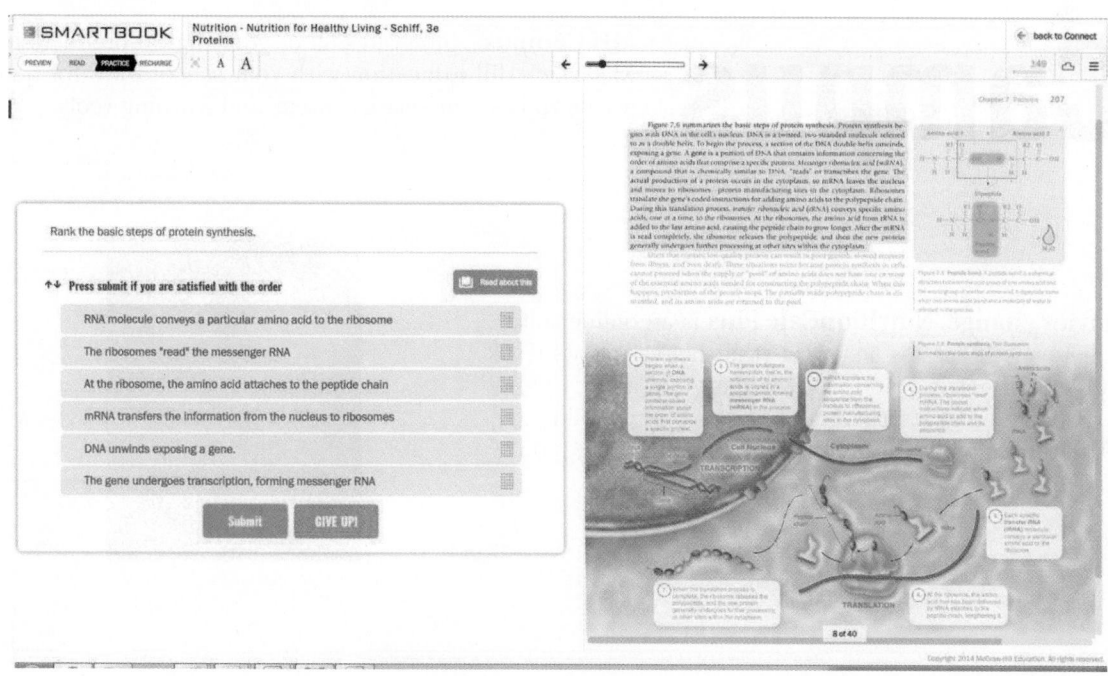

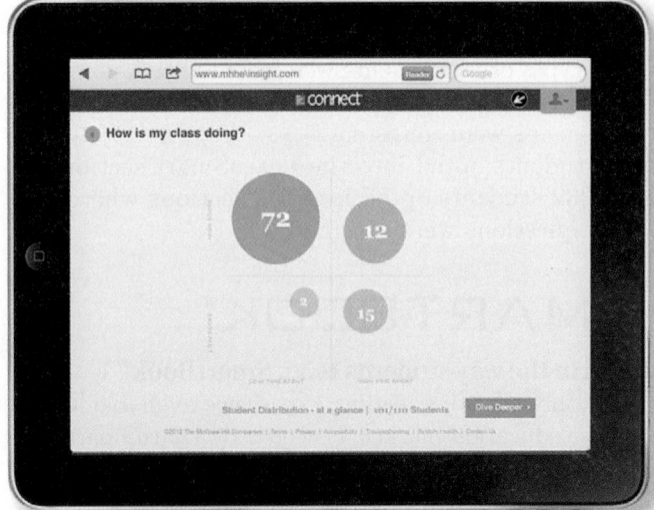

Connect® Insight is a powerful data analytics tool that allows instructors to leverage aggregated information about their courses and students to provide a more personalized teaching and learning experience.

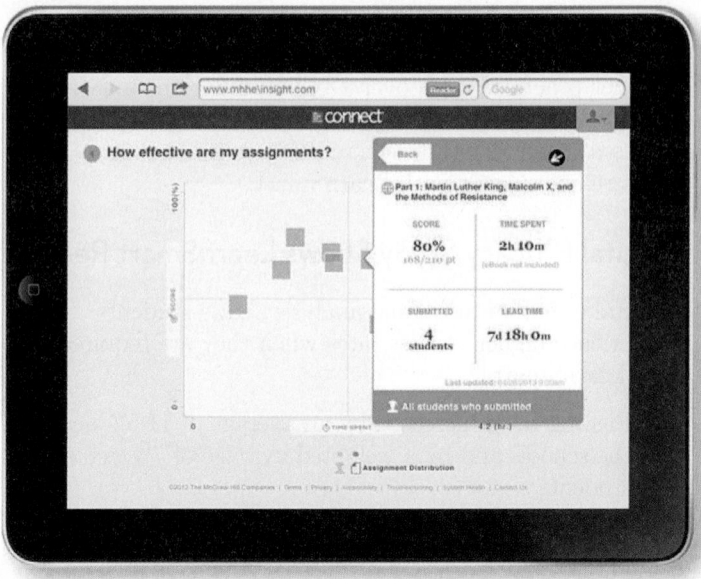

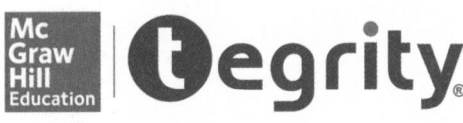

Deliver your lecture online quickly and easily. Tegrity® Campus is a fully automated lecture capture solution used in traditional, hybrid, "flipped classes" and online courses to record lessons, lectures, and skills.

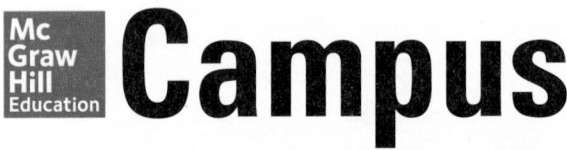

MH Campus® integrates all of your digital products from McGraw–Hill Education with your school LMS for quick and easy access to best–in–class content and learning tools.

Inspire behavior change. NutritionCalc Plus is an online suite of powerful dietary self–assessment tools that help students track their food intake and activity and analyze their diet and health goals. Students and instructors can trust the reliability of the ESHA database while interacting with a robust selection of reports.

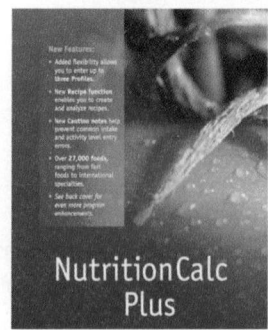

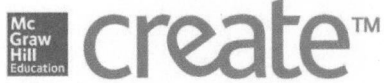

McGraw–Hill Create™ is a self–service website that allows you to create customized course materials using McGraw–Hill Education's comprehensive, cross–disciplinary content and digital products.

Acknowledgments

The preparation of a superior majors—level nutrition textbook is a lengthy, daunting task. During its development, *Human Nutrition: Science for Healthy Living* benefited from the content contributions and constructive suggestions of numerous nutrition experts, including many college instructors and emeriti.

We thank the following nutrition educators who contributed content:

Hawley Almstedt
Loyola Marymount University

Janet Colson
Middle Tennessee State University

Mary Dean Coleman
The Pennsylvania State University

Lauren Cromer
Middle Tennessee State University

Elizabeth Kirk
Bastyr University

We also offer our sincerest thanks to the following colleagues who provided a wide range of valuable input such as reviewing manuscript and artwork; serving on the textbook's Advisory Board blog; and preparing supplemental materials, including *LearnSmart* and *Connect* content and other ancillary materials.

Clinton Allred
Texas A&M University

Hope Bilyk
Rosalind Franklin University of Medicine and Sciences–Chicago Medical School

Angelina Boyce
Hillsborough Community College

Wendy Buchan
California State University– Sacramento

L. Nicholle Clark
College of the Desert

Mary Dean Coleman
The Pennsylvania State University

Janet Colson
Middle Tennessee State University

Smruti Desai
Lone Star College–CyFair

Kelly Eichmann
University of Phoenix

Elizabeth Eilender
Montclair State University

Nicolle Fernandes
Ball State University

Connie Fisk

Linden C. Haynes
Hinds Community College

Kevin D. Hall
National Institutes of Health

Jasminka Ilich–Ernst
Florida State University

Marilynn Kish–Molina
College of the Mainland

Barbara Konopka
Oakland Community College

Tony Lamanna
Paradise Valley Community College

Lynne Lohmeier
Mississippi Gulf Coast Community College

Megan Murphy
Southwest Tennessee Community College

Sarah Panarello
Yakima Valley Community College

Karen Peterkin
Rogue Community College

Jeffery Peterson
Hill College

Barbara B. Rabsatt
Brevard Community College

Larry Reichard
Metropolitan Community College– Maple Woods

Lisa Ritchie
Harding University

Christian Roberts
University of California– Los Angeles

Francis A. Tayie
Central Michigan University

Teresa Weir
Portland Community College

Heidi Wengreen
Utah State University

Najat Yahia
Central Michigan University

We owe a great deal of gratitude to the people who helped make *Human Nutrition: Science for Healthy Living* more personal by sharing their "real stories" to chapters. Thanks to Katie Adams, Paul Appelbaum, Dallas Clasen, Amanda Croker, Jan Haapala, Matthew Lang, Sarah Marie, Stephanie Patton, Ali Ritto, Justin Steinbruegge, Kelly Strosnider, and Andy Tonkin.

Finally, our heartfelt thanks extends to everyone at McGraw−Hill Education who worked on the development and production of this updated edition *Human Nutrition: Science for Healthy Living*. Developing such an innovative and superior nutrition majors' textbook was not an easy task, but our role as authors was made less challenging and more enjoyable by the talented and creative professionals who were assigned to the book. The book team consulted us when making important decisions that directly affected the textbook's features, layout, design, pedagogy, and even the cover. We appreciate their willingness to seek our input and consider us as valuable members of the team.

A few members of our McGraw−Hill team deserve to be recognized for their hard work and commitment to this textbook's development and production. Amy Reed and Marija Magner oversaw the development and production of the text. Michelle Whitaker and Matt Backhaus coordinated the creation and production of the textbook's unique and visually appealing design. Our production managers, April Southwood and MaryJane Lampe, had some of the most difficult jobs in ensuring that production deadlines were met, as well as overseeing the creation of the illustration program and the composition process. April and MaryJane did an amazing job managing the many details that were necessary to produce this textbook.

We also want to thank Marty Lange, Vice−President, and Michael Hackett, Managing Director, for providing the financial support necessary for the production of a comprehensive and elaborate new textbook. Kristine Rellihan, Marketing Manager, did a superb job promoting this textbook. Last, but not least, Product Developers, Angie Fitzpatrick, Darlene Schueller, and Donna Nemmers, deserve our sincerest gratitude for the hard work, long hours, and extraordinary dedication they invested in the production of *Human Nutrition: Science for Healthy Living* and the *Connect* and *LearnSmart* digital programs that support the textbook. We look forward to working with this team on future editions of *Human Nutrition: Science for Healthy Living*.

Wendy J. Schiff

Tammy J. Stephenson

Additionally, I would like to thank my introductory nutrition students who challenge and inspire me to be an excellent educator. Their thoughtful comments and willingness to try innovative learning activities in new learning environments provided the basis for many of the pedagogical features of this textbook. I also thank my colleagues and administrators at the University of Kentucky for supporting student−centered learning environments and allowing faculty to think "outside of the box" when developing courses.

Tammy J. Stephenson

1 Introduction to Nutrition

CASE STUDY

Healthy eating while on campus

EACH CHAPTER IN THE TEXTBOOK is introduced with a real-life application "Case Study" that describes a person's background, including his or her health and food choices. Begin by reviewing the case study and writing down potential responses to the case study questions. Then, after reading and studying the chapter, review your initial answers and make changes, if necessary. Compare your responses with the suggested responses to the case study that are provided at the end of each chapter.

Jorge has become concerned about his eating practices since he started college last month. He lives in a residence hall that has an all-you-can-eat dining facility in the basement and the Student Union is nearby. Several fast-food chain restaurants are in the Student Union, including burger, sandwich, and smoothie shops.

After moving in, Jorge began a daily routine of eating a fast-food breakfast sandwich at the Student Union before his 10 A.M. class, drinking sugary soft drinks between classes, then eating three slices of pizza or a couple of hamburgers and a large portion of French fries in the cafeteria at night. He knows he should eat more nutritious foods, but he thinks he does not have enough time to eat fresh salads or fresh fruit. Jorge wants your advice concerning how he can improve his food choices.

- Consider Jorge's current eating practices. Do his food choices reflect a nutritionally adequate pattern?

- What steps can Jorge take to improve his eating practices?

The suggested Case Study Response can be found on page 20.

connect NUTRITION Check out the Connect site at www.mcgrawhillconnect.com to further explore this case study.

QUIZ Yourself

Each chapter of this textbook begins with "Quiz Yourself," a brief true-or-false quiz to test your knowledge of the material covered in the chapter. Before reading Chapter 1, test your basic nutrition knowledge by taking the following quiz. The answers are found on page 24.

1. There are six classes of nutrients: carbohydrates, lipids, proteins, vitamins, minerals, and water. __T __F

2. Vitamins and minerals are sources of energy. __T __F

3. A healthy diet is one that contains no sugar or fat. __T __F

4. Heart disease is the leading cause of death in the United States. __T __F

5. The Food and Drug Administration regulates the safety and effectiveness of dietary supplements that are sold in the United States. __T __F

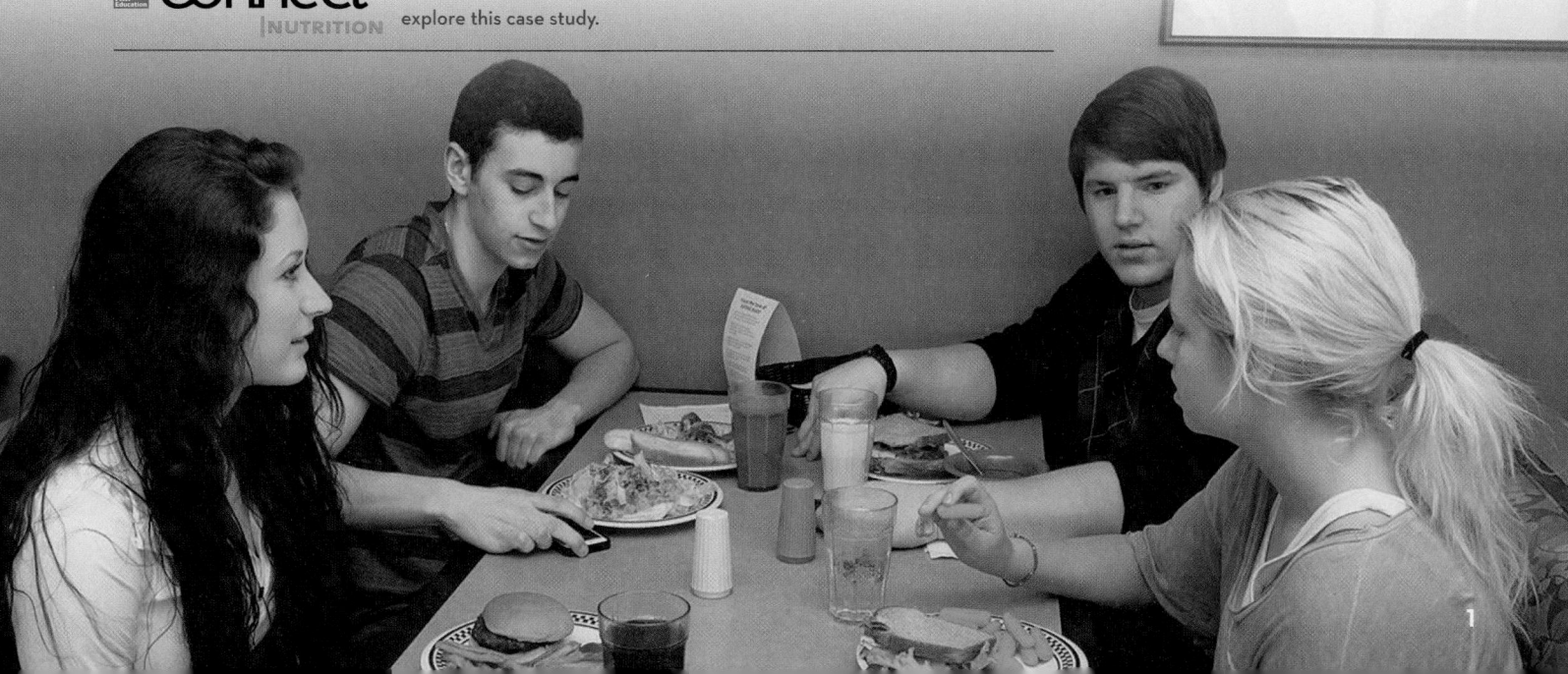

1.1 The Importance of Nutrition

LEARNING OUTCOMES

1 *Explain why it is important to study nutrition.*
2 *Describe Americans' current food-buying practices and how they compare to dietary recommendations.*

Many college students do not pay much attention to the foods they consume regularly, possibly because they are healthy now and they think poor health is unlikely to affect them until they are much older. When hungry, the typical college student may just want to eat "good food," which is something that tastes good, is inexpensive, and requires little preparation. Why should young adults focus more on what and how much they eat? What is nutrition? In this textbook, we will provide a framework of understanding nutrition and making healthy food choices.

Why Study Nutrition?

Food is a basic human need for survival: people become hungry and search for something to eat when their body needs **nutrients**, the life—sustaining substances in food. Nutrients are necessary for the growth, maintenance, and repair of the body's cells. **Nutrition** is the scientific study of nutrients and how the body uses them.

Humans have no instinctive drive that enables them to select the appropriate mix of nutrients their body requires for proper functioning. To eat well, people need to learn about the nutritional value of foods and the effects that their **diet**, their usual pattern of food choices, can have on health.

Simply having information about nutrients and their importance to good health may not be enough for people to change ingrained food—related behaviors and purchase healthier foods: a person must be motivated to make such changes. Some people strive to improve their diets because they want to lose or gain weight. Others are so concerned about their health, they are motivated to change their eating habits in specific ways, such as by eating fewer salty foods or more whole—grain products.

What People Eat in America

According to a recent analysis of food spending patterns, most Americans do not purchase recommended amounts of fruits, vegetables, whole grains, fish, and low—fat dairy products.[1] Americans, however, tend to buy more than recommended amounts of red meats; candies; cheese; sugary beverages, such as sweet—ened fruit and soft drinks; and *refined* grain products. In general, the more refined a food is, the more processing it has undergone before it is consumed, and as a result, the food has lost many vitamins, minerals, and other beneficial substances.[2]

Public health experts are concerned with Americans' eating habits, because many serious diseases, including obesity and type 2 diabetes, are associated with certain dietary practices. Over the past 30 years, these disorders have become increasingly more common, not only among Americans, but also among populations of other countries. People may be able to live longer, healthier lives by improving the nutritional quality of their diets.

How to Use This Textbook

Every major section of a chapter begins with a set of "Learning Outcomes" and ends with "Assess Your Progress" questions for you to evaluate your knowledge of the material. Key terms that you need to know when learning about nutrition are displayed in bold type within the narrative. The terms and their definitions are in the margins, but you can also look up the definitions in the Glossary.

nutrients life-sustaining substances in food

nutrition scientific study of nutrients and how the body uses them

diet a person's usual pattern of food choices

At the end of each chapter, you will find a summary of key points; a set of "Critical Thinking" questions; and "Practice Test," a group of multiple—choice questions that check your understanding of the material in the chapter. Answers to the "Practice Test" questions are provided at the end of the test. Many chapters also have a "Personal Dietary Analysis" activity and "Test Kitchen," a case study in which you modify a recipe to accommodate a client's special dietary needs.

ASSESS YOUR PROGRESS

① *Why is it important to learn about nutrition?*

② *Which foods do Americans tend to buy in amounts that are higher than recommended?*

1.2 The Nutrients

LEARNING OUTCOMES

1 *List the six classes of nutrients, and identify major roles of each class of nutrient in the body.*

2 *Identify the key features of an essential nutrient.*

3 *Categorize nutrients based on whether they are essential, and their designation as a micronutrient or macronutrient.*

4 *Identify rich food sources of phytochemicals.*

To understand nutrition, students need to learn about and use information from biology, anat—omy, physiology, and chemistry. This chap—ter introduces the nutrients and their general functions. Chapter 4 focuses on the struc—tures and functions of the human digestive system. Appendices B and C provide brief reviews of basic chemistry and physiol—ogy concepts that form the foundation for understanding the science of nutrition.

The Six Classes of Nutrients

There are six classes of nutrients: carbohy—drates, lipids (such as fats and oils), proteins, vitamins, minerals, and water. Both food and the human body are comprised of these nutrients. Although the percentage varies with age and sex, about 50 to 70% of the body's total weight is water. On average, healthy young men and women have similar amounts of vitamins, minerals, and car—bohydrates in their bodies, but the young women have less water and protein, and considerably more fat (Fig. 1.1). Bodies with high fat content tend to have less water in them than bodies with less fat.

Each nutrient typically has more than one physiological role, that is, function in the body (Table 1.1). In general, the body uses cer—tain nutrients for energy, growth and development, and regulation of processes, including the repair and maintenance of cells. Cells do not need food to survive, but they need the nutrients *in* food to

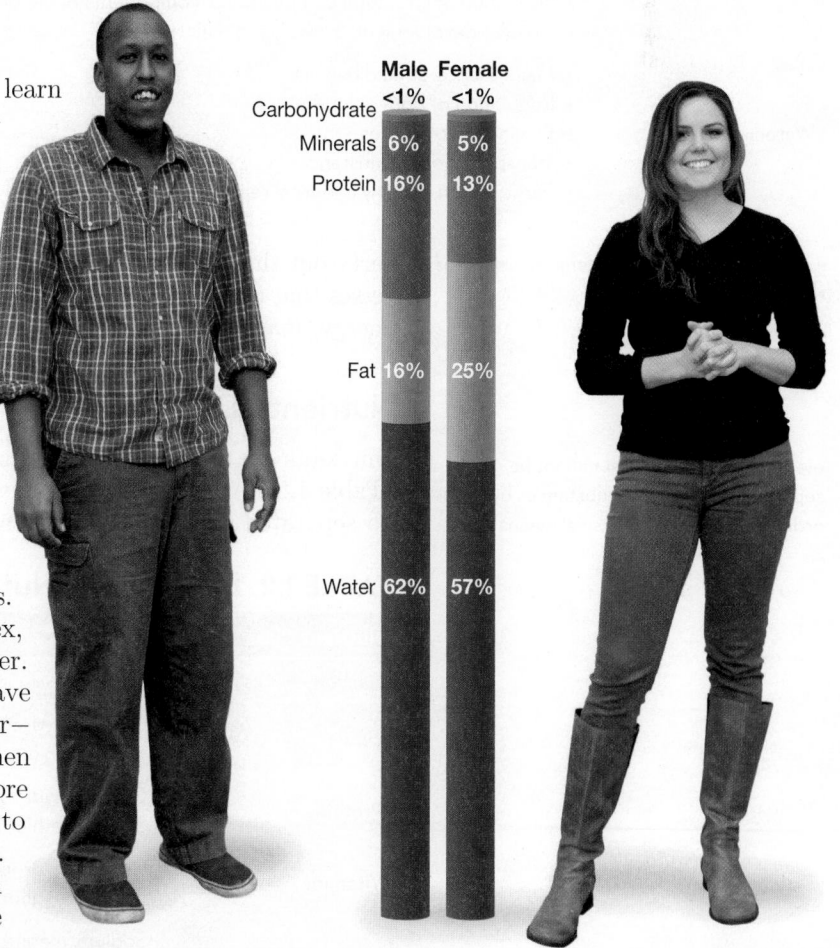

	Male	Female
Carbohydrate	<1%	<1%
Minerals	6%	5%
Protein	16%	13%
Fat	16%	25%
Water	62%	57%

FIGURE 1.1 Comparing body composition. These illustrations present the approximate percentages of nutrients that comprise the bodies of a healthy man and woman. Note that the amount of vitamins in the human body is so small, it is not shown.

TABLE 1.1 Nutrients

Nutrient Class	Major Functions
Carbohydrates	• Major source of energy (most forms) • Maintenance of normal blood glucose levels • Elimination of solid waste from gastrointestinal tract (fiber)
Lipids	• Major source of energy (fat) • Cellular development, physical growth and development • Regulation of body processes (certain hormones, for example) • Growth and development of the brain • Absorption of fat-soluble vitamins
Proteins	• Production of structural components, such as cell membranes, and functional components, such as enzymes • Cellular development, growth, and maintenance • Regulation of body processes (certain hormones, for example) • Transportation of substances within the blood • Energy (normally a minor source)
Vitamins	• Regulation of body processes • Immune function • Production and maintenance of cells • Protection against agents that can damage cellular components
Minerals	• Regulation of body processes, including fluid balance and energy metabolism • Formation of certain chemical messengers • Formation of structural and functional components of various substances and tissues • Cellular development, growth, and maintenance
Water	• Maintenance of fluid balance • Regulation of body temperature • Elimination of wastes • Transportation of substances • Participation in many chemical reactions

metabolism total of all chemical processes that occur in living cells

carry out their metabolic activities. **Metabolism** is the total of all chemical pro—cesses that occur in living cells, including chemical reactions involved in supplying energy, making proteins, and eliminating waste products.

Nutrients: Elements

element substance that cannot be separated into simpler substances by ordinary chemical or physical means

Nutrients are sources of elements that the body needs to carry out its activities (Table 1.2). An **element** is a substance, such as carbon and oxygen, that cannot be separated into simpler substances by ordinary chemical or physical means.

TABLE 1.2 Elements in Nutrients

Nutrient Class	Elements*
Carbohydrates	Carbon, hydrogen, and oxygen
Lipids	Carbon, hydrogen, and oxygen; phosphorus (phospholipids); nitrogen (certain phospholipids)
Proteins	Carbon, hydrogen, oxygen, nitrogen Sulfur (methionine and cysteine)
Vitamins	Carbon, hydrogen, oxygen Nitrogen, sulfur, phosphorus, cobalt
Minerals	Sodium, magnesium, potassium, calcium, chromium, manganese, iron, cobalt, copper, zinc, molybdenum, phosphorus, sulfur, chlorine, selenium, iodine, fluorine
Water	Hydrogen, oxygen

* Not every element listed may be a component of a particular nutrient in each class.

Elements are the basic substances that make up all things, including life forms such as human beings. Note that almost 98% of the human body (by weight) is composed of only five elements: oxygen, carbon, hydrogen, nitrogen, and calcium (Fig. 1.2).[3]

In chemistry, the term **organic** refers to compounds that contain carbon. Carbohydrates, lipids, proteins, and vitamins are organic nutrients, because they contain carbon. **Inorganic** nutrients, such as minerals and water, are substances that do not contain carbon.

Essential Nutrients

All nutrients are important for health, but the body can use the "raw materials" from food to synthesize (make) many nutrients, such as cholesterol and fats (types of lipids). The remaining nutrients, about 50 of them, are dietary essentials. An **essential nutrient** must be supplied by food, because the body does not synthesize the nutrient or make enough to meet its needs. Water is the most essential nutrient, because the body can survive for only a few days without it.

Nutrition scientists use the following factors to help determine whether a nutrient is essential:

- If the nutrient is missing from the diet, a deficiency disease occurs as a result. A **deficiency disease** is a state of health characterized by certain abnormal physiological changes. Changes that are observable or measurable are **signs** of disease. Disease signs include rashes, failure to grow properly, and elevated blood pressure. **Symptoms** are subjective complaints of ill health that are difficult to observe and measure, such as dizziness, fatigue, and headache.

- When the missing nutrient is added to the diet, the abnormal physiological changes are corrected. As a result, signs and symptoms of the deficiency disorder resolve as normal functioning is restored and the condition is cured.

- After scientists identify the nutrient's specific roles in the body, they can explain why the abnormalities occurred when the substance was missing from the diet.

To test an adult male human's need for vitamin C, for example, scientists would have the subject avoid consuming foods or vitamin supplements that contain the vitamin. When the amount of vitamin C in the subject's white blood cells (leukocytes) became too low for them to function normally, the person would develop physical signs of scurvy, the vitamin C deficiency disease. When the person brushed his teeth, his gums would bleed from the pressure of the toothbrush (Fig. 1.3). If he cut himself, the wound would heal slowly or not at all.

If the scientists began to feed foods that contain vitamin C to the subject again, the man's deficiency signs and symptoms would disappear within a few days, because his body was recovering. Chapter 10 provides information about the physiological roles of vitamin C. One of those roles is maintaining *collagen*, the protein in the body that holds cells together, including the cells that form tiny blood vessels in skin. Collagen is also needed to produce scar tissue for wound healing. When the vitamin is lacking, the tiniest blood vessels in the gums begin to leak blood where they are compressed, and even minor cuts have difficulty healing. Thus, vitamin C meets all the required features of an essential nutrient. Table 1.3 lists nutrients that are generally considered to be essential.

Some nutrients that are normally nonessential can become essential under certain conditions, such as in metabolic disorders or serious diseases, and during prenatal (before birth) development. In these conditions, **conditionally essential nutrients** may be made by the body but in amounts that are inadequate and must be supplemented by the diet. Chapter 7 discusses some amino acids that are

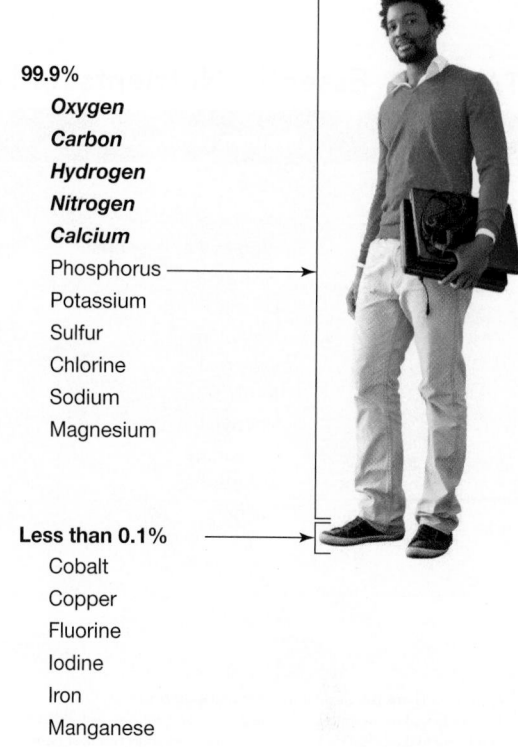

99.9%
Oxygen
Carbon
Hydrogen
Nitrogen
Calcium
Phosphorus →
Potassium
Sulfur
Chlorine
Sodium
Magnesium

Less than 0.1% →
Cobalt
Copper
Fluorine
Iodine
Iron
Manganese
Zinc

FIGURE 1.2 Nutrient-related elements in the human body.

organic (chemistry) refers to compounds that contain carbon

inorganic refers to substances that do not contain carbon

essential nutrient nutrient that must be supplied by food

deficiency disease state of health characterized by certain abnormal physiological changes that occur when the body lacks a nutrient

signs physical changes associated with a disease state that are observable or measurable

symptoms subjective complaints of ill health that are difficult to observe and measure

conditionally essential nutrients nutrients that are normally not essential but become essential under certain conditions, such as during a serious illness

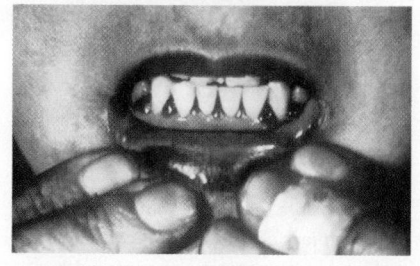

FIGURE 1.3 Sign of scurvy.

TABLE 1.3 Essential Nutrients for Humans

Carbohydrates	Proteins (Amino Acids*)	Lipids	Vitamins	Minerals	Water
Glucose	The following amino acids are generally recognized as essential: Histidine Leucine Isoleucine Lysine Methionine Phenylalanine Threonine Tryptophan Valine	Fats that contain: Linoleic acid Alpha-linolenic acid	A Thiamin Riboflavin Niacin Pantothenic acid Biotin Folic acid (folate) B-6 B-12 C D† E K Choline‡	**Major minerals:** Calcium Chloride Magnesium Phosphorus Potassium Sodium Sulfur **Trace minerals:** Chromium Copper Iodine Iron Manganese Molybdenum Selenium Zinc	Water

* Amino acids are the basic units that make up proteins.
† The body makes vitamin D after exposure to sunlight, but a dietary source of the nutrient is often necessary.
‡ The body makes choline but may not make enough to meet needs. Therefore, choline is classified as a *vitamin-like* compound.

conditionally essential. Amino acids are the nitrogen—containing compounds that make up protein molecules.

Macronutrients and Micronutrients

So far, we have organized nutrients based on their chemical composition and essentiality. A third way to classify nutrients is based on amounts that the body needs. Carbohydrates, fats, and proteins are **macronutrients**, because the body requires relatively large amounts of these nutrients daily (*macro* = large). Vitamins and minerals are **micronutrients**, because the body needs very small amounts of them to function properly (*micro* = small).

In general, a serving of food supplies grams (g) of carbohydrate, fat, and protein, and milligram (mg) or microgram (μg or mcg) quantities of vitamins and minerals. For example, a serving of a commercially prepared pumpkin pie (⅛ of a pie) provides about 57 g of carbohydrate, 16 g of fat, 6.5 g of protein, 740 mg of vitamin A, and 1.5 mg of iron.

Macronutrients supply energy for cells, whereas micronutrients are not sources of energy. Although the body requires large amounts of water, this nutrient does not provide energy and is not usually classified as a macronutrient.

Phytochemicals

Plants make hundreds of substances called **phytochemicals** (*phyto* = plant), which are not nutrients (nonnutrients), yet they may have healthful benefits. The stimulant caffeine, for example, is a phytochemical made by coffee plants. Beta—carotene is a phytochemical in many fruits and vegetables that the body can convert to vitamin A. Table 1.4 identifies rich food sources of several phy—tochemicals that scientists are studying. The table indicates some effects of the chemicals of the body, including possible health benefits.

Not all phytochemicals have beneficial effects on the body. Some phyto—chemicals, such as nicotine in tobacco leaves, ricin in castor beans, and oxalic acid in rhubarb leaves, are toxic or can interfere with the absorption of nutrients. Information about several phytochemicals that have known effects on human health is woven into chapters of this textbook where it is appropriate.

macronutrients nutrients that the body needs in large amounts

micronutrients nutrients that the body needs in very small amounts

phytochemicals substances in plants that are not nutrients but may have healthful benefits

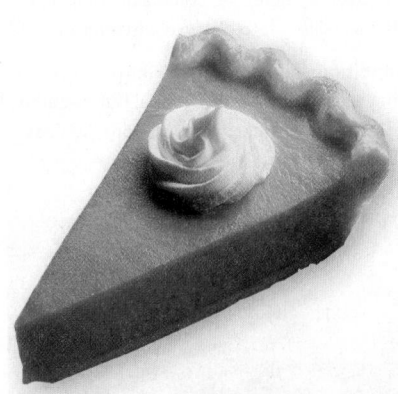

Most foods are mixtures of nutrients. Pumpkin pie is a rich source of carbohydrate and fat, but the dessert also contributes some protein, vitamin A, and iron to diets.

TABLE 1.4 Phytochemicals in Foods That Are of Scientific Interest

Classification and Examples	Biological Effects/Possible Health Benefits	Rich Food Sources
Carotenoids Alpha-carotene, beta-carotene, lutein, lycopene, zeaxanthin	May reduce risk of certain cancers and macular degeneration (a major cause of blindness in the United States)	Orange, red, yellow fruits and vegetables; egg yolks
Phenolics	Antioxidant activity; may inhibit cancer growth and reduce risk of heart disease	
Quercetin		Apples, tea, red wine, onions, olives, raspberries, cocoa
Catechins		Green and black tea, chocolate, plums, apples, berries, pecans
Anthocyanins		Red, blue, or purple fruits and vegetables
Resveratrol		Red wine, purple grapes and grape juice, dark chocolate, cocoa
Isoflavonoids		Soybeans and other legumes
Tannins		Tea, coffee, chocolate, blueberries, grapes, persimmons
Monterpenes		Oranges, lemons, grapefruit, cherries
Organosulfides Isothiocyanates, indoles, allylic sulfur compounds	Antioxidant effects; may improve immune system functioning and reduce the risk of heart disease	Garlic, onions, leeks, cruciferous vegetables (broccoli, cauliflower, cabbage, kale, bok choy, collard and mustard greens)
Alkaloids Caffeine	Stimulant effects	Coffee, tea, "energy drinks," kola nuts, cocoa
Capsaicinoids Capsaicin	May provide some pain relief	Chili peppers

ASSESS YOUR PROGRESS

3 *List the six major classes of nutrients, and identify at least one physiological role for each class.*

4 *Explain the meaning of organic in the context of chemical compounds.*

5 *What are three key factors that determine whether a substance is an essential nutrient?*

6 *Distinguish between macronutrients and micronutrients, and provide examples of each.*

7 *List at least seven foods that are rich sources of phytochemicals.*

1.3 Food as Fuel

LEARNING OUTCOMES

1 *Distinguish between calorie and kilocalorie.*

2 *Estimate the amount of energy (kcal) in a serving of food based on the grams of carbohydrate, protein, fat, and alcohol present.*

Most foods are sources of biological fuels, because they provide energy for cells. The human body uses energy while running, sitting, studying, and even sleeping. Every cell in the body needs energy to carry out its various activities. Therefore, people need to consume energy—containing foods and beverages to survive.

A **calorie** is the amount of heat (a form of energy) necessary to raise the temperature of 1 g (1 mL) of water 1° Celsius (C). A calorie is such a small unit of measurement that the amount of energy in food is reported in 1000—calorie units called kilocalories or *C*alories. Thus, a **kilocalorie (kcal)** or **Calorie** is the heat energy needed to raise the temperature of 1000 g (1 liter) of water 1° Celsius (C).

calorie amount of heat necessary to raise the temperature of 1 g (1 mL) of water 1° Celsius (C)

kilocalorie (kcal) or **Calorie** the heat energy needed to raise the temperature of 1000 g (a liter) of water 1° Celsius (C)

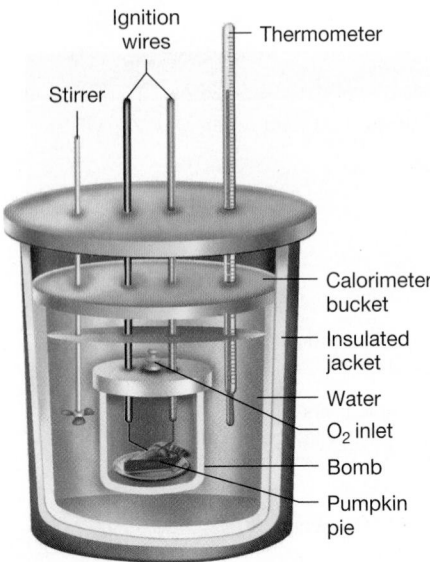

FIGURE 1.4 Bomb calorimeter.

bomb calorimeter device used to measure the calories in a sample of food

A small apple, for example, supplies 40,000 calories or 40 kcal or 40 Calories. If no number of kilocalories is specified, it is appropriate to use *calories*. In this textbook, the term *kilocalories* (kcal) is interchangeable with *food energy* or simply *energy*. Appendix I is a food composition table that lists energy and nutrient contents of many commonly consumed foods and beverages.

Direct Calorimetry

The calorie content of a food or beverage can be determined through direct calo–rimetry, which involves placing a specific amount of food in a **bomb calorimeter** (*kal–oh–rim'–eh–ter*). As shown in Figure 1.4, the "bomb" is a small chamber surrounded by a jacket of water. An electrical spark ignites the food and, under the conditions inside the bomb, the food burns completely. As the food burns, it releases heat, which raises the temperature of the water in the surrounding chamber. A ther–mometer measures the increased water temperature, and scientists use this informa–tion to determine the number of calories in the food.

Compared to the human body, a bomb calorimeter is much more efficient at using the energy–yielding nutrients in foods as fuel. Therefore, scientists must cor–rect for this difference in efficiency when developing food composition tables, such as the one in Appendix I.

Calculating Food Energy

Consumers can calculate the number of kcal in their diets by knowing amounts of macronutrients and the nonnutrient alcohol in their foods and beverages. A gram of carbohydrate and a gram of protein each supply about 4 kcal; a gram of fat provides about 9 kcal (Fig. 1.5). Alcohol is not a nutrient, because the

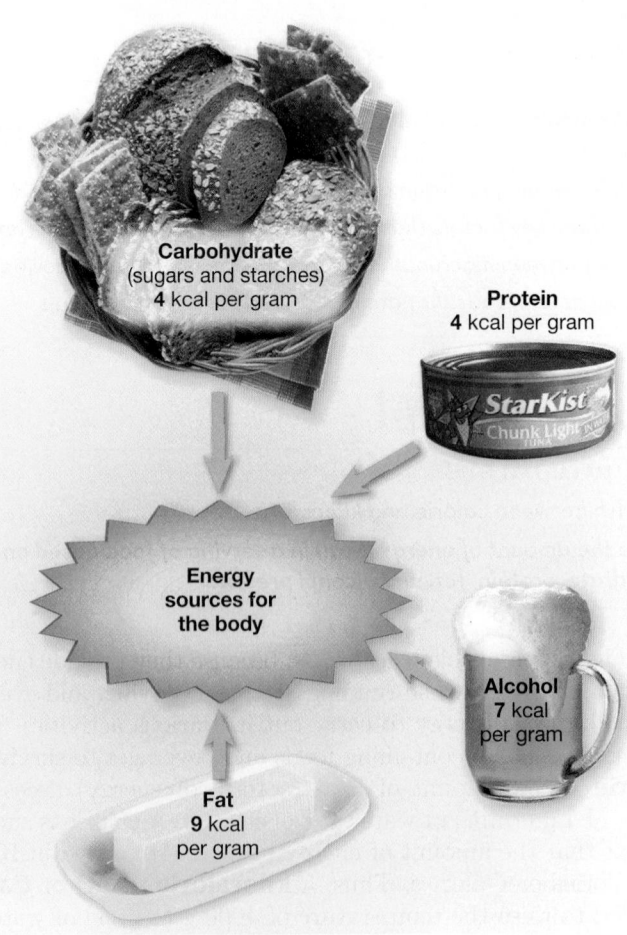

FIGURE 1.5 Energy sources for the body.

human body does not need the chemical to survive. Alcohol, however, is a source of energy; a gram of pure alcohol supplies 7 kcal. Chapter 8 discusses alcohol, including its effects on health.

Let us use the serving of pumpkin pie that we mentioned earlier as an exam—ple for estimating the caloric content of a food. The piece of pie contains about 57 g of carbohydrate, 16 g of fat, and 6.5 g of protein. To estimate the number of kcal provided in a serving of this food:

STEP 1: Determine how many kcal are provided by each type of macronutrient.

57 g carbohydrate	×	4 kcal/g carbohydrate	=	228 kcal
16 g fat	×	9 kcal/g fat	=	144 kcal
6.5 g protein	×	4 kcal/g protein	=	26 kcal

STEP 2: Add the individual kcal from carbohydrate, fat, and protein together to determine the total kcal per serving of the food.

Total kcal = 228 kcal (carbohydrate) + 144 kcal (fat) + 26 kcal (protein) = 398 kcal

This food provides almost 400 kcal per serving.

ASSESS YOUR PROGRESS

8 What is the difference between a calorie and a kilocalorie?

9 A slice of whole-wheat bread supplies approximately 13 g of carbohydrate, 1 g of fat, 3 g of protein, and 11 g of water. Based on this information, estimate the number of kilocalories this serving of food provides.

10 An alcoholic beverage contains 4 g of carbohydrate and 10 g of alcohol. In this drink, how many kilocalories are provided by the alcohol?

1.4 Does Diet Matter?

LEARNING OUTCOMES

1 Identify the leading causes of death in the United States.
2 Describe lifestyle factors that contribute to the leading causes of death in the United States.
3 Identify nutrition-related objectives of Healthy People 2020.

In the beginning of this chapter, we mentioned that public health officials are concerned about the impact that poor food choices can have on the health of Americans. The graph shown in Figure 1.6 indicates the 10 leading causes of deaths in the United States and the approximate percentages of deaths that were attributed to each of them in 2011. Note that heart disease was the leading cause of death for all Americans and cancer was the second leading cause of death. In 2011, these two diseases accounted for almost 50% of all deaths.[4] Also note that several of the leading causes of death are diet—related and responsible for the premature (early) deaths of thousands of adult Americans.

Risk Factors

Heart disease, diabetes, and cancer are chronic diseases. **Chronic** diseases are long—term conditions that usually take many years to develop and have complex causes.

chronic long-term

FIGURE 1.6 Ten leading causes of U.S. deaths (preliminary 2011). Lifestyle factors contribute to many of the 10 leading causes of death in the United States.

Source: Hoyert DL, Jiaquan X: Deaths: Preliminary data for 2011. National Vital Statistics Reports 61(6), 2012.

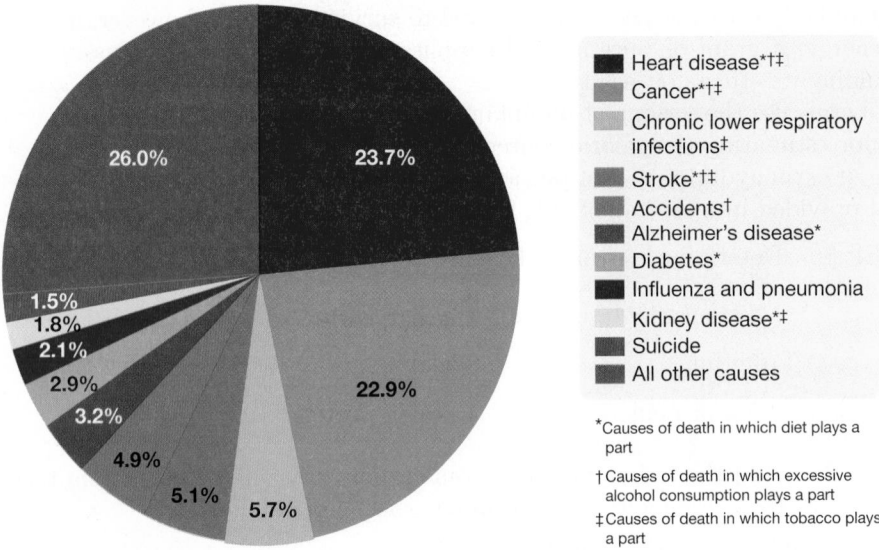

Legend:
- Heart disease*†‡
- Cancer*†‡
- Chronic lower respiratory infections‡
- Stroke*†‡
- Accidents†
- Alzheimer's disease*
- Diabetes*
- Influenza and pneumonia
- Kidney disease*‡
- Suicide
- All other causes

*Causes of death in which diet plays a part

†Causes of death in which excessive alcohol consumption plays a part

‡Causes of death in which tobacco plays a part

risk factor personal characteristic that increases a person's chances of developing a chronic disease

lifestyle a routine way of living

A **risk factor** is a personal characteristic that increases a person's chances of developing a chronic disease. For example, genetic background or family history is an important risk factor for heart disease. If your grandfather had a heart attack before he was 55 years old and your mother is being treated for having high blood pressure and high blood cholesterol levels (risk factors for heart disease), your family history indicates you have a higher-than-average risk of having a heart attack.

DID YOU KNOW?

A person's genetic makeup influences the effects that a person's diet may have on his or her health, as well as the individual's likelihood of developing most diseases. Nutritional genomics is a relatively new area of nutrition research that explores complex interactions among gene functioning, diet and other lifestyle choices, and the environment.[5] For example, your genetic makeup plays a major role in determining the levels of chemicals produced by your body, including those that influence hunger and appetite control. If your body makes abnormal amounts of these chemicals, you might overeat and gain excess body fat as a result. While you cannot change your genes, you can control or change many other factors that influence your health. Chapter 7 provides more information about nutritional genomics.

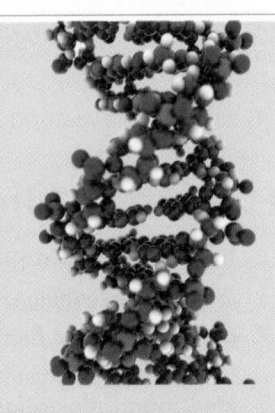

Model of a section of DNA.

DID YOU KNOW?

Smoking is a lifestyle choice. In the United States, cigarette smoking is the primary cause of preventable cancer deaths.[6]

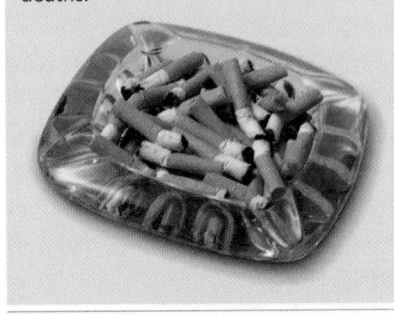

Lifestyle Choices

For many people, having a family history of a chronic disease does not mean that they will develop the condition. Other risk factors that contribute to ill health are unsafe environmental conditions; psychological factors, such as excess emotional stress; lack of access to health care; advanced age; and unhealthy lifestyle. **Lifestyle** is a routine way of living, which includes one's usual dietary practices and exercise habits.

A person's lifestyle may increase or reduce his or her chances of developing many chronic diseases or delay their occurrence for years, even decades. People who choose to consume fat-free or low-fat dairy products, fruits, vegetables, nuts, and whole-grain cereals, as well as exercise regularly, may reduce their chances of developing serious diseases that contribute to premature deaths, particularly heart disease, type 2 diabetes, certain cancers, and excess body fat.[7] On the other hand, people who consume more calories than needed and perform too little physical activity can develop *obesity*, a condition characterized by excessive and unhealthy amounts of body fat. Obesity is a risk factor for numerous chronic health problems, including heart disease and type 2 diabetes. Thus, preventing obesity is a major public health objective in the United States. Chapter 13 discusses obesity and its effects on health.

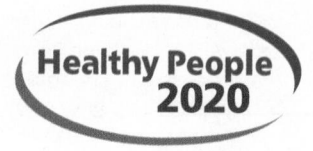

Healthy People 2020 In the United States, public health officials monitor the state of Americans' health. A major focus of the government's efforts is the development of educational programs designed to prevent obesity and other chronic health problems. In early 2011, the U.S. Department of Health and Human Services (DHHS) issued *Healthy People 2020*, a report that includes national health promotion and disease prevention objectives that Americans should meet by 2020.[8]

    Healthy People 2020 has several major nutrition–related objectives, some of which are listed in Table 1.5. These objectives include specific target goals. For example, under Objective NWS–9, no more than 30.5% of American adults should be obese by 2020.[9] In 2005–2008, almost 34% of adults in the United States were obese. In 2009–2010, almost 36% of American adults were obese, so the proportion of adults who are obese had not declined since 2005–2008.[9] To access more information about these objectives, visit the government's website: http://www.healthypeople.gov/2020/topicsobjectives 2020/default.aspx.

TABLE 1.5 *Healthy People 2020 Selected Objectives for Topic Area: Nutrition and Weight Status (NWS)*

Objective Number	Objective
NWS–9	Reduce the proportion of adults who are obese.
NWS–14	Increase the contribution of fruits to the diets of the population aged 2 years and older.
NWS–16	Increase the contribution of whole grains to the diets of the population aged 2 years and older.
NWS–17.3	Reduce consumption of calories from solid fats and added sugars.

ASSESS YOUR PROGRESS

11 What is lifestyle?

12 Identify the leading causes of death in the United States that are associated with dietary practices.

13 List at least three nutrition-related objectives of Healthy People 2020.

1.5 Factors That Influence Eating Habits

LEARNING OUTCOMES

1 Identify factors that influence a person's usual food selections.

2 Discuss the influence that biological, physiological, cognitive, and psychological factors can have on a person's food choices.

3 Discuss ways that food marketing efforts can influence an individual's food selections.

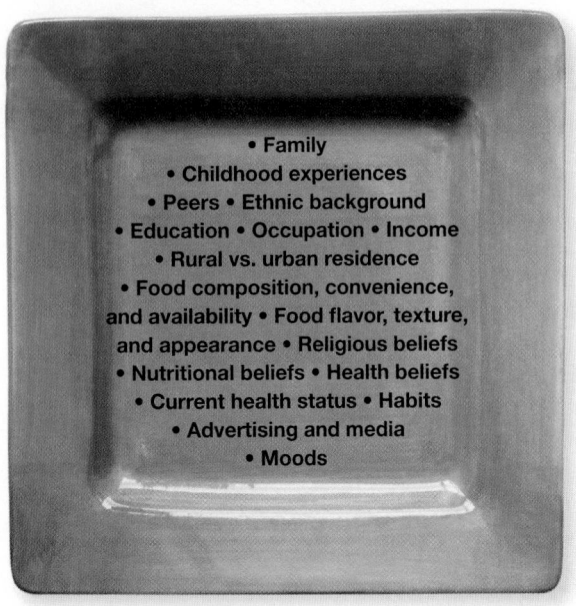

- Family
- Childhood experiences
- Peers • Ethnic background
- Education • Occupation • Income
- Rural vs. urban residence
- Food composition, convenience, and availability • Food flavor, texture, and appearance • Religious beliefs
- Nutritional beliefs • Health beliefs
- Current health status • Habits
- Advertising and media
- Moods

FIGURE 1.7 What influences your eating practices?

Food is more than just a collection of nutrients and "something to eat." Food also has personal meaning and significance, evokes feelings and sensations, and conveys status and ethnicity. Figure 1.7 displays many factors that influence a person's usual food selections. This section examines some of the biological, physiological, cognitive (involving thought processes), psychological, and environmental factors that play important roles in determining what people consider as food and when they choose to eat it.

Biological and Physiological Factors

Biological and physiological factors that often influence food selections include age; ability to perceive external sensory information, such as taste, smell, and texture of foods; and internal sensations of hunger and thirst. For example, very hungry persons who are in desperate conditions often must resort to eating things they would not consider consuming in better times, such as insects, boiled leather, and even the dead bodies of people.

Effects of Aging

Age is a major biological factor that influences food choices. Infants and young children rely on adult caregivers ("gatekeepers") for their food. Gatekeepers choose what the children eat and prepare it. Older children, particularly teenagers, typically have more control over their diets. When young adults leave home and associate with people from diverse geographical and ethnic backgrounds, they often broaden their usual food choices. Older adults with certain age-related health problems, such as swallowing difficulties or excessive tooth loss, may find their food choices are limited to soft or liquid foods.

In addition to age, other factors, such as stage of life (during pregnancy or older adult years, for example) and health problems, are likely to affect food selections. If a person develops a chronic disease, managing the condition may include changing his or her food choices, as well as the ways the food is prepared and how much can be eaten. Making such modifications may be necessary for an individual to maintain a sense of well-being as he or she grows older. Chapters 16, 17, and 18 provide information about nutritional recommendations during various stages of life.

Sensory Information

Would it be difficult for you to resist walking past a bakery shop without stopping to purchase some of the items? Humans rely on various types of sensory information, particularly the taste, texture, odor, and appearance of food, to develop personal food likes and dislikes. Chapter 4 includes information about the senses of taste and odor, and features a young woman who was born with a condition that greatly reduces her ability to taste foods.

Cognitive and Psychological Factors

Cognitive factors that influence food choices involve learning processes. People learn which foods are acceptable to eat from past experiences, cultural practices, and religious teachings. Learning about foods and nutrition also takes place at home; in the classroom; and from media, including the Internet. Individuals can use the information to build a personal food-belief system that may encourage them to try new foods or adopt a better diet.

Although learning which foods are healthy may influence a person's dietary practices, at times, psychological factors, especially emotional stress level and

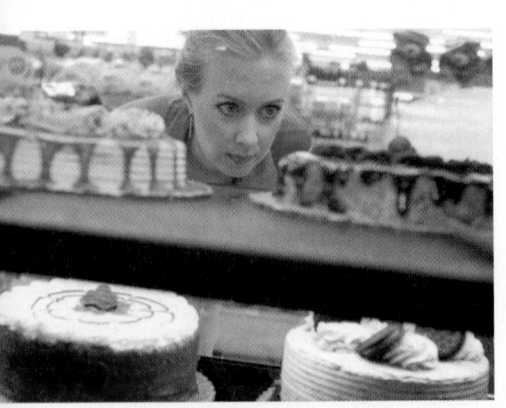

Senses, particularly sight, smell, and taste, contribute to the appeal of certain foods.

mood, also play important roles in what the individual chooses to eat. Pregnant women often experience increased desire for particular foods (food cravings). It is not clear whether a physiological need for certain nutrients is the stimulus for cravings. Some people, however, crave chocolate when they are depressed, anxious, or irritable.[10] By eating chocolate, such persons may reduce their anxiety level and improve their mood.[11,12]

Experiences with food can result in positive or negative associations. Children, for example, generally prefer the taste of sweet foods, and caregivers often use sugary snacks or desserts as rewards for children who display good behavior. Therefore, it is possible that as adults, people reward themselves with sweets to obtain the same positive feelings. In a similar way, "comfort foods" may provide desirable feelings for adults. Eating such foods may evoke a sense of being in a safe haven, such as at home.

Some food–related experiences are negative. A 6–year–old boy, for example, who enjoys macaroni and cheese eats a bowl of the food and about an hour later becomes "sick to his stomach" and vomits. Although the macaroni and cheese did not cause the vomiting, this child may be unwilling to eat that particular food for several years, and possibly for the rest of his life, because he associates the food with a stomach–related illness.

Environmental Factors

Environmental factors play a major role in what people eat. Such influences include income, location of one's home, availability of food on campus or in the workplace, and relationships. If you have access to grocery stores and a kitchen, you may prepare most of your meals with fresh ingredients and pack lunches and snacks to take with you to class. In contrast, if one of your favorite fast–food restaurants is near your home, you may find it easier to eat meals at the restaurant than to prepare them. If you must rely primarily on your campus's dining facilities for your meals, your food choices may be limited to what is offered.

Consumers may not realize the impact that food marketing has on their diets. Food manufacturers often develop food packaging intended to attract buyers, and the layout of most major supermarkets is designed to encourage consumers to purchase foods—in many instances, pricier items. Attractive displays at the ends of aisles, the positioning of products on shelves, and even the flooring material are intentionally designed to stimulate the senses, direct shoppers to more profitable items, and increase sales. Food marketing efforts also include media advertising, which relies heavily on the visual sense to attract people to try food products, regardless of their nutritional value. Such factors often make it difficult for nutrition educators to help their clients make wiser, healthier food choices.

ASSESS YOUR PROGRESS

14 *Identify two biological or physiological factors that influence food choices.*
15 *Give an example of a cognitive or psychological factor that could affect food choices.*
16 *Describe how food marketing influences food choices.*

1.6 Key Nutrition Concepts

LEARNING OUTCOMES

1 *Discuss the importance of the six key nutrition concepts to the study of nutrition.*
2 *Compare an empty-calorie food to a nutrient-dense food.*
3 *Explain energy density and provide examples of energy-dense food choices.*
4 *Describe a dietary supplement according to the Dietary Supplement and Health Education Act of 1994.*

TABLE 1.6 Key Nutrition Concepts

Concept 1: Most foods are mixtures of nutrients.
Concept 2: Variety, moderation, and balance can help ensure a diet's nutritional adequacy.
Concept 3: Food is the best source of nutrients.
Concept 4: Foods and the nutrients they contain are not cure-alls.
Concept 5: Malnutrition includes *overnutrition* as well as *under*nutrition.
Concept 6: Nutrition is a dynamic science.

Before you study nutrition, it is important to grasp some key basic concepts (Table 1.6). The content in the chapters that follow will build upon these key concepts and can help you make more informed choices concerning your dietary practices.

nutrient-dense describes a food that supplies more vitamins and minerals in relation to total calories

energy density refers to the amount of energy a food provides per given weight of the food

Concept 1: Most Foods Are Mixtures of Nutrients

Most foods are mixtures of nutrients, and in many instances, water is the major nutrient in foods. For example, an 8–fluid–ounce serving of fat–free milk is about 91% water by weight, but it is an excellent source of protein and supplies carbohydrate, very little fat, and several vitamins and minerals. Although sugar comprises about 44% of the weight of a chocolate–with–almonds candy bar, over one–third of the sweet snack's energy is from fat. The candy bar also contains small amounts of protein and a few vitamins and minerals. Because all foods have some nutritional value, no food deserves the label of "bad" or "junk." Some foods, however, are healthier to consume than others.

Nutrient-Dense Foods

Nutrition experts recommend including certain foods in diets because they are rich sources of micronutrients. A **nutrient—dense** food supplies more vitamins and minerals in relation to total calories. Broccoli, leafy greens, fat—free milk, oranges, lean meats, and whole—grain cereals are examples of nutrient—dense foods.

Energy-Dense Foods

Energy density (or calorie density) is the amount of energy a food (kcal) provides per given weight (grams) of the food. Both of these values are listed on most food labels (see Fig. 3.13). According to one rule of thumb, an energy—dense food has a kilocalorie—to—weight ratio of 4.0 or higher.[13] When compared to carbohydrate, protein, and alcohol, fat supplies the most energy per gram. Thus, fatty foods tend to be more energy dense than foods with lower fat contents. Water provides no energy for the body, so watery foods, such as most fruits and vegetables, tend to be low in calories and have low energy densities.

Figure 1.8 compares two foods that supply similar amounts of calories but differ in their energy densities. The chocolate, yeast—type frosted doughnut, which weighs about 3.5 ounces (approximately 100 g) and is about 4 inches in diameter, provides almost 400 kcal. This doughnut's energy density is 4.0 (400 kcal/100 g). Eight medium strawberries also weigh about 100 g, but the fruit provides only 32 kcal. The strawberries' energy density is 0.32 (32 kcal/100 g). A person would have to eat 100 strawberries to obtain the same amount of

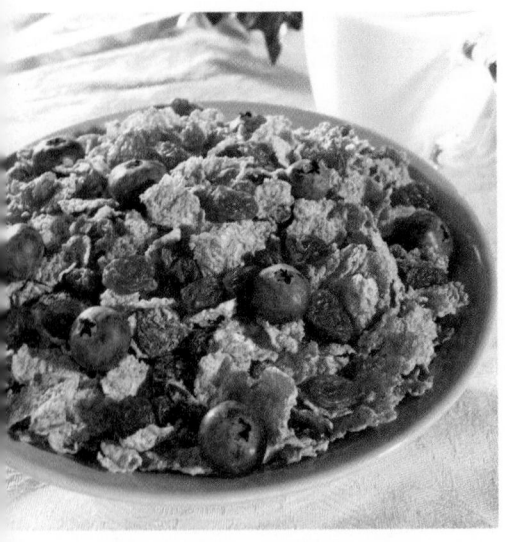

Whole-grain cereals, especially those that have added vitamins and minerals, are nutrient-dense foods.

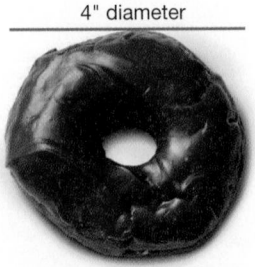

4" diameter

400 kcal

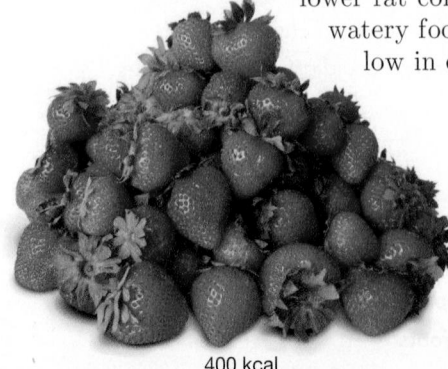

400 kcal

FIGURE 1.8 Energy density. Although each of these portions of food supplies about 400 kcal, they differ in their energy densities.

food energy that is in the chocolate doughnut. Therefore, the doughnut is an energy–dense food in comparison to the berries.

It is important to note that not all energy–dense foods are empty–calorie foods. Nuts, for example, are high in fat and, therefore, energy dense. However, nuts are also nutrient dense because they contribute protein, vitamins, minerals, and fiber to diets.

Empty-Calorie Foods

Some foods and beverages, such as candy, snack chips, and alcoholic or sugar–sweetened drinks, are sources of "empty calories." An **empty–calorie** food supplies a lot of calories from unhealthy types of fat, added sugar, and/or alcohol.[14] Additionally, an empty–calorie food is not a good source of vitamins and minerals. Eating too many empty–calorie foods may displace more nutritious foods from the diet. Thus, empty–calorie foods can contribute to an unhealthy diet. Chapter 3 provides more information about empty–calorie foods.

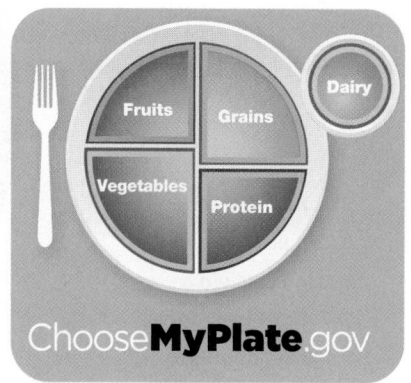

FIGURE 1.9 MyPlate food groups. People can add variety to their diets by choosing different foods from each of these five food groups. Chapter 3 provides more information about MyPlate.

Concept 2: Variety, Moderation, and Balance Can Help Ensure a Diet's Nutritional Adequacy

The human body is designed to obtain the nutrients it needs from a wide **variety** of foods. No *natural* (minimally processed) food is "perfect" in that it contains all nutrients in amounts that are required by the body. To help ensure the nutritional adequacy of their diets, people should eat several different kinds of foods from each food group that is shown in Figure 1.9. People should also consume each food in reasonable amounts **(moderation)**. Dietary moderation involves obtaining enough nutrients from food to meet one's needs while avoiding excessive amounts. By balancing caloric intake with physical activity, people can maintain a healthy weight **(balance)**. Chapter 3 provides more information about food groups, including recommendations for serving sizes.

Figure 1.10 compares amounts of energy and certain nutrients provided by 8–ounce servings of fat–free milk and a cola–type, sugar–sweetened ("regular") soft drink. Although the drinks supply similar amounts of calories, the milk provides more protein, calcium, phosphorus, riboflavin, and vitamin A. A nutritionally balanced diet contains a variety of nutrient–dense foods and limits empty–calorie items. If a diet is comprised primarily of nutrient–dense foods and meets a healthy individual's nutritional needs, then occasionally including some empty–calorie items can add enjoyment to living—when the foods are consumed in moderation.

empty-calorie describes a food that supplies excessive calories from unhealthy types of fat, added sugar, and/or alcohol

variety refers to a diet that contains foods from each food group

moderation refers to eating reasonable amounts of each food

balance refers to a level of caloric intake that enables a person to maintain a healthy weight

DID **YOU** *KNOW?*

Fat comprises about 3-5% of the volume of a serving of whole milk. When compared to whole milk, fat-free ("skim") milk is more nutrient-dense and less energy-dense. One cup of fat-free milk supplies about 80 kcal and 300 mg of calcium, whereas 1 cup of whole milk supplies about 150 kcal and 280 mg of calcium. Thus, fat-free milk has about the same amount of calcium per serving, but almost half the kcal of an equivalent serving of whole milk.

Concept 3: Food Is the Best Source of Nutrients

The most reliable and economical way for people to obtain nutrients and beneficial phytochemicals is to base their diet on a variety of "whole" and minimally processed foods. Plant foods often contain a variety of nutrients and phytochemicals, but processing (refining) food often removes some of the most healthful parts.

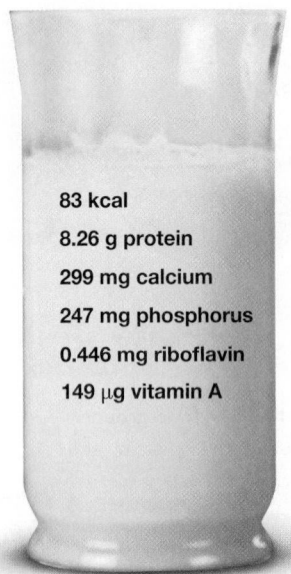

83 kcal

8.26 g protein

299 mg calcium

247 mg phosphorus

0.446 mg riboflavin

149 µg vitamin A

8 fluid ounces

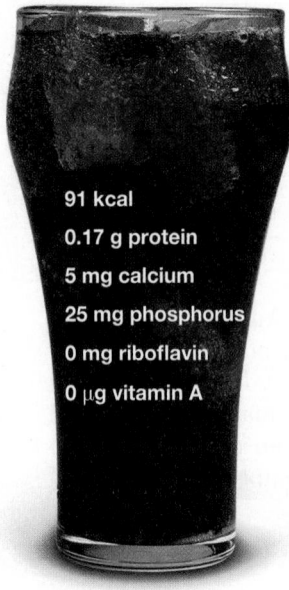

91 kcal

0.17 g protein

5 mg calcium

25 mg phosphorus

0 mg riboflavin

0 µg vitamin A

8 fluid ounces

FIGURE 1.10 Beverage comparison.
Although equivalent amounts of fat-free milk and a sugar-sweetened soft drink have similar calorie contents, the milk contains considerably more protein, riboflavin, vitamin A, and the minerals calcium and phosphorus.

dietary supplement product (excluding tobacco) that contains a vitamin, a mineral, an herb or other plant product, an amino acid, or a dietary substance that supplements the diet by increasing total intake

Dietary Supplement and Health Education Act of 1994 (DSHEA) federal legislation that allows manufacturers to classify nutrient supplements and herbal products as foods

Some individuals need higher amounts of vitamins and other nutrients than those found in food. A few people, for example, have inherited defects that increase their needs for certain nutrients, particularly vitamins. Older adults and people who have chronic illnesses, digestive disorders that interfere with nutrient absorption, and certain other, genetic disorders may also require supplemental nutrients. Because it is often difficult to plan and eat nutritious meals and snacks each day, taking a supplement that contains a variety of vitamins may be advisable, even for healthy adults.[15]

Dietary Supplements

A **dietary supplement** is a product (excluding tobacco) that contains a vitamin, a mineral, an herb or other plant product, an amino acid, or a dietary substance that supplements the diet by increasing total intake.[16] The **Dietary Supplement and Health Education Act of 1994 (DSHEA)** allows manufacturers to classify nutrient supplements and herbal products as foods.[16] As a result of this legislation, dietary supplements do not undergo the rigorous testing of safety and effectiveness that medications must undergo before being marketed.

Results of one study indicated about 52% of Americans adults reported taking a supplement in the past month.[17] The most commonly used dietary supplements are multivitamin/mineral (MVM) products. In general, taking a MVM supplement that provides 100% of recommended amounts of the micronutrients daily has little associated risk.[18] However, healthy adults should consider taking such supplements as an "insurance policy" and not a substitute for eating a variety of nutrient–dense foods.

Among American adults, the most popular nonvitamin, nonmineral dietary supplements are fish oil, glucosamine, echinacea, and flaxseed oil and pills.[17] Results of scientific research indicate that some dietary supplements, such as vitamins and certain herbs, have beneficial effects on health. Results of other studies, however, provide evidence that many popular dietary supplements are not helpful and may even be harmful. Information about specific dietary supplements is included in various chapters where it is appropriate.

At present, the Food and Drug Administration (FDA) does not regulate dietary supplements as strictly as prescription medications. When the FDA determines that a particular supplement presents a significant or unreasonable risk of harm, the agency alerts consumers about the risk and seeks to recall the product; that is, the FDA initiates efforts to have it removed from the market. In most instances, the manufacturer voluntarily recalls the product after determining there is a problem with it or being notified by the FDA about the problem.[19] In some cases, however, the FDA requests a recall.

Nutrient supplements do not contain everything one needs for optimal nutrition. Although supplements that contain phytochemicals are available, they may not provide the same healthful benefits as consuming the plants that contain these compounds. Why not? People may need to consume nutrients and phytochemicals together to provide desirable effects in the body. Minimally processed food often contains combinations of these chemicals in very small amounts and certain proportions that the body can use safely. There is nothing "natural" about gulping down handfuls of dietary supplements.

FRESH TIPS

Consider these guidelines to help you make informed choices about the use of dietary supplements:

- Determine whether the supplement is necessary. Discuss your need for the supplement with your physician or a dietitian before you purchase or use the product, especially if you are pregnant, are breastfeeding, or have a chronic condition such as diabetes or heart disease.

- If you are experiencing symptoms of a serious illness, consult a physician. Using supplements instead of seeking conventional medical care can be a risky practice. Delaying or forgoing medical evaluation and treatment may result in an illness becoming worse or even life-threatening.

- The following government websites provide reliable information about dietary supplements: U.S. National Library of Medicine www.nlm.nih.gov/medlineplus/herbalmedicine.html U.S. Food and Drug Administration http://www.fda.gov/Food/DietarySupplements/default.htm Office of the Dietary Supplements https://od.nih.gov/

- If you experience negative side effects after using a particular dietary supplement, consult a physician immediately. Furthermore, you and your physician should report the problem to the FDA's MedWatch program by calling (800) FDA-1088 or visiting the agency's website: http://www.fda.gov/Safety/MedWatch/HowToReport/default.htm.

For Each Nutrient, There Is a Range of Safe Intake

"More is not always better" when it relates to optimal nutrition. The **physiological dose** of a nutrient is the amount that is within the range of safe intake and enables the body to function optimally. Consuming less than the physiological dose can result in a marginal nutritional status. In other words, the person's body has just enough of the nutrient to function adequately, but that amount is not sufficient to overcome the added stress of infection or injury. If a person's nutrient intake falls below the marginal level, the individual is at risk of developing the nutrient's deficiency disease. The diagram shown in Figure 1.11 illustrates the general concept of deficient, safe, and toxic intake ranges for nutrients such as vitamins and minerals. Chapter 3 discusses nutrient needs and the *Dietary Reference Intakes*, which include standards for safe intakes of nutrients. Chapters 9–12 provide more information about micronutrients, including deficiencies and toxicities.

Most commonly eaten foods do not contain toxic levels of vitamins and minerals. A **megadose** is an amount of a vitamin or mineral that is at least 10 times the recommended amount of the nutrient.[20] When taken in high amounts, many vitamins behave like drugs and can produce unpleasant and even toxic side effects. Some physicians prescribe megadoses of the B–vitamin niacin to treat high blood cholesterol levels, but such amounts can cause serious side effects, including liver damage. Compared to vitamins, minerals generally have very narrow ranges of safe intakes.

Concept 4: Foods and the Nutrients They Contain Are Not Cure-Alls

Although specific nutrient deficiency diseases, such as scurvy, can be cured by eating foods that contain the nutrient that is missing or in short supply, nutrients do not "cure" other ailments. Diet is only one aspect that influences a person's health. By making certain dietary changes, however, a person may be able to

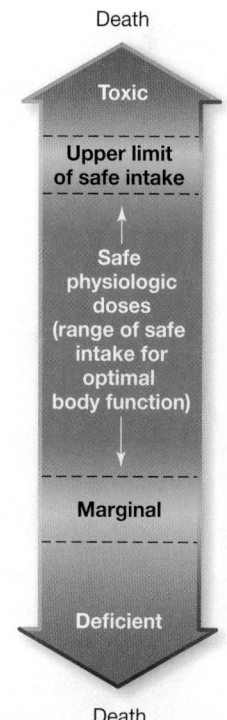

Death

Toxic

Upper limit of safe intake

Safe physiologic doses (range of safe intake for optimal body function)

Marginal

Deficient

Death

FIGURE 1.11 Nutrient intake continuum. For each nutrient, there is a range of safe intake.

physiological dose amount of a nutrient that is within the range of safe intake and enables the body to function optimally

megadose amount of a vitamin or mineral that is very high, generally at least 10 times the recommended amount of the nutrient

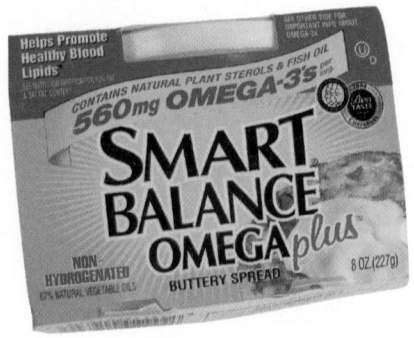

This substitute for butter is a functional food because it may lower blood cholesterol levels.

medical nutrition therapies nutritionally modified diets for people with chronic health conditions

malnutrition state of health that occurs when the body is improperly nourished

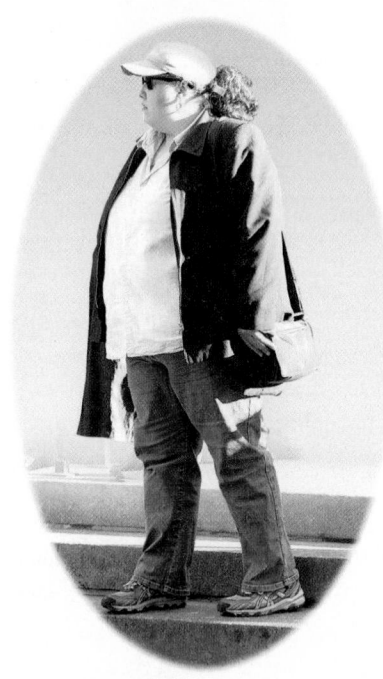

Obesity is a form of malnutrition.

prevent or forestall the development of certain diseases or possibly lessen their severity if they occur.

Each year, food manufacturers introduce new products into the market—place that are designed to attract health—conscious consumers. Many of these foods are referred to as "functional foods," because they contain nutrient and/or phytochemical ingredients that may provide health benefits. Functional foods are often manufactured to boost nutrient intakes or help manage specific health problems. For example, consumers who want to increase their calcium intake can purchase orange juice that has the mineral added to it. Various chapters present information about functional foods and their roles in health.

What About Special Diets?

Registered dietitians and registered dietitian nutritionists, who are specially trained nutrition experts, often plan modified ("special") diets **(medical nutrition therapies)**, for people with chronic health conditions such as diabetes. Dietitians must consider many factors regarding a patient's situation, including current health status, occupation, food likes and dislikes, budget, family and peer support systems, and ability to access and prepare foods. Information about special diets is included in the chapters where it is appropriate.

Concept 5: Malnutrition Includes Overnutrition as Well as Undernutrition

Malnutrition (*mal* = bad) is a state of health that occurs when the body is improperly nourished. Although many people associate malnutrition with under—nutrition and starvation, overnutrition—the long—term excess of energy or nutrient intake—is also a form of malnutrition. Chronic overnutrition results in obesity. Chapter 13 provides information about overnutrition; Chapters 7 and 20 include discussions about undernutrition.

Some people select nutritionally inadequate diets because they lack knowl—edge about nutritious foods or the importance of nutrition to health. People with low incomes and older adults living on fixed incomes are often at risk for mal—nutrition because they have limited financial resources for making healthy food purchases. Other people who are at risk of malnutrition include those who have severe eating disorders, are addicted to drugs such as alcohol, or have certain serious medical problems.

Concept 6: Nutrition Is a Dynamic Science

As researchers continue to explore the complex relationships between diet and health, nutrition information constantly changes. The public may expect medical researchers to provide definite answers to their nutrition—related questions and rigid advice concerning optimal dietary practices. However, nutrition is not an exact science, especially when the research involves human subjects. As a result, dietary practices and recommendations undergo revision as new scientific evidence becomes available and the information is reviewed and accepted by nutrition experts. Chapter 2 discusses how nutrition scientists collect information and report their findings.

ASSESS YOUR PROGRESS

17 Discuss the importance of variety, moderation, and balance in terms of a person's diet.

18 Provide at least three examples of an empty-calorie food, a nutrient-dense food, and an energy-dense food.

19 Explain why an herbal tea made from echinacea is a dietary supplement according to the Dietary Supplement and Health Education Act of 1994.

SUMMARY

SECTION 1.1 The Importance of Nutrition

- The human body needs nutrients for the growth, maintenance, and repair of cells. Nutrition is the scientific study of nutrients and how the body uses them.
- Public health experts are concerned with Americans' eating habits, because rates of certain serious chronic diseases are associated with certain dietary practices. People may be able to live longer, healthier lives by improving the nutritional quality of their diets.

SECTION 1.2 The Nutrients

- The six classes of nutrients are carbohydrates, lipids, proteins, vitamins, minerals, and water. The human body can synthesize many nutrients, but about 50 nutrients are dietary essentials that must be supplied by food.
- Carbohydrates, fats, proteins, and vitamins are organic nutrients; minerals and water are inorganic nutrients. Carbohydrates, fats, and proteins are macronutrients; vitamins and minerals are micronutrients.
- Plant foods contain a variety of phytochemicals. Many phytochemicals are beneficial antioxidants, but some phytochemicals are toxic.

SECTION 1.3 Food as Fuel

- A Calorie is the heat energy needed to raise the temperature of 1 liter of water 1° Celsius (C).
- A gram of carbohydrate and a gram of protein each supply about 4 kcal; a gram of fat provides about 9 kcal. Although alcohol is not a nutrient, a gram of pure alcohol furnishes 7 kcal.

SECTION 1.4 Does Diet Matter?

- Heart disease and cancer are the two leading causes of death for all Americans. Such chronic diseases are complex conditions that have multiple risk factors.
- People may live longer and healthier by modifying their lifestyles.
- Improving the health status of Americans is the focus of *Healthy People 2020*.

SECTION 1.5 Factors That Influence Eating Habits

- Biological, physiological, cognitive, psychological, and environmental factors influence a person's food choices.

SECTION 1.6 Key Nutrition Concepts

- Most foods are mixtures of nutrients.
- Variety, moderation, and balance can help ensure a diet's nutritional adequacy.
- Food is the best source of nutrients.
- Foods and the nutrients they contain are not cure-alls.
- Malnutrition includes overnutrition as well as undernutrition.
- Nutrition is a dynamic science.

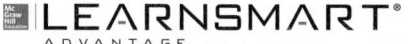

CASE STUDY RESPONSE

HEALTHY EATING WHILE ON CAMPUS

JORGE'S EATING PRACTICES do not reflect a nutritionally adequate pattern. His diet is nutritionally imbalanced because it lacks fruits, vegetables, and dairy products. His food choices do not include a variety of more nutrient-dense foods. Furthermore, his diet lacks moderation in that he chooses large portion sizes, particularly of empty-calorie foods. Jorge can:

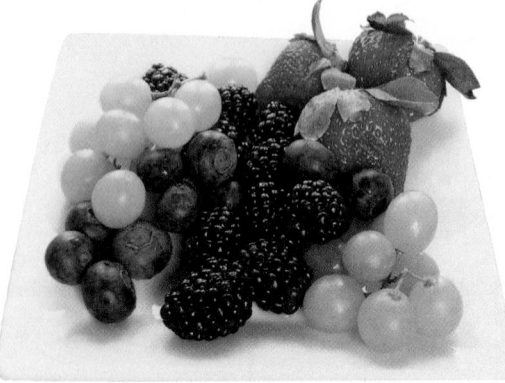

- Consider choosing more nutrient-dense foods. On busy class days, for example, he can carry light snacks with him, such as a bag of almonds or walnuts, carrot sticks, fresh fruit, or peanut butter spread on whole-grain crackers.

- Be more careful when choosing which foods to eat in his dorm's dining hall. He can learn to broaden his food likes to include more variety of foods, especially fruits and vegetables.

- Practice moderation by reducing his food portions, especially of the many energy-dense options that are available at the dining hall. Jorge can choose smaller portions and not return to the buffet for "seconds."

TEST KITCHEN

Modifying Recipes for Healthy Living

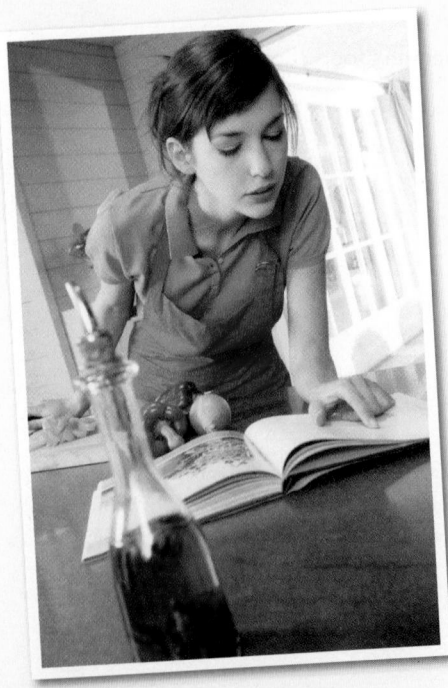

Most chapters include a "Test Kitchen" exercise that is related to the content of that chapter. You will be provided with a basic recipe and instructed to modify the recipe to make it healthier. By making minor changes to a recipe, such as replacing solid fat with canola oil, eliminating salt, or reducing the amount of sugar by 25%, you can improve the product's nutritional quality.

Table 1.7 provides suggestions for common ingredient substitutions and indicates how the changes improve the nutritional quality of the products. Modifying the type of milk in a waffle recipe, for example, can significantly decrease the product's fat content. As you modify recipes, keep the following tips in mind:

- Do not change every ingredient. Make one or two minor changes each time you try the recipe. For example, if you are making a cake for the first time, do not eliminate all the sugar and fat. These are ingredients that add flavor, color, texture, and moisture to the cake. A cake with no sugar or fat would be dry and almost tasteless.

- Recipes can often be made healthier simply by slightly reducing the fat, sugar, or salt. You probably will not notice a significant difference in taste or quality if you use ¾ cup of sugar instead of 1 cup or ½ teaspoon of salt instead of 1 teaspoon. Appendix A provides information about household measures, such as cups and teaspoons.

TABLE 1.7 Recipe Substitutions for Better Nutrition

Recipe Calls for	Modification or Substitution	Nutritional Effects of the Change
All-purpose (white) flour or bread flour	Use ½ whole-wheat flour and ½ all-purpose flour for each cup of all-purpose or bread flour.	Adds fiber
Butter or margarine (in baking)	Replace each quantity of butter or margarine with an equivalent amount of applesauce. Use ½ cup mashed cooked carrots, sweet potato, pumpkin, or squash for each 1 cup butter or margarine in baked goods.	Reduces calories and undesirable types of fat ("unhealthy fat"); adds some fiber and vitamins Reduces calories and unhealthy fat; adds some fiber, vitamins, and phytochemicals
Cream	Use whole milk or half-and-half.	Reduces calories and unhealthy fat
Cream cheese, regular	Use fat-free or reduced-fat ("Neufchatel") cream cheese.	Reduces calories and unhealthy fat
Cheese, regular	Use low-fat or nonfat cheese. NOTE: Do not use nonfat cheese in cooked foods, because it will not melt properly.	Reduces calories and unhealthy fat
Enriched pasta or rice	Whole-grain pasta or brown rice. Mix ½ whole-grain pasta with ½ regular pasta.	Adds fiber
Eggs	Use 2 egg whites or ¼ cup egg substitute for each whole egg.	Reduces calories and unhealthy fat
Evaporated milk	Use fat-free evaporated milk.	Reduces calories and unhealthy fat
Condensed milk	Use fat-free evaporated milk. NOTE: Products will not be as sweet.	Reduces calories from unhealthy fat and added sugar
Fruit canned in heavy sugar syrup	Use fresh or frozen fruit. Use fruit canned in "own juice" or light syrup, or rinse sugar syrup from fruit before using.	Reduces calories and sugar; adds vitamins and phytochemicals Reduces calories and sugar
Herbs with added salt (i.e., "garlic salt")	Use salt-free ground herbs and spices or fresh herbs and spices such as basil, cilantro, dill, oregano, or paprika.	Reduces sodium
Salt	Do not add to water before cooking vegetables or pasta. Do not add salt to foods before serving them.	Reduces sodium
Sour cream, regular	Use fat-free or low-fat sour cream. Use plain fat-free yogurt.	Reduces calories and unhealthy fat
Sugar, white or brown	Reduce the amount of sugar by 25 to 50%. Use sugar-substitute that is appropriate for preparing baked products.	Reduces calories and sugar
Vegetable oil	Reduce amount by 25%. Use ¾ cup mashed cooked carrots, sweet potato, pumpkin, or squash for 1 cup oil in baked goods.	Reduces calories and fat Reduces calories and fat and adds fiber, vitamins, and phytochemicals
Whole milk, 2% milk	Use fat-free or low-fat milk.	Reduces calories and unhealthy fat

PERSONAL Dietary Analysis

1. For 1 week, keep grocery and convenience store receipts.

    a. How much money did you spend on foods purchased at these markets? ____

    b. Which foods were the most expensive items purchased? ____

    c. How much money did you spend on empty-calorie foods and beverages such as cookies, salty snacks, soft drinks, and candy? ____

    d. What percentage of your food dollars were spent on empty-calorie foods? ____
    (Divide the amount of money spent on empty-calorie foods by the total cost of food for the week. Move the decimal point over two places to the right and place a percent sign after the number.)

    e. How much money did you spend on nutrient-dense foods such as whole-grain products, fruits, and vegetables? ____

    f. What percentage of your food dollars were spent on nutrient-dense foods? ____
    (Divide the amount of money spent on nutrient-dense foods by the total cost of food for the week. Move the decimal point over two places to the right and place a percent sign after the number.)

2. For 1 week, keep a detailed log of your usual vending machine purchases, including the item(s) purchased and amount of money spent for each purchase.

    a. What types of foods and beverages did you buy from the machines? ____

    b. How many soft drinks did you consume each day? ____

    c. How much money did you spend on vending machine foods and beverages? ____

    d. Based on this week's vending machine expenditures, estimate how much money you spend on such purchases in a year. ____

3. For 1 week, keep a detailed log of your usual fast-food consumption practices, including fast-food purchases at convenience stores. List the types of food and beverages you purchased and amount of money you spent.

    a. According to your weekly record, how often do you buy food from fast-food places and convenience stores? ____

    b. What types of foods did you usually buy? ____

    c. How much money did you spend on fast foods? ____

    d. Based on this week's expenditures, estimate how much money you spend on fast-food purchases in a year. ____

4. If you take dietary supplements, estimate the amount of money that you spend on such products each month. ____

Critical Thinking

1. Identify at least six factors that influence your food and beverage selections. Which of these factors is the most important? Explain why.

2. Analyze your current eating habits. Based on your analysis, is your diet nutritionally adequate? Explain why your diet is or is not nutritionally adequate.

3. "Everything in moderation." Explain what this statement means in terms of your diet.

4. Consider your parents' and grandparents' health (or causes of death). Based on your family history, which chronic health conditions do you have a higher than average risk of developing? If you were at risk of developing a chronic health condition that could be prevented by changing your diet, would you make the necessary changes at this stage of your life? Explain why or why not.

5. Eric spends about $100 each month on purchases of dietary supplements, including protein powders, vitamin pills, and herbal extracts. He thinks it is necessary to take the products to achieve optimal health and prevent chronic illnesses. Based on the information in this chapter, what would you tell Eric about his use of the supplements?

Practice Test

Select the best answer.

1. Diet is a
   a. practice of restricting energy intake.
   b. usual pattern of food choices.
   c. method of reducing portion sizes.
   d. technique to reduce carbohydrate intake.

2. Which of the following conditions is one of the 10 leading causes of death in the United States in which diet plays a role in its development?
   a. tuberculosis   c. hepatitis
   b. cancer   d. influenza

3. The nutrients that provide energy are
   a. proteins, fats, and carbohydrates.
   b. lipids, proteins, and minerals.
   c. vitamins, minerals, and proteins.
   d. carbohydrates, vitamins, and lipids.

4. Metabolism
   a. occurs as an end-product of energy transfer.
   b. is the process used to measure the amount of energy in a food.
   c. has a specific energy state.
   d. refers to all chemical processes that occur in living cells.

5. Which of the following substances is an essential nutrient?
   a. cholesterol   c. tyrosine
   b. vitamin C   d. beta-carotene

6. Which of the following foods is nutrient dense?
   a. unsalted butter   c. fat-free milk
   b. sugar-sweetened soft drink   d. iceberg lettuce

7. Which of the following foods is a rich source of phytochemicals?
   a. hamburger   c. peaches
   b. fish   d. chicken

8. Which of the following conditions is a chronic disease?
   a. heart disease   c. scurvy
   b. common cold   d. influenza

9. In the United States, the primary cause of preventable cancer deaths is
   a. physical inactivity.   c. high-fat diet.
   b. tobacco use.   d. excessive alcohol intake.

10. According to recent studies, most Americans do not purchase adequate amounts of
    a. sugary foods.   c. red meat.
    b. whole-fat milk.   d. whole grains.

11. A serving of food contains 12 g carbohydrate, 4 g protein, and 10 g fat. Based on this information, a serving of this food supplies
    a. 94 kcal.   c. 154 kcal.
    b. 184 kcal.   d. 294 kcal.

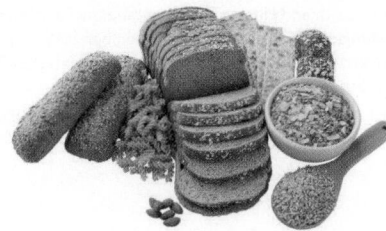

12. A serving of food supplies 20 g carbohydrate, 4 g protein, 10 g fat, 50 g water, 2 mg iron, and 50 mg vitamin C. Which of the following statements is true about a serving of the food?
    a. Fat provides the most food energy.
    b. Carbohydrate provides the most food energy.
    c. Water and vitamin C provide the most food energy.
    d. Fat provides about 25% of total calories.

13. Which of the following foods is the most nutrient dense?
    a. French fries   c. chicken broth
    b. mineral water   d. peanut butter

14. Which of the following statements is false?

    a. A megadose of vitamins provides no calories.
    b. Megadoses of nutrients may behave like drugs in the body.
    c. In general, megadoses of nutrients are safe to consume.
    d. A physiological dose of a vitamin is less than a megadose of the vitamin.

15. Which of the following substances is classified as a dietary supplement according to the DSHEA of 1994?

    a. St. John's wort
    b. mineral oil
    c. red wine
    d. chewing tobacco

ANSWERS TO THE PRACTICE TEST

1-b; 2-b; 3-a; 4-d; 5-b; 6-c; 7-c; 8-a; 9-b; 10-d; 11-c; 12-a; 13-d; 14-c; 15-a

ANSWERS TO CHAPTER 1 QUIZ Yourself

1. There are six classes of nutrients: carbohydrates, lipids, proteins, vitamins, minerals, and water. **True** (p. 3)
2. Vitamins and minerals are sources of energy. **False** (p. 6)
3. A healthy diet is one that contains no sugar or fat. **False** (p. 14)
4. Heart disease is the leading cause of death in the United States. **True** (p. 9)
5. The Food and Drug Administration regulates the safety and effectiveness of dietary supplements that are sold in the United States. **False** (p. 16)

References

1. Guthrie J and others: Americans' food choices at home and away: How do they compare with recommendations? *Amber Waves*. February 2103. Economic Research Service, U.S. Department of Agriculture. http://www.ers.usda.gov/amber-waves/2013-february/americans-food-choices-at-home-and-away.aspx#.UYmjOsotWSo Accessed: March 4, 2014

2. Sun Q and others: White rice, brown rice, and risk of type 2 diabetes in US men and women. *Archives of Internal Medicine* 170(11):961, 2010.

3. Shier D and others: *Hole's Human Anatomy & Physiology*, 12th ed. 2010. New York: McGraw-Hill.

4. Hoyert DL, Xu J: Deaths: Preliminary data for 2011. *National Vital Statistics Reports* 61(6), 2012. http://www.cdc.gov/nchs/fastats/deaths.htm Accessed: March 4, 2014

5. Simopoulos AP: Nutrigenetics/Nutrigenomics. *Annual Review of Public Health.* 31:53–68, 2010.

8. Centers for Disease Control and Prevention: *Tobacco use.* Last updated 2012. http://www.cdc.gov/chronicdisease/resources/publications/AAG/osh.htm Accessed: March 4, 2014

7. U.S. Department of Health and Human Services, U.S. Department of Agriculture: *2015–2020 Dietary Guidelines for Americans.* 2015. www.health.gov/dietaryguidelines/2015/guidelines/executive-summary Accessed: January 21, 2016.

8. U.S. Department of Health and Human Services: *Healthy People.gov: About Healthy People.* Last updated 2012. http://www.healthypeople.gov/2020/about/default.aspx Accessed: March 4, 2014.

9. U.S. Department of Health and Human Services: *Healthy People.gov: Nutrition and weight status: Objectives.* Last updated September 2013. http://www.healthypeople.gov/2020/topicsobjectives2020/nationaldata.aspx?topicId=29 Accessed: March 4, 2014

10. Parker G, Crawford J: Chocolate craving when depressed: A personality marker. *British Journal of Psychiatry* 191:312, 2007.

11. Rose N and others: Mood food: Chocolate and depressive symptoms in a cross-sectional analysis. *Archives of Internal Medicine* 170(8):699, 2010.

12. Martin FJ and others: Everyday eating experiences of chocolate and non-chocolate snacks impact postprandial anxiety, energy and emotional states. *Nutrients* 4(6): 554, 2012.

13. Rolls B: Don't be dense: Trim calories per bite to trim pounds. *Nutrition Action Healthletter,* March 2012, pp. 3–6.

14. U.S. Department of Agriculture, ChooseMyPlate.gov: SuperTracker and other tools, empty calories chart. Last modified June 2011. http://www.choosemyplate.gov/supertracker-tools/empty-calories-chart.html Accessed: March 4, 2014

15. Buhr G, Bales CW: Nutritional supplements for older adults: Review and recommendations—part II. *Journal of Nutrition for the Elderly* 29(1):42, 2010.

16. Dietary Supplement Health and Education Act of 1994. Public Law 103–417, 103rd Congress. http://www.fda.gov/RegulatoryInformation/Legislation/FederalFoodDrugandCosmeticActFDCAct/SignificantAmendmentstotheFDCAct/ucm148003.htm Accessed: March 4, 2014

17. National Center for Complementary and Alternative Medicine: The use of complementary and alternative medicine in the United States. Last updated: February 2013 http://nccam.nih.gov/news/camstats/2007/camsurvey_fs1.htm Accessed: March 4, 2014

18. Huang H-Y and others: The efficacy and safety of multivitamin and mineral supplement use to prevent cancer and chronic disease in adults: A systematic review for a National Institutes of Health State-of-the-Science Conference. *Annals of Internal Medicine* 145(5):372, 2006.

19. Food and Drug Administration: FDA 101: product recalls. May 2010. http://www.fda.gov/downloads/ForConsumers/ConsumerUpdates/UCM143332.pdf Accessed: March 4, 2014

20. Murphy SP and others: Multivitamin-multimineral supplements' effect on total nutrient intake. *American Journal Clinical Nutrition* 85(Suppl 1):280, 2007.

2 Evaluating Nutrition Information

CASE STUDY

Evaluating nutrition-related information

BEFORE SHE LEFT CAMPUS FOR THE SUMMER, Jeannie decided to lose the 8 pounds she gained during her sophomore year in college. She noticed an advertisement in a fashion magazine for a "revolutionary" blend of green teas that was guaranteed to cause rapid weight loss. Jeannie considered purchasing and using the green tea mix to lose weight. She asked friends about the supplement to find out whether any of them had used it. Her friend Shelly had followed the green tea diet plan and lost 10 pounds in just 2 weeks. Furthermore, Shelly had kept the weight off for 6 months, so the green tea mix seemed to be effective.

- What questions should Jeannie answer before she purchases and takes the green tea blend product?
- List three examples of websites where Jeannie could search for reliable health-related information about the green tea product?
- Who would be a source of reliable information concerning ways to lose excess weight safely?

The suggested Case Study Response can be found on page 42.

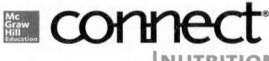 **connect** | NUTRITION

Check out the Connect site at www.mcgrawhillconnect.com to further explore this case study.

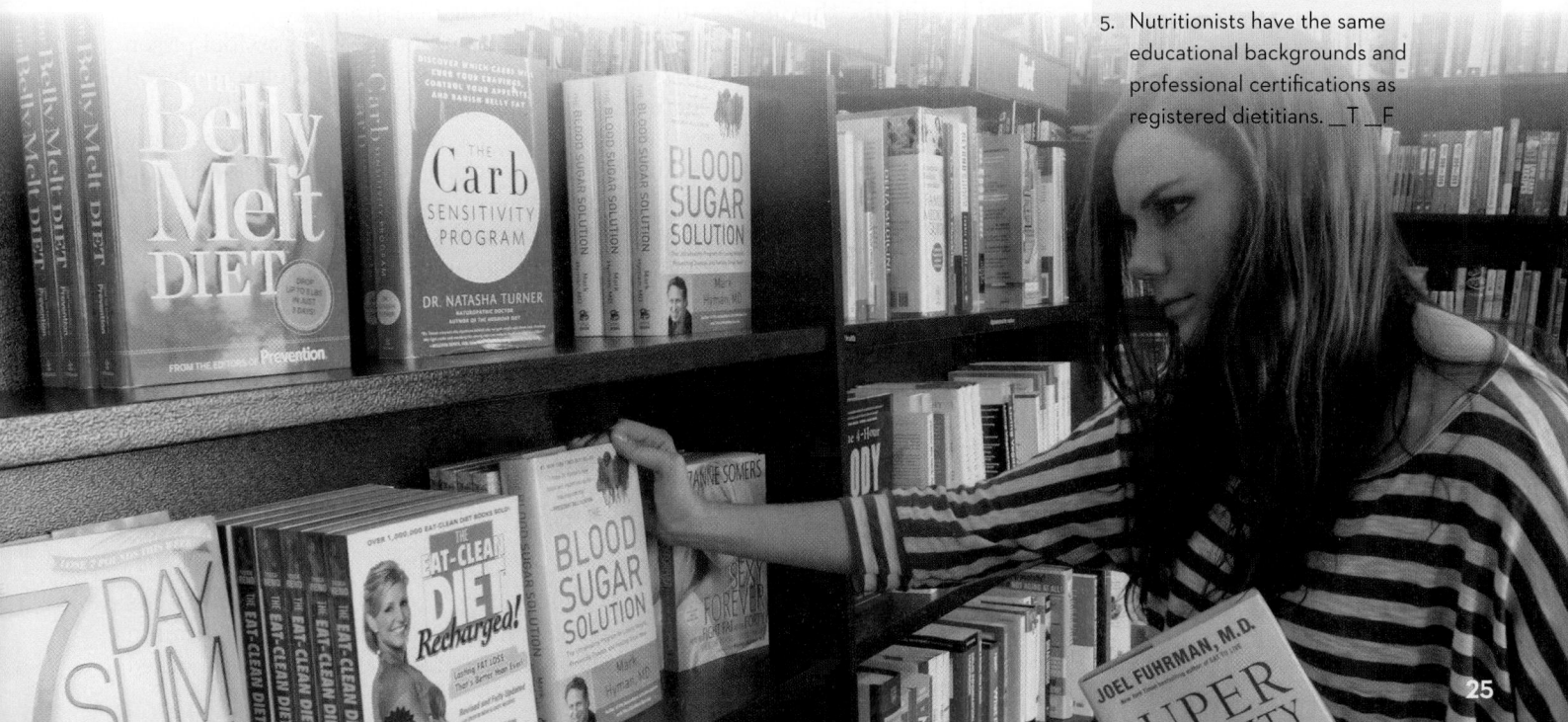

25

2.1 Dr. Goldberger's Discovery

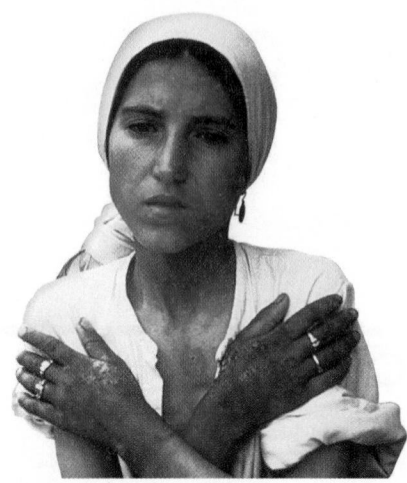

Dry skin and scaly skin sores are characteristic signs of pellagra.

LEARNING OUTCOMES

1 *Explain how Joseph Goldberger developed a hypothesis for the cause of pellagra.*
2 *Explain why it can be difficult for a novel hypothesis to be accepted by the scientific community.*

The woman in this photo has *pellagra* (*peh–lah'–grah* or *peh–lay'–grah*). In the early 1900s, pellagra was widespread in the United States, especially in southern states. Individuals with the disease had scaly skin sores, were weak, and developed diarrhea and mental confusion. Thousands of Americans died from this dreaded illness. In 1914, the U.S. surgeon general assigned Joseph Goldberger, a physician, to study pellagra. Most medical experts thought pellagra was an infectious disease because it often occurred where people lived in close quarters, such as prisons and orphanages.

While investigating factors associated with pellagra, Goldberger observed that not everyone who was exposed to people suffering from pellagra developed the condition. For example, many prisoners had pellagra, but none of their guards or prison administrators had the disease, even though they associated closely with the affected inmates. Based on his observations, Goldberger rejected the notion that pellagra was an infectious disease.

Dr. Goldberger noted that prisoners ate a diet that was typically eaten by other people with pellagra. The diet emphasized corn bread, hominy grits (a corn product), molasses, potatoes, cabbage, and rice. At the time, this low–protein diet was associated with poverty throughout the southern United States. He also observed that people who did not develop pellagra had higher incomes and ate more meat, milk, and fresh vegetables. After considering this information, Goldberger developed the hypothesis that pellagra resulted from the lack of something in people's diet. A **hypothesis** is a possible explanation for an observation that guides scientific research. Goldberger hypothesized that the missing dietary factor was in meat, milk, and other foods eaten regularly by people with higher incomes. To test his hypothesis, Goldberger gave these foods to people who had pellagra, and they were cured of the disease. Despite the results of Goldberger's experiment, many members of the medical establishment rejected his finding that a poor diet was the cause of pellagra.

hypothesis possible explanation for an observation that guides scientific research

To satisfy his critics, Goldberger enrolled a group of healthy Mississippi prison inmates in an experiment that involved consuming the corn– and molasses–based diet commonly eaten in the southern states at the time. After a few months, more than half of the inmates developed cases of pellagra. Once again, however, many of Goldberger's critics rejected his finding that poor diet was the cause of pellagra.

In 1916, Dr. Goldberger decided to experiment on himself and some volunteers during what they called a "filth party." The group applied secretions taken from inside the nose and throat of a patient with pellagra to their noses and throats; they also swallowed pills made with flakes of skin scraped from the rashes of people with the disease. Additionally, Goldberger and one of his colleagues gave each other an injection of blood from a person who had pellagra. If pellagra were infectious, filth–party participants should have contracted the disease—but none of them did. Despite the results of Dr. Goldberger's extraordinary experiment, a few physicians still resisted the idea that pellagra was associated with diet.[1]

Identification of the Missing Dietary Substance

Dr. Goldberger died in 1929—8 years before Dr. Conrad Elvehjem and his team of scientists at the University of Wisconsin isolated a form of the vitamin *niacin* from liver extracts. Elvehjem and his colleagues discovered niacin cured

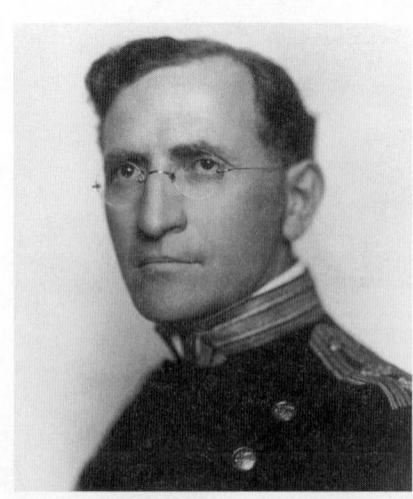

Dr. Joseph Goldberger

"black tongue," a condition affecting dogs that was similar to pellagra.[2] Not long after Elvehjem's findings were published, niacin was determined to be effective in treating pellagra, and the medical establishment finally accepted the fact that the disease was the result of a dietary deficiency. Today, the idea that something missing in diets can cause a nutrient deficiency disease is widely accepted.

This historical event illustrates how researchers use scientific methods to solve medical mysteries relating to nutrition. Even today, scientists can have difficulty gaining the support of their colleagues for unusual ideas or solutions to problems. Health experts often refrain from making quick judgments about a novel nutrition hypothesis until it undergoes repeated testing. Thus, it often takes many years before a scientific discovery becomes widely accepted by other experts in the nutrition field. This chapter focuses on how scientists determine facts about foods, nutrients, and diets. It also provides practical ways for consumers to evaluate the reliability of nutrition information and its sources.

ASSESS YOUR PROGRESS

1 *A group of low-income older adults avoids fruits and vegetables for economic reasons. You observe that many of these people have bleeding gums. State a hypothesis about the cause of bleeding gums in this group of older adults.*

2.2 Understanding the Scientific Method

LEARNING OUTCOMES

1 *Describe the typical steps that scientists generally use to investigate whether a disease has a nutrition-related cause.*

2 *Explain the importance of having controls when performing experiments.*

3 *Describe and provide examples of a case-control study and a cohort study.*

4 *Distinguish between correlation and causation in regard to interpreting the results of scientific studies.*

5 *Discuss the importance of peer review.*

In the past, nutrition facts and dietary practices were often based on intuition, common sense, "conventional wisdom" (tradition), or **anecdotes** (reports of personal experiences). Today, nutrition experts base dietary recommendations on the results of scientific research. Scientists ask questions about the natural world and follow generally accepted, standardized methods to obtain evidence—based answers to these questions. Figure 2.1 presents the general steps nutrition researchers usually take when conducting scientific investigations to collect nutrition information and establish nutrition facts. The following sections describe some of the ways scientists conduct research to find answers to their hypotheses.

anecdotes personal reports concerning a treatment's effectiveness

Animal Research: Laboratory Experiments

An **experiment** is a systematic way of testing a hypothesis. Because of safety and ethical concerns, nutrition scientists often conduct experiments on small mammals ("animal models") before performing similar research on humans. Certain kinds of mice and rats are raised for experimentation purposes, because the rodents

experiment systematic way of testing a hypothesis

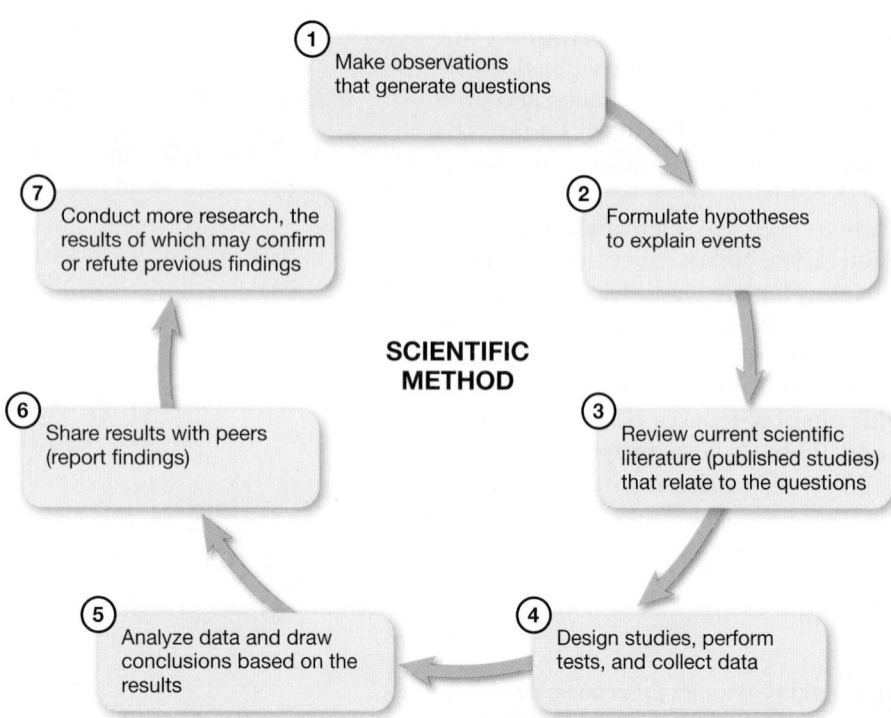

FIGURE 2.1 Scientific method.

in vivo describes experiments that use whole living organisms

in vitro describes experiments on cells or other components derived from living organisms

treatment (or experimental) group in a controlled study, group that receives a treatment

control group in a controlled study, group that does not receive a treatment

are inexpensive to house in laboratories, and their food and other living conditions can be carefully controlled. Researchers must follow government guidelines concerning the ethical care and treatment of laboratory animals.

An experiment that uses whole living organisms, such as mice, is called an ***in vivo*** experiment. Nutrition researchers also perform controlled laboratory experiments on cells or other components derived from living organisms. These studies are ***in vitro*** or "test tube" experiments.

Experiments generally include the basic steps shown in Figure 2.1. A team of nutrition scientists, for example, observes that people who eat high amounts of charcoal–grilled meat seem to have higher rates of stomach cancer than people who rarely eat grilled meat. The scientists generate a hypothesis based on this observation. According to their hypothesis, consuming "chemical X" in charcoal–grilled meat is harmful. Then the team of researchers reviews recent articles written by scientists who have investigated the effects of consuming chemical X.

To test their hypothesis using an animal model, the scientists divide 100 genetically similar, 3–week–old laboratory mice into two groups of 50 mice. Researchers feed the rodents in the **treatment (or experimental) group** a certain amount of chemical X daily for 52 weeks; the second group, the **control group**, does not receive the treatment during the period (Fig. 2.2).

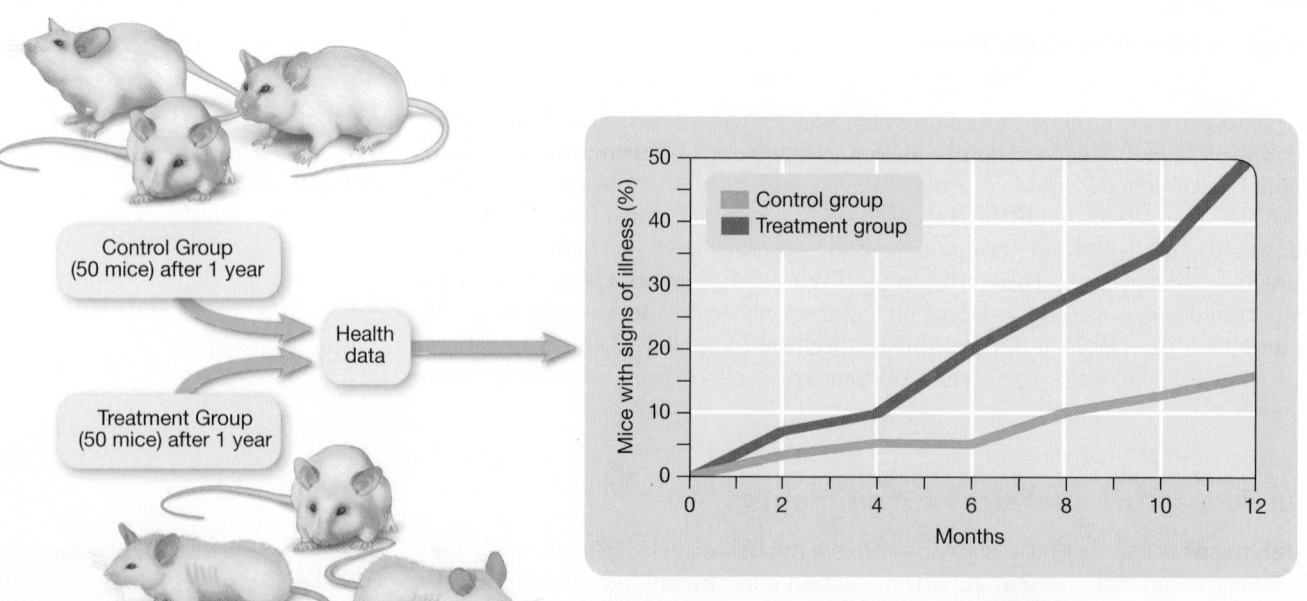

FIGURE 2.2 Interpreting results of an experiment. Based on the findings shown in the graph, is it safe for mice to consume chemical X daily for a year?

Why is a control group necessary? Having a control group enables scientists to compare results between the two study groups to determine whether the treatment had any effect. Many variables can influence the outcome of an experimental study. A **variable** is a factor, such as environment, that can change and influence an outcome. Scientists who want to determine the effect or effects of a single variable, such as chemical X intake, need to control the influence of other variables. Therefore, all other conditions, including the amount of exercise the animals obtain and the extent of their handling by technicians, must be the same for both groups of mice. If researchers design an experiment in which they fail to control variables that are not being tested, then their findings are likely to be unclear, inaccurate, or questionable.

For the duration of this study, the scientists examine the mice regularly for signs of health problems and record their results. If the mice in the treatment group are as healthy as the mice in the control group at the end of this experiment, the researchers may conclude that the rodents can safely consume the amount of chemical X used in the study on a daily basis for a year.

Medical researchers must be careful when applying the results of *in vivo* animal studies to people, because of the physiological differences between humans and other animals. Nevertheless, scientists are often able to determine the safety and effectiveness of treatments by conducting research on laboratory animals before engaging in similar testing on humans.

Human Research: Experimental (Intervention) Studies

Most nutrition–related research involving human subjects incorporates the basic steps of the scientific method (see Fig. 2.1). In many instances, however, it is not practical to conduct research on humans in laboratory settings, so scientists enroll subjects who are "free–living." Free–living subjects are able to participate in studies without experiencing much disruption to their usual routines.

When conducting an experimental study involving human subjects, researchers usually randomly divide a large group of people into treatment (intervention) and control groups. Random assignment helps ensure that the members of the treatment and control groups have similar variables, such as age and other characteristics. Then the scientists provide all study participants with the same instructions and a form of intervention, such as a dietary supplement or experimental food. However, only members of the treatment group actually receive the treatment.

Subjects in the control group are given a **placebo**. Placebos are not just "sugar pills"; they are a fake treatment, such as a pill, injection, or medical procedure. The placebo mimics the treatment. For example, a team of researchers is conducting a study involving human adults to test whether a dietary supplement that contains vitamin C is effective in shortening the duration of the common cold. The scientists provide placebo pills to members of the control group that look, taste, and smell like the supplement pills that contain vitamin C, which are provided for subjects in the treatment group. The placebo pills, however, have *inert* ingredients; that is, the pills contain substances that do not produce any measurable physical changes. Giving placebos to members of the control group enables scientists to compare the extent of the treatment's response with that of the placebo.

Double-Blind Studies

Human experimental studies are usually **double–blind**; that is, neither the investigators nor the subjects are aware of the subjects' group assignments. Codes are used to identify a subject's group membership, and this information is not revealed until the end of the study. Concealing group membership is important during the course of an experiment, because both researchers and subjects may

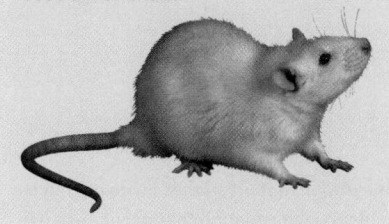

variable factor that can change and influence an outcome of a study

placebo fake treatment

double-blind describes human studies in which neither the investigators nor the subjects are aware of the subjects' group assignments

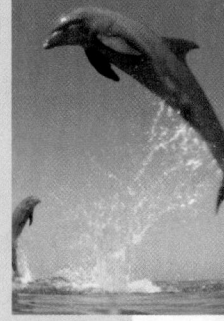

try to predict group assignments based on their expectations. If the investigators are aware of their subjects' individual group assignments during the study (a single–blind study), they may unwittingly convey clues to each subject, perhaps in the form of body language that could influence the subject's belief about being in the experimental or control group. Subjects who suspect they are in the control group and taking a placebo may report no changes in their condition, because they expect a placebo should have no effect on them. On the other hand, subjects who think they are in the treatment group could insist that they are experiencing physical reactions as a result of the treatment, even though the treatment may not be producing any measurable changes in their bodies. Ideally, subjects should not be able to figure out their group assignment while researchers are collecting information from them.

The Placebo Effect If a patient believes a medical treatment will improve his or her health, the patient is more likely to report positive results for the therapy. In intervention studies involving humans, subjects may report positive or negative reactions to a treatment even though they received the placebo. Such thinking is called the **placebo effect**. Even though a placebo contains inert ingredients, it may produce beneficial physiological and psychological changes, particularly in conditions that involve pain or depression.[4,5] Because subjects in the control group believe they are receiving a real treatment, their faith in the "treatment" can stimulate the release of chemicals in the brain that alter pain perception, reducing their discomfort. Therefore, when people report that a treatment was beneficial, they may not have been imagining the positive response, even when they were taking a placebo.

People who use unconventional medical therapies, such as herbal products, to prevent or treat diseases often report that the products and treatments are effective, despite the general lack of scientific evidence to support their beliefs. Such personal reports (anecdotes) may be examples of the placebo effect.

placebo effect in studies involving human subjects, the situation that occurs when a subject reports having positive results even though he or she is taking a placebo

epidemiology study of the occurrence, distribution, and causes of health problems in populations

Human Research: Epidemiological Studies

For decades, medical researchers have noted differences in rates of chronic diseases and causes of death among various human populations. For example, type 2 diabetes, the most common type of diabetes, occurs more frequently among Asian American, Hispanic, and non–Hispanic African–American adults than among non–Hispanic white American adults.[6] Additionally, breast cancer is more common among non–Hispanic white females than among females who are members of other American racial or ethnic groups.[7] To understand why these differences exist, medical researchers often rely on the findings of epidemiological studies. **Epidemiology** (*ehp–eh–dee'–me–all'–o–jee*) is the study of the occurrence, distribution, and causes of health problems in populations.[8] By conducting studies that explore differences in dietary practices and disease occurrences among populations, nutrition scientists may learn much about the influence of diet on health.

Epidemiologists often use physical examinations of people to obtain health data (Fig. 2.3). Additionally, they may collect information by conducting surveys. Such surveys question people about their personal and family medical histories, diets, environmental exposures, health practices, and attitudes. Surveys often rely on people remembering details about their past lifestyle practices, which can be inaccurate or incomplete. However, epidemiologists can obtain much useful information concerning a population's typical dietary practices by conducting surveys of large numbers of people.

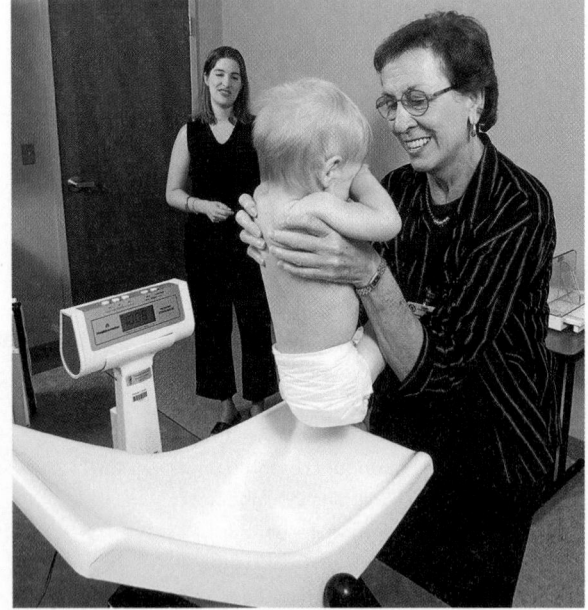

FIGURE 2.3 Collecting nutrition-related information.
Epidemiologists and dietitians often rely on physical examinations of people to obtain health data. In this photo, a U.S. Department of Agriculture staff member prepares to weigh a 1-year-old boy while his mother watches.

Since its introduction in the early 1960s, the **National Health and Nutrition Examination Survey (NHANES)** has provided information about the health and nutritional status of adults and children in the United States. This survey is unique, because it combines interviews and physical examinations. The interview includes dietary, health–related, and *demographic* questions. Demographics are characteristics of a particular population that might affect health, such as income, age, and education level.

Researchers use findings from the NHANES to assess nutritional status of the population and determine the prevalence of major diseases and risk factors for diseases. Such information is useful for educational programs designed to promote health and prevent disease. Medical experts also use the NHANES findings to establish national standards for assessing height, weight, and blood pressure (see Appendix F).

Observational Studies

Most nutrition research involving human subjects is observational and involves either case–control study or cohort study designs (Fig. 2.4). In a **case–control study**, individuals with a health condition (cases) such as heart disease or breast cancer are matched to persons with similar characteristics who do not have the condition (controls). Information such as personal and family medical histories, eating habits, and other lifestyle behaviors is collected from each participant in the study. By analyzing the results of case–control studies, researchers identify factors that may have been responsible for the illness. For example, scientists may be able to identify dietary practices that differ between the two groups, such as long–term fruit and vegetable intakes.

In a **cohort study**, epidemiologists collect and analyze various kinds of information about a large group of people over time. The scientists are generally interested in making associations between exposure to a specific factor and the subsequent development of health conditions.

Cohort studies can be retrospective or prospective. Retrospective means "to look back" and prospective means "to look forward" in time (Fig. 2.5). In a **retrospective cohort study**, researchers collect information about a group's past exposures and identify current health outcomes. For example, nutrition epidemiologists might examine whether a group of people who have stomach cancer consumed more charcoal–broiled meat (the exposure) in the past than a group of people with similar characteristics who do not have stomach cancer. In a **prospective cohort study**, a group of initially healthy people are followed over a time period and any diseases that eventually develop are recorded. Scientists then try to identify links between exposures and diseases that occurred between the beginning and end of the study period (see Fig. 2.5).

The Framingham Heart Study that began in 1949 in Framingham, Massachusetts, is one of the most well–known prospective studies. At the beginning of the study, over 5200 healthy participants (men and women) underwent extensive physical examinations and questioning about their family and personal medical histories, as well as their lifestyle practices. Over the following years, a group of medical researchers periodically collected data concerning each participant's health and, if the person died, the cause of death. Today, medical researchers are still collecting information from the original study participants, as well as their descendants.[9]

Limitations of Nutrition-Related Studies

Nutrition researchers use a variety of statistical methods to analyze data (information) collected from observations and experiments. As a result, scientists can determine whether their hypotheses are supported by the data. During

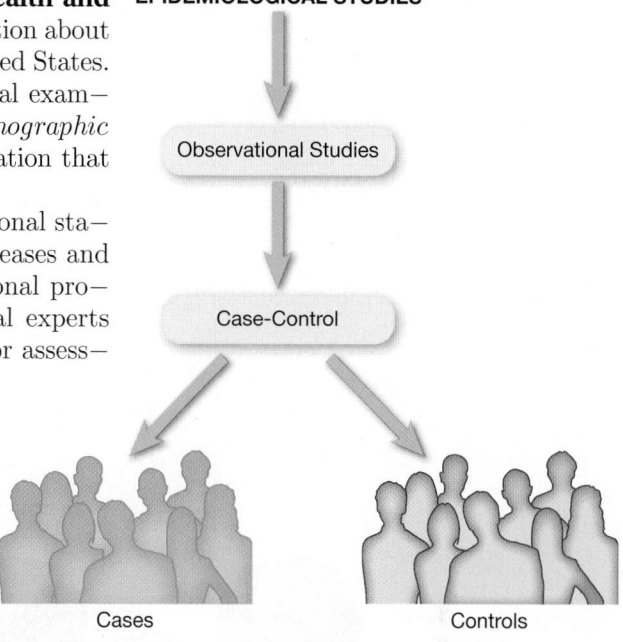

EPIDEMIOLOGICAL STUDIES

FIGURE 2.4 Case-control study. People with a health condition (cases) are matched with persons who have similar characteristics but are healthy (controls).

National Health and Nutrition Examination Survey (NHANES) survey that uses interviews and physical examinations to assesses the health and nutritional status of adults and children in the United States

case-control study study in which individuals with a health condition (cases) are matched to persons with similar characteristics who do not have the condition

cohort study epidemiological study in which researchers collect and analyze various kinds of information about a large group of people over time

retrospective cohort study study in which researchers collect information about a group's past exposures and identify current health outcomes

prospective cohort study study in which a group of initially healthy people are followed over a time period and any diseases that eventually develop are recorded

FIGURE 2.5 Cohort studies.
Epidemiological research often involves cohort studies that may be retrospective or prospective.

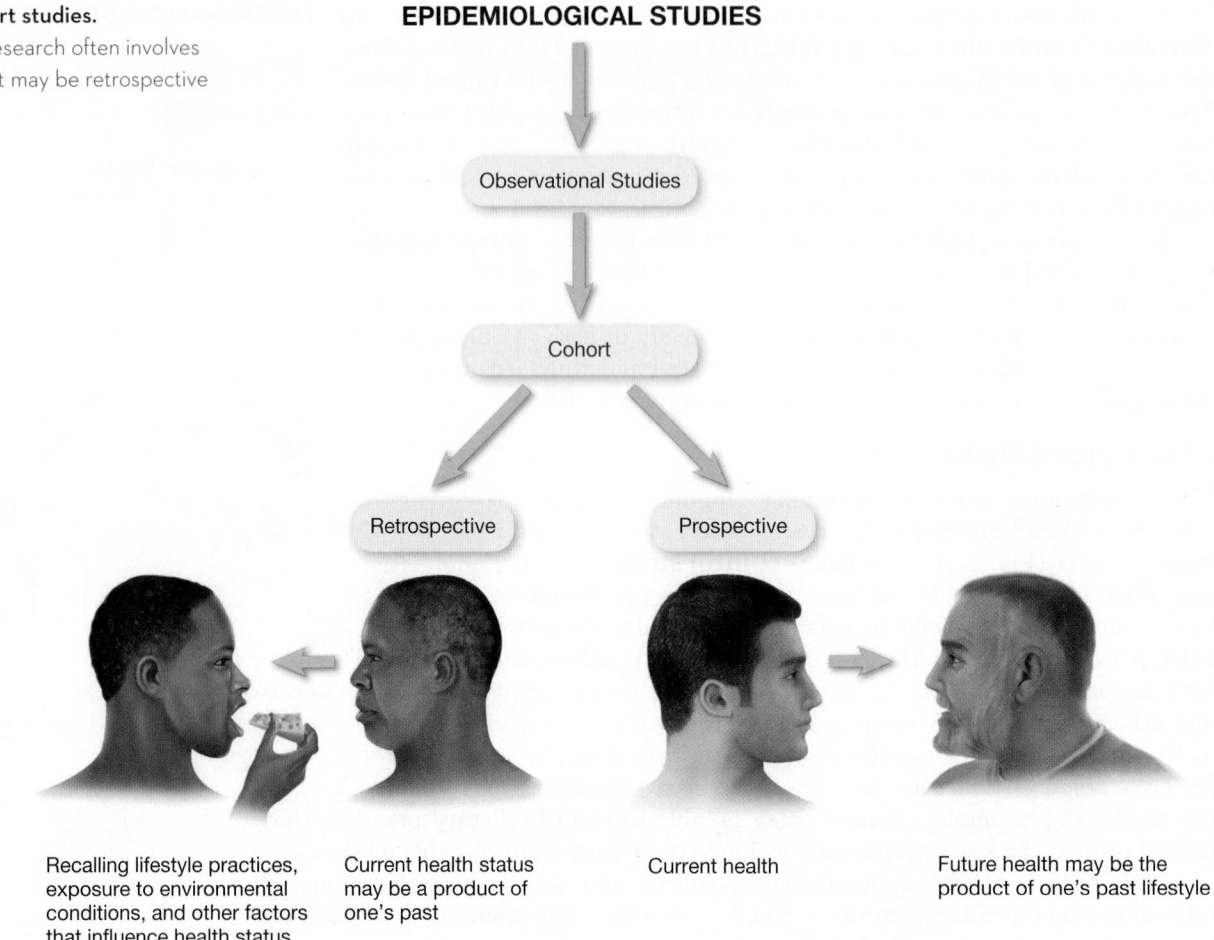

EPIDEMIOLOGICAL STUDIES

Observational Studies

Cohort

Retrospective

Prospective

Recalling lifestyle practices, exposure to environmental conditions, and other factors that influence health status

Current health status may be a product of one's past

Current health

Future health may be the product of one's past lifestyle

correlation relationship between variables

direct or **positive correlation** describes the relationship that occurs when two variables increase or decrease in the same direction

inverse or **negative correlation** describes the relationship that occurs when one variable increases and the other one decreases

causation specific practice that is responsible for an effect

their analysis, nutrition scientists often look for **correlations** (relationships) between variables and health outcomes. A correlation occurs when two variables change over the same period; for example, when a population's intake of sugar—sweetened soft drinks increases, the percentage of overweight people in the population also increases (Fig. 2.6a). In this case, the correlation is **direct** or **positive**, because the two variables—body weight and regular soft drink consumption—are changing in the same direction; they are both increasing. An **inverse** or **negative correlation** occurs when one variable increases and the other one decreases (the variables change in opposite directions). An example of an inverse correlation is the relationship between fruit intake and hypertension; as a population's fruit consumption increases, the percentage of people with hypertension in that population decreases (Fig. 2.6b).

When analyzing their results, nutrition scientists who conduct studies on free—living groups of people must also consider the effects of *confound—ers* on their results. Confounders are factors that were not being studied but could have influenced the outcomes of the research. For example, a group of scientists investigating the effects of alcohol consumption on bone health may determine that there is a positive relationship between the consumption of alcohol—containing beverages and risk of *osteoporosis*, a condition characterized by loss of bone tissue. However, many people who drink alcohol also smoke ciga—rettes. If the scientists did not adjust their results for their study population's use of tobacco, the results of their research may be weak or false.

Epidemiological studies cannot establish **causation**; that is, whether a spe—cific practice is responsible for an effect ("cause and effect"). When two different natural events occur simultaneously within a population, it does not necessarily mean they are related. What appears to be a correlation between a behavior and

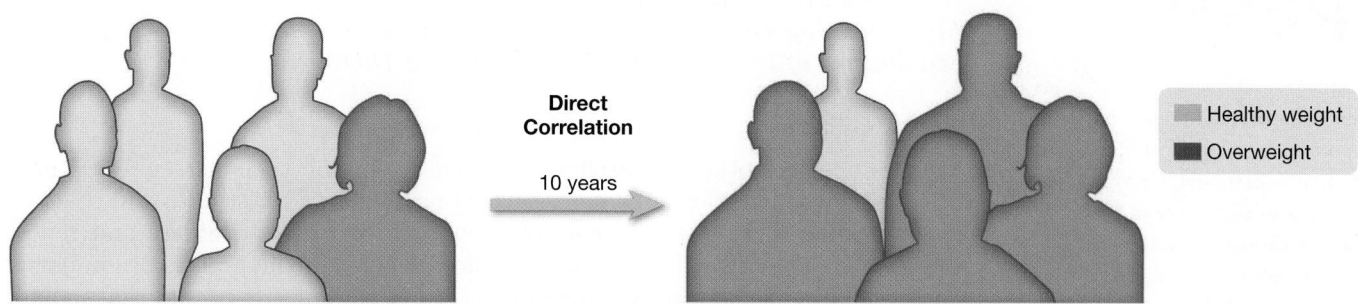

(a) As a population's intake of sugar-sweetened soft drinks increases (⋏), the percentage of overweight people in that population increases (⋏).

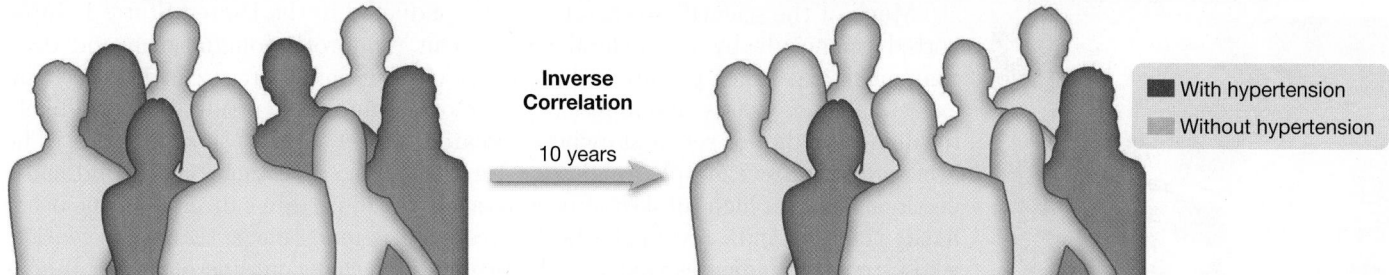

(b) As a population's fruit intake increases (⋏), the percentage of people in that population with hypertension decreases (⋎).

FIGURE 2.6 **Examples of direct and inverse correlations.** (*a*) Direct (positive) correlation. (*b*) Inverse (negative) correlation.

an outcome could be a coincidence, that is, a chance happening, and not an indi-cation of a cause—and—effect relationship between the two variables. For exam-ple, in a survey of lemonade consumption in Colorado over a 10—year period, we might observe that fewer people drank lemonade during the winter than during the summer months. In a survey of snow skiing accidents in Colorado during the same 10—year period, we might also find that snow skiing accidents were more likely to occur during the winter than in the summer. Thus, as lemonade con-sumption declined, snow skiing accidents increased. Does this mean that people who do not drink lemonade have a greater risk of having a skiing accident at this time of year? In Colorado, is lemonade consumption inversely correlated to skiing accidents? Probably not. It is more likely that the relationship between snow skiing and lemonade drinking is coincidental, because both activities are associated with seasonal weather conditions. Although this example is obviously far—fetched, it illustrates the problems scientists can have when analyzing results of epidemiological and other kinds of studies involving human subjects.

peer review critical analysis of an article about a study submitted to a journal that is conducted by a group of investigators who were not part of the study but are experts involved in related research

Reporting Findings

When an experiment or study is completed and the results analyzed, researchers summarize the findings and seek to publish articles with information about their investigation in scientific journals. Before arti-cles are accepted for publication, they undergo **peer review**, a critical analysis conducted by a group of "peers." Peers are investigators who were not part of the study but are experts involved in related research. It is important to note that peers are not selected by the researchers who submit their papers for publication. Editors of scientific journals choose the experts, and the researchers are usually not aware of the peers' identities.

If peers agree that a study was well conducted, its results are fairly represented, and the research is of interest to the journal's readers, these scientists are likely to recommend that the journal's editors publish the article. Examples of peer—reviewed medical and nutrition journals include the *Journal of*

Examples of peer-reviewed medical and nutrition journals.

FRESH TIPS

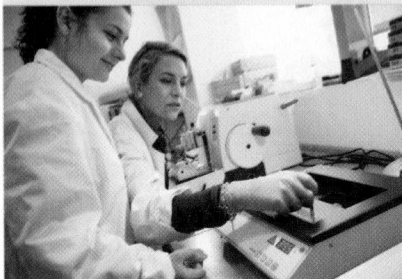

Nutrition, American Journal of Clinical Nutrition, New England Journal of Medicine, Journal of the American Medical Association, Nutrition Reviews, and *Journal of the Academy of Nutrition and Dietetics.*

Research Bias

Scientists expect other researchers to avoid relying on their personal attitudes and *biases* (points of view) when selecting participants for studies and collecting and analyzing data. Furthermore, researchers should evaluate and report their results objectively and honestly. These aspects of the process are important because personal biases can result in faulty findings or results that cannot be generalized to larger populations.

Much of the scientific research that is conducted in the United States is supported financially by the federal government, nonprofit foundations, and drug companies and other private industries. Some funding sources can have certain expectations or biases about research outcomes, and as a result, they are likely to finance studies of scientists whose research efforts support their interests. The beef industry, for example, might not fund scientific investigations to find connections between high intakes of beef and the risk of certain cancers. On the other hand, the beef industry might be interested in supporting a team of scientists whose research indicates that a high–protein diet that contains plenty of beef is useful for people who are trying to lose weight. Peer–reviewed journals usually require authors of articles to disclose their affiliations and sources of financial support. Such disclosures may appear on the first page or at the end of the article. By having this information, readers can decide on the reliability of the findings.

Following Up with More Research

The results of one study are rarely enough to gain widespread acceptance for new or unusual findings or to provide a basis for nutritional recommendations. Thus, the findings obtained by one research team must be supported by those generated in other studies. If the results of several scientific investigations conducted under similar conditions confirm the original researchers' conclusions, then these findings are more likely to be accepted by other nutrition scientists.

After the results of a study are published in a nutrition–related journal or reported to health professionals attending a meeting of a nutrition or medical society, the media (e.g., newspapers, magazines, Internet news sources) may receive notice of the findings. If the information is simplistic and sensational, such as a finding that drinking green tea can result in weight loss, it is more likely to be reported in the popular press. In many instances, people learn about the study's results when they are reported in a television or online news broadcast as a 15– or 30–second "sound bite." Such sources generally provide very little information concerning the way the study was conducted or how the data were collected and analyzed. Therefore, sensational media coverage of a medical "breakthrough" is not necessarily an indication of the value or quality of research that resulted in the news story or magazine article.

Confusion and Conflict

One day, the news highlights dramatic health benefits from eating garlic, dark chocolate, brown rice, or cherries. A few weeks later, the news includes reports of more recent scientific investigations that do not support the earlier findings. When consumers become aware of conflicting results generated by nutrition studies, they often become confused and disappointed. As a result, some people may mistrust the scientific community and think nutrition scientists do not know what they are doing.

Consumers need to recognize that conflicting findings often result from differences in the ways various studies are designed. Even when investigating the same question, different groups of scientists often conduct their studies and analyze the results differently. For example, the numbers, ages, and physical conditions of subjects; the type and length of the study; the amount of the treatment provided; and the statistical tests used to analyze results typically vary among studies. Additionally, individual genetic differences often contribute to a person's response to a treatment. Not only are people genetically different, but they also have different lifestyles, and they typically recall dietary information and follow instructions concerning health care practices differently. These and other factors can influence the results of nutrition research, especially studies involving human subjects.

The science of nutrition is constantly evolving: Old beliefs and practices are discarded when they are not supported by more recent scientific evidence, and new principles and practices emerge from the new findings. Science involves asking questions, developing and testing hypotheses, gathering and analyzing data, drawing conclusions from data, and, sometimes, accepting change.

ASSESS YOUR PROGRESS

2 *Distinguish between a control group and a treatment group in an experiment.*

3 *Explain the differences between a survey and an intervention study.*

4 *What is the major difference between a prospective study and a retrospective study?*

5 *Why is peer review a critical step in the scientific method?*

6 *Explain why results of similar studies involving human subjects may provide different findings.*

2.3 Nutrition Information: Fact or Fiction

LEARNING OUTCOMES

1 *List features of unreliable sources of nutrition information.*

2 *List characteristics of reliable sources of nutrition information.*

3 *Describe how the Internet can be used to access reliable nutrition information.*

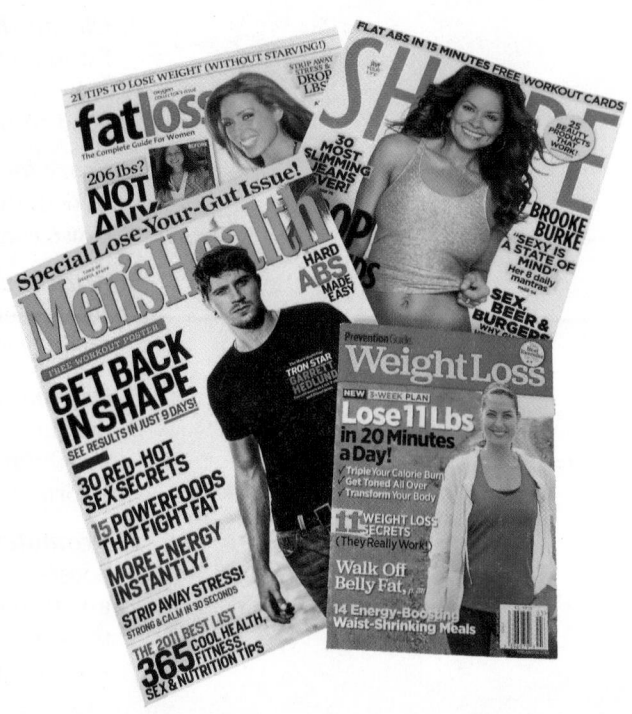

To be careful consumers, people should not assume that all nutrition information presented in the popular media is reliable. The U.S. Food and Drug Administration (FDA) can regulate nutrition- and health-related claims on product labels, but the agency cannot prevent the spread of health and nutrition misinformation published in books or pamphlets or presented in television or radio programs. The First Amendment to the U.S. Constitution guarantees freedom of the press and freedom of speech, so people can provide nutrition information that is not true. Thus, the First Amendment does not protect consumers with freedom from nutrition misinformation or false nutrition claims. Consumers are responsible for questioning and researching the accuracy of nutrition information, as well as the credentials of the people making nutrition-related claims.

Promoters of worthless nutrition-related products often use sophisticated marketing methods to lure consumers. For example, some promoters of dietary supplements claim their products are "scientifically tested," or they include citations for what appear to be scientific journal articles in their ads or articles. Consumers, however, cannot be certain this information is true. Few dietary supplements have been thoroughly evaluated by reputable scientists. In some instances, these products have been scientifically tested, but the bulk of the research has shown that most dietary supplements, other than vitamins and minerals, provide little or no measurable health benefits. Nevertheless, promoters of nonnutrient dietary supplements usually ignore the scientific evidence and continue to sell their goods to an unsuspecting, trusting public.

Ask Questions

Most people do not want to waste their money on things they do not need or that are useless or potentially harmful. How can a person become a more care—ful, critical consumer of nutrition—related information or products? To evaluate various sources of nutrition information, a person can ask:

- *What motivates the authors, promoters, or sponsors that provide the information?* Could they be more interested in helping people achieve better health and well—being or in selling their products?

- *Who is the source?* Is the source a nutrition expert who has reliable credentials?
  - Nutrition experts introduced or identified as "Doctor" may not be physicians or scientists. Their "doctoral" degree may be in a field that is unrelated to nutrition or a bogus degree purchased from the Internet.

- *What is the source?* Is the source a scientific (*evidence—based*), such as an article from a peer—reviewed nutrition journal?
  - Nutrition information in popular sources, such as magazines, generally has not been peer reviewed.
  - Articles and programs that promote nutrition information may actually be sophisticated advertisements for nutrition—related products.
  - Promoters may also refer to phony scientific journals to convince people that their information is reliable.

Look for Red Flags

To become more critical consumers of nutrition information, people need to be aware of "red flags," clues that indicate a source of information is unreliable. Common red flags include the following:

1. *Promises of quick and easy remedies:* "Our product helps you lose weight without exercising or dieting."

2. *Claims that sound too good to be true:* "Our all—natural product blocks fat and calories from being absorbed, so you can eat everything you like and still lose weight." Claims such as this are rarely true. If the claim sounds too good to be true, it probably is false.

3. *Scare tactics:* Sensational, frightening, false, or misleading statements about a food, dietary practice, or health condition, such as "Dairy products cause cancer."

4. *Attacks on conventional scientists and nutrition experts:* "Medical researchers don't want you to know the facts." Such statements indicate unsupported biases against the scientific community.

5. *Testimonials and anecdotes:* "I lost 50 pounds in 30 days using this product." A **testimonial** is a personal endorsement of a product. People usually receive payment for their endorsements. Reliable nutrition information is based on scientific evidence.

6. *Promotes benefits while overlooking risks:* "All—natural supplement boosts your metabolism naturally, so it won't harm your system." Anything a person consumes, even water, can be toxic in high doses. Consumers need to be wary of any source of information that fails to mention the possible side effects of using a dietary supplement or nutrition—related treatment.

testimonial personal endorsement of a product

7. *Vague, meaningless, or scientific—sounding terms:* "Our all—natural, scientifically tested, patented, chelated dietary supplement detoxifies your liver fast."

8. *Vague sources:* "Clinical research performed at a major university proves this revolutionary new dietary supplement cures diabetes." *Which* clinical study and at *which* "major university"?

9. *Pseudoscience:* **Pseudoscience** is the presentation of information masquerading as factual and scientific. Examples include: "Learn how to combine certain foods based on your blood type," or "Most diseases are caused by undigested food that gets stuck in your guts." Promoters of nutrition misinformation often try to confuse people by weaving false information with facts into their claims, making the untrue material seem credible, too.

10. *Disclaimers:* A disclaimer is a statement that modifies a claim or denies responsibility for it (Fig. 2.7). For example, an ad for a weight—loss product claims, "Lose 30 pounds in 30 days." However, the ad includes a disclaimer that is in small print and states, "Results not typical." Disclaimers are often clues that the product may not live up to consumers' expectations or the manufacturer's claims.

FIGURE 2.7 Results disclaimer. This disclaimer may be a red flag indicating the product has limited effectiveness, despite its promoter's claims.

Using the Internet Wisely

People can find plenty of sites with nutrition information, including ads for dietary supplements, on the Internet. However, consumers must be careful and question the sources before accepting the information as being reliable.

Be wary of websites that are authored or sponsored by one person or that promote or sell products for profit (.com), because such sources of information may be biased. Even many websites using the .org domain suffix are actually sources of unreliable nutrition formation because they have a hidden agenda. In general, websites sponsored by nationally recognized health associations such as the Academy of Nutrition and Dietetics (www.eatright.org) and nationally respected nonprofit organizations such as the National Osteoporosis Foundation (www.nof .org) are reliable sources of nutrition information. Government agencies (.gov), such as the Centers for Disease Control and Prevention (www.cdc.gov) and the Food and Drug Administration (www.fda.gov), are also excellent sources of credible nutrition information. The Fresh Tips box on page 38 presents some tips for using the Internet to obtain reliable nutrition information.

Scientific Nutrition-Related Literature: Searching Online

Health care professionals should refer to peer—reviewed scientific literature when searching for nutrition—related information. Many colleges and universities sub-scribe to a wide variety of online journals, enabling faculty and students to have free access to articles. To conduct an online review of scientific literature, visit the U.S. National Library of Medicine and National Institutes of Health "PubMed" website. The site provides abstracts of and links to full—text articles about various medical conditions. An abstract is a brief summary of an article that emphasizes key aspects of the research, that is, the "take—away" messages. To practice using PubMed, visit the website at http://www.ncbi.nlm.nih.gov/pubmed/ and enter a nutrition—related topic such as "anorexia" in the search box.

Not every journal that has articles cited by PubMed is a reliable source of nutrition or health information. In some cases, journals have been established and supported by groups with biases. Such journals provide a way of publishing articles

pseudoscience presentation of information masquerading as factual and scientific

Federal Trade Commission (FTC) federal government agency that protects consumers against "unfair and deceptive acts or practices" by businesses in the United States

DID **YOU** KNOW?

The **Federal Trade Commission (FTC)** is the federal government agency that protects consumers against "unfair and deceptive acts or practices" by businesses in the United States. The FTC can challenge promoters who use false and misleading claims to market their health care products and services. Despite FTC enforcement, misleading and deceptive advertisements continue to saturate the market. To learn how to avoid becoming a target of fraudulent health and nutrition marketing practices, visit the FTC's website (www.ftc.gov) and search for "miracle health claims." To complain about a product, consumers can complete and submit the FTC's complaint form at the website or call the agency's toll-free line (1-877-382-4357).

FRESH TIPS

To be careful consumers of Internet sources of information, people can:

- Compare information by using multiple sites, especially government sites as well as the sites of nationally recognized nutrition- or health-related organizations.

- Be wary of sites that have surveys to complete, advertisements for diet-related products, and promotions in pop-up windows.

- Rely primarily on sites that are managed or reviewed by a group of qualified health professionals. Blogs might be fun and interesting to read, but they tend to be anecdotal and not necessarily reliable.

- Look for the Health on the Net symbol at the bottom of the main page of the website. The Health on the Net Foundation is a nonprofit, international organization that promotes the *HONcode*, a set of principles for standardizing the reliability of health information on the Internet. Currently, adherence to the code is optional. For more information about HONcode, you can visit the organization's website (www.hon.ch/).

- Avoid sites that provide online diagnoses and treatments.

For more tips, visit: http://ods.od.nih.gov/Health_Information/
How_To_Evaluate_Health_Information_on_the_Internet
_Questions_and_Answers.aspx.

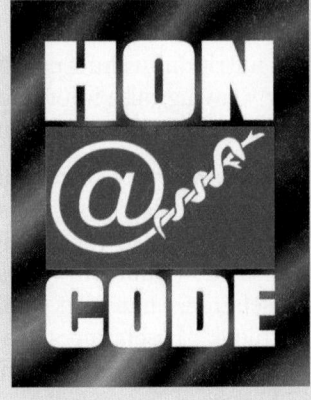

registered dietitian (RD) or registered dietitian nutritionist (RDN) college-trained health care professional who has extensive knowledge of foods, nutrition, and dietetics

dietetics application of nutrition and food information to achieve and maintain optimal health and to treat many health-related conditions

that would be rejected by editors of reliable journals, because peer reviewers would indicate that the studies are poorly designed or have questionable findings. Therefore, it is important to search for information in more than one journal and compare research designs and results. Scientific journals that have long histories of publishing peer—reviewed articles are usually reliable sources.

Directing Questions at Reliable Experts

If people have questions about food or nutrition, where can they find factual answers? People cannot always rely on someone who refers to himself or herself as a "nutrition expert" or "nutritionalist" for reliable nutrition information, because there are no standard legal definitions for these descriptors. Many states have licensure laws for someone using the title "nutritionist." In other states, however, people can refer to themselves as "nutritionists" regardless of their education or training. Be wary if the so—called nutrition expert has "cre—dentials" that lack credibility among members of the scientific community, such as RNC ("registered nutrition consultant"), ND ("doctor of naturopathy"), CNC ("certificate in nutritional counseling"), and MH ("master herbalist").

Universities and colleges that have nutrition or dietetics departments are likely to employ nutrition experts, including instructors and researchers who have advanced degrees in foods, nutrition, and dietetics. Many of these faculty members are also registered dietitians. A **registered dietitian (RD)** or **registered dietitian nutritionist (RDN)** is a college—trained health care professional who has extensive knowledge of foods, nutrition, and **dietetics**, the application of nutrition and food information to achieve and maintain optimal health, and to treat many health—related conditions. The titles "registered dietitian" and "reg—istered dietitian nutritionist" are legally protected and require certain credentials.

People can also locate registered dietitians by consulting online directories, contacting local dietetic associations or dietary departments of local hospitals, or visiting the Academy of Nutrition and Dietetics' website (www.eatright.org) or the Dietitians of Canada's website (www.dietitians.ca).

FRESH TIPS

To obtain information about a nutrition expert's credentials, consumers can enter the person's name at an Internet search engine and evaluate the results. If the person is associated with an accredited school of higher education or a government agency, such as the University of Kentucky or U.S. Department of Agriculture, the person is probably a reliable source of information. Consumers can also visit www.quackwatch.org and submit an "Ask a Question" e-mail requesting information about a person's credentials from the site's sponsors.

ASSESS YOUR PROGRESS

7 What is the difference between a testimonial and an anecdote?

8 List at least three "red flags" that may indicate a questionable source of nutrition information.

9 List at least three tips for using the Internet as a reliable source of nutrition information.

10 Explain why a person who uses the title "nutritionist" may not be a reliable source of nutrition information.

2.4 Nutrition Experts: Registered Dietitians

LEARNING OUTCOMES

1 Describe the roles that registered dietitians play as members of the health care team.

2 Discuss steps a person must take to become a registered dietitian nutritionist.

A registered dietitian (RD) or registered dietitian nutritionist (RDN) is a health care professional who is "a food and nutrition expert."[10] *Clinical* dietitians can work as members of medical teams that include other health professionals, such as physicians, nurses, and physical therapists, in hospitals or clinics. A clinical dietitian helps evaluate the health status of a patient and determines the patient's dietary deficiencies and needs. Dietitians plan dietary treatments (interventions), as well as appropriate and nutritious meals for hospitalized patients.

Dietitians can also work as community nutritionists in public health settings or as directors of food service systems, such as cafeterias in hospitals and schools. Although most registered dietitians work in health care settings, some RDs are educators, researchers, or dietary counselors in private practice.

Becoming a Registered Dietitian/Nutritionist

To become a registered dietitian or registered dietitian nutritionist, a person needs to meet specific educational and certification requirements that are approved by the Accreditation Council for Education in Nutrition and Dietetics of the *Academy of Nutrition and Dietetics*. To obtain the RD/RDN credential, a person has to earn at least a bachelor's degree in an approved or accredited plan of study, such as "nutrition or dietetics major" at an accredited college or university in the United States.

In addition to taking the required college coursework, the student dietitian must complete a *supervised practice program* that provides professional training in a health care facility such as a hospital, a food service company, or a community health care agency such as a state or local government health department. Finally, this individual has to pass the national registration examination to become certified as an RD/RDN. After becoming certified, RDs and RDNs are also required to fulfill continuing education requirements to maintain their certification. For more information about the dietetics profession, visit the Academy's website at www.eatright.org.

ASSESS YOUR PROGRESS

11 Discuss how dietitians work with other health care professionals in clinical settings.

12 What steps would you take to become an RD/RDN?

SUMMARY

SECTION 2.1 Dr. Goldberger's Discovery

- In the early 1900s, Dr. Joseph Goldberger developed a dietary hypothesis for the cause of pellagra. Goldberger tested his hypotheses and determined that poor diet was the cause of the disease. The scientific community eventually accepted the notion that dietary deficiencies caused illnesses that could be deadly.

SECTION 2.2 Understanding the Scientific Method

- Nutrition research relies on generally accepted scientific methods. Other scientists can test the findings to confirm or reject them. Nutrition experts discard conventional beliefs, explanations, and practices when the results of current scientific research no longer support them.

- In experimental studies, nutrition scientists can investigate whether a health condition results from a certain dietary practice. In human experimental studies, subjects are divided into treatment (intervention) and control groups. Members of the control group receive a placebo. Controls are important for comparing results.

- Epidemiology is the study of the occurrence, distribution, and causes of health problems in populations. By conducting studies that explore differences in dietary practices and disease occurrences among populations, nutrition scientists may learn much about the influence of diet on health.

- Observational research involves either case-control or cohort study designs. Cohort studies can be either retrospective or prospective. A correlation is a relationship between variables and can be direct (positive) or indirect (negative). Epidemiological studies cannot establish cause and effect, because the relationship between two variables could be a coincidence.

- When a study is completed and the results analyzed, researchers summarize the findings and seek to publish articles about their investigations in scientific journals. Before articles are accepted for publication, they undergo peer review. Scientists generally do not accept a hypothesis or the results of a study until they are supported by considerable research evidence.

- Conflicting findings often result because different teams of researchers use different study designs when investigating the same hypothesis. Furthermore, each team of scientists may analyze the results differently. Other factors, such as genetic and lifestyle differences, also can influence the results of nutrition research involving human subjects.

SECTION 2.3 Nutrition Information: Fact or Fiction

- Testimonials and anecdotes are typically used to promote nutrition-related products, but consumers cannot be sure that this information is reliable or based on scientific facts. Anecdotal reports are not scientific evidence.

- The media and the Internet are often unreliable sources of nutrition information. People who promote nutrition misinformation often take advantage of freedom of the press and freedom of speech to make their claims. Consumers need to be critical of various sources of nutrition information and ask questions to help determine its reliability.

SECTION 2.4 Nutrition Experts: Registered Dietitians

- A registered dietitian (RD) or a registered dietitian nutritionist (RDN) is a food and nutrition expert who has graduated from accredited degree programs in nutrition and dietetics, completed a supervised practice program, and passed a comprehensive national exam.

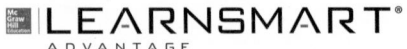

Get the most out of your study of nutrition with McGraw-Hill's innovative suite of adaptive learning products including McGraw-Hill LearnSmart®, SmartBook®, McGraw-Hill LearnSmart Achieve®, and McGraw-Hill LearnSmart Prep®. Visit www.learnsmartadvantage.com.

TEST KITCHEN
Modifying Recipes for Healthy Living

According to nutrition experts, Americans may obtain certain health benefits by increasing their whole-grain intake. You are a member of a research team that has developed this hypothesis: "Adding 15 g of fiber/day in the form of whole grains to diets will reduce blood sugar levels by at least 5% after a 6-month period." To evaluate whether consuming this amount of whole grains has an effect on blood sugar, your team plans to conduct a prospective study. The subjects of the study will be randomly assigned to eat either two "regular" muffins or two whole-grain muffins daily for 6 months, while maintaining their usual lifestyles. The following muffin recipe will be used to prepare the regular (control) muffins. Modify this recipe so it can be used to make the experimental (whole-grain) muffins.

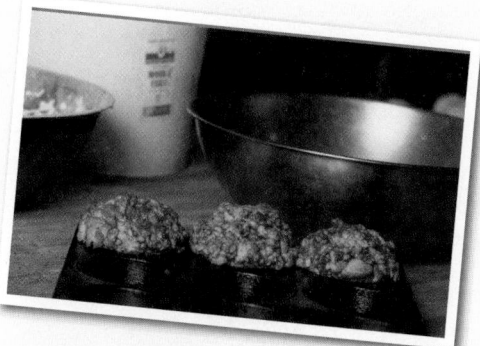

APPLESAUCE MUFFINS

PREPARATION STEPS

1. Preheat oven to 400°F. Spray vegetable oil spray lightly on the bottom of each cup of the muffin tin.
2. Combine flour, baking powder, baking soda, and spices in a large bowl. Stir until well mixed. By using a large spoon, form a depressed area (a "well") in the center of the dry ingredients.
3. In another bowl, break the egg and use a fork to beat the egg to blend the white and yolk into a yellow mixture.
4. Add applesauce, milk, brown sugar, and oil to the beaten egg, and stir with a large spoon until ingredients are well mixed.
5. Pour the applesauce-containing mixture into the "well" of dry ingredients in the first bowl. Stir gently and just until the dry ingredients have been moistened by the applesauce mixture. Do not beat or overmix the ingredients.
6. Spoon batter into muffin cups until each cup is half full of batter.
7. Bake 20 minutes or until muffins are golden brown. Cool muffins for about 5 minutes before removing them from the tin. Recipe makes 12 muffins.

INGREDIENTS

2 ¼ cups all-purpose flour

1 tsp baking powder

¾ tsp baking soda

1 tsp ground cinnamon

¼ tsp ground nutmeg

1 cup unsweetened applesauce

½ cup fat-free milk

½ cup brown sugar

3 Tbsp vegetable oil

1 medium egg

vegetable oil cooking spray

STEP 1 Brainstorm

Refer to Table 1.7 for recipe substitution suggestions.

1. Which ingredient of the control muffin recipe will you replace with a whole-grain product? Which whole-grain product will you add? Explain why you chose this whole-grain product.
2. How much of the whole-grain product will you add?

STEP 2 Develop the experimental muffin recipe

3. List ingredients and amounts needed.
4. List the preparation steps.

STEP 3 Evaluate the nutrients in the original and the modified recipes

5. Use a dietary analysis software program, the food composition table in Appendix I, or a food analysis website to evaluate the nutrient content of the original and modified recipes.
6. Develop a table to compare the amounts of fiber, protein, sugar, and fat in each muffin recipe.
7. Did your modification(s) change the nutrient composition of the muffin? If the change(s) made to the recipe altered the muffins' nutrient composition, describe these changes.

OPTIONAL ACTIVITIES

STEP 4 Test your new recipe

Take notes on any changes you make to ingredient amounts as you prepare the muffins.

STEP 5 Reflect on the modified recipe

Describe the appearance and taste of the experimental muffins. Based on your findings, explain how you would alter the ingredients to improve the product to make it more acceptable to subjects and more comparable to the control muffins.

CASE STUDY RESPONSE

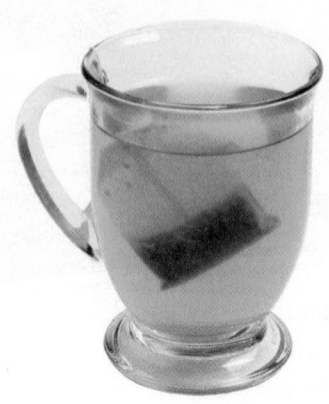

EVALUATING NUTRITION-RELATED INFORMATION

AN ANECDOTE IS A REPORT OF A PERSONAL experience, such as Jeannie's friend's personal experience of losing weight by using the green tea diet plan. Before trying the revolutionary new blend of green tea, Jeannie should ask the following questions:

1. What factors are likely to motivate the people who promote the use of green tea for weight loss?

2. Does the green tea manufacturer cite scientific evidence from peer-reviewed journal articles to support claims regarding the product's usefulness for losing weight?

3. If a study was cited, what was the design of the study? Was the research conducted through a controlled double-blind experiment?

4. What are the credentials of the individuals promoting the green tea? Are these individuals reliable sources of evidence-based information?

Jeannie should consider accessing websites that provide reliable sources of information about green tea and weight loss. Three of these websites are:

- www.eatright.org
- www.nih.gov (specifically, https://nccih.nih.gov/health/greentea)
- www.cdc.gov

Critical Thinking

1. A news broadcaster reports the results of a study in which male physicians who took vitamin E supplements every other day for 8 years did not reduce their risk of heart attack. Moreover, subjects in the experimental group experienced a significantly increased risk of bleeding in the brain. Explain how you would determine whether this information is reliable.

2. Search the Internet for information about a nonvitamin, nonmineral dietary supplement, such as *echinacea* or *melatonin*. Identify the website and record at least two claims regarding the benefits of the supplement. Visit *PubMed* (http://www.ncbi.nlm.nih.gov/pubmed/) and search for at least three peer-reviewed research articles that studied the usefulness of the particular supplement within the past 5 years. Explain whether the claims made about the supplement's benefits at the website are supported by scientific research.

3. A nutrition professor teaches morning and afternoon sections of a nutrition course. She observes that the students in her afternoon

section consistently obtain higher grades than the students in her morning section. Both sections of students take the same exams. Explain whether her observation is a correlation. How would you determine whether her observation indicates causation?

4. Browse through popular health-related magazines to find an article or advertisement that relates to nutrition, and make a copy of the article or advertisement. Analyze each sentence or line of the article or advertisement for signs of unreliability. Explain why the article or advertisement is or is not a reliable source of information.

5. Choose a popular nutrition or "diet" book to read. While reading the book, take notes concerning nutrition-related claims that seem "too good to be true." Investigate at least two of the claims to determine whether they are evidence based. Investigate the credentials of the book's author, and determine whether the author has bona fide nutrition credentials.

Practice Test

Select the best answer.

1. The first step of the scientific method usually involves
   a. gathering data.
   b. developing a hypothesis.
   c. identifying relationships between variables.
   d. making observations.

2. A team of scientists observes a large population of college students over 4 years to determine which of their characteristics leads to weight gain. This study is an example of a(n) _____ study.
   a. case-control
   b. prospective
   c. retrospective
   d. experimental

3. An aspect of _____ involves studying causes of health problems in a population.
   a. epidemiology
   b. technobiology
   c. pathology
   d. sociology

4. Comparing the diets of individuals with iron-deficiency anemia to the diets of persons who have very similar characteristics but are healthy would be an example of
   a. a prospective study.
   b. an anecdotal study.
   c. a retrospective study.
   d. a case-control study.

5. Generally, epidemiological studies

 a. establish causation.

 b. prove correlations.

 c. cannot determine cause-and-effect relationships.

 d. are experimentally based research efforts that examine two variables.

6. Which of the following journals does not have peer-reviewed articles?

 a. *Journal of the American Medical Association*

 b. *American Journal of Clinical Nutrition*

 c. *Journal of the Academy of Nutrition and Dietetics*

 d. *Ladies' Home Journal*

7. The government agency that enforces consumer protection laws by investigating false or misleading health-related claims that appear at an Internet website is the

 a. Federal Trade Commission (FTC).

 b. Environmental Protection Agency (EPA).

 c. Agricultural Research Service (ARS).

 d. Centers for Disease Control and Prevention (CDC).

8. A testimonial is a(n)

 a. unbiased report about a product's value.

 b. scientifically valid claim.

 c. personal endorsement of a product.

 d. form of scientific evidence.

9. Which of the following websites is most likely to provide biased or unreliable nutrition information?

 a. eatright.org

 b. nutritionhealthandfitness4you.com

 c. usda.gov

 d. psu.edu

10. A sham treatment is a(n)

 a. anecdote.

 b. double-blind study.

 c. biased experiment.

 d. placebo.

11. All registered dietitians have

 a. an associate's degree in human nutrition.

 b. passed a certification examination.

 c. the same certifications as nutritionists.

 d. a degree in biology from an accredited institution.

1-d, 2-b, 3-a, 4-d, 5-c, 6-d, 7-a, 8-c, 9-b, 10-d, 11-b

ANSWERS TO PRACTICE TEST

ANSWERS TO CHAPTER 2 QUIZ Yourself

1. The Food and Drug Administration regulates nutrition information in books and other forms of popular media. **False** (p. 35)

2. Popular health-related magazines typically publish articles that have been peer reviewed. **False** (p. 36)

3. By conducting a prospective epidemiological study, medical researchers can determine risk factors that may influence health. **True** (p. 31)

4. A placebo is a sham treatment that does not provide measurable effects. **True** (p. 29)

5. Nutritionists have the same educational backgrounds and professional certifications as registered dietitians. **False** (p. 38)

References

1. Kraut A: Dr. Joseph Goldberger & the war on pellagra. Office of NIH History. http://history.nih.gov/exhibits/goldberger/docs/intro_2.htm Accessed: March 4, 2014

2. Simoni RD and others: Copper as an essential nutrient and nicotinic acid as the anti-black tongue (pellagra) factor: The work of Conrad Arnold Elvehjem. *Journal of Biological Chemistry* 277(34):e22, 2002.

3. Venn-Watson S and others: Dolphins as animal models for type 2 diabetes: Sustained, post-prandial hyperglycemia and hyperinsulinemia. *General and Comparative Endocrinology* 170(1):193, 2011.

4. Hetrick SE and others: Combined pharmacotherapy and psychological therapies for post- traumatic stress disorder (PTSD). *Cochrane Database of Systematic Reviews* (7): CD007316. DOI: 10.1002/14651858.CD007316. pub2, 2010.

5. de la Fuente-Fernández R: The placebo-reward hypothesis: Dopamine and the placebo effect. *Parkinsonism & Related Disorders* 15 (Suppl 3):S72, 2009.

6. Centers for Disease Control and Prevention, Diabetes Public Health Resource: *2011 National Diabetes Fact Sheet 2011.* Last updated October 2013. http://www.cdc.gov/diabetes/pubs/estimates11.htm#4 Accessed: March 4, 2014

7. National Center for Health Statistics: *Breast cancer rates by race and ethnicity.* Last updated August 2013. http://www.cdc.gov/cancer/breast/statistics/race.htm Accessed: March 4, 2014

8. Rossignol A: *Principles and practice of epidemiology.* Boston: McGraw-Hill, 2007.

9. National Heart, Lung and Blood Institute and Boston University: *Framingham Heart Study.* ND. http://www.framinghamheartstudy.org/ Accessed: March 4, 2014

10. Academy of Nutrition and Dietetics: *Frequently asked questions.* http://www.eatright.org/Public/content.aspx?id=6713 Accessed: Accessed: March 4, 2014

3 Basis of a Healthy Diet

Planning a 1-day healthy menu

ERIC WEIGHS 170 POUNDS AND IS 5-FEET, 10-inches tall. He's a 23-year-old college graduate who has spent the past year working in sales, which involves traveling by car out of town for 3 to 4 days per week. Because of his job, he gets less than 30 minutes of exercise daily. Although he has access to several supermarkets and a farmers' market, he eats about 80% of his meals at fast-food places. Eric is concerned about the effects that his lifestyle may have on his health, and he is motivated to reduce his fast-food consumption and improve his diet.

- Go to www.choosemyplate.gov to determine recommended amounts of total calories, foods from each food group, and oils for Eric to consume daily.

- Using MyPlate recommendations, plan a 1-day nutritionally adequate menu for Eric. When planning the menu:

  - List the foods and beverages that Eric will eat during the day and identify them by a particular meal or snack.

  - Include serving sizes and specifics on food preparation, when necessary (e.g., grilled, baked, or fried chicken).

  - Identify where each food and beverage fits into MyPlate.

  - List the calories provided by each food or beverage (see Appendix I or use a nutrient analysis software program, or the "SuperTracker" at http://www.choosemyplate.gov/supertracker-other-tools).

The suggested Case Study Response can be found on page 74.

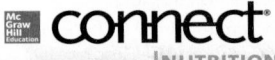

INUTRITION

Check out the Connect site at www.mcgrawhillconnect.com to further explore this case study.

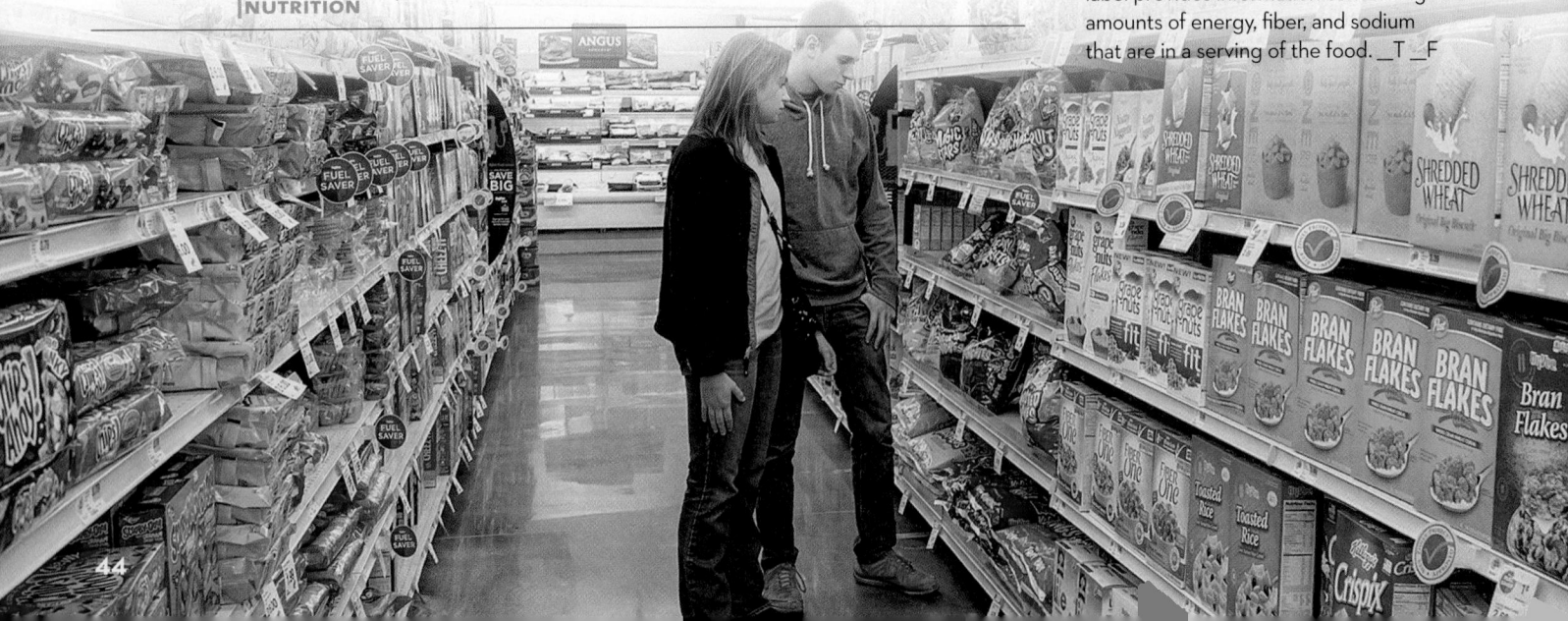

3.1 What Is a Nutrient Requirement?

LEARNING OUTCOMES

1 *Explain why a person's diet should supply recommended amounts of nutrients.*

2 *Discuss why nutrient needs vary among individuals.*

Lifestyle, age, sex, general health status, and use of medications are among the numerous factors that influence an individual's nutrient needs. Although human nutrient needs vary from person to person, scientists have been able to estimate the healthy human body's nutritional requirements by using research methods that were discussed in Chapter 2. A **nutrient requirement** is the smallest amount of a nutrient that maintains a defined level of nutritional health.[1] In general, this amount saturates certain cells with the nutrient or prevents the nutrient's deficiency disease.

    Many nutrients are stored in the body, primarily in the liver, body fat, and bones. For optimal nutrition, a person needs to consume enough of those nutrients to maintain optimal storage levels. When one's intake of a stored nutrient is low, or his or her need for this nutrient becomes increased, such as during recovery from illness, the body withdraws some from storage. By having optimal levels of stored nutrients, the person may avoid or delay developing the nutrients' deficiency disorders.

nutrient requirement smallest amount of a nutrient that maintains a defined level of nutritional health

ASSESS YOUR PROGRESS

1 *Define nutrient requirement.*

2 *List four factors that influence a person's nutrient requirements.*

3.2 Dietary Reference Intakes: Nutrient and Calorie Standards

LEARNING OUTCOMES

1 *Identify each of the dietary standards included in the Dietary Reference Intakes (DRIs).*

2 *Explain the differences between Estimated Average Requirement (EAR), Recommended Daily Allowance (RDA), Adequate Intake (AI), and Upper Level (UL).*

3 *Discuss how the Dietary Reference Intake standards are used to evaluate diets and plan menus.*

Dietary Reference Intakes (DRIs) are a set of energy and nutrient intake standards that nutrition experts can use as references when making dietary recommendations. The DRI standards are the Estimated Average Requirement (EAR), which includes the Estimated Energy Requirement (EER); Recommended Dietary Allowance (RDA); Adequate Intake (AI); Tolerable Upper Intake Level (UL); and Acceptable Macronutrient Distribution Range (AMDR) (Fig. 3.1). DRIs are intended to help health professionals evaluate the nutritional adequacy of diets and plan nutritious diets for healthy people.[2]

    In the United States, the **Food and Nutrition Board (FNB)** of the Institute of Medicine develops DRIs. Periodically, members of the board adjust DRIs as new information concerning human nutritional needs and the adequacy of the American diet becomes available. DRI tables can be found at the back of this textbook. The following sections provide basic information about the various DRI standards. It is important to become familiar with these standards, because they are used in this and other chapters.

Dietary Reference Intakes (DRIs) set of energy and nutrient intake standards that can be used as references when making dietary recommendations

Food and Nutrition Board (FNB) group of scientists who develop DRIs

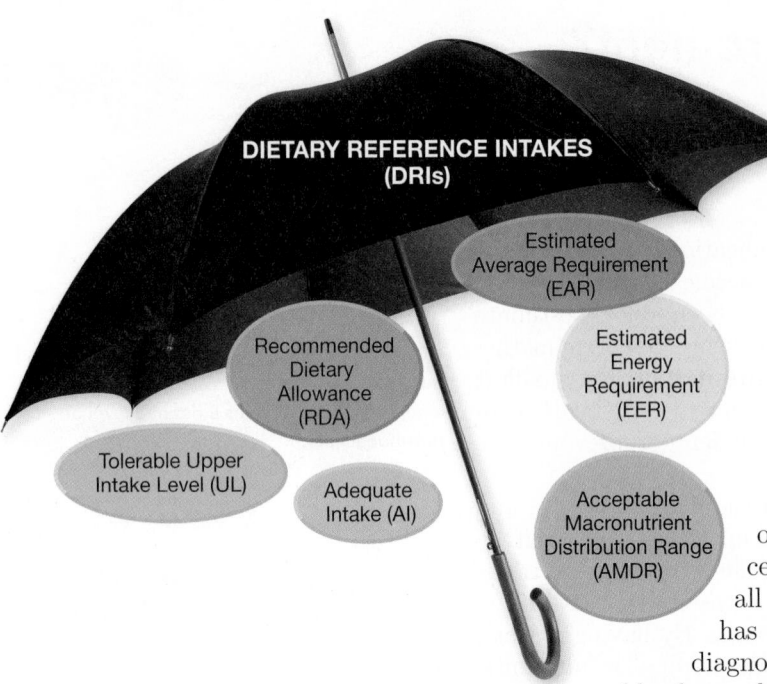

FIGURE 3.1 Dietary Reference Intakes (DRIs).

Estimated Average Requirement (EAR) amount of a nutrient that should meet the needs of 50% of healthy people who are in a particular life-stage/sex group

Estimated Energy Requirement (EER) average daily energy intake that meets the needs of a healthy person who is maintaining his or her weight

Recommended Dietary Allowances (RDAs) standards for recommended daily intakes of several nutrients

Adequate Intakes (AIs) dietary recommendations that assume a population's average daily nutrient intakes are adequate because no deficiency diseases are present

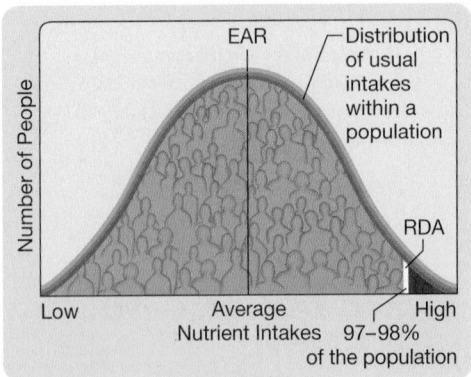

FIGURE 3.2 The Estimated Average Requirement and Recommended Dietary Allowance.

Estimated Average Requirement

An **Estimated Average Requirement (EAR)** is the amount of the nutrient that meets the needs of 50% of healthy people who are in a particular life–stage/sex group. (Fig. 3.2).[3] Life–stage groups classify people according to age and whether females are pregnant or breastfeeding. A typical 20–year–old female college student, for example, would be classified as female, between 19 and 30 years of age, and not pregnant or breastfeeding.

To establish an EAR for a nutrient, the Food and Nutrition Board identifies a physiological marker, a substance in the body that reflects proper functioning and can be measured. This marker indicates whether the level of a nutrient in the body is adequate. A marker of vitamin C, for example, is the amount of the vitamin in certain white blood cells. When these cells contain nearly all the vitamin C they can hold, this is a sign that the body has an optimal supply of the vitamin. Thus, a physician can diagnose whether a patient is vitamin C deficient by having a blood sample analyzed. Physiological markers may also be enzymes or products of metabolism (*metabolites*) in blood or urine.

Estimated Energy Requirement

The **Estimated Energy Requirement (EER)** is the average daily energy intake that meets the needs of a healthy person who is maintaining his or her weight. The EER takes into account the person's physical activity level, height, and weight, as well as sex and life stage. The EER, however, does not include an additional number of calories to serve as a "margin of safety." Thus, the EER may be higher or lower than some people's energy needs. Chapter 13 provides formulas for estimating a person's energy requirement.

Recommended Dietary Allowances

The **Recommended Dietary Allowances (RDAs)** are standards for recommended daily intakes of several nutrients. RDAs meet the nutrient needs of nearly all healthy individuals (97–98%) in a particular life–stage or sex group (Fig. 3.2). Thus, for most people, the RDAs are higher than the required amounts of nutrients.

To establish an RDA for a nutrient, nutrition scientists first determine its EAR. Then scientists add a "margin of safety" amount to the EAR. This additional amount allows for individual variations in nutrient needs and helps maintain stores of the nutrient in the body's tissues (Fig. 3.2). For example, the adult EAR for vitamin C is 60 mg for women who are not pregnant or breastfeeding and 75 mg for men.[1] However, the adult RDA for vitamin C is 75 mg for women who are not pregnant or breastfeeding and 90 mg for men. Thus, the margin of safety for vitamin C is 15 mg. Because smoking cigarettes increases the need for this micronutrient, smokers should add 35 mg to their RDA for the nutrient.

Adequate Intakes

In some instances, nutrition scientists are unable to develop RDAs for nutrients because there is not enough information available to determine human requirements. Until such information becomes known, scientists set **Adequate Intakes (AIs)** for these nutrients (Table 3.1). Dietitians use AIs along with RDAs as nutrient intake goals in planning diets.

TABLE 3.1 Nutrients Assigned Adequate Intakes (Adult AIs)

Vitamins	Minerals	Carbohydrates	Lipids	Water
Pantothenic acid	Sodium	Fiber	Total fat (infants)	Water
Biotin	Chloride		Linoleic acid	
Vitamin K	Potassium		Linolenic acid	
Choline*	Fluoride			
	Manganese			
	Chromium			

*Classified as a "vitamin-like" nutrient.

To establish an AI, scientists record the diets of a group of healthy people and estimate the group's average daily intake of the nutrient. If this group of people shows no evidence of the nutrient's deficiency disorder, the researchers assume that their typical intake is adequate and use that value as the AI (Fig. 3.3). As more scientific evidence becomes available, nutrients originally given AIs may be assigned RDAs.

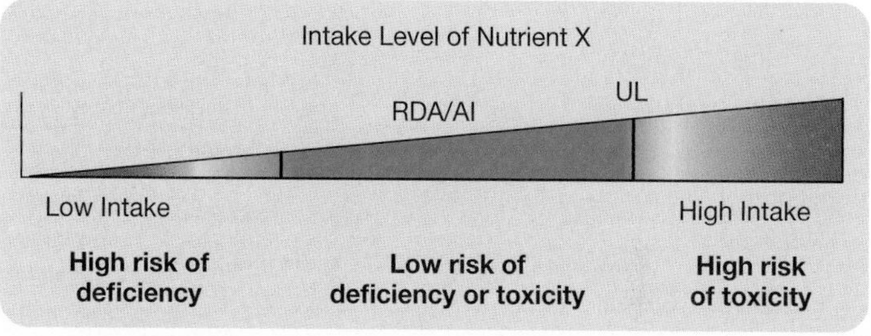

It is important to note that the RDA or AI for a nutrient is the "goal" intake for a healthy person. Failure to regularly consume the RDA or AI for a particular nutrient increases the like-lihood of developing the nutrient's deficiency symptoms. Furthermore, chronic disease may increase or decrease a person's nutrient needs; thus, the RDAs or AIs may not be appropriate to use under such conditions.

FIGURE 3.3 RDAs, AIs, and ULs.

Tolerable Upper Intake Level

Nutrition scientists establish a **Tolerable Upper Intake Level (Upper Level or UL)** for many vitamins and minerals. The UL is the highest average amount of a nutrient that is unlikely to harm most people when the amount is consumed daily (Fig. 3.3). The risk of a toxicity disorder increases when a person regularly consumes amounts of a nutrient that are greater than its UL. The UL for vita-min C, for example, is 2000 mg/day for adults. For most people, it is difficult to consume 2000 mg of vitamin C daily from foods that are natural sources of the micronutrient, such as oranges, broccoli, and baked potatoes. However, a person can easily reach or exceed the UL by taking a dietary supplement that provides vitamin C.

Tolerable Upper Intake Level (Upper Level or UL) highest average amount of a nutrient that is unlikely to harm most people when the amount is consumed daily

Acceptable Macronutrient Distribution Ranges (AMDRs) ranges of carbohydrate, fat, and protein intakes that provide adequate amounts of vitamins and minerals, and may reduce the risk of diet-related chronic diseases

Acceptable Macronutrient Distribution Ranges

In addition to the DRIs, nutrition experts with the FNB have established **Acceptable Macronutrient Distribution Ranges (AMDRs)**. AMDRs are ranges of carbohydrate, fat, and protein intakes that provide adequate amounts of vita-mins and minerals and may reduce the risk of developing certain diet-related chronic diseases, such as heart disease and type 2 diabetes. Additionally, people can use the AMDRs to determine whether their diets have a healthful balance of macronutrients. Table 3.2 lists AMDRs for adults.

Applying Nutrient Standards

Table 3.3 provides a summary of the various DRIs. Dietitians and other health care professionals refer to the DRIs to evaluate the nutritional adequacy of a population's diet and to plan nutritious diets for groups of people. Additionally,

TABLE 3.2 AMDRs for Adults

Macronutrient	Percent of Total kcal
Carbohydrate	45–65
Fat	20–35
Protein	10–35

Source: Adapted from: Otten JJ and others: *Dietary Reference Intakes: The essential guide to nutrient requirements.* Institute of Medicine of the National Academies. Washington, DC: National Academies Press, 2006.

TABLE 3.3 Summary of Dietary Reference Intakes

Standard	Definition	Example
Estimated Average Requirement (EAR)	Amount of a nutrient that meets the needs of 50% of healthy people who are in a particular life-stage and sex group	Vitamin C 75 mg/day for males and 60 mg/day for females ages 19 through 50 years
Recommended Dietary Allowance (RDA)	Amount of a nutrient that meets the needs of nearly all healthy individuals in a particular life-stage and sex group	Vitamin C 90 mg/day for males and 75 mg/day for females ages 19 through 50 years
Adequate Intake (AI)	Amount of a nutrient that is considered to be adequate based on the population's typical intakes, but there is not enough scientific information available to determine an RDA for the nutrient at this time	Vitamin C 40 mg/day for infants from birth through 6 months of age
Tolerable Upper Intake Level or Upper Level (UL)	Highest average amount of a nutrient that is unlikely to harm most people when the amount is consumed daily	Vitamin C 2000 mg/day for adults
Acceptable Macronutrient Distribution Range (AMDR)	Ranges of carbohydrate, fat, and protein intakes that provide adequate amounts of micronutrients and may reduce the risk of developing certain diet-related chronic diseases	See Table 3.2

DRIs can be used to assess the nutritional quality of a person's daily food intake and plan the individual's diet.[4] The U.S. Department of Agriculture (USDA) has developed an interactive DRI tool to help people evaluate and plan diets (http://fnic.nal.usda.gov/interactiveDRI/).

A person's diet is likely to be nutritionally adequate if the average daily intake for each nutrient meets the nutrient's RDA or AI value. If a person's diet consistently supplies less than the EAR for a nutrient, the individual may be at risk of developing the nutrient's deficiency disorder. On the other hand, if a person's intake of a nutrient is consistently above its UL, this individual is at risk of developing that nutrient's toxicity disorder. People who regularly take high doses of individual micronutrient nutrient supplements are more likely to develop nutrient toxicity disorders than people who do not use these products often.

Nutritional standards also have commercial applications. Pharmaceutical companies refer to DRIs when developing formulas that replace breast milk for infants and special formulas for people who cannot consume regular foods, such as a person who is in a coma and cannot chew food. As a result, babies can grow well by consuming commercially prepared formulas, and adults who are unable to eat solid food can survive for years on formula feedings that are administered through tubes inserted into their bodies.

ASSESS YOUR PROGRESS

3 *What is the difference between an RDA and an AI?*

4 *How does the EER differ from the EAR?*

5 *Describe the importance and applications of ULs.*

6 *Calculate ranges of caloric intakes for macronutrients by using the AMDRs for a healthy 22-year-old adult who consumes 2500 kcal/day.*

7 *Describe how dietitians and pharmaceutical companies use DRIs.*

3.3 Major Food Groups

LEARNING OUTCOMES

1 *List the major USDA food groups and identify foods that are typically classified in each group.*

2 *Provide examples of USDA standard serving sizes ("equivalents") of representative foods from each food group.*

3 *Explain the difference between enrichment and fortification.*

DRIs are complex lists of numerical values that are not translated into amounts of foods that contain the nutrients listed; therefore, they have limited use—fulness for the average consumer. Furthermore, the DRIs do not provide rec—ommendations concerning the role of diet and chronic—disease prevention. Most people need practical suggestions that can help them select a nutritious, healthy diet. A · **dietary guidance system** ("food guide") translates the DRIs and evidence—based information concerning the effects of certain foods and food components on health into basic dietary recommendations. A food guide provides a meaningful way for consumers to evaluate the nutritional quality of their diets and make modifications to improve it, if necessary.

Before developing a food guide, nutrition experts classify foods into major food groups, according to their natural origins and key nutrients. According to the USDA, the major food groups are: grains; dairy (milk and milk products); fruits; vegetables; and protein—rich foods, such as meat, nuts, and eggs. Other dietary guides may also include a group for oils. In most instances, dietary guides provide recommendations concerning amounts of foods from each group that should be eaten daily.

It is important to note that the nutritional content of foods within each group often varies widely. For example, 3.5 ounces of fresh sliced apples and 3.5 ounces of fresh orange slices each supply about 50 kcal. However, the apples contribute about 4 mg of vitamin C, whereas oranges supply about 46 mg of the vitamin to diets (Fig. 3.4). Therefore, dietary guides generally recommend that peo—ple choose a variety of foods from each food group when planning daily meals and snacks. The following points provide information about each food group, as well as oils.

Grains

Grains include products made from wheat, rice, and oats. Pasta, bread, and flour tortillas are members of this group, because wheat flour is usually their main ingredient. Table 3.4 lists foods that supply about the same amount of energy as 1 ounce of a grains food, according to the USDA.

Carbohydrate (starch) and protein are the primary macronutrients in grains. In the United States, refined grain products can also be good sources of several vitamins and minerals when they have undergone enrichment or fortification. **Enrichment** is the addition of specific amounts of iron and the B vitamins thi—amin, riboflavin, niacin, and folic acid to specific refined (processed) grain prod—ucts such as wheat flour and white rice. The federal government has established standards for amounts of these particular micronutrients that can be added after refinement. In general, enrichment replaces some of the nutrients that grains lose during refining. **Fortification** is the addition of nutrients to any food, such as adding calcium to orange juice, vitamins A and D to milk, and numerous vita—mins and minerals to ready—to—eat breakfast cereals.

Dietary guides generally recommend choosing foods made with **whole grains** instead of refined grains. According to the FDA, whole grains are the intact,

dietary guidance system food guide that translates the DRIs and evidence-based information concerning the effects of certain foods and food components on health into dietary recommendations

enrichment addition of specific amounts of iron and the B vitamins thiamin, riboflavin, niacin, and folic acid to specific refined grain products

fortification addition of nutrients to any food

whole grains intact, ground, cracked, or flaked seeds of cereal grains

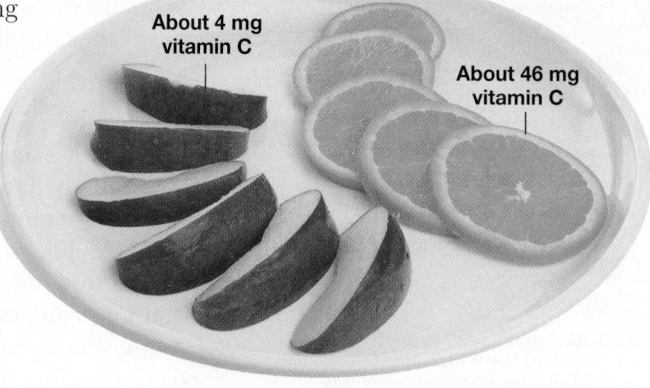

About 4 mg vitamin C

About 46 mg vitamin C

FIGURE 3.4 Comparing apples to oranges. The nutritional content of foods within each group often varies widely.

TABLE 3.4 Grain Foods Equivalents

1 regular slice bread or a small tortilla (6-in diameter)
1 cup ready-to-eat cereal (flakes)
½ English muffin or small bagel
½ cup cooked rice, pasta, or cereal such as oatmeal
3 cups popped popcorn
5 small whole-wheat crackers

Source: U.S. Department of Agriculture: Grains: What counts as an ounce equivalent of grains? http://www.choosemyplate.gov/food-groups/grains-counts.html Accessed: January 13, 2014

TABLE 3.5 Dairy Food Equivalents

1 cup milk calcium-fortified soy milk (soy beverage)

1 cup plain yogurt, frozen yogurt, or pudding

½ cup evaporated milk

2 cups cottage cheese

½ cup ricotta cheese

1 ½ oz natural cheese such as Swiss or cheddar

⅓ cup shredded cheese

2 oz processed cheese

Source: U.S. Department of Agriculture: What counts as a cup in the dairy group? http://www.choosemyplate.gov/food-groups/dairy-counts.html Accessed: January 13, 2014

TABLE 3.6 Protein Foods Equivalents

1 oz cooked lean pork, ham, poultry (without skin), tempeh (a soybean product), or fish or shellfish

1 egg

1 Tbsp peanut or almond butter

½ oz nuts (e.g., 12 almonds or 24 pistachios) or seeds

¼ cup cooked beans, cooked dried peas, roasted soybeans, baked or refried beans, or tofu

2 Tbsp hummus

Source: U.S. Department of Agriculture: Protein foods: What foods are in the protein foods group? http://www.choosemyplate.gov/food-groups/protein-foods-counts.html Accessed: January 13, 2014

TABLE 3.7 Fruit Equivalents

1 small apple

1 medium grapefruit, pear

1 large banana, orange, peach

8 large strawberries

1 cup diced melon, grapes, pineapple

1 cup applesauce or 100% fruit juice

½ cup dried fruit (e.g., raisins, apricots, prunes)

Source: U.S. Department of Agriculture: Fruits: What counts as a cup of fruit? http://www.choosemyplate.gov/food-groups/fruits-counts.html Accessed: January 13, 2014

ground, cracked, or flaked seeds of cereal grains.[5] Whole grains include whole wheat, oatmeal, whole-grain cornmeal, brown rice, whole-grain barley, whole rye, buckwheat, and spelt. Compared to refined grain products, foods made from whole grains naturally contain more fiber, as well as micronutrients that are not replaced during enrichment.

Dairy Foods

Dairy foods include milk and products made from milk that retain their calcium content, such as yogurt and hard cheeses. Dairy foods are also excellent sources of protein, phosphorus (a mineral), and riboflavin (a B vitamin). Additionally, most of the milk sold in the United States is fortified with vitamins A and D. Beverages made from soy beans (soy "milks") can substitute for cow's milk, if they are fortified with calcium and other micronutrients.

Ice cream, pudding, frozen yogurt, and ice milk are often grouped with dairy foods, even though they often have high sugar and fat contents. To obtain about the same amount of calcium as in 1 cup of fat-free milk, a person would have to eat about 1 ⅔ cups of regular vanilla ice cream. This amount of ice cream provides about 300 kcal and about 27 g of fat, whereas the fat-free milk supplies 90 kcal and less than 1 g of fat. Although cream cheese, cream, and butter are dairy products, they are not included in this group, because they have little or no calcium and are high in fat.[6] Table 3.5 lists foods that have about the same amount of protein and calcium as 1 cup of fat-free milk, according to the USDA.

Most dietary guides recommend choosing dairy products that have most of the fat removed, such as *fat-free* or low-fat milk. (Fat-free milk may also be referred to as nonfat or "skim" milk.) Compared to whole milk, which is about 3.25% fat by weight, low-fat milk contains only 1% fat by weight and is often called "1% milk."

Protein Foods

Protein-rich foods include beef, pork, fish, liver, and poultry. Protein foods also include beans, eggs, nuts, tofu, and seeds. Table 3.6 lists foods that have about the same amount of protein as 1 ounce (oz) of lean beef, according to the USDA. Foods in the protein group are also rich sources of micronutrients, especially iron, zinc, and B vitamins. In general, the body absorbs minerals, such as iron and zinc, more easily from animal foods than from plants.

Some dietary guides use fat content to categorize meats and other protein-rich foods. According to these guides, low-fat cottage cheese and the white meat of turkey are very lean protein foods; ground beef that is not more than 15% fat by weight and tuna are lean protein foods. Pork sausage, bacon, regular cheeses, and hot dogs are examples of high-fat protein foods.

Fruits

Fruits include fresh, dried, frozen, sauced, and canned fruit, as well as 100% fruit juice. Most fruits are low in fat and good sources of phytochemicals and micronutrients, especially potassium, vitamin C, and folate. Additionally, whole or cut-up fruit is a good source of fiber. Table 3.7 lists foods that are similar in nutritional value to one serving of fruit, according to the USDA. Although 100% juice is a source of phytochemicals and can count toward your fruit intake, the majority of your choices from this group should be whole or cut-up fruits.[7] Whole or cut-up fruits are healthier options than juices because they contain more dietary fiber.

Vegetables

Vegetables include fresh, cooked, canned, frozen, and dried/dehydrated vegetables and 100% vegetable juice. Guides may also group vegetables into dark green, orange, and starchy categories. Some guides include dried beans and peas in the vegetable group, as well as in the protein foods group. When planning diets, people should consider a serving of dried beans and peas as either a vegetable or a protein food, but count it in one group only.

Vegetables are usually low in fat and rich sources of potassium, vitamin A, vitamin C, folate, and fiber. In general, vegetables are good sources of micronu-trients, fiber, and phytochemicals, and many vegetables are naturally low in fat and energy. Table 3.8 lists foods that are equivalent nutritionally to one serving of vegetables, according to the USDA.

Oils

Oils include canola, corn, and olive oils, as well as other fats that are liquid at room temperature. Certain spreadable foods made from vegetable oils, such as mayonnaise, tub or soft margarine, and salad dressing, are also classified as oils. Because nuts, olives, avocados, and some types of fish have high fat contents, a dietary guide may group these foods with oils. Oils are often sources of vitamin E and essential fatty acids; cod liver oil is a rich source of vitamin D and "healthy fats," including omega−3 fatty acids. In general, one serving is 1 tablespoon (Tbsp) of oil. Table 3.9 lists foods that contain about the same amount of fat as 1 tablespoon of oil, according to the USDA.

TABLE 3.8 Vegetable Equivalents

1 cup raw or cooked vegetables, whole or mashed beans, mashed potatoes, bean sprouts
1 cup vegetable juice
2 cups leafy greens
1 large sweet potato, ear of corn, tomato

Source: U.S. Department of Agriculture: Vegetables: What counts as a cup of vegetables? http://www .choosemyplate.gov/food-groups/vegetables-counts .html Accessed: January 13, 2014

TABLE 3.9 Oil Equivalents

1 Tbsp vegetable oil (including canola, corn, olive, peanut, and soybean oils)
1 Tbsp soft, trans fat-free margarine
1 Tbsp mayonnaise
2 Tbsp Italian salad dressing or Thousand Island dressing
4 large olives
½ medium avocado
2 Tbsp peanut butter
1 oz nuts or sunflower seeds

Source: U.S. Department of Agriculture: Oils: What counts as a tablespoon of oil? http://www.choosemyplate.gov/food-groups/oils.html Accessed: January 13, 2014

Empty-Calorie Foods or Beverages

Dietary guides may also have a group for "empty−calorie" foods or beverages. In Chapter 1, we described empty−calorie foods as having a lot of added sugar and "unhealthy" types of fat, and/or alcohol. Sugary foods ("sweets") include candy, regular soft drinks, jelly, and other foods that contain high amounts of sugar added during processing or preparation. Alcoholic beverages generally con-tribute calories without adding much vitamins and minerals to diets.

DID **YOU** KNOW?

Early in 1981, President Ronald Reagan challenged Congress to cut federal spending. Congress responded by proposing drastic cost reductions for many programs, including slashing the USDA's budget for the school lunch program. Among the USDA's money-saving proposals, catsup and pickles would count as vegetable servings. The notion that foods derived from vegetables but generally considered condiments could replace more nutritious items in children's lunches was widely criticized, opposed, and ridiculed by nutrition and public health experts, as well as the general public. By October 1981, President Reagan withdrew the USDA's plans to water down the nutritional requirements of the school lunch program.

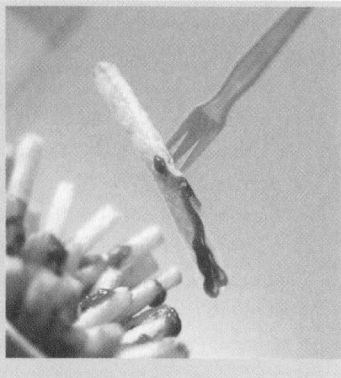

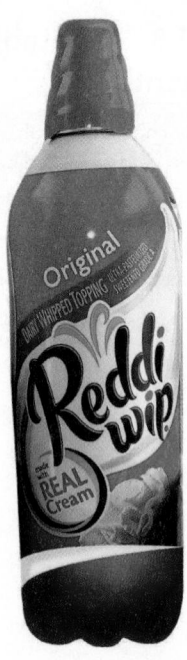

This food is a source of solid fat.

solid fats fats that are fairly hard at room temperature

Solid fats, such as beef fat, butter, stick margarine, lard (pork fat), and shortening, are fairly hard at room temperature. Although cream, whipped cream, cream cheese, and coconut oil are liquid or soft at room tempera‐ ture, these foods are sources of solid fats.[8] Solid fats are generally considered unhealthy fats, because diets that contain too much solid fat (dietary sources of saturated fat and trans fat) are associated with increased risk of developing cardiovascular disease (CVD). Chapter 6 discusses dietary fats and how these lipids can affect health.

ASSESS YOUR PROGRESS

8 *List at least three foods that are generally classified as grain products.*

9 *Explain why white flour is often enriched, and identify the nutrients that have been added to it.*

10 *List at least four foods that are generally classified as dairy foods.*

11 *Explain why most dietary guides include eggs, nuts, and seeds with meats, fish, and poultry products.*

12 *List at least four foods that are generally considered sources of empty calories.*

3.4 U.S. Dietary Guidelines

LEARNING OUTCOMES

1 *List and describe the key guidelines of the 2015–2020 Dietary Guidelines for Americans.*

2 *Apply the Dietary Guidelines when planning healthful diets.*

A considerable amount of scientific evidence associates the risk of developing heart disease, type 2 diabetes mellitus, and chronically elevated blood pres‐ sure (hypertension) with lifestyles, particularly poor dietary choices and lack of regular physical activity. The *Dietary Guidelines for Americans* ("Dietary

DID **YOU** KNOW?

The Dietary Guidelines form the basis of the federal government's nutrition policy, which serves as a framework for national, state, and local health promotion as well as food and nutrition pro‐ grams. Dietary Guidelines are also used for menu planning by individuals and health care pro‐ fessionals.[9] Furthermore, food and beverage manufacturers can apply the guidelines to develop healthier products that appeal to consumers.

To revise the 2010 version of the dietary guidelines, officials with the U. S. Department of Health and Human Services (USDHHS) and USDA appointed a Dietary Guidelines Advisory Committee (DGAC) comprised of nationally recognized medical and nutrition experts. DGAC members reviewed the scientific evidence concerning the role of foods in health, before pre‐ paring the *Scientific Report of the 2015 Dietary Guidelines Advisory Committee.*[9] This publica‐ tion contained recommendations for the development of the *2015–2020 Dietary Guidelines for Americans.* In February 2015, the overseeing government agencies made the DGAC report avail‐ able for the public to read and provide input.

According to the DGAC report, a healthy diet contains more fruits, vegetables, whole grains, low- or nonfat dairy products, seafood, legumes and nuts than the typical diet of the general American population.[9] Additionally, a healthy diet contains fewer refined grains, red and pro‐ cessed meats, sodium, and sugar-sweetened foods and beverages than the typical American eating pattern. Such eating patterns should be flexible so food choices can be varied and indi‐ vidualized to meet a person's preferences, medical needs, and economic situation. The federal government incorporated some but not all of the DGAC's recommendations into the *2015–2020 Dietary Guidelines for Americans.*[10]

Guidelines") incorporates scientific knowledge about the influence that dietary choices can have on health into a set of recommended eating and physical activity practices for healthy people over 2 years of age. About every 5 years, the USDHHS and the USDA revise and publish the Dietary Guidelines as new information about the role of diet in health becomes available. Government agencies and nutrition and food organizations use the Dietary Guidelines to develop and guide food and nutrition policies, as well as educational materials.

Summary of the *2015–2020 Dietary Guidelines for Americans*

The overarching guidelines of the Dietary Guidelines are listed in Table 3.10. These general recommendations "encourage healthy eating patterns."[10] According to the Dietary Guidelines, a healthy eating pattern includes foods from all five food groups and oils, but limits saturated fats, trans fats, added sugars, and sodium.[10] The following five sections provide basic dietary recommendations as stated in the Dietary Guidelines. For more information about the Dietary Guidelines and healthy eating patterns, visit http://health.gov/dietaryguidelines/2015/guidelines/ .

Follow a Healthy Eating Pattern Across the Lifespan

- All food and beverage choices matter.
  - Choose a healthy eating pattern that is at an appropriate calorie level to help achieve and maintain a healthy body weight, support nutrient adequacy, and reduce the risk of chronic disease.

Other recommendations include the following points.

Cholesterol intake should be as low as possible while following a healthy dietary pattern.

Adults who consume alcohol should limit their intake to fewer than two drinks per day (men) and no more than one drink per day (females who are not pregnant). For more information about alcohol, see Chapter 8.

Caffeine consumption should be limited to less than 400 mg/day (three to five 8-oz cups of coffee/day).

Focus on Variety, Nutrient Density, and Amount

- To meet nutrient needs within calorie limits, people should choose a variety of nutrient-dense foods across and within all food groups, and consume them in recommended amounts.

- Vegetable choices should vary, be nutrient dense, and include many different vegetables.

- At least half of the recommended fruit intake should be from whole fruits. When juices are consumed, they should be 100% juice, without added sugars.

- At least half of recommended amounts of grains foods should be whole grains.

- Choose a variety of protein foods, including dried beans and peas.

Limit Calories from Added Sugars and Saturated Fats and Reduce Sodium Intake

- Limit added sugar intake to less than 10% of total daily calories.

- Limit saturated fat intake to less than 10% of total daily calories.

- Limit daily sodium intake to less than 2300 mg.

TABLE 3.10 *2015–2020 Dietary Guidelines for Americans* Overarching Guidelines

- Follow a healthy eating pattern across the lifespan
- Focus on variety, nutrient density, and amount
- Limit calories from added sugars and saturated fats and reduce sodium intake
- Shift to healthier food and beverage choices
- Support healthy eating patterns for all

DID **YOU** *KNOW?*

Edamame (*e-deh-ma'-me*) are unripened (green) soybeans that may be purchased frozen or fresh in pods. Edamame are an excellent source of protein, many minerals, vitamin K, and fiber. One-half cup of prepared edamame provides about 100 kcal and over 8 g of protein.

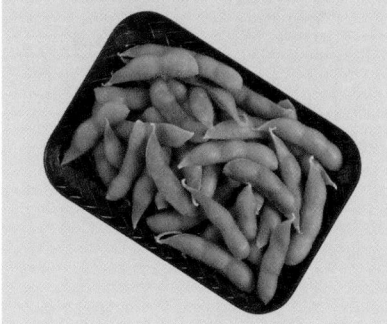

FRESH TIPS

Although sugary foods and products made from refined grains can be less expensive than produce, fruits and vegetables are more nutritious.[11] To eat more fruits and vegetables on a tight budget:

- Use canned or frozen fruits and vegetables.

- Visit farmer's markets and choose locally grown produce. Many farmers sell their slightly damaged or day-old fruits and vegetables at a discount. Furthermore, purchasing fresh foods at farmer's markets supports the local economy.

- Buy fruits and vegetables when they are in season; that is, when they are plentiful and their cost is lowest.

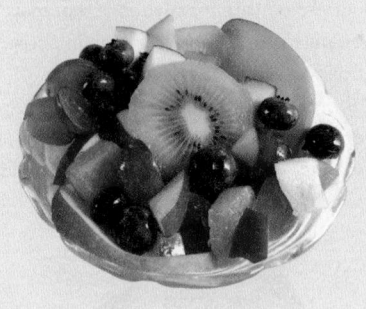

Shift to Healthier Food and Beverage Choices

- Dairy food choices should emphasize fat—free and low—fat (1%) products, including milk, yogurt, cheese, or fortified soy dairy substitutes (i.e., "soy milk").

- The general population should consume at least 8 ounces of various seafood per week.

- Use oils to replace solid fats.

- Choose foods that provide more potassium, dietary fiber, calcium, and vitamin D, which are "nutrients of public health concern" that Americans tend to consume in limited amounts. Iron is an additional nutrient of public health concern for pregnant females.

Support Healthy Eating Patterns for All

- Everyone has a role in helping to create and support healthy eating patterns nationwide.

- Health professionals and policymakers should use multiple strategies to promote healthy eating and physical activity behaviors across all segments of society. Such strategies can include developing educational resources that inspire individuals to take appropriate actions with regard to their food and beverage choices.

Applying the Dietary Guidelines

Table 3.11 (see page 55) suggests practical ways people can apply the Dietary Guidelines' recommendations to their usual food choices.

FRESH TIPS

The Dietary Guidelines also include specific recommendations for certain groups of Americans.

Women who are capable of becoming pregnant should:

- Choose foods that contain iron and foods that enhance iron absorption (see Chapter 12).

- Consume 400 µg per day of synthetic folic acid/day (from fortified foods and/or supplements) in addition to dietary sources of folate (see Chapter 10).

Women who are pregnant or breastfeeding should:

- Consume 8 to 12 ounces of seafood per week from a variety of seafood, but not eat tilefish, shark, swordfish, and king mackerel, because they may contain high amounts of the toxic substance *methylmercury*.

ASSESS YOUR PROGRESS

Respond to the following points according to recommendations of *2015-2020 Dietary Guidelines for Americans*.

13 *What kinds of dairy products should Americans consume?*

14 *Phil estimates that his average intake of sodium is 6025 mg/day. Explain how his intake of sodium compares to the recommendations of the Dietary Guidelines.*

15 *What percentage of a person's intake of grains should be whole grains?*

16 *Provide two examples of dietary modifications that a person can make to meet the recommendations of the Dietary Guidelines.*

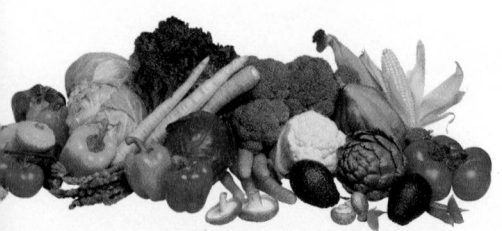

Consume a variety of vegetables.

TABLE 3.11 Applying the Dietary Guidelines to Usual Food Choices

If One Usually Eats:	Consider Replacing With:
White bread and rolls	Whole-wheat bread and rolls
Sugary breakfast cereals	Low-sugar high-fiber cereal sweetened with berries, bananas, peaches, or other fruit
Cheeseburger, French fries, and a regular (sugar-sweetened) soft drink	Roasted chicken or turkey sandwich, baked beans, fat-free or low-fat milk, or soy milk
Potato salad or cole slaw	Leafy greens or three-bean salad
Doughnuts, chips, or salty snack foods	Small bran muffin or whole-wheat bagel topped with peanut butter or soy nut butter, unsalted nuts, and dried fruit
Regular soft drinks	Water, fat-free or low-fat milk, or 100% fruit juice
Boiled vegetables	Raw or steamed vegetables (often retain more nutrients than boiled)
Canned vegetables	Frozen vegetables (retain more nutrients during processing)
Breaded and fried meat, fish, or poultry	Broiled or roasted meat, fish, or poultry
Fatty meats such as barbecued ribs, sausage, and hot dogs	Chicken, turkey, or fish; lean meats such as ground round
Whole or 2% milk, cottage cheese with 4% fat, or yogurt made from whole milk	1% or fat-free milk, low-fat cottage cheese (1% fat), or low-fat yogurt
Ice cream	Frozen yogurt or ice milk
Cream cheese	Low-fat cottage cheese (mashed) or reduced-fat cream cheese
Creamy salad dressings or dips made with mayonnaise or sour cream	Oil and vinegar dressing, reduced-fat salad dressings, or dips made from low-fat sour cream or plain yogurt
Chocolate chip or cream-filled cookies	Fruit-filled bars, oatmeal cookies, or fresh fruit
Salt added to season foods	Herbs, spices, or lemon juice

3.5 Food Guides for Dietary Planning

LEARNING OUTCOMES

1 *Explain how to use MyPlate to develop nutritionally adequate daily menus for healthy adults and children.*

2 *Describe educational resources available at www.choosemyplate.gov.*

3 *Identify tools people with diabetes can use for diet planning.*

For over 100 years, the USDA has issued specific dietary recommendations as food guides for Americans. The USDA refines these recommendations periodically as food availability, nutrition research, and tools for nutrition education efforts.

In 1943, the USDA introduced the first food guide based on RDAs for the gen—eral public to use. The guide grouped foods into seven categories and was designed to help Americans plan nutritious menus despite shortages of certain foods that often occurred during World War II. By the mid—1950s, the USDA simplified the original food guide to include only four food groups: milk, meat, fruit and vegeta—ble, and bread and cereal. In 1992, the USDA introduced the Food Guide Pyramid (Fig. 3.5). Unlike earlier dietary guides, the Food Guide Pyramid incorporated knowledge about the health benefits and risks associated with certain foods, and ranked food groups according to their emphasis in menu planning. The Food Guide Pyramid displayed the groups in a layered format with grain products at the base to establish the foundation for a healthy diet. Fatty and sugary foods formed the small peak of the Pyramid, a visual reminder that people should limit their intake of these foods. In 2005 the USDA released the MyPyramid Plan (Fig. 3.6). The

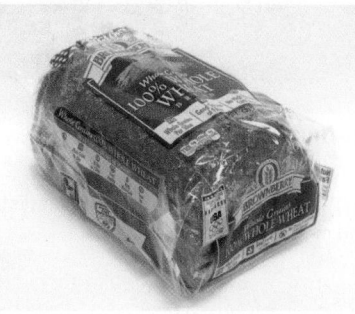

DID **YOU** KNOW?

"Wheat" bread does not necessarily contain whole grains. When purchasing breads and rolls, ignore the term *wheat bread* that may appear on labels. Look for products with "whole grain" as the first item in the ingredient list and "100 percent whole grains" on the product label. Bread made with whole grains are rich sources of fiber, B vitamins, and vitamin E.[12]

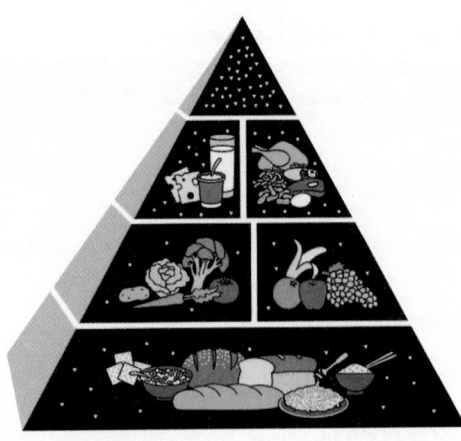

FIGURE 3.5 The Food Guide Pyramid.

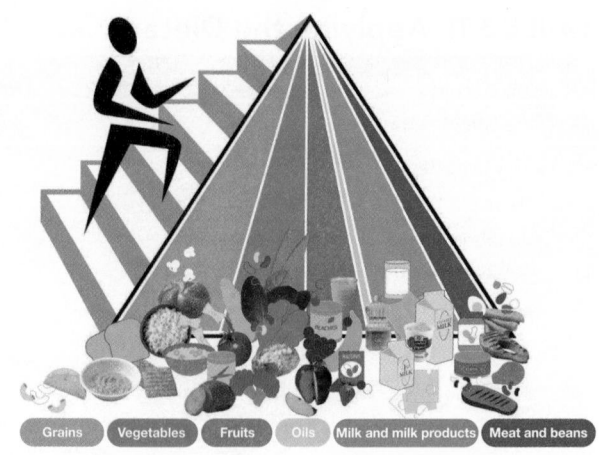

Grains   Vegetables   Fruits   Oils   Milk and milk products   Meat and beans

FIGURE 3.6 MyPyramid.

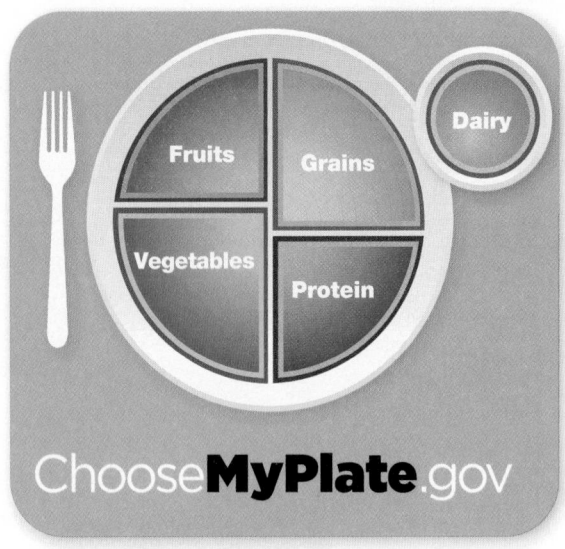

FIGURE 3.7 MyPlate.

MyPlate USDA's interactive Internet dietary and menu-planning guide

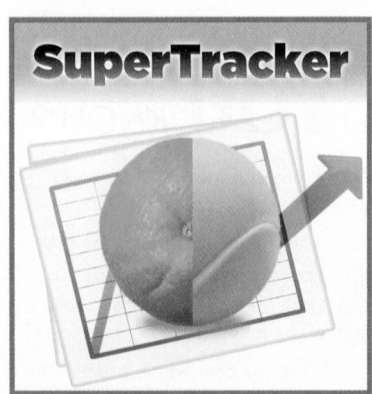

SuperTracker can be accessed at www.choosemyplate.gov.

MyPyramid Plan was an online interactive food guidance system based on *Dietary Guidelines for Americans, 2005.*

MyPlate

In 2011, the USDA replaced the MyPyramid Plan with **MyPlate**, another interactive dietary and menu–planning guide accessible at the website www.choosemyplate.gov. MyPlate includes a variety of food, nutrition, and physical activity resources for consumers that are based on the recommendations of the *2015–2020 Dietary Guidelines for Americans.*

MyPlate differs from the two previous USDA food guides in that it no longer has six food groups depicted by boxes or stripes within a pyramid (Fig. 3.7). MyPlate focuses on five different food groups: fruits, vegetables, protein foods, grains, and dairy. According to the USDA, "oils" do not comprise a food group.[13] The government agency, however, notes the need to include some fat in diets.

The choosemyplate.gov website has useful interactive tools, including:

- "SuperTracker" for assessing daily energy and food group needs, and recording and monitoring daily diet and physical activity habits.

- Information about each food group, including general recommendations, foods that fit into each category, how much of the food should be eaten, scientifically supported health benefits of foods, and recipes that incorporate foods from the group.

- Guidelines for incorporating physical activity into daily living.

- Dietary recommendations for specific population groups, including children and pregnant women.

Major Sources of Empty Calories

Empty calories include energy from alcoholic beverages and foods that contain high amounts of added sugars and/or solid fats. Many commonly eaten foods include various amounts of empty calories. According to the USDA, foods and beverages that contribute the most empty calories to Americans' diets are:

- Cakes, cookies, pastries, and donuts (added sugars and solid fat)
- Sugar–sweetened drinks, including carbonated, energy, sports, and fruit drinks (added sugars)
- Cheese and pizza (sources of solid fat)
- Ice cream (source of added sugar and solid fat)
- Sausage, bacon, hot dogs, and "ribs"[13]

Recommended Intakes

MyPlate has 12 different nutritionally adequate daily food plans that supply from 1000 to 3200 kcal/day (http://www.choosemyplate.gov/MyPlate–Daily–Checklist). Each food plan can be individualized to accommodate a person's age, sex, height, weight, physical activity level, and food preferences, as well as certain life stages, such as pregnancy. The system includes estimates of a person's daily energy needs and indicates how much food one should eat from each of the food groups daily to meet the recommended energy level.

MyPlate dietary patterns include foods and beverages that contain little or no solid fats, added sugars, and alcohol. After a person consumes recommended amounts of nutritious foods from each food group (and oils), a small number of calories remain. The 2000–kcal dietary pattern, for example, has only 260 kcal remaining, which is less than the energy in two 12–ounce sugar–sweetened soft drinks. People can use up these remaining calories by choosing foods that contain a lot of solid fat and/or added sugars, or healthy foods such as fresh fruits and vegetables.

Individualizing MyPlate Meal Plans

To use MyPlate as a personalized menu–planning guide, visit www.choosemyplate.gov and click on Online Tools, SuperTracker, and then "Create Your Profile." Fill in boxes that request information, including your age, sex, and estimated level of physical activity. After you provide and register this information, MyPlate provides a daily food plan that is based on an estimate of your daily energy needs and indicates how much food you should eat from each of the food groups and oils daily to meet your recommended energy level. Table 3.12 indicates MyPlate's food intake recommendations for average healthy young adults who consume 1800 to 3200 kcal per day.

TABLE 3.12 MyPlate: Recommendations for Average, Healthy 20-Year-Old Adults

MyPlate Guidelines (Daily)	Women	Men
Kilocalories	1800–2400	2600–3200
Fruits	2 cups	2–2.5 cups
Vegetables	2.5–3 cups	3.5–4 cups
Grains	6–8 oz	9–10 oz
Protein foods	5.0–6.5 oz	6.5–7 oz
Dairy	3 cups	3 cups
Oils	5–7 tsp	8–11 tsp

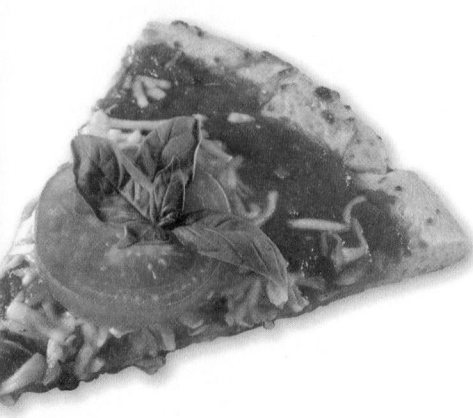

This slice of pizza has ingredients from more than one food group.

Overall, MyPlate can be helpful for planning menus because it promotes food variety, nutritional adequacy, and moderation. You can also use MyPlate's SuperTracker to evaluate the nutritional quality of your daily diet and the "Food Tracker" feature to analyze calorie and nutrient contents of recipes.

Classifying Mixed Dishes How do you classify menu items that combine small amounts of foods from more than one group, such as pizza, sandwiches, and cas—seroles? A slice of pizza, for example, has crust made with wheat flour (grains), tomato sauce (vegetable), and cheese (dairy). The first step is to determine the ingredients and classify each into an appropriate food group. Estimate the number of cups or ounces of each ingredient, and record the amounts contributed from a particular food group. Instead of relying on a set of measuring cups and a food scale to estimate portion sizes, consumers can judge amounts of foods by using familiar objects, including a tennis ball and a bar of soap (Fig. 3.8). By estimating amounts of ingredients, you may determine that a slice of pizza provides ¼ cup of vegetable, 2 ounces of grains, and ¼ cup of dairy.

FRESH TIPS

The MyPlate website includes some general tips to help consumers make healthier food selections, including:

- Make half your grains whole grains.
- Eat your food but eat less.
- Focus on fruits.
- Vary your protein routine.
- Make better beverage choices.
- Add more vegetables to your day.

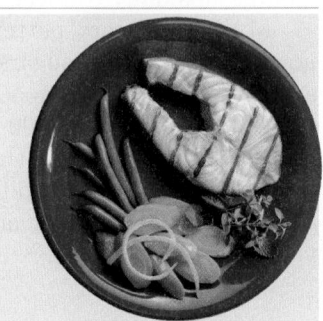

MyPlate: Losing Weight

The "My Weight Manager" page at www.choosemyplate.gov provides individual—ized information about planning nutritionally adequate diets for persons who are

FIGURE 3.8 Estimating portion sizes. People can use familiar items such as these to estimate portion sizes.

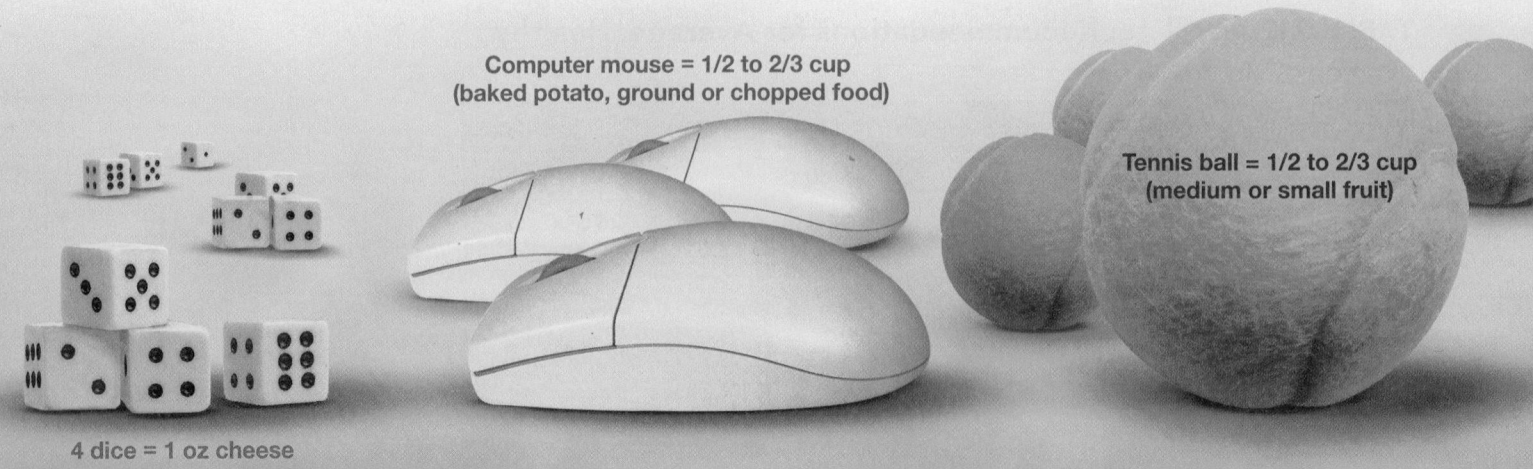

Computer mouse = 1/2 to 2/3 cup (baked potato, ground or chopped food)

Tennis ball = 1/2 to 2/3 cup (medium or small fruit)

4 dice = 1 oz cheese

trying to lose weight. If you would like to lose weight, start by obtaining your personalized daily food plan using SuperTracker. If you are too heavy for your height, the program will let you know and provide a food plan that will help you reach a healthy weight for your height. Chapter 13 provides information about body weight and its management.

Physical activity is particularly important for people who want to lose weight or who have lost weight and need to maintain their current weight. MyPlate includes information about physical activity, including recommendations for how much activity is necessary for promoting good health. Chapter 15 provides information about nutrition and physical activity, including the health benefits of regular physical activity and recommendations to achieve a physically active lifestyle.

Other Dietary Guides

The USDA's original Food Guide Pyramid inspired the development of other food pyramids for people who follow cultural and ethnic food traditions that differ from the mainstream American ("Western") diet. Section 3.7 discusses some cultural, ethnic, and religious influences on American dietary practices. Health Canada, the federal agency responsible for helping Canadians achieve better health, also has a dietary guide, "Eating Well with Canada's Food Guide" (see Appendix H). To use this interactive guide, go to http://www.hc−sc.gc.ca/fn−an/food−guide−aliment/index−eng.php.

Do Americans Follow Dietary Recommendations?

Analysis of government food consumption data indicates that most Americans do not follow the USDA's dietary advice.[14] In 2010, the typical diet of Americans did not provide recommended amounts of foods from the fruit, vegetables, and dairy groups (Fig. 3.9). Furthermore, the diet generally contained more added sugars and fats than in 1970. It is apparent that the public needs to learn more about the importance of choosing a variety of foods and applying the MyPlate guide to everyday menu planning.

Other Menu-Planning Tools

Many chronic diseases require special diets to prevent or delay complications. Diabetes, for example, is easier to control when the person's diet has about the same macronutrient composition from day to day. The **Exchange System** is a

Exchange System tool for estimating the energy, protein, carbohydrate, and fat contents of foods

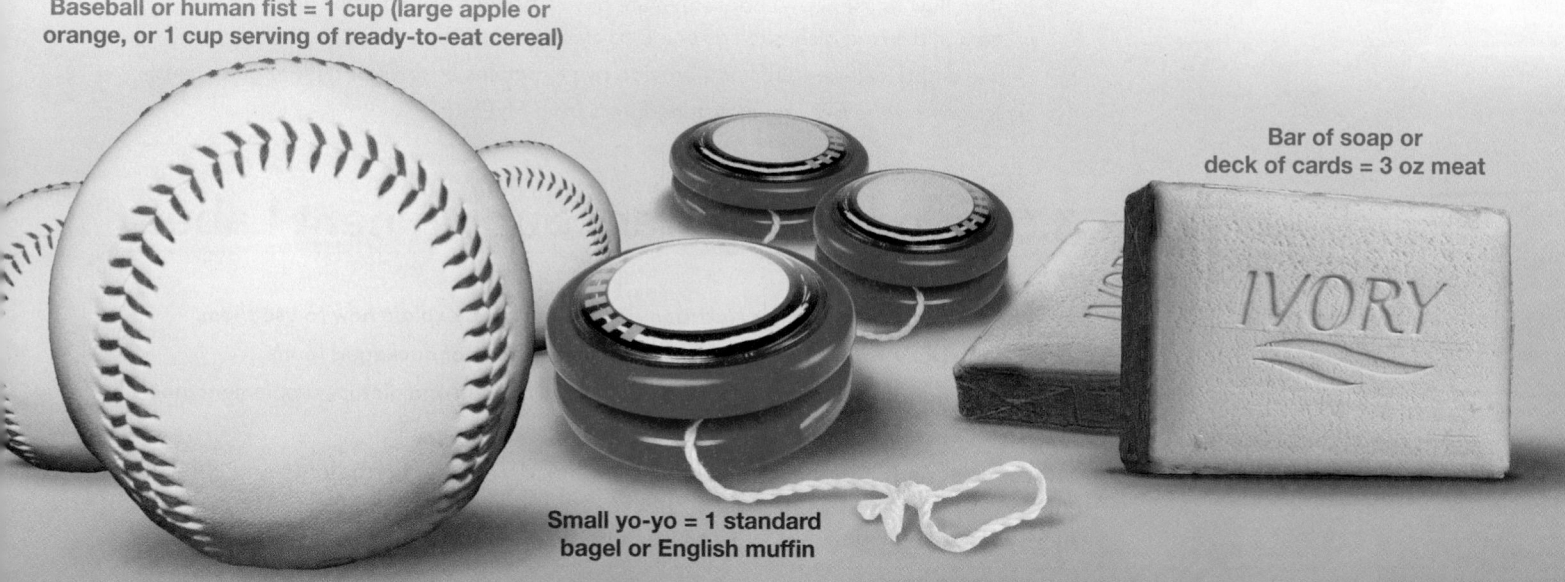

Baseball or human fist = 1 cup (large apple or orange, or 1 cup serving of ready-to-eat cereal)

Bar of soap or deck of cards = 3 oz meat

Small yo-yo = 1 standard bagel or English muffin

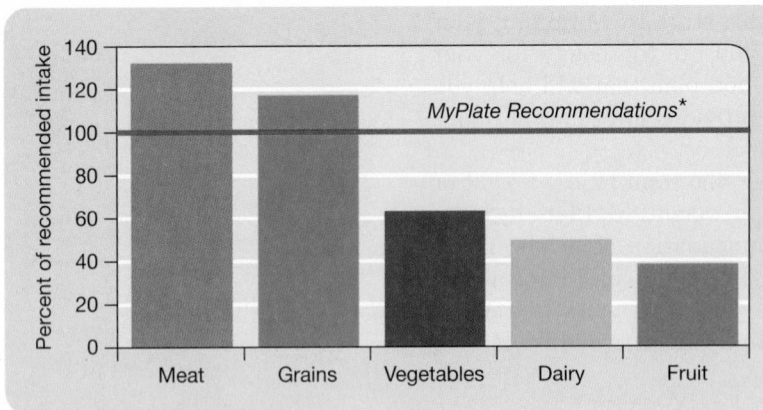

*Data based on a 2000-calorie diet.

Source: Calculated by ERS/USDA based on data from various sources (see Loss-Adjusted Food Availability Documentation). U.S. Department of Agriculture, Agricultural Research Service: *Food availability (per capita) data system*. Data as of February 2013.

FIGURE 3.9 Many Americans' diets do not meet MyPlate recommendations.

useful tool for estimating the energy, protein, carbohydrate, and fat contents of foods. Because the Exchange System makes it relatively easy to plan nutritious, calorie–reduced meals and snacks, it is also useful for people who are trying to manage their weight.

The Exchange System categorizes foods into three broad groups: carbohydrates, meat and meat substitutes, and fats. The foods within each group have similar macronutrient composition, regardless of whether the food is from a plant or animal. For example, the carbohydrate group includes fruits, vegetables, and grains, as well as milk products. Nuts and seeds are grouped with fats. Meats and meat substitutes are grouped according to their fat content. Cheeses are in the meat and meat substitutes group, because of their high protein and fat content. Thus, the Exchange System classifies foods in a different way than does MyPlate.

Within each of the three major food groups, the Exchange System provides exchange lists of specific types of foods. The amount of a food specified in an exchange list provides about the same amount of macronutrients and calories as each of the other specified amounts of foods in that list. According to the fruit list, for example, an orange is equivalent to a small apple, a kiwifruit, or one–half of a large grapefruit. This comparison allows people to plan a wide variety of nutritious menus by exchanging one food for another within each list. To learn more about the Exchange System, people can visit the Academy of Nutrition and Dietetics' website (www.eatright.org) to order the *Guide to Eating Right When You Have Diabetes*. The American Diabetes Association website (www.diabetes.org) also has publications about diabetes and menu planning for consumers and health professionals.

Counting carbohydrates ("counting carbs") is another meal planning technique that people with diabetes can use to control their blood sugar levels. The American Diabetes Association website also includes information about counting carbohydrates. Chapter 5 provides information about diabetes.

ASSESS YOUR PROGRESS

17 List four recommendations for healthy eating according to MyPlate.

18 Explain how to use www.choosemyplate.gov to find the food groups and calories present in a mixed dish, such as one 8-oz chicken pot pie.

19 Define empty-calorie foods and provide two examples based on MyPlate guidelines.

20 Describe how the Exchange System differs from MyPlate.

3.6 Food and Dietary Supplement Labels

LEARNING OUTCOMES

1 List the components of the Nutrition Facts panel, and explain how to use them.

2 Use the Daily Values to compare nutritional contents of packaged foods.

3 Identify nutrition-related claims the FDA allows on food and dietary supplement labels.

Information on food labels can help consumers determine ingredients and compare energy and nutrient contents of packaged foods and beverages. According to survey data collected by the FDA in 2008, 54% of Americans reported that they "often" read food labels when they consider buying a food for the first time.[15] Consumers who pay attention to the information on food labels are most interested in learning about amounts of calories, sodium, vitamins, and fat in the products.

In the United States, the FDA regulates and monitors information that can be placed on food labels, including claims about the health benefits of ingredients. Today, nearly all foods and beverages sold in grocery stores must have labels that provide the product's name, manufacturer's name and address, and amount of product in the package. Furthermore, products that have more than one ingredient must display a list of the ingredients in descending order according to weight. The package shown in Figure 3.10, for example, is for a product that has whole–wheat flour, water, and brown sugar as the first three ingredients. Thus, this food probably contains higher amounts of whole–wheat flour, water, and brown sugar than it does of the remaining ingredients listed.

Consumers can determine where certain foods were produced or grown by reading food labels. Producers and sellers of fresh and frozen fruits and vegetables, chicken, fish and shellfish, ginseng, and pecans, peanuts, and macadamia nuts must declare the product's country of origin either on the packaging or at the site where the product is located in stores (Fig. 3.11).

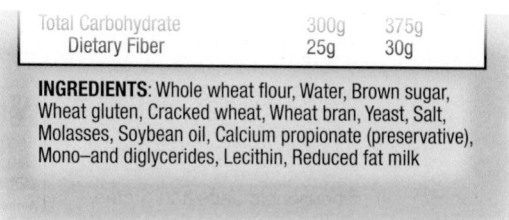

FIGURE 3.10 What's in a food?

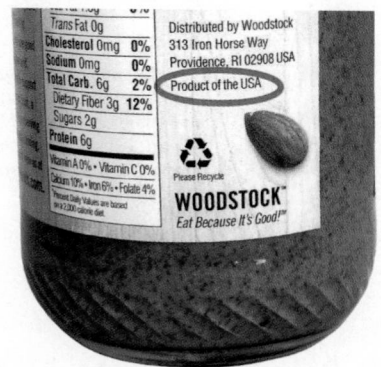

FIGURE 3.11 Country of origin.

Daily Values

To help consumers evaluate the nutritional content of food products, the FDA used RDAs to develop the **Daily Values (DVs)** for labeling purposes. Compared to the RDAs, the DVs are a more simplified and practical set of nutrient standards. The adult DV for a nutrient is based on a standard diet that supplies 2000 kcal/day. Not all nutrients have DVs, but DVs have been established for macronutrients, fiber, and several vitamins and minerals. Appendix G lists the set of DVs for people over 4 years of age for 2015. Three other sets of DVs are used on labels of foods intended for infants, children between 1 and 4 years of age, and pregnant or breastfeeding women.

When evaluating or planning nutritious menus, a person's goal is to obtain at least 100% of the DVs for fiber, vitamins, and minerals each day. On the other hand, one may need to limit his or her intake of foods that have high %DVs of total fat, saturated fat, and sodium (Fig. 3.12). High intakes of these nutrients may have negative effects on a person's health. Thus, people should consume less than 100% of the DV for total fat, saturated fat, and sodium each day. The general rule of thumb is: A food that supplies 5%DV or less of a nutrient is a low source of the nutrient, and a food that provides 20%DV or more is a high source of the nutrient.

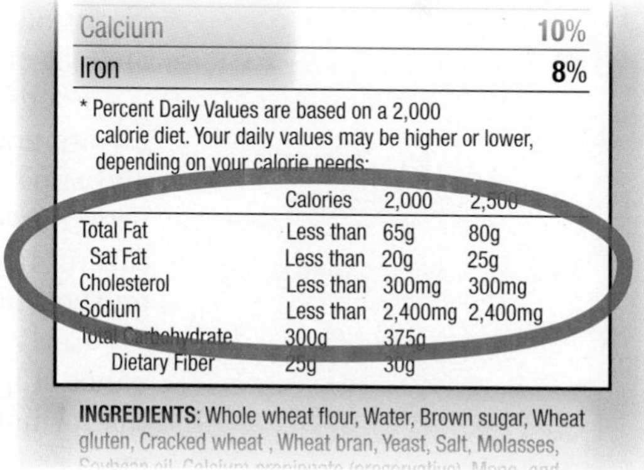

Nutrition Facts Panel

Consumers can find specific nutrition–related information about many packaged foods simply by reading the products' labels. The FDA requires food manufacturers to use a special format, the **Nutrition Facts panel**, to display information about the energy and nutrient contents of products (Fig. 3.13). The Nutrition Facts panel indicates the amount of a serving size, in household units as well as grams, and the number of servings in the entire container. Serving sizes must be consistent among similar foods; for example, all brands of ice cream must use the same serving size (½ cup) in the Nutrition Facts panel to describe the product's nutritional content.

As of 2015, the FDA requires food manufacturers to provide information about the food's total fat, saturated fat, trans fat, cholesterol, sodium, total carbohydrate, fiber, sugars, protein, vitamin A, vitamin C, calcium, and iron contents in the

FIGURE 3.12 Daily Value standards (as of February 1, 2016).

Daily Values (DVs) set of nutrient intake standards developed for labeling purposes

Nutrition Facts panel nutrition information about a food's nutrient contents that is displayed in a specific format on the food's package

Current Label

Serving size is shown in household units and grams.

% Daily Values relate to 2000 kcal/day diet.

To reduce risk of heart disease, choose foods that are low in saturated fat, trans fat, and sodium.

As of January 2016, there is no % Daily Value for sugar, but limit your intake of foods with **added** sugars included among the first few items in the ingredients list.

Consume adequate amounts of fiber and these micronutrients.

Proposed Label

Nutrition Facts

Serving Size 2/3 cup (55g)
Servings Per Container About 8

Amount Per Serving

Calories 230 Calories from Fat 40

% Daily Value*

Total Fat 8g — 12%
Saturated Fat 1g — 5%
Trans Fat 0g
Cholesterol 0mg — 0%
Sodium 160mg — 7%
Total Carbohydrate 37g — 12%
Dietary Fiber 4g — 16%
Sugars 1g
Protein 3g

Vitamin A — 10%
Vitamin C — 8%
Calcium — 20%
Iron — 45%

* Percent Daily Values are based on a 2,000 calorie diet. Your daily value may be higher or lower depending on your calorie needs.

	Calories:	2,000	2,500
Total Fat	Less than	65g	80g
Sat Fat	Less than	20g	25g
Cholesterol	Less than	300mg	300mg
Sodium	Less than	2,400mg	2,400mg
Total Carbohydrate		300g	375g
Dietary Fiber		25g	30g

(a)

Nutrition Facts

8 servings per container
Serving size — 2/3 cup (55g)

Amount per 2/3 cup
Calories — **230**

% DV*

12% **Total Fat** 8g
5% Saturated Fat 1g
Trans Fat 0g
0% **Cholesterol** 0mg
7% **Sodium** 160mg
12% **Total Carbs** 37g
14% Dietary Fiber 4g
Sugars 1g
Added Sugars 0g
Protein 3g

10% **Vitamin D** 2mcg
20% **Calcium** 260mg
45% **Iron** 8mg
5% **Potassium** 235mg

* Daily Values (DV) and calories reference to be inserted here.

(b)

FIGURE 3.13 Understanding the Nutrition Facts panel. (*a*) Current Label and (*b*) Proposed Label (as of February 1, 2016).

Nutrition Facts panel (Fig. 3.13a). Additionally, the panel must display the total amount of energy and energy from fat, indicated as numbers of calories, in a serving.

Foods such as fresh fruits and vegetables, fish and shellfish, meats, and poultry are not required to have Nutrition Facts labels. However, many food suppliers and supermarket chains provide consumers with information about their products' nutritional content on posters or shelf tags displayed near the foods. In the future, fresh foods such as raw meats are likely to include Nutrition Facts panels on their labels.

Early in 2014, the FDA proposed an updated version of the Nutrition Facts panel (Fig. 3.13b). The proposed panel format has some significant changes to the format that was used in early 2016. The new panel, for example, displays the number of calories per serving in very bold print, so it is highly visible. Under "Sugars," a new component, "Added sugars," differentiates between ingredients that are added to foods or beverages to sweeten them, such as high-fructose corn syrup, from sugars that are naturally in a food or beverage, such as those in fruit juice and cow's milk. Such information is helpful for people who want to monitor their empty-calorie intakes and compare foods for their added sugar contents. The proposed Nutrition Facts panel no longer provides information about the number of calories from fat. This is because FDA officials recommend that consumers should be more concerned about eating less unhealthy saturated and trans fats instead of choosing foods that are low in total fat. Furthermore, the FDA no longer requires manufacturers to include information about the vitamin A and C contents of packaged foods, but they must indicate amounts of potassium and vitamin D in their products. This change reflects public health concerns that many Americans have less-than-adequate intakes of these micronutrients.

What About Restaurant and Vending Machine Foods?

Percentages of DVs are designed to help consumers compare nutrient contents of packaged foods to make more healthful choices. However, most people do not eat just packaged foods. Fresh fruits and vegetables, as well as many restaurant meals, do not have labels or menus with information about %DVs per serving. Therefore, many consumers will underestimate their nutrient intakes if they do not consider the contribution that unlabeled foods make to their diets.

A section of the Patient Protection and Affordable Care Act of 2010 requires restaurants and similar retail food establishments with 20 or more locations to list calorie content information for standard menu items on restaurant menus and menu boards.[16] Information about total calories, fat, saturated fat, cholesterol, sodium, total carbohydrates, sugars, fiber, and total protein contents of menu items must be available in writing when the customer requests it. According to this act, companies that maintain 20 or more vending machines must disclose calorie contents of certain items for consumers to see.

The goal of listing calories is to help consumers make healthier choices, but how accurate are the caloric counts listed by restaurants? According to results of a study at Tufts University, calorie levels were *underreported* an average of 18% of the time on items sold at restaurants.[17] Although the nutrition information that is displayed may provide a close estimate of the values, portions are not exactly the same every time a food is served. Therefore, consumers should consider the calorie levels posted at restaurants as a rough guide.

Rating Foods for Nutritional Value

Standardized food labeling that includes Nutrition Facts panels on most packaged foods has been in use since 1994, but many Americans do not read and use this information.[19] To provide unbiased, science–based nutrition information that consumers can understand and use, public health experts have developed reliable **food rating systems**. Food rating systems use a variety of methods to evaluate the nutritional value of foods and then rank the products from highly nutritious and healthful to low in nutritional value or unhealthy. Products that contain unhealthy amounts of added sugars, salt, and solid fat generally receive low ratings, whereas foods that have less of these ingredients are likely to have higher ratings. The presence of micro–nutrients, omega–3 fat, dietary fiber, and phytochemicals can raise a food's score or ranking.

Food rating systems often use easy–to–understand formats, such as a color or a numerical score, to convey valuable information about the nutritional value of foods. Such systems can be displayed on the product's shelf tag in a super–market where shoppers can easily see them.

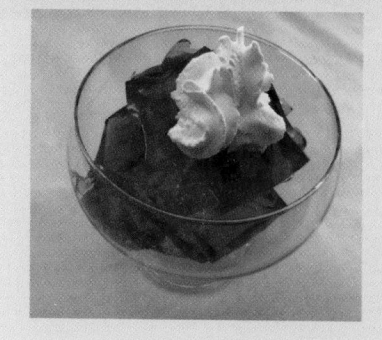

food rating systems variety of methods that evaluate the nutritional value of foods and display this information to consumers

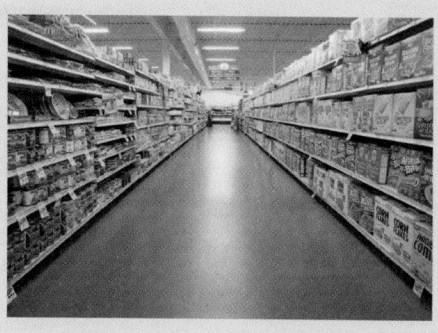

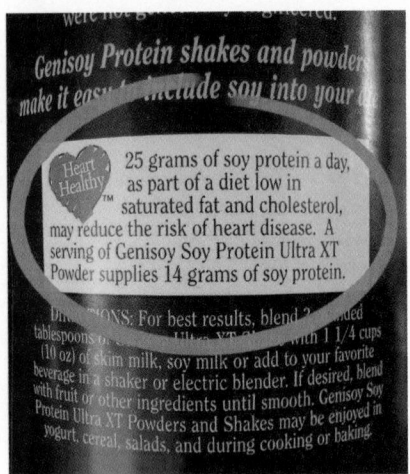

FIGURE 3.14 Health claim (2016).

Health Claims

The FDA permits food manufacturers to include health claims on food labels (Fig. 3.14). The FDA, however, limits the kinds of claims that manufacturers can use. Manufacturers cannot claim that the food can be used in the "... diagnosis, cure, mitigation, or treatment of disease."[22] An allowable health claim, for example, may state, "Diets low in saturated fat and cholesterol may reduce the risk of heart disease." The FDA would not permit a claim such as "Eating Fluffy Brand Margarine each day prevents heart disease" to appear on the product's label.

The FDA requires specific wording for certain health claims that are allowed on labels. For information about qualified health–related claims that can be used on labels, visit FDA's website at www.fda.gov and search for "qualified health claims."

As of 2015, the FDA would not approve health claims for foods that contain more than 13 g of fat, 4 g of saturated fat, 60 mg of cholesterol, or 480 mg of sodium per serving. For example, calcium is a mineral that strengthens bones and protects them from osteoporosis, a condition in which bones become brittle and break easily. Milk is a rich source of calcium. Nevertheless, the label on a carton of *whole* milk cannot include a health claim about calcium and osteoporosis, because whole milk contains more than 4 g of saturated fat per serving. In addition, the product must meet specific conditions that relate to the health claim. For example, a claim regarding the benefits of eating a low–fat diet is allowed only if the product contains 3 g or less of fat per serving, which is the FDA's standard definition of a low–fat food.

Structure/Function Claims

A structure/function claim describes the role a nutrient or dietary supplement plays in maintaining a structure, such as bone, or promoting a normal bodily function, such as digestion. The FDA allows structure/function claims such as "calcium builds strong bones" or "fiber maintains bowel regularity" (Fig. 3.15). Structure/function statements cannot claim that a nutrient or dietary supplement can be used to prevent or treat a disease. For example, the FDA would not permit a claim that a product "promotes low blood pressure," because that claim implies the product has druglike effects and can be used treat high blood pressure.

Nutrient Content Claims

The FDA permits labels to include claims about levels of nutrients in processed foods. Nutrient content claims can use terms such as *free*, *high*, or *low* to describe how much of a nutrient is in the product. Additionally, nutrient content claims can use terms such as *more* or *reduced* to compare amounts of nutrients in a product to those in a similar product. This claim is often used for an item that substitutes for a *reference food*, a similar and more familiar food. For example, a "reduced–fat" salad dressing has considerably less fat than its reference food, regular salad dressing.

Table 3.13 lists some legal definitions for common nutrient content claims that may be used on labels as of 2015. Note that a product may contain a small amount of a nutrient (less than 0.5 g), yet the Nutrition Facts panel (2015) can indicate the amount as "0 g." For example, the Nutrition Facts panel may indicate that a serving of food supplies "0" grams of saturated fat, even though the food actually supplies 0.3 g of saturated fat, because that amount is less than 0.5 g. Furthermore, manufacturers are allowed to claim that the product is "free" of the nutrient. As a result, it is possible to consume some saturated fat from processed foods even though

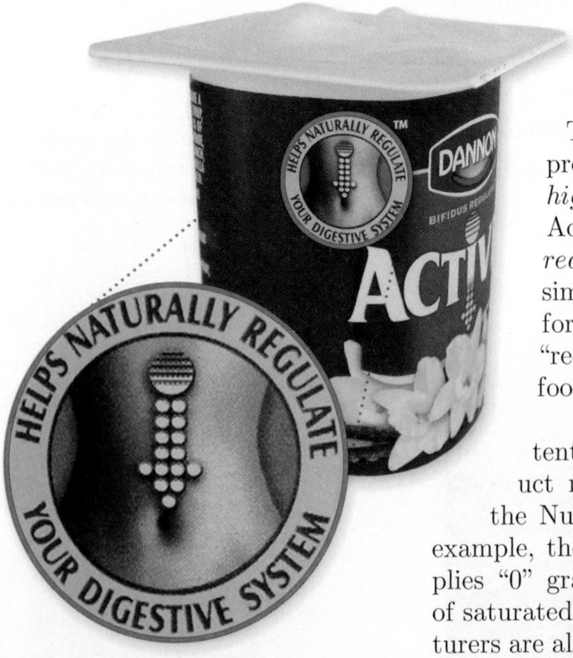

FIGURE 3.15 Structure/function statement.

TABLE 3.13 Legal Definitions for Common Nutrient Content Claims (2015)

Sugar	• **Sugar free:** The product provides less than 0.5 g sugar per serving. • **Reduced sugar:** The food contains at least 25% less sugar per serving than the reference food.
Calories	• **Calorie free:** The food provides fewer than 5 kcal per serving. • **Reduced or fewer calories:** The food contains at least 25% fewer kcal per serving than the reference food.
Fat	• **Fat free:** The food provides less than 0.5 g fat per serving. • **Low fat:** The food contains 3 g or less fat per serving. Two percent milk is not "low fat," because it has more than 3 g fat per serving. The term *reduced fat* can be used to describe 2% milk. • **Reduced or less fat:** The food supplies at least 25% less fat per serving than the reference food.
Fiber	• **High fiber:** The food contains 5 g or more fiber per serving. Foods that include high-fiber claims on the label must also meet the definition for low fat. • **Good source of fiber:** The food supplies 2.5 to 4.9 g fiber per serving.
Meat and poultry products regulated by USDA	• **Extra lean:** The food provides less than 5 g fat, 2 g saturated fat, and 95 mg cholesterol per serving. • **Lean:** The food contains less than 10 g fat, 4.5 g saturated fat, and 95 mg cholesterol per serving.

labels indicate a serving of each food does not contain this type of fat. To learn more about the FDA's regulations concerning nutrient claims, visit the agency's website at www.fda.gov and search for "nutrient claims."

Other Descriptive Labeling Terms

The U.S. Food and Drug Administration and Department of Health and Human Services have established legal definitions and standard recipes for many commonly eaten foods, including milk and milk products, macaroni, ice cream, and salad dressing. Such *standards of identity* are intended to prevent manufacturers from producing substandard foods and marketing the items to consumers.

Food manufacturers often develop new items that simulate existing foods that have definitions and standards of identity. For example, a product that is labeled "Whipped Cream" must be made from whipping cream, according to the standard of identity. For example, Food Company A develops a product to replace whipped cream that is similar to the food topping made from cream but contains no animal fat. Therefore, the new food does not meet the definition and standard of identity for whipped cream, so it cannot be marketed as "whipped cream." Instead, the manufacturer can label and market the food as a "whipped topping."

To attract consumers, food manufacturers often include the term *natural* on their products' labels. At this time, the FDA has no legal definition for *natural*. The agency, however, permits food manufacturers to use the term on labels, if the product does not contain added color, artificial flavors, or other synthetic substances.

FRESH TIPS

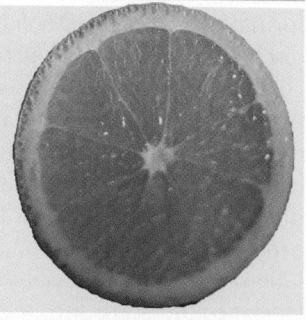

Often, the only difference between a creamy salad dressing, such as ranch or bleu cheese, and the "light" version of the dressing is the amount of water they contain. Instead of paying extra for calorie-reduced bottled salad dressings, make your own light salad dressing by adding about ¼ cup of water to a jar of regular creamy salad dressing, then stir the mixture well.

DID YOU KNOW?

A variety of factors, including genetic traits, age, growing conditions, and production methods, contribute to a plant's nutrient contents. Therefore, scientists generally analyze several samples of a particular food to determine its nutrient contents and then average the results. For example, if the amount of energy in three Valencia oranges that each weigh about 4 ounces (120 g) were 55, 60, and 62 kcal, respectively, the value listed in the food composition table for a Valencia orange weighing 4 ounces would be 59 kcal, the average of the three.

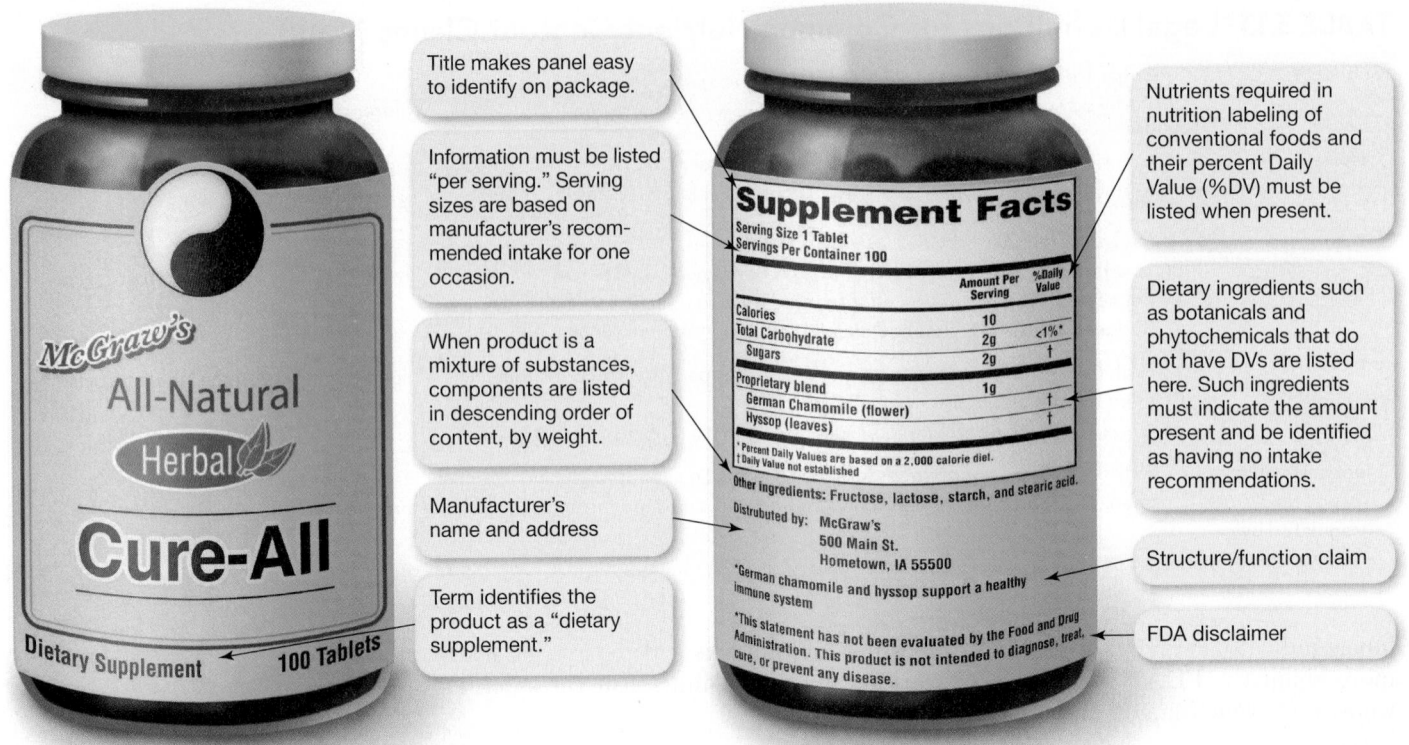

FIGURE 3.16 Dietary supplement label. Consumers can obtain information about the contents of a dietary supplement by reading the product's label.

Dietary Supplement Labels

According to federal law, every dietary supplement container must be properly labeled (Fig. 3.16). The label must include the term *dietary supplement* or a similar term that describes the product's particular ingredient, such as *herbal supplement* or *vitamin C supplement*. Dietary supplement labels are also required to display the list of ingredients, manufacturer's address, and suggested dosage. Furthermore, the label must include facts about the product's contents in a special format—the "Supplement Facts" panel (Fig. 3.16). The panel provides information about the serving size; amount per serving; and percent Daily Value (%DV) for ingredients, if one has been established. DVs have not been established for phytochemicals.

According to the FDA, dietary supplements are not intended to treat, diagnose, cure, or alleviate the effects of diseases. Therefore, the agency does not permit manufacturers to market a dietary supplement product as a treatment or cure for a disease or to relieve signs or symptoms of a disease. Although such products generally cannot prevent diseases, some can improve health or reduce the risk of certain diseases or conditions. Thus, the FDA allows supplement manufacturers to display structure/function claims on labels. Manufacturers of iron supplements, for example, may have a claim on the label that states: "Iron is necessary for healthy red blood cell formation." If the FDA has not reviewed a claim, the label must include the FDA's disclaimer indicating that the claim has not been evaluated by the agency (Fig. 3.17).

The FDA does not require dietary supplement manufacturers or sellers to provide evidence that labeling claims are accurate or truthful before they appear on product containers. However, manufacturers that include structure/function claims on labels must notify the FDA about the claims within 30 days after introducing the products into the marketplace. If FDA officials question the safety of a dietary supplement or the truthfulness of claims that appear on supplement labels, manufacturers are responsible for providing the agency with evidence that their products are safe and the claims on labels are honest and not misleading.

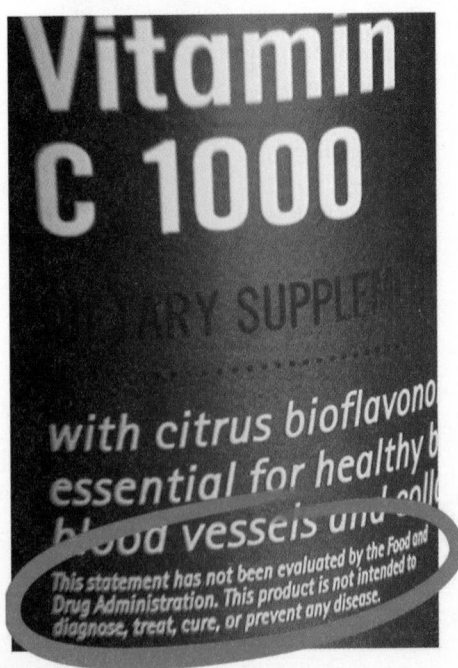

FIGURE 3.17 FDA disclaimer.

Organic Food

Technically, organic substances have the element carbon bonded to hydrogen in their chemical structures. Therefore, all foods are organic by this definition because they contain substances comprised of carbon bonded with hydrogen. The term *organic*, however, also refers to certain methods of food production. **Organically produced foods** are those that do not rely on the use of antibiotics, hormones, synthetic fertilizers and pesticides, genetic improvements, or ioniz-ing radiation.[23] An organic farming operation, for example, would use natural nonchemical methods to manage pests, such as those discussed in Chapter 20.

organically produced foods foods that are produced without the use of antibiotics, hormones, synthetic fertilizers and pesticides, genetic improvements, or ionizing radiation

Comparison of Organic and Conventional Farming Methods

Table 3.14 compares organic and conventional agricultural systems. Although organic farming techniques can benefit the environment, crop yields are typically lower than yields of similar crops grown conventionally.[24]

Over the past 40 years, the popularity of organic foods has increased in the United States as many Americans have become concerned about the environment and the safety and nutritional value of the food supply. Sales of organic foods have increased steadily since the 1990s, even though these products are usually more expensive than the same foods produced by conventional farming methods. In 2011, Americans spent an estimated $31.5 billion on organic foods and beverages.[25]

People who purchase organically grown foods often think the products are better for their health and more nutritious than conventionally produced foods. Few well-designed studies have compared nutrient and phytochemical con-tents of organically grown foods to their conventionally grown counterparts. Nevertheless, some general trends have emerged. In general, organic food crops are not more nutritious than conventionally grown food crops.[26] Organic foods, however, may contain fewer pesticides and antibiotic-resistant bacteria than conventionally grown crops.[27]

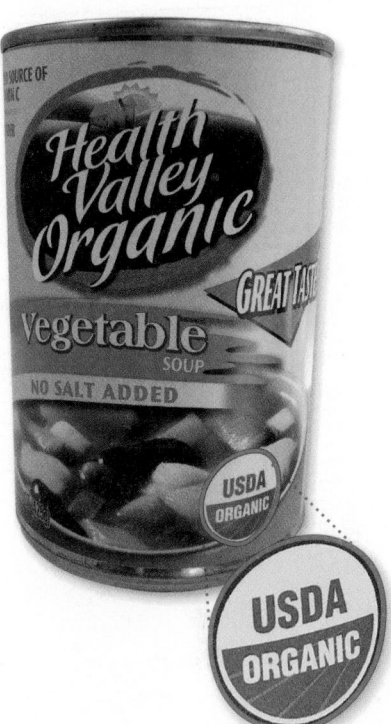

Labeling Organic Foods

To protect consumers, the USDA developed and implemented rules for the organic food industry. A food product cannot be labeled "organic" unless its production meets strict national standards. For labeling purposes, organic food manufac-turers can use the circular "USDA Organic" symbol on the package (Fig. 3.18).

FIGURE 3.18 USDA organic symbol.

TABLE 3.14 Comparing Organic and Conventional Farming Systems

Organic	Conventional
Synthetic fertilizers are not allowed.	Limited restrictions on fertilizers
Sewage sludge products are not allowed.	Sludge products may be used on some fields.
Restrictions on use of raw manure on fields used for food crops	Few restrictions on raw manure use for edible crop fields
Synthetic pesticides are not allowed; natural pest management practices are encouraged.	Any government-approved pesticide may be used according to label instructions. Natural pest management practices may also be used.
Genetically modified organisms (GMOs) are not allowed.	Government-approved GMOs are permitted.
Feeding livestock mammal and poultry by-products and manure is not allowed.	Certain mammal and poultry by-products are allowed in livestock feed.
Use of growth hormones and antibiotics in livestock production is not allowed.	Government-approved hormone and antibiotic treatments are permitted.
Food irradiation (a food safety method) is not allowed.	Food irradiation may be used.
Detailed recordkeeping and site inspections by regulators are required.	Some records are required, but no on-site checks by regulators are necessary.

TABLE 3.15 Organic Labeling Categories

"100% Organic" (may use USDA seal)	100% organic ingredients, including processing aids
"Organic" (may use USDA seal)	Contains at least 95% organic ingredients
	Remaining 5% of ingredients are on USDA's list of allowed ingredients.
"Made with organic ingredients"	Contains 70 to 95% organic ingredients

This symbol indicates the products meet USDA's standards for organic food. The USDA rules provide for three organic labeling categories (Table 3.15). Note that certain foods can have the organic symbol on the package, yet they may contain small amounts of nonorganic ingredients. For more information about the government's organic food standards, visit the USDA's National Organic Program's website (www.ams.usda.gov/nop).

ASSESS YOUR PROGRESS

21 List the categories of information included on the Nutrition Facts panel (as of 2015).

22 Distinguish between the RDA and the %DV for a nutrient.

23 Describe how supermarket shoppers can use food rating systems to make purchase decisions.

24 What is the difference between a health claim and a structure/function claim? What is a nutrient content claim? Give an example of each type of claim.

25 Give examples of how organic food production methods differ from conventional food production methods.

3.7 Food and Culture: The Melting Pot

LEARNING OUTCOMES

1 Describe the influence of particular ethnic and religious groups on Americans' food choices.

2 Compare and contrast dietary and lifestyle recommendations of MyPlate and the Latin American, Mediterranean, and Asian Diet Pyramids.

Wherever you live or travel in the United States, you're likely to find restaurants that serve a wide variety of ethnic fare, such as Italian, Mexican, Thai, Vietnamese, or Middle Eastern dishes. Traditional ethnic diets are often based on dishes containing small amounts of animal foods and larger amounts of locally grown fruits, vegetables, and unrefined grains. However, these foods are typically the first to be abandoned as ethnic population groups *assimilate*, that is, blend into the general population over time. After an ethnic population has assimilated fully, the prevalence of chronic diseases such as cardiovascular disease, type 2 diabetes, and high blood pressure often increases among them, partly as a result of adopting less healthy eating and food preparation practices.

Hispanic Diet

The Hispanic (people with Spanish ancestry) population is now the largest minority group in the United States. Many Hispanic–Americans migrated to the United States from Mexico. The traditional Mexican diet included corn, beans, chili peppers, avocados, papayas, and pineapples. Other plant foods that are often incorporated into Mexican meals include fresh chayote, cherimoya, jicama, plantains, and cactus leaves and fruit. Such fruits and vegetables add fiber and a variety of nutrients, phytochemicals, vivid colors, and interesting flavors to Mexican dishes. Figure 3.19 shows foods that are components of the traditional Latin American Diet Pyramid.

Authentic Mexican meals are based primarily on rice, tortillas, and beans, depending on the region. To appeal to people with more Western food prefer—ences, "Mexican" fast—food restaurants in the United States often serve dishes that contain large portions of high—fat beef topped with sour cream and cheese. Diets that contain high amounts of solid fats are associated with excess body fat, CVD, and type 2 diabetes.

Southern European Diet

The Mediterranean Diet Pyramid shown in Figure 3.20 is based on traditional dietary practices of Greece, southern Italy, and the island of Crete. Grains, fruits, and vegetables, particularly beans and potatoes, form the foundation of this diet. Red meat is rarely eaten. Main dishes often include seafood and poul—try, and wine may be included with meals. Although the Mediterranean Diet Pyramid allows as much as 35% of total calories as fat in the diet, much of the fat is from olive oil. Olive oil is a rich source of a type of fat that reduces rather than increases the risk of CVD. Chapter 6 provides more information about oils and fats and their roles in health.

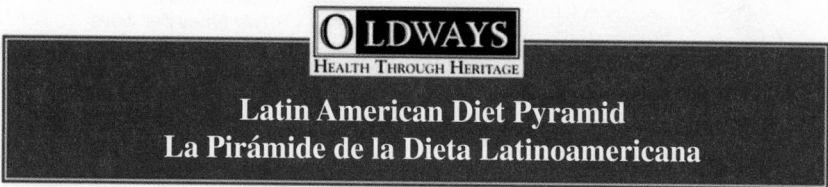

Latin American Diet Pyramid
La Pirámide de la Dieta Latinoamericana

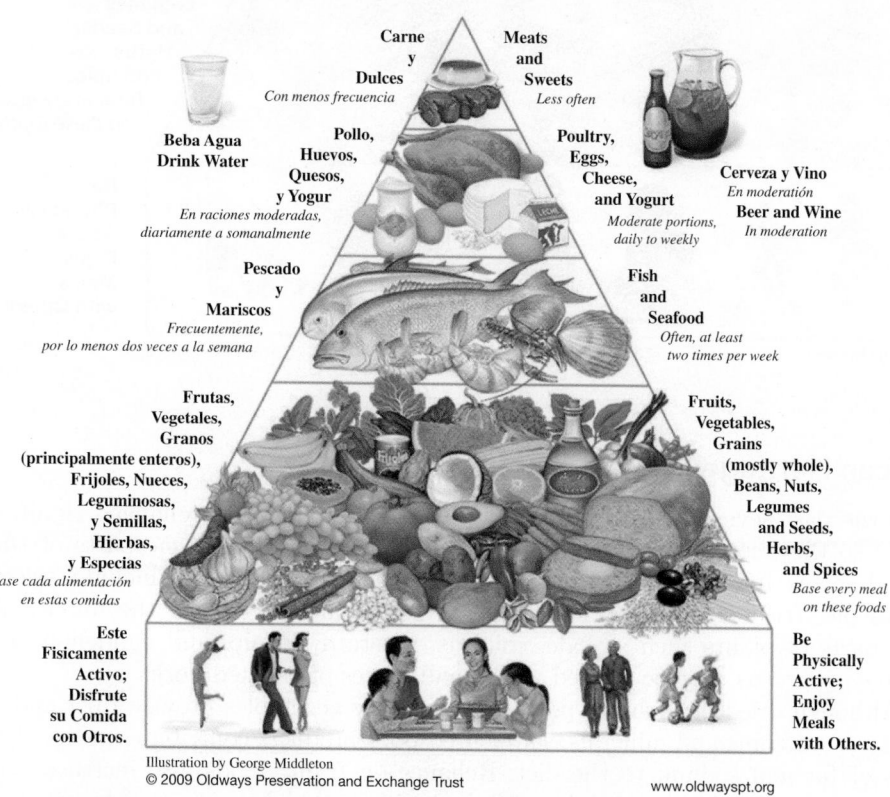

Illustration by George Middleton
© 2009 Oldways Preservation and Exchange Trust

www.oldwayspt.org

FIGURE 3.19 Latin American Diet Pyramid.

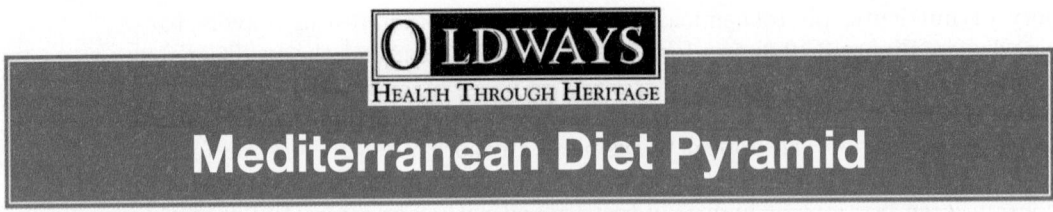

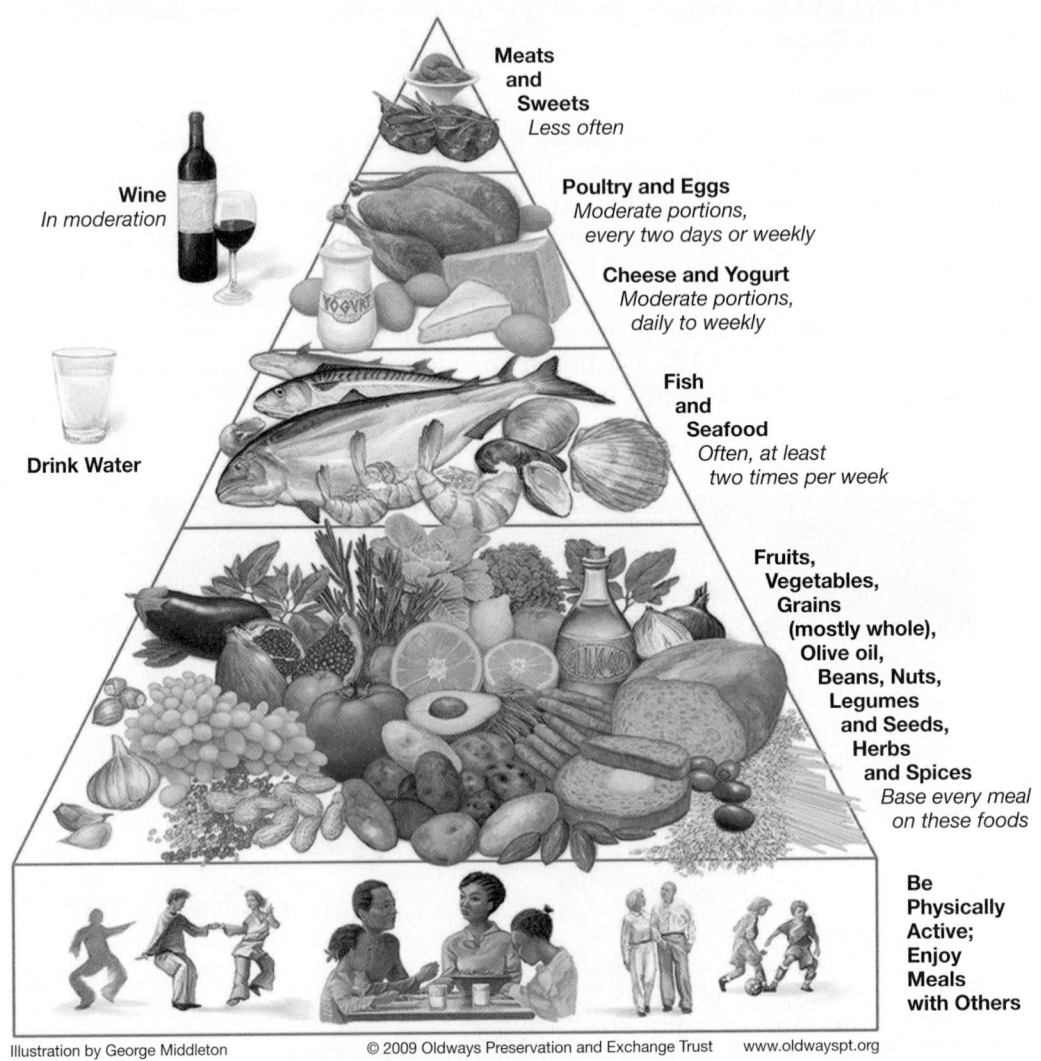

FIGURE 3.20 Mediterranean Diet Pyramid.

African Heritage Diets

Over the past several decades, the diets of African Americans changed significantly so they now incorporate regional food preferences. In some parts of the United States, for example, the traditional African–American diet includes sweet potato pie, fried chicken, pork, black–eyed peas, and "greens," the nutritious leafy parts of plants such as kale, collards, mustard, turnip, and dandelion. To add flavor, greens may be cooked with small pieces of smoked pork.

Although dried peas, sweet potatoes, and leafy vegetables provide fiber and a variety of vitamins and minerals, salt–cured pork products contribute undesirable levels of fat and sodium to the diet. Reliance on frying foods also increases fat intakes. High–fat diets are associated with obesity, and high–sodium diets raise the risk of hypertension. You will learn more about the role of diet in the development of hypertension in Chapters 6 and 9. For more information about African heritage diets and foods, visit http://oldwayspt.org/programs/african–heritage–health .

Asian Diet

Traditional Asian diets, such as Chinese, Japanese, Vietnamese, Thai, and Korean cuisines, are similar and generally feature large amounts of vegetables, rice, or noodles combined with small amounts of meat, fish, or shellfish. The variety of vegetables used in Asian dishes adds color, flavor, texture, phytochemicals, and nutrients to meals. Additionally, Asian dishes often include flavorful sauces and seasonings made from plants, such as soy sauce, rice wine, ginger root, garlic, scallions, peppers, and sesame seeds. The Asian Diet Pyramid, shown in Figure 3.21, illustrates the traditional Asian dietary pattern that generally provides inadequate amounts of calcium from milk and milk products. However, using calcium−rich or calcium−fortified foods can add the mineral to diets.

Traditional Chinese food preparation methods, particularly steaming and stir−frying, tend to preserve the vitamins and minerals in fresh vegetables. Stir−frying involves cooking foods in a lightly oiled, very hot pan for a short period of time. Unlike Western methods of deep−fat frying or boiling vegetables, stir−frying vegetables keeps them crisp and colorful. North American Chinese restaurants typically offer menu items that contain much larger portions of animal foods such as beef and chicken than authentic dishes. Furthermore, American−Chinese foods are often prepared with far greater amounts of fat than are used in true Chinese cooking.

Rice is the staple food in the traditional Japanese diet. Additionally, fish, poultry, pork, and foods made from soybeans provide protein in this diet. In the United States, American−Japanese restaurants often feature sushi, small pieces of raw fish or shellfish that are usually served rolled in or pressed into rice and served with vegetables and seaweed.

The traditional Japanese diet of fresh vegetables, minimal amounts of salt and animal protein (mainly from pork and fish), and moderate amounts of fat may protect people from premature heart disease and stroke. However, some Japanese consume high amounts of the mineral sodium, which may increase their risk of hypertension.

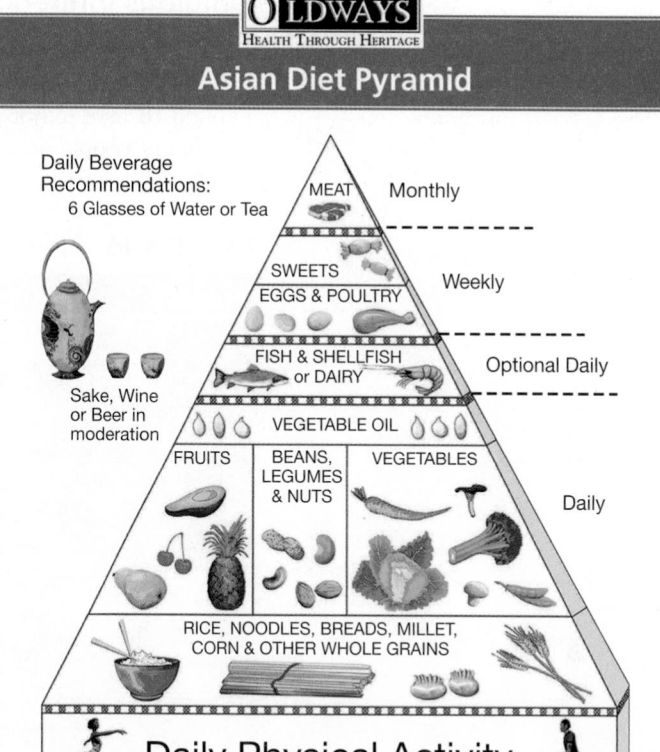

FIGURE 3.21 Asian Diet Pyramid.

Native American Indian Diets

In the past, many American Indian tribal members were hunter−gatherers who depended on wild vegetation, fish, and game for food. Other American Indians learned to grow vegetable crops, including tomatoes, corn, and squash. In general, the traditional American Indian diet was low in sodium and fat and high in fiber. During the last half of the twentieth century, many Americans Indians discontinued their traditional diets and followed the typical Western diet. The negative health effects of this lifestyle change have been significant. Before the 1930s, for example, members of the Pima tribe in the southwestern United States primarily ate native foods. By the end of the century, the Pima had adopted a more Western diet. Now, obesity and type 2 diabetes are extremely prevalent among the Pima, whereas in the past, these conditions rarely affected tribal members.[28] According to the Centers for Disease Control and Prevention, about 16% of the adult American Indian and Alaska Native population has diabetes.[29]

Religious Influences

Some religions have extensive rules governing food—related practices, some of which, such as forbidding the consumption of alcohol, may influence a person's health. Table 3.16 lists major religions and their dietary guidelines. It is important to note that many people do not follow their religion's dietary rules fully or at all.

TABLE 3.16 Traditional Dietary Practices of Common Religions

Religion	Dietary Practices
Buddhist	Meat is avoided; vegetarianism is encouraged.
Eastern Orthodox	Meat and fish restrictions; fasting and specific food abstinence during certain holidays
Hindu	Beef is forbidden, but dairy products are "pure" for consumption. Pork may be restricted. Alcohol is avoided. Fasting is often encouraged.
Islam	Pork; birds of prey; reptiles; insects, except locusts; most gelatins; and alcohol are prohibited (*ha-raam*). Ritual killing of animals that are permitted as food (*ha-lal*) Stimulant beverages (i.e., coffee and tea) are avoided. Fasting from all food and drink (daytime) during month of Ramadan and certain other religious holidays
Jewish	Only kosher foods are acceptable. *Tref* (*trayf*) refers to prohibited foods. Pork and shellfish are prohibited. Eating meat with dairy is prohibited. Consuming blood is forbidden. Raw meat is soaked in cold water to remove blood, salted for 1 hour, and then rinsed. Eggs, fruits, and vegetables can be eaten with either meat or dairy foods. Eggs, however, are inspected to make sure they do not contain blood specks. Only fish with fins and scales can be eaten. Only land animals that have split hooves and chew their cud can be eaten, and only the front half of the cud-chewing animal is used. Ritual killing of certain animals is required. Fasting and specific food restrictions for certain holidays
Mormon (LDS)	Avoid beverages containing alcohol or caffeine (tea, coffee, and caffeinated beverages) Fasting is practiced monthly.
Roman Catholic	Fasting before communion; fasting and specific food abstinence during certain holidays
Seventh Day Adventist	Animal product consumption generally limited to milk, milk products, and eggs (lacto-ovo vegetarianism). Alcohol and beverages containing stimulants are prohibited.

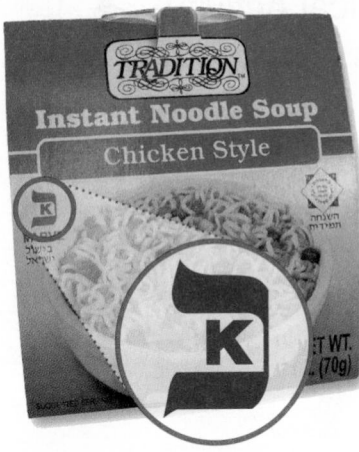

Symbol for kosher

ASSESS YOUR PROGRESS

26 *Describe general dietary characteristics of the following American subpopulation groups: Hispanic, Southern European, African-American, Asian, and American Indian.*

27 *Which food groups are emphasized in the Latin American Diet Pyramid?*

28 *Identify the major food groups in the Mediterranean Diet Pyramid.*

29 *Identify the major food groups in the Asian Diet Pyramid.*

30 *What are two specific examples of religious influences on diet?*

SUMMARY

SECTION 3.1 What Is a Nutrient Requirement?

- A requirement is the smallest amount of a nutrient that maintains a defined level of health. Numerous factors, including age and sex, influence an individual's nutrient needs.

SECTION 3.2 Dietary Reference Intakes: Nutrient and Calorie Standards

- Scientists use information about the body's energy needs, nutrient requirements, and nutrient storage capabilities to establish specific recommendations concerning energy and nutrient intakes.

- The Dietary Reference Intakes (DRIs) are standard values for nutrient recommendations that include the Estimated Average Requirement, Recommended Dietary Allowances, Adequate Intake, and Tolerable Upper Intake Level. The Estimated Energy Requirement is used to evaluate a person's energy intake. Acceptable Macronutrient Distribution Ranges may reduce the risk of chronic diseases.

- DRIs can be used for planning nutritious diets for groups of people and evaluating the nutritional adequacy of a population's diet. RDAs and AIs are often used to evaluate an individual's dietary practices.

SECTION 3.3 Major Food Groups

- Dietary guides generally classify foods into groups according to their natural origins and key nutrients. Major food groups usually include grains, dairy, fruits, vegetables, and protein-rich foods. Some dietary guides also include a group for oils. Empty-calorie foods or beverages contribute added sugars, solid fats, and alcohol to diets.

SECTION 3.4 U.S. Dietary Guidelines

- The Dietary Guidelines for Americans is a set of general nutrition-related lifestyle recommendations designed to promote adequate nutritional status and good health and to reduce the risk of major chronic health conditions. The U.S. Department of Health and Human Services and the U.S. Department of Agriculture revise the guidelines about every 5 years.

SECTION 3.5 Food Guides for Dietary Planning

- MyPlate is an online, interactive food intake and physical activity guide that is based on the Dietary Guidelines. The food guidance system provides individualized calorie and food group recommendations. Most Americans do not follow the government's dietary recommendations.

- The Exchange System is a tool for estimating the calorie and macronutrient contents of foods.

SECTION 3.6 Food and Dietary Supplement Labels

- Consumers can use information on food labels to determine ingredients and compare nutrient contents of packaged foods and beverages.

- The FDA regulates and monitors information that can be placed on food labels, including claims about the product's health benefits.

- Nearly all foods and beverages sold in supermarkets must be labeled with the product's name, manufacturer's name and address, amount of product in the package, and ingredients listed in descending order by weight. Furthermore, food labels must use a special format for listing specific information on the Nutrition Facts panel.

- The Daily Values (DVs) are a practical set of nutrient standards for labeling purposes. The nutrient content in a serving of food is listed on the label as a percentage of the DV (%DV). Not all nutrients have DVs.

- Organic foods are produced without the use of antibiotics, hormones, synthetic fertilizers and pesticides, genetic improvements, or spoilage-killing radiation. In general, organic food crops are not more nutritious than similar conventionally grown foods. More research is needed to determine whether there are health advantages to eating organic foods.

SECTION 3.7 **Food and Culture: The Melting Pot**

- Traditional ethnic diets are often based on dishes containing small amounts of animal foods and larger amounts of locally grown fruits, vegetables, and unrefined grains. After an immigrant population has assimilated fully, the prevalence of serious chronic diseases often increases among them, partly as a result of adopting unhealthy eating practices.
- Many religions require members to follow dietary practices that often include the prohibition of certain foods and beverages.

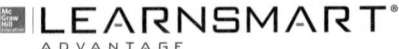 **LEARNSMART®** ADVANTAGE

Get the most out of your study of nutrition with McGraw-Hill's innovative suite of adaptive learning products including McGraw-Hill LearnSmart®, SmartBook®, McGraw-Hill LearnSmart Achieve®, and McGraw-Hill LearnSmart Prep®. Visit www.learnsmartadvantage.com.

CASE STUDY RESPONSE

PLANNING A 1-DAY HEALTHY MENU

Total calories:	2600 kcal
Grains	9 oz
Vegetables	3–5 cups
Fruits	2 cups
Dairy	3 cups
Protein foods	6–5 oz
Oils	8 tsp

These are MyPlate guidelines for Eric, a 23-year-old male who is 5-feet, 10-inches tall and 170 pounds and engages in less than 30 minutes of exercise daily.

ERIC HAS MANY OPTIONS FOR 1-DAY nutritionally adequate meal plans; the one shown in Table 3.17 is just an example. Principles discussed in Chapter 1 of the textbook, such as variety and nutrient density, are incorporated into the meal plan. Eric can eat several small, frequent meals and nutrient-dense snacks during the course of the day. Many fast-food restaurants offer fresh salads and roasted meats instead of fried meats, so Eric can choose more healthful options, if he must rely on fast food during his travels.

TABLE 3.17 Sample Day's Menu

	Food/Beverage	MyPlate Group	Kcal
Breakfast	1 cup oatmeal	Grains	266
	1 banana	Fruit	105
	1 cup nonfat milk	Dairy	83
	1 cup black coffee		
Mid-morning snack	6 oz Greek yogurt	Dairy	139
	½ cup blueberries	Fruits	44
	Water		
Lunch	2 slices whole-wheat bread	Grains	160
	2 oz sliced turkey	Protein foods	89
	2 slices tomato	Vegetables	10
	½ cup romaine lettuce	Vegetables	5
	2 Tbsp light mayonnaise	Oils	90
	Water		
Mid-afternoon snack	Apple	Fruits	72
	2 Tbsp peanut butter	Protein foods	200
	Water		
Dinner	3 oz baked salmon	Protein foods	425
	1 ½ cups broccoli	Vegetables	75
	2 whole-wheat dinner rolls	Grains	140
	1 cup spinach	Vegetables	7
	3 Tbsp olive oil dressing	Oils	300
	1 cup nonfat milk	Dairy	83
	3 small pieces dark chocolate	Empty calories	255

TEST KITCHEN
Modifying Recipes for Healthy Living

One of your clients is a healthy, physically active young man who wants to improve the nutritional quality of his diet and needs guidance in menu planning. He would eat a salad for his main meal if it contained fresh ingredients and was easy to prepare. To maintain his current weight, this client needs 3000 kcal/day. After you explain to the client how to use MyPlate as a meal planning guide, you ask him to use the food guidance system to develop a recipe for his special salad. His original recipe is described here.

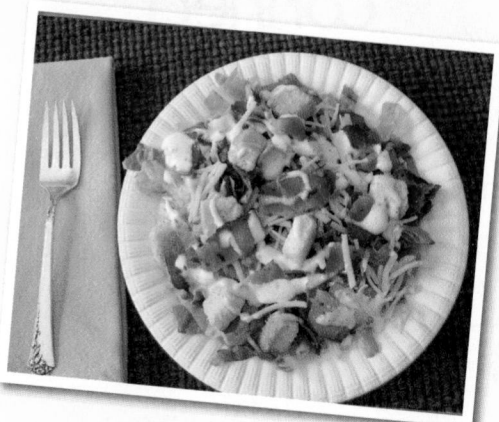

MAIN MEAL SALAD

PREPARATION STEPS

1. Wash and shred lettuce.
2. Top with shredded cheese, croutons, diced bacon, and dressing.
3. Serve immediately. Serves one.

INGREDIENTS

1 cup iceberg lettuce, shredded
¼ cup cheddar cheese, shredded
¼ cup croutons
2 Tbsp cooked bacon, diced
2 Tbsp ranch dressing

STEP 1 Brainstorm

Use SuperTracker https://supertracker.usda.gov/ to analyze the nutrient and calorie content of the "Main Meal Salad." Review the nutrient information. Would his salad substitute for a nutritionally well-balanced main meal? What suggestions, if any, should you make to the client that would improve the nutritional content of this salad?

STEP 2 Develop a modified version of this recipe

Develop a modified version of this recipe that would increase the salad's nutrient density.

1. List ingredients and amounts of each of them that are needed.
2. List the preparation steps.

STEP 3 Evaluate the modified recipe

Use SuperTracker to analyze the nutrient and calorie content of the modified "Main Meal Salad." Compare caloric contents and key nutrients in the original and modified recipes. Explain how the salads differ nutritionally.

STEP 4 Conduct MyPlate analysis

For each recipe, develop a table showing where each salad ingredient fits into MyPlate guidelines for a person who needs 3000 kcal/day.

OPTIONAL ACTIVITIES

STEP 5 Shop for your ingredients

Were the ingredients readily available at the supermarket?
List ingredients that you could not find or that were not available fresh.

STEP 6 Test your new recipe

Keep notes on any changes you make to ingredient amounts as you prepare the salad.

STEP 7 Reflect on the modified recipe

How does the salad look? How does the salad taste? Is the salad filling?

STEP 8 Serve the salad

Is this a recipe that you and others enjoyed? Would you feel comfortable recommending it to friends, family, and clients? Add the recipe to your collection, or continue to modify the recipe until it is acceptable.

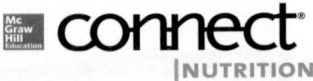

PERSONAL Dietary Analysis

1. Go to www.choosemyplate.gov to obtain your personalized My Plan. Use the SuperTracker option and enter in your age, sex, height, weight, and physical activity level. Save your profile and My Plan.

2. Record every food and beverage you eat over a 24-hour period. Recall how much you consumed and how it was prepared. Use the format shown in the sample (Table 3.18) to record your food and beverage intake.

TABLE 3.18 Sample Food Record

Time of Day	Foods and Beverages	Food Preparation Description (e.g., fried, baked, raw)	Estimated Amount Consumed
Breakfast – 7 A.M.	Whole-grain breakfast cereal	–	¾ cup
Breakfast – 7 A.M.	Fat-free milk	–	1 cup

3. Access your profile at www.choosemyplate.gov. Use the "FoodTracker" option at SuperTracker to enter your food and beverages.

4. Using Table 3.19, enter a minus sign (−) if your total intake is below the MyPlate recommendations and a plus sign (+) if it equals or exceeds the daily recommended amount for each food group.

TABLE 3.19 Rating Your Record

Energy, USDA Food Group, or Food Category	Actual Intake (from Question 3)	Recommended Intake (from Question 4)
Total kcal		
Grains		
Vegetables		
Fruits		
Protein foods		
Dairy		
Oils		

5. Evaluate the quality of your 24-hour food intake based on MyPlate guidelines.

   a. Did you consume enough, too many, or too few calories?

   b. Did you exceed your recommended intake of oils? If yes, by how many calories?

   c. Did your food intake meet MyPlate guidelines for all food groups? If it did not, list the food group(s) for which your intake(s) exceeded the recommendations. List food group(s) for which your intake(s) did not meet the guidelines.

   d. Rate the overall quality of your general diet based on MyPlate on a scale of 1 to 5, with 1 being "poor" and 5 being "excellent." Why did you give your diet this rating?

   e. If your usual intake of nutrients does not meet or exceeds daily calorie and food group recommendations on a regular basis, describe how you could modify your diet to improve your intakes.

Critical Thinking

1. Your friend takes several dietary supplements daily, and as a result, his vitamin B-6 intake is 50 times higher than the RDA for the vitamin. You would like to convince him to stop taking the supplements. To support your advice, which nutrient standard would you show him? Explain why.

2. You are working with a 25-year-old healthy female client. You have determined that she needs to consume 1800 kcal daily to maintain her present weight. Based on information the client has provided, you have calculated that she eats an average of 75 g of fat, 200 g of carbohydrates, and 80 g of protein each day. What is this woman's caloric intake? Are the amounts of her macronutrient intakes within AMDR guidelines? Explain your answers and include calculations.

3. Why should an individual use the MyPlate guidelines to plan menus instead of the DRIs?

4. Review Table 3.11. Which foods in the left-hand column do you eat regularly? Why are those foods listed in that column?

5. The ingredient list on a package of crackers includes vegetable oil. However, the Nutrition Facts panel on the package's label indicates "0 g" of fat is in the product, and a statement on the label claims the product is fat-free. Explain why this claim was permissible in 2015.

6. According to a newspaper article, an 8-oz serving of fat-free milk contains 15 mcg of folate (a B vitamin). Another source of nutrition information indicates that an 8-oz serving of fat-free milk contains 12 mcg of folate. Explain why both sources of information can be correct.

Practice Test

Select the best answer.

1. The amount of a nutrient that should meet the needs of half of the healthy people in a particular group is the
   a. Estimated Average Requirement (EAR).
   b. Recommended Dietary Allowance (RDA).
   c. Adequate Intake (AI).
   d. Tolerable Upper Intake Level (UL).

2. Which of the following statements is false?
   a. RDAs are standards for daily intakes of certain nutrients.
   b. RDAs meet the nutrient needs of nearly all healthy people.
   c. RDAs contain a margin of safety.
   d. RDAs are listed on food labels.

3. The Estimated Energy Requirement (EER)
   a. has a margin of safety.
   b. does not account for a person's height, weight, or physical activity level.
   c. is based on the average daily energy needs of a healthy person.
   d. reflects a person's actual daily energy needs.

4. A diet is highly likely to be safe and nutritionally adequate if
   a. average daily intakes for nutrients meet RDA or AI values.
   b. intakes of various nutrients are consistently less than EAR amounts.
   c. nutrient intakes are consistently above ULs.
   d. vitamin supplements are included.

5. Nutritional standards, such as the RDAs, are
   a. dietary recommendations for chronically ill adults.
   b. the basis for establishing DVs.
   c. used on Nutrition Facts labels.
   d. practical menu-planning guides.

6. According to the U.S. Department of Agriculture, which of the following foods is nutritionally equivalent to 1 ounce of a food from the grains group?
   a. 1 slice bread
   b. 1 cup cooked pasta
   c. 1 cup cooked rice
   d. 2 cups ready-to-eat cereal

7. Protein-rich food sources that also contain saturated fat and cholesterol include
   a. peanut butter.
   b. dry beans.
   c. nuts.
   d. beef.

8. Fruit is generally a good source of all of the following substances, except
   a. fiber.
   b. vitamin C.
   c. phytochemicals.
   d. protein.

9. The Dietary Guidelines for Americans is
   a. revised every year.
   b. a set of general nutrition-related recommendations.
   c. not concerned with physical activity.
   d. published by the Centers for Disease Control and Prevention.

10. Which of the following statements is false?
    a. Each dietary pattern of the MyPlate guidelines includes a recommendation for daily fruit intake.
    b. MyPlate can be individualized to meet a person's food preferences.
    c. A major weakness of MyPlate is its failure to emphasize the importance of regular physical activity.
    d. A person can use MyPlate to evaluate his or her diet's nutritional adequacy.

11. The Exchange System
    a. classifies foods in the same groups as the MyPlate system.
    b. has exchange lists within each food group.
    c. is useful only for people who have diabetes.
    d. incorporates high-protein foods with high-carbohydrate foods.

12. Which of the following information is not provided by the Nutrition Facts (2015) panel?
    a. percentage of total calories from fat
    b. amount of total carbohydrate per serving
    c. serving size
    d. amount of total fat per serving

13. Daily Values are

    a. for people who consume 1200 to 1500 kilocalorie diets.
    b. based on the lowest RDA or AI for each nutrient.
    c. dietary standards developed for food-labeling purposes.
    d. used to evaluate the nutritional adequacy of a population's diet.

14. Organically grown foods are

    a. nutritionally superior to conventionally produced foods.
    b. produced without the use of antibiotics, pesticides, or genetic improvements.
    c. usually less expensive than conventionally produced foods.
    d. easier to prepare than conventionally grown foods.

15. People who follow Islamic dietary rules will not consume

    a. pork.   c. beef.
    b. rice.   d. milk.

ANSWERS TO PRACTICE TEST

1-a, 2-d, 3-c, 4-a, 5-b, 6-a, 7-d, 8-d, 9-b, 10-c, 11-b, 12-a, 13-c, 14-b, 15-a

ANSWERS TO CHAPTER 3 QUIZ Yourself

1. According to expert dietary recommendations, carbohydrates should supply the majority of your daily calorie intake. **True** (p. 47)
2. The latest U.S. Department of Agriculture dietary guide combines fruits and vegetables into the produce food group. **False** (p. 49)
3. Last week, Colin didn't consume the recommended amount of vitamin C for a couple of days. Nevertheless, he is unlikely to develop scurvy, the vitamin C deficiency disease. **True** (p. 47)
4. MyPlate groups foods according to the amount of calories, carbohydrates, protein, and fat supplied per serving of a particular food. **False** (p. 56)

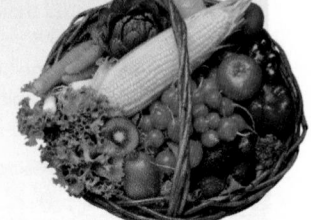

5. The Nutrition Facts panel on a food label provides information concerning amounts of energy, fiber, and sodium that are in a serving of the food. **True** (p. 62)

References

1. Institute of Medicine: *Dietary Reference Intakes for vitamin C, vitamin E, selenium, and carotenoids.* Washington, DC: National Academies Press, 2000.
2. Otten J J and others: *Dietary Reference Intakes: The essential guide to nutrient requirements.* Institute of Medicine of the National Academies. Washington, DC: National Academies Press, 2006.
3. Institute of Medicine: *Dietary Reference Intakes for energy, carbohydrate, fiber, fat, fatty acids, cholesterol, protein, and amino acids (macronutrients).* Washington, DC: National Academies Press; 2005.
4. Barr SI: Applications of dietary reference intakes in dietary assessment and planning. *Applied Physiology, Nutrition, and Metabolism* 31(1):66-73, 2006.
5. U.S. Food and Drug Administration: The scoop on whole grains. Last updated December 2013. http://www.fda.gov/ForConsumers/ConsumerUpdates/ucm151902.htm Accessed: January 13, 2014
6. U.S. Department of Agriculture: Food groups: Dairy: What foods are included in the dairy group? http://www.choosemyplate.gov/food-groups/dairy.html Accessed: January 13, 2014
7. U.S. Department of Agriculture: Food groups: fruits. http://www.choosemyplate.gov/food-groups/fruits.html Accessed: January 13, 2014
8. U.S. Department of Agriculture: What are solid fats? http://www.choosemyplate.gov/weight-management-calories/calories/solid-fats.html Accessed: January 13, 2014
9. U.S. Departments of Agriculture and Health and Human Services: *Scientific report of the 2015 Dietary Guidelines advisory committee.* 2015. http://health.gov/dietaryguidelines/2015-scientific-report/PDFs/Scientific-Report-of-the-2015-Dietary-Guidelines-Advisory-Committee.pdf Accessed: January 22, 2016
10. U.S. Department of Health and Human Services and U.S. Department of Agriculture. *2015-2020 Dietary Guidelines for Americans.* 8th Edition. December 2015. http://health.gov/dietaryguidelines/2015/guidelines/ Accessed: January 24, 2016
11. Drewnowski A: The cost of US foods as related to their nutritive value. *American Journal of Clinical Nutrition* 92(5):1181, 2010.
12. American Dietetic Association: Position of the American Dietetic Association: Health implications of dietary fiber. *Journal of the American Dietetic Association* 108:1716, 2008.
13. U.S. Department of Agriculture: Calories: What are empty calories? http://www.choosemyplate.gov/weight-management-calories/calories/empty-calories.html Accessed: January 13, 2014
14. U.S. Department of Agriculture, Economic Research Service: *Food availability (per capita) data system: Summary findings.* Last updated September 2013. http://www.ers.usda.gov/data-products/food-availability-%28per-capita%29-data-system/summary-findings.aspx#.UtVUp7T6ySo Accessed: January 14, 2014
15. U.S. Food and Drug Administration: *2008 Health and Diet Survey.* Updated June 2013. http://www.fda.gov/Food/FoodScienceResearch/ConsumerBehaviorResearch/ucm193895.htm#FOODLABELUSEALL Accessed: January 13, 2014
16. Department of Health and Human Services: Read the law: The Affordable Care Act, section by section. (ND). http://www.hhs.gov/healthcare/rights/law/index.html Accessed: January 13, 2014
17. Urban LE and others: The accuracy of stated energy contents of reduced-energy, commercially prepared foods. *Journal of the American Dietetic Association* 110(1):116, 2010.
18. Oliver L: *The food timeline,* http://www.foodtimeline.org/index.html#copyright Accessed: January 13, 2014
19. Ollberding NJ and others: Food label use and its relation to dietary intake among U.S. adults. *Journal of the American Dietetic Association* 110(10):1233, 2010.
20. FMI Food Marketing Institute: *Supermarket facts: Industry overview 2012.* http://www.fmi.org/research-resources/supermarket-facts Accessed: January 13, 2014
21. USDA, Economic Research Service: *Processing and marketing: New products.* Updated February 2013. http://www.ers.usda.gov/topics/food-markets-prices/processing-marketing/new-products.aspx#.UdwUVW3ZWSo Accessed: January 13, 2014
22. U.S. Food and Drug Administration: *Guidance for industry: A food labeling guide. (11. Appendix C: Health Claims).* 2009. Last updated November 2013. http://www.fda.gov/Food/GuidanceRegulation/GuidanceDocumentsRegulatoryInformation/LabelingNutrition/ucm064919.htm Accessed: January 14, 2014
23. Organic Foods Production Act of 1990: As amended through public law 109-97: Nov 10, 2005. http://www.ams.usda.gov/AMSv1.0/getfile?dDocName=STELPRDC5060370&acct=nopgeninfo Accessed: Accessed: January 14, 2014
24. Comis D: No shortcuts in checking soil health. *Agricultural Research* 55(6):4, 2007.
25. Organic Trade Association: 2012 press releases: *Consumer-driven U.S. organic market surpasses $31 billion in 2011.* http://www.organicnewsroom.com/2012/04/us_consumerdriven_organic_mark.html Accessed: January 14, 2014
26. Dangour AD: Nutrition-related health effects of organic foods: A systemic review. *American Journal of Clinical Nutrition* 92(1):203, 2010.
27. Smith-Spangler C and others: Are organic foods safer or healthier than conventional alternatives? A systematic review. *Annals of Internal Medicine.* 157(5):348, 2012.
28. Moore K: Youth-onset Type 2 diabetes among American Indians and Alaska Natives. *Journal of Public Health Management Practice* 16(5):388, 2010.
29. U.S. Centers for Disease Control and Prevention: National diabetes fact sheet 2011. Last updated 2011. http://www.cdc.gov/diabetes/pubs/estimates11.htm#4 Accessed: January 14, 2014

4 Human Digestion, Absorption, and Transport

CASE STUDY

Irritable bowel syndrome

ANNIE IS A 20-YEAR-OLD COLLEGE JUNIOR who is taking a full course load. She is also actively involved in three student organizations, and she volunteers over 10 hours a week at the local hospital. Six months ago, Annie experienced frequent bouts of diarrhea, followed by several days of constipation. At first, the diarrhea was mild, only once every few weeks, but over the past few days, the diarrhea has become daily, making it difficult for her to continue attending classes and volunteering at the hospital.

After examining Annie and taking her history, a physician at the university's Student Health Center tells the young woman that she has irritable bowel syndrome (IBS). The physician refers her to a registered dietitian who helps Annie understand how she can prevent and manage the symptoms of IBS.

• What is IBS, and how does it differ from inflammatory bowel disease (IBD)?

• What are the long-term consequences to untreated IBS?

• Are there certain foods and/or beverages that Annie should avoid?

• What lifestyle changes should Annie consider to manage IBS?

The suggested Case Study Response can be found on page 106.

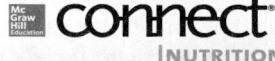

Mc Graw Hill Education **connect** | NUTRITION   Check out the Connect site at www.mcgrawhillconnect.com to further explore this case study.

Surface of a small intestinal cell.

QUIZ Yourself

What happens to food in your stomach? How much time does it take for food to be digested? What is acid reflux? To test your knowledge of the material covered in Chapter 4, take the following quiz. The answers are found on page 108.

1. The esophagus is the tube that connects the mouth to the stomach. __T __F

2. The stomach produces hydrochloric acid. __T __F

3. Most nutrient absorption occurs in the large intestine. __T __F

4. The gallbladder makes bile. __T __F

5. A type of bacteria is responsible for the development of most stomach ulcers. __T __F

4.1 Overview of the Digestive System

LEARNING OUTCOMES

1 *Identify the major components of the digestive system and the major functions of each component.*

2 *Describe the distinct layers of the gastrointestinal tract wall.*

3 *Identify the location, anatomical name, and function of each sphincter involved in the digestive system.*

4 *Explain the differences between chemical and mechanical digestion.*

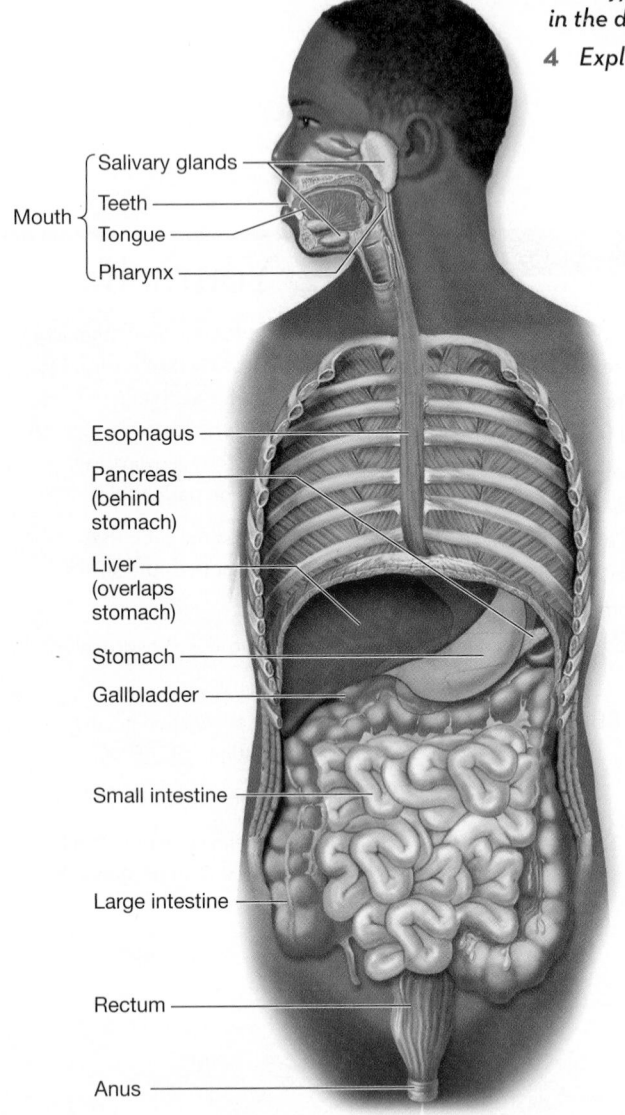

Mouth
- Salivary glands
- Teeth
- Tongue
- Pharynx

Esophagus

Pancreas (behind stomach)

Liver (overlaps stomach)

Stomach

Gallbladder

Small intestine

Large intestine

Rectum

Anus

FIGURE 4.1 Digestive system.

The cells of the body do not need food to carry out their metabolic activities; they need nutrients that are in food. The primary roles of the digestive system are the breakdown of food into smaller components (nutrients), absorption of nutrients, and elimination of solid waste products. **Digestion** is the process of breaking down large food molecules into nutrients that the body can use. **Absorption** is the uptake and removal of nutrients from the **digestive tract**, which may also be referred to as the **gastrointestinal tract (GI tract)**, alimentary canal, or gut.

The **digestive system** has two major components, the GI tract and accessory organs (Fig. 4.1). In a *living* person, the GI tract is a hollow, muscular tube that extends approximately over 16 feet in length.[1] The other major component of the digestive system, the accessory organs, assists the functioning of the GI tract. The digestive system functions in concert with the other organ systems of the body. If the digestive system is not functioning properly, the entire body eventually shows signs and symptoms of disease.

The Wall of the GI Tract

The wall of the GI tract has distinct layers (Fig. 4.2). The innermost layer, the **mucosa**, surrounds the **lumen** of the digestive tract, which is a hollow space through which food and fluids pass. Embedded within the mucosa are cells that secrete **mucus**, a watery slippery fluid. The muscular layer has two distinct types of tissue, the circular and the longitudinal muscles. The circular muscles are surrounded by the longitudinal muscles (Fig. 4.2).

The wall of the stomach is the thickest and strongest of the GI tract, because it has a third type of muscle, diagonal (oblique) muscle (Fig. 4.3). By relaxing and contracting, these muscles can mix substances that are within the lumen and control the movement (*motility*) of the material through the tract.

Sphincters Control the Flow of GI Contents

Intestinal **sphincters** (*sfink'–ters*) are thickened regions of circular muscle that function like valves to control the flow of contents at various points in the GI tract. When an intestinal sphincter relaxes, the passageway opens and the contents of the GI tract flow through it. When a sphincter contracts, it closes the passageway and restricts the flow at that point in the digestive tract. Intestinal sphincters are essential for normal digestion and absorption, because they help control

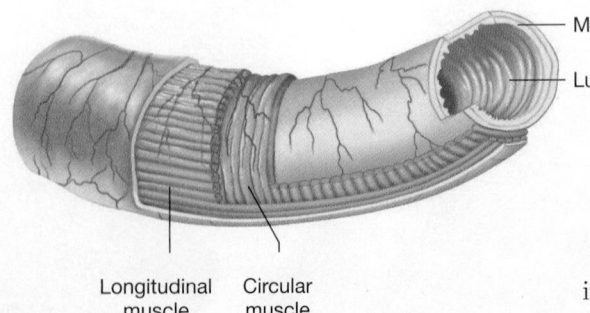

Mucosa

Lumen

Longitudinal muscle   Circular muscle

FIGURE 4.2 Wall of the GI tract.

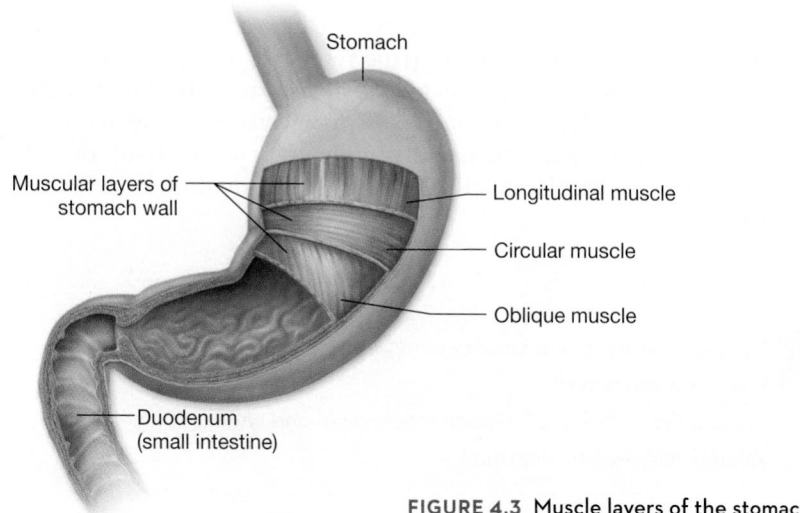

FIGURE 4.3 **Muscle layers of the stomach.**

Labels: Stomach; Muscular layers of stomach wall; Longitudinal muscle; Circular muscle; Oblique muscle; Duodenum (small intestine)

digestion process of breaking down large food molecules into nutrients that the body can use

absorption process of removing nutrients from the intestinal tract and enabling them to enter the circulatory or lymphatic systems

digestive tract or **gastrointestinal tract (GI tract)** alimentary canal or gut

digestive system body system that breaks down food into its components, absorbs nutrients, and eliminates the waste

mucosa innermost layer of the digestive tract wall

lumen hollow space through which food and fluids can pass (digestive tract)

mucus watery slippery fluid secreted by special cells

sphincters thickened regions of circular muscle that control the flow of contents at various points in the GI tract

mechanical digestion refers to physical treatments that food undergoes while it is in the intestinal tract

chemical digestion refers to the breakdown of large nutrient molecules in food into smaller components, primarily by the action of enzymes

enzyme protein that speeds up the rate of a chemical reaction without being altered in the process

rates of digestion and absorption by keeping the contents within the lumen in place. Figure 4.4 shows the locations of the lower esophageal and the pyloric sphincters.

Mechanical and Chemical Digestion

The digestive tract breaks down food by physical and chemical processes. **Mechanical digestion** refers to physical treatments that food undergoes while it is in the intestinal tract, such as being chewed into smaller pieces and mixed with various secretions. Mechanical digestion does not change the chemical composition of the food, but it facilitates chemical digestion.

Chemical digestion is the breakdown of large nutrient molecules in food into smaller components, primarily by the action of stomach acid and various enzymes. An **enzyme** is a protein that speeds up the rate of a chemical reaction without being altered in the process. Most digestive enzymes are *hydrolytic*;

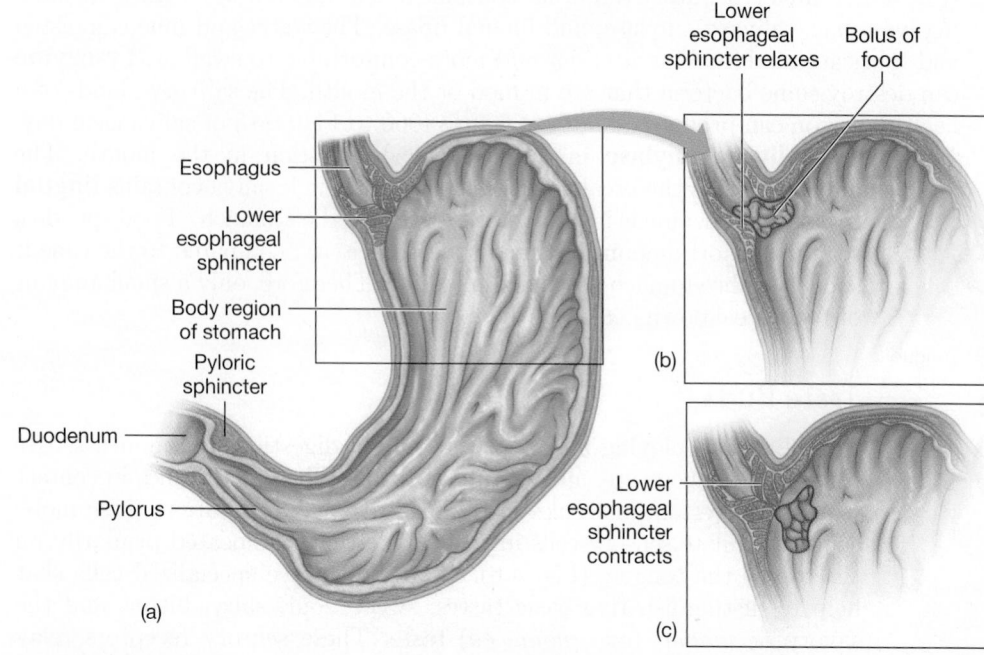

Labels: Esophagus; Lower esophageal sphincter; Body region of stomach; Pyloric sphincter; Duodenum; Pylorus; Lower esophageal sphincter relaxes; Bolus of food; Lower esophageal sphincter contracts; (a); (b); (c)

FIGURE 4.4 **Lower esophageal sphincter.** This illustration shows the position of the lower esophageal sphincter (*a*). When this sphincter relaxes, the bolus of food enters the stomach (*b*). The sphincter contracts to keep the bolus in the stomach (*c*).

that is, they require water. Lipases are hydrolytic enzymes that help break down fats into smaller molecules (*lipo* refers to "fat"). Proteases digest proteins into their components, amino acids. Nucleases initiate the breakdown of nucleic acids (DNA and RNA). The names of most enzymes end with *−ase*. The first part of an enzyme's name usually indicates the nutrient or other substance that the enzyme breaks down. Sections 4.2 through 4.6 describe digestion and absorption.

ASSESS YOUR PROGRESS

1. *List the primary and accessory components of the GI tract.*
2. *What is a sphincter?*
3. *Explain the difference between mechanical and chemical digestion.*
4. *What is a hydrolytic enzyme?*

4.2 The Mouth

LEARNING OUTCOMES

1. *Describe the mechanical and chemical digestion that occurs in the mouth.*
2. *Identify and explain the effects of smell and taste disorders in humans.*

Digestion starts in the mouth **(oral cavity)**. Teeth chew (*masticate*) food. Mastication is a physical activity that prepares solid foods for swallowing and chemical digestion. Such mechanical activity makes the food easier to swallow and increases its surface area, which enables enzymes to have greater access to nutrients. The tongue helps direct the mashed−up food to the back of the mouth and into the pharynx ("throat"), where it can be swallowed. The **pharynx** is the section of the alimentary canal that connects the nasal cavity with the top of the esophagus (see Fig. 4.1).

Salivary Glands

As a person chews, several **salivary glands** secrete **saliva** into the oral cavity (Fig. 4.5). Saliva is a watery fluid that contains mucus and a few enzymes, includ−ing lysozyme, salivary amylase, and lingual lipase. The water and mucus moisten and lubricate food, making it easier and more comfortable to swallow. **Lysozyme** can destroy some bacteria that are in food or the mouth. The salivary glands of a healthy person can produce about 4 to 6 cups (960 to 1440 mL) of saliva each day.

Salivary amylase initiates chemical digestion in the mouth. The amylase begins the breakdown of starch. Although saliva contains **lingual lipase**, the enzyme is inactive until it reaches the stomach.[1] Food spends a relatively short amount of time in the oral cavity, compared to the time it spends in the stomach and small intestine. Therefore, only a small amount of food breakdown occurs in the mouth.

Taste Buds

In addition to playing an important role in digestion, the mouth senses the taste, temperature, and texture of foods. When food comes in contact with saliva, certain molecules in the food dissolve. In solution, these mol−ecules stimulate sensory cells in taste buds that are located primarily on the top of the tongue. (Fig. 4.6). Taste buds have specialized cells that help to distinguish five basic tastes: sweet, sour, salty, bitter, and the savory or *umami* (*ew−mom′−ee*) taste. These sensory receptors relay

oral cavity mouth

pharynx section of the alimentary canal that connects the nasal cavity with the top of the esophagus

salivary glands structures that produce saliva and secrete the fluid into the oral cavity

saliva watery fluid that contains mucus and a few enzymes

lysozyme enzyme in saliva that can destroy some bacteria that are in food or the mouth

salivary amylase enzyme in saliva that begins starch digestion

lingual lipase enzyme secreted into saliva that begins fat digestion

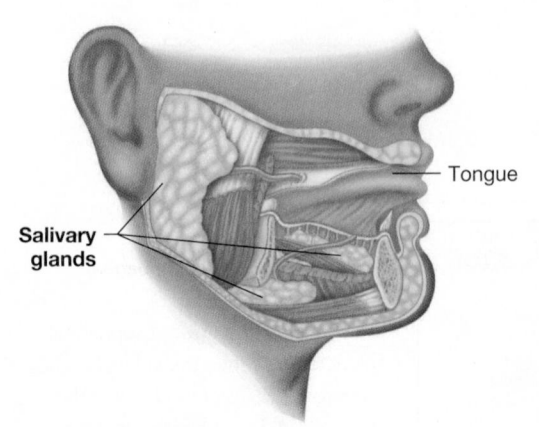

Tongue

Salivary glands

FIGURE 4.5 Salivary glands.

information from the oral cavity to a part of the brain that identifies the particular taste.

Although taste buds that can detect each kind of taste are distributed all over the tongue, some regions of the tongue are more sensitive to one type of taste and less sensitive to the others. The tip of the tongue, for example, is more likely to detect sweet tastes than the sides or back of the tongue, which may explain why people often sample a new food with just the tip of their tongue.

What benefits do people gain from being able to detect various tastes? The sense of taste is important, because:

- Foods that taste sweet usually contain carbohydrates, major energy sources for cells.

- Chemicals that elicit a bitter taste are often poisonous, so people are more likely to eat sweet—tasting foods and reject bitter—tasting ones.

- The sour taste can indicate the presence of ascorbic acid, more commonly known as vitamin C. Many people like foods that taste tart or sour, especially when they are included with sweet ingredients.

- Sodium stimulates taste buds to detect the salty taste; a food that tastes salty may contain other mineral nutrients as well.

The umami taste is detected when certain amino acids (the "building blocks" of proteins) stimulate taste buds. Foods that elicit the umami taste may be protein—rich.

Recently, scientists have identified a protein in the tongues of rodents that appears to help the animals detect fatty foods. However, researchers have not determined whether human taste buds are capable of sensing the presence of fat in food.[2]

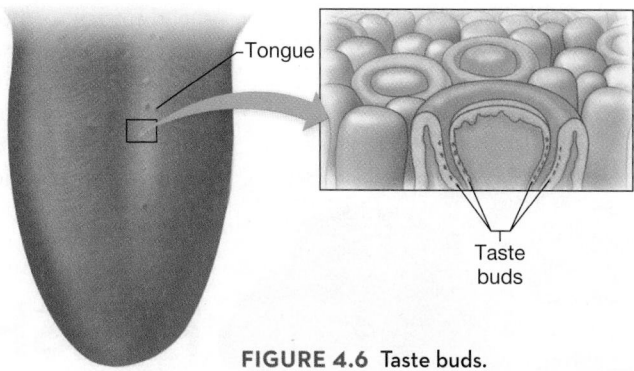

FIGURE 4.6 Taste buds.

Disorders of Taste and Smell

The sense of smell (*olfaction*) contributes to the ability to taste food. As food is chewed, it releases chemicals that become airborne and stimulate the olfactory region of the nasal passages (Fig. 4.7). This region signals the two *olfactory bulbs*, specialized structures in the brain that are essential for being able to sense odors (Fig. 4.7). The brain combines information about the smell of foods with taste sensations from the mouth to identify the food's flavors. When a person has an upper respiratory tract infection and the inside of the nose is congested, his or her favorite foods may seem tasteless and unappealing, because the olfactory region is unable to function properly.

Anosmia (*an—oz'—me—uh*) is the complete inability to detect odors. Nearly one—fourth of adults over the age of 50 have some degree of anosmia.[3] Obstruction of the nasal passageways; brain tumors; dental disease; and irritation of the inner lining of the nose due to the common cold or nasal allergies contribute to the partial or total loss of the sense of smell.

Hypogeusia (*hy—po—goo'—zhah*), the diminished ability to taste, and **ageusia** (*a—goo'—zhah*), the total loss of taste, affect approximately 1% of the U.S. population.[4] Very few individuals are born with a permanent taste disorder. Most taste disorders are temporary and develop as a result of upper respiratory or middle ear infections; radiation treatment; medications such as antibiotics or antihistamines;

anosmia complete inability to detect odors

hypogeusia diminished ability to taste substances

ageusia total loss of the ability to taste substances

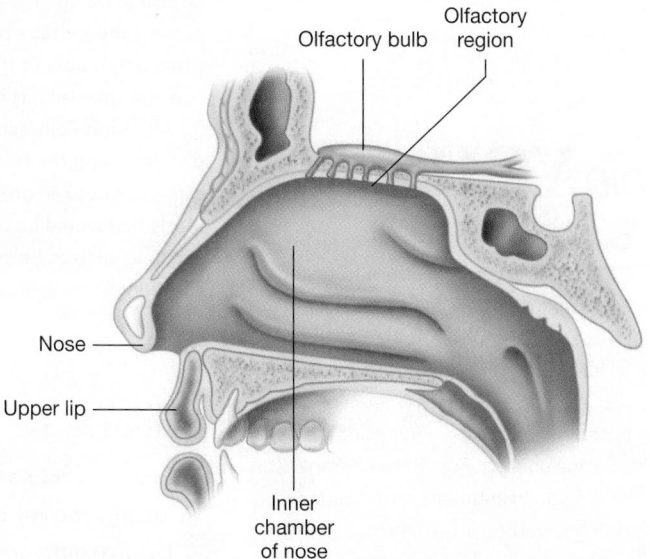

FIGURE 4.7 Detecting odors. The olfactory region of the oral cavity is responsible for sensing odors.

head injury; or poor dental health. Loss of taste can also be a sign of degenerative nerve diseases, such as Alzheimer's disease and Parkinson's disease.

Taste and smell disorders can negatively affect a person's appetite, weight, and quality of life. For many, a loss of these senses leads to the use of excessive amounts of salt and sugar in food preparation. The extra sugar and salt can contribute to serious health problems, such as high blood pressure and unwanted weight gain.

FRESH TIPS

People who are unable to taste foods can be encouraged to:

- Use a variety of spices.
- Add fruits and vegetables that have interesting textures (such as raw apples and carrots) or appealing colors to meals and snacks.
- Avoid casseroles or combination dishes that mix too many strongly flavored ingredients together.

REAL People, **REAL** Stories

Kelly Strosnider

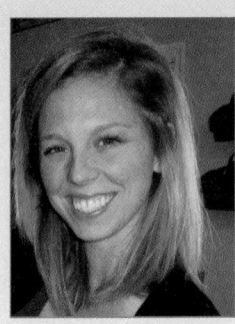

As a child, Kelly Strosnider and her parents knew something was abnormal about her ability to taste and smell things. Kelly added hot sauce to everything, including pizza, rice, mashed potatoes, vegetables, fish, and even cheese. While her friends watched in amazement, Kelly would eat whole lemons and limes, including the peels. When Kelly was 16 years old, she was diagnosed with complete anosmia, and her physicians determined that she had been born without olfactory bulbs.

Cases of total anosmia, such as Kelly's, are quite rare; approximately 5% of the American population has *functional* anosmia, or partial loss of smell.[6] Because the sense of smell is critical to being able to taste foods, Kelly can only taste about 30% of what the average person with a healthy sense of olfaction can taste. She is able to differentiate basic sweet, sour, salty, and bitter tastes, but only if they are intense; she also has hypogeusia.

Although Kelly can identify coffee, hummus, and grapefruit by their taste, she has difficulty distinguishing the tastes of different cooked vegetables. To Kelly, a cooked carrot tastes the same as a cooked green bean. She has an extremely high threshold for strong-tasting foods that would be rejected by people with a normal sense of taste. People who have total anosmia, such as Kelly, can obtain a nutritious, well-balanced diet by choosing their foods carefully.

ASSESS YOUR PROGRESS

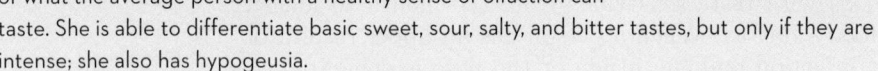

5. *Explain what normally happens to a piece of food that enters the mouth.*
6. *Identify the key components of saliva.*
7. *List five different taste sensations that human taste buds detect.*
8. *Discuss disorders of taste and smell, including their causes.*

4.3 The Esophagus

LEARNING OUTCOMES

1 *Describe the action of swallowing and what it accomplishes.*

2 *Identify the muscular activity that propels a mass of food through the esophagus.*

3 *Explain what happens when someone is choking on food and demonstrate the first aid techniques employed to save the person's life.*

4 *Identify the two esophageal sphincters and their functions.*

The mass of food that has been chewed as well as moistened and mixed with saliva is called a **bolus**. After being swallowed, the bolus travels through the **esophagus** (*e−sof'−ah−gus*), a muscular tube that extends about 10 inches from the pharynx to the upper portion of the stomach (see Fig. 4.1). The primary function of the esophagus is to transfer a bolus into the stomach.

The entrance to the esophagus is near the larynx ("voice box") and the opening of the trachea ("windpipe"). The **epiglottis** (*ep−eh−glot'−tis*) is a flap of tough tissue that prevents the food from entering the larynx and trachea (Fig. 4.8). When swallowing initiates, breathing automatically stops, and the bolus normally lands on the epiglottis, making it cover the opening of the larynx. These responses keep swallowed food from entering the trachea, which would lead to choking. When a person talks, the larynx is not covered by the epiglottis, so the trachea also remains open.

bolus mass of food that has been chewed, moistened, mixed with saliva, and swallowed

esophagus muscular tube that extends about 10 inches from the pharynx to the upper portion of the stomach

epiglottis flap of tough tissue that prevents the food from entering the larynx and trachea

Choking

When a small piece of food enters the trachea instead of the esophagus, the mate−rial irritates the airways and the body responds with vigorous coughing to expel it. If a larger piece of food enters the trachea, it can block the windpipe, preventing air from entering the lungs (Fig. 4.8). Because a choking person cannot speak or breathe, the victim usually grabs his or her throat to indicate there is a problem. Swift action must be taken to remove the chunk of food from the trachea; other−wise, the lack of oxygen will cause the person to lose consciousness and die.

"Abdominal thrusts" (also called the *Heimlich maneuver*) are a simple and effective first−aid technique that can dislodge a piece of food or other item from the trachea. Figure 4.9 shows how to perform the abdominal thrust maneuver on an adult, an infant, and oneself. The Fresh Tips box on page 86 provides some tips to reduce the likelihood of choking among young children.

FIGURE 4.8 What happens when you swallow? (*a*) While chewing, the epiglottis does not cover the larynx. (*b*) When swallowing, the epiglottis prevents the bolus from entering the larynx and trachea. (*c*) After swallowing, the epiglottis returns to its usual position and allows air to enter the larynx and trachea.

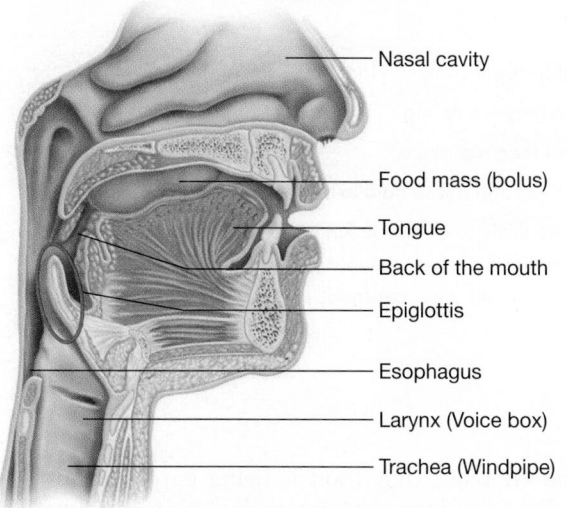

— Nasal cavity

— Food mass (bolus)

— Tongue

— Back of the mouth

— Epiglottis

— Esophagus

— Larynx (Voice box)

— Trachea (Windpipe)

(a)

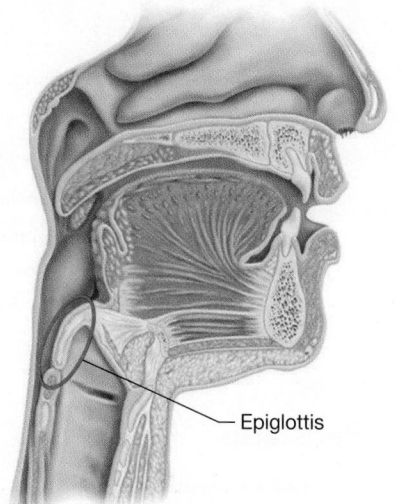

— Epiglottis

(b)

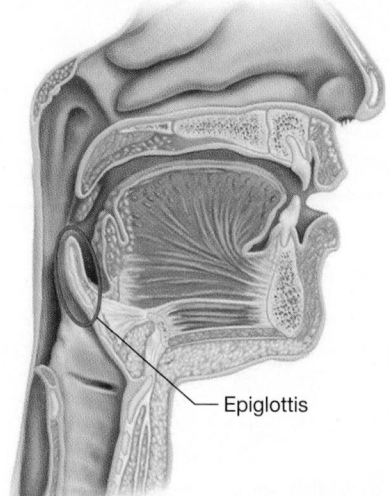

— Epiglottis

(c)

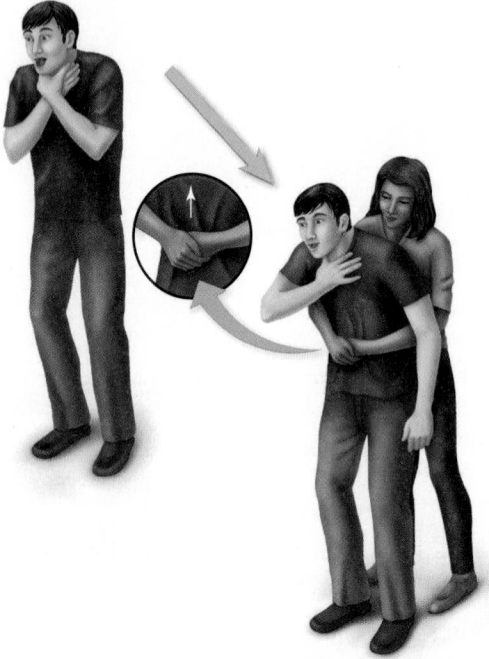

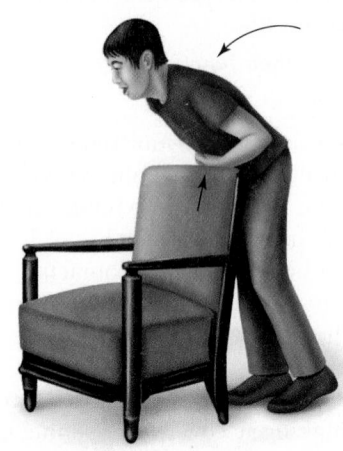

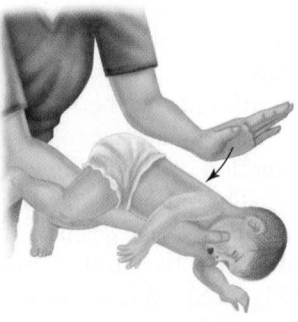

A **Choking treatment for adults and children:**

1. Stand behind the person and wrap your arms around his or her waist.
2. Make a fist and place the thumb side of your fist below the person's ribcage and above the navel.
3. Hold your fist with your other hand and press into his or her upper abdomen with a quick upward thrust. Do not squeeze the ribcage.
4. Repeat thrusts until the object is dislodged from the trachea and the person is breathing and able to talk.

B **Choking treatment for oneself:**

1. Lean over a heavy, fixed structure such as a chair, countertop, or railing.
2. Press your upper abdomen against the edge to produce a quick upward thrust.
3. Repeat thrusts until the object that is blocking the trachea is dislodged.

OR, if no fixed large object is available:

1. Make a fist and place the thumb side of your fist below the ribcage and above the navel.
2. Hold your fist with your other hand and press into your upper abdomen with a quick upward thrust.
3. Repeat thrusts until the object that is blocking the trachea is dislodged.

C **Choking treatment for infants:**

1. Lay the child facedown across your forearm.
2. Using the palm of your hand, give five forceful quick blows on the infant's back.
3. Repeat until the object is dislodged and the child is breathing.

FIGURE 4.9 First aid for choking.

FRESH TIPS

To reduce the likelihood that young children will choke on food, caregivers should:

- Not leave children unattended when they are eating.
- Not allow children to run with food in their mouths.
- Encourage children to take smaller bites and not to hold extra food in their mouths.
- Avoid giving foods to children that are likely to cause choking, such as grapes, raw carrots, hot dogs, nuts, minimarshmallows, popcorn, pretzels, peanut butter, hard candy, chewing gum, and large pieces of meat (such as steak). Also, cut foods into small pieces that can be chewed and swallowed easily.

Peristalsis

peristalsis waves of muscular contractions that help move material through most of the digestive tract

The act of swallowing signals the GI tract that food is being eaten and stim—ulates **peristalsis** ($per'-eh-stall'-sis$), waves of muscular contractions that help move material through most of the digestive tract. In the esophagus, each peristaltic muscular contraction is followed by a brief period of muscle relaxation that moves small amounts of food and beverage from the esophagus into the stomach (Fig. 4.10). Peristalsis is an involuntary response, which means the muscular activity happens without the need to think about it.

Esophageal Sphincters

Sphincters are located both at the top and bottom of the esophagus. The **upper esophageal sphincter (UES)** (*e−sof−ah−jee′−al sfink′−ter*) opens when a bolus is swal−lowed, allowing the mass of food to enter the esophagus. The **lower esophageal sphincter (LES)**, also known as the gastroesophageal sphinc−ter or cardiac sphincter, is located at the bottom of the esophagus and controls flow both in and out of the stomach. Normally, the LES is closed, preventing the backflow of acidic stomach contents into the esophagus. Heartburn ("acid reflux") occurs when the LES fails to close properly.

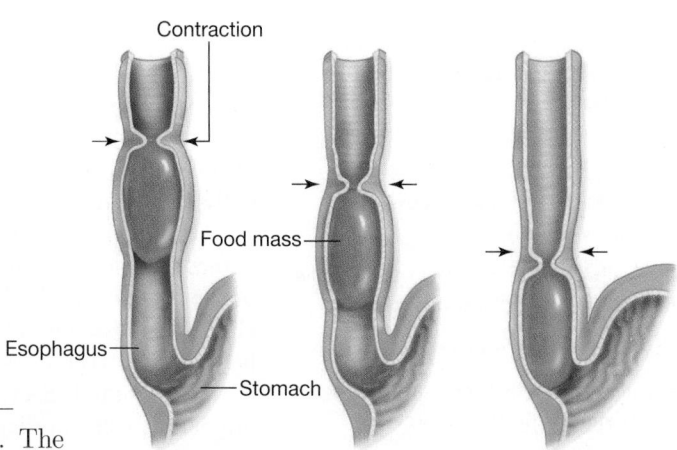

FIGURE 4.10 Peristalsis.

upper esophageal sphincter (UES) region of the upper part of the esophagus that opens to allow a mass of food to enter the esophagus

lower esophageal sphincter (LES) region of the lower part of the esophagus that controls flow of material into the upper part of the stomach; also known as the gastroesophageal sphincter

stomach muscular sac that stores and mixes food

gastric juice collection of stomach secretions that includes mucus, hydrochloric acid, intrinsic factor, and digestive enzymes

mucous cells cells that secrete mucus

ASSESS YOUR PROGRESS

9 *Describe peristalsis. Explain how peristalsis in the esophagus transfers a bolus of food from the throat to the stomach.*

10 *Explain why choking can occur while eating. What should you do to save a choking person's life?*

11 *What normally keeps stomach contents from reentering the esophagus?*

4.4 The Stomach

LEARNING OUTCOMES

1 *Identify the types of cells in gastric glands and what each secretes.*

2 *Describe the kinds of mechanical and chemical digestion that occur in the stomach.*

3 *List the components of gastric juice.*

After a bolus passes through the LES, it enters the **stomach**, a muscular sac that stores and mixes food (see Fig. 4.3). During a typical meal, an adult's stomach can stretch to hold about 4 to 6 cups (960 to 1440 mL) of semiliquid mate−rial. The maximum capacity of the stomach is about 16 cups (3840 mL)—the amount of food and fluids that an adult may consume during a traditional Thanksgiving dinner, which is followed by dessert!

Secretions of the Stomach

The upper part of the stomach has tiny gastric (*gas−tric* = stomach) glands that are lined with specialized cells. Certain gastric gland cells synthesize and secrete the pri−mary components of **gastric juice**, which are mucus, hydro−chloric acid (HCl), intrinsic factor, and digestive enzymes (Fig. 4.11). **Mucous cells** secrete *mucin*, a carbohydrate−rich

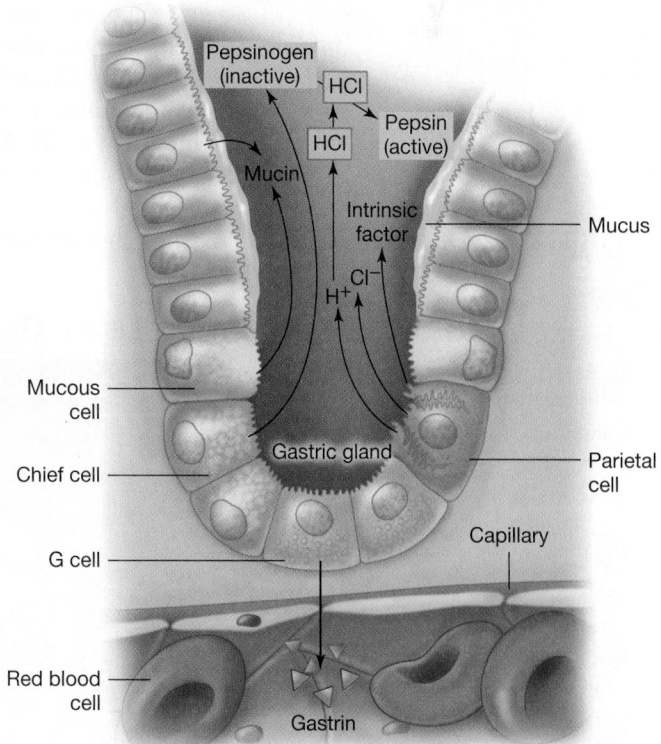

FIGURE 4.11 Gastric gland and its secretory cells.

parietal cells stomach cells that secrete intrinsic factor and the components of hydrochloric acid into the lumen of the stomach

intrinsic factor substance necessary for absorbing vitamin B-12

chief cells stomach cells that secrete some chemically inactive digestive enzymes

G cells stomach cells that secrete gastrin

gastrin hormone that stimulates stomach motility and gastric gland secretions

hormones chemical messengers secreted by organs of the endocrine system that convey information to target cells

chyme semiliquid mass that forms when food mixes with gastric juice

pyloric sphincter region of the stomach that regulates the flow of chyme into the small intestine

acidic solutions with pH values lower than 7

alkaline solutions with pH values higher than 7

pepsin active enzyme that begins the enzymatic digestion of proteins

substance that forms mucus when combined with water. **Parietal cells** secrete hydrogen and chloride ions, which form hydrochloric acid (HCl). Parietal cells also synthesize and release **intrinsic factor**, the substance that is necessary for absorbing vitamin B−12. **Chief cells** secrete *gastric lipase* and some chemi−cally inactive digestive enzymes, particularly *pepsinogen.*

Gastric glands also have cells **(G cells)** that secrete **gastrin**, a hormone that enters the bloodstream and stimulates stomach motility and the secretory activity of the gastric glands (Fig. 4.11). Organs of the endocrine system secrete **hormones**, chemical messengers that convey information to cells ("target" cells). Target cells have special receptors on their cell membranes that enable them to respond to a hormonal signal. Section 4.8 discusses gastrin and some other hormones that play important roles in digestion. Table 4.1 lists the four major kinds of cells in gastric glands, their secretions, and the major functions of the secretions.

The main function of the lower portion of the stomach is mixing food with gastric juice to form **chyme** (*kime*), a semiliquid mass. Chyme leaves the stom−ach through a canal called the pylorus. The **pyloric sphincter** that surrounds the pylorus regulates the flow of chyme into the small intestine (see Fig. 4.4).

Digestion in the Stomach

When stimulated by the presence of food, the stomach's muscular walls respond by producing waves of peristalsis. The churning movements mix food with gastric juice, and as a result, some protein and fat in the chyme break down. Although the stomach absorbs very few nutrients from chyme, a few drugs, including some aspirin and alcohol, can pass through the organ's walls and enter the bloodstream.

HCl is a strong acid that contributes to the low pH of gastric juice. Chemists measure the hydrogen ion (H$^+$) concentration of solutions by using the pH scale. This scale ranges from 0 to 14. A solution with a pH of 7 is neutral; solutions with pH values lower than 7 are **acidic**; solutions with pH values higher than 7 are **alkaline** (basic). After mixing with gastric juice, the pH of chyme is about 2.0, which is more acidic than lemon juice or vinegar (Fig. 4.12).

The enzymatic digestion of starch that began in the mouth stops in the stom−ach, because salivary amylase does not function when the pH is lower than 4.5. Although lingual lipase becomes active when exposed to the acidic environment of the stomach, the enzyme breaks down only about 10% of the fat in food. The majority of fat digestion occurs in the small intestine. The chemical digestion of proteins begins in the stomach. HCl converts the inactive gastric enzymes to their active forms. For example, inactive pepsinogen is converted into active **pepsin**, which begins the enzymatic digestion of proteins (see Fig. 4.11).

DID **YOU** KNOW?

When people eat foods or drink beverages, they swallow some air, too. Burping expels most of this air before it enters the stomach. If some air enters the stomach and small intestine, it mixes with chyme and bubbles through it, often producing rather loud, gurgling sounds called *borborygmus* (*bor-bo-rig'-mus*).

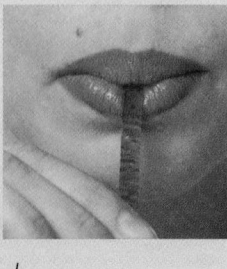

TABLE 4.1 Gastric Gland Cells

Gastric Gland Cells	Secretion	Major Functions
Mucous	Mucus	Protects stomach mucosa from HCl and enzymes
Parietal	Components that form HCl (hydrogen ions [H$^+$] and chloride ions [Cl$^-$])	Activates pepsinogen, destroys many food-borne microbes
	Intrinsic factor	Facilitates the absorption of vitamin B-12
Chief	Pepsinogen	Digests protein after conversion to pepsin
	Gastric lipase	Digests small amount of fat
G cell	Gastrin	Stimulates stomach motility and gastric gland activity

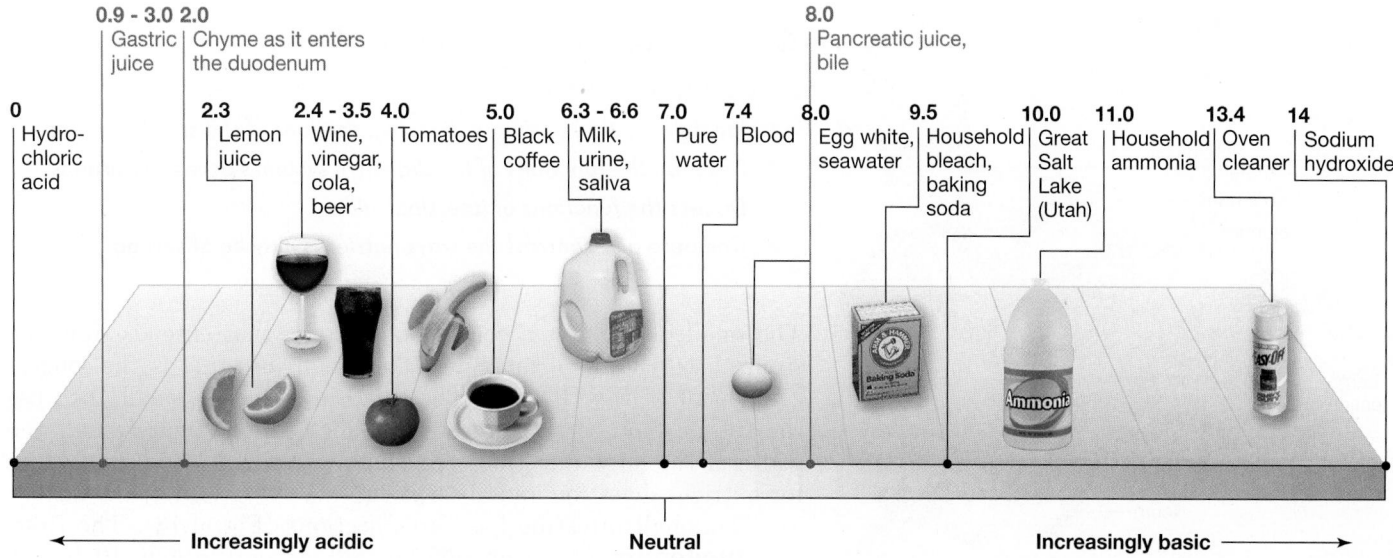

FIGURE 4.12 pH scale. This scale indicates the pH values of some substances, including foods.

Stomach walls consist of muscle proteins, so how does the stomach avoid digesting itself? The stomach's mucous cells produce a thick layer of mucus that protects the stomach from being damaged by its acid and digestive enzymes. If the layer of mucus breaks down, HCl and gastric enzymes can make contact with the stomach wall, destroying the tissue. Such destruction can cause one or more sores (*gastric* or *peptic ulcers*) to form. Section 4.9 provides more information about factors that increase the risk of developing gastrointestinal tract ulcers.

Normal Stomach Emptying and "Dumping Syndrome"

Following a meal, the stomach empties in about 4 hours, but the timing depends on the contents and size of the meal. Watery meals such as soups spend less time in the stomach; fatty and high–fiber meals spend more time there. Obviously, larger meals take longer to empty from the stomach than smaller meals. The pyloric sphincter regulates the passage of chyme through the pylorus at a rate of approximately ½ to 2 teaspoons/minute.

Dumping syndrome is a disorder that occurs when chyme flows too rapidly into the small intestine. When this happens, the chyme contains large particles of food that have not been broken down sufficiently and mixed with gastric juice. A person with dumping syndrome often experiences abdominal fullness, nausea, sweating, rapid heart rate, and weakness not long after eating a meal. These signs and symptoms may be followed with abdominal cramps and diarrhea. Poor nutrient absorption resulting in nutrient deficiency disorders can occur, if the condition is not treated effectively.

Dumping syndrome often occurs after surgeries of the esophagus or stomach, including bariatric procedures for rapid weight loss. Changing the types of food eaten, reducing the amount of food that is consumed at one time, and slowing the rate of food consumption during meals can help manage dumping syndrome.[7]

dumping syndrome disorder that occurs when chyme flows too rapidly into the small intestine

ASSESS YOUR PROGRESS

12 Identify the four different gastric glands cells and the secretions they produce.

13 Describe the digestive processes that occur in the stomach.

14 Explain how the stomach protects itself from digestion. What condition might occur if this protection fails?

15 Discuss the effects of eating a high-fiber meal on stomach emptying.

FRESH TIPS

The longer a food stays in the stomach, the more full the person will feel after eating. Plant foods that contain fiber often delay stomach emptying.[8] Therefore, people can consider eating a bowl of oatmeal, a whole-grain bagel, or other high-fiber food for breakfast as a way of increasing their sense of stomach fullness. Chapter 5 provides more information about foods that are sources of fiber.

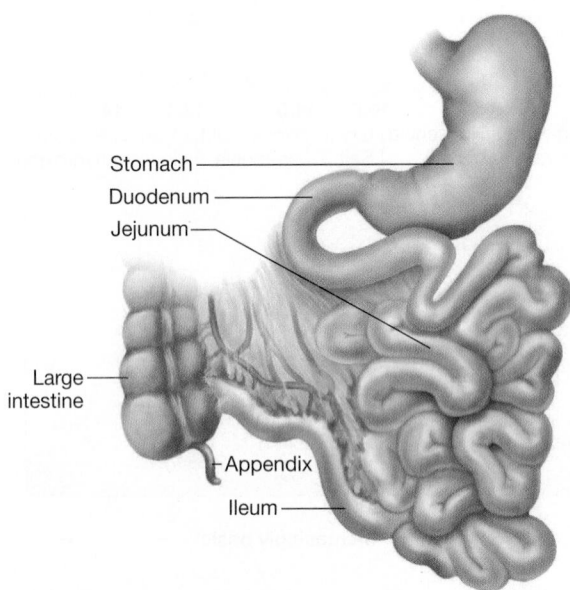

Stomach
Duodenum
Jejunum
Large intestine
Appendix
Ileum

FIGURE 4.13 Small intestine. The small intestine is tightly coiled within the abdominal cavity. Although the appendix may have immune function, you can live without it.

duodenum first segment of the small intestine

jejunum middle segment of the small intestine

ileum last segment of the small intestine

ileocecal sphincter region of ileum that controls the rate of emptying undigested material into the large intestine

bile fluid that is produced in the liver and stored in the gallbladder until it is needed for fat digestion and absorption

4.5 The Small Intestine

LEARNING OUTCOMES

1 *Identify the three primary digestive sections of the small intestine.*
2 *Describe the functions of the digestive system's accessory organs.*
3 *Discuss the functions of intestinal villi.*
4 *Compare and contrast the ways nutrients may be absorbed.*

The small intestine is a coiled, hollow tube that extends from the stomach to the large intestine. The small intestine is the longest component of the GI tract. The small intestine is "small" because the tube's diameter is only about 1 inch, approximately half the width of the large intestine. The small intestine is the primary site for nutrient digestion and absorption.

The small intestine has three sections (Fig. 4.13). The first, the **duodenum** $(do-wah-dee'-num)$, is only about 10 inches long. Within the duodenum, the acidic stomach contents mix with alkaline fluids secreted by the pancreas and gallbladder. The middle segment of the small intestine is the **jejunum** $(jeh-ju'-num)$. The jejunum is about 3 to 5.5 feet long. Most digestion and nutrient absorption occurs in the upper part of the small intestine, primarily in the duodenum and upper jejunum. The last portion of the small intestine, the **ileum** $(il'-lee-um)$, is about 5 to 9 feet long. Some nutrient absorption takes place in the ileum.[9]

As chyme moves out of the ileum and into the large intestine, it passes through the **ileocecal sphincter**. Similar to the pyloric sphincter, the ileocecal sphincter controls the rate at which the contents of the ileum empty into the large intestine. When it contracts, the ileocecal sphincter prevents the contents of the large intestine from flowing back into the small intestine.

Accessory Organs: The Liver, Gallbladder, and Pancreas

The liver, gallbladder, and pancreas are accessory organs of the gastrointestinal system that play major roles in digestion, even though chyme does not move through them. Figure 4.1 shows where these organs are located. Figure 4.14 provides a more detailed view of the liver, pancreas, and gallbladder, including the organs' major ducts.

Liver and Gallbladder

The liver processes and stores many nutrients. This organ also synthesizes cholesterol and uses this type of lipid to make **bile**, a greenish-yellow, bitter-tasting fluid that contains cholesterol, minerals, bile salts, and *bilirubin*. Bilirubin is a waste product that results from the breakdown of hemoglobin, the iron-containing pigment in red blood cells. The liver makes about 2 to 4 cups (480 to 960 mL) of bile daily. Bile flows from the liver into the gallbladder via ducts (Fig. 4.14). The gallbladder concentrates and stores bile until it is needed for fat digestion and absorption. Chapter 6 describes the role of bile in digestion and absorption in detail.

Pancreas

The pancreas is an accessory organ of the digestive tract that produces and secretes many of the enzymes that break down carbohydrates, protein, and fat in the GI tract. Additionally, the pancreas secretes *bicarbonate ions* (HCO_3^-). The pH of chyme is approximately 2.0 as it enters the duodenum. Pancreatic juice has an alkaline pH of approximately 8.5, so the juice neutralizes the highly acidic chyme when it enters the duodenum. This is a critical step in the digestion process, because the enzymes that function in the small intestine are not active in acidic conditions. Following bicarbonate secretion, the contents in the small intestine have a pH that is neutral or slightly alkaline—the pH at which the enzymes function best.

Digestion in the Small Intestine

The small intestine is the major site of chemical and mechanical digestion of nutri-ents. As mentioned, most digestion occurs in the duodenum and upper part of the jejunum. To accomplish digestion, the small intestine secretes approximately 1 ½ quarts (1440 mL) of watery fluids that contain mucus and enzymes each day. This fluid lubricates the walls of the small intestine, facilitating the passage of chyme and protecting the mucosa from being damaged by the material as it moves through the tract.

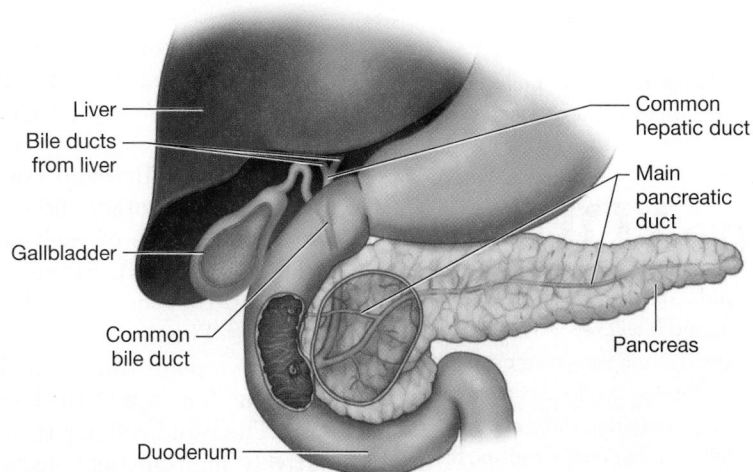

FIGURE 4.14 Liver, pancreas, and gallbladder. These accessory organs play important roles in digestion. Ducts are passageways that connect the liver, pancreas, gallbladder, and small intestine.

While chyme passes through the lumen of the small intestine, enzymes secreted by the pancreas and mucosa of the small intestine break down large nutrient molecules in the mass, as well as mucosal cells that have been shed into the lumen. Table 4.2 lists many of these enzymes and their functions. Information about nutrient–specific digestive enzymes is in Chapters 5, 6, and 7.

In addition to enzyme activity and peristalsis, the small intestine also relies on segmentation to facilitate digestion. **Segmentation** involves regular con-tractions of circular intestinal muscles followed by muscular relaxations to mix chyme within a short portion of the small intestine (Fig. 4.15). The alternating pressure exerted by the muscles forces chyme to move back and forth within the segment of intestine. Segmentation gradually moves chyme through the duodenum, jejunum, and ileum, providing adequate time for maximal nutrient absorption.

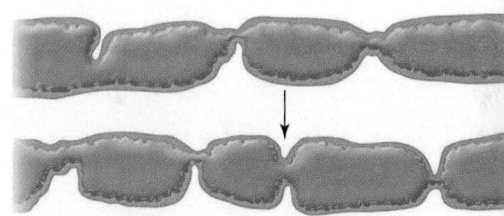

FIGURE 4.15 Segmentation. Segmentation helps mix chyme.

Villi and Surface Area

The mucosa of the small intestine is highly folded and covered by tiny, fingerlike projections called **villi** (*vill'–eye*). The villi and folds provide a healthy mucosa with a surface area of about 200 square meters, the size of a regulation, singles tennis court. This enormous surface area enables the small intestine to absorb nutrients very efficiently. Each villus (singular of villi) has an outer layer of absorptive cells that are also called **enterocytes** (Fig. 4.16).

TABLE 4.2 Major Pancreatic and Intestinal Enzymes

Enzyme	Source	Action
Pancreatic amylase	Pancreas	Digests starch
Pancreatic lipase	Pancreas	Digests fat into smaller components
Trypsin, chymotrypsin	Pancreas	Partially digest proteins
Carboxypeptidase	Pancreas	Breaks down certain partially digested proteins
Nuclease	Pancreas	Digests DNA and RNA into nucleotides
Peptidase	Small intestine	Breaks down certain partially digested proteins
Sucrase, maltase, lactase	Small intestine	Break down certain sugars into simpler sugars
Intestinal lipase	Small intestine	Breaks down fats into smaller components

segmentation regular contractions of circular intestinal muscles followed by muscular relaxations that mix chyme within a short portion of the small intestine

villi tiny, fingerlike projections of the small intestinal mucosa that are involved in digestion and nutrient absorption

enterocytes absorptive cells that form the outer layer of a villus

microvilli tiny hairlike projections that form the brush border of an enterocyte

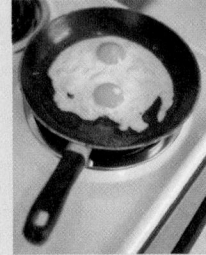

One end of an enterocyte is exposed to chyme (Fig. 4.16b). This end of the cell ("the brush border") has thousands of hairlike projections called **microvilli** (*my'–cro–vill'–eye*) that give the tissue a fuzzy appearance when it is viewed under a microscope. (The opener photo of the chapter shows microvilli on an enterocyte.) Microvilli contain "brush border enzymes" that participate in the digestion of protein and carbohydrates.

At the base of each villus is the *intestinal crypt*, the opening of a tubular gland (Fig. 4.16). Enterocytes develop in the bottom of the crypt, and as they mature, they move to the tip of the villus. Absorptive cells live for only 3 to 6 days.[1] The dead cells are shed into the lumen, and newer absorptive cells constantly replace those that have been sloughed off. The dead cells that were shed into the lumen add to the contents of chyme and eventually are digested.

The rapid cellular turnover rate of the small–intestinal mucosa leads to relatively high nutrient needs for these tissues. When the small intestine does not have an adequate supply of nutrients for energy or cell division, its mucosa cannot replace enterocyte cells. A reduction in the number of the absorptive cells results in less nutrient absorption, which makes nutrient deficiency disorders more likely.

Nutrient Absorption and Transport

The process of absorbing nutrients across the wall of the small intestine depends on several factors, including the type and amount of the nutrient. As shown in Figure 4.17, nutrient absorption can occur by:

- **Simple diffusion.** Simple diffusion occurs when the concentration of a particular nutrient is higher in the lumen of the small intestine than in an enterocyte. The nutrient moves down its *concentration gradient*; that is, it moves from a location where it is more highly concentrated, such as in the lumen, to a place where it is less concentrated, such as inside the absorptive cells. This form of transport does not require the input of energy. The digestive tract absorbs many water–soluble vitamins, lipids, and some minerals by simple diffusion (Fig. 4.17a).

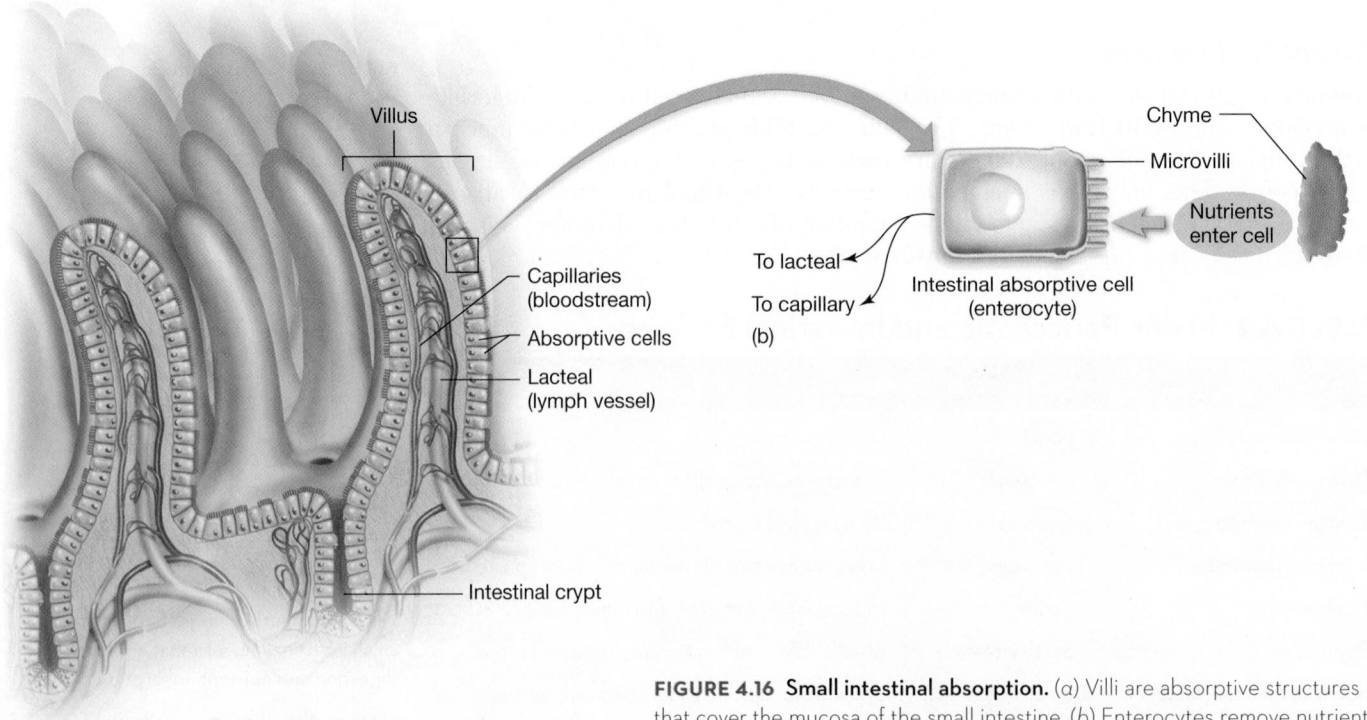

FIGURE 4.16 Small intestinal absorption. (*a*) Villi are absorptive structures that cover the mucosa of the small intestine. (*b*) Enterocytes remove nutrients from chyme and enable them to enter the intestinal blood or lymph vessels.

- *Facilitated diffusion.* Enterocytes absorb some nutrients by facilitated diffusion, a process that also does not require energy. Although the nutrient moves down its concentration gradient, it still needs to be carried by a special transport protein within the membrane of the enterocyte. Transport proteins are specific for the type of nutrient they are responsible for carrying. Absorption of the simple sugar fructose occurs by facilitated diffusion (Fig. 4.17b).

- *Active transport.* Some nutrients move from the lumen of the intestine and into an enterocyte *against* the concentration gradient; that is, the concentration of the nutrient is higher inside the absorptive cell than in the lumen. Absorption of these nutrients requires both a unique transport protein and energy. Enterocytes rely on active transport to absorb glucose and amino acids (Fig. 4.17c).

- *Osmosis.* Each day, about 7.6 to 8.5 quarts (1824 to 2040 mL) of water from ingested foods and beverages, as well as the watery secretions of intestinal cells, enter the lumen of the GI tract. Water moves freely across the cell membranes of enterocytes, because a concentration gradient is created by the absorption of water—soluble nutrients, such as sugars and minerals. A healthy body absorbs most of the water that enters the GI tract (Fig. 4.17d).

- *Endocytosis.* In a few instances, a segment of an absorptive cell's plasma membrane surrounds and "swallows" relatively large substances, such as entire protein molecules. This process enables an infant's intestinal tract to absorb whole proteins in human milk that provide immune benefits. Endocytosis, however, is not a common way for nutrients to enter enterocytes (Fig. 4.17e).

Within the core of a villus is a miniature circulatory system consisting of a tiny artery (*arteriole*), blood capillary network, and vein (*venule*). The core also contains a **lacteal**, a vessel of the lymphatic system (see Fig. 4.16a). As enterocytes absorb nutrients from chyme, the nutrients enter the capillary network or the lacteal. Whether a nutrient enters directly into the bloodstream or the lymphatic system depends on the type of nutrient. Water—soluble nutrients and certain fats pass directly from enterocytes into the capillary network of the villus. Eventually, these nutrients travel to the liver via the **hepatic portal vein** (Fig. 4.18); *hepatic* means "related to the liver." Most lipids must undergo

Membrane

(a) Low concentration   **Simple diffusion**   High concentration

Transporter Molecule

(b) Low concentration   **Facilitated diffusion**   High concentration

Transporter Molecule

(c) Low concentration   **Active transport**   High concentration

Solvent (e.g., Water)

(d)   **Osmosis**

Outside cell   Inside cell

(e)   **Endocytosis**

FIGURE 4.17 Nutrient absorption. Five different ways that nutrients can move into cells are shown: (*a*) simple diffusion, (*b*) facilitated diffusion, (*c*) active transport, (*d*) osmosis, and (*e*) endocytosis.

lacteal vessel of the lymphatic system

hepatic portal vein vein that transports absorbed nutrients to the liver

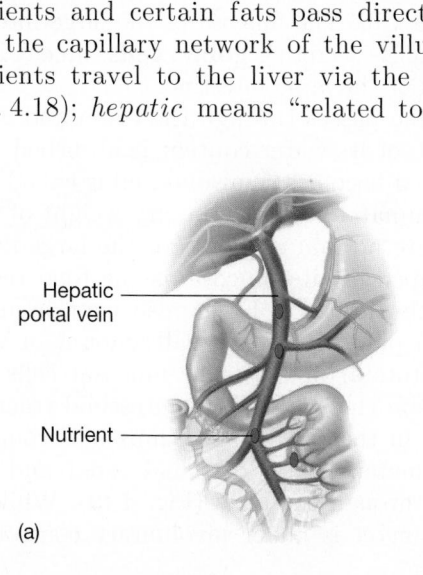

Hepatic portal vein

Nutrient

(a)

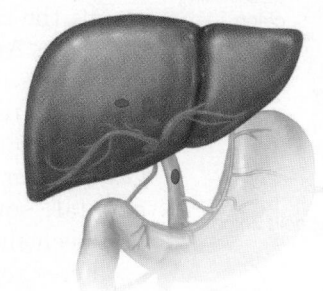

(b)

FIGURE 4.18 Transporting absorbed nutrients to the liver. (*a*) Certain nutrients travel in the hepatic portal vein to the liver. (*b*) The liver monitors the nutrient content of blood and stores various nutrients.

special processing within enterocytes before they enter lacteals. Chapter 6 provides a more detailed discussion of lipid absorption and transport.

By the time chyme reaches the middle part of the ileum, most of its nutrient contents have been digested and absorbed.[1] It takes about 3 to 10 hours for chyme to move from the duodenum to the end of the ileum.

ASSESS YOUR PROGRESS

16   List the three primary sections of the small intestine, and indicate their functions.
17   Where is bile synthesized and stored?
18   Where does most nutrient digestion and absorption occur?
19   Explain how the structure of villi increases the surface area available for absorption of nutrients.
20   Identify five ways that nutrients can enter enterocytes. Which of these transport methods require energy?

4.6 The Large Intestine

LEARNING OUTCOMES

1   *Identify the sections of the large intestine.*
2   *Describe the role of the large intestine in nutrient absorption and waste elimination.*

Under normal circumstances, very little carbohydrate, protein, or fat escape digestion and absorption in the small intestine. Any remaining water and the undigested material that reach the end of the small intestine must pass through the ileocecal sphincter before entering the large intestine (Fig. 4.19).

The large intestine is about 5 feet (1.5 meters) long and has a larger diameter than the small intestine. After moving through the ileocecal sphincter, unabsorbed water and undigested remains of chyme ("food residue") enter the **cecum** and then the *ascending colon* in the right side of the abdomen (Fig. 4.19). The residue then moves through the *transverse colon, descending colon,* and *sigmoid colon* before entering the **rectum** and finally, the *anus*.

cecum first segment of the large intestine

rectum last section of the large intestine

goblet cells intestinal cells that secrete mucus

Functions of the Large Intestine

Little additional absorption, other than of some water and minerals, takes place in the large intestine, because its mucosa has no villi. The mucosa of the large intestine has numerous mucus–secreting **goblet cells**; mucus is the primary secretion of the large intestine.

As food residue passes through the colon and enters the rectum, much of its water content is absorbed. As a result, the material becomes semisolid and is called feces or stools. Approximately 30% of the dry weight of feces is bacteria that are normal residents of the large intestine but are scraped off its mucosa as the food residue moves through the lumen.[10] Feces also contain undigested fiber from plant foods, a small amount of water and fat, some protein, mucus, and mucosal cells that had been shed from the walls of the intestinal tract.[10]

Feces remain in the rectum until muscular contractions move the material into the anal canal and then out of the body through the anus (Fig. 4.19). While the internal anal sphincter is under involuntary control, the

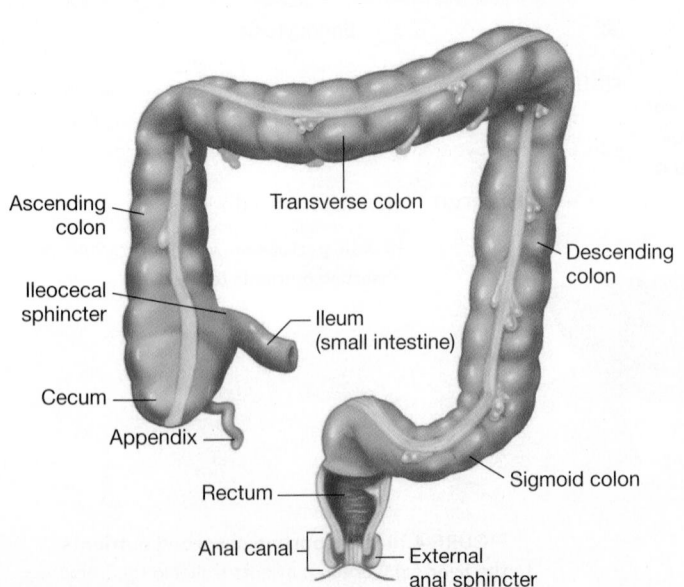

Ascending colon

Transverse colon

Ileocecal sphincter

Descending colon

Ileum (small intestine)

Cecum

Appendix

Rectum

Sigmoid colon

Anal canal

External anal sphincter

FIGURE 4.19 Large intestine.

external anal sphincter that allows feces to be expelled is under voluntary con—trol (defecation). Figure 4.20 provides a summary of digestion and absorption, including key organs involved in digestion and absorption.

external anal sphincter sphincter that allows feces to be expelled from the anus and is under voluntary control

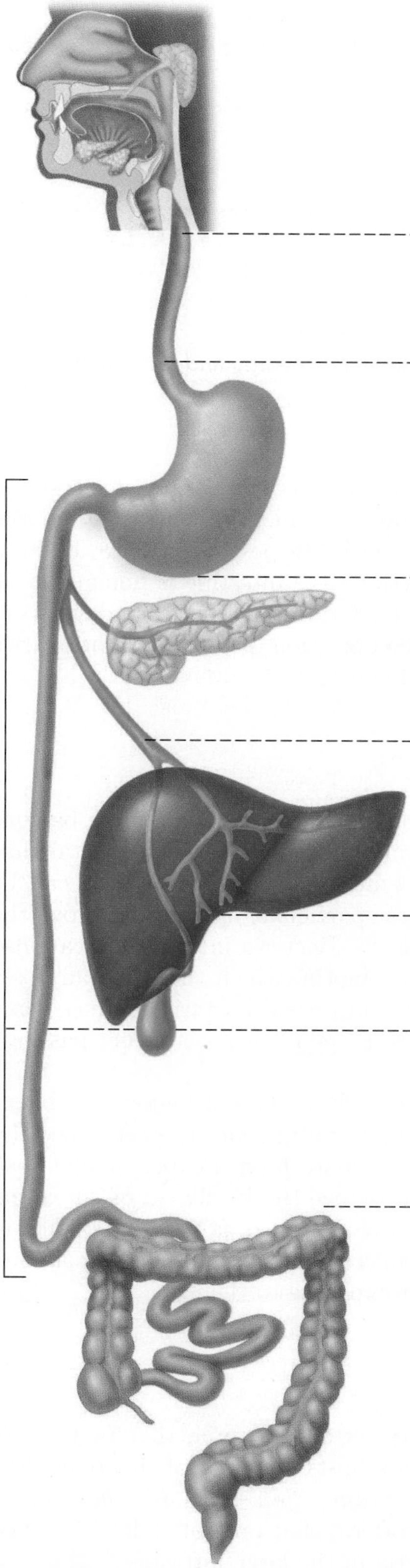

Organ	Secretions	Digestive Functions
Mouth and salivary glands	Saliva and water	Moisten food
	Mucus	Lubrication
	Amylase	Starch-digesting enzyme
Teeth		Chew
Esophagus		Moves food to stomach by peristaltic waves
	Mucus	Lubricates food
Stomach		Stores, mixes, dissolves, and continues digestion; regulates emptying of chyme into small intestine
	HCl	Kills microbes; activates pepsinogen to pepsin
	Pepsin	Digests proteins
	Mucus	Lubricates and protects stomach wall
Pancreas		Secretes enzymes and bicarbonate
	Enzymes	Digest carbohydrates, fats, proteins, and nucleic acids
	Bicarbonate	Neutralizes HCl entering small intestine from stomach
Liver		Receives water-soluble products of digestion from small intestine
		Synthesizes and secretes bile
	Bile salts	Emulsify water-insoluble fats
Gallbladder		Stores and concentrates bile between meals
		Releases bile during meals
Small intestine		Digests and absorbs most substances; mixes and propels contents
	Enzymes	Food digestion
	Water	Maintains fluidity of intestinal contents
	Mucus	Lubricates inner walls
Large intestine		Stores and concentrates undigested matter; absorbs salt and water; eliminates wastes
	Mucus	Lubricates mucosa

FIGURE 4.20 Summary of the primary and accessory organs of the GI tract and their functions.

ASSESS YOUR PROGRESS

21 *List the main sections of the large intestine from the ileocecal sphincter to the anus.*

22 *What happens to chyme when it is in the large intestine?*

23 *What is the typical composition of feces?*

24 *Trace the pathway of food from the mouth to the anus, including key organs and their functions.*

4.7 Microbes in the Digestive Tract

LEARNING OUTCOMES

1 *Discuss the importance of bacteria in the digestive tract.*

2 *Describe the role of prebiotics and probiotics in human health, and provide an example of each.*

The small intestine of a healthy person usually has few microorganisms residing in its lumen, particularly in the duodenum and jejunum.[10] In contrast, the large intestine is home to vast numbers of various species (types) of bacteria, because of its slower motility and neutral pH. A healthy large intestine is home to over 10 *trillion* bacteria, representing an estimated 400 different species and subspecies (**microflora**).[10] Interestingly, the usual composition of the microflora varies from person to person, because of dietary differences.

microflora population of several kinds of bacteria

probiotics live microorganisms that promote good health for their human hosts

Actions of Intestinal Bacteria

Under normal conditions, the microflora of the large intestine maintain a balance with each other that is beneficial to their human hosts. Bacteria can metabolize undigested food, such as dietary fiber, and synthesize certain fats that can be used for energy by the cells of the colon. These particular fats may improve the host's blood lipid levels and immune function.[11,12] Bacteria in the colon can also make the vitamins K, folate, B–6, B–12, and biotin, which their human hosts can absorb.[10] As a result of metabolic activity, intestinal bacteria produce gases that are expelled through the anus. *Flatulence* is the medical term for "passing" intestinal gas through the anus.

Large numbers of intestinal bacteria eventually become a major component of feces. Some species of these bacteria can be harmful (*pathogenic*), especially if they enter other parts of the body or contaminate food. People should wash their hands after having bowel movements to reduce the likelihood of spreading pathogens from their intestinal tract to themselves—such as through breaks in the skin—or to others. Chapter 19 discusses microorganisms that cause common food–borne infections and ways to limit your exposure to them.

Probiotics and Prebiotics

Probiotics are live microorganisms, primarily certain bacteria, that play a role in maintaining good health for their human hosts. Strains of *Lactobacillus* (*lak'–toe–bah'–sill–us*) and *Bifidobacterium* (*bih'–fih–doe–bak–ter'–e–um*) are among the kinds of bacteria (microflora) that promote a healthy balance between probiotic and pathogenic bacteria in the large intestine.

Many factors, including starvation, excessive emotional stress, and antibiotic use, can upset the normal balance of intestinal microflora. As a result of

DID **YOU** KNOW?

You may have seen celebrity-endorsed advertisements for colon cleansing to lose weight, prevent and treat cancer, and even for smoother, acne-free skin. Using "high colonics" and other types of enemas to "cleanse" and detoxify your colon is not necessary because the large intestine does not need to be cleansed. Furthermore, frequent enemas may deplete the body of vital minerals, including sodium and potassium. The beneficial bacteria that live in the colon are also lost through colon cleansing. Check with your physician before trying enema treatments.

the imbalance, an overgrowth of pathogenic bacteria can occur, increasing the likelihood of diarrhea and serious intestinal infections. Probiotics help control the growth of pathogenic bacteria that reside in the large intestine by competing successfully against them for available nutrients.

When an individual has a bacterial infection and takes an antibiotic to kill the pathogens, bacteria that normally reside in the colon are also destroyed. Results of some studies suggest that eating probiotic—containing foods, such as yogurt with "live and active cultures" of *Lactobacillus acidophilus*, can help restore the population of beneficial bacteria in the large intestine. People can also consume pills and solutions that contain the microbes. Certain probiotics may also be helpful for people with *ulcerative colitis*, a chronic condition charac-terized by an inflammation of the mucosa of the large intestine.[13] Furthermore, probiotics may be beneficial in regulating body weight and may reduce the risk of diarrheal diseases, as well as urinary tract infections, such as bladder infections, that commonly affect women.[14]

The acidic environment of the stomach kills both probiotic and pathogenic bacteria. Therefore, a person who is using probiotic therapy must ingest large amounts of the microbes to enable enough to survive and reach the large intes-tine.[13] Physicians who diagnose and treat digestive system disorders (gastroen-terologists) can administer a fluid that contains probiotics via an enema (rectal route), but patients generally prefer to obtain the microorganisms by taking pills or eating food. The process of colonizing the large intestine with probiotics takes at least 7 to 10 days. In some cases, however, the beneficial microorganisms may need to be consumed indefinitely.[13]

Prebiotics are food components, such as dietary fiber, that are not broken down by human digestive enzymes but are used as fuels by beneficial bacteria in the large intestine. Prebiotics are in a wide variety of foods, particularly fruits, vegetables, and whole grains. Soybeans, berries, garlic, barley, kale, and legumes are all rich sources of prebiotics.

Table 4.3 lists some health benefits that may be attributed to consum-ing probiotics and prebiotics regularly. Despite the reports of health benefits, many unanswered questions remain about the use of probiotics and prebiot-ics, including optimal doses, duration of treatment, and safety concerns.[15] Thus, medical researchers continue to explore the effects of probiotics and prebiotics on health.[16,17]

prebiotics food components that beneficial bacteria in the large intestine use for fuel

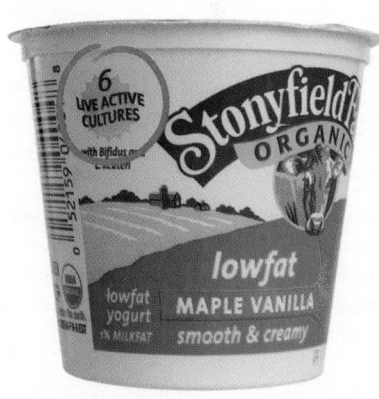

Some brands of yogurt contain live cultures of beneficial bacteria.

TABLE 4.3 Possible Health Benefits of Probiotics and Prebiotics

Probiotics (Live Bacteria)	Prebiotics (Often Fiber-Rich Foods)
Prevention and treatment of diarrhea	Alleviate constipation
Prevention and treatment of inflammatory bowel disease (IBD)	Improved immune function
Improved blood fat levels	Protection against colon cancer
Protection against ulcers	Alleviate allergy symptoms
Prevention and treatment of lactose intolerance	Prevention of obesity

Sources: Roberfroid M and others: Prebiotic effects: Metabolic and health benefits. *British Journal of Nutrition* 104 Suppl:S1, 2010; Verna EC, Lucak S: Use of probiotics in gastrointestinal disorders: What to recommend? *Therapeutic Advances in Gastroenterology* 3:307, 2010; Vandenplas Y and others: Probiotics and prebiotics in infants and children. *Current Infectious Disease Reports* 15:251, 2013.

ASSESS YOUR PROGRESS

25 *Summarize the roles intestinal bacteria play in human health.*

26 *Explain the difference between a probiotic and prebiotic, and give an example of each.*

4.8 Hormonal Regulation of Digestion

LEARNING OUTCOME

1 *Describe how gastrin, secretin, and cholecystokinin (CCK) regulate digestion.*

Three hormones play key roles in digestion: gastrin, secretin, and cholecystokinin ($ko'-le-sis'-toe-ki'-nin$). The information in Table 4.4 summarizes the role of each of these gut hormones in digestion and absorption.

Gastrin, Secretin, and Cholecystokinin

When food enters the stomach, G cells in the stomach's gastric glands secrete gastrin. As mentioned earlier in this chapter, gastrin hormone signals parietal cells to release H^+ and Cl^-, which results in the formation of HCl, and chief cells to secrete pepsinogen. Gastrin also stimulates the motility of the stomach and small intestine, and signals the ileocecal sphincter between the small and large intestines to relax.

When acidic chyme passes through the pyloric sphincter and enters the duo—denum, cells in the mucosa of the duodenum and first part of the jejunum release **secretin**. Secretin stimulates the pancreas and liver to release a bicarbonate—rich solution that raises the pH level of chyme. As a result, the mucosa of the small intestine is protected from the potentially harmful effects of HCl. Raising the pH of chyme also creates a more favorable environment for the activity of pancreatic and intestinal enzymes.

As fat and partially digested proteins enter the duodenum, the mucosa of the small intestine secretes **cholecystokinin (CCK)**. CCK stimulates the gallbladder to contract and release bile into the duodenum. Recall that bile is necessary for proper fat digestion and absorption. CCK also triggers the release of enzyme—rich pancreatic juice into the small intestine. Another action of CCK is reducing gastric secretions and motility, thus helping to control the flow of chyme from the stomach. As a result, nutrient digestion and absorption can proceed at a rea—sonable rate within the small intestine.

secretin hormone secreted by the duodenum and first part of the jejunum that stimulates the pancreas and liver to release a bicarbonate-rich solution into the small intestine

cholecystokinin (CCK) hormone secreted by the mucosa of the small intestine that stimulates the gallbladder to contract and the pancreas to release pancreatic juice into the small intestine

TABLE 4.4 Actions of Key Digestive Hormones in the GI Tract

Hormone	Primarily Released from	Responds to	Key Actions
Gastrin	Stomach	Food entering the stomach	Triggers parietal cells to release HCl and chief cells to release pepsinogen
			Stimulates stomach and small intestinal motility
Secretin	Small intestine	Acidic chyme entering the duodenum and first part of jejunum	Stimulates the release of a bicarbonate-rich solution from the liver and pancreas
Cholecystokinin (CCK)	Small intestine	Fat and breakdown products of proteins (peptides) entering the small intestine	Stimulates release of bile from the gallbladder into the small intestine
			Stimulates the release of pancreatic enzymes, decreases stomach secretions, and slows stomach motility

Identify the three major gut hormones, including the tissues from which they are released, the factors causing their release, and their key actions.

4.9 Common Digestive Tract Disorders

LEARNING OUTCOMES

1 *Identify and describe common gastrointestinal health problems.*

2 *Discuss preventative measures and treatments for constipation, diarrhea, vomiting, heartburn, ulcers, inflammatory bowel syndrome (IBS), and irritable bowel disease (IBD).*

Many people can eat and drink a variety of foods and beverages, and then regularly and easily eliminate the waste products. Most people have experienced an "upset stomach" occasionally and felt terrible as a result, but then they recovered within a day or two and returned to their usual diet. Some digestive disorders, however, are serious chronic illnesses that can make life difficult for those who have them.

In the United States, 60 to 70 million Americans suffer from digestive disorders.[18] Over 13 million of these individuals are hospitalized because of the disorder, and treating digestive disorders accounts for a significant percentage of all surgical procedures. This section focuses on some of the more common gastrointestinal disorders, including constipation, diarrhea, vomiting, and heartburn. Lactose intolerance, gallbladder disease, and celiac disease are intestinal disorders that are discussed in other chapters.

Constipation

Many Americans, especially older adults, think they are constipated if they do not have a bowel movement at least once a day. According to the American Gastroenterological Association, it is not necessary to have a daily bowel movement. For healthy people, the frequency of bowel movements can range from having three per day to three per week.[19] However, when bowel movements occur less frequently and feces are difficult to eliminate, the condition is called **constipation**.

Lack of dietary fiber; low water intake; anxiety, depression, and other psychological disturbances; and changes to typical routines, such as taking a long trip or having major surgery, can alter a person's usual pattern of bowel movements. Furthermore, constipation can result when a person regularly ignores the normal urge to have a bowel movement and avoids making a trip to the bathroom to defecate.

Although occasional constipation is common, *chronic* constipation can cause abdominal discomfort. Furthermore, straining while having a difficult bowel movement may increase pressure in the rectum and colon. The increase in pressure can force small areas of the mucosa to protrude through the walls of the colon, forming **diverticula**—tiny pouches (Fig. 4.21). **Diverticulosis**, a condition characterized by the presence of diverticula, is quite common in the United States, especially among older adults. About 50% of Americans who are older than 60 years of age have diverticulosis.[20] If diverticula become inflamed **(diverticulitis)**, antibiotics and, sometimes, surgery may be necessary to treat the condition.

constipation infrequent bowel movements and feces that are difficult to eliminate

diverticula tiny pouches that form in the wall of the colon

diverticulosis condition characterized by the presence of diverticula

diverticulitis condition characterized by inflamed diverticula

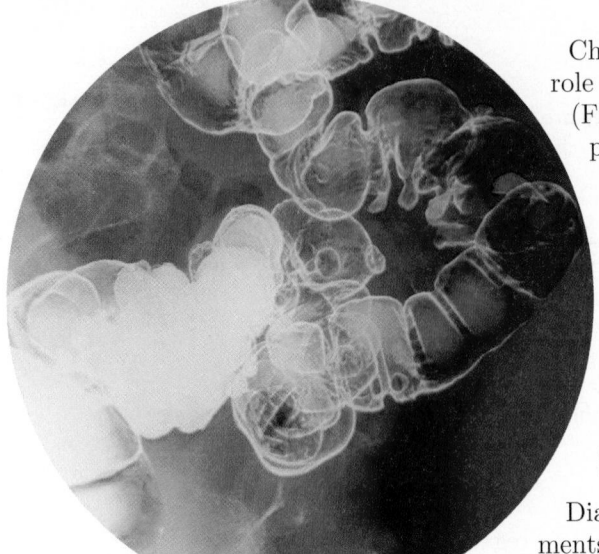

FIGURE 4.21 Diverticula. In this color-enhanced x-ray, the blue areas are diverticula.

Chronic constipation and straining during bowel movements also play a role in the development of **hemorrhoids**, swollen veins in the anal canal (Fig. 4.22). In some cases, hemorrhoids protrude out of the anus, causing pain, itching, and bleeding. Surgery is often necessary to remove troublesome hemorrhoids.

Individuals who feel uncomfortable because their bowel habits have changed and who have hard, dry feces that are difficult to eliminate should discuss the matter with a physician. In many instances, adding more fiber-rich foods to the diet is the first step to becoming more "regular." Chapter 5 provides information about dietary fiber, including rich food sources.

Diarrhea

Diarrhea is a condition characterized by frequent, watery bowel movements. Diarrhea occurs when more water than normal is secreted into the GI tract or the tract absorbs less water than normal. Most cases of diarrhea result from bacterial or viral infections of the intestinal tract. The infectious bacteria or viruses produce irritating or toxic substances that increase the movements (motility) of the GI tract. As a result, the GI tract propels chyme more rapidly through it, absorbing less water than normal in the process. Increased GI motility also helps the large intestine eliminate the watery feces and the toxic material it contains rapidly.

Loperamide, a medication that is available without a prescription, can be helpful for relieving an occasional bout of mild diarrhea. Cases of severe diarrhea, however, require more immediate medical attention. Frequent watery bowel movements can deplete the body's fluid volume, causing dehydration and excessive losses of the minerals sodium and potassium. Therefore, treatment of severe diarrhea generally includes drinking replacement fluids that contain sodium, potassium, and simple sugars such as glucose. It is also prudent to avoid eating solid foods until the condition resolves.

Prompt treatment of severe diarrhea—within 24 to 48 hours—is especially crucial for infants and older adults, because they can become dehydrated quickly by the loss of body water. In adults, diarrhea that is accompanied by bloody stools or lasts more than 7 days may be a sign of a serious intestinal disease, and a physician should be consulted.

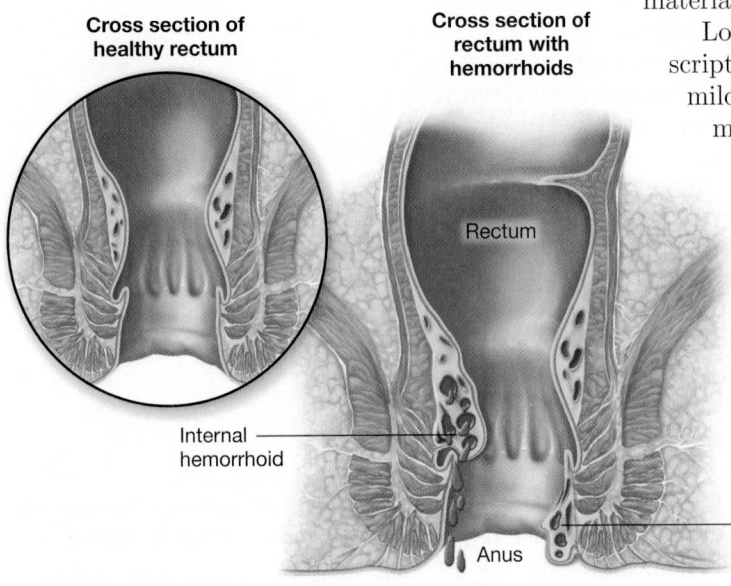

Cross section of healthy rectum

Cross section of rectum with hemorrhoids

Rectum

Internal hemorrhoid

External hemorrhoid

Anus

FIGURE 4.22 Hemorrhoids. Hemorrhoids are clusters of swollen rectal veins that can bleed, cause pain, and become itchy

hemorrhoids swollen veins in the anal canal

Vomiting

Not long after eating something toxic or drinking too much alcohol, a person may begin to feel queasy or "sick to his or her stomach." The individual soon becomes well aware that his or her body has an effective way of removing the harmful food or beverage: vomiting. Although vomiting is an unpleasant experience, it prevents toxic substances from entering the small intestine, where they can do more harm or be absorbed. Vomiting can also be a response to intense pain, head injury, rotating movements of the head (motion sickness), hormonal changes in pregnancy (morning sickness), and touching the back of the throat.[21] *Hyperemesis gravidarum*, excessive vomiting in pregnancy, will be discussed in more detail in Chapter 16.

Vomiting occurs when the vomiting center in the brain interprets information from various nervous system receptors, including those concerned with the physical and chemical conditions of the stomach, small intestine, and bloodstream. When the center detects a toxic chemical, it initiates vomiting by contracting the abdominal muscles, expelling the contents of the stomach and duodenum forcefully out of the body via the mouth.

Generally, vomiting does not last more than 24 hours. Repeated vomiting, however, can deplete body water, resulting in dehydration. Dehydration can be serious, especially if the vomiting is accompanied by diarrhea. Treatment includes avoiding solid food until the condition resolves. Additionally, sipping small amounts of water or clear liquids, including noncarbonated soft drinks such as sports drinks, can help prevent dehydration. If the affected person is able to retain small amounts of fluid, then he or she can try to drink increasing amounts of fluid until the vomiting subsides completely.

Adults should contact a physician if their vomiting lasts for more than a day and they have signs of dehydration, such as increased thirst, decreased urination, and dry lips and mouth.[21] Contacting a physician immediately is necessary if there is blood in the vomit (the vomit appears to have coffee grounds in it) or vomiting is accompanied by other signs and symptoms, such as diarrhea, weakness, confusion, fever, or severe abdominal pain (Table 4.5).

Children who suffer from vomiting and/or diarrhea are likely to develop dehydration more rapidly than adults who are suffering from these conditions. Signs of dehydration in young children include sunken eyes, dry lips and mouth, and decreased urination. Caregivers should contact a physician if the child has vomiting and diarrhea that persist for more than a few hours and shows signs of dehydration.

Heartburn

About half of American adults experience occasional **heartburn**, a gnawing pain or burning sensation generally felt in the upper chest, under the breastbone. Ten percent of the population has chronic heartburn that is characterized by symptoms occurring at least once a week. Heartburn is not the result of a heart problem but is caused by the passage of acidic contents from the stomach into the esophagus. Table 4.6 lists some of the factors that can contribute to heartburn or worsen the condition, including having excess body fat and smoking cigarettes.[22,23]

Gastroesophageal Reflux Disease

Although many people think heartburn is a trivial health problem, frequent chronic heartburn can be a symptom of **gastroesophageal reflux disease (GERD)**. In addition to heartburn, symptoms of GERD may include nausea, gagging, coughing, or hoarseness. If not treated properly, GERD irritates the lining of the esophagus and contributes to the development of esophageal ulcers (sores) (Fig. 4.23). Such ulcers can damage blood vessels in the walls of the esophagus, causing bleeding. Signs of bleeding from the esophagus include black, tarlike bowel movements and iron–deficiency anemia. In severe cases, the loss of blood from a bleeding ulcer can be deadly.

People who suffer from GERD have a higher risk of esophageal cancer than people who do not have a history of this condition. Typical dietary advice for treating the condition includes consuming smaller, more frequent meals that are low in fat; not overeating at mealtimes; and limiting intake of foods that relax the lower gastroesophageal sphincter, such as chili powder, onions, garlic, peppermint, caffeine, alcohol, and chocolate. Additionally, people should wait about 2 hours after meals before lying down, because remaining upright reduces the

TABLE 4.5 Vomiting Danger Signs

Contact a Physician When Vomiting:
1. Lasts longer than a few hours (children under 6 years of age)
2. Lasts longer than a day (people over 6 years of age)
3. Is accompanied by:
Blood in vomit (looks like coffee grounds)
Signs of dehydration
Diarrhea
Fever
Weakness
Headache or stiff neck
Severe abdominal pain
Confusion or decreased alertness

heartburn pain generally felt in the upper chest that results from the passage of acidic contents from the stomach into the esophagus

gastroesophageal reflux disease (GERD) chronic condition characterized by frequent heartburn that can damage the esophagus

TABLE 4.6 Factors That Contribute to or Worsen Heartburn

Having excess body fat, especially around the waistline
Drinking alcohol, coffee, carbonated beverages, and citrus juices
Overeating
Eating chocolate, peppermint, and greasy or spicy foods
Eating foods that contain tomatoes or vinegar
Smoking

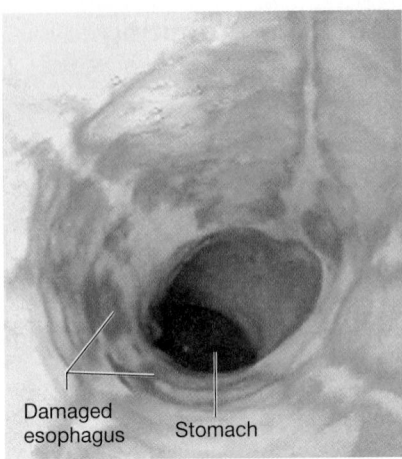

FIGURE 4.23 Acid reflux damage. An endoscopic view of the esophagus near the opening of the stomach. The reddened areas are signs of damage caused by acid reflux.

TABLE 4.7 Recommendations to Reduce the Risk of Heartburn

1. Lose excess body weight.
2. Do not lie down within 2 hours after eating a meal.
3. Do not overeat at mealtimes.
4. Avoid smoking cigarettes.
5. Elevate the head of the bed so it is about 6 inches higher than the foot of the bed.
6. Do not wear tight belts or clothes with tight waistbands.
7. Learn to recognize foods that cause heartburn.

likelihood that stomach contents will push against the lower gastroesophageal sphincter and move into the esophagus. Table 4.7 lists these and other recommendations for reducing the risk of heartburn and managing GERD. Taking over-the-counter antacids can neutralize excess stomach acid and relieve the discomfort of heartburn within minutes, but these products do not prevent heartburn. People suffering from GERD should ask their physicians to recommend other medications that are taken daily to inhibit stomach acid production, preventing heartburn.

Peptic Ulcer

A peptic ulcer is a sore that occurs in the lining of the stomach or the upper small intestine. The typical symptoms of a peptic ulcer are deep, dull upper abdominal pain and a feeling of fullness that occur about 2 hours after eating. The pain results when most of the chyme has left the stomach, and the HCl that remains comes in contact with and digests the lining of the mucosa of the organ, forming one or more sores. It is not unusual for the sores to damage the wall of a blood vessel, causing bleeding; thus, untreated peptic ulcers may result in iron-deficiency anemia. Furthermore, an ulcer may erode through the stomach or intestinal wall and allow GI contents to leak into the body cavities, resulting in a potentially life-threatening infection. Therefore, it is important to recognize ulcer symptoms and obtain treatment early.

Physicians detect gastrointestinal ulcers by performing a clinical examination called upper endoscopy. The first step of this procedure involves administering a medication that relaxes the patient. After the patient is sedated, the physician inserts a special flexible scope into the person's mouth, down the esophagus, and into the stomach and upper small intestine. The scope is equipped with a video camera that transmits images of the lining of the esophagus, stomach, and upper small intestine to a screen that the physician views for the presence of ulcers, eroded areas, or cancerous tumors. The scope also enables the physician to use tools to treat areas of bleeding or remove pieces of tissue (biopsy) for microscopic examination.

At one time, medical experts thought excessive emotional stress caused peptic ulcers. By the 1990s, however, researchers determined that *Helicobacter pylori* (*H. pylori*), a type of bacteria that can live in parts of the stomach, was responsible for the development of most stomach ulcers (Fig. 4.24). *H. pylori* infection makes the lining of the stomach more susceptible to being damaged by stomach acid. In addition to infection with *H. pylori*, other factors are associated with the development of peptic ulcers, particularly smoking cigarettes, heavy consumption of alcohol, and regular use of NSAIDs (nonsteroidal anti-inflammatory drugs) such as aspirin, ibuprofen, and naproxen. Table 4.8 lists these and other factors that increase a person's risk of peptic ulcers.

Stress is still considered to be a risk factor for ulcer formation. Chronic stress may reduce the normal functioning of the immune system, making *H. pylori* infection more likely. Having good stress management skills may explain why some people who are infected with *H. pylori* do not develop these ulcers.

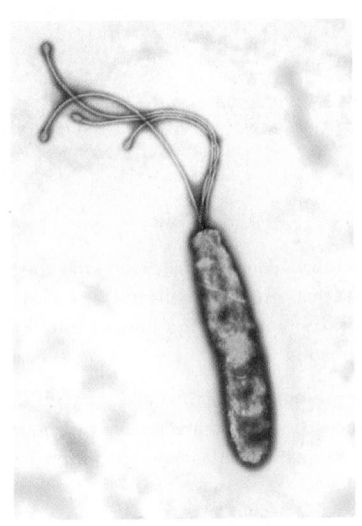

FIGURE 4.24 *H. pylori.*

TABLE 4.8 Factors That Increase the Risk of Peptic Ulcers

Infection with *H. pylori*
NSAIDs
Alcohol consumption
Genetics
Smoking
Emotional stress
Excess acid production

In the past, ulcer patients were advised to consume bland, low—fat diets that lacked spices to control their ulcer symptoms. Today, a combination of medical approaches is used for ulcer therapy. People infected with *H. pylori* are given antibiotics, as well as medications that reduce stomach acid production. This treatment is highly effective for combating *H. pylori* infections and healing peptic ulcers. The combination of medical treatment and lifestyle changes has minimized the need for peptic ulcer patients to make such drastic dietary changes. Current dietary approaches to treatment include avoiding foods that increase ulcer symp— toms. Such foods often vary among individuals. For example, a man who has a history of peptic ulcer may report that spicy foods irritate his stomach, whereas his friend who also has a gastric ulcer may be able to tolerate peppery foods.

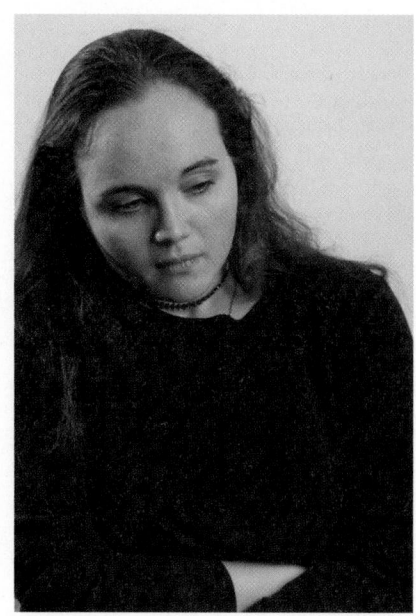

Irritable Bowel Syndrome

In the United States, as many as 15% of the adult population suffers from irritable bowel syndrome (IBS), a condition characterized by intestinal cramps and abnormal bowel function, particularly diarrhea, constipation, or alternating episodes of both.[24] Loose stools are often accompanied with mucus, and after bowel movements, the affected person feels as though his or her elimination of stools was incomplete. For reasons that are unclear, women are more likely than men to suffer from IBS.

The cause of IBS is unknown, but certain foods and beverages, as well as emotional stress, often trigger severe bouts of the disorder. The GI tract muscles of people with IBS may produce stronger contractions that last longer than the GI muscles of people who do not have this condition.[25] Researchers are investi— gating the role of the nervous system in stimulating these abnormal movements of the intestinal tract.

Therapy is individualized and may include elimination diets that focus on determining which foods are most likely to contribute to IBS symptoms. Foods often eliminated include dairy products, legumes, and certain vegetables, espe— cially cabbage and broccoli. Some fruits, particularly grapes, raisins, cherries, and cantaloupe, may also need to be avoided. Treatment may also include learn— ing stress management strategies, obtaining psychological counseling, and taking antidepressant and other medications.

It is important not to confuse IBS with IBD (inflammatory bowel disease). Although irritable bowel syndrome can be physically uncomfortable and emotionally upsetting, the condition does not appear to inflame the tissue of the small or large intestine or increase the risk of colorectal cancer. For more information about IBS, visit the website http://digestive.niddk.nih.gov/ddiseases/pubs/ibs/index.htm.

Inflammatory Bowel Disease

As many as 1.4 million Americans have **inflammatory bowel disease (IBD)**, which is characterized by chronic inflammation of the GI tract.[26] The inflam— mation causes the typical signs and symptoms of IBD: diarrhea, rectal bleeding, abdominal cramps, fever, and unintentional weight loss. In some cases, skin rashes or sores, blurry vision, and joint pain also develop. People with IBD typ— ically experience "flares," periods in which the signs and symptoms of the dis— ease occur, followed by periods of remission in which they are relatively healthy.

IBD commonly develops when people are in adolescence or young adulthood. Although the actual cause or causes of IBD are unknown, the disease results from an abnormal immune system response to an environmental or psycholog— ical trigger, such as an infection or a stressful situation.[27] *Crohn's disease* and *ulcerative colitis* are the two types of IBD.

No special diets are used to treat IBD. However, people with the conditions often find that certain foods seem to trigger flares, so they learn to avoid those items. Physicians generally prescribe medications to control IBD, but surgery may be necessary, especially in cases that do not respond to drug treatment.

inflammatory bowel disease (IBD) condition that is characterized by chronic inflammation of the GI tract

ulcerative colitis (UC) type of IBD that causes ulcers to form in the mucosa of the colon and rectum

Ulcerative Colitis

In cases of **ulcerative colitis (UC)**, the inflammatory process causes ulcers to form in the mucosa of the colon and rectum. These sores can spread in a continuous pattern from the rectum to the colon, but they do not occur elsewhere in the GI tract. As in cases of Crohn's disease, people with UC have an increased risk of colon cancer. The "Real People, Real Stories" feature in this section of the chapter highlights Matthew Lang, who has UC.

Crohn's Disease

Crohn's disease type of IBD; the body's immune system cells attack normal intestinal cells, damaging parts of the intestines

Crohn's disease is an autoimmune disorder, a chronic condition in which the body's immune system does not function properly and begins to attack normal cells. In cases of Crohn's disease, certain immune system cells invade the intestinal lining and cause patches of inflammation. The inflammation can affect all layers of the colon, as well as the ileum. However, any part of the GI tract, from the mouth to the anus, can become inflamed. The disease often results in the formation of intestinal *abscesses* (infected sores), blockages, and *fistulas*. An internal fistula is an abnormal opening or connection that forms between two regions of the intestinal tract or between a section of the GI tract and an abdominal organ. Such fistulas cause pain and swelling, and often require surgery to repair the abnormality. Additionally, people with Crohn's disease have a higher risk of developing cancer of the small intestine and colon than healthy people. In some cases, Crohn's disease causes such extensive destruction of intestinal tissue that the affected person needs to have surgery to remove the damaged part. Surgery is not a cure for Crohn's disease, because the inflammation eventually develops in other regions of the GI tract.

REAL People, **REAL** Stories

Matthew Lang

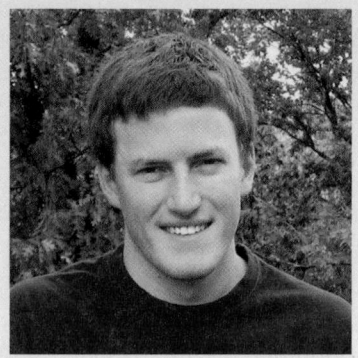

Matthew Lang is a college student who used to take the health of his intestinal tract for granted. When he was 20 and living on campus, he noticed a large amount of blood in his stools after having a bowel movement. Over the next few days, Matthew continued to pass blood in his bowel movements, and he had severe "stomach" cramps. He felt unusually tired, and his friends told him that he "looked pale." At the insistence of his parents, he visited the student health center on campus. The clinician took a sample of Matthew's blood to assess its components and a sample of his stools to test for the presence of blood.

Not long after Matthew returned to his dormitory, he received an urgent call from the clinician. She told him that he had blood in his stools, and there was evidence that the blood loss had been chronic. He also had *anemia*, a condition characterized by an insufficient number of red blood cells. Matthew's lack of energy and pale skin color were among the signs and symptoms of anemia. The clinician told Matthew to make an appointment immediately with a gastroenterologist, a physician who specializes in treating disorders of the digestive system.

Later that week, Matthew met with a gastroenterologist, and a few days after the appointment, the physician performed a colonoscopy on the young man. During this procedure, a colonoscope, a long, narrow, flexible tube with a video camera on the end, is inserted into the anal opening and carefully guided through the rectum and colon, allowing the physician to view the inside of the lower intestinal tract. Additionally, the physician can insert small surgical instruments through the colonoscope to perform *biopsies*, the removal of small pieces of abnormal-appearing or damaged intestinal tract tissues. These tissues are sent to a laboratory and studied microscopically for evidence of inflammation or disease. According to the results of Matthew's biopsy, his colon was inflamed and slightly ulcerated, which are signs of ulcerative colitis.

Medical experts are not certain about the causes of ulcerative colitis, but emotional stress and genetic factors play major roles in its development. Matthew recalls being very "stressed out" during his sophomore year in college, and his intestinal problem became severe enough to send him to the student health center around the time of his midterm exams. He notices that his symptoms seem to improve when he is able to relax.

Anti-inflammatory drugs are used to control ulcerative colitis. Matthew recognizes that he will need to monitor his intestinal health and probably take medication for the rest of his life. "It's annoying to take all these pills every day," he said, "but I'm getting used to it. I know it's necessary along with following a good diet for the rest of my life. Having ulcerative colitis has made me realize the benefits of a good diet. Even people who don't have IBD should improve their eating habits. They might feel better, too."

ASSESS YOUR PROGRESS

28 *What are potential long-term consequences of frequent untreated constipation?*

29 *Explain why vomiting for 24 hours and longer can be serious enough to require medical attention.*

30 *Identify potential health effects of untreated, frequent GERD.*

31 *What factors contribute to the development of peptic ulcers?*

32 *What dietary recommendations would you provide to a person experiencing irritable bowel syndrome (IBS)?*

33 *Describe the differences between Crohn's disease and ulcerative colitis.*

SUMMARY

SECTION 4.1 Overview of the Digestive System

- The primary roles of the digestive system are the breakdown of large food molecules into nutrients and the absorption of nutrients into the bloodstream.
- The GI tract includes the mouth, esophagus, stomach, and small and large intestines. The other component of the digestive system, the accessory organs, assists the functioning of the GI tract.

SECTION 4.2 The Mouth

- Mechanical and chemical digestion begin in the mouth. Taste buds distinguish sweet, sour, salty, bitter, and umami tastes.

SECTION 4.3 The Esophagus

- The esophagus conveys a bolus from the mouth to the stomach. The lower esophageal sphincter prevents reflux of stomach contents into the esophagus.

SECTION 4.4 The Stomach

- The stomach is a muscular sac that stores and mixes food. Gastric juice contains mucus, HCl, intrinsic factor, and enzymes, such as pepsinogen. The muscular action of the stomach mixes food with gastric juice to form chyme.

SECTION 4.5 The Small Intestine

- The three sections of the small intestine are the duodenum, jejunum, and ileum.

- In the small intestine, enzymes of the pancreas and those in the brush border of microvilli complete the process of digestion. Bile is made in the liver, stored in the gallbladder, and secreted into the duodenum, especially when fat enters the small intestine.
- Nutrients are absorbed into the bloodstream or lymphatic system, depending on the nutrient.

SECTION 4.6 The Large Intestine

- A minor amount of additional absorption, primarily some water and minerals, takes place in the large intestine, because its mucosa has no villi. Any remaining undigested material, some water, and intestinal bacteria eventually exit the body as feces.

SECTION 4.7 Microbes in the Digestive Tract

- Under normal conditions, the bacteria of the large intestine maintain a balance with each other that is beneficial for their human host. Probiotics are live microorganisms that promote good health. Prebiotics are food components that beneficial bacteria in the large intestine use for fuel.

SECTION 4.8 Hormonal Regulation of Digestion

- Gastrin stimulates release of HCl and pepsinogen, and stimulates stomach and small intestinal motility. Secretin stimulates the release of bicarbonate-rich pancreatic juice. Cholecystokinin slows stomach motility and stimulates the release of bile from the gallbladder and release of pancreatic enzymes.

SECTION 4.9 Common Digestive Tract Disorders

- Chronic constipation may contribute to the development of diverticula and hemorrhoids. Diarrhea and vomiting can lead to dehydration.
- Frequent chronic heartburn can be a symptom of GERD. People with GERD are at risk of esophageal cancer.
- Irritable bowel syndrome does not result in inflammation of the large intestine. Inflammatory bowel disease includes Crohn's disease and ulcerative colitis.
- Infection with *H. pylori,* smoking cigarettes, heavy consumption of alcohol, and regular use of nonsteroidal anti-inflammatory drugs increase the risk of developing a peptic ulcer.

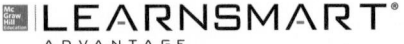

CASE STUDY RESPONSE

IRRITABLE BOWEL SYNDROME

IRRITABLE BOWEL SYNDROME (IBS) is a disorder of the GI tract that is characterized by bouts of diarrhea and constipation. Unlike inflammatory bowel disease (IBD), IBS does not seem to inflame the tissue of the small or large intestines. Furthermore, IBS does not appear to increase the risk of colorectal cancer.

Eating and drinking certain foods and beverages, such as pizza, can contribute to IBS. Annie should keep a food log to identify her trigger foods and avoid those foods or consume them only in moderation.

As a full-time college student who is also working and volunteering, Annie is probably experiencing a high level of stress. Therefore, she should determine how she can reduce or manage her stress, perhaps by not volunteering as much each week or by choosing only one student organization in which to remain active. If Annie cannot manage her stress on her own, she should obtain psychological counseling.

TEST KITCHEN
Modifying Recipes for Healthy Living

Arthur is a 25-year-old computer technician who smokes a pack of cigarettes a day and works approximately 60 hours per week. For the past 2 years, he has experienced episodes of heartburn that occur more than three times a week. Arthur loves pizza. He eats at fast-food restaurants frequently and exercises very little. Since graduating from college, Arthur has gained 30 pounds. He thinks that his diet contributes to his frequent bouts of heartburn.

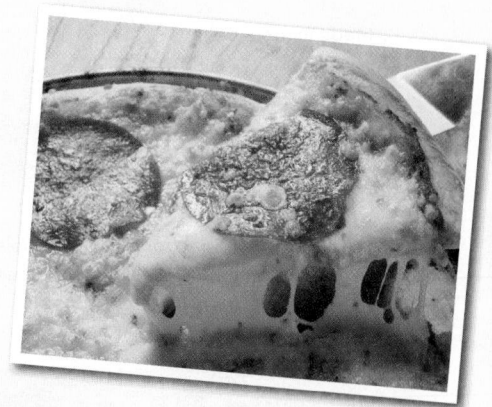

You ask Arthur to keep a small notebook in his shirt pocket at all times. He should use the notebook to record his activities during the week, as well as his food and beverage intakes for the period. Whenever he experiences heartburn, he should indicate the timing and degree of the discomfort in the notebook. A week later, Arthur returns to your office with his "heartburn" diary. According to one of his daily notes:

Tuesday, May 17

7 a.m.	2 cups regular coffee, 2 cigarettes
9 a.m.	Vending machines—2 chocolate doughnuts, 2 cups reg. coffee
12 noon	Lunch at Mickey's—double cheeseburger, fries, fried fruit pie
3 p.m.	(Break) 2 cups of reg. coffee, 2 cigarettes
7:00 p.m.	Got home from work. 3 cigarettes
7:00-8:00 p.m.	Watched TV
9:00 p.m.	Went out to Pizza Dive with friends. Dinner included: 5 slices of pepperoni, sausage, and ham pizza; 24 ounces of beer; 1 piece of chocolate cake with chocolate icing. Smoked 6 cigarettes
11:00 p.m.	Got home from dinner. Smoked a couple of cigarettes. Very tired. Went to bed
11:30 p.m.	Couldn't sleep. **Terrible heartburn**. Got up. Took some Pepto-Bismol® and smoked a couple of cigarettes.

STEP 1

Identify the foods and lifestyle factors that likely contributed to Arthur's episode of heartburn.

STEP 2

Plan a dinner menu that would minimize the chances that Arthur would suffer more episodes of heartburn. What kinds of foods would you recommend he avoid? With regard to the amount of food he consumes and its timing, what could he do to reduce the likelihood of developing heartburn?

STEP 3

Explain to Arthur how lifestyle and excess body weight contribute to heartburn. How can he rearrange his schedule and alter his habits to reduce his chances of experiencing heartburn and its more serious complications?

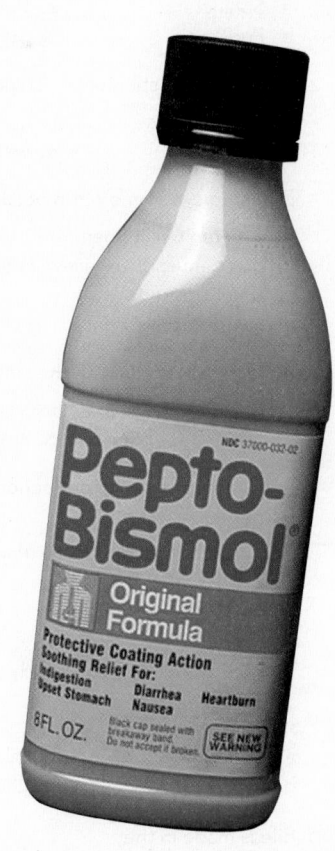

Critical Thinking

1. Meghan ate a peanut butter and jelly sandwich made with whole-wheat bread. Describe what happens to her sandwich as it passes through her GI tract.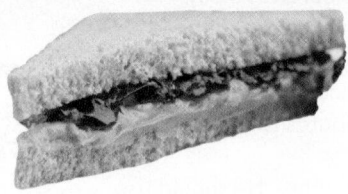

2. Eric's body makes abnormally low levels of gastrin. Explain how this condition affects his ability to digest and absorb nutrients.

3. Taylor had a serious condition that required removal of the upper third of his small intestine. Based on this information, is he at risk of developing multiple nutrient deficiencies? Explain why or why not.

4. Margaret has pancreatic cancer. Explain how this chronic disease can affect her ability to digest food.

5. Your mother complains of having persistent heartburn, but she does not think her discomfort is serious enough to be investigated by her physician. Do you agree or disagree with her attitude about heartburn? Explain your position.

Practice Test

Select the best answer.

1. Which of the following organs is an accessory organ of the digestive system?
   a. heart   b. kidney   c. liver   d. bladder

2. Mechanical digestion begins in the
   a. mouth.
   b. stomach.
   c. small intestine.
   d. liver.

3. ___ move(s) food from the back of the mouth, through the esophagus, and into the stomach.
   a. Sphincters
   b. Peristalsis
   c. Reflux
   d. Segmentation

4. Chemical digestion of ___ begins in the mouth.
   a. nucleic acids
   b. proteins
   c. carbohydrates
   d. water-soluble vitamins

5. Dumping syndrome often occurs after a person
   a. eats too much fiber.
   b. takes antacids to relieve heartburn.
   c. is dehydrated.
   d. has stomach surgery.

6. As food moves through the small intestine, the semiliquid mass is called
   a. bile.   b. bolus.   c. chyme.   d. bicarbonate.

7. ___ are tiny, fingerlike projections of the small intestine that absorb nutrients.
   a. Crypts   b. Villi   c. Papillae   d. Diverticula

8. Gastric glands secrete
   a. bile.
   b. intrinsic factor.
   c. salivary amylase.
   d. lysozyme.

9. Saliva contains
   a. lysozyme.
   b. hydrochloric acid.
   c. bile.
   d. cholecystokinin.

10. Bile is made in the
    a. pancreas.
    b. gallbladder.
    c. liver.
    d. small intestine.

11. What is the approximate pH of stomach's contents as it passes through the pylorus?
    a. 2.0   b. 4.5   c. 7.0   d. 9.5

12. Probiotics
    a. are bacteria that may benefit the intestinal tracts of their human hosts.
    b. cause diarrhea and intestinal bleeding in people with IBS and other chronic bowel diseases.
    c. are phytochemicals in citrus foods.
    d. contain live viruses.

13. Absorption of nutrients occurs primarily in the
    a. stomach.
    b. large intestine.
    c. small intestine.
    d. pancreas.

14. After being absorbed, which nutrients leave the GI tract through the lymphatic system?
    a. most fats and fat-soluble vitamins
    b. proteins and phytochemicals
    c. sugars and fiber
    d. water-soluble vitamins and minerals

15. Which of the following practices increases the risk of peptic ulcer?
    a. chewing gum
    b. smoking cigarettes
    c. drinking orange juice
    d. eating a low-fiber diet

ANSWERS TO PRACTICE TEST
1-c; 2-a; 3-b; 4-c; 5-d; 6-c; 7-b; 8-b; 9-a; 10-c; 11-a; 12-a; 13-c; 14-a; 15-b

ANSWERS TO CHAPTER 4 **QUIZ** Yourself

1. The esophagus is the tube that connects the mouth to the stomach. **True** (p. 85)
2. The stomach produces hydrochloric acid. **True** (p. 87)
3. Most nutrient absorption occurs in the large intestine. **False** (p. 90)
4. The gallbladder makes bile. **False** (p. 90)
5. A type of bacteria is responsible for the development of most stomach ulcers. **True** (p. 102)

References

1. Saladin KS: *Anatomy & physiology.* 7th ed. Boston: McGraw-Hill Publishing Company, 2015.

2. Widmaier E and others: *Vander's human physiology.* 12th ed. Boston: McGraw-Hill Publishing Company, 2010.

3. Smeets MA and others: Sense of smell disorder and health related quality of life. *Rehabilitation Psychology* 54:404, 2009.

4. National Institutes of Health: *Taste disorders.* Updated June 2011. http://www.nidcd.nih.gov/health/smelltaste/pages/taste.aspx Accessed: March 11, 2014

5. Fonk T and others: Characteristics of taste disorders. *European Archives of Otorhinolaryngology* 270:1855, 2013.

6. Welge-Lussen A and others: A study about the frequency of taste disorders. *Journal of Neurology* 258:386, 2010.

7. Tack J and others: Pathophysiology, diagnosis and management of postoperative dumping syndrome. *Nature Reviews: Gastroenterology and Hepatology* 6:583, 2009.

8. Russo F and others: Effects of a diet with inulin-enriched pasta on gut peptides and gastric emptying rates in healthy young volunteers. *European Journal of Nutrition* 50: 271, 2011.

9. Seeley RR and others: *Essentials of anatomy and physiology.* 9th ed. Boston: McGraw-Hill Publishing Company, 2011.

10. Prescott and others: *Microbiology.* 8th ed. Boston: McGraw-Hill Publishing Company, 2011.

11. Meijer K and others: Butyrate and other short-chain fatty acids as modulators of immunity: What relevance for health? *Current Opinions in Clinical Nutrition and Metabolic Care* 13:715, 2010.

12. Floch MH: The effect of probiotics on host metabolism: the microbiota and fermentation. *Journal of Clinical Gastroenterology* 44 Suppl 1:S19, 2010.

13. Dylag K and others: Probiotics in the mechanism of protection against gut inflammation and therapy of gastrointestinal disorders. *Current Pharmaceutical Design* 20:1149, 2014.

14. Angelakis E and others: The relationship between gut microbiota and weight gain. *Future Microbiology* 7:91, 2011.

15. Verna EC, Lucak S: Use of probiotics in gastrointestinal disorders: What to recommend? *Therapeutic Advances in Gastroenterology* 3:307, 2010.

16. Kale-Pradhan PB and others: Role of *Lactobacillus* in the prevention of antibiotic-associated diarrhea: A meta-analysis. *Pharmacotherapy* 30:119, 2010.

17. Roberfroid M and others: Prebiotic effects: Metabolic and health benefits. *British Journal of Nutrition* 104 Suppl:S1, 2010.

18. National Institutes of Health, National Institute of Diabetes and Digestive and Kidney Diseases: *Digestive disease statistics for the United States.* Last updated 2013. http://www.digestive.niddk.nih.gov/statistics/statistics.aspx Accessed: March 11, 2014

19. American Gastroenterological Association: *Understanding constipation.* January, 2013. http://www.gastro.org/patient-center/digestive-conditions/constipation Accessed: January 18, 2014

20. National Institutes of Health, National Institute of Diabetes and Digestive and Kidney Diseases: *Diverticulosis and diverticulitis.* http://digestive.niddk.nih.gov/ddiseases/pubs/diverticulosis/diverticulosis.pdf Accessed: January 18, 2014

21. Cleveland Clinic Information Center: *Nausea and vomiting.* http://my.clevelandclinic.org/symptoms/nausea/hic_nausea_and_vomiting.aspx Accessed: March 11, 2014

22. Djarv T and others: Physical activity, obesity and gastroesophageal reflux disease in the general population. *World Journal of Gastroenterology* 18: 3710, 2012.

23. American Gastroenterological Association: *Understanding heartburn and reflux disease.* http://www.gastro.org/patient-center/digestive-conditions/heartburn-gerd Accessed: March 11, 2014

24. American College of Gastroenterology: *Understanding irritable bowel syndrome.* http://patients.gi.org/gi-health-and-disease/understanding-irritable-bowel-syndrome/ Accessed: March 11, 2014

25. Chang JY, Talley NJ: An update on irritable bowel syndrome: From diagnosis to emerging therapies. *Current Opinions in Gastroenterology* 27:72, 2011.

26. Centers for Disease Control and Prevention: *Inflammatory bowel disease (IBD).* Updated January 2014. http://www.cdc.gov/ibd/ Accessed: March 11, 2014

27. Bernstein CN: Why and where to look in the environment with regard to the etiology of inflammatory bowel disease. *Digestive Disorders* 30:28, 2012.

5 Carbohydrates: Sugars, Starches, and Fiber

CASE STUDY

Carbohydrates for breakfast?

JERRY IS A GRADUATE STUDENT WORKING on his doctorate. Two months ago, Jerry read an article posted on an Internet website about the importance of limiting intakes of carbohydrates, particularly at breakfast. Since reading the article, Jerry has consumed only a fried egg, three pieces of bacon, and a glass of water for breakfast. He also avoids eating carbohydrate-containing foods at other meals. Although Jerry does not need to lose weight, he does have a family history of type 2 diabetes.

- Describe to Jerry the different categories of carbohydrates and how each of these classes may influence his health.
- Provide Jerry with two examples of breakfasts that incorporate healthy, nutrient-dense carbohydrates.
- Explain to Jerry why eating carbohydrates does not necessarily cause diabetes.

The suggested Case Study Response can be found on page 142.

connect | NUTRITION Check out the Connect site at www.mcgrawhillconnect.com to further explore this case study.

QUIZ Yourself

Would sweetening cereal with honey be a healthier choice than using table sugar? Is fiber good for one's health? Check your knowledge of carbohydrates by taking the following quiz. The answers are found on page 146.

1. The carbohydrate found in milk is called lactose. _T _F
2. Ounce per ounce, sugar provides more energy than starch. _T _F
3. Digestion of starch begins in the mouth. _T _F
4. Eating a high-fiber diet can improve the functioning of the large intestine and reduce blood cholesterol levels. _T _F
5. Individuals with diabetes should follow a carbohydrate-free diet. _T _F

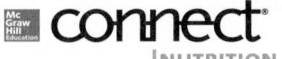

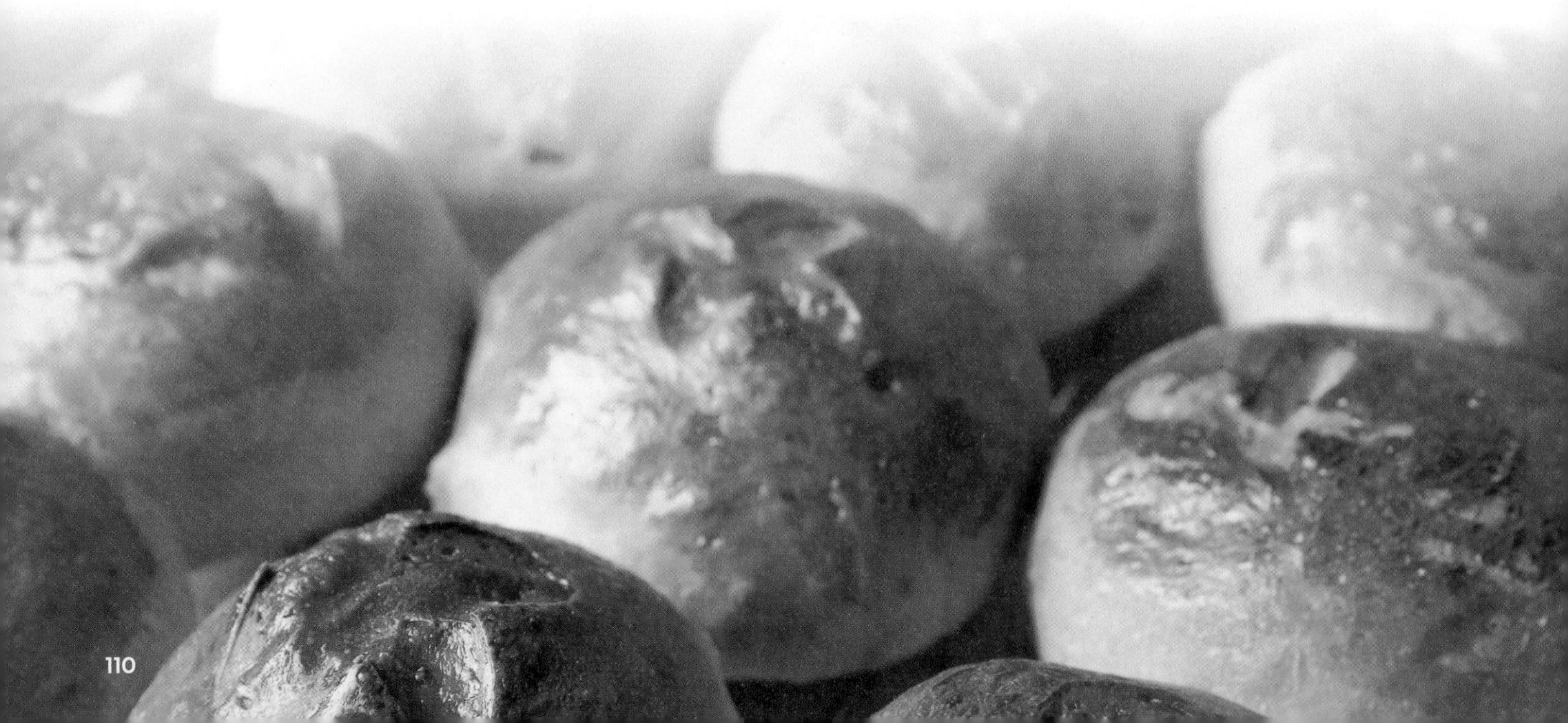

5.1 Introducing Carbohydrates

LEARNING OUTCOMES

1 *Explain why plant foods are sources of carbohydrates.*
2 *Identify the two general categories of carbohydrates.*

Can you imagine celebrating birthdays, weddings, or holidays without cakes, candies, or cookies? Many Americans enjoy eating sweets and even describe themselves as having a "sweet tooth." Why do humans, even newborn infants, prefer foods that taste sweet? The pleasant and sometimes irresistible taste of sugar is a clue that the food contains **carbohydrates**, a major source of energy for cells. Without a steady supply of energy, cells cannot function and they die.

Plants are rich sources of carbohydrates; they make these substances by using the sun's energy to combine carbon, oxygen, and hydrogen atoms from carbon dioxide and water (Fig. 5.1). Some of the energy from the sun is transferred to the bonds that hold the carbon and hydrogen atoms together. Human cells can release that energy and use it to power various forms of cellular work, including muscle contraction, bone formation, and hormone synthesis.

In addition to being a source of energy, carbohydrates play other import—ant roles in the body. Certain carbohydrates serve as the "glue" that holds cells together in tissues. Cell membranes have carbohydrates that signal the cell's identity to other cells. Saliva, mucus, and the fluid that lubricates skeletal joints contain mucins, a class of carbohydrates that are chemically associated with proteins.

Carbohydrates are often classified into two general categories: simple carbohydrates and complex carbohydrates, which include most forms of dietary fiber. Each class of carbohydrates has effects on health, which will be discussed in this chapter.

carbohydrates class of nutrients that is a major source of energy for the body

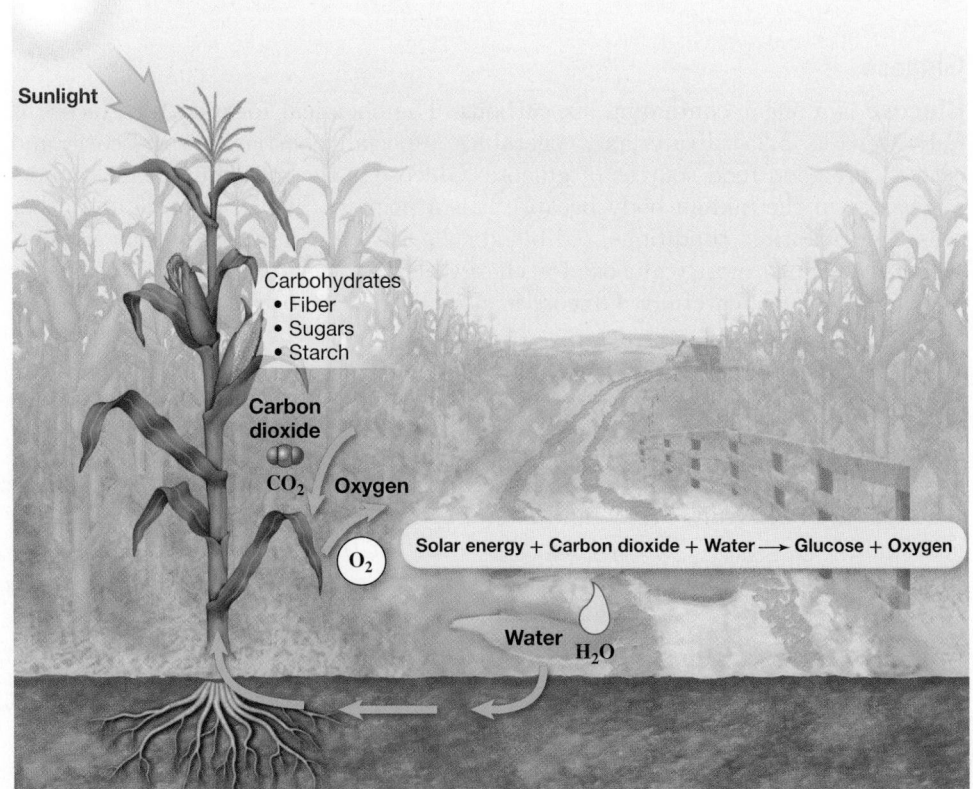

Sunlight

Carbohydrates
• Fiber
• Sugars
• Starch

Carbon dioxide

CO_2 **Oxygen**

O_2 **Solar energy + Carbon dioxide + Water ⟶ Glucose + Oxygen**

Water H_2O

FIGURE 5.1 Carbohydrates. Plants use the sun's energy to combine carbon, oxygen, and hydrogen atoms from carbon dioxide and water to make glucose. As a result of this process, oxygen gas is released. Plants can use glucose to make fiber, starch, and other sugars.

monosaccharide simple sugar that is the basic molecule of carbohydrates

glucose monosaccharide that is a primary fuel for muscles and other cells; "dextrose" or "blood sugar"

fructose monosaccharide in fruits, honey, and certain vegetables; "levulose" or "fruit sugar"

galactose monosaccharide that is a component of lactose

5.2 Simple Carbohydrates

LEARNING OUTCOMES

1 *Describe the three most important dietary monosaccharides and disaccharides.*

2 *Identify nutritive sweeteners that are often added to foods and beverages.*

3 *List FDA-approved nonnutritive sweeteners.*

Most Americans are familiar with sugar as the sweet, white, granulated crystals often sprinkled on cereal or into iced tea, but table sugar is only one type of sugar. There are many different types of sugars, or simple carbohydrates. Milk, blood, and *DNA*, the genetic material in cells, contain specific kinds of sugars. The simplest type of sugar, the **monosaccharide** (*mono* = one; *saccharide* = sugar), is the basic chemical unit of carbohydrates.

Monosaccharides

The three most important dietary monosaccharides are glucose, fructose, and galactose (Fig. 5.2). Glucose, fructose, and galactose all contain carbon, hydrogen, and oxygen in the ratio of 1 carbon: 2 hydrogen: 1 oxygen. The chemical names of carbohydrates, particularly sugars, often end in *ose*. Glu*cose*, fruc*tose*, and galac*tose* are sugars commonly found in foods such as table sugar, fruit, and cow's milk.

Glucose

Glucose is a sugar containing six carbons. The chemical formula for glucose is $C_6H_{12}O_6$ (Fig. 5.2a). Fruits and vegetables, especially berries, grapes, corn, and carrots, are good food sources of glucose. Glucose is the most important mono-saccharide in the human body because it is a primary fuel for muscle and other cells. Under normal conditions, red blood cells as well as brain and other nervous system cells burn mostly glucose for energy. Thus, a healthy body maintains its blood glucose level carefully. Glucose is also called *dextrose* and may be referred to as "blood sugar."

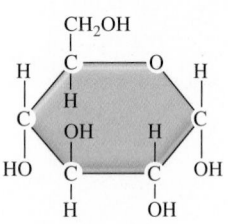

(a)   **Glucose**

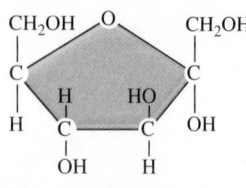

(b)   **Fructose**

Fructose

Fructose has the same chemical formula as glucose, but the monosaccharide has a slightly different structure (Fig. 5.2b). Fructose (fruit sugar or levulose) is naturally found in fruit, honey, and a few vegetables, particularly cabbage, green beans, and asparagus. The body has little need for fructose, but certain cells can convert fructose into glucose or into fat.

Galactose

(c)   **Galactose**

FIGURE 5.2 Monosaccharides. These chemical symbols for glucose, fructose, and galactose indicate the number and arrangement of carbon, hydrogen, and oxygen atoms.

Galactose also has the same formula as glucose and fructose, but the structure of galactose is slightly different from the structure of glucose (Fig. 5.2c). Galactose is not commonly found in foods. Galactose, however, is needed as a component of lactose, the form of carbohydrate in milk.

Disaccharides

A **disaccharide** is a simple sugar that has two monosaccharides linked (bonded) together. Major dietary disaccharides are maltose, sucrose, and lactose (Fig. 5.3). **Maltose** (malt sugar) has two glucose molecules bound together (Fig. 5.3a). Few foods naturally contain maltose. **Sucrose** (table sugar) consists of a molecule of glucose and one of fructose (Fig. 5.3b). **Lactose** (milk sugar) forms when a galactose molecule bonds to a glucose molecule (Fig. 5.3c). Disaccharides form as a result of *condensation reactions* (Fig. 5.4). An *alpha bond* holds the two monosaccharides together in sucrose and maltose (Fig. 5.4). A different kind of bond, a *beta bond*, holds together the two monosaccharides that form lactose (see Fig. 5.3c).

Sucrose

Although sucrose occurs naturally in honey, maple syrup, carrots, and pineapples, much of the sucrose in the American diet is refined from sugar cane and sugar beets. The refining process strips away the small amounts of vitamins and minerals in sugar cane and sugar beets. "Raw sugar," turbinado sugar, and some forms of brown sugar are not as fully processed from sugar cane as white sugar. These sweeteners contain a small amount of *molasses*, which contributes to their flavor, color, and nutritional value. Since refined sucrose has the reputation of being a "junk food," some manufacturers use creative names, such as "granulated cane juice," to disguise the presence of table sugar in their product's ingredient list.

Some people claim that refined white sugar is poisonous and honey is nutritionally superior to table sugar. However, these claims are not true. Table sugar does not contain toxic substances; in fact, it is almost 100% carbohydrate. Table 5.1 compares the nutritional value of honey with certain forms of sucrose. Note that none of the sweeteners is a good source of protein, fat, vitamins, or minerals. The monosaccharides in honey are not superior to the monosaccharides that comprise sucrose. When a person eats a food that contains the simple sugars in honey and table sugar, his or her body does not distinguish whether the end-products of digestion—glucose and fructose—came from sugar or honey.

A tablespoon of white table sugar is almost 100% sucrose; a tablespoon of honey has free glucose, free fructose, water, and a small amount of sucrose. Although the tablespoon of honey contains more protein and micronutrients than the tablespoon of white sugar, the amounts are insignificant. For example, a person would have to eat a cup of honey to obtain 1 g of protein, 2 mg of vitamin C, and 1.4 mg of iron. That amount of honey supplies over 1000 kcal! Although honey contains phytochemicals, substances in plant foods that may provide health benefits, the amounts are too small to make this sticky sweetener a valuable source of these compounds.

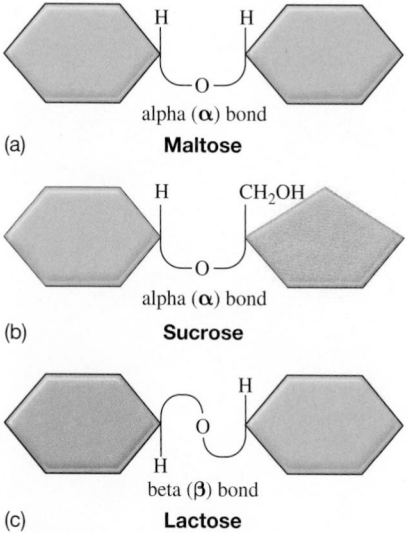

FIGURE 5.3 Disaccharides.

disaccharide simple sugar comprised of two monosaccharides

maltose disaccharide composed of two glucose molecules; "malt sugar"

sucrose disaccharide composed of a glucose and a fructose molecule; "table sugar"

lactose disaccharide composed of a glucose and a galactose molecule; "milk sugar"

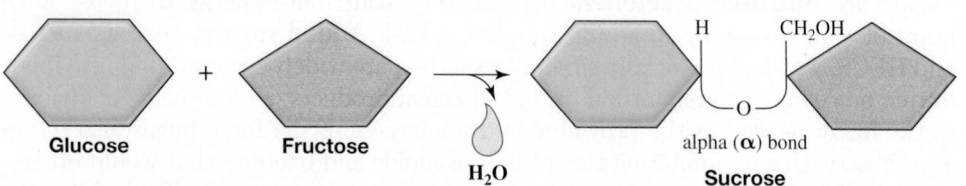

FIGURE 5.4 Condensation reaction. A condensation reaction is one where two molecules bond to form a larger molecule, releasing water in the process. Disaccharides are formed through condensation reactions. In this example, glucose and fructose combine to form sucrose.

DID **YOU** KNOW?

Bees make honey by consuming the sucrose-rich nectar from flowers and digesting most of it into glucose and fructose. The bees regurgitate this material within the beehive, and eventually, it is collected by beekeepers for processing and packaging.

TABLE 5.1 Nutritional Comparison of Selected Sweeteners

Sugar/Syrup 1 Tablespoon	Water %	Kcal	Protein g	Carb g	Vit. C mg	Calcium mg	Niacin mg	Potassium mg	Iron mg	Zinc mg
Honey	17	64	0.06	17.3	0.1	1	0.025	11	0.09	0.05
White granulated sugar	0	49	0	12.6	0	0	0	0	0.01	0
Maple syrup	32	52	0.01	13.4	0	20	0.016	42	0.02	0.29
High-fructose corn syrup	24	53	0	14.4	0	0	0	0	0.01	0
Brown sugar	1	52	0.02	13.5	0	11	0.015	18	0.10	0
Molasses	22	58	0	15.0	0	41	0.186	293	0.94	0.06

Source: Data from *USDA National nutrient database for standard reference, release 25.*

FRESH TIPS

Honey can contain spores (the inactive life stage) of the deadly bacterium *Clostridium botulinum* that resist being destroyed by food preservation methods. These spores can become active within an infant's intestinal tract because the baby's immature stomach does not produce acid strong enough to kill the spores. The bacteria can then produce a poison that is extremely toxic to nerves.[1] According to experts at the Centers for Disease Control and Prevention (CDC), honey should not be fed to children younger than 12 months of age or used to sweeten infant foods because it may cause botulism poisoning.[2] Older children and adults can eat honey without being concerned about botulism, because the mature stomach produces enough acid to destroy the bacterial spores.

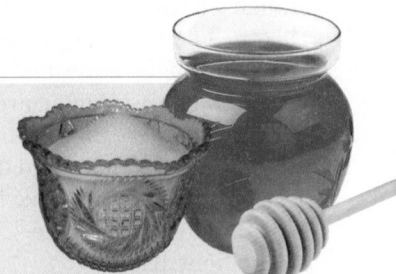

Honey and table sugar have similar nutritional value.

high-fructose corn syrup (HFCS) syrup obtained from the processing of corn

nutritive sweeteners substances that sweeten and contribute energy to foods

added sugars sugars added to foods during processing or preparation

What Is High-Fructose Corn Syrup?

Fructose tastes much sweeter than glucose and is easily obtained from the processing of corn, a crop readily available in the United States. Food manufacturers use large amounts of **high–fructose corn syrup (HFCS)** as a food additive. Despite the name, HFCS contains approximately the same amount of fructose as is found in sucrose. Although Americans' high intake of HFCS has been blamed for causing poor health and disease, there is no conclusive scientific evidence that consuming HFCS is more detrimental to health than consuming regular table sugar.[3,4] Consumption of foods and beverages sweetened with either HFCS or table sugar is associated with excess caloric intake. These excess calories can contribute to an increased risk for diabetes and heart disease.

Nutritive Sweeteners

Sugars are **nutritive sweeteners** because they contribute energy to foods. Each gram of a mono–or disaccharide supplies 4 kcal. **Added sugars**, such as sucrose and HFCS, which is chemically similar to sucrose, are widely incorporated into foods during processing or preparation. In baked cereal products, added sugars contribute to the flavor as well as the browning and tenderness of the food. Sugar also serves as a preservative by inhibiting the growth of molds and bacteria that would otherwise cause food spoilage. If one of the nutritive sweeteners listed in Table 5.2 is the first or second ingredient listed on a product's label, the food probably contains a high amount of added sugar. Table 5.3 indicates the amounts of added sugars that are in typical servings of commonly consumed foods and beverages.

TABLE 5.2 Names for Sugars

Raw sugar	High-fructose corn syrup (HFCS)	Polydextrose
Brown sugar	Cultured corn syrup	Fructose (levulose)
Table sugar	High-maltose corn syrup	Invert sugar
Turbinado sugar	Agave nectar	Lactose
Confectioner's or powdered sugar	Maple syrup	Maltose
Coconut sugar	Molasses	Maltodextrin
Date sugar	Honey	Sorbitol
Evaporated cane juice	Fruit juice concentrate	Mannitol
Granulated cane juice	Fruit juice sweetener	Xylitol
Corn sweeteners	Glucose	Erythritol
Corn syrup	Dextrose	

Alternative Sweeteners

Some people choose to control their caloric intake by reducing their consumption of foods and beverages sweetened with nutritive sweeteners such as sugar. **Alternative sweeteners** (also referred to as sugar substitutes or "artificial" sweeteners) are substances added to food that sweeten the item while providing few or no kcal.

Alternative nutritive sweeteners include **sugar alcohols**: *sorbitol*, *xylitol*, and *mannitol*. Unlike sugars, sugar alcohols do not promote dental decay.[6] Food manufacturers use sugar alcohols to replace sucrose in products such as sugar-free chewing gums, sugar-free breath mints, and some sugar-free candies. Sugar alcohols are not fully absorbed by the intestinal tract, and

alternative sweeteners substances that sweeten foods while providing few or no kilocalories

sugar alcohols alternative sweeteners used to replace sucrose in some sugar-free foods; sorbitol, xylitol, and mannitol

TABLE 5.3 How Much Added Sugar Is In That Food?

Food	Serving Size	Kcal	Approximate Teaspoons Added Sugars
Doughnut, cake, plain	3 ¼" diameter	226	2
Chocolate chip cookies, commercial brand	2 medium (50 g)	239	4
Sugar-frosted cornflakes	¾ cup	114	3
Chocolate-flavored 2% milk	1 cup	158	3
Ice cream, vanilla, light, soft-serve	½ cup	111	2
Chocolate candy bar with almonds	1.76 oz	235	5
Yogurt, vanilla low-fat	8 oz	193	4
Cola, canned	12 fl oz	136	8
Fruit punch drink	12 fl oz	175	10
Chocolate milkshake, fast food	16 fl oz	580	10

Source of data: Krebs-Smith SM: Choose beverages and foods to moderate your intake of sugars: Measurement requires quantification. *Journal of Nutrition* 131:527S, 2006.

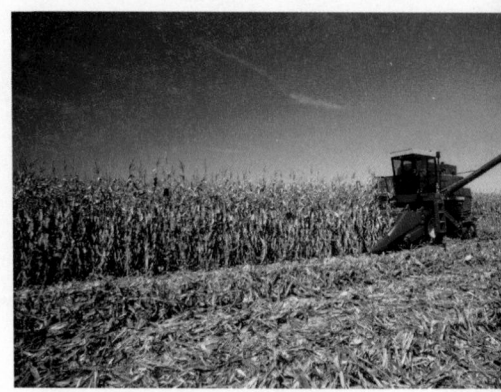

According to the U.S. Department of Agriculture (USDA), farmers in the United States produce over 13 billion bushels of corn annually. The majority of corn grown is used as an energy source in livestock feed. However, corn can also be processed to make high-fructose corn syrup (HFCS), a common sweetener.

TABLE 5.4 Comparing Nonnutritive Sweeteners

Sweetener	Comparison to Sugar/ Serving*	Brand Name	Kilocalories/ Serving
Aspartame	160–220 times sweeter	NutraSweet®, Equal®	Nearly 0
Saccharin	300 times sweeter	Sweet'N Low®, Sugar Twin®, Necta Sweet®	0
Acesulfame-K	200 times sweeter	Sunett®, Sweet One®	0
Neotame	7,000–13,000 times sweeter	Neotame	0
Sucralose	600 times sweeter	Splenda®	0
"Stevia," including stevia leaf extracts such as rebaudioside A	250 times sweeter	Truvia®, SweetLeaf®, Rebiana	0
Erythritol	60 to 80% as sweet	Nectresse™	<5

*Source: Position of the Academy of Nutrition and Dietetics: Use of nutritive and nonnutritive sweeteners. *Journal of the Academy of Nutrition and Dietetics*, 112(5): 739, 2012.

as a result, they supply an average of 2 kcal/g. Because sugar alcohols are incompletely absorbed, the alternative sweeteners may cause diarrhea when consumed.

Nonnutritive sweeteners are a group of synthetic compounds that elicit an intensely sweet taste when compared to the same amount of sugar (Table 5.4). Thus, very small amounts of nonnutritive sweeteners are needed to sweeten a food, and they supply no energy per serving. Nonnutritive sweeteners can help people control their energy intake.[7] Consumers, however, need to recognize that most "sugar–free" or "diabetic" foods are not calorie free. The Food and Drug Administration (FDA) has approved the use of the nonnutritive sweeteners listed in Table 5.4 as additives to sweeten foods as well as other products that may be swallowed, such as mouthwash and toothpaste.

nonnutritive sweeteners group of synthetic compounds that are intensely sweet tasting compared to sugar

The Safety of Nonnutritive Sweeteners

In the United States, the safety of nonnutritive sweeteners has been under public and scientific scrutiny for decades. In 1970, the FDA banned the nonnutritive sweetener *cyclamate* after research indicated that the substance caused bladder cancer in mice. In the 1980s, panels of experts at the FDA and the National Academy of Sciences reviewed the scientific evidence and determined that cycla–mate did not increase the risk of cancer in humans. Nevertheless, the ban on this food additive continues in the United States. Although *saccharin* has been in use for over 100 years, its safety has also been questioned.[7] Despite the concern, most of the scientific evidence indicates that saccharin is safe when consumed in amounts that are less than nine packets of saccharin–containing sweetener per day.

Aspartame consists of phenylalanine and aspartic acid, two amino acids (the molecules that comprise proteins). Some people must avoid aspartame and certain protein–rich foods because they have *phenylketonuria* (PKU) (*fen'–nul–keet'–en–yur'–e–ah*), a rare inherited disorder that results in abnormal phenylalanine metabolism. If an infant with PKU is not treated with a special diet, phenylal–anine and its metabolic by–products accumulate in the child's bloodstream and cause severe brain damage. All infants born in the United States and Canada are tested for PKU soon after birth. To alert people with PKU about the presence of aspartame in foods, the FDA requires manufacturers of products containing the nonnutritive sweetener to include a warning on the label (Fig. 5.5). One of the "Real People, Real Stories" features in Chapter 7 is about a young person who has PKU.

Since its approval for use as a food additive in 1981, aspartame has been blamed for causing a variety of health problems, including cancer, certain immune system diseases, and chronic headaches. Despite these claims, no scientifically reliable studies have linked aspartame to any health disorder.[7] In 2006, results of a European study involving rats concluded that aspartame increased the risk of cancer in the animals.[8] The European Food Safety Authority challenged the findings of this study when it determined the conclusions were not supported by the data. The safety of aspartame has been studied extensively, and at the present time, no links to cancer have been found.

Sucralose is made from a molecule of sucrose that has been chemically modified to become nondigestible. As a result, sucralose sweetens foods and beverages without increasing their caloric value. Because the sweetener is not digested or absorbed by the intestinal tract, it is excreted unchanged in feces. During normal cooking and storage conditions, sucralose resists destruction by heat, a feature that makes it better for sweetening baked products than aspartame, which breaks down when heated.

Some of the newest nonnutritive sweeteners are made from the leaves of the South American shrub *Stevia rebaudiana* Bertoni. For hundreds of years, people have used extracts of stevia leaves, called stevioside, as sweeteners. *Rebiana* is the common name for the chemical in stevia leaves (rebaudioside A) that is responsible for their intense sweetness.

A group of international health and safety organizations, including the FDA, have established *Acceptable Daily Intakes* (*ADIs*) for certain nonnutritive sweeteners (Table 5.5). According to the Academy of Nutrition and Dietetics, nonnutritive sweeteners are safe when consumed "within acceptable daily intakes, even during pregnancy."[7]

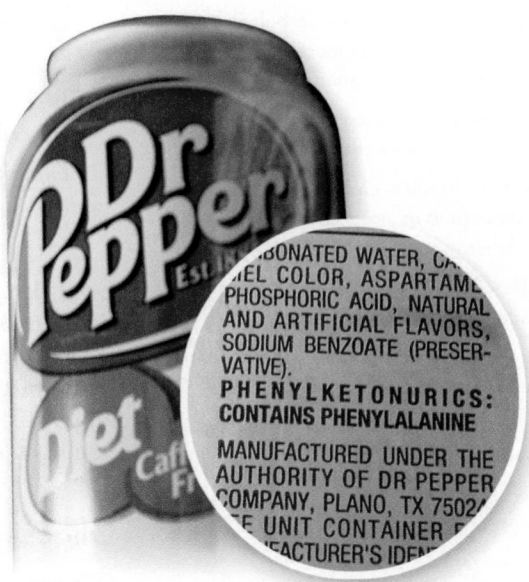

FIGURE 5.5 Warning label for people with PKU.

DID **YOU** KNOW?

Results of several studies suggest that stevioside and related compounds in the *stevia* leaf may offer therapeutic benefits such as improvement in blood glucose levels, blood pressure, and digestive function.[9,10] More research, however, is needed to determine the usefulness of stevia leaf extracts as treatments for various health problems.

TABLE 5.5 Acceptable Daily Intakes for Some Nonnutritive Sweeteners

Food/Beverage	Nonnutritive Sweetener	Amount
Diet cola	Aspartame	18 to 19 12-oz cans
Packets	Saccharin	9 to 12 packets
Lemon-lime soft drink	Acesulfame-K	30 to 32 12-oz cans
Diet cola	Sucralose	6 12-oz cans

Source: Mattes RD, Popkin BM: Non-nutritive sweetener consumption in humans: Effects on appetite and food intake and their putative mechanisms. *American Journal of Clinical Nutrition* 89(1):1, 2009.

ASSESS YOUR PROGRESS

4 List the chemical names for blood sugar, table sugar, milk sugar, and malt sugar.

5 Name the monosaccharides that comprise each molecule of maltose, lactose, and sucrose.

6 What is the difference between a nutritive sweetener and a nonnutritive sweetener?

7 Explain why consuming foods or beverages that contain aspartame may be dangerous for certain people.

complex carbohydrates carbohydrates comprised of three or more monosaccharides bonded together

polysaccharides carbohydrates comprised of 10 or more monosaccharides bonded together

oligosaccharides carbohydrates comprised of three to 10 monosaccharides bonded together

raffinose nondigestible oligosaccharide made of three monosaccharides

stachyose nondigestible oligosaccharide made of four monosaccharides

starch storage polysaccharide in plants; composed of amylose and amylopectin

glycogen highly branched storage polysaccharide in animals

5.3 Complex Carbohydrates

LEARNING OUTCOMES

1 *Describe the differences among oligosaccharides, starch, glycogen, and fiber.*

2 *Explain why starch is digestible and fiber is nondigestible in humans.*

3 *Compare soluble and insoluble fiber.*

Complex carbohydrates have three or more monosaccharides bonded together. **Polysaccharides** (*poly* = many) are complex carbohydrates comprised of more than 10 monosaccharides bonded together. Plants and animals use complex carbohydrates to store energy or make certain structural components such as stems and leaves. The most common dietary polysaccharides include digestible and nondigestible forms.

Oligosaccharides

Oligosaccharides (*oligo* = a few) are complex carbohydrates comprised of three to 10 monosaccharides. The most common oligosaccharides in foods are **raffinose** (*raf′−ih−nos*) and **stachyose** (*stack′−ee−os*). Food sources of raffinose and stachyose include onions, brussels sprouts, cabbage, broccoli, legumes, and whole grains. Other oligosaccharides include inulin and oligofructose. Chicory root, onions, garlic, leeks, legumes, asparagus, and wheat are among the richest natural sources of inulin and oligofructose.

Human digestive enzymes do not readily break down oligosaccharides, so most of these carbohydrates pass through the stomach and small intestine intact. In the large intestine, bacteria can use oligosaccharides as a source of energy, producing waste products (various gases) as a result. This explains why people often experience bloating and intestinal gas (*flatulence*) after consuming foods that contain oligosaccharides, especially legumes, whole grains, and other vegetables that are rich in raffinose and stachyose.

To reduce flatulence, people can take a product, such as Beano®, immediately before a meal that contains these oligosaccharides. Beano contains *alpha−galactosidase*, the enzyme that breaks down oligosaccharides, so fewer of them reach the colon to be metabolized by bacteria.

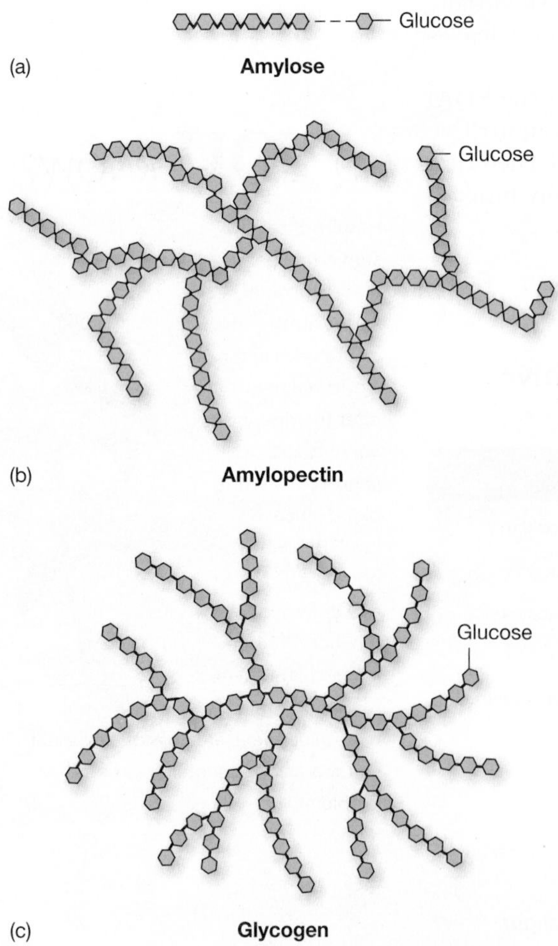

(a) **Amylose**

(b) **Amylopectin**

(c) **Glycogen**

FIGURE 5.6 Starch and glycogen. Starch and glycogen contain hundreds of glucose molecules bound together into large chainlike structures. (*a*) Amylose and (*b*) amylopectin are forms of starch made by plants. (*c*) The chains of glycogen are more highly branched than those of starch.

Starch and Glycogen

Starch and glycogen are polysaccharides that contain hundreds of glucose molecules bound together into large, chainlike structures (Fig. 5.6). As shown in Figure 5.6, **starch** is composed of amylose, a linear chain of glucose molecules, and amylopectin, a branched chain of glucose molecules. Plants store glucose as starch, particularly in their seeds, roots, and fleshy underground stems called tubers. Rich food sources of starch include bread and cereal products made from wheat, rice, barley, and oats; vegetables such as corn, squash, beans, and peas; and tubers such as potatoes, yams, taro, cassava, and jicama. Sports drinks and sports or energy bars often include modified starches such as *maltodextrin* and *dextrin*. Regardless of its source, each gram of starch supplies 4 kcal, the same as other digestible carbohydrate sources.

The human body stores limited amounts of glucose as **glycogen** (Fig. 5.6c). Muscles and the liver are the major sites for glycogen formation and storage. Although muscles contain glycogen, most animal foods (e.g., red meat or the flesh or muscle of fish and poultry) are not sources of this complex carbohydrate, because muscle glycogen breaks down soon after an animal dies.

Fiber

In addition to storing energy as starch, plants use complex carbo—hydrates to make supportive structures and protective seed coats that contribute to the fiber content of the diet. Most forms of **dietary fiber ("fiber")** are complex carbohydrates comprised of monosaccharides connected by bonds that humans cannot digest (Fig. 5.7). *Cellulose, hemicellulose, pectin, gums,* and *mucilages* are carbohydrate forms of fiber; *lignin* is the only type of fiber that is not carbohydrate. Because fiber is not digested, it moves through the human intestinal tract and contributes to the residue that is eventually eliminated in feces.

There are two types of dietary fiber, **soluble fiber** and **insoluble fiber**. Soluble types of fiber, such as pectins and gums, dissolve or swell in water. Insoluble forms of fiber, such as cellu—lose and lignin, generally do not dissolve in water. Oat bran and oatmeal, beans, apples, carrots, oranges and other citrus fruits, and psyllium (*sill'—e—um*) seeds are rich sources of soluble fiber; whole—grain products, including brown rice, contain high amounts of insoluble fiber. Table 5.6 provides information about the solubility of various types of fiber, effects of fiber in the body, and major food sources of soluble and insoluble fiber. Although the foods listed in Table 5.6 are rich sources of either soluble or insoluble fiber, plant foods usually contain both forms.

The FDA allows products made from ground, cracked, or flaked cereal grains to be labeled as "whole grain" only if they contain the starchy endosperm, oily germ, and fiber—rich bran seed components in the same relative proportions as they exist in the intact grain.[11] Refined grain products are generally low in fiber, because such foods lack the fiber—rich bran seed component (Fig. 5.8). To determine whether a product contains whole grains, review the ingredient list on the package label and look for "whole grain ..." in the name of a major ingredient (Fig. 5.9).

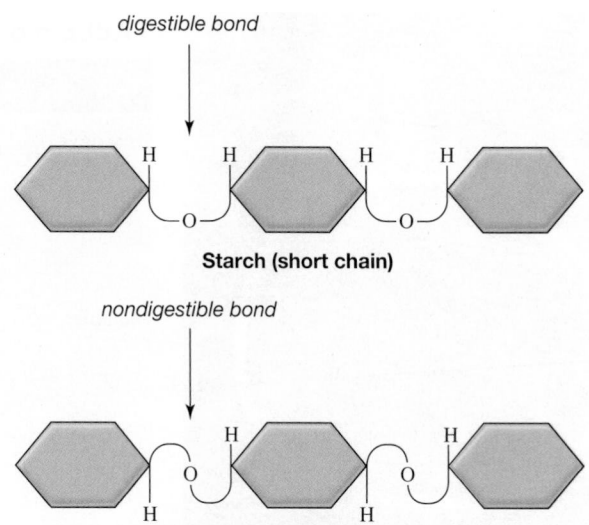

FIGURE 5.7 Starch and fiber bonds. The bonds that link glucose units together in starch are digestible. Enzymes in the human digestive tract cannot break apart the bonds between glucose molecules in fiber.

dietary fiber ("fiber") nondigestible plant material; most types are polysaccharides

soluble fiber forms of dietary fiber that dissolve or swell in water; include pectins, gums, mucilages, and some hemicelluloses

insoluble fiber forms of dietary fiber that generally do not dissolve in water; include cellulose, hemicelluloses, and lignin

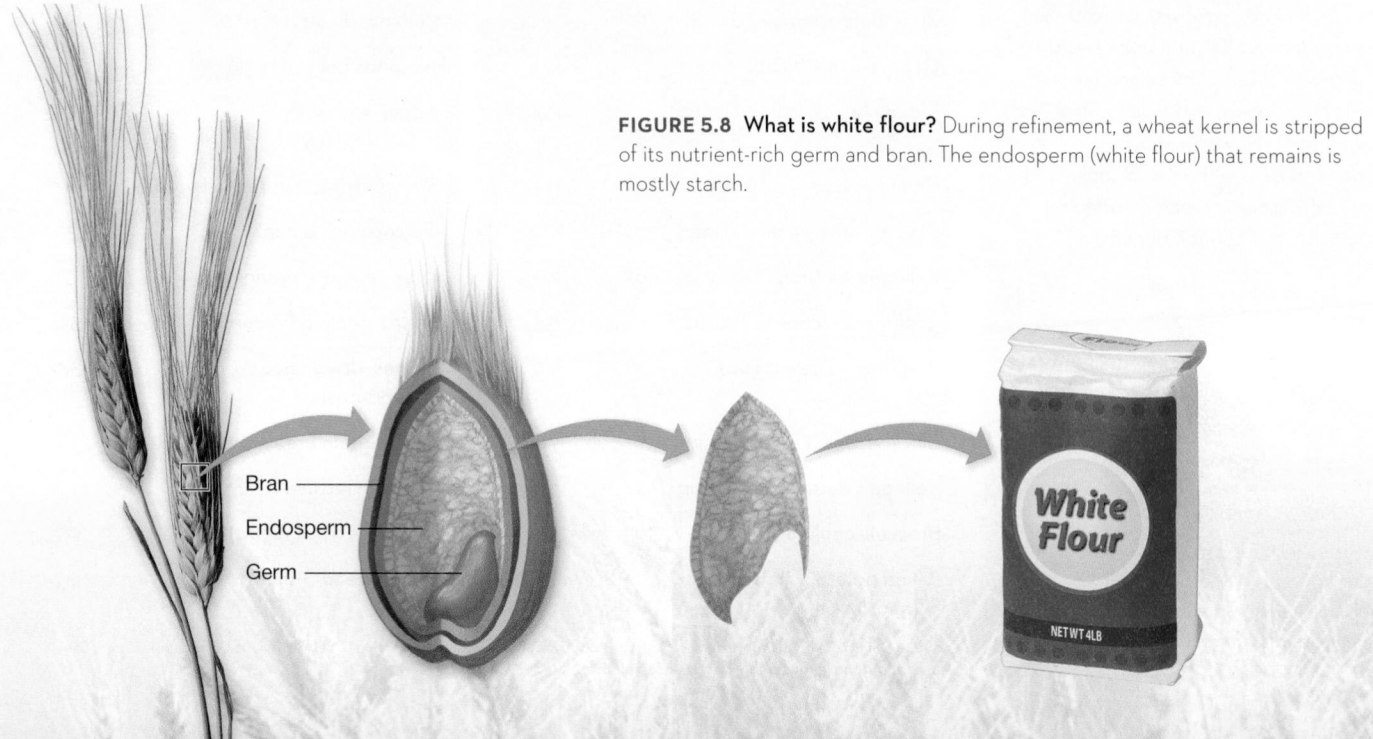

FIGURE 5.8 What is white flour? During refinement, a wheat kernel is stripped of its nutrient-rich germ and bran. The endosperm (white flour) that remains is mostly starch.

Bran
Endosperm
Germ

White Flour
NET WT 4 LB

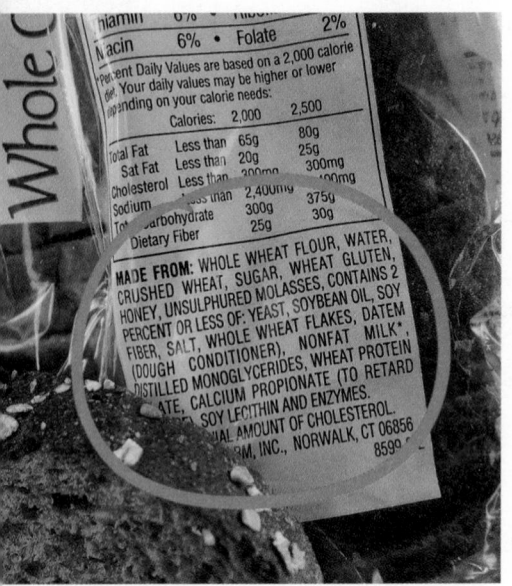

FIGURE 5.9 Whole grain. According to food-labeling guidelines issued by the FDA, whole grains are intact, ground, cracked, or flaked seeds of cereal grains.

TABLE 5.6 Classifying Fiber

Type	Component(s)	Physiological Effects	Food Sources
Insoluble	Cellulose, hemicelluloses	Increases fecal bulk and speeds fecal passage through GI tract	All plants, especially whole wheat, rye, brown rice, vegetables
	Lignin	Increases fecal bulk, may ease bowel movements	Whole grains, wheat bran
Soluble	Pectins, gums, mucilages, some hemicelluloses	Delays stomach emptying; slows glucose absorption; can lower blood cholesterol	Apples, bananas, citrus fruits, carrots, oats, barley, psyllium seeds, beans, and thickeners added to foods

Although fiber is not digested by humans, soluble and insoluble fiber provide important health benefits. Soluble fiber can help reduce blood cholesterol levels, and insoluble fiber may ease bowel movements. Section 5.8 on "Carbohydrates and Health" provides information about the benefits of adding more fiber to diets and practical ways to increase fiber intake.

Table 5.7 lists common foods that are sources of dietary fiber. Note that only plant foods provide dietary fiber; animal flesh contains muscle fibers, which are digestible proteins. The recommended Adequate Intakes (AIs) for fiber are 38 and 25 g/day for young men and women, respectively, but the typical American diet supplies only about 16 g of dietary fiber/day.

DID **YOU** KNOW?

Inulin and oligofructose are often the main ingredients in prebiotics, which promote growth of healthful bacteria in the large intestine. Consumption of inulin and oligofructose may also benefit heart, GI, and bone health; improve blood glucose and blood pressure levels; and help control body weight.[12,13] However, more research is needed before the use of inulin and oligofructose is recommended for specific therapeutic benefits.[14,15]

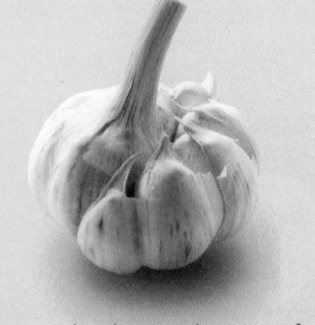

Onions and garlic are rich sources of inulin and oligofructoses.

TABLE 5.7 Dietary Fiber Content of Common Foods

Food	Fiber (g)	Food	Fiber (g)
Split peas, cooked (1 cup)	16.3	Beans, green snap, cooked (1 cup)	4.0
Black beans, cooked (1 cup)	15.0	Banana, sliced (1 cup)	3.9
Oat bran, raw (1 cup)	14.5	Almonds (24 almonds)	3.5
Kidney beans, canned (1 cup)	13.6	Apple, with skin (approx. 4.5 oz)	3.3
Chickpeas, cooked (1 cup)	12.5	Strawberries, raw, sliced (1 cup)	3.3
Baked beans, canned (1 cup)	10.4	Carrots, raw (1 cup)	3.1
Kellogg's All-Bran® cereal (½ cup)	8.8	Orange, raw (1 orange)	3.1
Green peas, cooked (1 cup)	8.8	Barley, cooked (½ cup)	3.0
Raspberries, raw (1 cup)	8.0	Prunes, dried uncooked (5 prunes)	3.0
Blackberries (1 cup)	7.6	Whole-grain bread (1 slice)	1.9
Kellogg's Raisin Bran® (1 cup)	6.8	Romaine lettuce (1 cup)	1.2
Broccoli, cooked (1 cup)	5.1	Iceberg lettuce (1 cup)	0.7
Baked potato, with skin (approx. 6.5 oz)	4.4	White bread (1 slice)	0.7

Source: Data from U.S. Department of Agriculture, Agricultural Research Service, USDA Nutrient Data Laboratory: *USDA Nutrient database for standard reference, release 25, 2012.*

FRESH TIPS

Many people do not eat beans because they want to avoid flatulence and other unpleasant GI side effects. To reduce the oligosaccharide content of beans, soak dried beans in room temperature water (3 parts water and 1 part beans) for 16 hours.[16] Then, discard the water before cooking the beans. Pretreatment soaking causes the oligosaccharides to dissolve and leach out into the water. This reduces the beans' oligosaccharide content and reduces the likelihood of experiencing unwanted GI side effects.

ASSESS YOUR PROGRESS

8 *Distinguish between glycogen and starch, including similarities and differences.*
9 *What is dietary fiber?*
10 *Identify at least two food sources of soluble fiber and two sources of insoluble fiber.*
11 *What is the FDA definition of a food product labeled "whole grain"?*

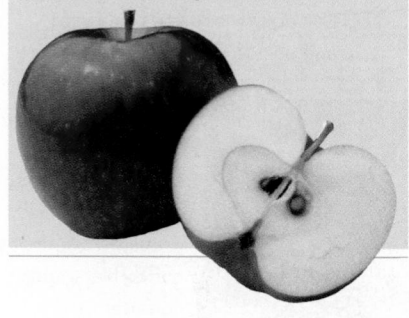

DID YOU KNOW?

Different forms of a food can have very different fiber contents. For example, an unpeeled raw apple that weighs 6 ounces (about 3 inches in diameter) has 4.8 g of fiber. However, 6 ounces of applesauce contains 2.0 g of fiber, and a 6-ounce serving of apple juice provides only 0.4 g of fiber.

5.4 Carbohydrate Consumption Patterns

LEARNING OUTCOMES

1 *Describe carbohydrate consumption patterns in the United States.*
2 *List strategies to reduce a person's intake of refined carbohydrates.*

In developing nations, millions of people rely on diets that supply 70% or more of energy from relatively unprocessed carbohydrates, especially complex carbohydrates in whole grains, beans, potatoes, corn, and other starchy vegetables. In industrialized nations, people tend to eat more highly refined starches and added sugars. The diet of the typical American (2 years of age and older) supplies about 51% of kcal from carbohydrates (Fig. 5.10). Nutritionally adequate diets provide 45 to 65% of total energy from carbohydrates, preferably from foods that are rich sources of unrefined carbohydrates.[17]

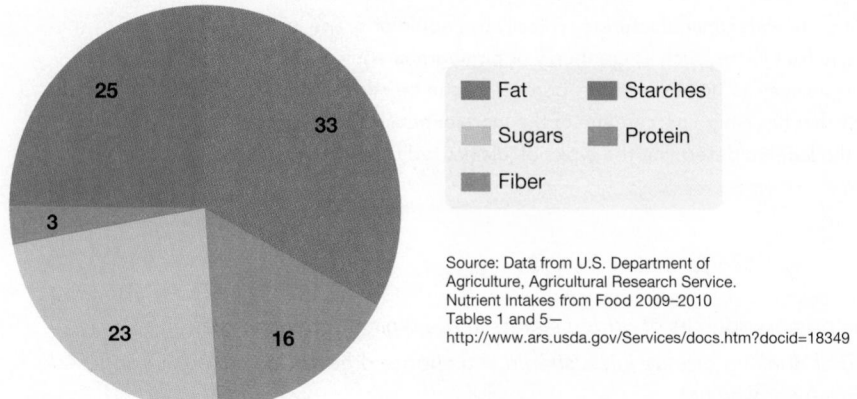

Fat   Starches
Sugars   Protein
Fiber

Source: Data from U.S. Department of Agriculture, Agricultural Research Service. Nutrient Intakes from Food 2009–2010 Tables 1 and 5— http://www.ars.usda.gov/Services/docs.htm?docid=18349

FIGURE 5.10 Macronutrient consumption in the United States. This graph shows the average American's (over 2 years of age) intake of macronutrients and alcohol as percentages of total kcal (2070 kcal) on one day in 2009–2010. (Percentage of total energy from alcohol is not included.)

DID **YOU** KNOW?

The typical 24-ounce commercial iced coffee beverage contains over 500 kcal and 70 g of sugars; a 16-ounce serving of a hot espresso-based chocolate drink provides nearly 400 kcal and 40 g of sugar! According to results of one study, college students who were regular drinkers of such gourmet coffee beverages consumed 206 more kcal and 32 more grams of sugar per day than those who did not consume such drinks.[22] If you drink commercially prepared gourmet coffee beverages, consider requesting a "skinny," that is, a coffee prepared with low-fat milk and without flavored syrups.

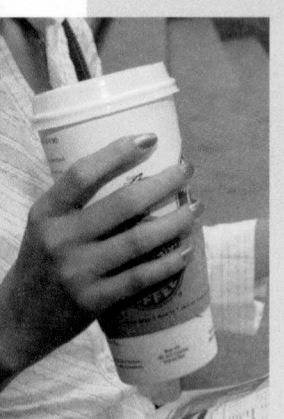

Added Sugar Consumption

In 2012, there were enough added sugars available for each American to consume almost 130 pounds of added sugars yearly.[18] This amount of added sugars provided over 30% of the energy, or 600 kcal per day, in a diet that supplies 2000 kcal/day. According to the Dietary Guidelines, people should limit their added sugar intake to less than 10% of total calories. A 12-ounce can of a cola-flavored, caffein-ated, sugar-sweetened soft drink contains 33 g of refined added sugars, primarily HFCS.[19] Each gram of sugar supplies 4 kcal, so the sugars in the soft drink con-tribute about 132 kcal to a person's diet. By drinking only one can of the cola, a person who needs 2000 kcal daily will almost meet two-thirds of his or her daily recommended limit for the intake of added sugars. (see Chapter 3).

A 12-ounce serving of 100% unsweetened orange juice supplies almost the same amount of sugars as 12 ounces of a sugar-sweetened cola. Because both beverages contain simple sugars, should a person drink regular soft drinks instead of fruit juices? Unlike colas and other soft drinks, 100% fruit juices, such as orange, grapefruit, and cranberry juice, contribute micronutrients and antioxi-dant phytochemicals to diets.

Regular soft drinks and energy drinks are major sources of added sugars in Americans' diets. While energy drink consumption has increased in the United States over the past few years, soft drink consumption declined from 1999 to 2010.[20] Still, the average American drank about 47 gallons of carbonated soft drinks in 2009, or about 16 fluid ounces of these beverages daily, most of which were sweetened with refined sugars.[21]

Regular soft drinks, cookies, chips, and many other types of processed snack foods contain large amounts of refined carbohydrates, including added sugars. Such foods can satisfy hunger, but they may be crowding out more nutritious items from the diet.

FRESH TIPS

- Replace soft drinks with a naturally calorie-free thirst-quencher: plain water.
- Make plain water more interesting to drink by adding to it a slice of lemon or lime, or a few fresh or frozen berries.
- Add 1 part club soda to 1 part orange or other 100% fruit juice to make a refreshing carbonated drink.
- Read the label carefully for information about juice content when selecting a fruit juice product. Fruit "drinks," "punches," "blends," "cocktails," or "ades" often contain added sugars and may provide only 10% fruit juice.
- In addition to water, manufacturers typically use apple or grape juice to dilute more expensive fruit juices, such as cranberry or pomegranate juice. Therefore, beverage descriptors such as "100% juice" or "pure juice" can be misleading, especially if you want a product that has a high percentage of the more expensive fruit juices. Read the ingredient list on the label to determine the types of juices used to prepare the product.

ASSESS YOUR PROGRESS

12 List the primary sources of added sugars in the typical American diet.

13 Instead of drinking orange juice, should you choose a beverage called "Orange-Ade"? Explain why or why not.

14 Explain the ways in which apple slices or whole-grain crackers that are topped with a tablespoon of peanut butter provide a more nutritious snack than a 1-½-ounce milk chocolate bar.

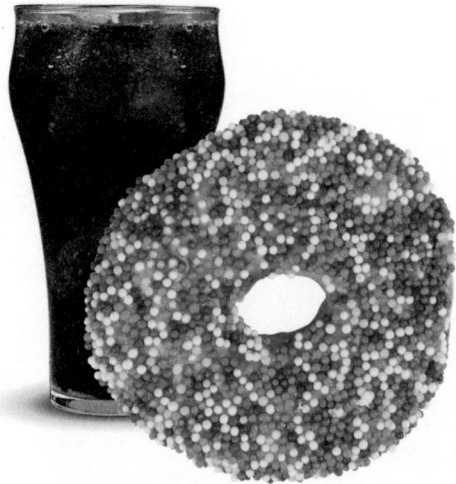

Sugar-sweetened beverages, pastries, and desserts are commonly consumed sources of added sugars.

5.5 Carbohydrates: Digestion and Absorption

LEARNING OUTCOMES

1 *List the sequence of carbohydrate digestion, beginning with the mouth.*
2 *Identify the part of the digestive tract in which carbohydrate absorption occurs and the organ in which carbohydrate breakdown is completed.*
3 *Explain how fiber affects bacterial growth in the colon.*

What happens to the carbohydrates in the body when a person eats a bowl of cooked oatmeal made with milk and sweetened with a little brown sugar for breakfast? The carbohydrates in oats are primarily starch and fiber; mixing milk and brown sugar with the cereal adds lactose and sucrose. All of these carbohydrates must be broken down into monosaccharides, primarily glucose, before they are absorbed in the small intestine.

pancreatic amylase enzyme secreted by pancreas that breaks down starch into maltose molecules

maltase enzyme that splits maltose molecule

sucrase enzyme that splits sucrose molecule

lactase enzyme that splits lactose molecule

Carbohydrate Digestion

The small intestine is the main site for carbohydrate digestion and absorption, but a minor amount of starch digestion begins in the mouth, as salivary amylase converts some of the oat starch molecules into maltose. Starch digestion, however, stops soon after the food enters the acidic environment of the stomach. The fiber in the oats slows the rate at which chyme empties from the stomach, and this delay promotes fullness and *satiety* (the feeling that one has eaten enough).

In the small intestine, an amylase secreted by the pancreas (**pancreatic amylase**) breaks down the remaining polysaccharides in oat starch into maltose molecules. The enzyme **maltase** digests maltose into glucose molecules. The small intestinal enzyme **sucrase** splits each sucrose molecule from the brown sugar, forming one glucose and one fructose molecule in the process. Additionally, the enzyme **lactase** breaks down the lactose from the milk into glucose and galactose molecules. At this point, the disaccharides and complex carbohydrates (except fiber) in the meal have been broken down into the monosaccharides glucose, fructose, and galactose (Fig. 5.11).

DID **YOU** KNOW?

Results of animal studies indicate that dietary fructose from high-fructose corn syrup enhances sodium absorption in the small intestine. If the body absorbs too much sodium, the excess mineral may contribute to the development of high blood pressure.[23] Research involving humans is needed to determine the effects of a high-HFCS diet on blood pressure.

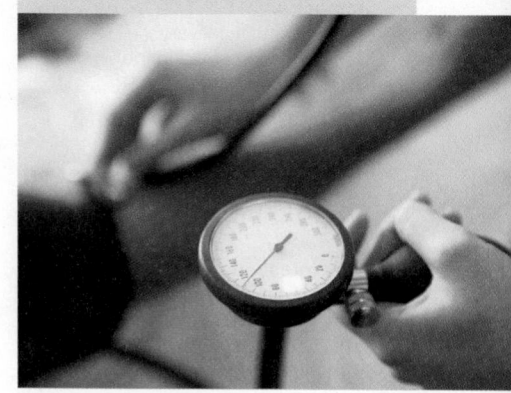

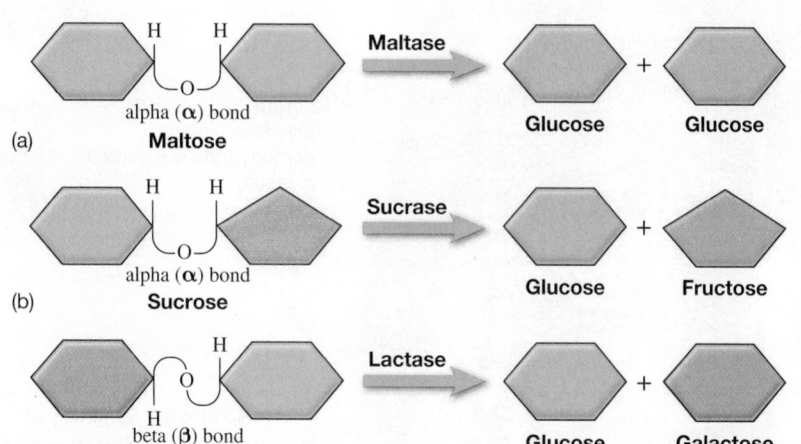

FIGURE 5.11 Digestion of disaccharides. The enzymes (*a*) maltase, (*b*) sucrase, and (*c*) lactase break down disaccharides into monosaccharides in preparation for absorption.

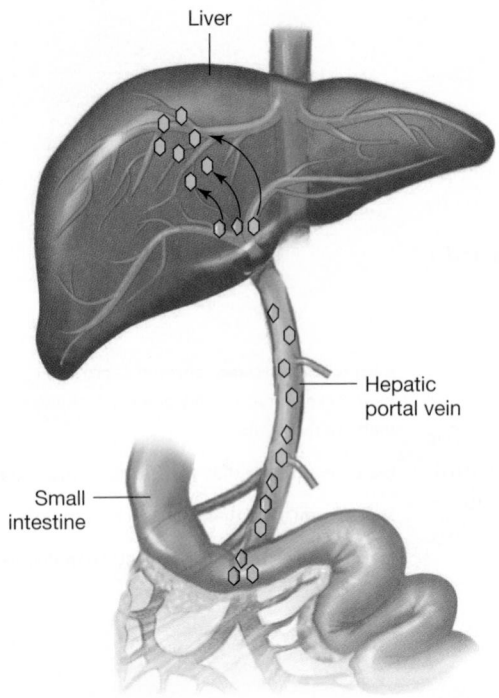

Liver

Hepatic portal vein

Small intestine

FIGURE 5.12 Transport of monosaccharides to the liver. Glucose, fructose, and galactose are absorbed from the small intestine and travel through the hepatic portal vein to the liver. In the liver, galactose and some fructose are converted into glucose.

Carbohydrate Absorption

Absorption of monosaccharides occurs almost exclusively in the small intestine. Intestinal cells absorb glucose and galactose by active transport; fructose is absorbed by facilitated diffusion (see Fig. 4.17). The monosaccharides enter the capillary network of the villus.

The hepatic portal vein transports the monosaccharides to the liver. The liver can use the simple sugars to make glycogen or fat, but if the body needs energy, the organ releases glucose into the bloodstream. Both galactose and some fructose are converted into glucose in the liver (Fig. 5.12). Figure 5.13 summarizes carbohydrate digestion and absorption.

Fiber

The fiber in oats is not digested by the human small intestine, so the fiber eventually enters the large intestine. Then "friendly" intestinal bacteria that reside in the large intestine can break down (*ferment*) the soluble fiber and metabolize the fermentation products for energy. Soluble fiber is sometimes referred to as *viscous fiber*, because it usually forms a semisolid mass in the intestinal tract that is rapidly fermented by bacterial action. In contrast, insoluble or fermentation-resistant fiber does not break down completely and, as a result, contributes to softer and easier-to-eliminate feces.[17]

① **Mouth**
Some starch is broken down to maltose by salivary amylase.

② **Stomach**
The activity of salivary amylase soon stops in the acidic environment of the stomach.

③ **Small intestine**
An amylase secreted by the pancreas (pancreatic amylase) breaks down starch into maltose. Maltase digests maltose into glucose. Sucrase digests sucrose into glucose and fructose. Lactase breaks down lactose into glucose and galactose.

④ **Liver**
Glucose, fructose, and galactose are absorbed by intestinal cells and transported to the liver by the hepatic portal vein.

⑤ **Large intestine**
Some soluble fiber is fermented by bacteria in the large intestine.

⑥ **Rectum**
Very little dietary carbohydrate is excreted in feces.

Salivary gland

Pancreas

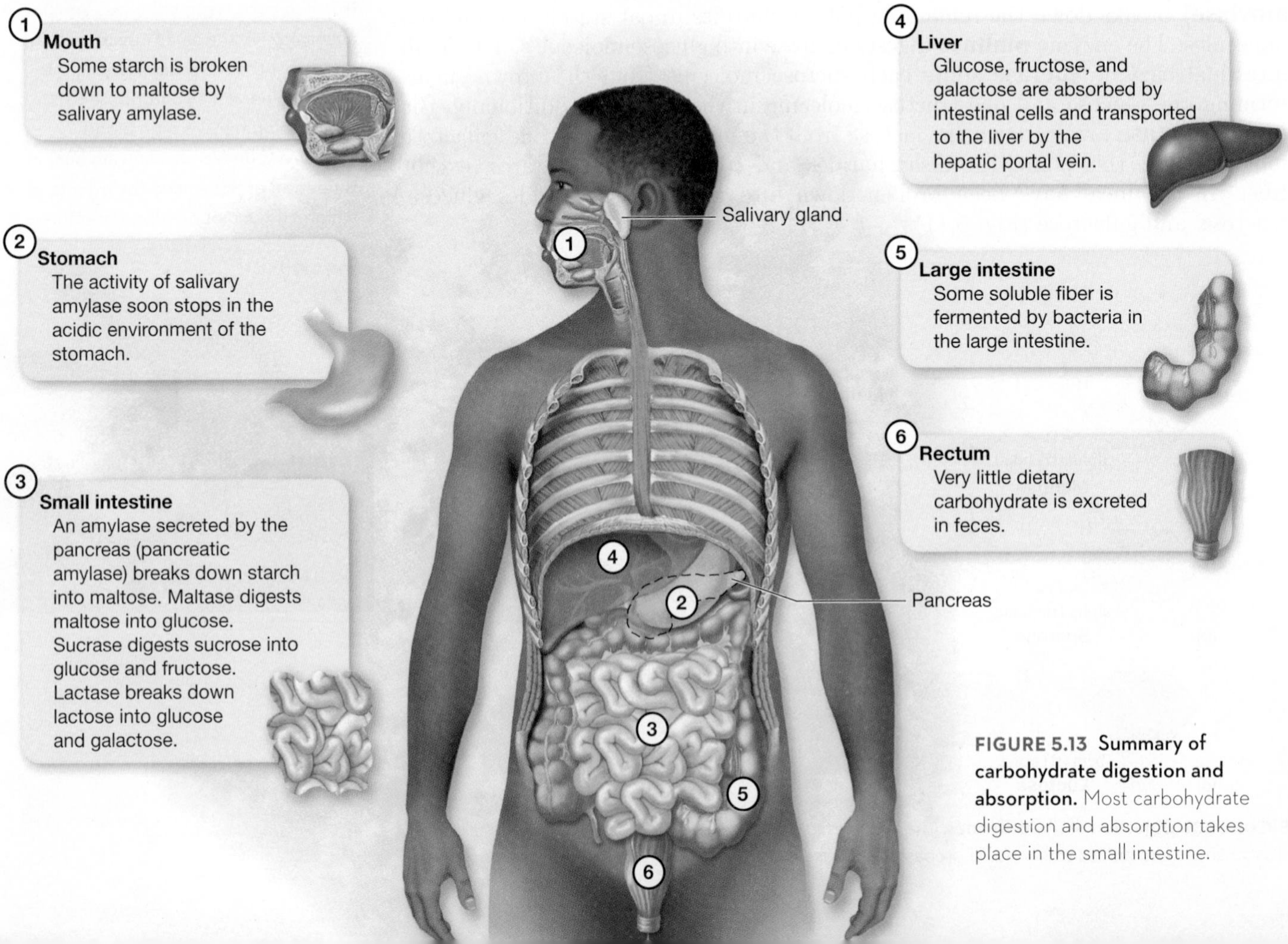

FIGURE 5.13 Summary of carbohydrate digestion and absorption. Most carbohydrate digestion and absorption takes place in the small intestine.

Resistant starches are not broken down in the human GI tract. Some resistant starches occur naturally in foods, such as seeds, legumes, unripened bananas, and raw potatoes, whereas others form by chemical changes that take place during cooking or processing. Food manufacturers are interested in making new products that contain resistant starch to provide health benefits that are similar to those of dietary fiber.

Scientists once thought fiber was a nonnutrient because it had no nutritional value. Recent scientific evidence indicates that the body, particularly the cells that line the large intestine, can use by-products of the bacterial metabolism of fiber for energy. A gram of fiber is estimated to add fewer than 3 kcal to human diets.[17] Fiber, however, contributes relatively little to a typical person's energy intake.[5]

resistant starches starches found in seeds, legumes, whole grains, and some fruits and vegetables that resist digestion and are not broken down in the human GI tract

ASSESS YOUR PROGRESS

15 *Sherita ate some whole-wheat crackers with grape jelly for a snack. As this snack passed through her digestive tract, discuss what happened to the starch, sucrose, and fiber in the food.*

16 *Describe the absorption of carbohydrates by the small intestine and their transport to the liver.*

17 *Explain the relationship between fiber and normal bacteria of the colon.*

5.6 Maintaining Normal Blood Glucose Levels

LEARNING OUTCOMES

1 *Compare the actions of insulin and glucagon.*

2 *Explain ketone body formation.*

Glucose is such an important cellular fuel, the body relies on hormones to maintain proper blood glucose levels. The pancreas, an accessory digestive system organ, contains *beta cells*, clusters of special cells that produce **insulin**, and groups of *alpha cells* that produce **glucagon**. These two hormones play key roles in regulating blood glucose levels.

In a healthy person, the body maintains blood glucose levels at between 70 and 99 milligrams per deciliter of blood (mg/dL). If a person has not eaten for a while, blood glucose levels begin to fall, the person starts to feel hungry, and the stomach likely growls. In this case, the individual may grab an apple or a cheese sandwich to eat, and as the carbohydrates in these foods are digested, the glucose from these foods is absorbed into the bloodstream and transported to the liver. As the blood glucose level begins to rise, the pancreas responds by secreting insulin into the bloodstream (Fig. 5.14). Insulin helps reduce blood glucose to normal levels, because the hormone enables glucose to enter most cells. The hormone also enhances energy storage by promoting cellular fat, glycogen, and protein production.

If an individual ignores the hunger signals and does not eat, the alpha cells in the pancreas secrete glucagon. Glucagon opposes insulin's effects by promoting the breakdown of glycogen. This process, called glycogenolysis (*lysis* = break) releases glucose into the bloodstream and, as a result, keeps blood glucose from dropping too low (Fig. 5.14). Glucagon also stimulates liver and kidney cells to

insulin hormone secreted from the beta cells of the pancreas that helps regulate blood glucose levels

glucagon hormone secreted from the alpha cells of the pancreas that helps regulate blood glucose levels

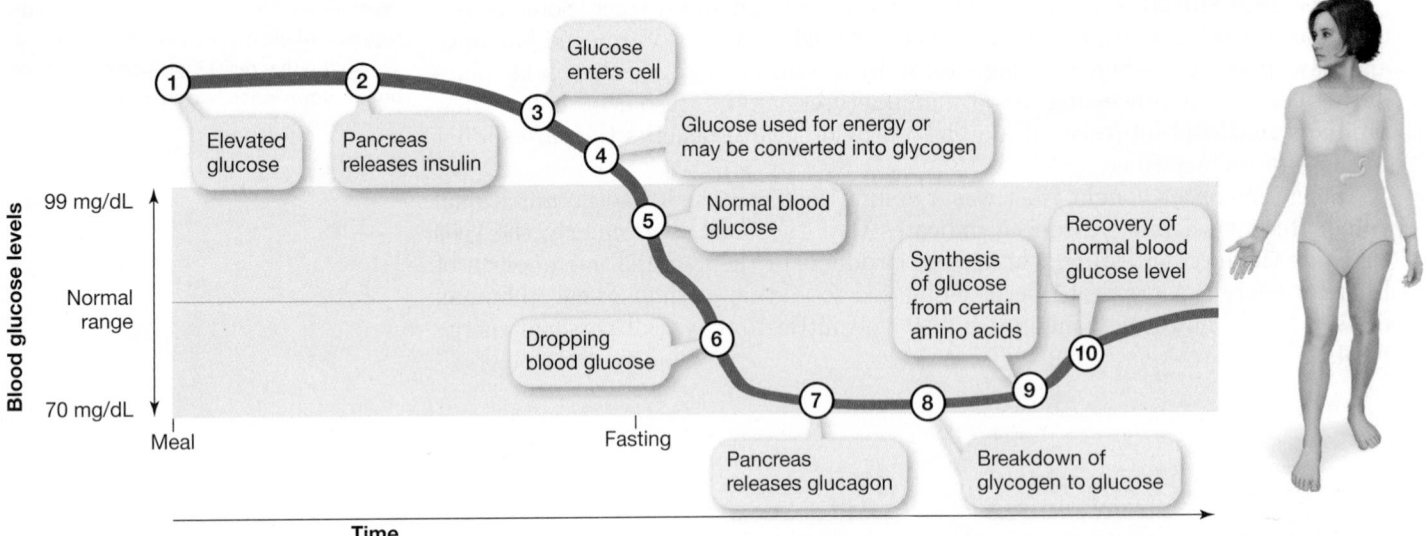

FIGURE 5.14 Regulating blood glucose. Insulin and glucagon are key hormones in maintaining normal blood glucose concentration.

lipolysis process by which triglycerides (fats) are broken down and glycerol and fatty acids are released into the bloodstream

produce glucose from certain *amino acids*, the basic molecules that make up proteins. Furthermore, glucagon stimulates **lipolysis** (*lipo* = fat), the breakdown of triglyceride (fat) into *glycerol* and *fatty acids*. As a result, glycerol and fatty acids rapidly enter into the bloodstream. The liver uses glycerol to produce glucose, and most cells, including muscle cells, can metabolize fatty acids for energy. Although the body can convert certain amino acids into glucose, it cannot use fatty acids to make glucose.

What happens to glucose? Its fate depends on the energy state of the body. If muscles and other cells that use glucose need energy, glucose enters the cells and is metabolized for energy. When an individual is well fed and resting ("fed state"), the body stores the extra glucose as glycogen. When glycogen storage reaches maximum capacity, the liver can convert excess glucose into fat.

Glucose for Energy

Cells metabolize glucose to release the energy stored in the molecule. Carbon dioxide and water form as a result of this process (Fig. 5.15).

ketone bodies chemicals formed from the incomplete breakdown of fat

ketosis condition in which ketone bodies accumulate in the blood; can result in loss of consciousness and death in severe cases

Cells need a small amount of glucose to properly metabolize fat for energy. When a person has poorly controlled diabetes, is fasting or starving, or follows a very low–carbohydrate/high–protein diet (e.g., the Atkins diet), his or her cells must use greater–than–normal amounts of fat for energy. Under these conditions, there is not enough glucose available for cells to metabolize the fat efficiently, and excessive amounts of **ketone bodies** ("ketones") form as a result. Ketone bodies are chemicals that result from the incomplete breakdown of fat. Muscle and brain cells can use ketone bodies for energy, but a condition commonly called **ketosis** occurs when these compounds accumulate in the blood. If not treated, severe ketosis can disrupt the body's ability to maintain normal blood chemistry, resulting in loss of consciousness and even death. Chapter 8 provides more information about glucose metabolism and ketone bodies.

The Recommended Dietary Allowance (RDA) for carbohydrate is 130 g/day.[17] This amount of carbohydrate is enough to prevent ketosis. (The RDAs and other DRIs were discussed in Chapter 3.) To estimate your daily carbohydrate intake, complete the "Personal Dietary Analysis" at the end of this chapter.

Glucose + Oxygen $\longrightarrow$ Carbon dioxide + Water + Energy

$$C_6H_{12}O_6 + 6O_2 \longrightarrow 6CO_2 + 6H_2O + Energy$$

FIGURE 5.15 Releasing energy from glucose. Cells use oxygen to release the energy stored in glucose. As a result of this process, cells produce carbon dioxide and water.

ASSESS YOUR PROGRESS

18 *Explain how insulin and glucagon regulate blood glucose levels.*

19 *What is a ketone body, and under what conditions does the body form excessive ketone bodies?*

5.7 Diabetes Mellitus

LEARNING OUTCOMES

1 *Describe type 1, type 2, and gestational diabetes.*

2 *Identify signs and symptoms of diabetes mellitus.*

3 *Discuss treatment options for diabetes.*

4 *Explain how hypoglycemia can occur.*

Diabetes mellitus ("diabetes") is a group of serious chronic diseases characterized by abnormal glucose, fat, and protein metabolism. Before the early 1920s, there was no effective treatment for diabetes. People with the disease often died soon after they were diagnosed with the condition.

In 1921, Canadian physician Dr. Frederick Banting and his assistant Charles Best conducted laboratory experiments on dogs to find a treatment for diabetes. The two researchers removed the pancreas of a dog and made an extract from the tissue. When the extract was injected into a diabetic dog, the animal's signs and symptoms of diabetes quickly disappeared. Soon after their success in treating diabetic dogs, Banting and his team of scientists began producing larger quantities of the extract from cattle pancreases. By January 1922, the team had prepared a highly refined version of the antidiabetes extract, which they named "insulin," for human testing.

Banting's first human subject was Leonard Thompson, a 14-year-old Canadian boy who was dying of diabetes.[24,25] After being injected with insulin, Thompson's blood glucose level returned to near normal within a 1-day period. Regular insulin injections enabled Leonard Thompson to live until the age of 27, when he died of complications of diabetes. The discovery of insulin was one of the most significant medical advances of the 20th century. Because of Banting and Best's pioneering efforts to find a useful treatment for diabetes, millions of people with the disease are able to live productive lives.

What Is Diabetes?

In 2014, 29.1 million Americans, 9.3% of the U.S. population, had diabetes.[26] Of these Americans, 21.1 million had been diagnosed with diabetes, but an estimated 8.1 million had the disease but had not been diagnosed.

There are two major types of diabetes mellitus: type 1 and type 2 diabetes. About 5% of people with diabetes have type 1; in the past, this form of diabetes was called "juvenile diabetes" because it was diagnosed more often in children and young adults. Type 1 diabetes, however, can develop at any age.[26] The majority of Americans with diabetes have type 2, which used to be called "adult-onset diabetes." Compared to children, Americans who are 20 years of age and older are more likely to develop type 2 diabetes.[26]

Regardless of the type of diabetes, the primary sign of the disease is **hyperglycemia** (*hyper* = excess; *glycemia* = blood glucose), abnormally elevated blood glucose levels (Table 5.8). Some people with diabetes experience hyperglycemia because their beta cells do not produce any insulin or do not produce enough

diabetes mellitus (diabetes) group of serious chronic conditions characterized by abnormal glucose, fat, and protein metabolism

hyperglycemia abnormally elevated blood glucose levels

DID **YOU** KNOW?

Obesity and diabetes are not just a concern in humans. In the United States, at least one-third of dogs are obese.[27] Like their human masters, obese companion animals often develop high blood pressure, cancer, breathing problems, arthritis, and diabetes. The symptoms of diabetes in cats and dogs are similar to those in humans and include excessive thirst, excessive urination, and weight loss. Certain breeds of dogs (Australian terriers and beagles) and cats (Burmese) are more prone to develop diabetes than other breeds.[28] Treating an animal with diabetes involves both diet modification and insulin therapy.

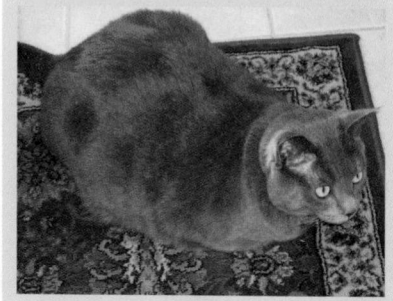

TABLE 5.8 Classifying Diabetes Mellitus

Blood Glucose Level (Fasting)	Classification
70–99 mg/dL	Normal
100–125 mg/dL	Pre-diabetes
126 mg/dL or more	Diabetes

type 1 diabetes autoimmune disease that results in destruction of the beta cells of the pancreas; as a result, insulin must be supplied to the affected person regularly through exogenous sources

type 2 diabetes most common type of diabetes; beta cells of the pancreas produce insulin, but the hormone's target cells are insulin-resistant, leading to elevated blood glucose levels

to meet their needs. In other cases, the affected person produces some insulin, but his or her body does not respond properly to the hormone, and hyperglycemia results. Major signs and symptoms of hyperglycemia include excessive thirst, frequent urination, blurred vision, and poor wound healing (Table 5.9).

Over time, untreated or poorly controlled hyperglycemia damages nerves, organs, and blood vessels. In fact, poorly controlled diabetes is a major cause of heart disease; kidney failure; blindness; and poor blood circulation, particularly of the lower limbs, which can require amputation. In 2010, over 69,000 Americans died from diabetes; the chronic disease was the seventh leading cause of death in the United States.[29] Public health officials are very concerned about the increasing number of Americans who have diabetes (Fig. 5.16).

Type 1 Diabetes

Type 1 diabetes is an autoimmune disease that occurs when certain immune system cells malfunction and do not recognize the body's own beta cells. As a result, the immune system cells attack and destroy the beta cells, and the affected person must obtain an *exogenous* ("outside the body") source of insulin regularly. It is not clear why the immune cells of some individuals malfunction, but genetic susceptibility and environmental factors, particularly exposure to certain viral intestinal infections, are associated with the development of type 1 diabetes.[30]

Stephanie Patton has type 1 diabetes. You can learn about her and how she manages her diabetes by reading the "Real People, Real Stories" feature on page 129.

Type 2 Diabetes

The most common form of diabetes is **type 2 diabetes**. Beta cells of people with type 2 diabetes usually produce insulin, but the hormone's target cells are *insulin-resistant*, which means they do not respond properly to the hormone and do not allow glucose to enter them. As a result, the level of glucose in the bloodstream rapidly becomes abnormally elevated, and the signs and symptoms of diabetes occur.

Over the past 20 years, the number of adults and children with type 2 diabetes has reached epidemic proportions in the United States.[26] Certain people have greater risk of type 2 diabetes than others. Individuals who are physically inactive (sedentary), overweight, and genetically related to a close family member with type 2 diabetes are more likely to develop the disease than persons who do not have these characteristics. Additionally, Americans who have Hispanic, Native American, Asian, African, or Pacific Islander ancestry are more likely to develop type 2 diabetes than Americans who are not members of these racial or ethnic groups.[26] The American Diabetes Association (ADA) has an online questionnaire that people can take to assess their risk of type 2 diabetes (www.diabetes.org).

Diabetes During Pregnancy

During pregnancy, a woman with poorly controlled diabetes and her developing offspring (*embryo* or

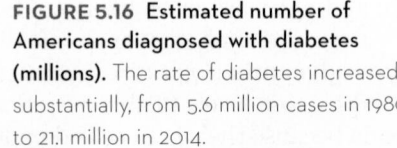

2014 (21.1)
2005 (15.8)
2000 (12.0)
1995 (8.0)
1990 (6.6)
1985 (6.2)
1980 (5.6)

FIGURE 5.16 Estimated number of Americans diagnosed with diabetes (millions). The rate of diabetes increased substantially, from 5.6 million cases in 1980 to 21.1 million in 2014.

TABLE 5.9 Signs and Symptoms of Diabetes Mellitus

Elevated blood glucose levels	Impotence (male)
Excessive thirst	Sores that do not heal
Frequent urination	Increased appetite with weight loss *
Blurry vision	Breath that smells like fruit *
Vaginal yeast infections (adult women)	Fatigues easily *
Foot pain, abdominal pain	Confusion *
Numbness	

* Typical symptoms of poorly controlled type 1 rather than type 2 diabetes.

REAL People, REAL Stories

Stephanie Patton

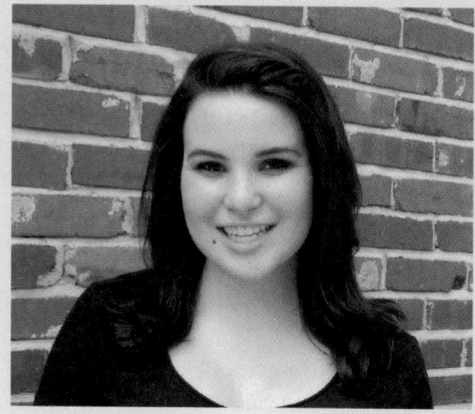

Although she is only 18 years old, college freshman Stephanie Patton has a long list of accomplishments. "When I was little, I took singing, dancing, and acting lessons. I loved being on the stage, so I had my parents take me to auditions for local talent shows and theatrical performances. Since I was 7 years old, I've been in over 50 musicals and plays. I appeared in my first beauty pageant at age 10, and I recently competed for the Miss Missouri title. I placed in the top 11, won the preliminary talent award and two college scholarships for community service." Stephanie is majoring in Health Sciences at the University of Missouri-Columbia. While in college, she plans to continue competing for the title of Miss Missouri.

Stephanie manages to balance her college life with her extracurricular activities, but she also has to manage her health and diet. This impressive young lady has type 1 diabetes. "Just before my fifth birthday, I lost weight and began drinking gallons of juice, water, and milk. At night, I wet the bed. My parents became alarmed, because I have some cousins with type 1 diabetes, and they were worried that I had the disease, too." On Stephanie's fifth birthday, her parents took her to the doctor's for a check-up, and her physician told the child's parents to have her admitted immediately to the local children's hospital. While she was in the hospital, Stephanie's parents learned about diabetes and how to take care of their daughter's condition. "At first, my parents gave the insulin shots to me, but in a few months, I learned to inject myself and 'count carbs.' An apple was 15 carbs, and my body needed 1 unit of insulin to handle every 15 carbs. I also learned that I had to eat on a set schedule because of the way insulin worked in my body.

"In first grade, the kids avoided me. They didn't understand that you don't 'catch' diabetes like the flu. I was miserable, so my parents placed me in a new school. Since then, I learned that I'm different, and that's OK. I also became determined to educate my friends and the public about diabetes. I was always a very outgoing kid, so after I was diagnosed, my parents started volunteering for the Juvenile Diabetes Research Foundation, and I became one of the organization's child ambassadors. I gave speeches about the importance of finding a cure for diabetes, and I raised thousands of dollars for this cause. Diabetes doesn't get in my way; I don't let diabetes define who I am."

fetus) can develop serious health problems. If a woman with diabetes lacks good control of her blood glucose level, her embryo can develop birth defects as a result. By managing her blood glucose properly, however, the pregnant woman with diabetes can reduce her chances of giving birth to a baby with birth defects. Additionally, she will be less likely to experience serious health problems, such as high blood pressure, during pregnancy.

gestational diabetes type of diabetes that develops in some pregnant women

As many as 10% of pregnant American women develop a form of diabetes called **gestational diabetes**, usually after the 24th week of pregnancy.[31] Pregnant women who have a family history of type 2 diabetes, are overweight, or have high blood pressure are more likely to experience gestational diabetes than pregnant women who do not have these characteristics.[32] The fetus of a woman with gestational diabetes receives too much glucose from its hyperglycemic mother. As a result of obtaining the excess glucose, the fetus gains weight rapidly and can be abnormally heavy at birth, weighing 9 pounds or more. Giving birth to such a large infant is risky for the mother as well as the infant, because it may prolong the birth process and cause the baby to be injured during delivery.

After giving birth, 5 to 10% of women who had gestational diabetes continue to have diabetes, most often type 2 diabetes.[26] The remaining new mothers are healthy, but they have a 35 to 60% increased risk of developing type 2 diabetes within the following 5 to 10 years, compared to women who did not develop gestational diabetes.

A healthy pregnancy typically lasts about 40 weeks. Women with poorly controlled diabetes or gestational diabetes are more likely to have miscarriages (death of an embryo/fetus before the 20th week of pregnancy), stillbirths (delivery of a dead baby), and premature (born before the 37th week of pregnancy) deliveries than women with diabetes who manage their blood glucose properly. Furthermore, women with poorly controlled diabetes or gestational diabetes are more likely to give birth to babies who have difficulty controlling their own blood glucose levels than mothers who do not have diabetes or develop the condition during pregnancy. Thus, pregnant women who have diabetes are encouraged to monitor blood glucose levels carefully to minimize risks to both themselves and their fetuses.

hemoglobin A1c (HbA1c) glycosylated hemoglobin; blood test used to measure a person's average blood glucose over several months' period of time

Women who have adequate *prenatal* (before birth) medical care during pregnancy usually undergo screening to detect gestational diabetes at 20 to 24 weeks of pregnancy. Treatment for woman who are diagnosed with gestational diabetes generally includes a special, carbohydrate-controlled diet to help manage blood glucose levels and regular physical activity. Some mothers-to-be will also need to monitor their blood glucose levels and give insulin injections to themselves regularly.

Adequate prenatal care is important for women who have diabetes.

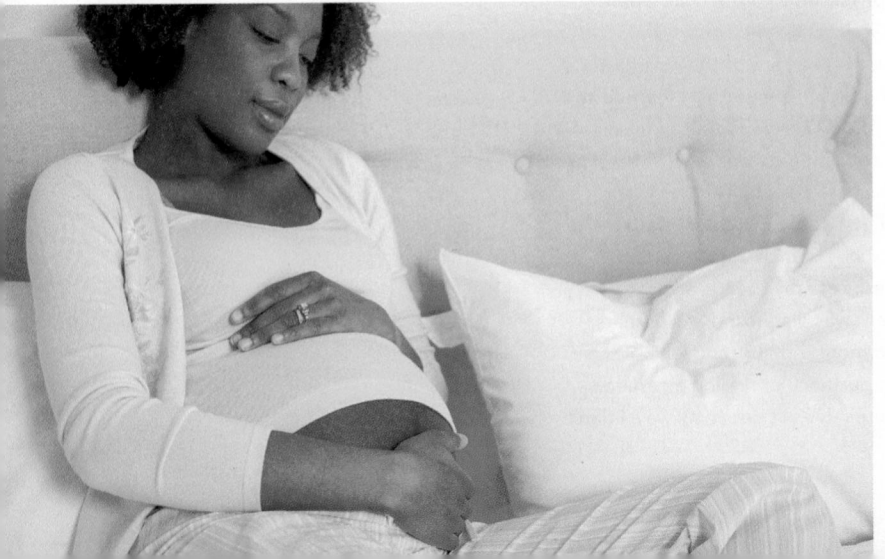

Testing for Diabetes

To avoid or delay serious health complications, people who have diabetes need to achieve and maintain normal or near-normal blood glucose levels. Many people with diabetes rely on daily blood testing to monitor their blood glucose levels (Fig. 5.17). Additionally, physicians can measure *glycated* hemoglobin, also called *glycosylated* hemoglobin or **hemoglobin A1c (HbA1c)**, to determine their patients' average blood glucose levels over longer periods. This can provide information about a patient's long-term management of the condition.

Hemoglobin is the compound in red blood cells that carries oxygen. A1c is a component of hemoglobin that attracts some glucose that is in blood. About 5% of a healthy person's hemoglobin

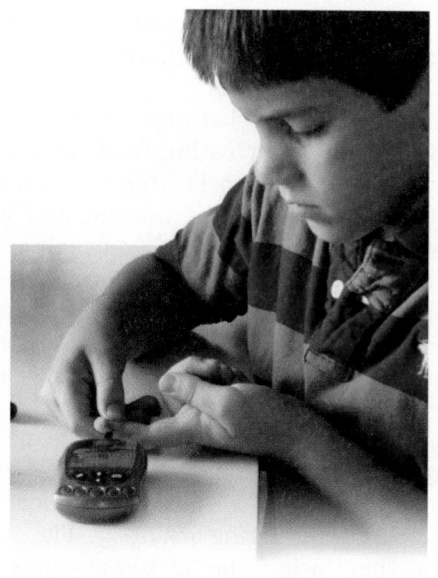
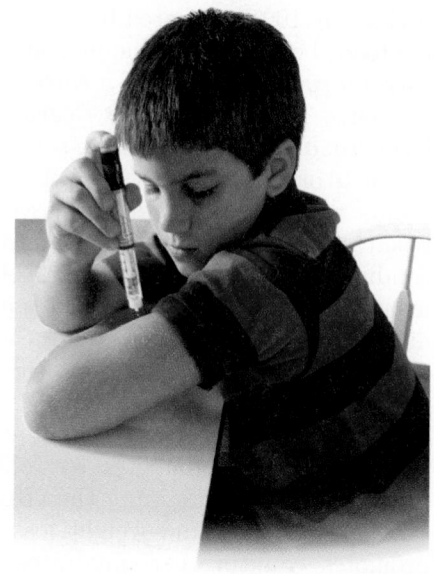

(a)   (b)

FIGURE 5.17 Managing diabetes. Nine-year-old Carson Smith was diagnosed with type 1 diabetes when he was 5 years of age. (*a*) Carson checks his blood glucose at least four times a day. (*b*) After obtaining information about Carson's blood glucose level, his parents determine the amount and type of insulin he needs, and Carson uses a special device to inject the insulin into his body.

is HbA1c. A person with poorly controlled diabetes often has blood glucose levels that are much higher than normal. As a result, this individual's hemoglobin will have a higher percentage of HbA1c. According to the ADA, people with diabetes should strive to maintain their HbA1c level below 7% (Table 5.10).[33]

Controlling Diabetes

Treatment for diabetes may include diet, exercise, insulin injections, and oral medications. Which treatment option a person receives depends on a variety of factors, including his or her type of diabetes, age, and current health status.

Diet

Proper blood glucose management generally involves monitoring blood glucose levels regularly and following a special diet carefully. The patient's diabetes meal plan should focus on whole grains, vegetables, fruits, legumes, poultry, fish, and low–fat dairy foods. Additionally, the patient's simple sugar and starch con–sumption should be consistent and should be monitored to help regulate his or her blood glucose levels.

The Exchange System and **carbohydrate counting** are tools that people with diabetes can use to plan their diets (for information about the Exchange System, see Chapter 3). Carbohydrate counting involves determining a maximum daily carbohydrate intake that is appropriate for the individual. Then, the person tracks his or her carbohydrate intake by recording grams of carbohydrate con–sumed per meal and for the day. Most health care professionals who treat people with diabetes recommend having meals that supply 45 to 60 grams of carbohy–drates. However, this amount of carbohydrate may need to be adjusted based on results of regular blood glucose testing.

Glycemic Index and Glycemic Load Different carbohydrates undergo different rates of digestion and absorption, which affect the body's insulin response. The **glycemic index (GI)** and **glycemic load (GL)** are standards that reflect the body's insulin response to a carbohydrate–containing food. Glycemic index is a way of classifying foods by comparing the rise in blood glucose that occurs after eating a sample of food that supplies 50 g of digestible carbohydrate to the rise that occurs after eating a standard source of carbohydrate, such as 50 g of glucose or white bread.[34] A related value, the glycemic load, is the grams of carbohydrate in a serving of food multiplied by the food's GI; this figure is then

TABLE 5.10 Classifying Diabetes According to Hemoglobin A1c Values

Diagnosis*	A1c Level
Normal	4.5–5.7%
Pre-diabetes	5.7–6.4%
Diabetes	6.5% or above

*Any test for diagnosing diabetes requires a second test to confirm the diagnosis, unless the patient has signs and symptoms of diabetes.

carbohydrate counting diabetes management tool in which an individual tracks his or her daily carbohydrate intake

glycemic index (GI) tool to measure the body's insulin response to a carbohydrate-containing food

glycemic load (GL) tool to measure the body's insulin response to a carbohydrate-containing food; similar to the glycemic index, but also factors in a typical serving size of the food

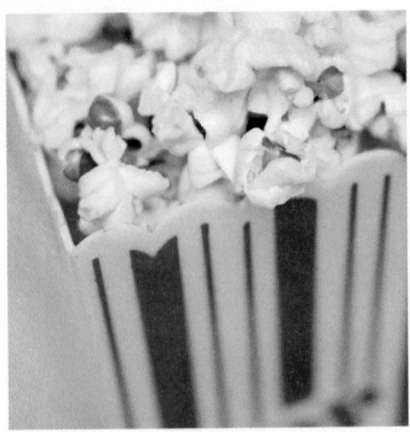

Popcorn has a high glycemic index (GI) but a low glycemic load (GL). Most health professionals recommend focusing more on GL than on GI.

hyperinsulinemia condition in which the pancreas releases an excessive amount of insulin; over time, condition may contribute to the development of type 2 diabetes

divided by 100. Compared to the GI, the GL may be a more realistic way of rating foods because the value indicates the relative rise in blood glucose levels after eating a *typical* serving of a carbohydrate-containing food.

Some people may be "carbohydrate-sensitive," because they develop **hyperinsulinemia** (*insulinemia* = blood insulin) after eating foods that have GIs of 70 or more, such as some of the foods listed in Table 5.11. Hyperinsulinemia occurs when the pancreas releases an excessive amount of insulin, and as a result, cells remove too much glucose from the bloodstream. Eventually, this condition may overtax the beta cells' ability to produce adequate amounts of insulin. Thus, hyperinsulinemia may contribute to the development of type 2 diabetes, particularly in people who are genetically prone to develop the disease.[35] Tumors of the pancreas, the organ that produces insulin, may also cause hyperinsulinemia.

Promoters of certain weight-reduction diets claim that people can lose weight or control diabetes by following low glycemic index diets. However, research studies examining the effects of glycemic index and glycemic load on glycemic response and weight loss have found conflicting results.[36] The ADA promotes counting carbohydrates rather than using the glycemic index for choosing foods. According to the ADA, the amount of total carbohydrate consumed is more important than the GI of foods for maintaining healthy blood glucose levels.[37]

Insulin Injections

Over 20 different types of insulin are sold in the United States. The forms of insulin differ in how quickly they act, how long they last, and the period of time during which their activity in the body is greatest.

TABLE 5.11 Glycemic Index and Load: Average Values of Selected Foods

Food	Glycemic Index*	Glycemic Load†	
		Serving Size	Value
Potato, Russet, baked	158	150 g	33
Jelly beans	114	30 g	22
White rice, medium-grain, boiled	107	150 g	29
Bagel, white plain	99	70 g	24
French fries	90	150 g	21
Cola drink	90	1 cup	16
Banana	89	120 g	16
Cornflakes cereal	80	30 g	21
Popcorn, microwave, plain	79	20 g	6
Spaghetti, cooked	68	180 g	23
Orange juice	66	1 cup	12
Ice cream, vanilla, low-fat	66	50 g	7
Snickers® candy bar	61	60 g	15
Apple, raw	56	120 g	6

* Compared to white bread (GI = 100)

† Per serving

Source: Data from Atkinson FS and others: International tables of glycemic index and glycemic load values: 2008. *Diabetes Care* 31(12):2281, 2008.

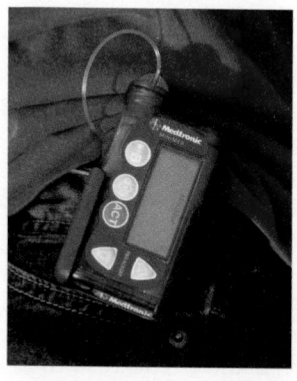

(a)

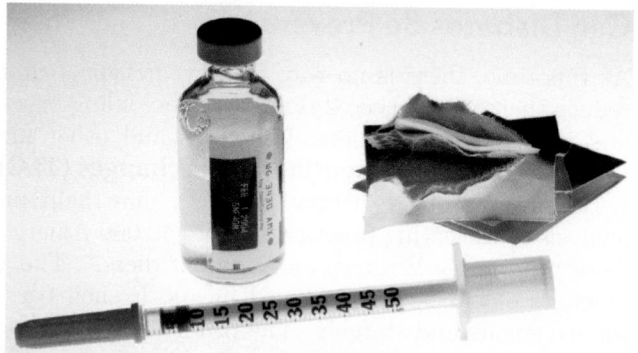

(b)

FIGURE 5.18 Insulin therapy. Insulin injections through either an insulin pump (*a*) or multiple daily insulin injections (*b*) are necessary for those with type 1 diabetes.

People with type 1 diabetes rely on daily insulin injections, either by the use of multiple daily insulin shots or an insulin pump (Fig. 5.18). The insulin pump, which is usually worn on a waistband or belt, has a container for insulin. The device is pro—grammed to deliver the hormone into the patient's body through a small tube that is inserted under the patient's skin. Either multiple daily insulin injections and insulin pumps enable people with type 1 diabetes to manage their condition efficiently.[38]

Pancreas Transplants At present, people with type 1 diabetes must receive insulin, either through injections or the pump device, for the rest of their lives. Since the late 1960s, medical researchers have tested various surgical treatments for type 1 diabetes, particularly pancreas transplantation.[39] However, the risks associated with a pancreas transplant often outweigh the benefits. In over half of the surgeries, the patient's body rejects the donor pancreas not long after the procedure, and 10 to 20% of those receiving a pancreas die within a year of the transplant.[40] People who receive a transplanted pancreas must take *immuno—suppressive* drugs to reduce the chances that their bodies will reject the organ. However, survival rates following pancreas transplantation have improved significantly over the past 50 years, and the procedure is an option for some individuals with diabetes.[41] In the future, scientists may find ways to treat or cure type 1 diabetes by implanting beta cells into patients with the condition.

Oral Medications

Some people with type 2 diabetes can take oral medication to stimulate their bodies' insulin production. Oral medications are most effective for people who have had type 2 diabetes for less than 10 years.[42] In general, such medications help patients control their blood glucose levels when they are combined with a healthy lifestyle that includes monitoring carbohydrate intake and engaging in regular physical activity.

Physical Activity

Regular physical activity improves diabetes control as well as overall health and well—being.[43] Physical activity increases glucose uptake by muscles, reducing blood glucose levels and improving the body's insulin response. Regular physical activity also can also help overweight people with type 2 diabetes lose weight. By losing even a small amount of excess body fat, people with type 2 diabetes can often reduce their insulin resistance.[44] People with diabetes, however, should consult their health care team before starting an exercise program.

With proper management of their disease, athletes with diabetes can excel in their sport. Athletes with type 1 diabetes must monitor blood glucose levels before, during, and after exercise, and follow a diet that maximizes their physical performance while minimizing the likelihood of fatigue.[45]

DID **YOU** *KNOW?*

In 1999, doctors told Gary Hall Jr. that he had type 1 diabetes and he would not be able to continue swimming competitively.[46] Hall had won two gold and two silver medals at the 1996 Olympics and was at the peak of his athletic abilities. Instead of letting the diagnosis of diabetes end his promising swimming career, the young athlete continued to train, and in the 2000 and 2004 Olympics, he won six more medals, including three gold ones. In 2012, Hall was inducted into the U.S. Olympic Hall of Fame.

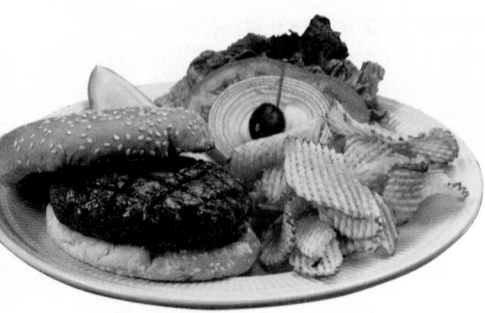

A hamburger with chips is an example of a typical meal for a Western diet.

therapeutic lifestyle changes (TLC) actions, such as avoiding excess body fat, exercising daily, and improving the diet, that promote health and reduce risk for chronic disease

hypoglycemia condition that occurs when blood glucose level is too low

epinephrine (adrenaline) hormone produced by the adrenal glands; secreted in response to declining blood glucose levels

reactive hypoglycemia (postprandial hypoglycemia) low blood glucose that occurs within 4 hours of eating

Can Diabetes Be Prevented?

At this time, there is no way to prevent type 1 diabetes. However, people may reduce their risk of type 2 diabetes by avoiding excess body fat, exercising daily, and improving their diets. Dietitians and other medical practitioners refer to these actions as **therapeutic lifestyle changes (TLC)**.

Improving one's dietary practices may help prevent type 2 diabetes. An analysis of the eating practices of over 40,000 American men identified two major dietary patterns: Western and prudent diets.[47] The Western diet contained high amounts of red meat, processed meats, French fries, high–fat dairy foods, and refined sugars and starches. The prudent diet had more poultry, fish, and fiber–rich whole grains, fruits, and vegetables than the Western diet. The results of this study indicated that men who ate Western diets had almost twice the risk of developing type 2 diabetes compared with those who followed prudent diets. Results of another study indicated that high red meat and processed meat intakes may increase the risk of type 2 diabetes in men.[48]

High–fiber diets, particularly those containing cereal fiber and whole grains, may protect against diabetes.[49] Dietary factors seem to have the greatest impact on type 2 diabetes risk in persons who have a *genetic predisposition* for this form of diabetes, that is, a family history of the disease.[50]

What Is Hypoglycemia?

If a person is healthy and has not eaten for a while, his or her blood glucose levels decline, and the individual becomes hungry. Eating a meal or snack raises this person's blood glucose. **Hypoglycemia** (*hypo* = low) is a condition that occurs when the blood glucose level is too low to provide enough energy for cells.

Hypoglycemia may be diagnosed when the blood glucose level is less than 70 mg/dL.[51] In response to rapidly declining blood glucose levels, the body responds by secreting **epinephrine**, a hormone (sometimes called adrenaline) that is produced by the adrenal glands. Like glucagon, epinephrine increases the supply of glucose and fatty acids in the bloodstream, but the hormone can also make a person with hypoglycemia feel irritable, restless, shaky, and sweaty. If the blood glucose level drops too low, the affected person can become confused, and he or she may lose consciousness and die.

Several years ago, popular books and magazine articles warned Americans about the dangers of hypoglycemia and its signs and symptoms. Many people became convinced that they suffered from the condition. Although hypoglycemia is a serious disorder that can affect people with diabetes mellitus and certain tumors of the pancreas, it rarely affects otherwise healthy persons. Some people develop **reactive hypoglycemia**, also called **postprandial hypoglycemia**, which is low blood glucose that occurs within 4 hours of eating. Typically, the indi–vidual consumed too much highly refined carbohydrates, and his or her pancreas responded by releasing too much insulin. However, these individuals generally have normal fasting blood glucose levels. People with reactive hypoglycemia may feel better if they avoid eating large amounts of sugary foods and eat smaller, more frequent meals that contain a mixture of macronutrients.

ASSESS YOUR PROGRESS

20 *Compare type 1, type 2, and gestational diabetes.*

21 *What are the signs and symptoms of type 1 and type 2 diabetes?*

22 *Identify the consequences of untreated gestational diabetes.*

23 *Describe the roles of diet, exercise, and medication in the treatment of diabetes.*

24 *What is reactive hypoglycemia and how can it be treated?*

5.8 Carbohydrates and Health

LEARNING OUTCOMES

1 *Explain the relationship between carbohydrates and obesity.*
2 *Describe metabolic syndrome and list major signs of the condition.*
3 *Discuss ways in which people may avoid tooth decay (dental caries).*
4 *Explain what causes lactose intolerance, and list strategies to avoid its symptoms.*
5 *Describe the role of fiber in preventing certain chronic diseases.*

Carbohydrates, especially sugar and white flour, get a lot of "bad press." Promoters of low–carbohydrate/high–protein diets often blame sugars and starches for causing obesity and diabetes. Many Americans think consuming sugary foods causes depression and hyperactive behavior. On the other hand, "carbs" are welcomed by athletes as an inexpensive and efficient source of energy. What have scientists learned about the roles carbohydrates play in health?

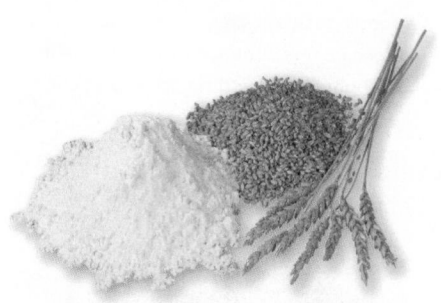

Grains are used to make breads, cereal, and pasta, foods that may have a negative effect on health when consumed in excess. Choose whole grains when possible.

Are Carbohydrates Fattening?

Americans are fatter now than they were 20 years ago. In their efforts to lose weight, millions of Americans follow *fad* low–carbohydrate diets, such as the Atkins, Sugar Busters!, or the Zone diet. A fad is a practice that gains wide–spread popularity rapidly and then loses its appeal quickly when people tire of the behavior or follow a newer trend. Are carbohydrates responsible for the epidemic of excess body fat in the United States?

"Calories do count," because people gain body fat when their intake of food energy from macronutrients and the nonnutrient alcohol consistently exceeds their output of energy for various physiological needs. Regardless of whether people consume a high–carbohydrate, high–fat, or high–protein diet, they will maintain their weight as long as their energy intake matches their energy output.

Foods that contain large amounts of refined carbohydrates, however, do not satisfy hunger as well as those that contain more protein or fat. As a result, hunger occurs sooner after eating a meal or snack that contains high amounts of added sugars and refined starches than after a high–protein, high–fat meal or snack. Thus, a person following a low–carbohydrate, high–protein, high–fat diet can lose weight in the short term, because the diet keeps his or her appetite under control by reducing hunger. Eating a diet rich in fiber can also contribute to weight loss because fiber–rich foods tend to be filling, contributing to a reduced food intake.[52]

Over the past 35 years, the percentage of overweight and obese Americans rose dramatically. During this same period, Americans substantially increased their consumption of fructose in HFCS. Some nutrition scientists think Americans' love of foods and beverages sweetened with HFCS is largely responsible for the population's rising rate of obesity. The prevalence of obesity among children is a major public health concern; regular soft drinks are the primary source of added sugar in the diets of American children.[53] School boards in some communities are so concerned about the epidemic of childhood obesity that some have banned empty–calorie foods, including soft drinks, from school vending machines.

Is there a connection between consumption of regular soft drinks and excess body weight? The role that regular soft drink consumption plays in the develop–ment of obesity is controversial.[54] Findings from some scientific studies suggest that people who drink regular soft drinks do not reduce their energy intake from solid food accordingly.[55] The reasons are unclear, but the fructose in these bever–ages may not reduce the urge to eat as does solid food. As a result, consumers of regular soft drinks ("liquid candy") are likely to overeat and have excessive energy intakes that contribute to weight gain. By contributing to unwanted weight gain, consumption of regular soft drinks may increase the risk of type 2 diabetes.[56]

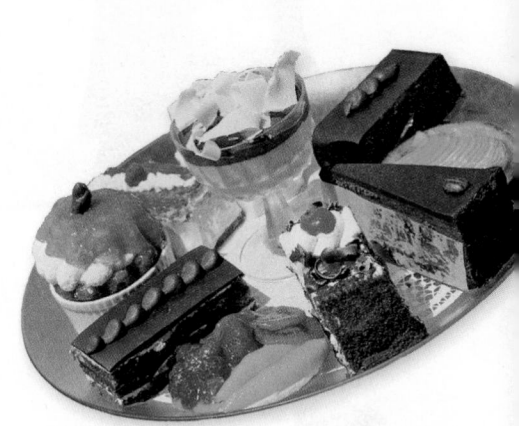

Many people find it difficult to resist foods that contain a lot of sugar and fat, such as cheesecake and pastries.

DID **YOU** KNOW?

Many people think sucrose is addictive. An addiction is characterized by an uncontrolled need (compulsion) to consume a substance and the development of withdrawal signs and symptoms when the substance is not consumed. Many people report cravings, extreme preferences for certain foods, especially sweet fatty foods, such as cakes and pastries. Researchers continue to investigate if carbohydrates, and sugars in particular, are truly addictive.[59]

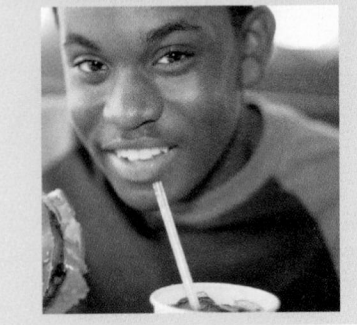

metabolic syndrome condition that increases risk of type 2 diabetes and CVD

syndrome group of signs and symptoms that occur together and indicate a specific health problem

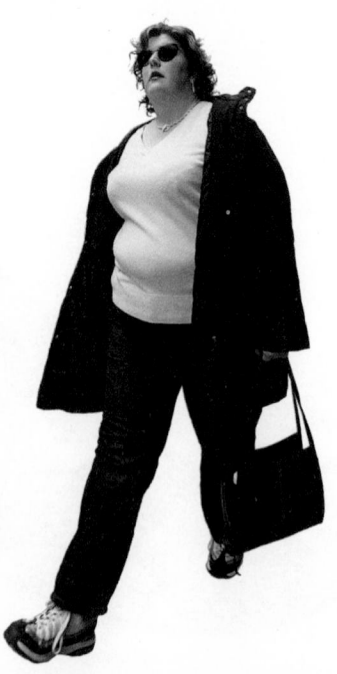

Having excess abdominal fat can be dangerous, especially when it is accompanied by hypertension and elevated blood lipid levels.

In general, Americans consume an excess of calories from all foods, and the higher intake contributes to the increased prevalence of obesity in the United States.[57,58] Therefore, Americans' overall dietary habits may be partly to blame for rising rates of overweight and obesity among the U.S. population.

Metabolic Syndrome

People who are too fat often have excess abdominal fat, which can be dangerous, especially when it is accompanied by hypertension and elevated blood lipid (triglyceride and cholesterol) levels.[60]

An estimated 47 million Americans have **metabolic syndrome**, a condition characterized by three or more of the signs listed in Table 5.12.[61,62] A **syndrome** is a group of signs and symptoms that occur together and indicate a specific health problem. Compared to people who do not have metabolic syndrome, individuals with this condition have about five times the risk of type 2 diabetes and almost twice the risk of certain diseases of the heart and blood vessels (cardiovascular disease or CVD).[63]

Although genetic factors play a major role in the development of metabolic syndrome, excess abdominal fat and insulin resistance are the primary risk factors for the condition.[63] Poor diet, cigarette smoking, and lack of physical activity also contribute to the development of the syndrome. By exercising more than three times/week, high-risk people may reduce their risk of metabolic syndrome.[63] Furthermore, people may lower their likelihood of developing metabolic syndrome by increasing their intake of fruits and vegetables and other fiber-rich foods, such as whole-grain cereals.[64] Older adults are more likely to have metabolic syndrome than younger adults.[62]

Individuals who already have metabolic syndrome may reduce their risk of CVD by losing excess weight, exercising regularly, and reducing intakes of saturated fat and simple sugars,[63] particularly sucrose and fructose.[65,66] If such therapeutic lifestyle changes do not help patients with metabolic syndrome, medication may be necessary to manage blood pressure and blood lipid levels. Chapter 6 provides more information about CVD.

TABLE 5.12 Signs of Metabolic Syndrome

Sign	Defining Value
Large waist circumference*	≥ 40 inches (men) ≥ 35 inches (women)
Chronically elevated blood pressure (hypertension)	≥ 130 mm Hg systolic (upper value) or ≥ 85 mm Hg diastolic (lower value) or Drug treatment for hypertension
Chronically elevated fasting blood fats (triglycerides)	≥ 150 mg/dL or Drug treatment for elevated triglycerides
Low fasting high-density lipoprotein cholesterol (HDL cholesterol)	< 40 mg/dL (men) < 50 mg/dL (women) or Drug treatment for reduced HDL
High fasting blood glucose	≥ 100 mg/dL or Drug treatment for elevated glucose

* To measure your waist circumference, remove clothing from the midsection of your body. Locate the top of your hip bones and place a flexible measuring tape around your abdomen at the top of the bones. Exhale normally and take the measurement. (The measuring tape should fit snugly around your waist without pinching the skin and be parallel to floor.)

Source: Data from Grundy SM and others: Diagnosis and management of the metabolic syndrome: An American Heart Association/ National Heart, Lung, and Blood Institute scientific statement: Executive summary. *Circulation* 112:e285, 2005.

Tooth Decay (Dental Caries)

Tooth decay is clearly associated with consuming carbohydrates, particularly simple sugars that stick to teeth. If a person does not follow good dental hygiene practices, the debris becomes food for bacteria that live on teeth. As the bacteria metabolize carbohydrate for their energy needs, they produce acid that damages tooth enamel and results in decay.

Tooth decay and lack of adequate dental care may result in tooth loss. Tooth loss often has negative effects on a person's facial structure, speech, and diet. The typical diet of an individual with several missing teeth consists of liquids and soft foods that are easily swallowed.

Lactose Intolerance

An estimated 30 to 50 million Americans suffer from **lactose intolerance** (also referred to as *lactose maldigestion*), the inability to digest lactose completely.[68] Lactose—intolerant people do not produce enough lactase, the enzyme that breaks lactose into glucose and galactose. Lactose intolerance is not the same as milk allergy, which is an immune system response to cow's milk proteins affect— ing less than 5% of the population.[69] Milk allergy is most likely to occur during infancy, whereas lactose intolerance is more likely to occur in adulthood.[68]

When a lactose—intolerant person consumes lactose, the disaccharide is not completely digested and absorbed by the time it enters the large intes— tine. Bacteria that reside in the large intestine break down lactose and produce irritating gases and acids as metabolic by—products. As a result, a lactose— intolerant person usually experiences intestinal cramps, bloating, flatulence, and diarrhea within a couple of hours after consuming milk or other lactose— containing products.

Normally, infants produce lactase, but by the time children are 2 years old, their small intestine begins to produce less of the enzyme. Many older children and adults, particularly those with African, Asian, Eastern European, and Native American ancestry, are lactose intolerant and experience some degree of abdom— inal discomfort after drinking milk.

Dietary Modifications

Milk and milk products are excellent sources of protein, many vitamins, and the minerals calcium and phosphorus. What can people with lactose intolerance do to achieve a nutritionally adequate diet without drinking milk? Lactose— intolerant people are often able to eat hard cheeses and yogurt without expe— riencing any digestive tract discomfort. Milk loses most of its lactose content when it is processed to make aged cheeses, such as cheddar and Swiss. The bacteria used to make yogurt convert much of the lactose in milk to lactic acid, and the microbes assist with the digestion of the remaining lactose even after the yogurt is eaten.[70]

Some people with lactose intolerance discover through trial and error that they can consume small amounts of milk without experiencing intestinal discom— fort. Most lactose—intolerant individuals can consume 12 to 15 g of lactose per day (about 1 cup of milk) without experiencing unpleasant side effects.[71]

People who cannot tolerate even limited amounts of fresh fluid milk can often drink milk that has been pretreated with lactase to reduce its lactose content. Most large supermarkets sell fresh lactase—treated milk in the dairy food section (Fig. 5.19). Also, lactase—containing solutions and pills are available without prescription. A lactose—intolerant person simply adds a small amount of the solution to fresh milk before drinking the beverage or takes one of the pills with lactose—containing food. Lactose—intolerant people can substitute soy milk for cows' milk, because soy milk does not contain lactose. Table 5.13 lists the amount of lactose in some commonly consumed foods.

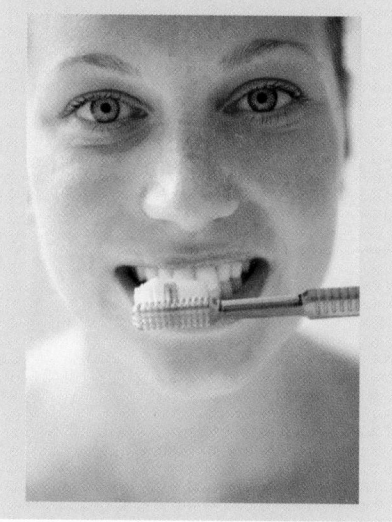

DID **YOU** KNOW?

Tooth decay is common among American college students, because of their poor dental hygiene practices and frequent consumption of sugar-sweetened beverages and other sweet foods.[67] Female college students tend to practice better oral hygiene habits than their male counterparts. If you have not begun to practice good oral hygiene, being in college is a good time to start.

lactose intolerance inability to digest lactose properly because of a deficiency in the enzyme lactase

DID **YOU** KNOW?

Many nondairy foods contain lactose. People who have severe lactose intolerance should read food labels carefully, because lactose-containing substances may be listed as ingredients. Products contain lactose if they include whey, curds, milk by-products, dry milk solids, or nonfat dry milk powder. In addition to a variety of foods, over 20% of prescription medications are sources of lactose.

FIGURE 5.19 Lactase-treated milk. Fresh lactase-treated milk is often available near soy milk in the dairy section of supermarkets.

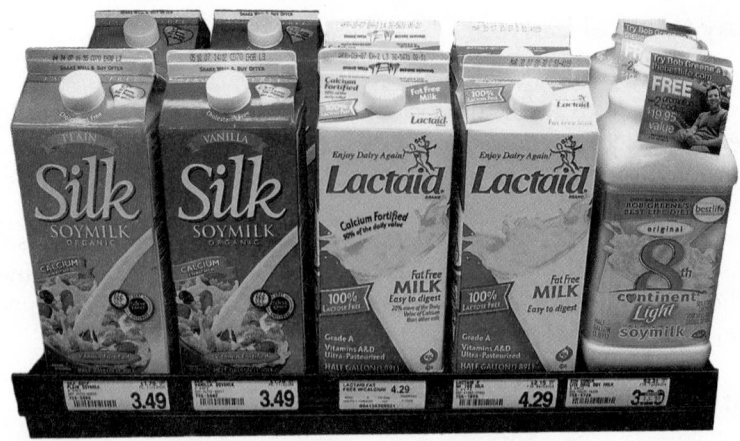

TABLE 5.13 Lactose Content of Selected Foods

Food	Value
Milk, 1 cup	10–12 g
Yogurt, 1 cup	5 g
Cheese, 1 ounce	1–2 g
Ice cream, ½ cup	6–9 g
Half-and-half, ½ cup	5 g
Butter, 1 tsp	2–3 g
Cottage cheese, ½ cup	2–3 g
Lactose-reduced milk, 1 cup	2–4 g

Does Sugar Cause Hyperactivity?

If you have ever been in charge of a 7–year–old child's birthday party or observed third graders preparing for their Halloween celebration, you can understand why people often blame sugary foods for causing unruly and "hyperactive" behavior. Attention deficit hyperactivity disorder (ADHD) is characterized by impulsivity and difficulty controlling behavior and/or pay–ing attention.[72] According to the reports of parents, 9.5% of children ages 4 to 17 years in the United States have ADHD; boys (13.2%) are more likely to be diagnosed with ADHD than girls (5.6%).[73]

Although the causes of ADHD are uncertain, they probably involve genetic and environmental factors. Eating sweets can produce pleasurable sensations, but the results of scientific studies do not indicate that sugar increases chil–dren's physical activity levels, causes ADHD, or otherwise negatively affects their behavior.[72] Birthday and school parties are exciting and happy occasions that typically involve a radical change from a child's usual routine. In these situations, a youngster's excitement and higher–than–usual activity level are more likely to result from the occasion than from a particular food.

Fiber and Health

Fiber is not an essential nutrient, because the human body can live with–out it. People may live better, however, by adding fiber–rich foods to their diets. Eating high–fiber foods may reduce a person's risk of obesity, type 2 diabetes, certain intestinal tract disorders, and cardiovascular disease, which

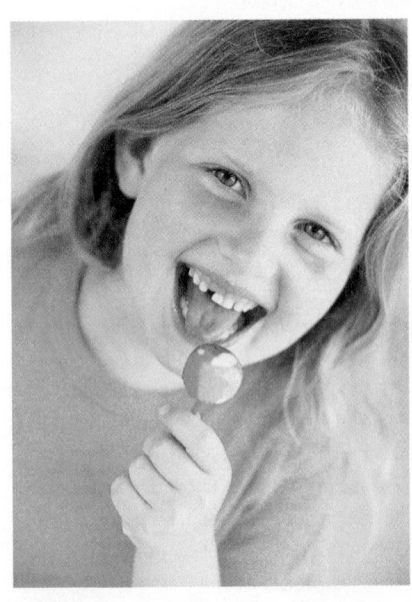

Contrary to popular belief, eating sugary foods does not cause hyperactive behavior.

includes heart disease and stroke. Because many Americans consume low—fiber diets, the Dietary Guidelines refer to fiber as a "nutrient of public health concern."

Fiber and the Digestive Tract

A person's diet, particularly its fiber content, affects bowel habits. The insoluble fiber in food contributes to the formation of a large, soft fecal mass that applies pressure to the inner muscular walls of the large intestine. This pressure stimulates the muscles to push the residue through the colon and into the rectum. People who often eat foods that contain insoluble fiber have easier and more regular bowel movements, and they are less likely to strain while having bowel movements than people whose diets lack fiber. Thus, people generally do not need to rely on over—the—counter laxatives or fiber supplements to treat constipation. Eating more fiber—rich foods is the natural way to become "regular."

Fiber and Colorectal Cancer Throughout the world, colon or *colorectal* cancer (cancer of the last portion of large intestine) is a common type of cancer.[74,75] In the early 1970s, a group of scientists noted that rural African populations that typically ate high—fiber diets rarely developed colorectal cancer. When these populations moved to urban areas and adopted relatively low—fiber Western diets, their risk of colorectal cancer increased. As a result of these observations, the scientists hypothesized that high—fiber diets were protective against colorectal cancer. By 2005, however, an analysis of the results of several large epidemiological studies indicated that diets high in dietary fiber did not reduce the risk of colorectal cancer.[76]

Although total fiber intake is not associated with lower colon cancer risk, a diet rich in whole grains,[77] fruits, and vegetables can reduce the likelihood of developing the disease.[75] Nutrition experts recommend that people eat a variety of high—fiber foods because they provide other important health benefits, such as reducing the risk of cardiovascular disease.[78]

Fiber and Heart Health Diets rich in fiber, particularly soluble types of fiber, can reduce the risk of cardiovascular disease by reducing blood cholesterol levels.[78] High blood levels of cholesterol are associated with increased risks of cardiovascular disease. The liver uses cholesterol to make bile, a substance that helps digest fats. The gallbladder stores bile and releases it into the small intestine during meals. Instead of eliminating bile along with fecal matter in bowel movements, the intestinal tract breaks down the bile and absorbs its components, which eventually enter the liver. The liver recycles bile components to make new bile.

When oat cereal is consumed, the soluble fiber in oats interferes with the bile recycling process, because it binds to the bile components in the intestinal tract and prevents them from being absorbed. Thus, the bile components are eliminated in feces. As a result, blood cholesterol levels drop as the liver removes cholesterol from the blood to make new bile. The healthful benefits of soluble fiber in oats are so important, the FDA permits manufacturers of oat cereals to use the American Heart Association's heart—healthy symbol (Fig. 5.20).

Fiber and Weight Control People who are trying to lose excess body fat may find it helpful to add more fiber—rich foods to their diets. High—fiber foods tend to be "filling" by increasing the volume of food eaten, which results in satiety. Additionally, a serving of a high—fiber food generally has a lower energy content than the same volume of a low—fiber food.[78] As a result, energy intakes usually decrease when people switch from consuming low—fiber to high—fiber diets.

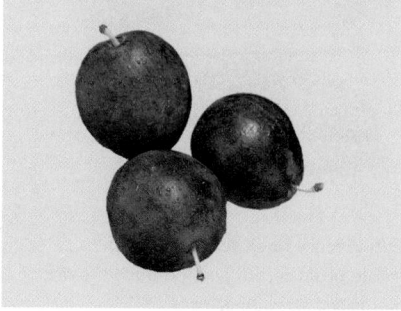

DID **YOU** *KNOW?*

Dried plums (*Prunus domestica* L.) are commonly called prunes. The fruit contains fiber, the sugar alcohol sorbitol, and other substances that are mild natural laxatives. Prune juice provides the laxative effect of prunes but lacks the whole fruit's fiber content.

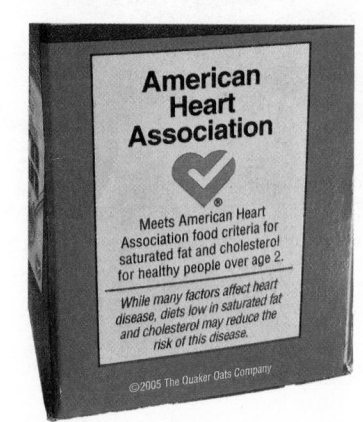

FIGURE 5.20 Soluble fiber in oats. The FDA permits oat cereal manufacturers to include the American Heart Association's heart-healthy symbol.

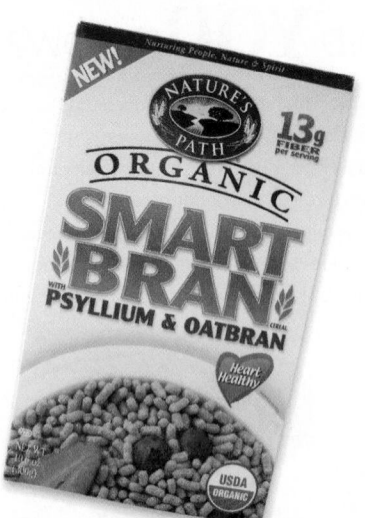

Eating more fiber-rich foods, such as whole-grain cereals, may reduce the risk of metabolic syndrome.

Increasing Fiber Intake

You can estimate your daily fiber intake by completing the "Personal Dietary Analysis" at the end of this chapter. The following "Fresh Tips" feature provides tips for increasing the fiber content of your diet. Scientists have not determined a Tolerable Upper Intake Level (UL) for fiber. However, eating excessive amounts of fiber may produce severe intestinal gas and interfere with the intestinal absorption of certain minerals. In rare instances, consuming too much dietary fiber results in intestinal blockage, especially if fluid intake is low.

Intestinal bacteria produce gases when they metabolize fiber; therefore, dietitians recommend that people gradually increase their fiber intake to reduce the likelihood of having uncomfortable and embarrassing flatulence. Practices that result in swallowing air, such as eating quickly; drinking carbonated bev—erages, especially with a straw; and chewing gum, also contribute to flatulence.

FRESH TIPS

- For healthy breakfasts or snacks, eat whole-grain, bran, or oatmeal breads and cereals. Read the ingredient label to find out if a bread or cereal product is whole grain; whole grain or bran should be the first ingredient.

- When comparing bread or cereal products, do not rely on the product's name or appearance. Check the ingredients. Terms such as "100% wheat," "multigrain," or "stone-ground wheat" are misleading, because the product may contain little or no whole grains.

- Brown rice has more fiber and flavor than white rice. If you are concerned about convenience, instant-cooking brown rice takes less time to cook than regular brown rice.

- Substitute whole-wheat pasta for regular pasta or use pasta products that contain 50% whole grain in pasta dishes.

- Snack on pieces of fresh, frozen, or dried fruit.

- Instead of removing them, eat the edible peels, pulp, and seeds of fruits and vegetables. Eat vegetables as snacks.

- Include more nuts, beans, and seeds in your diet.

- Spread peanut or soy butter on whole-grain crackers for a fiber-filled snack.

- Sprinkle unsalted nuts or hulled unsalted sunflower seeds on pancakes, waffles, or salads.

- Add frozen, dried, or fresh fruit such as berries, raisins, or bananas instead of sugar or honey to sweeten cereal or plain yogurt.

- Add a small amount of uncooked oatmeal and wheat germ to raw ground meats when making hamburgers or meatloaf.

- Add bran, wheat germ, or uncooked oatmeal to pancake or waffle batter to enhance the batter's fiber content.

- Good dietary sources of fiber contain at least 2.5 g of fiber per serving.

- You can determine the amount of fiber in a serving of food by reading the Nutrition Facts panel on the product label.

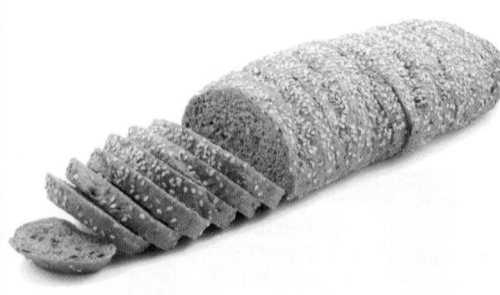

Whole-grain bread options are available in many supermarkets and restaurants, especially those that serve sandwiches.

ASSESS YOUR PROGRESS

25 *Does drinking sugar-sweetened soda contribute to obesity? Explain.*

26 *Identify at least three signs of metabolic syndrome.*

27 *Explain why some lactose-intolerant individuals are able to consume yogurt, cheese, and small amounts of milk without experiencing intestinal discomfort.*

28 *List at least three ways to increase one's fiber intake.*

29 *Discuss the health benefits of including soluble and insoluble fiber in diets.*

SUMMARY

SECTION 5.1 Introducing Carbohydrates

- Carbohydrates are an important source of energy for the body. Plants use carbon dioxide, water, and the sun's energy to make carbohydrates. Human cells break down the bonds in carbohydrates, releasing energy for cellular work.

SECTION 5.2 Simple Carbohydrates

- The three most important dietary monosaccharides are glucose, fructose, and galactose.
- Glucose is a primary fuel for muscles and other cells; nervous system and red blood cells rely on glucose for energy under normal conditions.
- Alternative sweeteners provide few or no kcal while sweetening foods and beverages.

SECTION 5.3 Complex Carbohydrates

- Oligosaccharides are complex carbohydrates comprised of three to 10 monosaccharides bonded together.
- Polysaccharides are complex polysaccharides comprised of more than 10 monosaccharides bonded together.
- Starch, glycogen, and most forms of dietary fiber are polysaccharides.
- Fibers are categorized as soluble or insoluble based on their solubility in water. Whole-grain products are rich sources of fiber, particularly insoluble fiber.

SECTION 5.4 Carbohydrate Consumption Patterns

- Healthy Americans should consume diets that furnish 45 to 65% of energy from carbohydrates, primarily complex carbohydrates. Intake of added sugars should be limited to less than 10% of total calories.

SECTION 5.5 Carbohydrates: Digestion and Absorption

- Salivary amylase initiates starch digestion in the mouth. Starch digestion halts in the stomach before resuming in the small intestine through the activity of pancreatic amylase. Maltase, sucrase, and lactase complete carbohydrate digestion.
- Glucose, fructose, and galactose are absorbed by the small intestine and travel through the hepatic portal vein to the liver.
- Humans cannot digest dietary fiber.

SECTION 5.6 Maintaining Normal Blood Glucose Levels

- Insulin and glucagon play major roles in maintaining normal blood glucose levels. Insulin allows glucose to enter cells, where it is metabolized for energy. Insulin also stimulates glycogen production. Glucagon stimulates the liver to break down glycogen into glucose molecules and release them into the bloodstream.
- Ketosis occurs when cells have an inadequate supply of glucose to metabolize for energy and they begin to break down considerable amounts of fat as an alternative fuel source.

SECTION 5.7 Diabetes Mellitus

- Diabetes mellitus ("diabetes") is characterized by elevated blood glucose levels. Poorly treated diabetes can result in cardiovascular disease, kidney failure, blindness, and lower limb amputations.
- Type 1 diabetes is an autoimmune disease that results from the lack of insulin production by the pancreas. In type 2 diabetes, beta cells of the pancreas usually produce insulin, but cells are insulin resistant. Type 2 is the more common form of the disease. People who are sedentary, are overweight, eat Western diets, and have a close relative with type 2 diabetes are at risk of developing type 2 diabetes.
- Gestational diabetes develops during pregnancy. If untreated, this form of diabetes can be dangerous to both mother and fetus.
- Regular blood glucose monitoring is important for diabetes management. Physicians treating diabetes evaluate both daily blood glucose measurements as well as hemoglobin A1c in determining treatment options.

- Medications, diet, and physical activity are important in the management of diabetes. People with type 1 diabetes require insulin through either multiple daily injections or insulin pumps. Type 2 diabetes can often be managed through diet and physical activity but may also require medications to improve insulin sensitivity.

- Carbohydrate counting, the Exchange System, and glycemic index and glycemic load are tools that people with diabetes can use to control their dietary intakes of carbohydrates.

SECTION 5.8 **Carbohydrates and Health**

- Tooth decay is the only health problem that is clearly associated with eating carbohydrates.

- Many adults are lactose intolerant because they do not produce enough lactase. People with lactose intolerance can often consume small amounts of yogurt and hard cheeses without experiencing intestinal discomfort. Enzyme pills, lactase-treated milk and milk products, and lactose-free products are also available.

- Eating fiber-rich foods may reduce the risk of obesity, type 2 diabetes, cardiovascular disease, and certain intestinal tract disorders.

Get the most out of your study of nutrition with McGraw-Hill's innovative suite of adaptive learning products including McGraw-Hill LearnSmart®, SmartBook®, McGraw-Hill LearnSmart Achieve®, and McGraw-Hill LearnSmart Prep®. Visit www.learnsmartadvantage.com.

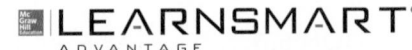

CASE STUDY RESPONSE

CARBOHYDRATES FOR BREAKFAST?

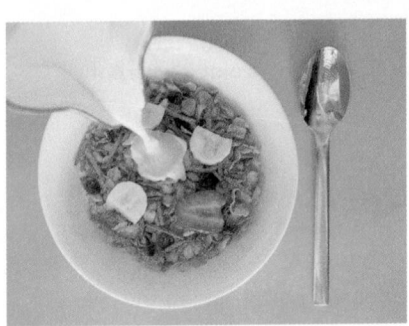

MANY AMERICANS CONSUME EXCESSIVE AMOUNTS of sucrose. Eating sugary foods can cause one's blood glucose concentration to rise rapidly and then drop quickly. By replacing simple sugars with oligosaccharides and polysaccharides, a person may reduce his or her risk of developing serious chronic diseases, particularly obesity and type 2 diabetes.

Jerry should focus on eating foods that are rich sources of complex carbohydrates, particularly dietary fiber. Nutrient-dense, carbohydrate-rich breakfast options include:

- Low-fat yogurt mixed with fresh berries, granola, and nuts
- "Quick-cooking" oatmeal mixed with berries, raisins, and nuts
- Whole-grain, ready-to-eat cereal with fresh fruit and low-fat milk
- Whole-grain waffles or pancakes sprinkled with wheat germ and topped with fresh fruit

Results of scientific studies indicate that carbohydrates as a nutrient category are not a direct cause of diabetes. Consuming too much of any digestible macronutrient and excessive weight gain can contribute to one's risk of developing type 2 diabetes.

Critical Thinking

1. One of your friends thinks honey is more nutritious and safer to eat than table sugar. He wants to avoid table sugar and use only honey as a sweetener. What would you tell this person about the nutritive value and safety of honey compared to sugar?

2. Your roommate experiences bloating, nausea, and upset stomach after drinking milk and eating ice cream. She thinks that she might be lactose intolerant, but she is confused because she can eat yogurt and cheese without having any GI side effects. Explain why your roommate is probably lactose intolerant. What steps can your roommate take to obtain key nutrients in dairy foods without experiencing the GI discomfort caused by consuming lactose?

3. Prepare a pamphlet that describes the health benefits of dietary fiber. In addition to English, you may prepare the pamphlet in Spanish, Vietnamese, or another modern language.

4. Your 30-year-old, overweight cousin was recently diagnosed with type 2 diabetes. Describe the condition to your cousin, and explain why his blood glucose level is elevated.

5. An advertisement for a very low-carbohydrate diet claims that "Carbs make you fat!" Discuss whether this claim is a true statement.

TEST KITCHEN
Modifying Recipes for Healthy Living

You are working with a client who has recently been diagnosed with type 2 diabetes. Your client is concerned about the high amounts of sugar that are in many of her favorite desserts. She would like to know how to reduce the sugar content of this strawberry cobbler recipe. Indicate how to modify the recipe so that it is more "heart healthy" and does not contain as much sucrose.

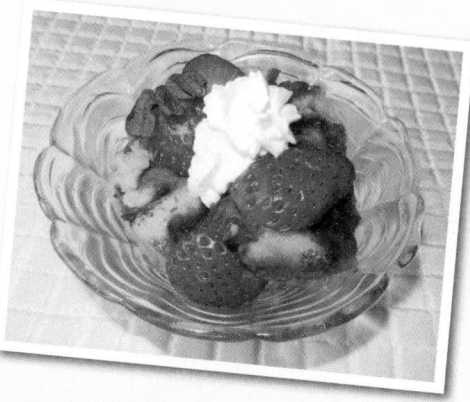

STRAWBERRY COBBLER

PREPARATION STEPS

1. Preheat oven to 375° F.
2. Grease the inside of an 8" square baking dish with melted butter.
3. Combine sugars, flour, baking powder, and salt in a small bowl. Add milk and blend well to form a batter.
4. Pour batter into the baking dish and add strawberries to the top of the batter. Sprinkle with tablespoon of white sugar.
5. Bake for 50 to 55 minutes; batter will be golden brown and a toothpick will come out of the batter clean when the cobbler is done.
6. Serve warm with whipped cream or a scoop of vanilla ice cream.

STEP 1 Brainstorm

Examine the recipe. What ingredients can you use to reduce the added sugar content of the recipe? What ingredients can you add or substitute to boost the recipe's soluble fiber content? (Refer to Table 1.7 for substitutions.)

STEP 2 Develop a modified version of this recipe

List ingredients and amounts needed.

List the preparation steps.

STEP 3 Analyze nutrient contents of the original and modified recipes by using a computer software program

Develop a table that compares the number of kcal and amounts of total carbohydrate, saturated fat, protein, fiber, and sugar in each strawberry cobbler recipe.

How did your modifications change the nutrient composition of the cobbler?

OPTIONAL ACTIVITIES

STEP 4 Test your new recipe

Keep notes on any changes you make to ingredient amounts as you prepare, bake, and garnish the cobbler.

STEP 5 Reflect on your findings

How did the cobbler look and taste?

STEP 6 Add the recipe to your collection or repeat steps to improve the product

INGREDIENTS

3 Tbsp melted butter

½ cup white sugar

¼ cup brown sugar

¾ cup all-purpose flour

¾ cup whole milk

1 tsp baking powder

Pinch of salt

2 cups frozen or fresh hulled strawberries, sliced into halves

1 Tbsp white sugar

PERSONAL Dietary Analysis

1. Keep a 3-day food log in which you record everything you eat over a 3-day period. One of the days should be Friday or Saturday. Use nutritional analysis software or the food composition table in Appendix I to analyze your daily food intakes. List the total number of kcal you consumed for each day of record keeping. Add the figures to obtain a total, divide the total by 3, then round the figure to the nearest whole number to obtain your average daily energy intake for the 3-day period.

Sample Calculation:

Day 1	<u>2500</u> kcal	
Day 2	<u>3200</u> kcal	
Day 3	<u>2750</u> kcal	
Total kcal	<u>8450</u> ÷ 3 days = <u>2817</u> kcal/day	

(average kcal intake, rounded to the nearest whole number)

Your Calculation:

Day 1	___ kcal	
Day 2	___ kcal	
Day 3	___ kcal	
Total kcal	___ ÷ 3 days = ___ kcal/day	

(average kcal intake, rounded to the nearest whole number)

2. Add the number of grams of carbohydrate eaten each day of the period. Divide the total by 3 and round to the nearest whole number to calculate the average number of grams of carbohydrate consumed daily.

Sample Calculation:

Day 1	<u>300</u> g
Day 2	<u>495</u> g
Day 3	<u>475</u> g
Total grams	<u>1270</u> ÷ 3 days = <u>423</u> g/day

(average, rounded to the nearest whole number)

Your Calculation:

Day 1	___ g
Day 2	___ g
Day 3	___ g
Total grams	___ ÷ 3 days = ___ g of carbohydrate/day

(average, rounded to the nearest whole number)

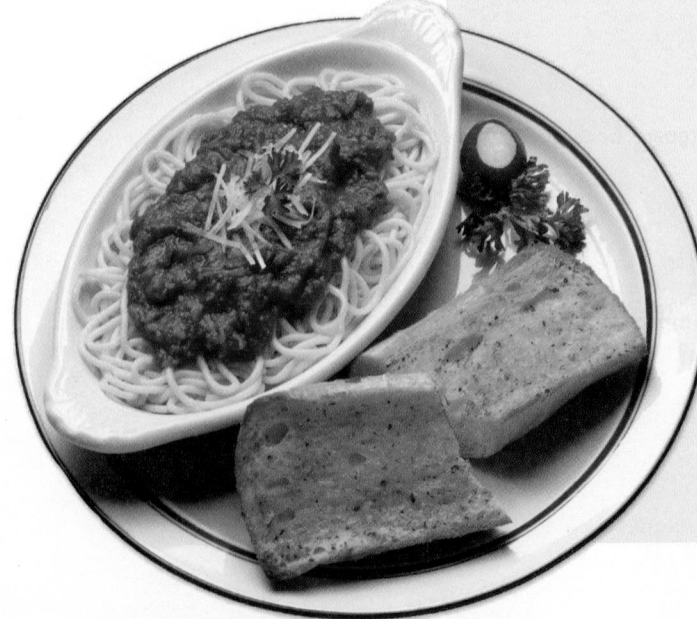

3. Each gram of carbohydrate provides about 4 kcal; therefore, you must multiply the average number of grams of carbohydrate obtained in step 2 by 4 to obtain the number of kcal from carbohydrates.

Sample Calculation:

423 g/day $\times$ 4 kcal/g = 1692 kcal from carbohydrates

Your Calculation:

___ g/day $\times$ 4 kcal/g = ___ kcal from carbohydrates

4. To calculate the average daily percentage of kcal that carbohydrates contributed to your diet, divide the average number of kcal from carbohydrate obtained in step 3 by the average total daily kcal intake obtained in step 1; round figure to the nearest one-hundredth. Multiply the value by 100, drop the decimal point, and add the percent symbol.

Sample Calculation:

1692 kcal $\div$ 2817 kcal = 0.60

0.60 $\times$ 100 = 60% of total daily kcals supplied by carbohydrates

Your Calculation:

___ kcal $\div$ ___ kcal = ___

___ $\times$ 100 = ___ 60% of total daily kcals supplied by carbohydrates

5. On average, did you consume at least the RDA of 130 g of carbohydrate? Yes ___ No ___

6. Did your average carbohydrate intake meet the recommended 45 to 65% of total energy? Yes ___ No ___

   a. If your average carbohydrate intake was less than 130 g or below 45% of total kcal, list five nutrient-dense, carbohydrate-rich foods you could eat that would boost your intake of carbohydrates.

7. Review the log of your 3-day food intake. Calculate your average daily intake of fiber by adding the grams of fiber consumed over the 3-day period and dividing the total by 3.

Your Calculation:

Day 1	___	g
Day 2	___	g
Day 3	___	g
Total g	___	g

Total grams ___ $\div$ 3 days = ___ g of fiber daily

   a. What was your average daily fiber intake? ___ g

   b. Did your average daily fiber intake meet the recommended Adequate Intake (38 and 25 g/day for young men and women, respectively)? Yes ___ No ___

   c. If your response is yes, list foods that contributed to your fiber intake.

   d. If you did not meet the recommended level of fiber intake, list at least five foods that you would eat to increase your fiber intake to the recommended level.

Practice Test

Select the best answer.

1. Which of the following substances is a disaccharide?
   - a. fructose
   - b. sucrose
   - c. galactose
   - d. glycogen

2. _____ is a primary fuel for muscles and other cells.
   - a. Protein
   - b. Cholesterol
   - c. Glucose
   - d. HFCS

3. Which artificial sweetener must be avoided by a person with PKU?
   - a. saccharin
   - b. sucralose
   - c. aspartame
   - d. stevioside

4. Which of the following substances is not a polysaccharide?
   - a. glycogen
   - b. lactose
   - c. cellulose
   - d. starch

5. The human body stores glucose in the form of
   - a. glycogen.
   - b. galactose.
   - c. adrenaline.
   - d. insulin.

6. Raffinose and stachyose are examples of
   - a. monosaccharides.
   - b. disaccharides.
   - c. oligosaccharides.
   - d. starch.

7. Dietary fiber
   - a. supplies more energy, gram per gram, than fat.
   - b. is not digested by the human intestinal tract.
   - c. promotes tooth decay.
   - d. is only in animal sources of food.

8. Insoluble fiber
   - a. is in beef and pork.
   - b. dissolves or swells in water.
   - c. is in whole-grain products, including brown rice.
   - d. increases the risk of heart disease.

9. _____ is the hormone that enables glucose to enter cells.
   - a. Glucagon
   - b. Insulin
   - c. Glycerin
   - d. Thyroxine

10. _____ is the enzyme that breaks down starch.
    - a. Sucrase
    - b. Amylase
    - c. Lactase
    - d. Starchase

11. Type 2 diabetes is
    - a. a disease that primarily affects young children.
    - b. characterized by severe hypoglycemia.
    - c. often associated with excess body weight.
    - d. caused by eating refined sugars.

12. Gestational diabetes
    - a. should not be treated until after the fetus is born.
    - b. can result in a newborn baby who is too small.
    - c. increases a woman's risk of developing type 2 diabetes.
    - d. is most common in underweight pregnant women.

13. Which of the following foods has the highest glycemic index?
    - a. nonfat milk
    - b. cornflakes cereal
    - c. salted peanuts
    - d. apple

14. Which of the following signs is associated with metabolic syndrome?
    - a. low blood pressure
    - b. high fasting blood glucose
    - c. low hemoglobin
    - d. high fasting HDL cholesterol

15. Which of the following foods would be recommended for preventing constipation?
    - a. cheddar cheese
    - b. whole-grain bread
    - c. pizza
    - d. lean ground beef

ANSWERS TO PRACTICE TEST
1-b; 2-c; 3-c; 4-b; 5-a; 6-c; 7-b; 8-c; 9-b; 10-b; 11-c; 12-c; 13-c; 14-b; 15-b

ANSWERS TO CHAPTER 5 QUIZ Yourself

1. The carbohydrate found in milk is called lactose. **True** (p. 113)
2. Ounce per ounce, sugar provides more energy than starch. **False** (p. 118)
3. Digestion of starch begins in the mouth. **True** (p. 123)
4. Eating a high-fiber diet can improve the functioning of the large intestine and reduce blood cholesterol levels. **True** (p. 139)
5. Individuals with diabetes should follow a carbohydrate-free diet. **False** (p. 131)

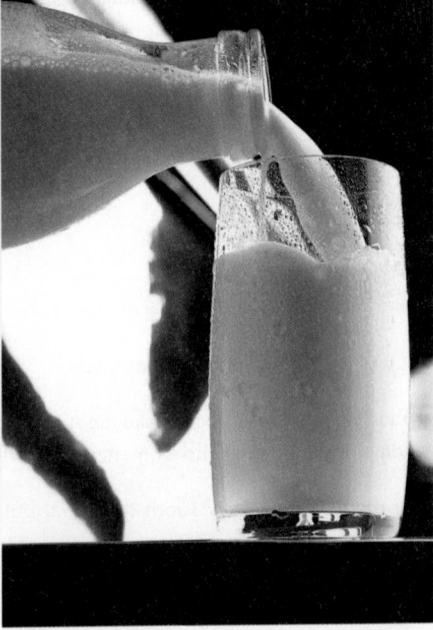

References

1. Grant KA and others: Infant botulism: Advice on avoiding feeding honey to babies and other possible risk factors. *Community Practitioner* 86(7):44, 2013.

2. Centers for Disease Control and Prevention, Division of Bacterial and Mycotic Diseases: *Botulism.* Updated July 2011. http://www.cdc.gov/nczved/divisions/dfbmd/diseases/botulism/ Accessed: January 10, 2014

3. Yu Z and others: High-fructose corn syrup and sucrose have equivalent effects on energy-regulating hormones at normal human consumption levels. *Nutrition Research* 33(12):1043, 2013.

4. Rippe JM, Angelopoulos TJ: Sucrose, high-fructose corn syrup, and fructose, their metabolism and potential health effects: What do we really know? *Advances in Nutrition* 4(2):236, 2013.

5. United States Department of Agriculture Agricultural Research Service: *What We Eat in America 2009–2010.* http://www.ars.usda.gov/Services/docs.htm?docid=13793 Accessed: January 10, 2014

6. Makinen K: Sugar alcohols, caries incidence, and remineralization of caries lesions: A literature review. *International Journal of Dentistry* 2010:1, 2010. Published online 2010 January 5. DOI: 10.1155/2010/981072

7. Academy of Nutrition and Dietetics: Position of the Academy of Nutrition and Dietetics: Use of nutritive and nonnutritive sweeteners. *Journal of the Academy of Nutrition and Dietetics* 112(5):739, 2012. Erratum vol. 112(8):1279, 2012.

8. Soffritti M and others: First experimental demonstration of the multi-potential carcinogenic effects of aspartame administered in the feed to Sprague-Dawley rats. *Environmental Health Perspectives* 114(3):379, 2006.

9. Chatsudthipong V, Muanprasat C: Stevioside and related compounds: Therapeutic benefits beyond sweetness. *Pharmacology and Therapeutics* 121:41, 2009.

10. Brahmachari G and others: Stevioside and related compounds—molecules of pharmaceutical promise: A critical overview. *Archives of Pharmacology* 344: 5, 2011.

11. FDA provides guidance on "whole grain" for manufacturers. FDA News, P06-23, 2006. http://www.fda.gov/Food/GuidanceRegulation/GuidanceDocumentsRegulatoryInformation/LabelingNutrition/ucm059088.htm Accessed: January 10, 2014

12. Raninen K and others: Dietary fiber type reflects physiological functionality: Comparison of grain fiber, inulin, and polydextrose. *Nutrition Reviews* 69:9, 2011.

13. Kelly G: Inulin-type prebiotics—a review: part 1. *Alternative Medicine Reviews* 13:315, 2008.

14. Bonsu NK and others: Can dietary fructans lower serum glucose? *Journal of Diabetes* 3:58, 2011.

15. Martin BR and others: Fructo-oligosaccharides and calcium absorption and retention in adolescent girls. *Journal of the American College of Nutrition* 29:382, 2010.

16. De Oliveira AC and others: The domestic processing of the common bean resulted in reduction in the phytates and tannins, antinutritional factors, in the starch content and in the raffinose, stachiose, and verabascose flatulence factors. [article in Portuguese] *Archivos Latinoamericanos de Nutrición* 51(3):276, 2001.

17. Otten JJ and others, eds.: *Dietary Reference Intakes: The essential guide to nutrient requirements.* Washington, DC: National Academies Press, 2006.

18. Economic Research Service, U.S. Department of Agriculture: *Sugar and sweeteners yearbook tables, Table 50.* June 2013. http://www.ers.usda.gov/data-products/sugar-and-sweeteners-yearbook-tables.aspx#.Ubsvs5zZWSo Accessed: January 10, 2014

19. U.S. Department of Agriculture, Agricultural Research Service, Nutrient Data Laboratory: *USDA national nutrient database for standard reference, Release 26.* Updated 2013. http://ndb.nal.usda.gov/ Accessed: January 10, 2014

20. Kit BK and others: Trends in sugar-sweetened beverage consumption among youth and adults in the United States: 1999–2010. *American Journal of Clinical Nutrition* 98(1):180, 2013.

21. O'Leary N: Soft drink consumption continues to decline. *AdWeek*, March 30, 2010. http://www.adweek.com/news/advertising-branding/soft-drink-consumption-continues-decline-107218 Accessed: January 10, 2014

22. Shielders DH and others: Gourmet coffee beverage consumption among college women. *Journal of the American Dietetic Association* 104:650, 2004.

23. Soleimani M: Dietary fructose, salt absorption and hypertension in metabolic syndrome: Toward a new paradigm. *Acta Physiologica* 201(1):55, 2011.

24. Sattley M: The history of diabetes. *Diabetes Health*, December 2008.

25. Dean L, McEntrye J: The Genetic Landscape of Diabetes. *National Center for Biotechnology Institute of Health*, 2004.

26. Centers for Disease Control and Prevention: *National Diabetes Statistics Report, 2014.* Updated June 2014. http://www.cdc.gov/diabetes/pubs/statsreport14.htm Accessed: June 11, 2014

27. Zoran DL: Obesity in dogs and cats: A metabolic and endocrine disorder. *The Veterinary Clinics of North America—Small Animal Practice* 40(2):221, 2010.

28. Rucinsky R and others: American Animal Hospital Association Diabetes Management Guidelines for Dogs and Cats. *Journal of the American Animal Hospital Association* 46:215, 2010.

29. Murphy SL and others: Deaths: Final data for 2010. *National Vital Statistics Reports* 61(4):1, 2013.

30. van Belle TL and others: Type 1 diabetes: Etiology, immunology, and therapeutic strategies. *Physiological Reviews* 91(1):79, 2011.

31. *Centers for Disease Control and Prevention: Diabetes & Pregnancy.* 2012. http://www.cdc.gov/Features/DiabetesPregnancy/ Accessed: June 11, 2014

32. Poston L and others: Obesity in pregnancy: Implications for the mother and lifelong health of the child: A consensus statement. *Pediatric Research* 69(2):175, 2011.

33. American Diabetes Association: Living with diabetes, A1C. Last revised December 2013. http://www.diabetes.org/living-with-diabetes/treatment-and-care/blood-glucose-control/a1c/ Accessed: January 10, 2014

34. Webb D: Glycemic index: Gateway to good health or grand waste of time? *Environmental Nutrition* 25(1):1, 6, 2002.

35. Muntoni S, Muntoni S: Insulin resistance—Pathophysiology and rationale for treatment. *Annals of Nutrition and Metabolism* 58(1):25, 2011.

36. Larsen TM and others: Diets with high or low protein content and glycemic index for weight-loss maintenance. *New England Journal of Medicine* 363(22):2102, 2010.

37. American Diabetes Association: Glycemic index and diabetes. Updated January 2014. http://www.diabetes.org/food-and-fitness/food/planning-meals/glycemic-index-and-diabetes.html Accessed: January 10, 2014

38. Nathan DM: The diabetes control and complications trial/epidemiology of diabetes interventions and complications study at 30 years: overview. *Diabetes Care* 37:1, 2014.

39. Jahansouz C and others: Evolution of β-cell replacement therapy in diabetes mellitus: Pancreas transplantation. *Diabetes Technology and Therapy* 13:395, 2011.

40. American Diabetes Association: Pancreas transplantation. Updated January 2014. http://www.diabetes.org/living-with-diabetes/treatment-and-care/transplantation/pancreas-transplantation.html Accessed: January 10, 2014

41. Mittal S, Gough SC: Pancreas transplantation: a treatment option for people with diabetes. *Diabetic Medicine* Published online before in print, 2013. DOI: 10.1111/dme.12373

42. American Diabetes Association: *Living With Diabetes—Treatment and Care—Oral Medications.* ND. http://www.diabetes.org/living-with-diabetes/treatment-and-care/medication/oral-medications/ Accessed: January 10, 2014

43. Jalilian M and others: Physical activity stage-matched intervention: Promoting metabolic control in type 2 diabetes. *Journal of Education and Health Promotion* 2:18, 2013.

44. American Diabetes Association: *Diabetes—Lower Your Risk—Overweight.* Updated December 2013. http://www.diabetes.org/are-you-at-risk/lower-your-risk/overweight.html?loc=atrisk-slabnav Accessed: January 10, 2014

45. Gallen IW and others: Fueling the athlete with type 1 diabetes. *Diabetes and Obesity Metabolism* 13(2):130, 2011.

46. Juvenile Diabetes Research Foundation: Athletes with diabetes—Gary Hall Jr. Updated 2013. http://kids.jdrf.org/index.cfm?fuseaction=home.viewpage&page_id=0552132C-2A5E-7B6E-198EDD7B51645FF0 Accessed January 10, 2014

47. van Dam RM and others: Dietary patterns for type 2 diabetes mellitus in U.S. men. *Annals of Internal Medicine* 136(3):201, 2002.

48. de Koning L and others: Low-carbohydrate diet scores and risk of type 2 diabetes in men. *American Journal of Clinical Nutrition* 93:844, 2011.

49. Psaltopoulou T and others: The role of diet and lifestyle in primary, secondary, and tertiary diabetes prevention: a review of meta-analyses. *The Review of Diabetic Studies* 7(1):26, 2010.

50. Qi L and others: Genetic predisposition, Western dietary pattern, and the risk of type 2 diabetes in men. *American Journal of Clinical Nutrition* 89(5):1453, 2011.

51. National Institute of Diabetes and Digestive and Kidney Diseases: *Hypoglycemia.* Publication No. 09–3926 Updated November 2012. http://diabetes.niddk.nih.gov/dm/pubs/hypoglycemia/ Accessed January 10, 2014

52. Rosen LA and others: Effects of cereals on postprandial glucose, appetite regulation and voluntary energy intake at subsequent lunch; focusing on rye products. *Nutrition Journal* 10:7, 2011.

53. Jennings A and others: Diet quality is independently associated with weight status in children aged 9–10 years. *Journal of Nutrition* 141:153, 2011.

54. Kaiser KA and others: Will reducing sugar-sweetened beverage consumption reduce obesity? Evidence supporting conjecture is strong, but evidence when testing effect is weak. *Obesity Reviews* 14(8):620, 2013.

55. Dennis EA and others: Beverage consumption and adult weight management: A review. *Eating Behaviors* 10(4):237, 2009.

56. Basu S and others: Relationship of soft drink consumption to global overweight, obesity, and diabetes: A cross-national analysis of 75 countries. *American Journal of Public Health* 103(11):2071, 2013.

57. Rizkalla SW: Health implications of fructose consumption: A review of recent data. *Nutrient Metabolism* 4(7):82, 2010.

58. Johnson RK, Yon BA.: Weighing in on added sugars and health. *Journal of the American Dietetic Association* 110(9):1296, 2010.

59. Ventura and others: Neurobiologic basis of craving for carbohydrates. *Nutrition* Published online before in print, 2013. DOI: 10.1016/j.nut.2013.06.010

60. Carmienke S and others: General and abdominal obesity parameters and their combination in relation to mortality: A systematic review and meta-regression analysis. *European Journal of Clinical Nutrition* 67(6):573, 2013.

61. Bakris GL: Current perspectives on hypertension and metabolic syndrome. *Journal of Managed Care Pharmacy* 13(5):S3, 2007.

62. Ford ES and others: Prevalence and correlates of metabolic syndrome based on a harmonious definition among adults in the US. *Journal of Diabetes* 2(3):180, 2010.

63. Grundy SM and others: Diagnosis and management of the metabolic syndrome: An American Heart Association/National Heart, Lung, and Blood Institute scientific statement: Executive summary. *Circulation* 112:e285, 2005.

64. Baik I and others: A healthy dietary pattern consisting of a variety of food choices is inversely associated with the development of metabolic syndrome. *Nutrition Research and Practice* 7(3):233, 2013.

65. O'Keefe JH, Abuannadi M.: Dietary strategies for the prevention and treatment of metabolic syndrome. *Missouri Medicine* 107(6):406, 2010.

66. Lichtenstein AH and others: Diet and lifestyle recommendations revision 2006: A scientific statement from the American Heart Association Nutrition Committee. *Circulation* 114(1):82, 2006.

67. Daly B and others: Dental tooth surface loss and quality of life in university students. *Primary Dental Care* 18:31-5, 2011.

68. National Institute of Diabetes and Digestive and Kidney Diseases: *Lactose intolerance.* NIH Publication No. 09–2751, Updated April 2012. http://digestive.niddk.nih.gov/ddiseases/pubs/lactoseintolerance/index.htm Accessed: January 10, 2014

69. Bahna SL: Cow's milk allergy versus cow milk intolerance. *Annals of Allergy, Asthma, and Immunology* 89(6 Suppl 1):56, 2002.

70. Montalto M and others: Management and treatment of lactose malabsorption. *World Journal of Gastroenterology* 12(2):187, 2006.

71. Wilt TJ and others: Lactose intolerance and health. *Evidence report/technology assessment* 192:1, 2010.

72. National Institute of Mental Health: *Attention deficit hyperactivity disorder.* ND. http://www.nimh.nih.gov/health/topics/attention-deficit-hyperactivity-disorder-adhd/index.shtml Accessed: January 10, 2014

73. Centers for Disease Control and Prevention: Increasing prevalence of parent-reported attention-deficit/hyperactivity disorder among children—United States, 2003 and 2007. *Morbidity and Mortality Weekly Report* 59(44);1439, 2010.

74. World Health Organization: *Cancer: key facts.* Reviewed January 2013. http://www.who.int/mediacentre/factsheets/fs297/en/index.html Accessed: January 10, 2014

75. Centers for Disease Control and Prevention: *Colorectal (colon) cancer.* Updated January 2014. http://www.cdc.gov/cancer/colorectal/ Accessed: January 10, 2014

76. Park Y and others: Dietary fiber intake and risk of colorectal cancer: A pooled analysis of prospective cohort studies. *Journal of the American Medical Association* 294(22):2849, 2005.

77. Egeberg R and others: Intake of whole-grain products and risk of colorectal cancers in the Diet, Cancer, and Health cohort study. *British Journal of Cancer* 103(5):730, 2010.

78. American Dietetic Association: Position of the American Dietetic Association: Health implications of dietary fiber. *Journal of the American Dietetic Association* 108(10):1716, 2008.

6 Lipids: Triglycerides, Phospholipids, and Sterols

CASE STUDY

Lipids and heart health

ALTHOUGH SHE WAS OVERWEIGHT, 45-year-old Samantha was surprised to learn at her last doctor's appointment that she had high blood pressure. Additionally, her blood lab values indicated that some of her blood lipids were not within the desirable range. Her total cholesterol level was 230 mg/dL; her LDL cholesterol was 140 mg/dL; her HDL cholesterol was 35 mg/dL; and her triglycerides were 90 mg/dL. The physician told Samantha she had a high risk for developing heart disease. As a result of her physician's advice, Samantha is ready to make lifestyle changes to lower her risk of heart disease.

- What are normal blood lipid concentrations for adult females?

- Explain the differences between HDL cholesterol and LDL cholesterol.

- Describe how blood lipid concentrations contribute to the development of the disease.

- List five dietary recommendations to help Samantha to lower her risk of developing heart disease.

The suggested Case Study Response can be found on page 181.

Mc Graw Hill Education **connect** | NUTRITION Check out the Connect site at www.mcgrawhillconnect.com to further explore this case study.

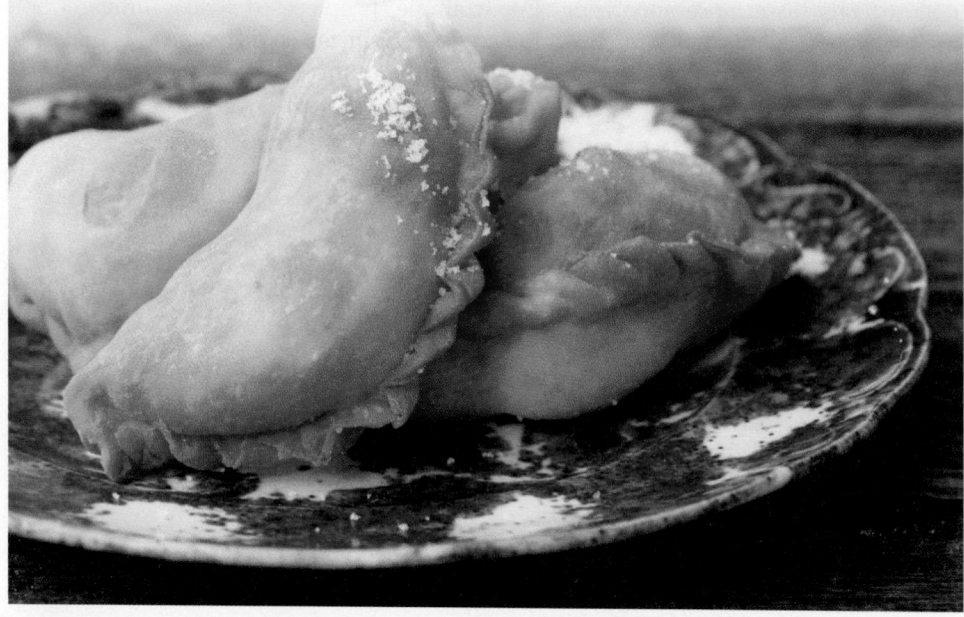

6.1 Introducing Lipids

LEARNING OUTCOMES

1 *Identify the three major classes of lipids.*
2 *Describe major functions of lipids in the body.*

Numerous studies conducted over the past 60 years indicate that consuming high amounts of certain lipids may increase the risk of developing serious health conditions, including obesity,[1] certain cancers,[2] and cardiovascular disease (CVD), which includes heart disease and stroke.[3,4] However, some fat is essential for good health, and certain types of fats may actually decrease the risk of developing chronic disease and promote optimal health.

In this chapter, we will show that not all lipids are "bad" and that lipids are an essential part of a well-balanced diet. We will review how the different types of lipids affect health and wellness, and which types of lipids should be emphasized in diets.

Classes of Lipids

lipids class of nutrients that do not dissolve in water; triglycerides, phospholipids, and sterols

Lipids include triglycerides (*try–glis'–er–eyeds*), phospholipids (*fos–foe–lip'–ids*), and sterols, such as cholesterol. Lipids dissolve in organic solvents such as alcohol and acetone, but most lipids are insoluble in water. Consider what happens when you mix vinegar and olive oil to make a vinaigrette salad dressing. Vinegar is 95% water; oil is 100% lipid. Therefore, the oil does not dissolve in the water to make a solution. Additionally, oil is less dense than water, so it rises to the top of the vinegar in small globules. The oil globules join together to form an oily layer that floats on the vinegar until the mixture is shaken. Shaking the ingredients mixes them temporarily. When left undisturbed, the oil and vinegar separate; hence the saying, "Oil and water don't mix."

Major Functions of Lipids

Lipids are structural components of the plasma membrane that surrounds each cell. The layer of fat under the skin (*subcutaneous fat*) stores energy, insulates against cold temperatures, protects against minor bruising, and contributes to the body's contours. Table 6.1 lists these and some other major roles of lipids in the body.

Lipids also provide nonnutritional benefits such as enhancing food flavor, texture, and aroma. Whether fat occurs naturally in food or is added to it, this nutrient often makes foods taste more appetizing. For example, people used to consuming whole milk, which is about 3.25% fat by volume, will recognize the difference fat makes to "mouthfeel" when they drink fat–free milk that contains less than 0.5% fat.

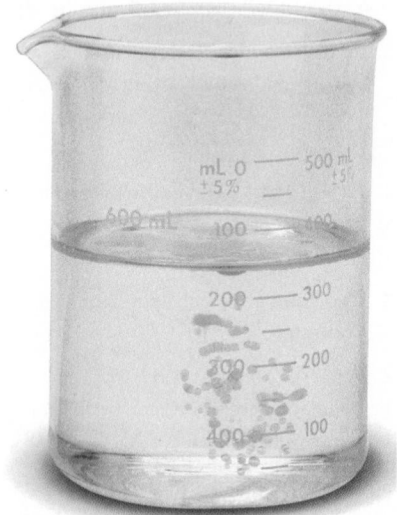

Oil and water do not mix.

TABLE 6.1 Major Functions of Lipids in the Body

The body uses fats and other lipids to:
• Provide and store energy (triglycerides)
• Form and maintain cell membranes
• Produce steroid hormones
• Insulate the body against cold temperatures
• Cushion the body against bumps and blows
• Form body contours
• Absorb fat-soluble vitamins and phytochemicals

ASSESS YOUR PROGRESS

1 *List the three major classes of lipids.*
2 *What are four functions of lipids in the body?*

6.2 Fatty Acids

LEARNING OUTCOMES

1 *Distinguish between saturated, monounsaturated, and polyunsaturated fatty acids.*

2 *Identify the two essential fatty acids and explain their nutritional importance.*

3 *Describe trans fats, including how they are made and how they are different from most other fats.*

Most lipids have **fatty acids** in their structures. Fatty acids provide energy for muscles and most other types of cells. As Figure 6.1 illustrates, a fatty acid is comprised of a **hydrocarbon chain**, a chain of carbon atoms bonded to each other and to hydrogen atoms. One end of the fatty acid chain has a carbon molecule with three hydrogen atoms attached to it. This part of the molecule is called the **omega** or the **methyl end**. The other end of fatty acid molecule forms a **carboxylic acid**.

In biological systems, common fatty acids have an even number of carbon atoms. *Short−chain* fatty acids have 2 to 4 carbons; *medium−chain* fatty acids have 6 to 12 carbons; and *long−chain* fatty acids have 14 to 24 carbons. The molecules shown in Figure 6.1 contain 18 carbons; thus, they are long−chain fatty acids. Chemists identify a fatty acid by (1) its number of carbon atoms and (2) the type of bond between carbon atoms in the hydrocarbon chain. These two characteristics influence how fatty acids can affect health.

Saturation

Fatty acids can be saturated or unsaturated. The carbons in the fatty acid chain shown in Figure 6.1a have single bonds between them. Note that each carbon in the chain has two hydrogen atoms attached to it. This is a **saturated fatty acid (SFA)**, because each carbon within the chain is saturated, that is, completely filled with hydrogen atoms.

An **unsaturated fatty acid** has at least two neighboring carbons within the chain that are missing two hydrogen atoms, and a double bond holds the two particular carbons together (Fig. 6.1b). The fatty acid illustrated in Figure 6.1b has only one double bond linking two carbon atoms; therefore, it is referred to as a ***mono*unsaturated fatty acid (MUFA)**. The fatty acids shown in Figures 6.1c and 6.1d are also unsaturated, but they have two or more double bonds in their hydrocarbon chains; so, they are ***poly*unsaturated fatty acids (PUFAs)**.

Most foods contain fats with both saturated and unsaturated fatty acids, including those listed in Table 6.2. Some commonly consumed fats have 18−carbon fatty acids in their hydrocarbon chain. **Stearic acid** is an 18−carbon SFA (Fig. 6.1a). **Oleic** (*oh−lay'−ik*) **acid** is also an 18−carbon fatty acid, but it is a MUFA because it has one double bond (Fig. 6.1b). **Linoleic** (*lin'−o−lay'−ik*) **acid** and **alpha (α)−linolenic** (*al'−fah−lin'−o−len'−ik*) **acid** are 18−carbon PUFAs. Linoleic acid has two double bonds (Fig. 6.1c). Alpha−linolenic acid has three double bonds (Fig. 6.1d).

Omega Fatty Acids

Fatty acids are identified not only by their chain length and number of double bonds, but also by the location of the double bonds in the carbon chain. A particular group of PUFAs, the "omega fats," are very important in human nutrition. To name these molecules, begin at the omega end of the fatty acid chain and note the position of the first double bond. An **omega−3 fatty acid** is a PUFA with its first double bond at the third carbon from the omega end

fatty acid hydrocarbon chain found in lipids; one end of the chain forms a carboxylic acid, and one end forms a methyl group

hydrocarbon chain chain of carbon atoms bonded to each other and to hydrogen atoms

omega (methyl) end end of a fatty acid containing a methyl ($-CH_3$) group

carboxylic acid organic molecule with a carboxyl ($-COOH$) group

saturated fatty acid (SFA) fatty acid that has each carbon atom within the chain filled with hydrogen atoms

unsaturated fatty acid fatty acid that is missing hydrogen atoms and has one or more double bonds within the carbon chain

monounsaturated fatty acid (MUFA) fatty acid that has one double bond within the carbon chains

polyunsaturated fatty acid (PUFA) fatty acid that has two or more double bonds within the carbon chain

stearic acid 18-carbon saturated fatty acid

oleic acid 18-carbon monounsaturated fatty acid

linoleic acid 18-carbon polyunsaturated fatty acid with two double bonds; an essential fatty acid

alpha-linolenic acid 18-carbon polyunsaturated fatty acid with three double bonds; an essential fatty acid

omega-3 fatty acid type of polyunsaturated fatty acid with the first double bond at the third carbon from the omega end of the molecule

DID **YOU** KNOW?

What is the difference between fats and oils? Although both have fatty acids, fats tend to be solid and oils liquid at room temperature. Compared to foods that contain high amounts of unsaturated fatty acids, foods that are rich sources of long-chain SFAs tend to be more solid at room temperature. Butter, for example, contains more long-chain SFAs than vegetable oil, which contains more long-chain unsaturated fatty acids.

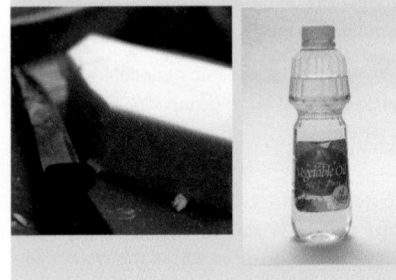

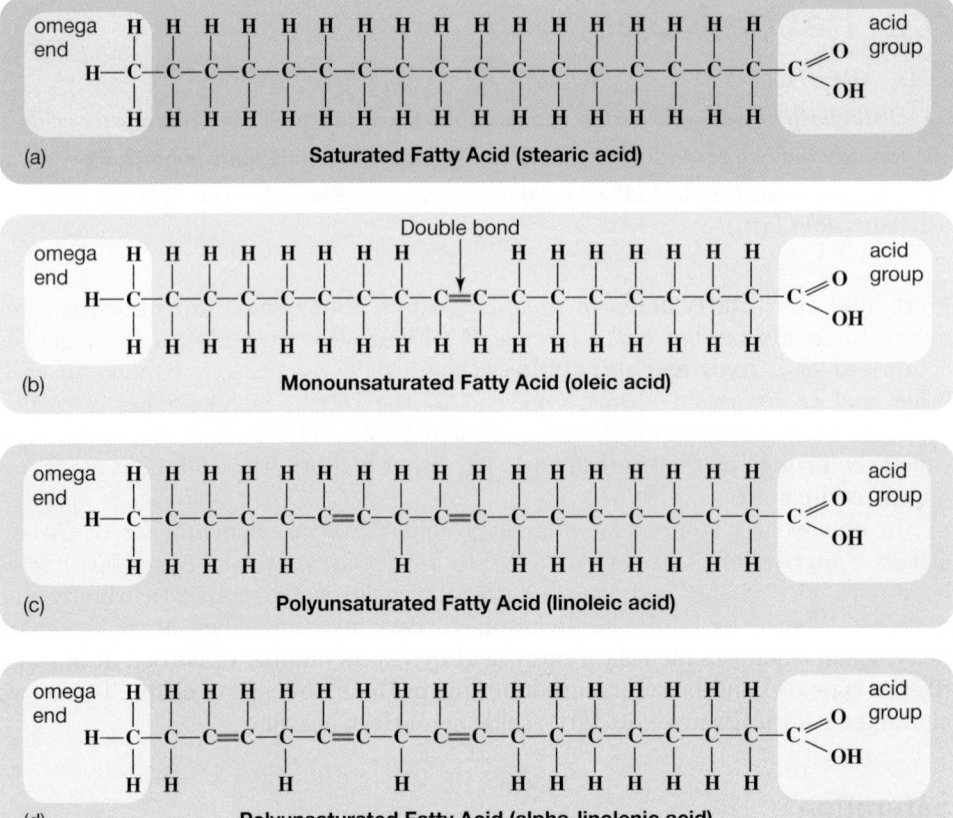

FIGURE 6.1 Fatty acids. Each of these fatty acids has 18 carbons, but they differ in the number of double bonds. (*a*) A saturated fatty acid has single bonds between the carbon atoms in the hydrocarbon chain. (*b*) An unsaturated fatty acid has at least two neighboring carbons within the chain that are missing two hydrogen atoms with a double bond holding those particular carbons together. Oleic acid is a monounsaturated fatty acid because it has one double bond. (*c*) A polyunsaturated fatty acid has two or more double bonds between carbons in the hydrocarbon chain. Linoleic acid has two double bonds. (*d*) Alpha-linolenic acid is a polyunsaturated fatty acid with three double bonds in the hydrocarbon chain.

omega-6 fatty acid type of polyunsaturated fatty acid with the first double bond at the sixth carbon from the omega end of the molecule

of the molecule (Fig. 6.1d). Alpha–linolenic acid is an omega–3 fatty acid. An **omega–6 fatty acid** is also a PUFA, but its first double bond occurs at the sixth carbon from the omega end of the chain (Fig. 6.1c). Linoleic acid is an omega–6 fatty acid. In section 6.9, we discuss the roles of omega–3 and omega–6 fatty acids in health.

TABLE 6.2 Common Fatty Acids

	Fatty Acid Name	Number of Carbon Atoms	Number of Double Bonds
Saturated fatty acids	Myristic acid	14	0
	Palmitic acid	16	0
	Stearic acid	18	0
Unsaturated fatty acids	Oleic acid	18	1
	Linoleic acid	18	2
	Alpha-linolenic acid	18	3
	Arachidonic acid	20	4

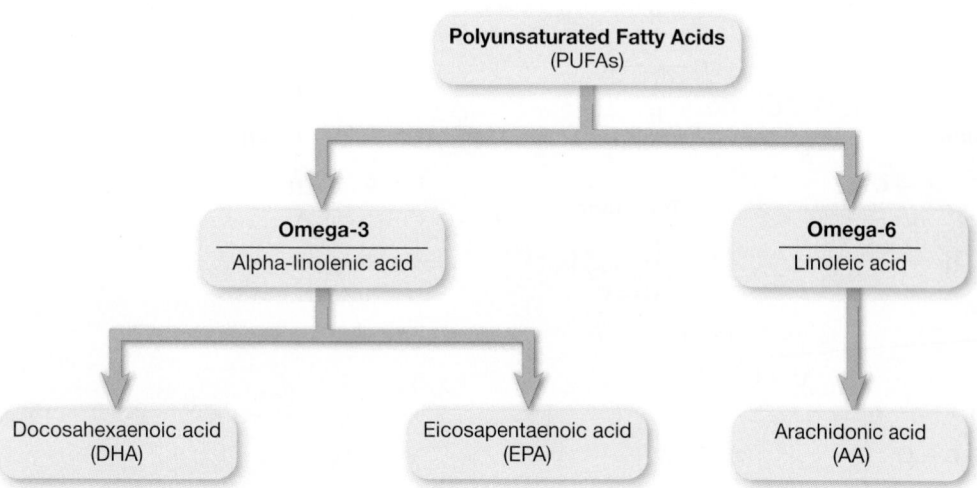

FIGURE 6.2 Essential fatty acids. Alpha-linolenic acid and linoleic acid are not synthesized by the body; they must be supplied in the diet. The body uses these essential fatty acids to make DHA, EPA, and AA.

Essential Fatty Acids

The body cannot synthesize linoleic acid and alpha−linolenic acid, so the diet must supply these two **essential fatty acids**. The body converts linoleic acid to **arachidonic** ($ar'−a−keh−don'−ik$) **acid (AA)** and alpha−linolenic acid to two other omega−3 fatty acids, **eicosapentaenoic** ($eye'−ko−seh−pen'−tah−e−no'−ik$) **acid (EPA)** and **docosahexaenoic** ($doe'−ko−seh−hek'−seh−e'−no'−ik$) **acid (DHA)**. Figure 6.2 shows relationships among essential fatty acids.

The body needs AA, EPA, and DHA to make **eicosanoids** ($eye−koh'−sah−noids$), a group of long−chain fatty acids that have hormonelike functions. Prostaglandins ($pros−tah−glan'−dins$), thromboxanes ($throm−bok'−sanes$), and leukotrienes ($loo−ko−try'−eens$) are classes of eicosanoids. **Prostaglandins** produce a variety of important effects on the body, such as stimulating uterine contractions, regulating blood pressure, and mediating the immune system's inflammatory response.

Essential fatty acids are necessary in small amounts for good health. Infants require DHA and EPA for nervous system development, and babies do not grow properly when their diets lack essential fatty acids. Other signs of essential fatty acid deficiency include scaly skin, hair loss, and poor wound healing. The Adequate Intake (AI) for alpha−linolenic acid is 1.6 g/day for men and 1.1 g/day for women. The AI for linoleic acid is 17 g/day for men and 12 g/day for women who are between 19 and 50 years of age.[5] These amounts can be met with foods made with 2 to 3 tablespoons of vegetable fat daily, especially products made with canola and soybean oils, and meals that contain fatty fish, such as salmon and tuna, at least twice a week.

What Are Trans Fats?

Most naturally occurring unsaturated fatty acids are cis fatty acids. A cis fatty acid has the two carbon atoms that are connected by a double bond, each having a hydrogen atom on the same side of the hydrocarbon chain (Fig. 6.3). **Trans fats** are unsaturated fatty acids that have at least one trans double bond in their chemical structure, rather than the more common cis configuration. The hydrogen atoms of the double−bonded carbons within the hydrocarbon chain are on opposite sides of the chain (Fig. 6.3b). The trans configuration at the double bond enables the hydrocarbon chain to be relatively straight, which

essential fatty acids fatty acids that must be supplied by the diet; linoleic and alpha-linolenic acid are essential fatty acids

arachidonic acid (AA) essential fatty acid; precursor to some eicosanoids;

eicosapentaenoic acid essential fatty acid; precursor to some eicosanoids

docosahexaenoic acid essential fatty acid; precursor to some eicosanoids

eicosanoids group of long-chain fatty acids with hormonelike functions

prostaglandins class of eicosanoids that produce a variety of important effects on the body

trans fats unsaturated fatty acids that have a trans double bond

FIGURE 6.3 Cis and trans double-bond arrangements. (*a*) Oleic acid, a cis fatty acid, has the hydrogen atoms of the double-bonded carbons on the same side of the molecule, resulting in a kink. (*b*) Elaidic acid, a trans fatty acid, has the hydrogen atoms of the double-bonded carbons on opposite sides, resulting in a straighter arrangement of the fatty acid chain. For simplicity, most of the hydrogen atoms in these molecules are not shown.

is similar to a SFA molecule's structure. Fats that contain a high proportion of trans fatty acids are more solid at room temperature than those with a high proportion of cis fatty acids.

Trans Fats in Foods

Whole milk and whole—milk products, butter, and meat naturally contain small amounts of trans fats. Processed foods and margarines contribute the largest share of trans fatty acids in the American diet. Most of the trans fatty acids in processed food result from the **hydrogenation** process. Partial hydrogenation is a food manufacturing process that adds hydrogen atoms to some unsaturated fatty acids in liquid vegetable oil, which results in the formation of SFAs. The hydrogenation process also converts many of the oil's naturally occurring cis fatty acids into trans fatty acids. Partially hydrogenated vegetable oil, because it is more solid at room temperature, can be made into shortening or shaped into sticks of margarine. Shortening is often used to prepare deep—fat fried foods and cakes, pastries, and frostings.

Foods made with partially hydrogenated fat can be stored for longer periods of time—for some products, over a year—than foods that contain cis fatty acids. The reason is that trans fatty acids are less likely to undergo *oxidation*, a chem—ical process that alters the compound's structure. Unsaturated fatty acids that have the cis double—bond arrangement, especially PUFAs, are very susceptible to oxidation. When oxidized, the fat in food becomes rancid and develops an unappetizing odor and taste. Instead of relying on trans fatty acids to extend the shelf life of products, manufacturers can preserve PUFAs and other ingredients in foods by adding antioxidants to them.

In the body, trans fatty acids raise "bad" blood cholesterol levels and lower "good" blood cholesterol levels, which may increase the risk of heart disease.[6] The Food and Drug Administration (FDA) requires food manufac—turers to include information about trans fatty acid content on their prod—ucts' Nutrition Facts panels. In 2013, information in a Nutrition Facts panel could indicate that a serving of food has "0 g" trans fat, but the serving could still provide a small amount of trans fat (less than 0.5 g). Therefore, a person could consume several grams of trans fatty acids daily, depending on food choices and portion sizes.

hydrogenation food manufacturing process that adds hydrogen atoms to liquid vegetable oil, forming trans fats

DID **YOU** *KNOW?*

Cooks often use shortening to make pie crust because the partially hydrogenated fat in shortening results in a flaky tender crust. When making pie dough, oil can be substituted for shortening, but it produces a crumbly texture that may be undesirable.

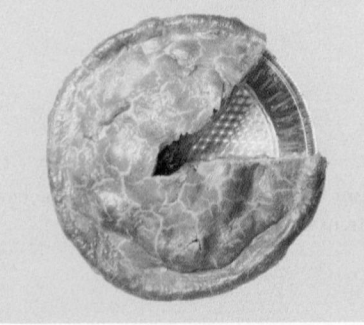

As American consumers have become more aware of the potential health problems associated with trans fat consumption, many food manufacturers have removed ingredients that contain trans fatty acids from their products. In 2013, officials with the FDA announced a ban on the addition of trans fats to processed foods.[7] The FDA, however, will allow food manufactures to gradually phase out their use of trans fats.

The use of a synthetic lipid, *interesterified* (*in′ −ter−eh−ster′−rih−fide′*) oil, to replace trans fats in processed foods may also have undesirable health effects, including raising blood glucose levels.[8] More research is needed to determine the long−term safety of consuming foods that contain interesterified oil. Processed foods that include "fully hydrogenated" or "interesterified" oil in their ingredient lists are sources of interesterified fat.

ASSESS YOUR PROGRESS

③ *What are the definitions of saturated, monounsaturated, and polyunsaturated fatty acids?*

④ *How does an omega-3 fatty acid differ from an omega-6 fatty acid?*

⑤ *Identify the two essential fatty acids, and describe key signs of an essential fatty acid deficiency.*

⑥ *What structural characteristic distinguishes a trans fatty acid from a cis fatty acid?*

FRESH TIPS

Margarine, butter, oil, and shortening have higher fat contents than as "lite" spreads that may have water as the first ingredient. Therefore, replacing some or all of the fat in a recipe with a reduced-fat spread could alter the product's taste, texture, and appearance. It is a good idea to read the reduced-fat spread's label to determine whether the product is suitable to use in recipes.

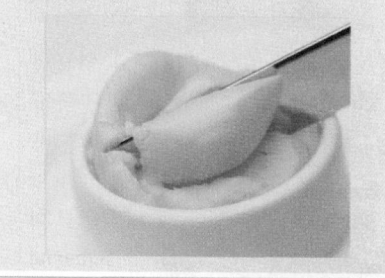

6.3 Triglycerides

LEARNING OUTCOMES

1 *Describe the basic structure of a triglyceride.*

2 *Compare the percentages of saturated, monounsaturated, and polyunsaturated fatty acids in animal-derived fats with those in most plant-derived fats.*

3 *Name two plant oils that are high in saturated fats.*

Triglycerides comprise about 95% of lipids in food and in the human body. Body fat is largely composed of stored triglycerides. A **triglyceride** has three fatty acids bonded to **glycerol** (*glis′−er−ol*), a three−carbon alcohol that is often referred to as the "backbone" of the triglyceride (Fig. 6.4). Each glycerol backbone can bond with up to three fatty acids. A glycerol molecule bonded to one, two, or three fatty acids is called a **monoglyceride**, **diglyceride**, and triglyceride, respectively.

Triglycerides in Foods

Most triglycerides contain mixtures of unsaturated and saturated fatty acids (Fig. 6.5). In a particular food, such as olives or cheese, the unsaturated and saturated fats occur in different proportions, but one type of fatty acid (SFA, MUFA, or PUFA) often predominates.

Figure 6.5 compares the percentages of SFAs, MUFAs, and PUFAs in commonly eaten fats. Note that the fat in beef and dairy products contains more saturated than unsaturated fatty acids; olive oil is a rich source of MUFAs; and liquid corn oil contains a greater proportion of unsaturated than saturated fatty acids. Certain animal foods, especially beef and dairy foods, contain higher percentages of SFAs than most plant fats. Important exceptions are tropical oils such as coconut and palm oils. Tropical oils contain more saturated than unsaturated fatty acids.

triglyceride lipid that has three fatty acids attached to a three-carbon compound called glycerol

glycerol three-carbon alcohol that forms the "backbone" of fatty acids

monoglyceride lipid that has one fatty acid attached to a three-carbon compound called glycerol

diglyceride lipid that has two fatty acids attached to a three-carbon compound called glycerol

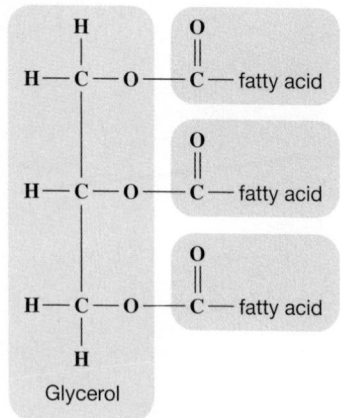

FIGURE 6.4 Triglycerides. A triglyceride has three fatty acids attached to a glycerol "backbone."

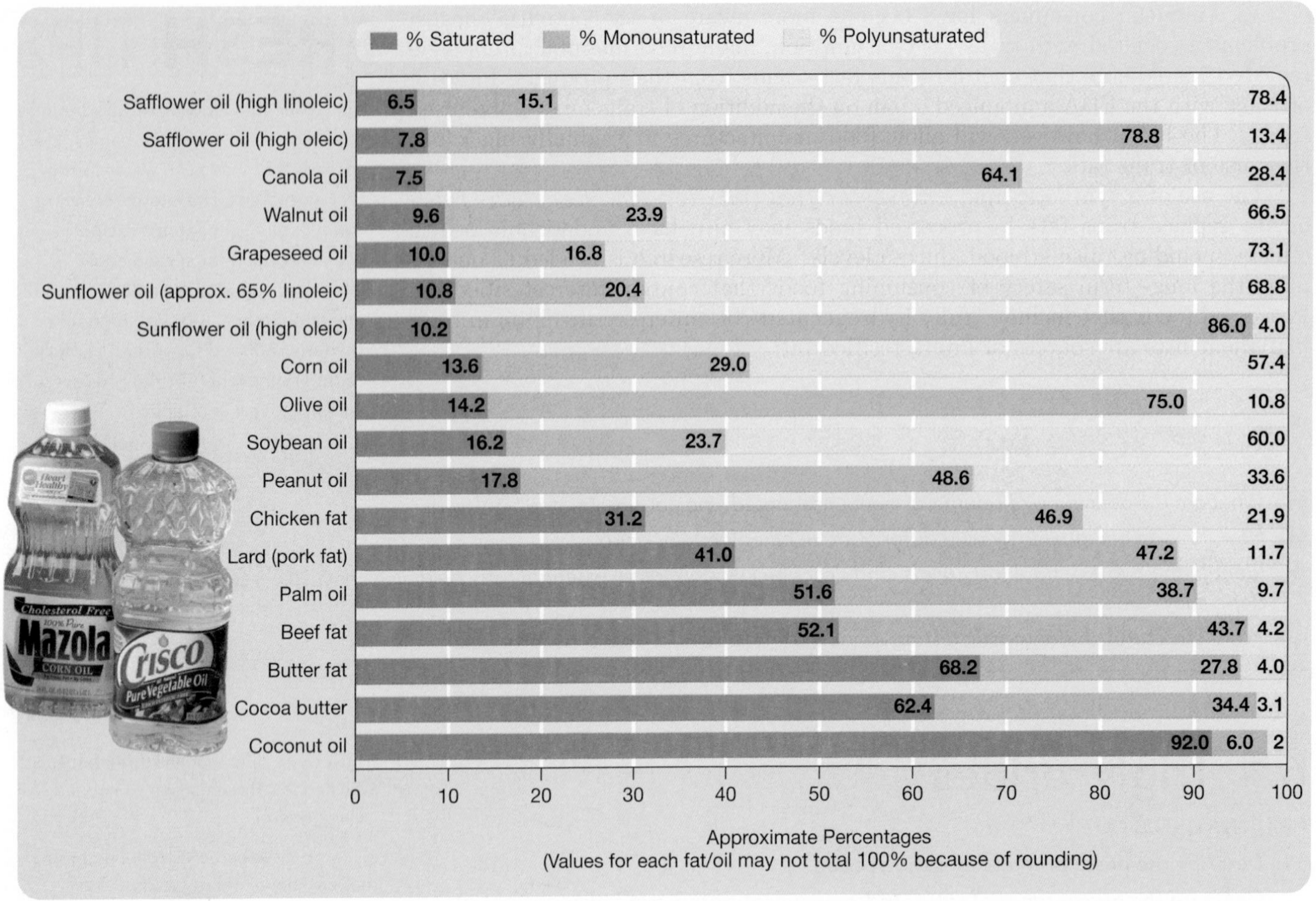

	% Saturated	% Monounsaturated	% Polyunsaturated

Oil/Fat	Saturated	Monounsaturated	Polyunsaturated
Safflower oil (high linoleic)	6.5	15.1	78.4
Safflower oil (high oleic)	7.8	78.8	13.4
Canola oil	7.5	64.1	28.4
Walnut oil	9.6	23.9	66.5
Grapeseed oil	10.0	16.8	73.1
Sunflower oil (approx. 65% linoleic)	10.8	20.4	68.8
Sunflower oil (high oleic)	10.2	86.0	4.0
Corn oil	13.6	29.0	57.4
Olive oil	14.2	75.0	10.8
Soybean oil	16.2	23.7	60.0
Peanut oil	17.8	48.6	33.6
Chicken fat	31.2	46.9	21.9
Lard (pork fat)	41.0	47.2	11.7
Palm oil	51.6	38.7	9.7
Beef fat	52.1	43.7	4.2
Butter fat	68.2	27.8	4.0
Cocoa butter	62.4	34.4	3.1
Coconut oil	92.0	6.0	2

Approximate Percentages
(Values for each fat/oil may not total 100% because of rounding)

Source: Data from U.S. Department of Agriculture, Agricultural Research Service, USDA Nutrient Data Laboratory: *USDA national nutrient database for standard reference, release* 26. 2013.

FIGURE 6.5 Fats and oils. This figure shows approximate percentages of the three major types of fatty acids in common fats and oils.

Why is it important to understand the differences between saturated, unsat—urated, and trans fats and to identify foods that contain high amounts of these fats? Because populations that consume diets rich in saturated fat and trans fat have higher incidence of developing CVD than populations whose diets contain more unsaturated than saturated fat.[9] For more information about this topic, see section 6.9, "Reducing Risk of Developing Atherosclerosis: Dietary Changes."

DID **YOU** KNOW?

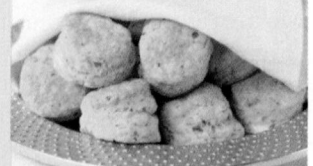

Lard is pork fat. In some parts of the United States, lard is used to make biscuits, pie dough, and refried beans. Lard is high in saturated fat (41%), but it is not as highly saturated as butter (66%). The consumption of lard in the United States has decreased significantly in the past 40 years.[10]

ASSESS YOUR PROGRESS

7 *Identify at least two foods that are rich sources of (a) saturated fat, (b) monounsaturated fat, and (c) polyunsaturated fat.*

6.4 Phospholipids

LEARNING OUTCOMES

1 *Explain how a phospholipid differs in structure from a triglyceride.*
2 *List the key roles of phospholipids in foods and in the body.*

A **phospholipid** is chemically similar to a triglyceride, except that one of the fatty acids is replaced by a chemical group that contains phosphorus and, often, nitrogen (Fig. 6.6a). Phospholipids are naturally found in foods derived from plants and animals.

Unlike triglycerides, phospholipids are partially water soluble because the phosphorus–containing portion of the molecule is **hydrophilic** (*hydro* = water; *philic* = loving); that is, it attracts water (Fig. 6.6b). A phospholipid molecule also has a **hydrophobic** (*phobic* = fearing) portion that avoids watery substances. By having both hydrophilic and hydrophobic regions, a phospholipid can serve as an **emulsifier**, a substance that keeps water–soluble and water–insoluble compounds mixed together (Fig. 6.7).

In the body, phospholipids are major structural components of cell membranes. Cell membranes are composed of a double layer that is mostly phospholipids (Fig. 6.8). The chemical structure of the phospholipids enables the membrane to be flexible and function properly. Phospholipids are also needed for normal functioning of nerve cells, including those in the brain.

Phospholipid deficiencies among adults are uncommon, because these lipids occur in a variety of foods and healthy adults synthesize these compounds. Egg yolks, liver, wheat germ, peanut butter, and soybeans are rich sources of *lecithin* (*less′–eh–thin*), the most abundant phospholipid in food. Lecithin contains **choline** (*co′–leen*), a water–soluble, vitamin–like compound that has

phospholipid type of lipid needed to make cell membranes and for proper functioning of nerve cells; chemically similar to a triglyceride except that one of the fatty acids is replaced by a chemical group that contains phosphorus

hydrophilic part of a molecule that attracts water

hydrophobic part of a molecule that avoids water and attracts lipids

emulsifier substance that helps water-soluble and water-insoluble compounds mix with each other

choline water-soluble, vitamin-like compound; component of lecithin

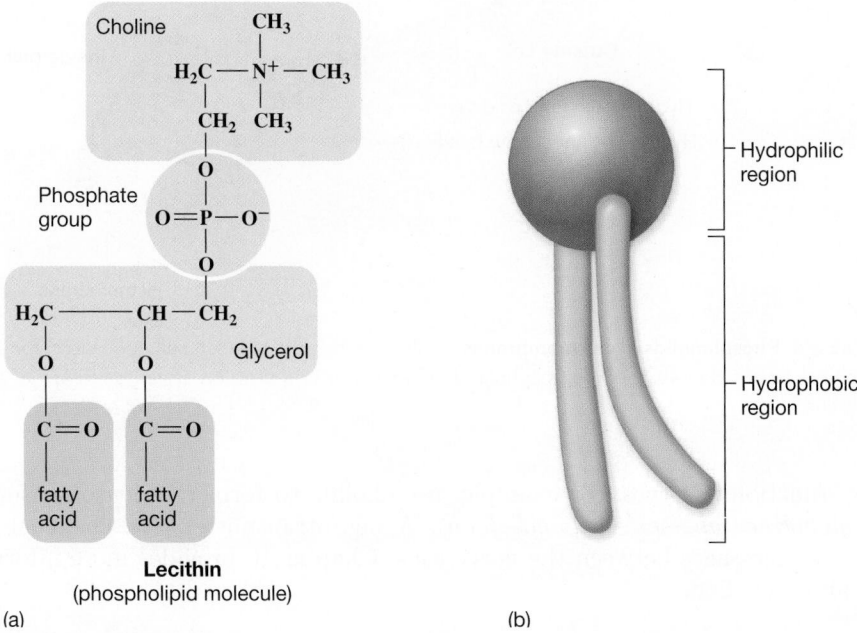

(a)   (b)

FIGURE 6.6 Phospholipids. A phospholipid molecule such as lecithin has a chemical structure that is similar to that of a triglyceride molecule. (*a*) The chemical structure of lecithin has a glycerol backbone, a phosphorus (P)-containing phosphate group, and a nitrogen (N)-containing compound called choline. (*b*) Phospholipids have hydrophilic and hydrophobic portions. As a result, a phospholipid can serve as an emulsifier.

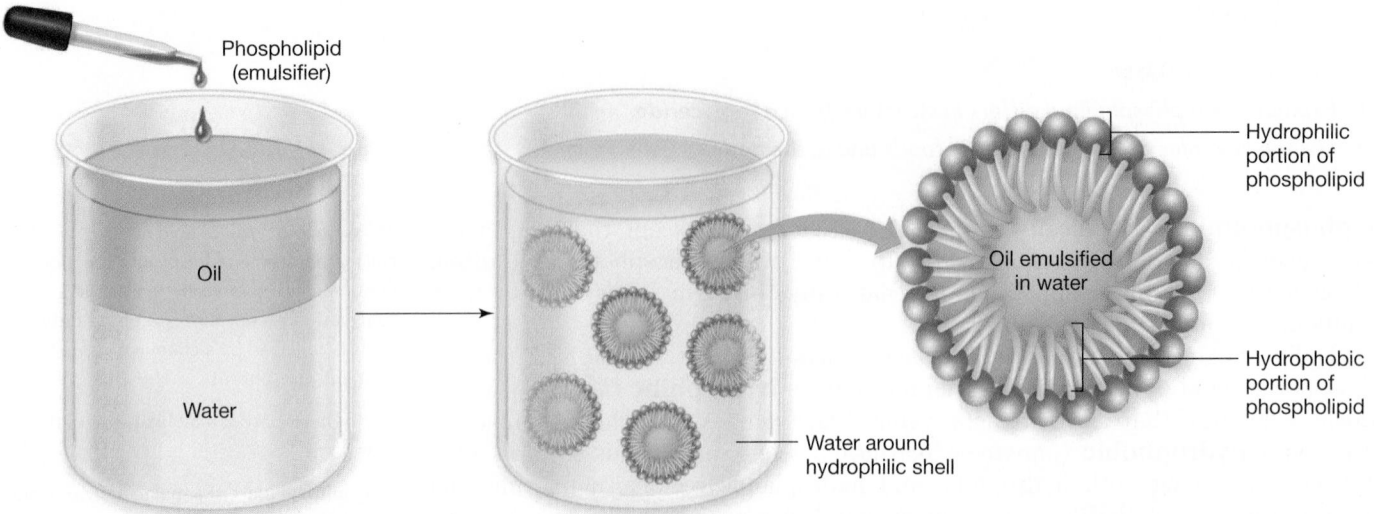

FIGURE 6.7 Emulsification. Emulsification keeps lipids dispersed in small particles, increasing their surface area.

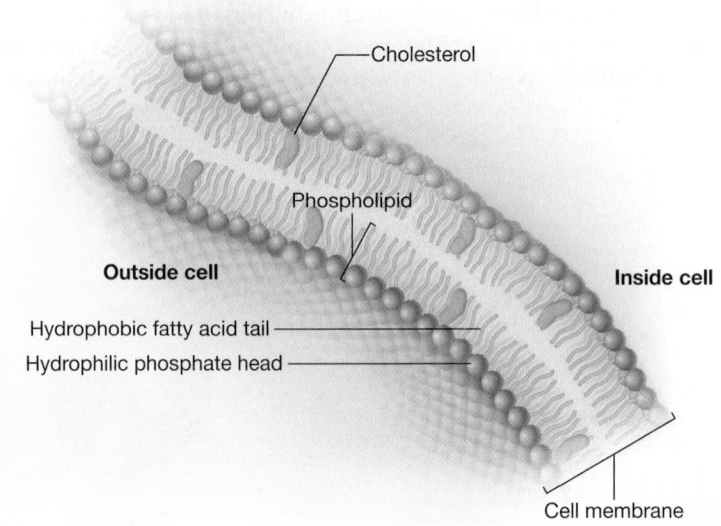

FIGURE 6.8 Phospholipids in cell membranes. In all cells, including human cells, cell membranes are comprised of a double layer of phospholipids. Cholesterol and proteins are embedded in the membrane.

many functions. Nerves, for example, use choline to form the neurotransmitter *acetylcholine (ah—see'—till—co'—leen)*. A neurotransmitter is a chemical that transmits messages between the nerve cells. Chapter 10 provides more information about choline.

ASSESS YOUR PROGRESS

8 *What are the components of a phospholipid?*

9 *Explain the function of an emulsifier in food preparation and manufacturing.*

6.5 Cholesterol and Other Sterols

LEARNING OUTCOMES

1 *Describe key roles of cholesterol in the body.*

2 *Explain how plant sterols and stanols may lower blood cholesterol levels.*

Cholesterol is the most well−known *sterol*. **Sterols** are lipids that have a more chemically complex structure than a triglyceride or phos−pholipid (Fig. 6.9). Many people think cholesterol is unhealthy and foods that contain choles−terol should be avoided. Cholesterol, however, is essential to health as it is an integral component of every cell membrane in the body. Although cholesterol is not metabolized for energy, cells use it to synthesize a variety of substances, including *steroid hormones*, such as vitamin D, cortisol, aldosterone, testosterone, estrogen, and progesterone.

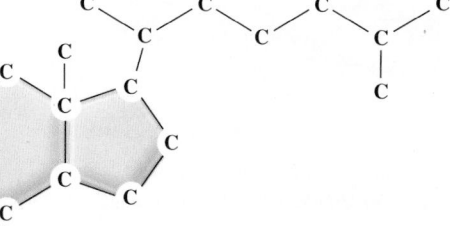

FIGURE 6.9 Cholesterol. Cholesterol is a complex organic molecule synthesized by animals. For simplicity, this illustration shows cholesterol's carbon atoms and HO group.

Cholesterol is found only in foods derived from animals. Egg yolk, liver, meat, poultry, and dairy products made from cream or whole milk are rich sources of the lipid (Table 6.3). Most adults do not need to consume dietary sources of cho−lesterol because the liver can make enough cholesterol to satisfy the body's needs. For average adults, about two−thirds of their total body cholesterol is made in their liver and one−third is consumed through food sources.

cholesterol lipid found in animal foods; precursor for steroid hormones, bile, and vitamin D

sterols type of lipid that has a more complex chemical structure than triglycerides and phospholipids

TABLE 6.3 Approximate Cholesterol Content of Some Foods/Serving

Food	Serving Size	Cholesterol (mg)
Liver	3 oz	234
Egg	1 large	186
Egg yolk	1	186
Sardines	3 oz	121
Single-patty cheeseburger	1	111
Beef	3 oz	88
Turkey, ground	3 oz	84
Danish fruit-filled pastry	2 ½ oz	81
Shrimp	6 large	80
Ham	3 oz	80
Ice cream, soft-serve	½ cup	78
Ground beef, lean (15% fat)	3 oz	77
Salmon	3 oz	75
Turkey, dark meat	3 oz	71
Egg noodles	1 cup	53
Chicken breast	3 oz	49
Hot dog	1	44
Chocolate milkshake	16 oz	43
Whole milk	1 cup	34

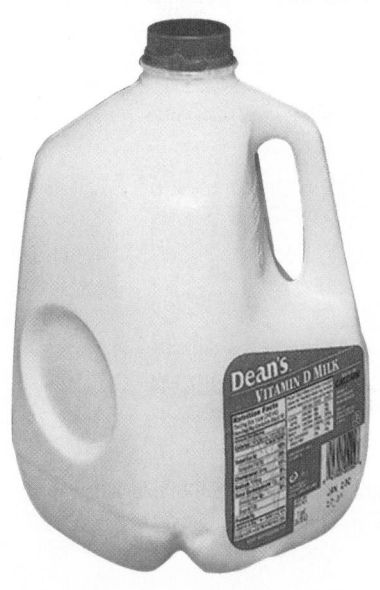

One cup of whole milk supplies approximately 34 mg of cholesterol.

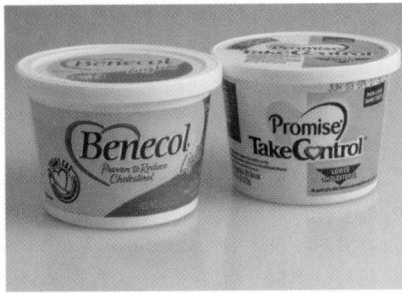

Take Control® and Benecol® spreads contain added plant sterols and stanols.

plant sterols/stanols chemicals found in plants that are structurally similar to cholesterol

Plant Sterols and Stanols

Plant sterols and **stanols**, including *sitostanol*, are structurally similar to cholesterol. These lipids occur naturally in small amounts in many grains, fruits, vegetables, nuts, seeds, and legumes. Because their chemical structures are similar to cholesterol's, plant sterols and stanols compete with cholesterol for intestinal absorption, which reduces the amount of cholesterol that is absorbed. As a result, consuming foods that contain plant sterols and stanols may be an effective way to lower elevated blood cholesterol levels, a risk factor for developing heart disease.[11,12]

ASSESS YOUR PROGRESS

10 *Explain why cholesterol is necessary for health.*

11 *List three food sources of cholesterol.*

12 *What effect do plant sterols and stanols have on cholesterol absorption?*

6.6 Lipid Digestion, Absorption, and Transport

LEARNING OUTCOMES

1 *Summarize the major steps of lipid digestion and absorption, and identify the major digestive organs involved in the process.*

2 *Describe gallstones and strategies for dietary management.*

3 *Identify the function of lipoproteins.*

The average American consumes 77 g of fat per day.[13] Most lipids are completely insoluble in water. This characteristic makes lipid digestion, absorption, and transport more complicated than that of carbohydrates, because these three processes involve considerable amounts of water. Despite the added challenges, the average healthy adult digests, absorbs, and utilizes about 98% of fat that is consumed.

Lipid Digestion

lipases enzymes that break down lipids

Triglycerides and phospholipids need to be broken down by **lipases**, fat-digesting enzymes, before they can be absorbed. When a person eats a cheeseburger and French fries, an inactive lipase in his or her saliva mixes with the food. As the food enters the stomach, the organ's acidic environment activates the lipase, enabling some lipid breakdown to occur. The small intestine, however, is the primary site of lipid digestion.

As the fatty chyme leaves the stomach and enters the small intestine, it stimulates certain intestinal cells to secrete the hormones cholecystokinin (*kol'−e−sis'−toe−kye'−nin*) (CCK) and secretin. Secretin stimulates the liver to produce bile and causes the pancreas to secrete bicarbonate−rich pancreatic juice, which is necessary to create an alkaline environment in the small intestine. CCK signals the pancreas to secrete digestive enzymes, including **pancreatic lipase**, into the duodenum of the small intestine. CCK also triggers the gallbladder to release stored bile and the sphincter that controls the flow of bile and pancreatic juice into the duodenum to open.

pancreatic lipase digestive enzyme that removes two fatty acids from each triglyceride molecule

Bile contains **bile salts**, compounds that enhance digestion and absorption by emulsifying lipids in the watery environment of the small intestine. Emulsification keeps lipids dispersed in small particles, which increases their surface area and enables lipase to gain greater access to the individual lipid molecules (Fig. 6.10). Without bile's action, lipids would collect in a greasy film or aggregate into large globules within the lumen of the small intestine.

bile salts component of bile; aid in lipid digestion

Pancreatic lipase digests triglycerides by removing two fatty acids from each triglyceride molecule. This action converts most triglycerides into monoglycerides (Fig. 6.10). Some triglycerides are completely broken down into glycerol and fatty acid molecules.

The process of digesting phospholipids is similar to that of digesting tri—glycerides. A pancreatic phospholipase removes the fatty acid from the second position of the phospholipid molecule. The remaining structure is a phospholipid fragment (see Fig. 6.6).

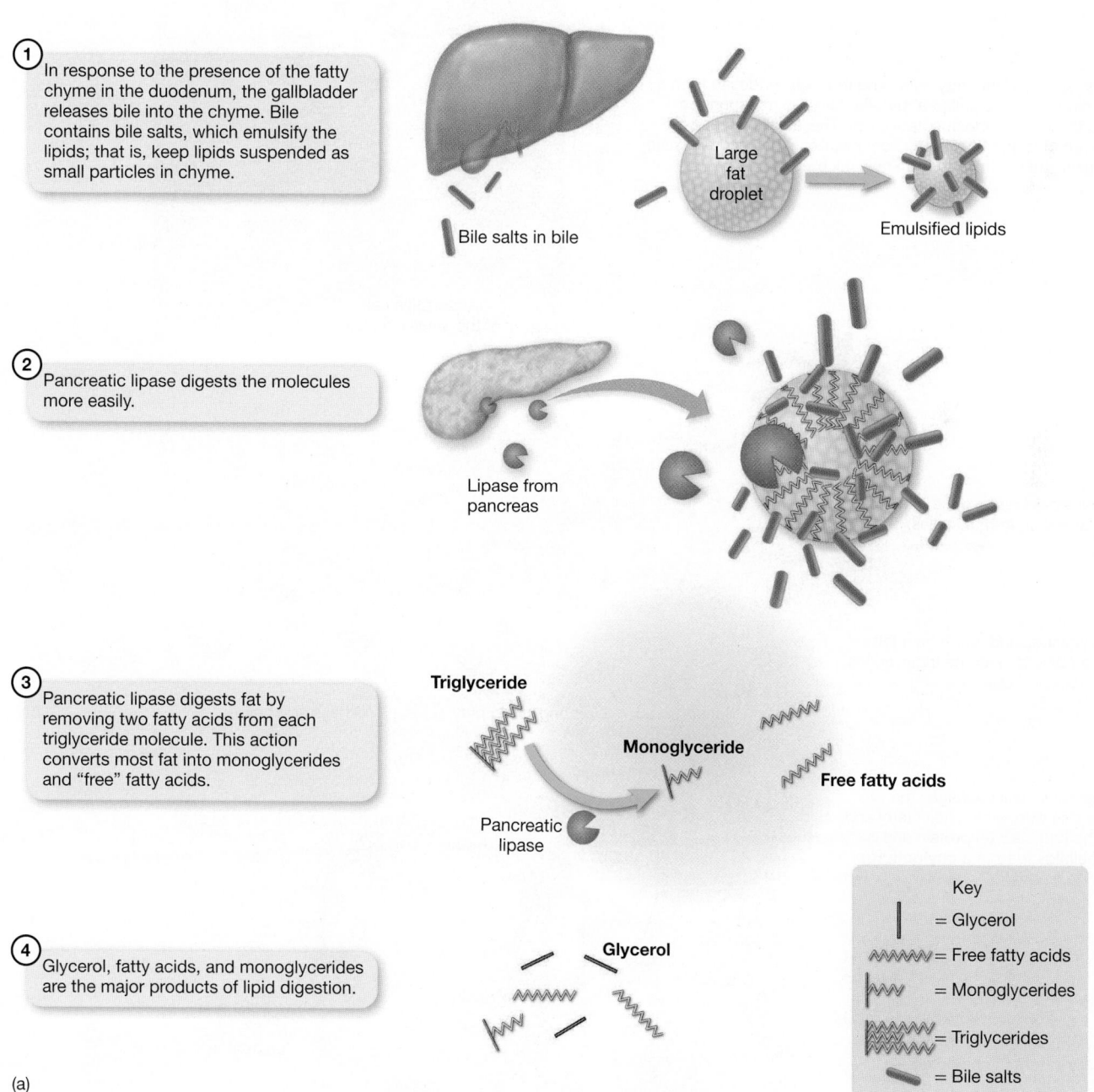

1 In response to the presence of the fatty chyme in the duodenum, the gallbladder releases bile into the chyme. Bile contains bile salts, which emulsify the lipids; that is, keep lipids suspended as small particles in chyme.

Bile salts in bile

Large fat droplet

Emulsified lipids

2 Pancreatic lipase digests the molecules more easily.

Lipase from pancreas

3 Pancreatic lipase digests fat by removing two fatty acids from each triglyceride molecule. This action converts most fat into monoglycerides and "free" fatty acids.

Triglyceride

Monoglyceride

Free fatty acids

Pancreatic lipase

4 Glycerol, fatty acids, and monoglycerides are the major products of lipid digestion.

Glycerol

Key

| = Glycerol

ᴧᴧᴧᴧ = Free fatty acids

= Monoglycerides

= Triglycerides

= Bile salts

(a)

FIGURE 6.10 Lipid digestion and absorption. Pancreatic lipase and bile acids facilitate lipid digestion. (a) After the lipid digestive products enter absorptive cells of the small intestine, triglycerides are re-formed. Triglycerides and other lipids are surrounded with a layer of protein, phospholipids, and cholesterol to form chylomicrons. (b) Chylomicrons are a type of lipoprotein.

micelle water-soluble spherical lipid cluster; bile salts create a shell around each cluster, allowing for the structure to be suspended in watery digestive juices

Lipid Absorption

The majority of lipid absorption occurs in the small intestine, particularly in the duodenum and jejunum. Glycerol, fatty acids, monoglycerides, cholesterol, and phospholipid fragments are the end products of lipid digestion. Short— and medium—chain fatty acids diffuse into the absorptive cells of villi, where they enter the capillary network (bloodstream). Absorption of long—chain fatty acids, however, requires additional steps.

Fig. 6.10, *continued*

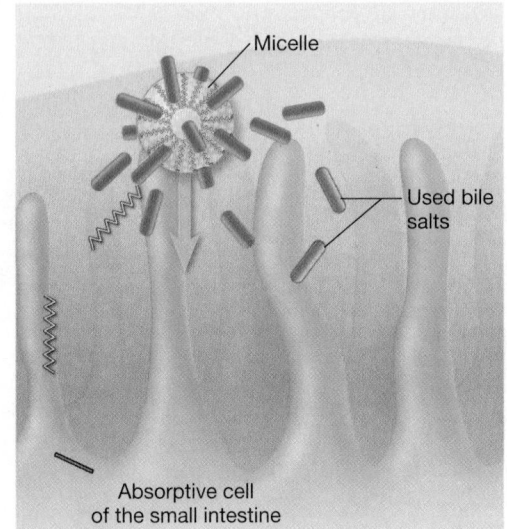

Micelle

Used bile salts

Absorptive cell of the small intestine

(5) Bile salts surround the fatty acids and monoglycerides to form a water-soluble particle called a **micelle**. Micelles transport the lipids to the edge of the absorptive cell. These cells remove the monoglycerides and fatty acids from micelles. The used bile salts that remain can continue to form new micelles.

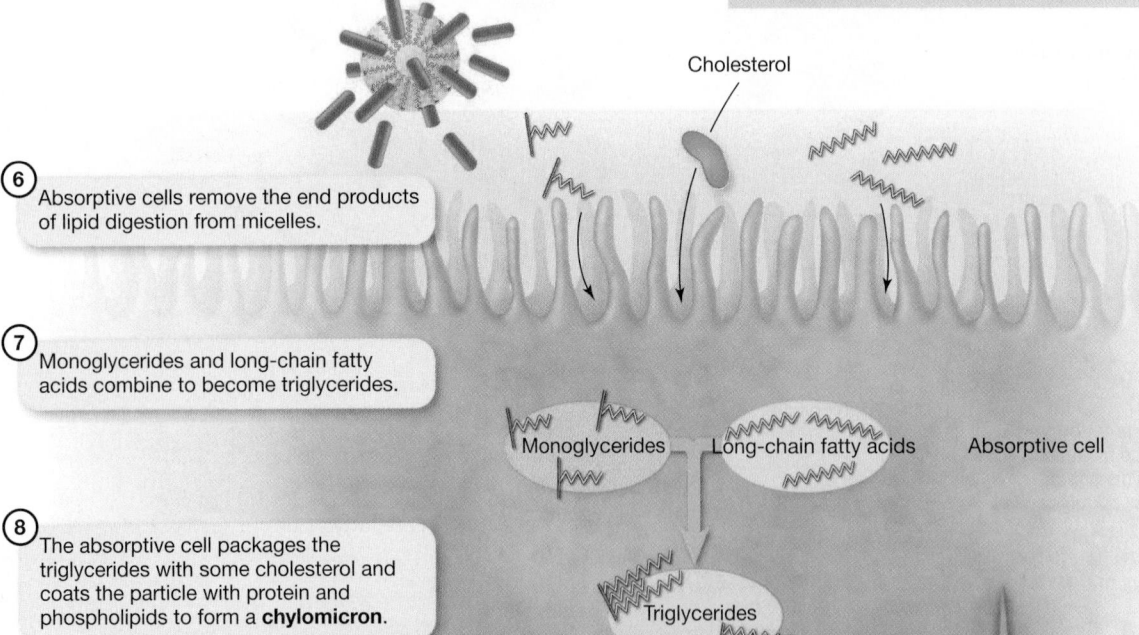

Cholesterol

(6) Absorptive cells remove the end products of lipid digestion from micelles.

(7) Monoglycerides and long-chain fatty acids combine to become triglycerides.

Monoglycerides   **Long-chain fatty acids**   **Absorptive cell**

(8) The absorptive cell packages the triglycerides with some cholesterol and coats the particle with protein and phospholipids to form a **chylomicron**.

Triglycerides

Phospholipid

Protein

(9) The chylomicron enters the lacteal and eventually enters the bloodstream (see Fig. 4.16).

Lacteal

Chylomicron

(b)

When exposed to watery digestive juice, hydrophobic long–chain fatty acids, along with bile, cholesterol, fat–soluble vitamins, and other products of lipid digestion, pack together into round structures called micelles (*my'–cells*). The bile salts create a shell around each micelle, which allows the small lipid clusters to remain suspended in the watery digestive juices (Fig. 6.10). When micelles come close to the villi, their contents diffuse into absorptive cells (enterocytes).

Under normal conditions, the small intestine digests and absorbs nearly all of the triglycerides and phospholipids in food, but only about 50% of dietary cholesterol is absorbed. Diseases that affect the intestinal tract can interfere with digestion and cause poor absorption of fat, called **fat malabsorption**. Diarrhea, steatorrhea, and rapid weight loss are the most common signs of fat malabsorption.

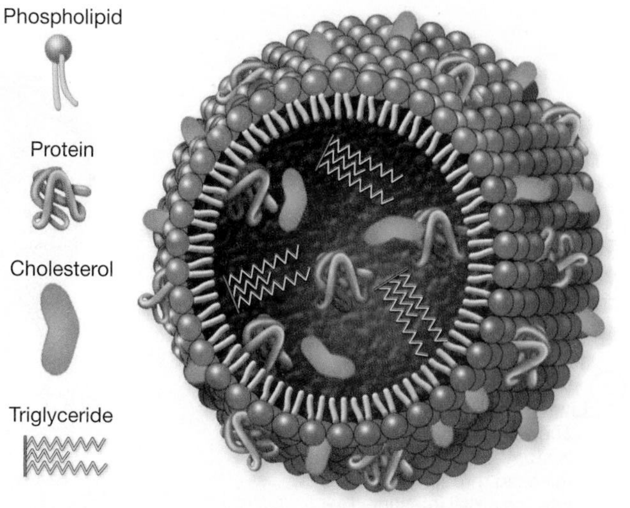

Phospholipid

Protein

Cholesterol

Triglyceride

FIGURE 6.11 Lipoproteins. A section of a lipoprotein (a chylomicron) is cut away in this illustration to show its contents.

Lipid Transportation

After absorption, fatty acids, glycerol, monoglycerides, and phospholipid fragments are reassembled into triglycerides and phospholipids within the absorptive cells of the small intestine. Cholesterol and the reassembled triglycerides are coated with a thin layer of protein, phospholipids, and cholesterol to form chylomicrons (Fig. 6.11). A **chylomicron** (*ky'–low–my'–kron*) is a specific type of lipoprotein formed in enterocytes. **Lipoproteins** are water–soluble structures that transport lipids through the bloodstream. Chylomicrons are too large to leave the villus via the bloodstream, so they pass through the larger openings of a lacteal (*lak–te'–al*), the lymph vessel located in the center of each villus (see Fig. 4.16).

The lymphatic system transports chylomicrons to the thoracic duct, where they enter the bloodstream through the *left subclavian* vein in the chest (Fig. 6.12). As chylomicrons circulate through the body, **lipoprotein lipase (LPL)**, an enzyme in the walls of capillaries, breaks down their load of triglycerides into fatty acids and glycerol. Nearby cells can pick up the fatty acids and glycerol molecules to use for energy. Chapter 8 provides an in–depth discussion of lipid and energy metabolism.

fat malabsorption impaired fat absorption; symptoms include diarrhea, steatorrhea, and rapid weight loss

chylomicron type of lipoprotein formed in enterocytes to transport lipids away from the GI tract

lipoproteins water-soluble structure that transports lipids through the bloodstream

lipoprotein lipase (LPL) enzyme in capillary walls that breaks down triglycerides

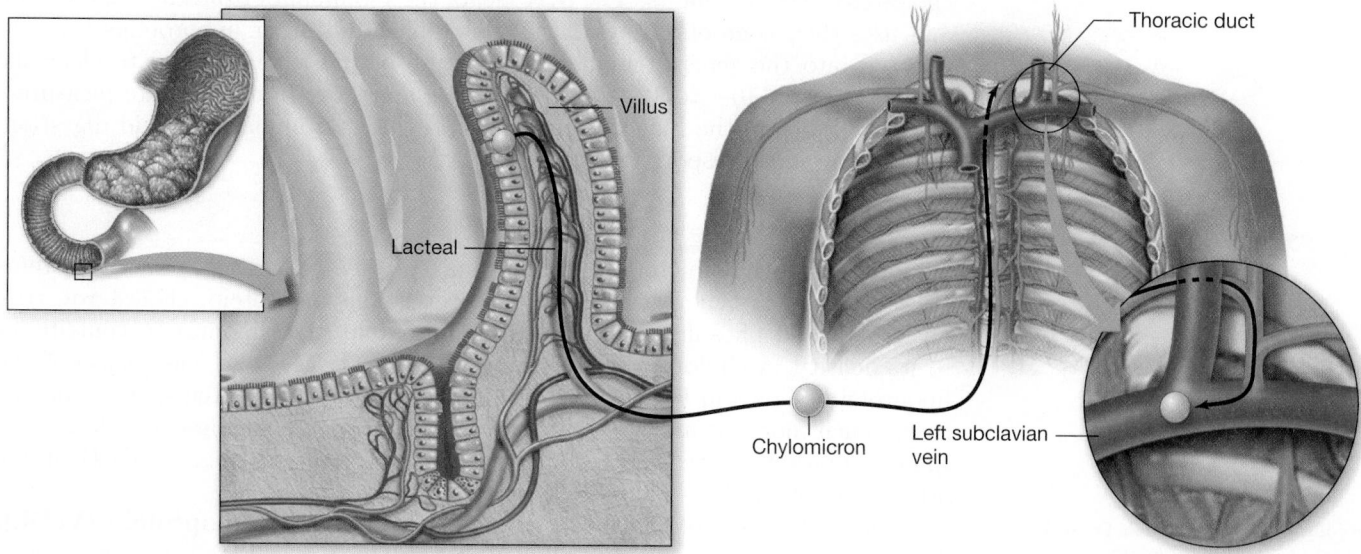

Thoracic duct

Villus

Lacteal

Chylomicron

Left subclavian vein

FIGURE 6.12 Journey into the general circulation. Chylomicrons are too large to move directly into the bloodstream, so they must pass through the larger openings of lacteals, lymphatic system vessels in each villus. The lymphatic system transports chylomicrons to the thoracic duct, where they enter the bloodstream via the left subclavian vein in the chest.

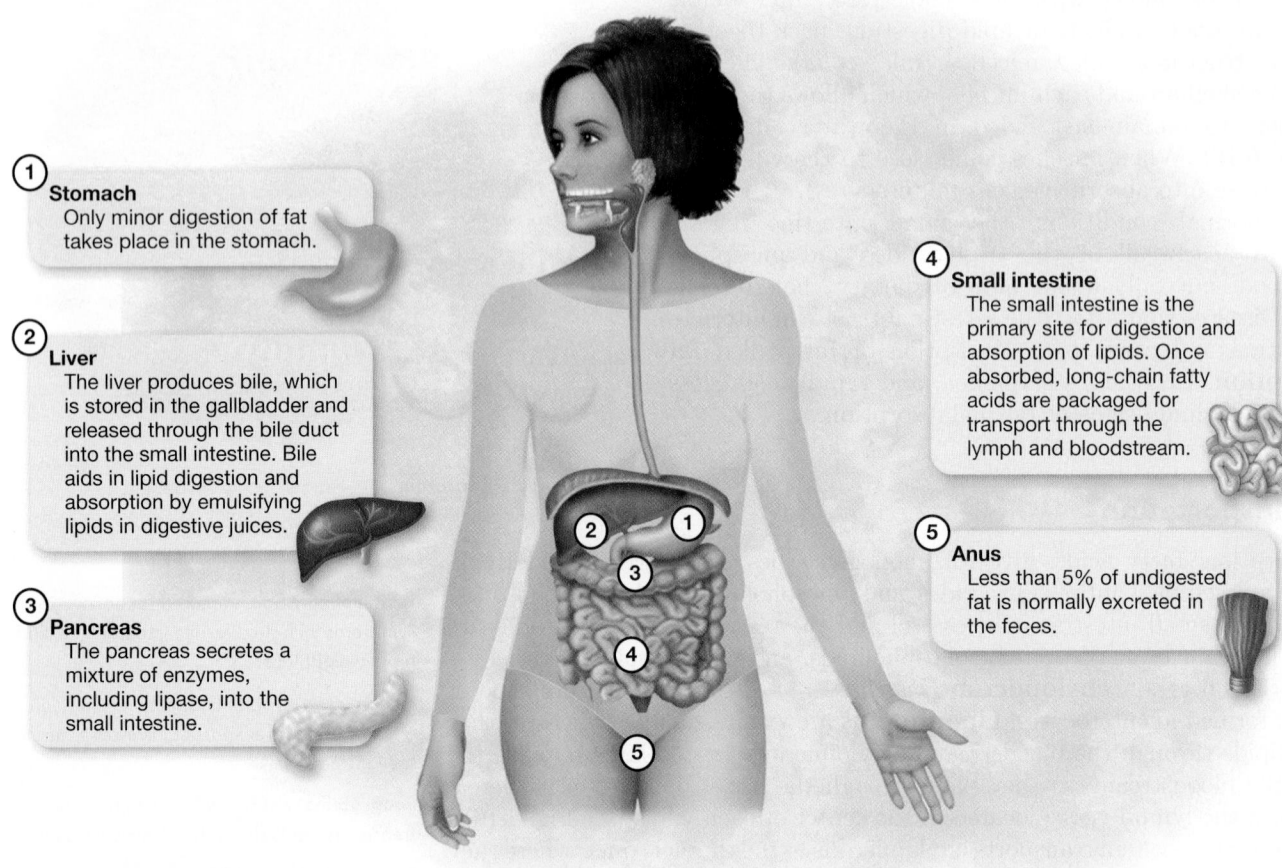

1 Stomach
Only minor digestion of fat takes place in the stomach.

2 Liver
The liver produces bile, which is stored in the gallbladder and released through the bile duct into the small intestine. Bile aids in lipid digestion and absorption by emulsifying lipids in digestive juices.

3 Pancreas
The pancreas secretes a mixture of enzymes, including lipase, into the small intestine.

4 Small intestine
The small intestine is the primary site for digestion and absorption of lipids. Once absorbed, long-chain fatty acids are packaged for transport through the lymph and bloodstream.

5 Anus
Less than 5% of undigested fat is normally excreted in the feces.

FIGURE 6.13 Summary of lipid digestion and absorption.

Ten to 12 hours after a meal, most chylomicrons have been reduced to small cholesterol—rich remnants. The liver clears these remnants from the bloodstream and uses their contents to synthesize new lipids and other lipoproteins that are released into the general circulation. Because of the time required to clear the chylomicrons, a 10— to 12—hour fast is necessary to obtain accurate measure— ments of lipids in the blood. Figure 6.13 provides a summary of lipid digestion, absorption, and transport.

Lipoproteins

In addition to chylomicrons, the body makes three major types of lipoproteins (Fig. 6.14). Each type carries different proportions of protein, cholesterol, tri— glycerides, and phospholipids. The protein content of a lipoprotein contributes to its density. A chylomicron, for example, is the largest and least dense of the lipoproteins shown in Figure 6.14. Compared to other lipoproteins, chylomicrons carry much more fat and very little protein. HDL is the smallest and densest of these lipoproteins, because it transports more protein and less lipids than the other lipoproteins.

The liver uses cholesterol to form **very—low—density lipoprotein (VLDL)**. Triglycerides comprise most of a VLDL's volume (Fig. 6.14). The liver releases VLDL into the bloodstream, and the cells that line capillaries release LPL that breaks down the triglycerides into fatty acids and glycerol. Most cells can use the fatty acids and glycerol for energy or production of body fat.

very-low-density lipoprotein (VLDL)
lipoprotein made in the liver and that carries much of the triglycerides in the bloodstream

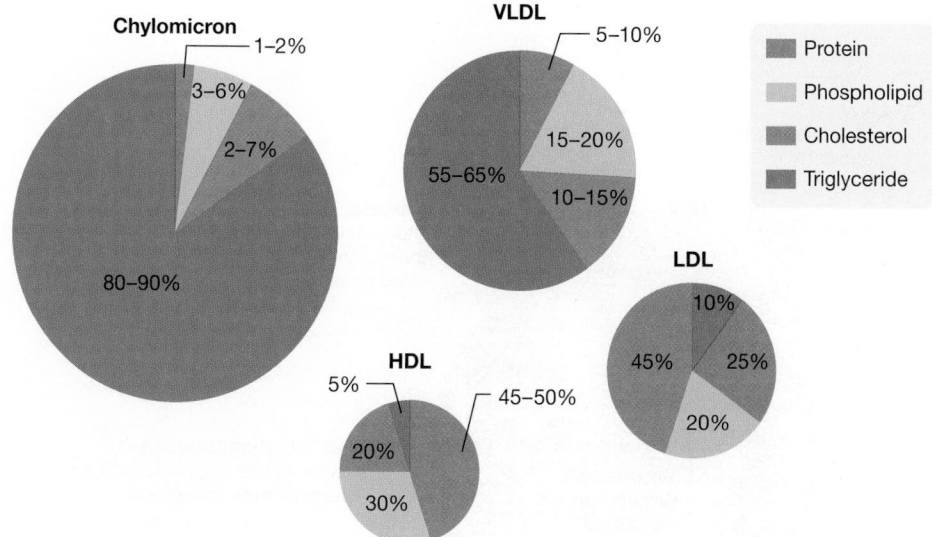

FIGURE 6.14 Major lipoproteins. Lipoproteins contain different percentages of lipid and protein. Low-density lipoprotein (LDL) carries more cholesterol in the bloodstream than the other lipoproteins. In comparison, chylomicrons carry the most triglycerides.

After being stripped of most of its fat, VLDL becomes **low—density lipoprotein (LDL)**. About 45% of the volume of a low—density lipoprotein is cholesterol. LDL transports cholesterol and other lipids to tissues. Cells remove LDL from the bloodstream and use its lipids to make vital substances and structures.

The liver releases protein "shells" into the bloodstream that pick up cholesterol and other lipids that are released from cells. When they are filled with lipids, the shells are called **high—density lipoprotein (HDL)**. Compared to the other lipoproteins, HDL has the most protein.

Certain lipoproteins carry lipids from the liver to cells. Other lipoproteins convey lipids from cells to the liver, where they may be converted into new compounds. Section 6.8 provides more information about lipoproteins and their effects on cardiovascular health.

low-density lipoprotein (LDL) lipoprotein that carries cholesterol into tissues; elevated LDL is strongly linked to increased risk of cardiovascular disease

high-density lipoprotein (HDL) lipoprotein that transports cholesterol away from tissues and to the liver, where it can be eliminated; low HDL is linked to increased risk for cardiovascular disease

Enterohepatic Circulation of Bile

Approximately 98% of the bile salts in bile are reabsorbed in the ileum, where they enter the bloodstream and travel to the liver. The liver incorporates the bile salts into new bile. The process of recycling bile from the intestinal tract is called **enterohepatic** (*ent'—eh—roe—hih—pah'—tik*) **circulation** (Fig. 6.15). Interfering with enterohepatic circulation can reduce blood cholesterol levels, because the liver must use cholesterol to make new bile salts.

Plants contain substances, such as soluble fiber, that interfere with cholesterol and bile absorption (see Table 5.7 for common food sources of soluble fiber). Soluble fiber in the GI tract binds with bile in the jejunum and ileum, preventing the bile salts from being reabsorbed. Because the bile salts are then excreted in feces, new bile must be made from cholesterol, reducing blood cholesterol levels.

enterohepatic circulation process that recycles bile salts in the body

Gallstones

Twenty million Americans suffer from **gallstones** that develop in their gallbladders or bile ducts, making gallstones one of the most common digestive diseases in the United States.[14] Gallstones usually consist primarily of cholesterol. Gallstones can be small and grainy or as large as a dime and lumpy (Fig. 6.16). When a gallbladder that contains stones contracts or when a large gallstone lodges in one of the ducts that carry bile from the gallbladder to the small intestine, the person feels considerable pain in the right upper part of

gallstones hard particles that can accumulate in the gallbladder or become lodged in one of the ducts carrying bile from the gallbladder to the small intestine

FIGURE 6.15 Enterohepatic circulation of bile. As a result of recycling bile salts, the liver conserves cholesterol. Soluble fiber, however, interferes with bile salt reabsorption. When the ileum absorbs less bile salts, the liver has to use cholesterol to form new bile salts.

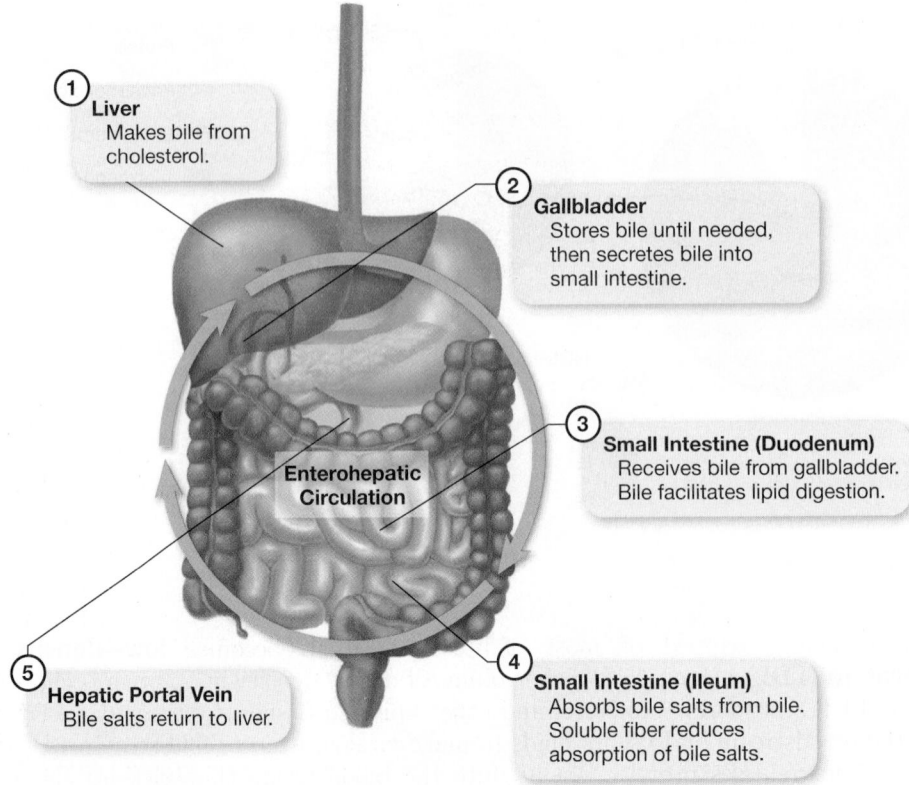

① **Liver**
Makes bile from cholesterol.

② **Gallbladder**
Stores bile until needed, then secretes bile into small intestine.

③ **Small Intestine (Duodenum)**
Receives bile from gallbladder. Bile facilitates lipid digestion.

Enterohepatic Circulation

④ **Small Intestine (Ileum)**
Absorbs bile salts from bile. Soluble fiber reduces absorption of bile salts.

⑤ **Hepatic Portal Vein**
Bile salts return to liver.

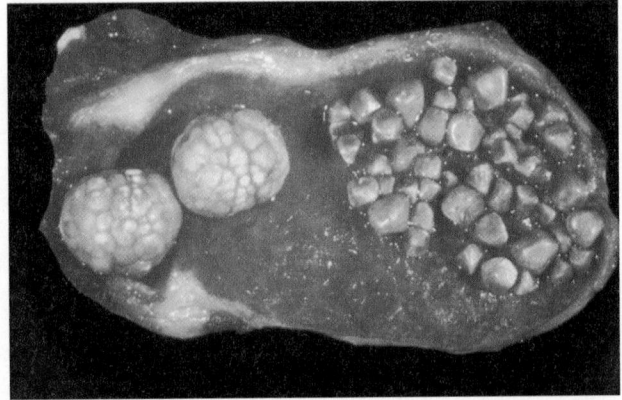

FIGURE 6.16 Gallstones. Gallstones can form in the gallbladder. The stones usually consist of cholesterol.

cholecystectomy surgery to remove a diseased gallbladder

steatorrhea presence of lipid in the stool

the abdomen ("gallbladder attack"). If the stone moves out of the duct, the discomfort ends, but in some cases, the duct remains blocked and bile backs up into the liver or pancreas. **Cholecystectomy** (*coll'–lee'–sis–tek'–toe–me*), a surgical procedure that removes the diseased gallbladder, is often necessary.

People who have high risk of gallstones include those who are overweight or obese and those who lose weight rapidly. Maintaining a healthy body weight is particularly important for American Indians and Mexican–Americans, because members of these ethnic groups have the highest rates of gallbladder disease in the United States.[14]

When the gallbladder is removed or does not function properly, the affected individual digests fat less efficiently. If the gallbladder is damaged or removed, bile drips directly from the liver into the duodenum. Thus, if a person eats a high–fat meal, there will not be enough bile available in the GI tract to digest all the fat. The undigested fat is excreted in the feces. **Steatorrhea** (*stee'–at–or–ree'–ah*) is the presence of lipid in the stool. To prevent steatorrhea and maximize fat absorption, an individual with a missing or damaged gallbladder should eat smaller, more frequent meals; and avoid high–fat meals.

Lipid Storage Diseases

Lipid storage diseases (singular *lipidosis*, plural *lipidoses*) are genetic conditions that cause lipid accumulation in cells, which damages tissues. Some signs of lipid storage diseases include an enlarged spleen or liver, swollen abdomen, skeletal disorders, and swollen lymph nodes. The most common lipid storage disorder, which affects between 1 in 50,000 and 1 in 100,000 Americans, is

Gaucher (*gow'–chur*) disease. Gaucher disease is caused by a deficiency of an enzyme involved in lipid metabolism. The lack of the enzyme results in lipid accumulation in bone marrow and some organs, including the liver, kidneys, and brain.[15] Although Gaucher disease is fatal, some individuals with the inherited condition survive to the early teenage years and young adulthood.

Gaucher disease most common lipid storage disease; caused by a deficiency of the enzyme glucocerebrosidase

ASSESS YOUR PROGRESS

13 *Describe what happens to the fat in a piece of fried chicken as it undergoes digestion and absorption; include the roles of bile, CCK, pancreatic lipase, villi, and micelles.*

14 *Compare the composition of a chylomicron, VLDL, LDL, and HDL.*

15 *Explain the relationship between fat malabsorption and steatorrhea.*

6.7 Lipid Consumption Patterns

LEARNING OUTCOMES

1 *Summarize current lipid consumption patterns in the United States.*

2 *List total dietary fat, saturated fat, trans fat, and cholesterol intake recommendations.*

In 2009–2010, the typical American consumed about 62 pounds of fat per year, which was an increase of almost 15% of the amount consumed by the average American in 1987–1988.[16,17] Today, fat contributes 33% of the average American's daily energy intake.[13] Although the DRI committee has not established an RDA or AI for total fat intake (for people over 1 year of age), the Acceptable Macronutrient Distribution Range (AMDR) for fat is 20 to 35% of total caloric intake.[5] According to the Dietary Guidelines, adults should emphasize foods that are rich sources of polyunsaturated and monounsaturated fatty acids, such as fish, nuts, and vegetable oils.[18] Eating low–fat foods is not the only way to meet this recommendation. By balancing intakes of low–fat and high–fat foods, daily fat intake can average less than 35% of total energy intake. For example, based on a 2000–kcal diet and eating 30% of total energy from fat, a person can consume up to 67 grams of fat daily. For reference, a slice of bacon provides approximately 2 g of total fat and a quarter of a cup of sliced avocado has 5 g of total fat.

According to the Dietary Guidelines, adults should consume less than 10% of their total calories from saturated fatty acids, and limit their trans fat and cholesterol intakes to as little as possible.[18] In 2009–2010, Americans 2 years of age and older consumed about 11% of their total daily energy from saturated fat, 12% from monounsaturated fat, 7% from polyunsaturated fats, and 3% from trans fats.[13] Average cholesterol intake during that same period was 333 mg/day for males and 224 mg/day for females.

AMDRs have been established for the essential fatty acids (see the last pages of this book). In adults, linoleic acid should provide 5 to 10% and alpha–linolenic acid 0.6 to 1.2% of total daily kcal.[5] Americans consuming a typical Western diet regularly meet these essential fatty acid recommendations.[13]

Table 6.4 summarizes the Dietary Guidelines' and DRI committee's dietary fat and cholesterol recommendations. To estimate the average percentage of your total daily energy from total fat and saturated fat intake, complete the "Personal Dietary Analysis" activity at the end of this chapter.

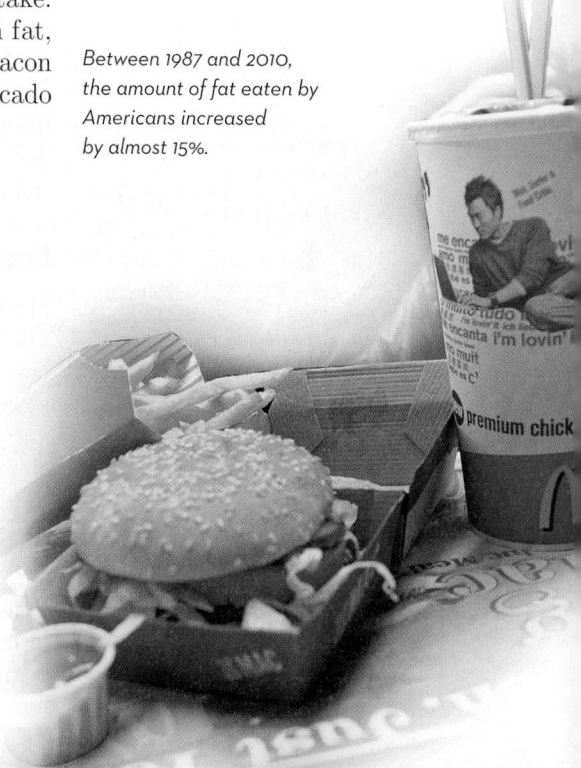

Between 1987 and 2010, the amount of fat eaten by Americans increased by almost 15%.

TABLE 6.4 Dietary Fat and Cholesterol Recommendations

Total fat	20–35% of total calories (45–75 g total fat for a 2000-kcal diet)
Saturated fat	Less than 10% of total calories (22 g saturated fat for a 2000-kcal diet)
Linoleic acid	5–10% of total calories (11–22 g linoleic acid for a 2000-kcal diet)
Alpha-linolenic acid	0.6–1.2% of total calories (1–3 g alpha-linolenic acid for a 2000-kcal diet)
Cholesterol	As little as possible while consuming a healthy diet
Trans fat	Keep intake as low as possible

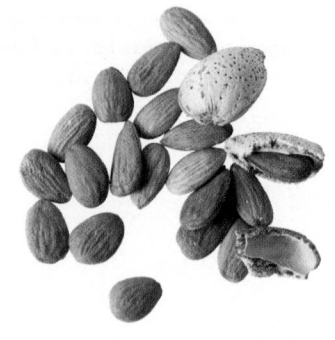

Almonds are a rich source of monounsaturated fatty acids. Bulk and prepackaged roasted almonds are sold in many supermarkets.

ASSESS YOUR PROGRESS

16 *What percentage of total energy intake does fat contribute in the "average" American's diet?*

17 *According to the Dietary Guidelines, how much saturated fat, cholesterol, and trans fat should an adult consume?*

18 *Calculate how many grams of total fat, saturated fat, linoleic acid, and alpha-linolenic acid an adult should consume who is eating 2300 kcal daily.*

6.8 Lipids and Cardiovascular Disease

LEARNING OUTCOMES

1 *Explain the process and health effects of atherosclerosis.*

2 *List at least six risk factors for developing cardiovascular disease.*

3 *Distinguish between high-density lipoprotein (HDL) and low-density lipoprotein (LDL).*

cardiovascular disease (CVD) group of diseases that affect the heart and blood vessels; includes coronary artery disease, stroke, and disease of the blood vessels

Cardiovascular disease (CVD) includes heart disease (coronary artery disease, or CAD), stroke, and diseases of the blood vessels. More than one in three adult Americans has one or more forms of CVD.[19] In 2010, heart disease, stroke, and hypertension were among the top four leading causes of death in the United States.[20] CVD does not just affect the elderly people: About 32% of Americans who die of heart disease are younger than 75 years of age.[19] This section focuses on dietary and other lifestyle practices that set the stage for developing heart disease and other forms of cardiovascular disease. Although people often establish poor lifestyle practices early in life, changing these practices at any age can reduce their chances of developing CVD.

From Atherosclerosis to Cardiovascular Disease

atherosclerosis long-term disease process in which plaque builds up inside arterial walls

arteriosclerosis condition that results from atherosclerosis and is characterized by loss of arterial flexibility

Most cases of heart disease and stroke result from **atherosclerosis** (*athero* = lipid containing; *sclerosis* [*skleh–ro'–sis*] = hardening), a chronic process that negatively affects artery function. Atherosclerosis results in decreased arterial blood flow and **arteriosclerosis**, reduced arterial wall flexibility ("hardening of the arteries"). *Atherosclerosis* and *arteriosclerosis* are terms that are often used interchangeably; however, arteriosclerosis is actually a symptom or by–product of atherosclerosis.

How Atherosclerosis Develops

Healthy arteries have a smooth lining (Fig. 6.17.1). When the arterial lining is injured (e.g., by oxidation, infection, or nutrient deficiency), a cascade of events begins that, over time, results in atherosclerosis (Fig. 6.17.2). The immune system responds by producing inflammation of the injured arterial lining. Under

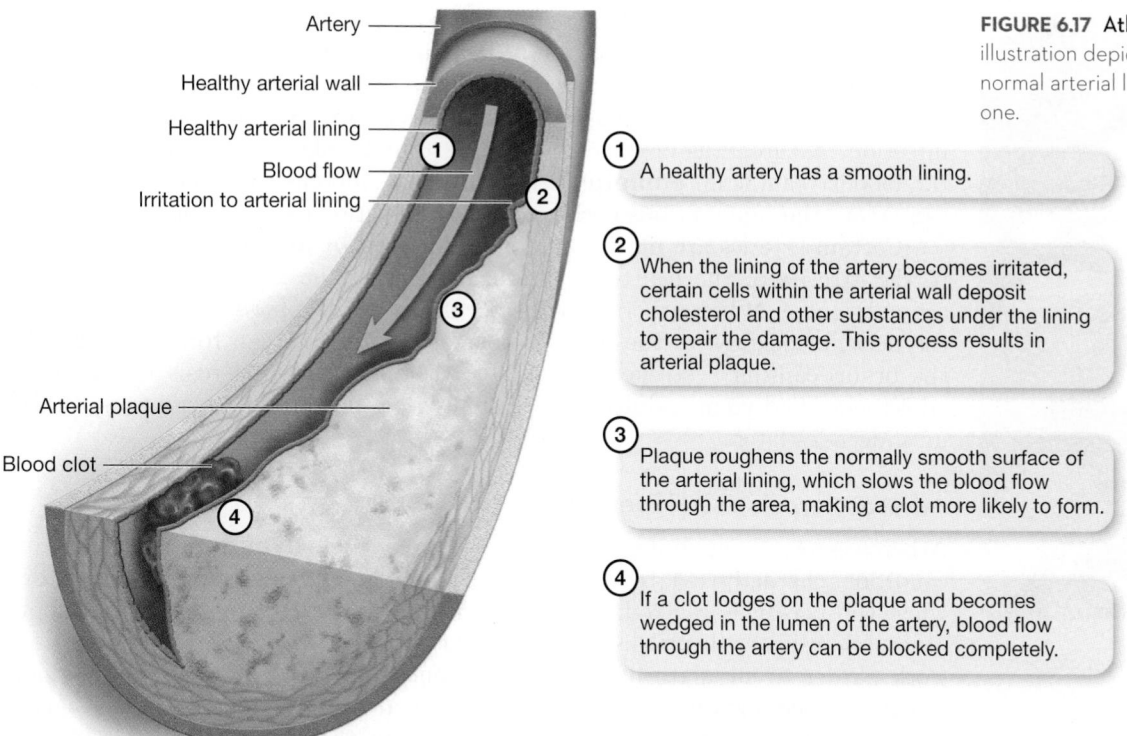

Artery

Healthy arterial wall

Healthy arterial lining

Blood flow

Irritation to arterial lining

Arterial plaque

Blood clot

① A healthy artery has a smooth lining.

② When the lining of the artery becomes irritated, certain cells within the arterial wall deposit cholesterol and other substances under the lining to repair the damage. This process results in arterial plaque.

③ Plaque roughens the normally smooth surface of the arterial lining, which slows the blood flow through the area, making a clot more likely to form.

④ If a clot lodges on the plaque and becomes wedged in the lumen of the artery, blood flow through the artery can be blocked completely.

FIGURE 6.17 Atherosclerosis. This illustration depicts the progression from a normal arterial lining to an atherosclerotic one.

conditions in which blood LDL concentration is high, inflammation triggers certain white blood cells in arteries to become heavily laden with oxidized LDL particles ("foam cells"). The cholesterol—rich foam cells become trapped in the artery wall and over time, contribute to the formation of **arterial plaques** (Fig. 6.17.3). An arterial plaque is a fatty buildup in the artery.

Arterial plaque interferes with circulation because it narrows the artery and may even block its entire opening (lumen). Furthermore, plaque roughens the normally smooth arterial endothelial surface, which slows blood flow to the area supplied by the artery. This makes clots more likely to form (Fig. 6.17.4). When a plaque *ruptures* (tears open), repairing the rupture also involves clot formation, and such blood clots can be life threatening. Figure 6.18 shows cross sections of a healthy artery and an artery almost completely blocked by plaque.

Blood clotting is a healthy response to blood vessel injury that prevents excessive bleeding. When a blood clot forms too easily, it can result in a **thrombus**, a fixed bunch of clots that remain in place and disrupt blood flow. The thrombus partially closes off an artery's lumen. If this condition occurs in an artery that nourishes the heart, the heart muscle supplied by the artery does not receive enough oxygen and nutrients to function properly. As a result, the affected person experiences bouts of chest pain, especially when the heart beats faster, such as during intense emotional states or physical activities. When a thrombus completely blocks blood flow to a section of the heart muscle, the muscle dies, resulting in a **myocardial infarction** (*my'—oh—card'—e—al in—farc'—shun*), which is commonly called a "heart attack." Sudden death can result from a severe myocardial infarction.

arterial plaque fatty buildup in the artery

thrombus fixed bunch of clots that remain in place and disrupt blood flow

myocardial infarction heart attack

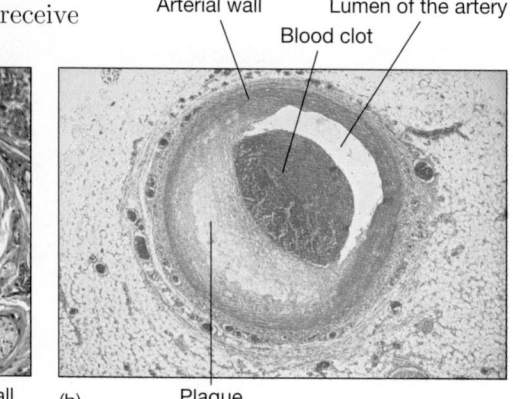

Arterial wall

Lumen of the artery

Blood clot

(a) Lumen of the artery | Arterial wall

(b) Plaque

FIGURE 6.18 Healthy and atherosclerotic arteries. Note the differences between the cross section of a healthy artery (*a*) and that of an artery nearly completely blocked by atherosclerosis (*b*).

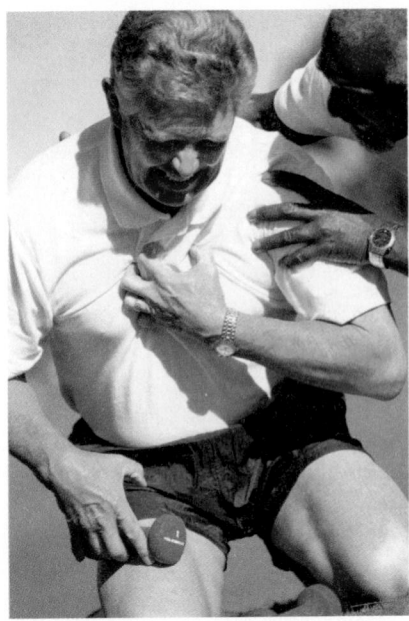

The most common sign of a heart attack is chest pain or discomfort. Shortness of breath, light-headedness, and pain or discomfort in the arms, back, neck, jaw, or stomach are also warning signs of a heart attack.

stroke clot blocks an artery in the brain; brain cells that are nourished by the vessel die

embolus thrombus or part of a plaque that breaks free and travels through the bloodstream

hypertension abnormally high blood pressure levels that persist even when the person is relaxed

A **stroke** can happen when a clot blocks an artery in the brain and brain cells that are nourished by the vessel die. When an artery to a limb is blocked, the tissue in the extremity dies, causing *gangrene* to occur. If the affected area is large, amputation of the gangrenous limb is often necessary to prevent life-threatening infection. A thrombus or part of a plaque that breaks free and travels through the bloodstream is an **embolus** (Fig. 6.19). An embolus that lodges in an artery can create the same serious consequences as a stationary thrombus.

Certain arteries are more commonly damaged by atherosclerosis; in addition to the arteries of the heart and brain, arteries of the kidneys, retina, and legs are vulnerable. When atherosclerosis occurs in the *common carotid arteries* in the neck, blood flow to the brain is decreased and clots can form that travel to the brain, causing a stroke (Fig. 6.20). Although atherosclerosis begins during adolescence and young adulthood, it usually does not produce symptoms of CVD until decades later.

Atherosclerosis and Hypertension

Atherosclerosis contributes to the development of **hypertension**, a chronic condition characterized by abnormally high blood pressure that persists even when the person is relaxed. Hypertension is a major risk factor for developing atherosclerosis and heart disease. The heart of a person with hypertension must work harder to circulate blood through abnormally stiff arteries. Furthermore, elevated blood pressure can cause hardened arteries to tear or burst, causing serious bleeding or sudden death, depending on the artery's size and location. According to the American Heart Association, an estimated 78 million American adults have hypertension, which is typically a result of a poor diet, lack of physical activity, stress, and family history.[19]

CVD: Major Risk Factors

The American Heart Association has identified major risk factors for developing CVD.[19] The more risk factors a person has, the greater his or her likelihood of

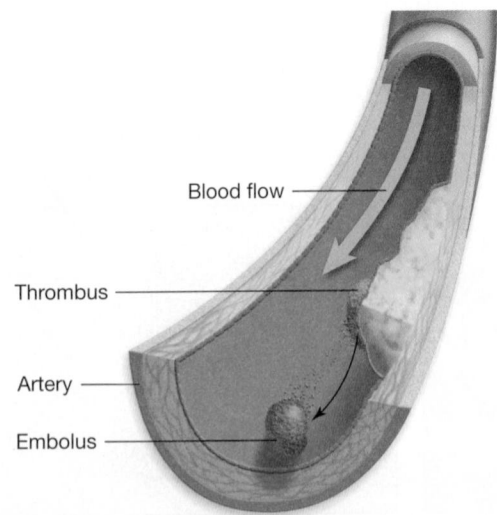

FIGURE 6.19 Embolus formation. A thrombus, or part of a plaque, that breaks free from where it formed and travels through the bloodstream is an embolus.

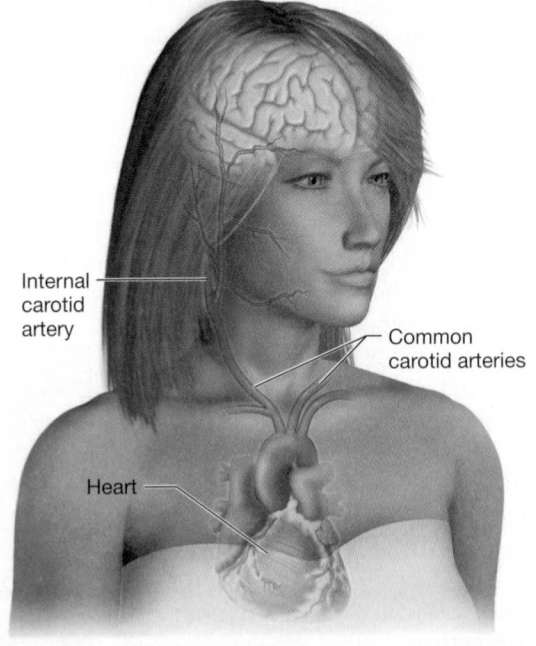

FIGURE 6.20 Carotid arteries. The carotid arteries convey blood to the brain. Atherosclerosis in these arteries can result in reduced blood flow to the brain and increase the risk of stroke.

TABLE 6.5 Atherosclerosis: Major Risk Factors

Nonmodifiable Risk Factors
Family history of CVD (especially before 60 years of age)
Increasing age
Race/ethnic background
Male sex

Modifiable Risk Factors
Hypertension
Diabetes mellitus
Elevated blood cholesterol (especially LDL cholesterol)
Excess body fat
Physical inactivity
Tobacco use or exposure to tobacco smoke
Untreated sleep apnea

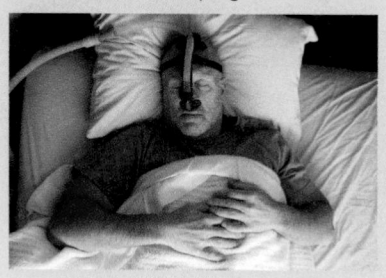

CVD. Table 6.5 lists these major CVD risk factors and indicates which are non—modifiable or modifiable. A person cannot change a nonmodifiable risk factor, such as age and genetics. Modifiable risk factors generally involve lifestyle practices that can be changed, such as smoking and lack of physical activity.

Unmodifiable Risk Factors

Age, sex, racial/ethnic ancestry, and family history are major, nonmodifiable risk factors for developing CVD, including heart disease. The risk of heart disease increases as people grow older, and men are more likely to have heart attacks than women. Although a woman's risk of developing CVD increases after menopause, her risk is still less than that of a man of the same age. Americans of African, Mexican, or Native American ancestry are more likely to have heart disease than those of other racial or ethnic backgrounds. Another trait people cannot change is their family history. For example, if your father had his first heart attack when he was 42 years old, you have a greater risk of developing heart disease prematurely (too soon) than someone whose father had his first heart attack at 75 years of age.

Genetics and CVD Genetics (family history) is a major risk factor for atheroscle—rosis and CVD that cannot be modified. A person's genes, for example, may code for various physical conditions that increase risk of heart disease, such as hyper—tension and diabetes. Additionally, genes may influence the way in which the cir—culatory and immune systems respond to diet. Thus, some people may be protected against the development of CVD, whereas other persons with similar diets develop serious arterial plaques early in life and die prematurely of CVD as a result.

The amino acid **homocysteine** (*ho'—mo—sis—teen*) may be associated with CVD. Amino acids are the chemical units that comprise proteins. Although homo—cysteine is an amino acid, it is not found in human proteins, but the substance is a toxic by—product of protein metabolism. Cells use three vitamins—B—6, folate, and B—12—to convert homocysteine into safer compounds (details of this relationship are provided in Chapter 10). Some people have **homocysteinuria**, a group of conditions caused by gene mutations that result in the accumulation of homocysteine in their bloodstream. Higher—than—normal blood levels of homo—cysteine may injure arterial walls. Thus, people with homocysteinuria have a higher risk of developing CVD than persons who do not have the condition.

Scientists are searching the entire set of human genes (*genome*) to locate genes involved in the development of atherosclerosis and to develop blood tests that identify biomarkers produced by the mutated genes. In the future, young people could undergo genomic testing to determine their risk of developing ath—erosclerosis well before the symptoms of the condition appear.

homocysteine amino acid that may play a role in the development of atherosclerosis

homocysteinuria group of conditions caused by gene mutations that cause homocysteine to accumulate in the blood

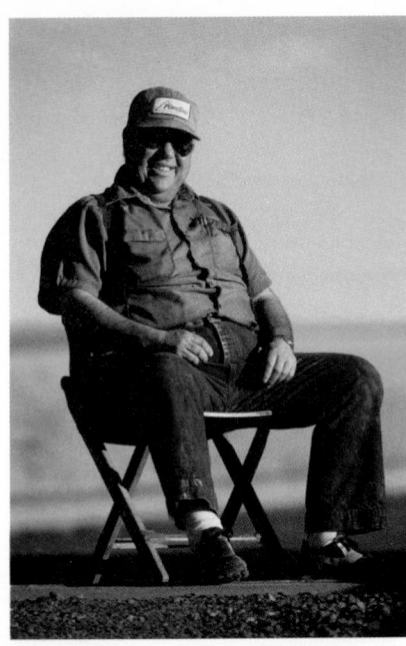

Major risk factors for developing CVD include male sex, increasing age, excess body fat, and physical inactivity.

oxidized LDL LDL that has been damaged by free radicals

adipose (fat) cells cells that store triglycerides

Modifiable Risk Factors

Several major risk factors for atherosclerosis involve lifestyle choices that can be modified, including hypertension, diabetes, and smoking (Table 6.5).

Nearly one in three adult Americans has hypertension.[19] Hypertension is often referred to as a "silent disease," because people with the condition frequently feel healthy and do not have obvious symptoms that indicate trouble within their circulatory system. The condition, however, is quite serious because it damages arterial walls and increases the risk of stroke, heart failure, and kidney disease. Chapter 11 presents information about hypertension, including healthy blood pressure values (see Table 11.12) and ways to reduce the likelihood of developing the condition.

Diabetes and obesity are other modifiable risk factors for developing CVD. According to the American Diabetes Association, two–thirds of the people who have diabetes die of heart disease or stroke.[25] Chapter 5 discusses diabetes in detail. Excess body fat, especially in the abdominal region, increases the risk of type 2 diabetes and hypertension; Chapter 13 focuses on sensible ways to lose body fat. Physical inactivity also contributes to excess body fat. Chapter 15 provides suggestions for becoming more physically active.

Tobacco use is another major and modifiable risk factor for atherosclerosis. Compared to nonsmokers, smokers have two to four times the likelihood of developing heart disease and having a stroke.[26] Exposure to "secondhand" smoke is also a risk factor for heart disease. Simply improving a smoker's diet is unlikely to reduce his or her risk of developing atherosclerosis; therefore, smokers should make every effort to quit using tobacco products.[27] Furthermore, those who do not smoke should avoid breathing secondhand smoke.

Having one or more risk factors increases a person's chances of developing the condition. It is important to understand that a risk factor is not the same as a *cause* of disease. AIDS, for example, is caused by human immunodeficiency virus (HIV); a person cannot develop AIDS without being infected with HIV. Atherosclerosis, however, is an extremely complex disease process. In most cases, no single cause for the condition can be identified.

Lipoproteins and Atherosclerosis

Lipoproteins play major roles in the development of atherosclerosis. HDL conveys lipids away from tissues and to the liver, where they can be processed and eliminated. Thus, the cholesterol carried by HDL (*HDL cholesterol*) is often called "good" cholesterol because it does not contribute to plaque formation.

The cholesterol carried by LDL (*LDL cholesterol*) is often referred to as "bad" cholesterol, because LDL conveys the lipid to tissues, including cells in the arterial walls that make atherosclerotic plaques. However, there are different types of LDL, and not all forms of the lipoprotein are unhealthy. LDL is needed to transport lipids to tissues, where the nutrients are used to make cell structures and vital compounds. Some LDLs are smaller and denser than others. People with high levels of small, dense LDLs are more likely to develop atherosclerosis than people with low levels of these LDLs.[28] Additionally, chemically unstable substances (radicals) can damage LDL, forming **oxidized LDL**. This particular type of LDL is not beneficial because it is taken up by immune system cells called macrophages, which over time, become "foam" cells. Foam cells form plaque. Thus, oxidized LDL contributes to atherosclerosis. Several lifestyle behaviors, including cigarette smoking, increase the oxidation of LDL.[29] Figure 6.21 illustrates the roles of HDL, LDL, and oxidized LDL.

VLDL contains only about 15% of the cholesterol in the bloodstream, but this lipoprotein carries a larger share of triglycerides than cholesterol. VLDLs shuttle lipids to **adipose (fat) cells**, which remove the triglycerides from VLDL and store them. As blood triglyceride levels increase, concentrations of HDL tend to decrease. Some medical researchers think elevated triglyceride levels contribute to the development of CVD, but the mechanisms are unclear at this point.[30]

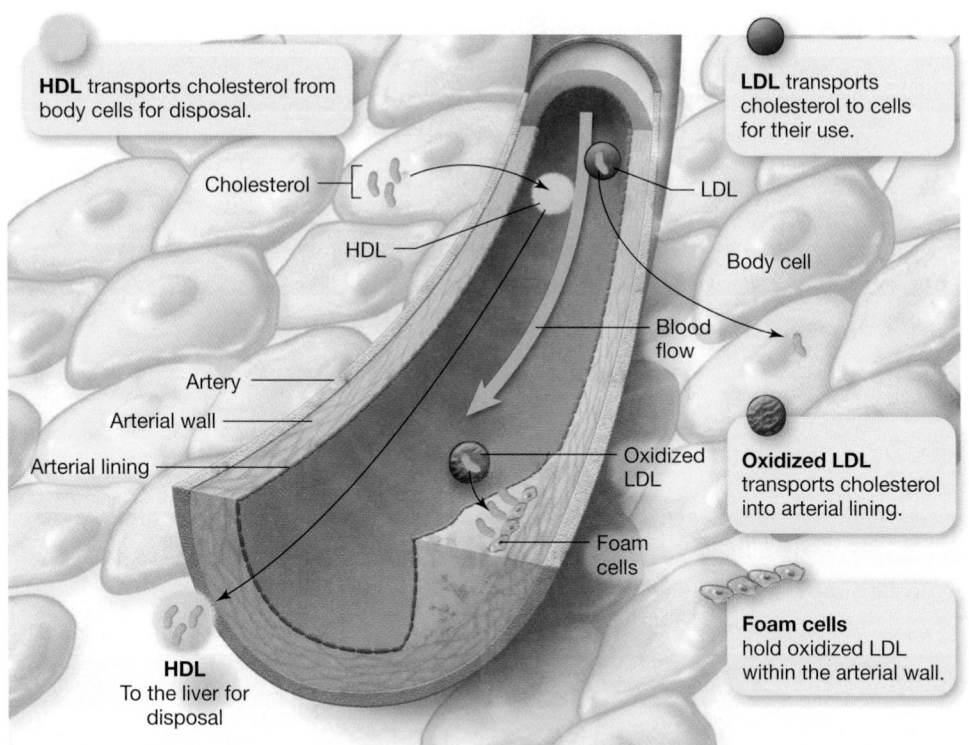

HDL transports cholesterol from body cells for disposal.

LDL transports cholesterol to cells for their use.

Cholesterol

HDL

LDL

Body cell

Blood flow

Artery

Arterial wall

Arterial lining

Oxidized LDL

Oxidized LDL transports cholesterol into arterial lining.

Foam cells

HDL To the liver for disposal

Foam cells hold oxidized LDL within the arterial wall.

FIGURE 6.21 HDL, LDL, and oxidized LDL. A particular form of LDL, oxidized LDL, is harmful. Oxidized LDL is taken up by *macrophages,* a type of immune system cell. Over time, the cholesterol-laden macrophages become "foam" cells that build up and contribute to atherosclerosis.

Assessing Risk of Atherosclerosis

A person may be able to forestall CVD and live a longer, more satisfying life by reducing or eliminating modifiable risk factors for developing atherosclerosis. Diet, for example, influences the likelihood of developing atherosclerosis and is highly modifiable.

To determine a person's risk of developing atherosclerosis, it is a good idea to have regular medical checkups in which a physician checks the patient's blood pressure and listens to blood flow in the carotid arteries. Such tests assess whether the arteries are becoming blocked. Furthermore, the physician may request a **lipoprotein profile**, a specific series of blood tests, to evaluate total serum cholesterol levels, as well as serum HDL cholesterol, LDL cholesterol, and triglyceride levels. Patients should request a copy of the laboratory results and keep them along with others in their personal "medical file" for future reference.

Classifying Blood Lipid Levels

Table 6.6 presents classifications for healthy and unhealthy blood lipid levels. According to the American Heart Association and the National Cholesterol Education Program, the desirable range for total blood cholesterol is less than 200 mg/dL.[31,32] In 2012, an estimated 32 million American adults, 14% of the population, had total blood cholesterol levels greater than 240 mg/dL.[19]

Even if a person's total cholesterol level is below 200 mg/dL, he or she may still have a high risk of developing atherosclerosis. The reason is that the amounts of certain lipoproteins in blood, particularly LDL and HDL, are more critical risk factors than is total cholesterol. It is healthier to have higher levels of HDL cholesterol, compared to normal ranges, than to have higher levels of LDL cholesterol, compared to normal ranges.

People with a high ratio of total cholesterol to HDL cholesterol usually have too much LDL cholesterol in their blood and an increased risk of heart disease and stroke. For example, a young man has a total blood cholesterol level of 180 mg/dL. Of that amount, only 30 mg/dL are carried by high-density lipoprotein. This man's ratio of total cholesterol to HDL cholesterol is 6:1 (180 mg/30 mg). A healthy ratio of total cholesterol to HDL cholesterol is less than 4:1.[19] If this

DID **YOU** *KNOW?*

Although this textbook generally refers to "blood cholesterol" or "blood lipids," the amount of lipids in *serum* or *plasma,* rather than in whole blood, is usually measured. **Serum** is the liquid portion of blood that has had the cells and clotting factors removed; **plasma** is similar to serum except that it contains clotting factors.

lipoprotein profile series of blood tests to evaluate total cholesterol, HDL cholesterol, LDL cholesterol, and triglyceride levels

serum liquid portion of blood that has had the cells and clotting factors removed

plasma liquid portion of blood that has had the cells removed; contains clotting factors

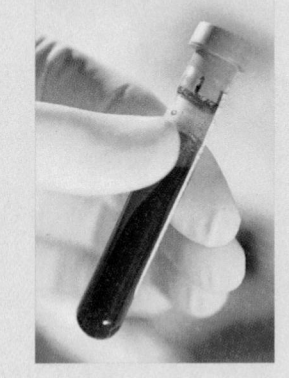

high-sensitivity C-reactive protein (hs-CRP) protein produced primarily by the liver in response to inflammation; a marker of CVD

TABLE 6.6 Classification of Blood Lipid Levels

Total Cholesterol (mg/dL)	Classification
< 200	Desirable
200–239	Borderline high
≥ 240	High
LDL Cholesterol (mg/dL)	**Classification**
< 100	Optimal
100–129	Near optimal/Above optimal
130–159	Borderline high
160–189	High
≥ 190	Very high
HDL Cholesterol (mg/dL)	**Classification**
< 40 (for men); < 50 (for women)	Low
≥ 60	High
Triglycerides (mg/dL)	**Classification**
< 150	Normal
150–199	Borderline high
≥ 200	High

Source of data: American Heart Association: *Levels of cholesterol.* Updated August 2012. http://www.heart.org/HEARTORG/Conditions/Cholesterol/AboutCholesterol/What-Your-Cholesterol-Levels-Mean_UCM_305562_Article.jsp Accessed: January 19, 2014

man thinks his risk of developing atherosclerosis and CVD is low because his blood cholesterol level is less than 200 mg/dL, he is incorrect.

The ratio of blood LDL to HDL cholesterol in blood may also predict the risk of CVD,[33] because it is healthier to have a higher blood level of HDL cholesterol than LDL cholesterol. To calculate risk of having a heart attack during the next 10 years, use the risk assessment tool at www.heart.org.

C-Reactive Protein

The development of CVD involves chronic inflammation.[34] The liver responds to infection and inflammation by producing and releasing **high–sensitivity C–reactive protein (hs–CRP)**, simply referred to as *C–reactive protein* or *CRP*, into the bloodstream. People with elevated CRP are more likely to develop CVD and hypertension than people who have lower levels of the protein.[35] Thus, elevated CRP may be a biomarker for atherosclerosis, like homocysteine. Individuals with a family history of CVD should consider having their hs–CRP levels measured.

ASSESS YOUR PROGRESS

19 *Discuss the series of physiological changes that occur in arteries and contribute to the development of CVD.*

20 *What are the recommendations concerning healthy blood lipoprotein levels?*

21 *List at least three major risk factors for developing CVD that are nonmodifiable and at least five that are modifiable.*

22 *Discuss the possible connection between elevated blood homocysteine levels and CVD.*

23 *Bernard's total blood cholesterol level is 195 mg/dL, and his HDL cholesterol level is 62 mg/dL. Based on this information, does Bernard have a high risk or low risk of developing CVD? Explain your answer.*

24 *What is "hs-CRP"? How does it relate to the risk of developing CVD?*

6.9 Reducing Risk of Atherosclerosis: Dietary Changes

LEARNING OUTCOMES

1 *Explain dietary factors that can reduce risk for developing atherosclerosis.*
2 *Summarize lifestyle factors that can reduce risk for developing atherosclerosis.*

Populations that consume diets rich in saturated fats (SFAs) generally have higher rates of CVD than populations that eat less saturated fat. SFA alters the structure of liver cell membranes so they no longer function properly. As a result, the liver removes less cholesterol from the bloodstream.[38] Thus, most SFAs increase total blood cholesterol levels by raising concentrations of both LDL and HDL cholesterol. Trans fats also raise blood cholesterol levels.[39] However, trans fats raise LDL cholesterol while reducing beneficial HDL cholesterol.[38] Cholesterol intake may also raise some individuals' blood LDL cholesterol levels.

Monounsaturated fatty acids (MUFAs) generally lower blood LDL cholesterol without reducing HDL cholesterol levels. Similar to MUFAs, diets containing high amounts of polyunsaturated fatty acids (PUFAs) may reduce blood levels of total cholesterol and blood LDL cholesterol. In some individuals, however, PUFAs also reduce beneficial HDL cholesterol. Nevertheless, PUFAs tend to be healthful because they do not promote atherosclerosis.

To reduce the risk of developing CVD, Dietary Guidelines and American Heart Association guidelines recommend limiting saturated fat intake to less than 10% of total energy by replacing foods that are rich sources of long-chain saturated fat with foods that contain high amounts of unsaturated fat.[18,19] People should limit their trans fat intake as much as possible. This can be accomplished by eating fewer solid fats, especially foods made with partially hydrogenated oils, such as stick margarine.

What About Omega-6 and Omega-3 Fats?

The typical American eats far more omega-6 foods than foods that contain omega-3 fatty acids.[43] The essential omega-6 fatty acid, linoleic acid, is found in vegetable oils used for frying and for making margarines and salad dressings. Cells use linoleic acid to make certain eicosanoids that increase inflammation and blood clotting. Some inflammation is necessary because it attracts immune system cells to disease-causing microorganisms. Clotting is an important function of blood, but having blood that clots too readily can increase the risk of heart attack and stroke. In 2009, the American Heart Association issued an advisory statement indicating that consuming 5 to 10% of total energy intake in the form of omega-6 fatty acids *reduces* the risk of developing heart disease.[44] The role of omega-6 fats in preventing heart disease is controversial among medical experts. Thus, more research is needed to clarify the pros and cons of following diets that contain high amounts of omega-6 fatty acids.

Eating foods that supply omega-3 fatty acids reduces the risk of developing heart disease to a greater extent than does eating foods that supply omega-6 fatty acids.[43] The body incorporates omega-3 fatty acids into cell membranes and uses these fatty acids to synthesize eicosanoids.[45] To obtain beneficial long-chain omega-3 fatty acids such as DHA, the Dietary Guidelines recommend that Americans eat at least 8 ounces of seafood (fish and shellfish) a week, such as sardines, salmon, tuna, and trout (see Chapter 3).[18] Table 6.7 lists possible health benefits of omega-3 fatty acids, and Table 6.8 presents foods that are rich sources of omega-3 fats.

For those who dislike or do not want to eat seafood, fish oil supplements can reduce elevated triglyceride levels; however, doses higher than 3 g/day may interfere with blood clotting and increase the risk of strokes. Therefore, consumers should check with their physician before taking fish oil supplements.

DID **YOU** *KNOW?*

In many parts of the world, coconuts and coconut oil are important components of diets. For example, coconut oil comprises 80% of the fat consumed in the southeastern Asian country of Sri Lanka.[40] Although coconut oil is highly saturated, the oil is rich in medium-chain saturated fatty acids that are metabolized differently in the body than long- and short-chain fatty acids. Medium-chain fatty acids may be beneficial to health.[41,42]

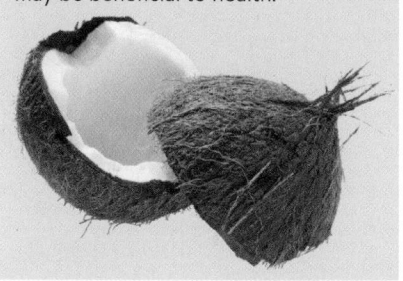

TABLE 6.7 Possible Health Benefits of Omega-3 Fatty Acids

Omega-3 Fats May Reduce the Risk of Developing:
• Heart disease
• Preterm birth
• Depression, including postpartum depression
• Dental disease
• Alzheimer's disease
• Certain cancers
• Arthritis
Omega-3 Fats May Improve:
• Immune function
• Cognitive development in infants

TABLE 6.8 Rich Food Sources of Omega-3 Fats

Fish/Shellfish (DHA and EPA)	Oils*	Nuts and Seeds*	Other
Herring, salmon, sablefish, anchovies, tuna, bluefish, sardines, catfish, striped bass, mackerel, trout, shark, swordfish, halibut, pollock, flounder, shrimp, mussels, crab	Flaxseed, walnut, canola, soybean	Walnuts, flaxseeds	Algae

*The human body is not as efficient at converting the omega-3 fatty acids from these foods into EPA, compared to the omega-3 fatty acids found in seafood.

DID **YOU** KNOW?

In 2008, actor Jeremy Piven was scheduled to appear in a Broadway play in New York City. A few weeks before the play's opening night, Piven began to experience extreme fatigue, dizziness, and nausea. He was diagnosed with mercury toxicity, and he was forced to drop out of the play to give his body time to recover. Mercury toxicity occurs when the organic form of the heavy metal (methylmercury) accumulates in the body over time. Piven's mercury toxicity was attributed primarily to his daily consumption of sushi. Treatment for methylmercury toxicity involves avoiding foods that contain fish, which allows the body to eliminate the mercury gradually. Farmed fish usually have higher methylmercury concentrations than wild fish.[46] However, the amount of methylmercury in farmed and wild fish is generally below the upper tolerable daily intake levels.[47]

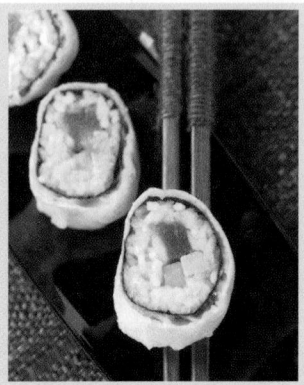

Sushi often contains raw fish, including tuna, salmon, and other fatty fish. Excessive consumption of these fish may lead to methylmercury toxicity.

FRESH TIPS

- Eat seafood, especially fatty fish, two times a week. Before cooking, marinate fresh fish in olive or canola oil that has been seasoned with a small amount of garlic, pepper, and lemon juice. The light coating of oil on fish can help keep the fish from drying out during cooking.

- Bake, grill, or broil fish.

- Add drained, water-packed tuna to salads, or mix the tuna with a little olive oil and pickle relish, and spread on whole-wheat toast.

- When olive oil is not desired, use canola oil, soybean oil, or soft margarines made from these oils for frying or sautéing.

- Sprinkle chopped walnuts on salads, yogurt, or cereal, or eat the nuts as a snack.

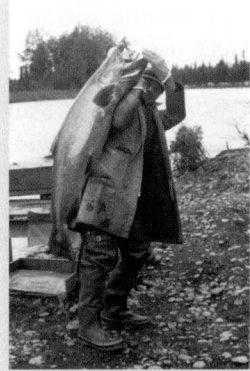

A fisherman in Kenai, Alaska, carrying a king salmon. Alaskans consume significantly more omega-3 fatty acids than the general U.S. population.

What about Dietary Cholesterol?

Often foods (or food ingredients) derived from animals are high in cholesterol, and they are also high in saturated fat. Thus, limiting consumption of animal foods can help reduce dietary cholesterol and saturated fat intakes.

Eggs are a relatively economical and rich source of high–quality protein and many micronutrients. However, egg yolks are the most concentrated source of cholesterol in the typical American's diet. One yolk, from a large egg, contains about 5 g of fat and 186 mg of cholesterol. To reduce cholesterol consumption, many Americans eat fewer fresh eggs than in the past. Whole eggs, however, are often ingredients in commonly eaten foods such as salad dressings, noodles, frozen custards, sauces, and baked goods.

Does eating egg yolks and other cholesterol–rich animal–derived foods raise the risk of developing CVD? Studies designed to determine the effects of dietary cholesterol on blood cholesterol levels have had mixed results.[48,49] In general, scientific evidence suggests that dietary cholesterol does not have as much effect on blood cholesterol levels as dietary saturated fat. The reason appears to be that in a healthy person, the liver synthesizes less cholesterol when dietary cholesterol intake is higher. On the other hand, eating large amounts of saturated fat increases the liver's cholesterol production.

Is It Safe to Eat Butter?

Many Americans have replaced butter with partially hardened vegetable oil margarines because of concern over butter's cholesterol and saturated fat content. Compared to butter, a serving of margarine provides more unsaturated fat, less saturated fat, and less cholesterol. However, margarine made from partially hydrogenated vegetable oil contains considerable amounts of unhealthy trans fatty acids.[51] The amount of saturated and trans fat in soft margarines is less than the amount in hard margarines or butter. Consumers can reduce their intakes of trans fats by using soft (tub) or liquid margarines, or trans fat–free spreads that resemble margarine, instead of stick margarine. People who use soft or liquid spreads can lower their blood LDL cholesterol more than those who use butter.[52,53] Using butter occasionally is unlikely to clog one's arteries. The "Fresh Tips" feature on page 178 suggests ways to reduce trans fatty acid intake.

Food Selection and Preparation

People can modify their food selection and preparation practices to reduce their intakes of dietary fat, especially "unhealthy" fats. Fatty red meats such as beef rib steaks are often more tender and expensive than leaner cuts such as chuck roasts. Certain cooking methods, however, can increase the tenderness of lean cuts of meat. Moist cooking methods, such as pot roasting or tightly covering the baking dish with foil, help tenderize meats without adding fat. After cooking, avoid eating the visible fat that remains. For example, trim away much of the fat from the meat and do not use pan drippings to make sauces or gravies.

Steaming meats and vegetables is a cooking method that does not require adding fat during preparation. Stir–frying pieces of raw vegetables, meat, fish, shellfish, and poultry in small amounts of hot vegetable oil cooks them quickly and preserves micronutrients. Additionally, when ground beef is browned in a pan, much of the fat can be drained before adding other ingredients to the meat.

Although it is easy to peel greasy breading from fried fish or chicken, much of the fat that we eat is hidden in foods and beverages. For example, fat comprises only 2% of the milk's volume but contributes 37% of the beverage's calories. Fat–free milk actually contains less than 0.5% fat by volume, and fat contributes essentially no energy to the beverage. What about the fat content of the cream cheese, margarine, or butter that you spread on a piece of toast? About 90% of the calories in cream cheese and about 100% of the calories in butter and margarine are from fat. Fried foods, chips, and salad dressings are high in fat;

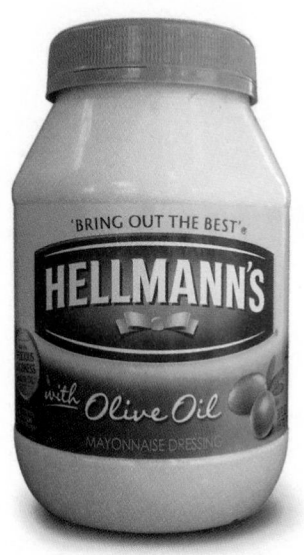

Spreads made with olive oil offer a rich source of monounsaturated fatty acids.

bacon, sausage, hot dogs, luncheon meats, and hard cheeses are also fatty foods. Nuts, including peanuts and almonds, have high fat content, but they generally contain high amounts of healthier monounsaturated fats. The "Fresh Tips" features on this and the following page provide some practical suggestions for reducing saturated and trans fat intakes.

People who are trying to reduce their energy intake should recognize that fat-reduced and fat-free foods are not "calorie-free." Food manufacturers often increase the amounts of added sugars in these products to improve taste and to compensate for reduced fat content.

Other Dietary Modifications

People may also reduce their risk of developing CVD by making other dietary changes. Eating foods that are rich sources of fiber, particularly soluble fiber (see Chapter 5), can reduce LDL cholesterol levels without lowering beneficial HDL cholesterol levels. When blood triglyceride levels are too high (>150 mg/dL), people should consider reducing their intakes of refined carbohydrates, such as candy, pastries, and sugar-sweetened soft drinks. Alcohol intake also increases the concentration of triglycerides in blood, so consuming less alcohol may help reduce a person's blood level of this lipid in blood.

Weight Loss and Physical Activity

Excess body fat, especially around the midsection of the body, is associated with unhealthy blood LDL cholesterol and triglyceride levels. Physical inactivity and excess energy consumption contribute to weight gain. Engaging in moderate-intensity physical activity at least 5 days a week and balancing energy intake with energy expenditure each day can help people achieve and maintain healthy body weights. Taking these steps can also reduce blood LDL and triglyceride levels and raise blood HDL levels. Chapter 13 provides more information concerning the role of physical activity in achieving and maintaining a healthy weight.

FRESH TIPS

- Read the Nutrition Facts panel and the ingredient list on the label when choosing processed foods, especially margarine. Compare margarines to find the product with 0 g of trans fat. Margarines that have "liquid" vegetable oil as the first ingredient generally have less trans fat than stick margarines.

- Avoid products that include interesterified (fully hydrogenated) oil, partially hydrogenated fat, or shortening in the ingredient list.

- Eat fewer commercially prepared baked goods, snack foods, and fried fast-food items.

- Purchase brands of microwave popcorn that have little added fat or no trans fats. Buy plain popcorn and pop the kernels using a small amount of hot oil in a covered saucepan or use a hot-air machine.

- Commercial frostings that are made with vegetable shortenings are likely to be high in hydrogenated oils. Remove most of the frosting from a serving of cake before eating it. (Frosting is primarily sugar and fat, a rich source of empty calories.) You can make your own frosting by mixing soft margarine or smooth peanut butter with a little milk, powdered sugar, and vanilla flavoring.

- Pastry dough may be made with shortening. Replace shortening with oil or soft margarine to make your own pastry dough from scratch.

What If Lifestyle Changes Do Not Work?

Some people are unable to lower their risk of CVD significantly by making dietary changes, exercising regularly, and losing excess body fat. If a person's blood lipid levels are too high and the levels have remained elevated even after making these lifestyle modifications, he or she should discuss additional treatment options with his or her physician. Millions of Americans take a class of prescription drugs called statins to reduce their elevated blood lipid levels. Statins interfere with the liver's metabolism of cholesterol, effectively reducing LDL cholesterol and tri–glyceride levels as a result. Statins are relatively safe when taken as directed and with regular monitoring by one's physician.

Zetia® is a drug that works differently from a statin. Zetia inhibits intestinal absorption of cholesterol and, as a result, lowers LDL cholesterol levels. However, questions have been raised about the medication's safety, particularly when it is taken with other cholesterol–lowering medications.[55]

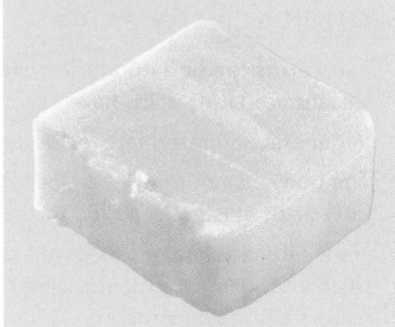
FRESH TIPS

- Reduce intake of fried foods.

- Purchase lean meats and trim visible fat from meat before cooking. Before eating cooked meat, trim and discard any remaining visible fat.

- Try replacing some fatty foods with reduced-fat or fat-free alternatives. For example, substitute plain, fat-free yogurt in recipes that call for sour cream. Place a spoonful of the yogurt, instead of butter or sour cream, on a baked potato.

- Because most nuts are rich sources of healthy unsaturated fats, replace foods that contain saturated fat with nuts. For example, use peanut or soy nut butters instead of cheese or luncheon meat in sandwiches. Some nut butters contain trans fats and added sugars, so read the Nutrition Facts panel and ingredients list before selecting these products.

- Pretzels, air-popped popcorn, and most fruits and vegetables are low fat and generally more nutrient dense than chips, cookies, pastries, and candy bars.

- Patronize fast-food restaurants that offer low-fat menu items such as meatless salads, baked or broiled chicken and fish, low-fat yogurt, and bean burritos.

- Use less creamy salad dressings on salads. When in restaurants, order oil-and-vinegar salad dressings or creamy dressings "on the side" so the amount added is easy to control.

- Use one-quarter less butter, oil, or margarine than is indicated in recipes. Use olive or canola oils in recipes that call for vegetable oil.

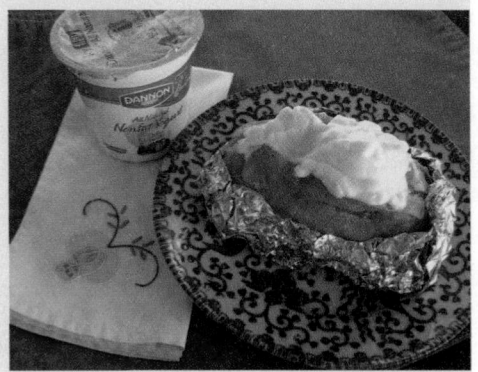

ASSESS YOUR PROGRESS

25. *Suggest at least four ways people can reduce their intakes of saturated fats and increase their intakes of unsaturated fats.*

26. *List at least two strategies for reducing trans fat intake.*

27. *Describe four health benefits of omega-3 fatty acid consumption.*

28. *List five rich food sources of omega-3 fatty acids.*

29. *Describe how prescription medications may improve blood lipid levels.*

SUMMARY

SECTION 6.1 Introducing Lipids

- Major lipids are triglycerides, phospholipids, and sterols. The body needs lipids for energy (triglycerides), proper growth and development, nerve functioning, maintenance of healthy skin and hair, and the production of bile and several hormones.

SECTION 6.2 Fatty Acids

- Fatty acids can be saturated or unsaturated, and unsaturated fatty acids can be either monounsaturated or polyunsaturated. Unsaturated fatty acids have one or more double bonds in their chemical structure.
- In general, saturated fatty acids are solid at room temperature and unsaturated fatty acids are liquid.
- The body cannot synthesize the omega-6 fatty acid linoleic acid or the omega-3 fatty acid alpha-linolenic acid; these essential fatty acids must be supplied by the diet.
- Trans fatty acid molecules have a different configuration than cis fatty acid molecules. Most of the trans fat in food results from the hydrogenation process. Diets that contain high amounts of trans fats are associated with an increased risk of developing heart disease and stroke.

SECTION 6.3 Triglycerides

- A triglyceride has three fatty acids attached to a glycerol backbone. Triglycerides comprise about 95% of lipids in the body and in food.
- Triglycerides usually contain mixtures of unsaturated and saturated fatty acids, but one type of fatty acid tends to predominate.

SECTION 6.4 Phospholipids

- Phospholipids have both hydrophilic and hydrophobic regions, and as a result, they are partially soluble in water and can serve as emulsifiers. Phospholipids are the major structural component of cell membranes and are needed for proper functioning of nerve cells. Lecithin is the major phospholipid in food.

SECTION 6.5 Cholesterol and Other Sterols

- The sterol cholesterol is a component of every cell membrane. Cells use cholesterol to make a variety of substances, including bile and vitamin D. Cholesterol is found only in animal foods. Plants synthesize sterols and stanols that are not well absorbed by humans.

SECTION 6.6 Lipid Digestion, Absorption, and Transport

- The triglycerides and phospholipids in food undergo digestion primarily in the duodenum. The GI hormone CCK stimulates secretion of pancreatic lipase and bile. Bile emulsifies fat molecules, and pancreatic lipase removes two fatty acids from the triglyceride.
- Following digestion and absorption of fats, bile salts are reabsorbed in the ileum. Soluble fiber can interfere with this enterohepatic circulation of bile.
- The digestion of phospholipids results from phospholipase removing two fatty acids from each phospholipid molecule.
- Cholesterol is not broken down and is packaged in micelles along with monoglycerides, fatty acids, and phospholipid fragments. After entering absorptive cells, monoglycerides and two fatty acids reform triglycerides.
- Within small intestinal absorptive cells, lipids are coated with a layer that contains protein to form chylomicrons. Chylomicrons enter the lymphatic system of the small intestine and eventually reach the bloodstream. The liver uses lipids from chylomicrons to make other lipoproteins.

SECTION 6.7 Lipid Consumption Patterns

- During the last century, the amount of fat eaten by Americans increased, primarily because of increased consumption of fast foods and high-fat commercial food products.
- Recommended diets for healthy people generally limit fat to 30 to 35% of total energy intake; the AMDR for fat is 20 to 35% of total calories.
- According to the Dietary Guidelines, saturated fat should account for less than 10% of total calories, and people should limit their cholesterol intake to as little as possible while following a healthy diet pattern.

SECTION 6.8 **Lipids and Cardiovascular Disease**

- Heart disease, stroke, and hypertension are major forms of CVD. In the United States, heart disease is the leading cause of death in both males and females. Atherosclerosis is a long-term process that can result in CVD.

- Numerous risk factors are associated with atherosclerosis; some risk factors are difficult to modify, but many are related to lifestyle practices that can be altered.

- Blood lipid levels can have a major influence on a person's risk of CVD. It is better to have high blood levels of HDL cholesterol than high blood LDL cholesterol levels, because elevated LDL cholesterol contributes to development of atherosclerosis. Elevated HDL cholesterol is associated with lower risk of this condition.

SECTION 6.9 **Reducing Risk of Atherosclerosis: Dietary Changes**

- Physical activity and replacing saturated fats with monounsaturated fats may reduce LDL levels and increase HDL levels. In the body, trans fats raise blood cholesterol levels.

- Omega-3 fatty acids may protect the heart from CVD. Fatty fish, including salmon and tuna, are good sources of omega-3 fatty acids. Although omega-3 and fish oil capsules are sources of omega-3 fatty acids, overconsumption of the fat can be dangerous.

- People with elevated blood cholesterol and/or triglyceride levels may reduce their risk of developing CVD by modifying their diets, losing excess weight, and engaging in regular physical activity.

Get the most out of your study of nutrition with McGraw-Hill's innovative suite of adaptive learning products including McGraw-Hill LearnSmart®, SmartBook®, McGraw-Hill LearnSmart Achieve®, and McGraw-Hill LearnSmart Prep®. Visit www.learnsmartadvantage.com.

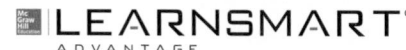

CASE STUDY RESPONSE

LIPIDS AND HEART HEALTH

ACCORDING TO SAMANTHA'S LIPOPROTEIN PROFILE, she has borderline high total cholesterol, borderline high LDL cholesterol, low HDL cholesterol, and normal triglycerides. Desirable blood lipid levels for women are:

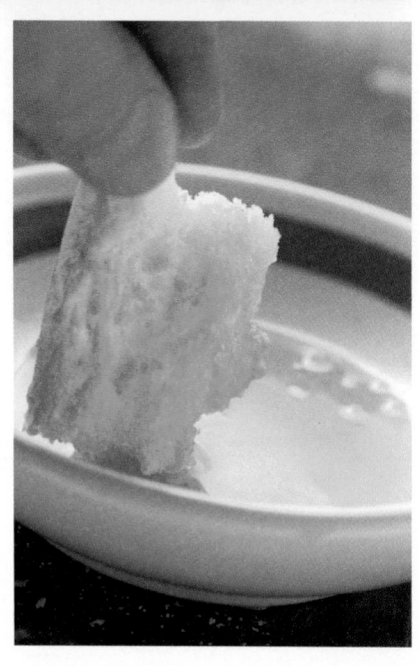

Total cholesterol	< 200 mg/dL
LDL cholesterol	< 100 mg/dL
HDL cholesterol	> 50 mg/dL
Triglycerides	< 150 mg/dL

HDL and LDL are both lipoproteins that transport fat in the blood. HDL transports lipids from tissues and back to the liver; it is often referred to as "good" cholesterol. LDL transports lipids to tissues, including blood vessel walls, which can lead to plaque formation. Abnormal lipoprotein levels, such as HDL and LDL cholesterol, contribute to arterial plaque formation. LDL may therefore be termed "bad" cholesterol. Family history and lifestyle factors, such as diet and exercise, contribute to blood levels of HDL and LDL cholesterol.

Dietary recommendations to improve Samantha's health and lower her risk for heart disease include:

- Choose fatty fish, such as salmon and tuna, lean meats, and plant-based proteins, such as beans and nuts, to meet protein needs.

- Replace food that are sources of solid fat with reduced-fat or fat-free alternatives. For example, instead of dipping carrots in a creamy dip, use hummus or fat-free Greek yogurt.

- Use olive oil for sautéing vegetables and mix with her favorite herbs as a dip for whole-wheat bread.

Modifying Recipes for Healthy Living

Andrea is a 21-year-old, slightly overweight (5-feet, 10-inches tall and 185 pounds) college student. According to her physician, Andrea's total and LDL cholesterol levels are too high. She is aware of her family history of heart attacks and strokes, so she is very concerned about her risk of CVD. She lives in an off-campus apartment that has a fully equipped kitchen. One of her favorite dishes is fettuccini Alfredo that she serves with beef. Advise Andrea on ways to modify this recipe to make it "heart-healthy."

FETTUCCINI ALFREDO

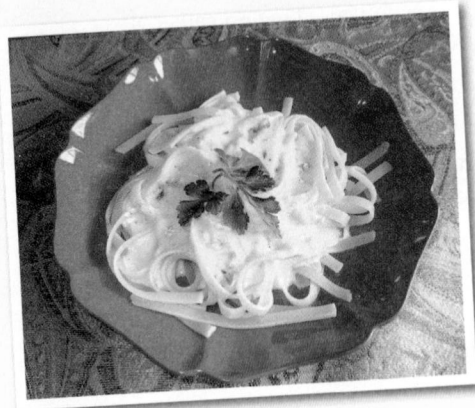

PREPARATION STEPS

1. Bring a large pot of lightly salted water to a boil. Add fettuccini and cook for 8 to 10 minutes, drain.
2. In a large skillet, melt the butter and add the garlic. Cook on low for 3 to 5 minutes, stirring often.
3. Slowly add cream to butter mixture. Add salt and pepper.
4. Raise heat to medium and slowly stir in cheeses until melted.
5. Immediately remove from the stove and serve over cooked pasta as a side dish for the steak. Serves four.

STEP 1 Brainstorm

Examine the recipe. What ingredients can you change to lower the total fat, reduce the sources of saturated fat, and lower the calories in the recipe? (Refer to Table 1.7 for substitutions.)

STEP 2 Develop a modified version of this recipe

List ingredients and amounts needed.
List the preparation steps.

STEP 3 Analyze nutrient contents of the original and modified recipes by using a computer software program

Develop a table that compares the number of calories and amounts of total fat, saturated fat, monounsaturated fat, polyunsaturated fat, and trans fat in each recipe. How did your modifications change the nutrient composition of the Alfredo dish?

OPTIONAL ACTIVITIES

STEP 4 Test your new recipe

Keep notes on any changes you make to ingredient amounts as you prepare the Alfredo dish.

STEP 5 Reflect on your findings

How did the Alfredo dish look and taste? Was the sauce too runny, too thick, or acceptable?

STEP 6 Add the recipe to your collection or repeat steps to improve the product

INGREDIENTS

12 oz dry fettuccini pasta

½ cup butter

2 cloves garlic, chopped

1 cup heavy cream

¼ tsp salt

¼ tsp pepper

¼ cup Parmesan cheese

¾ cup Romano cheese

1 lb broiled flank steak, cut into strips

PERSONAL Dietary Analysis

1. Refer to the 3-day food log from the "Personal Dietary Analysis" feature in Chapter 5. List the total number of kilocalories you consumed for each day of recordkeeping. Add the figures to obtain a total, divide the total by 3, then round the figure to the nearest whole number to obtain your average daily energy intake for the 3-day period.

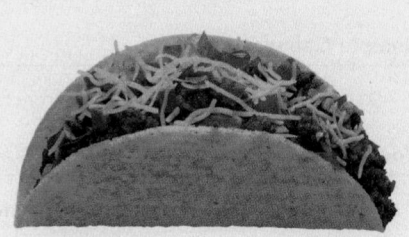

connect | NUTRITION

Complete the Personal Dietary Analysis activity online at www.mcgrawhillconnect.com, where you will also find McGraw-Hill LearnSmart®, SmartBook®, NutritionCalc Plus, and many other dynamic learning tools.

Sample Calculation:

Day 1	<u>2000</u> kcal
Day 2	<u>1700</u> kcal
Day 3	<u>2350</u> kcal
Total kcal	<u>6050</u> ÷ 3 days = <u>2017</u> kcal/day (average kilocalorie intake, rounded to the nearest whole number)

Your Calculation:

Day 1	___ kcal
Day 2	___ kcal
Day 3	___ kcal
Total kcal	___ ÷ 3 days = ___ kcal/day

(average kilocalorie intake, rounded to the nearest whole number)

2. Add the number of grams of fat eaten each day of the period. Divide the total by 3 and round to the nearest whole number to calculate the average number of grams of fat consumed daily.

Sample Calculation:

Day 1	<u>50</u> g
Day 2	<u>57</u> g
Day 3	<u>42</u> g
Total grams	<u>149</u> ÷ 3 days = <u>50</u> g/day (average)

Your Calculation:

Day 1	___ g
Day 2	___ g
Day 3	___ g
Total grams	___ ÷ 3 days = ___ g of fat/day

(average, rounded to the nearest whole number)

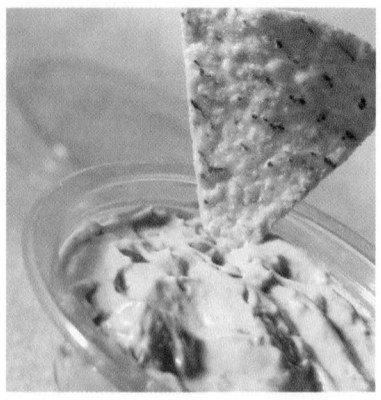

Guacamole is made from avocados, which are an excellent source of monounsaturated fatty acids. While the fats in the guacamole are healthy fats, it still contains significant calories.

3. Each gram of fat provides about 9 kcal; therefore, you must multiply the average number of grams of fat that you ate daily (step 2) by 9 to obtain the average number of kilocalories from fat.

Sample Calculation:

<u>50</u> g/day × <u>9</u> kcal/g = <u>450</u> kcal from fat

Your Calculation

___ g/day × <u>9</u> kcal/g = ___ kcal from fat

4. To calculate the average percentage of calories that fat contributed to your diet, divide the average number of calories from fat obtained in step 3 by the average total daily calorie intake obtained in step 1, and round to the nearest one-hundredth. Multiply the value by 100, drop the decimal point, and add the percent symbol.

Sample Calculation:

<u>450</u> kcal ÷ <u>2017</u> kcal = <u>0.22</u>

<u>0.22</u> × <u>100</u> = <u>22%</u>

Your Calculation

___ kcal ÷ ___ kcal = ___

___ × <u>100</u> = ___ %

5. Did your average daily fat intake meet the recommended 20 to 35% of total energy? Yes ___ No ___

6. If your average fat intake was more than 35% of your total energy intake, which foods contributed to your intake of fats?

Foods: _____

7. Review the log of your 3-day food intake. Calculate your average daily intake of saturated fat by adding the grams of saturated fat consumed over the 3-day period and dividing the total by 3.

Your Calculation:

Day 1   ___ g

Day 2   ___ g

Day 3   ___ g

Total g   ___ ÷ 3 days = ___ g of saturated fat daily

a. What was your average daily saturated fat intake? ___ grams

b. Did your average daily saturated fat intake meet the Dietary Guidelines recommended level for a healthy adult (less than 10% of total calories)?

c. If your average saturated fat intake was greater than the recommended level, list foods that contributed to your high intake.

Assessment: Evaluating Your Solid Fat Intake

Do You Consume:	Rarely or Never	1 to 2 Times/Week	3 to 5 Times/Week	Daily
1. Bacon, hot dogs, sausage, salami, bologna, or other fatty luncheon meat?	O	1	2	3
2. Whole milk?	O	1	2	3
3. 2% milk?	O	1	2	3
4. Ice cream or milkshakes?	O	1	2	3
5. Sour cream or cream cheese?	O	1	2	3
6. Fatty cuts of pork or beef?	O	1	2	3
7. Hard cheeses, such as cheddar or Swiss?	O	1	2	3
8. Butter?	O	1	2	3
9. Stick margarine?	O	1	2	3
10. Gravy, cheese sauce, or cream-based sauce?	O	1	2	3
11. Buttered popcorn or "rinds"?	O	1	2	3
12. Biscuits, croissants, doughnuts, Danish pastries, pies, cakes, or cookies?	O	1	2	3
13. Products made with lard?	O	1	2	3
14. Cream in your coffee or tea?	O	1	2	3
15. Pizza?	O	1	2	3
16. Creamed soups such as cream of potato soup or New England clam chowder?	O	1	2	3
TOTAL	__	__	__	__

Scoring: Add points in each column and then add those figures together. (The higher the total points, the higher your solid fat intake.)

My "Solid Fat Score" is ___

If your score is 30 or more: Your solid fat intake is probably too high. Note which of these fatty foods you eat more than three times per week. Consider reducing your intake of these items and replacing them with foods that do not contain solid fat.

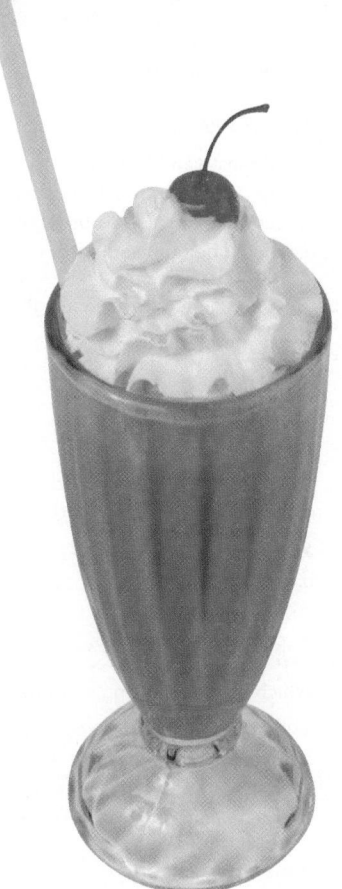

Critical Thinking

1. George is a 45-year-old, overweight college professor who had his gallbladder removed recently. Since having the surgery, George has experienced frequent bouts of diarrhea and steatorrhea. What dietary recommendations can you give George that will reduce his likelihood of having these signs of fat malabsorption?

2. Geri would like to make her family's favorite recipes healthier. She has heard that some sources of fat are more healthful than others. What kinds of advice would you give to Geri that can help her chose such fats? Explain how these fats can be incorporated into her recipes.

3. Develop a lesson for middle school–aged children that describes how atherosclerosis develops and the role that lifestyle choices play in the development of the disease.

4. According to results of his lipoprotein profile, Alex has elevated total cholesterol, LDL cholesterol, and homocysteine levels. Furthermore, his serum HDL cholesterol level was low. Explain to Alex what his test results mean in regard to his risk of developing CVD and steps he can take to reduce his risk.

5. Sophia is pregnant with her first child. At Sophia's last prenatal appointment, her obstetrician recommended that she eat a diet rich in omega-3 fatty acids, including 2 or 3 servings of tuna or salmon per week. She does not like to eat fish, so based on the information in this chapter, what would you tell her concerning the importance of consuming a diet rich in omega-3 fatty acids during pregnancy?

Practice Test

Select the best answer.

1. Fats in foods
   a. add taste and contribute to satiety.
   b. are rapidly digested and absorbed.
   c. carry water-soluble nutrients.
   d. should be removed before cooking.

2. Solid fats generally have a high proportion of _____ fatty acids.
   a. unsaturated
   b. saturated
   c. polyunsaturated
   d. monounsaturated

3. Which of the following foods is the richest source of monounsaturated fatty acids?
   a. whipped butter
   b. whole milk
   c. olive oil
   d. coconut oil

4. Which of the following statements is true?
   a. Certain fish are rich sources of omega-3 fatty acids.
   b. Omega-3 fatty acids increase the risk of cardiovascular disease.
   c. Trans fats are rich sources of omega-3 fatty acids.
   d. The human body converts dietary fiber into omega-3 fatty acids.

5. Trans fatty acids are
   a. naturally found in many foods.
   b. a by-product of the partial-hydrogenation process.
   c. essential for good health.
   d. eliminated in urine and feces.

6. Which of the following statements is false?
   a. Phospholipids are in cell membranes.
   b. Phospholipids act as emulsifiers.
   c. Phospholipids are partially water soluble.
   d. Phospholipids act as antioxidants.

7. Cholesterol is
   a. not synthesized by the human body.
   b. found only in animal foods.
   c. toxic to human cells.
   d. metabolized for energy.

8. The primary site of triglyceride digestion and absorption is the
   a. stomach.
   b. liver.
   c. small intestine.
   d. gallbladder.

9. Intestinal absorptive cells package triglycerides, cholesterol, and phospholipids into _____ for transport in blood.
   a. chylomicrons
   b. bile salts
   c. emulsifiers
   d. stanols

10. Lipoproteins
    a. are water insoluble.
    b. transport lipids in the bloodstream.
    c. contain glucose.
    d. cause heart attacks.

11. The _____ is the main site of bile salt reabsorption.
    a. colon
    b. jejunum
    c. duodenum
    d. ileum

12. Homocysteine is a(n)
    a. form of folate, a B vitamin.
    b. nondigestible lipid.
    c. possible risk factor for CVD.
    d. essential amino acid in dairy products.

13. HDL cholesterol is

    a. made in the large intestine.
    b. commonly called "bad" cholesterol.
    c. a lipoprotein that carries lipids away from tissues.
    d. an essential fatty acid.

14. Egg yolks

    a. are a concentrated source of cholesterol.
    b. should be eliminated from the diet.
    c. may decrease one's risk for steatorrhea.
    d. provide little nutritional value.

15. Which of the following foods is most likely to be contaminated with methylmercury?

    a. apple
    b. beef
    c. celery
    d. salmon

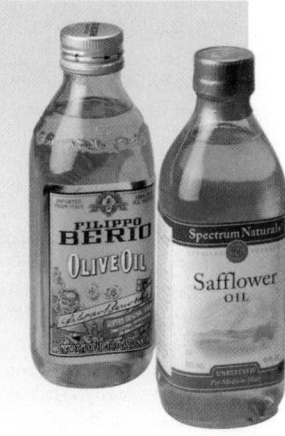

ANSWERS TO CHAPTER 6 QUIZ Yourself

1. To lose weight, use regular, stick margarine instead of butter because it has 25% fewer calories per teaspoon. **False** (p. 179)
2. Eating a diet rich in olive oil may lower one's risk for developing heart disease. **True** (pp. 155, 175)
3. Egg yolks are a rich source of cholesterol. **True** (p. 177)
4. A person who has had his or her gallbladder removed can no longer digest fats. **False** (p. 166)
5. Taking too many fish oil supplements may be harmful to health. **True** (p. 175)

ANSWERS TO PRACTICE TEST
1-a; 2-b; 3-c; 4-a; 5-b; 6-d; 7-b; 8-c; 9-a; 10-b; 11-d; 12-c; 13-c; 14-a; 15-d

References

1. Shikany JM and others: Is dietary fat "fattening"? A comprehensive research synthesis. *Critical Reviews in Food Science and Nutrition* 50(8):699, 2010.

2. Pericleous M and others: Nutrition and pancreatic cancer. *Anticancer Research* 34(1):9, 2014.

3. Foroughi M and others: Stroke and nutrition: A review of studies. *International Journal of Preventative Medicine* 4(Suppl 2):S165, 2013.

4. Hunter JE and others: Cardiovascular disease risk of dietary stearic acid compared with trans, other saturated, and unsaturated fatty acids: A systemic review. *American Journal of Clinical Nutrition* 91(1):46, 2010.

5. Otten JJ and others (eds.): *Dietary Reference Intakes: The essential guide to nutrient requirements.* Washington, DC: National Academies Press, 2006.

6. Brouwer IA and others: Effect of animal and industrial *trans*-fatty acids on HDL and LDL cholesterol levels in humans—A quantitative review. *PLoS One* 5(3):e9434, 2010.

7. U.S. Food and Drug Administration: *FDA targets trans fat in processed food.* Updated November 2013. http://www.fda.gov/ForConsumers/ConsumerUpdates/ucm372915.htm Accessed January 18, 2014.

8. Sundram K and others: Stearic-acid rich interesterified fat and trans fat raise the LDL/HDL ratio and plasma glucose relative to palm olein in humans. *Nutrition & Metabolism* 4:3, 2006.

9. Willett WC: Dietary fats and coronary heart disease. *Journal of Internal Medicine* 272(1):13, 2012.

10. U.S. Department of Agriculture, Economic Research Service: *Dietary Assessment of Major Trends in U.S. Food Consumption 1970–2005.* Updated May 2012. Bulletin Number 33, 2008. http://www.ers.usda.gov/Publications/EIB33/EIB33.pdf Accessed: January 19, 2014.

11. Scholle JM and others: The effect of adding plant sterols or stanols to statin therapy in hypercholesterolemic patients: A systematic review and meta-analysis. *Journal of the American College of Nutrition* 28(5):517, 2009.

12. Talati R and others: The comparative efficacy of plant sterols and stanols on serum lipids: A systemic review and meta-analysis. *Journal of the American Dietetic Association* 110(5):719, 2010.

13. U.S. Department of Agriculture, Agricultural Research Service: *What We Eat in America.* 2009–2010. 2012. http://www.ars.usda.gov/Services/docs.htm?docid=18349 Accessed: January 19, 2014.

14. National Institutes of Health, National Institute of Diabetes and Digestive and Kidney Disorders: *Gallstones.* Updated November 2013. http://digestive.niddk.nih.gov/ddiseases/pubs/gallstones/index.htm Accessed: January 19, 2014.

15. National Institutes of Health, National Institute of Neurological Disorders and Stroke: *Lipid Storage Diseases Fact Sheet.* Updated October 2012. http://www.ninds.nih.gov/disorders/lipid_storage_diseases/detail_lipid_storage_diseases.htm Accessed: January 19, 2014.

16. U.S. Department of Agriculture: Nationwide food consumption survey, food and nutrient intakes by individuals in the United States, 1 day, 1987–88. Updated July 2012. http://www.ars.usda.gov/SP2UserFiles/Place/12355000/pdf/8788/nfcs8788_rep_87-i-1.pdf Accessed: January 19, 2014.

17. U.S. Department of Agriculture. Agricultural Research Service: NHANES, 2009–2010, What we eat in America. Table 1: Nutrient intakes from food: Mean amounts consumed per individual, by gender and age, in the United States, 2009–2010. http://www.ars.usda.gov/SP2User-Files/Place/12355000/pdf/0910/Table_1_NIN_GEN_09.pdf Accessed: July 23, 2014.

18. U.S. Departments of Health and Human Services and Agriculture: *2015-2020 Dietary Guidelines for Americans.* 2015. http://health.gov/dietaryguidelines/2015/guidelines/ Accessed: January 22, 2016.

19. Go AS and others: Heart disease and stroke statistics—2013 update: A report from the American Heart Association. *Circulation* 127(1):143, 2013.

20. Murphy SL and others: Deaths: Final data for 2010. *National Vital Statistics Reports* 61(4):1, 2013.

21. National Heart Lung and Blood Institute: *Atherosclerosis: Who is at risk for atherosclerosis?* Updated July 2011. http://www.nhlbi.nih.gov/health/health-topics/topics/atherosclerosis/atrisk.html Accessed: January 19, 2014.

22. Snowdon DA and others: Serum folate and the severity of atrophy of the neocortex in Alzheimer's disease: Findings from the Nun Study. *American Journal of Clinical Nutrition* 71(4):993, 2000.

23. Gallucci M and others: Serum folate, homocystein, brain atrophy, and auto-CM system: The Treviso Dementia (TREDEM) study. *Journal of Alzheimers Disease* 38(3):581, 2014.

24. Herrmann W, Obeid R: Homocysteine: A biomarker in neurodegenerative diseases. *Clinical, Chemistry, and Laboratory Medicine* 49(3):435, 2011.

25. American Diabetes Association: *American Diabetes Month® 2012 overview.* www.diabetes.org Accessed: January 19, 2014.

26. Centers for Disease Control and Prevention: *Health effects of cigarette smoking.* Updated December 2013. http://www.cdc.gov/tobacco/data_statistics/fact_sheets/health_effects/effects_cig_smoking/index.htm#overview Accessed: January 19, 2014.

27. Erhardt L: Cigarette smoking: An undertreated risk factor for cardiovascular disease. *Atherosclerosis* 205(1):23, 2009.

28. Shoji T and others: Small dense low-density lipoprotein cholesterol concentration and carotid atherosclerosis. *Atherosclerosis* 202(2):582, 2009.

29. Thanassoulis G and others: Association of long-term and early adult atherosclerosis risk factors with aortic and mitral valve calcium. *Journal of the American College of Cardiology* 55 (22):2491, 2010.

30. Miller M and others: Triglycerides and cardiovascular disease: A scientific statement from the American Heart Association. *Circulation* 123(20):2292, 2011.

31. American Heart Association: *Levels of cholesterol.* Updated August 2012. http://www.heart.org/HEARTORG/Conditions/Cholesterol/AboutCholesterol/What-Your-Cholesterol-Levels-Mean_UCM_305562_Article.jsp Accessed: January 19, 2014.

32. National Cholesterol Education Program (National Institutes of Health): *High blood cholesterol: What you need to know.* Revised June 2005. http://www.nhlbi.nih.gov/health/public/heart/chol/wyntk.htm Accessed: January 19, 2014.

33. Fernandez ML, Webb D: The LDL to HDL cholesterol ratio as a valuable tool to evaluate coronary heart disease risk. *Journal of the American College of Nutrition* 27(1):1, 2008.

34. Wang Z, Nakayama T: Inflammation, a link between obesity and cardiovascular disease. *Mediators of Inflammation* 2010:535918, 2010.

35. Kaptoge S and others: C-reactive protein concentration and risk of coronary heart disease, stroke, and mortality: An individual participant meta-analysis. *Lancet* 375(9709):132, 2010.

36. Thanassoulis G and others: Associations of long-term and early adult atherosclerosis risk factors with aortic and mitral valve calcium. *Journal of the American College of Cardiology* 55(22):2491, 2010.

37. Kawada T: Effect of coronary artery calcium as a subclinical atherosclerosis measure on cardiovascular disease events or causes of death. *American Journal of Cardiology* 113(3):571, 2014.

38. Fernandez ML, West KL: Mechanisms by which dietary fatty acids modulate plasma lipids. *Journal of Nutrition* 135(9):2075, 2005.

39. Eckel RH and others: Understanding the complexity of trans fatty acid reduction in the American diet. *Circulation* 115(16):2231, 2006.

40. Amarasiri WA, Dissanayake AS: Coconut fats. *Ceylon Medical Journal* 51(2):47, 2006.

41. Labarthe F and others: Medium-chain fatty acids as metabolic therapy in cardiac disease. *Cardiovascular Drugs and Therapy* 22(2):97, 2008.

42. Huang CB and others: Short- and medium-chain fatty acids exhibit antimicrobial activity for oral microorganisms. *Archives of Oral Biology* 56(7):650, 2011.

43. De Caterina R: N-3 fatty acids in cardiovascular disease. *New England Journal of Medicine* 64:2439, 2011.

44. Harris WS and others: Omega-6 fatty acids and risk for cardiovascular disease: A science advisory from the American Heart Association Nutrition Subcommittee of the Council on Nutrition, Physical Activity, and Metabolism; Council on Cardiovascular Nursing; and Council on Epidemiology and Prevention. *Circulation* 119(6):902, 2009.

45. National Institutes of Health, National Center for Complementary and Alternative Medicine: *Omega-3 supplements: An introduction.* Updated June 2013. http://nccam.nih.gov/health/omega3/introduction.htm#jump4 Accessed: January 19, 2014.

46. Easton MD and others: Preliminary examination of contaminant loadings in farmed salmon, wild salmon and commercial salmon feed. *Chemosphere* 46(7):1053, 2002.

47. Kelly BC and others: Mercury and other trace elements in farmed and wild salmon from British Columbia, Canada. *Environmental Toxicology and Chemistry* 27(6):1361, 2008.

48. Djousse L, Gaziano JM: Egg consumption and risk of heart failure in the Physician's Health Study. *Circulation* 117(4):512, 2008.

49. Spence JD, others: Dietary cholesterol and egg yolks: Not for patients at risk of vascular disease. *Canadian Journal of Cardiology* 26(9):E336, 2010.

50. Raloff J: *Cholesterol medicine for eggs?* Science News Online, 164(2), 2003. http://www.sciencenews.org/view/generic/id/4036/title/Food_for_Thought_Cholesterol_Medicine_for_Eggs%3F Accessed: January 19, 2014.

51. Mayo Clinic: *Butter vs. margarine: Which is better for my heart?* Updated June 2012. http://www.mayoclinic.com/health/butter-vs-margarine/AN00835 Accessed: January 19, 2014.

52. Tonstad S and others: Serum cholesterol response to replacing butter with a new trans-free margarine in hypercholesterolemic subjects. *Nutrition, Metabolism, and Cardiovascular Disease* 11(5):320, 2001.

53. Gagliardi AC and others: Effects of margarines and butter consumption on lipid profiles, inflammation markers and lipid transfer to HDL particles in free-living subjects with the metabolic syndrome. *European Journal of Clinical Nutrition* 64(10):1141, 2010.

54. Thompson GR, Grundy SM. History and development of plant sterol and stanol esters for cholesterol-lowering purposes. *American Journal of Cardiology* 96(1A):3D, 2005.

55. Ballantyne CM and others: Efficacy, safety and effect on biomarkers related to cholesterol and lipoprotein metabolism of rosuvastatin 10 or 20 mg plus ezetimibe 10 mg vs. simvastatin 40 or 80 mg plus ezetimibe 10 mg in high-risk patients: Results of the GRAVITY randomized study. *Atherosclerosis* 232(1):86, 2014.

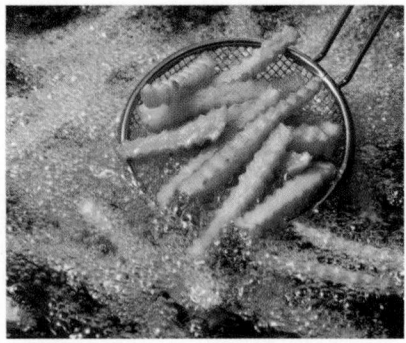

7 Proteins:
Amino Acids

CASE STUDY
Meeting protein needs

COLLEGE SENIOR MANUEL IS 6-FEET, 2-INCHES tall and weighs 175 pounds. Manuel is a former high school baseball player. Although he does not play the sport in college, he stays in shape by working out for 30 to 40 minutes three or four times per week. His workout program involves jogging 2 days per week and lifting weights 1 or 2 days per week.

Manuel eats a protein-rich diet that includes meat, poultry, or eggs at every meal. According to his calculations, his diet supplies between 120 and 150 g of protein daily. Despite his high intake of animal protein, he is considering adding a protein shake for snacks, twice a day. The protein shake he would like to add to his diet provides 20 g of protein per serving.

- Calculate Manuel's RDA for protein. How does his current daily consumption compare to this recommendation?

- Provide Manuel with five meatless food choices that supply at least 15 g of high-quality protein per serving of such foods.

- Do you recommend that Manuel drink the protein shake twice a day? Why or why not?

The suggested Case Study Response can be found on page 220.

connect | NUTRITION Check out the Connect site at www.mcgrawhillconnect.com to further explore this case study.

QUIZ Yourself

How much protein should a healthy adult consume daily? Can people obtain enough protein by eating only plant foods? What happens if you eat more protein than your body needs? Before reading Chapter 7, take the following quiz to test your knowledge of protein. The answers are found on page 224.

1. Red meat is the only source of high-quality protein. __T __F

2. Americans typically consume inadequate amounts of protein. __T __F

3. Certain hormones and enzymes are proteins. __T __F

4. Vegetarian diets are often lower in saturated fat and calories than typical "Western" diets. __T __F

5. To maintain good health, individuals with celiac disease should follow a gluten-free diet. __T __F

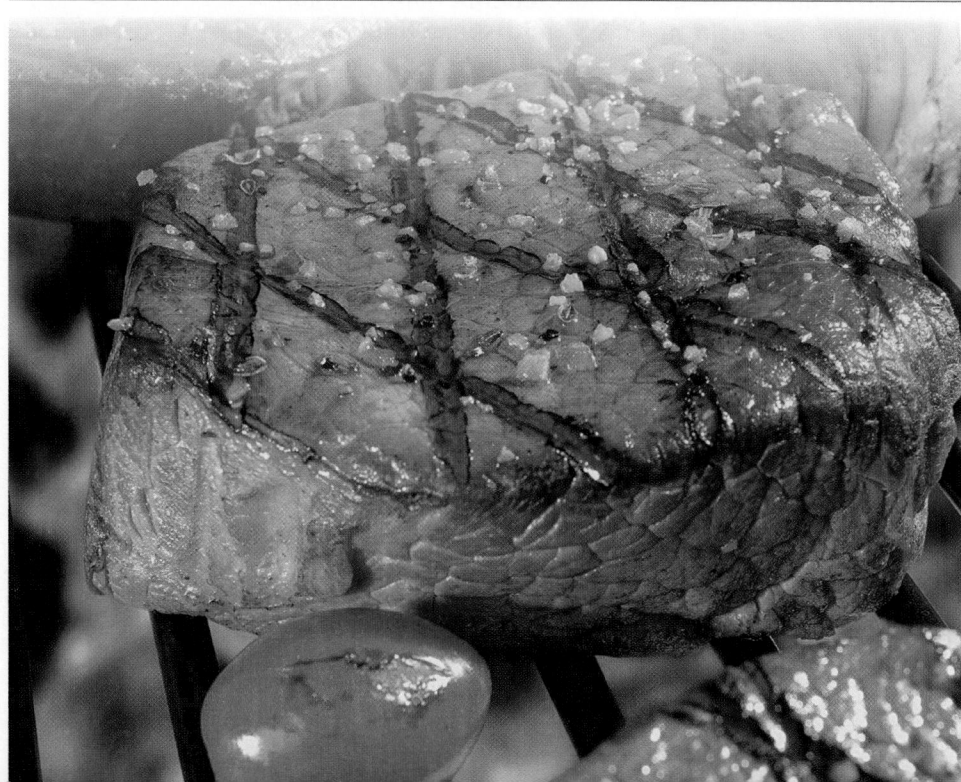

7.1 Introducing Proteins

LEARNING OUTCOMES

1 *Name the elements that are found in all proteins.*

2 *List the primary functions of proteins in the body.*

proteins large, complex organic molecules made up of amino acids

Proteins are complex organic molecules that are chemically similar to lipids and carbohydrates because they contain carbon, hydrogen, and oxygen atoms. Proteins, however, also contain nitrogen, an element cells need to make a wide array of important biological compounds such as enzymes and hormones. Plants, animals, bacteria, and even viruses contain proteins.

By reading this chapter, you will learn about the roles of proteins in the body and major food sources of proteins. You will also learn how proteins influence health, including celiac disease, phenylketonuria, food allergy, weight loss, and heart disease.

Proteins' Major Functions in the Body

Proteins are necessary for muscle development and maintenance, but the estimated 100,000 proteins in the body have a wide variety of functions (Table 7.1). Skin, blood, nerve, bone—all cells in the body—contain proteins. Structural proteins such as *collagen* are in cartilage, ligament, and bone tissues. *Keratin* is another structural protein; it is in hair, nails, and skin. Contractile proteins in muscles enable movement. Proteins in the retina of the eye enable sight, and other proteins in blood are necessary for blood to clot properly.

edema accumulation of fluid in tissues; "swelling"

acid-base balance maintaining the proper pH of body fluids

buffer substance that can protect the pH of a solution

Proteins in blood, such as *albumin*, also help maintain the proper distribution of fluids in blood and body tissues (Fig. 7.1). The force of blood pressure moves watery fluid out of the bloodstream and into tissues. Blood proteins help counteract the effects of blood pressure by attracting the fluid and returning it to the bloodstream. During starvation (a state in which the body lacks food energy and/or protein), the level of protein in blood decreases, and as a result, some water leaks out of the bloodstream and enters spaces between cells. The resulting accumulation of fluid in tissues is called **edema** (*eh–dee'mah*).

Proteins also help maintain **acid–base balance**, the proper pH of body fluids. To function properly, blood and tissue fluids need to maintain a pH of 7.35 to 7.45, which is slightly basic.[1] Metabolic processes can produce acidic or basic by-products. If a particular body fluid becomes too acidic or too basic, cells can have difficulty functioning and may die. A **buffer** can protect the pH of a solution. Proteins can act as buffers, because they have acidic and basic components. For example, if cells form an excess of hydrogen ions (H^+), the pH of tissues decreases (becomes more acidic). To help restore the pH level to within the normal range, the basic portions of protein molecules bind to the excess H^+, neutralizing the excess ions and raising the pH (becoming less acidic). Table 7.1 lists these and other basic functions of proteins in the body.

TABLE 7.1 Major Functions of Proteins in the Body

The Body Uses Proteins:
• To build new cells and many functional components of cells
• As a component of hardened structures, such as hair and nails
• As enzymes to speed chemical reactions
• As lubricants to ease movement
• In clotting compounds in blood
• To build antibodies that fight disease organisms
• As compounds that help maintain fluid and pH balance
• As transporters and to make certain hormones
• As an energy source (a minor function, under usual conditions)

ASSESS YOUR PROGRESS

1 *How are proteins chemically different from carbohydrates or lipids?*

2 *List at least four different functions of proteins in the body.*

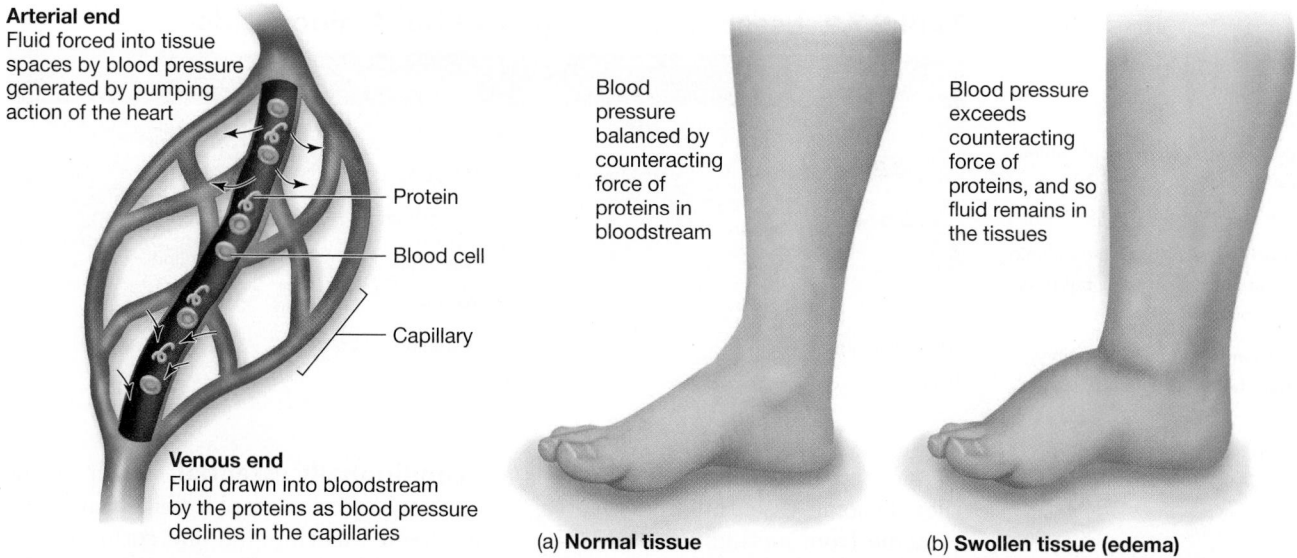

Arterial end
Fluid forced into tissue spaces by blood pressure generated by pumping action of the heart

Protein

Blood cell

Capillary

Venous end
Fluid drawn into bloodstream by the proteins as blood pressure declines in the capillaries

Blood pressure balanced by counteracting force of proteins in bloodstream

Blood pressure exceeds counteracting force of proteins, and so fluid remains in the tissues

(a) **Normal tissue**

(b) **Swollen tissue (edema)**

FIGURE 7.1 Normal fluid balance and edema. (*a*) As a result of the balance between blood pressure and proteins in the bloodstream, the tissues contain normal amounts of fluid. (*b*) When blood pressure is greater than the counteracting force of the proteins in the bloodstream, fluid remains in the tissues, causing edema.

7.2 Amino Acids

LEARNING OUTCOMES

1 *Describe the basic chemical structure of an amino acid.*

2 *Distinguish between essential, conditionally essential, and nonessential amino acids.*

Proteins are comprised of smaller chemical units called **amino acids**. The human body contains proteins made from 20 different amino acids. Each amino acid has a carbon atom that anchors a hydrogen atom and three different groups of atoms: the **amino** or **nitrogen–containing group**, the **R group** (sometimes called the **side chain**), and the **carboxylic acid group**. The chemical structure of the amino acid *alanine* shown in Figure 7.2 indicates these three groups. Note that the nitrogen atom is in the amino group. The R group identifies the molecule as a particular amino acid, such as *ser-ine* or *lysine*. When the nitrogen–containing group is removed, the R group, carboxylic acid group, and anchoring carbon atom form the "carbon skeleton" of an amino acid (Fig. 7.2). Appendix D shows has the chemical structures of amino acids.

Essential Amino Acids

Traditionally, amino acids as either nonessential or essential according to the body's ability to make them. A healthy human body can make 11 of the 20 amino acids. These compounds are the **nonessential amino acids**. The remaining nine amino acids are **essential amino acids** that must be supplied by foods, because the body cannot synthesize them or make enough to meet its needs. Sometimes, nonessential and essential amino acids are referred to as "dispensable" and "indispensable" amino acids, respectively.

amino acids nitrogen-containing chemical units that comprise proteins

amino or **nitrogen-containing group** portion of an amino acid that contains nitrogen

R group (side chain) part of an amino acid that determines the molecule's physical and chemical properties

carboxylic acid group carboxylic acid portion of a compound

nonessential amino acids group of amino acids that the body can make

essential amino acids amino acids the body cannot make or cannot make enough of to meet its needs

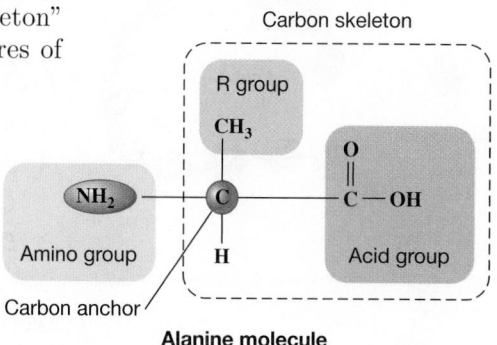

Carbon skeleton

R group

CH_3

NH_2

Amino group

C

Carbon anchor

H

$\overset{O}{\overset{\|}{C}} - OH$

Acid group

Alanine molecule

FIGURE 7.2 Amino acid: Basic chemical structure. Alanine has the typical chemical features of an amino acid.

conditionally essential amino acid amino acids that are normally nonessential but become essential under certain conditions

amino acid derivatives nitrogen-containing compounds that are not proteins but have important physiological roles

amines compounds that include amino groups in their chemical structure

TABLE 7.2 Essential and Nonessential Amino Acids

Essential		Nonessential	
Histidine	Threonine	Alanine	Cysteine*
Isoleucine	Tryptophan	Aspartic acid	Glutamine*
Leucine	Valine	Asparagine	Glycine*
Lysine		Glutamic acid	Proline*
Methionine		Serine	Tyrosine*
Phenylalanine		Arginine*	

*Under certain conditions, this amino acid can become essential.

Several nonessential amino acids are **conditionally essential**, which means they become essential under certain conditions. For example, cells can make cysteine from methionine and serine. If a person's methionine and serine intake is inadequate, however, his or her body cannot make enough cysteine to meet its needs, and dietary sources of the amino acid are necessary. Table 7.2 lists amino acids according to their classification as essential and nonessential, and identifies nonessential amino acids that can be conditionally essential.

Derivatives of Amino Acids

The body uses amino acids to form nitrogen—containing compounds that are not proteins but have important physiological roles. Examples of such **amino acid derivatives** include creatine; melanin; and *regulatory amines* such as serotonin, epinephrine, and histamine. **Amines** are compounds that include amino groups in their chemical structures. For example, epinephrine is made from the amino acid tyrosine, and serotonin is made from the amino acid tryptophan (Fig. 7.3). Thus, tryptophan and tyrosine are *precursors* for these amines.

(a) Tryptophan ⟹ Serotonin

(b) Tyrosine ⟹ Epinephrine

FIGURE 7.3 Amino acids as precursors. The amino acid tryptophan is a precursor for (*a*) serotonin, whereas the amino acid tyrosine is a precursor for (*b*) epinephrine.

ASSESS YOUR PROGRESS

③ *List the major components of an amino acid.*

④ *Explain the difference between essential, conditionally essential, and nonessential amino acids.*

⑤ *List the essential amino acids.*

7.3 Protein Synthesis and Structure

LEARNING OUTCOMES

1 *Explain the basic steps of protein synthesis.*

2 *Compare the primary, secondary, tertiary, and quaternary structures of a protein.*

3 *Describe protein denaturation, and identify factors that cause proteins to denature.*

Every organism synthesizes proteins that are unique to that specific organism. To help visualize the process of protein synthesis, imagine proteins as various chains made from 20 different amino acid "beads." Figure 7.4 illustrates this analogy. Note that each bead is connected to another bead to form a chain. To make a copy of a particular beaded chain, you would follow directions for connecting the beads in a specific order and length by stringing each bead together. In living things, the

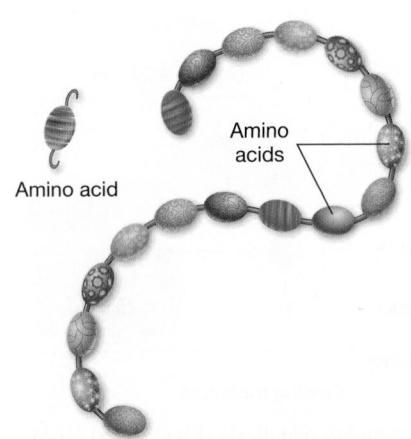

Amino acids

Amino acid

FIGURE 7.4 Amino acids form proteins. Each type of bead represents a specific amino acid in human proteins.

beaded chains are proteins that contain numerous amino acids ("beads"). Consider the vast variety of beaded chains comprised of different bead sequences and chain lengths that you could make from just 20 different beads.

The human body makes proteins by following information coded in **DNA**, or **deoxyribonucleic** $(de-ox'-e-rye'-bow-new-klay'-ik)$ **acid**, the hereditary material in a cell's nucleus that are in **genes**. To make proteins, cells assemble the 20 amino acids in specific sequences according to the information pro-vided by DNA. The connection between two amino acids is a **peptide bond**, a chemical link between the acid group of one amino acid and the amino group of another amino acid (Fig. 7.5). A dipeptide forms when two amino acids bond, and a molecule of water is released in the process. **Peptides** contain two or more amino acids. Most naturally occurring proteins are **polypeptides** $(poly =$ many; $peptides =$ amino acids) comprised of 50 or more amino acids. Figure 7.6 sum-marizes the basic steps of protein synthesis.

Diets that do not supply adequate amounts of essential amino acids can result in poor growth, slowed recovery from illness, and even death. These situations occur because protein synthesis in cells cannot proceed when the supply ("pool") of amino acids is lacking in one or more of the essential amino acids. When an amino acid is not available, production of a protein stops. The partially made polypeptide chain is dismantled, and its amino acids are returned to the pool.

Protein Structure

When assembly of the new protein has been completed, the polypeptide acid chain coils and folds into a three-dimensional shape that is characteristic of that particular protein. The structure of a protein can be specified at the primary, secondary, tertiary, and quaternary level.

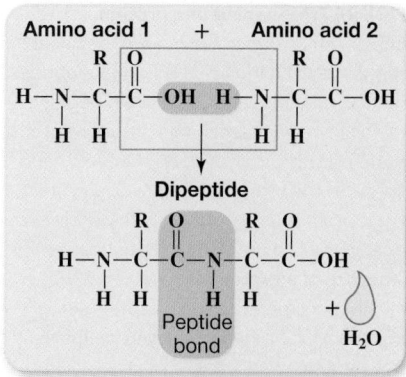

FIGURE 7.5 Peptide bond. A peptide bond is a chemical attraction between the acid group of one amino acid and the amino group of another amino acid. A dipeptide forms through a condensation reaction.

DNA (deoxyribonucleic acid) hereditary material that provides instructions for making proteins

gene portion of DNA

peptide bond chemical attraction that connects two amino acids together

FIGURE 7.6 Protein synthesis.

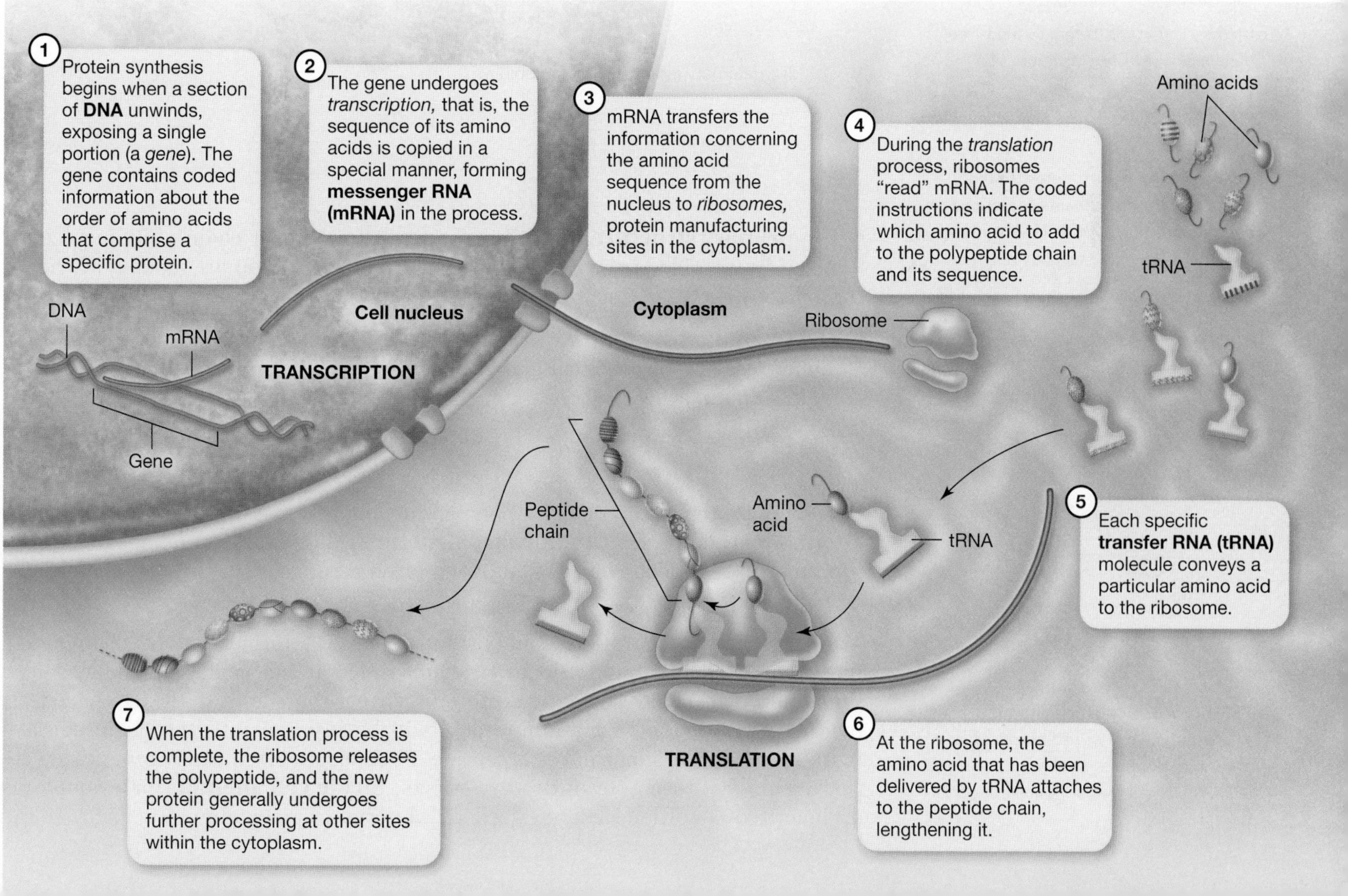

① Protein synthesis begins when a section of **DNA** unwinds, exposing a single portion (a *gene*). The gene contains coded information about the order of amino acids that comprise a specific protein.

② The gene undergoes *transcription,* that is, the sequence of its amino acids is copied in a special manner, forming **messenger RNA (mRNA)** in the process.

③ mRNA transfers the information concerning the amino acid sequence from the nucleus to *ribosomes,* protein manufacturing sites in the cytoplasm.

④ During the *translation* process, ribosomes "read" mRNA. The coded instructions indicate which amino acid to add to the polypeptide chain and its sequence.

⑤ Each specific **transfer RNA (tRNA)** molecule conveys a particular amino acid to the ribosome.

⑥ At the ribosome, the amino acid that has been delivered by tRNA attaches to the peptide chain, lengthening it.

⑦ When the translation process is complete, the ribosome releases the polypeptide, and the new protein generally undergoes further processing at other sites within the cytoplasm.

DNA
mRNA
Cell nucleus
TRANSCRIPTION
Gene
Cytoplasm
Ribosome
Amino acids
tRNA
Peptide chain
Amino acid
tRNA
TRANSLATION

FIGURE 7.7 Shaping of a protein. (*a*) The primary structure of a protein is the linear sequence of amino acids linked by peptide bonds. (*b*) The polypeptide chain begins to coil, forming a secondary structure of a protein. (*c*) The polypeptide then folds and coils into the tertiary structure of a protein. Most proteins in foods and in the body exist in the tertiary form. (*d*) The quaternary structure of a protein is characterized by multiple polypeptide chains aggregating. For example, hemoglobin contains four polypeptide chains, each chain associated with an iron-containing unit.

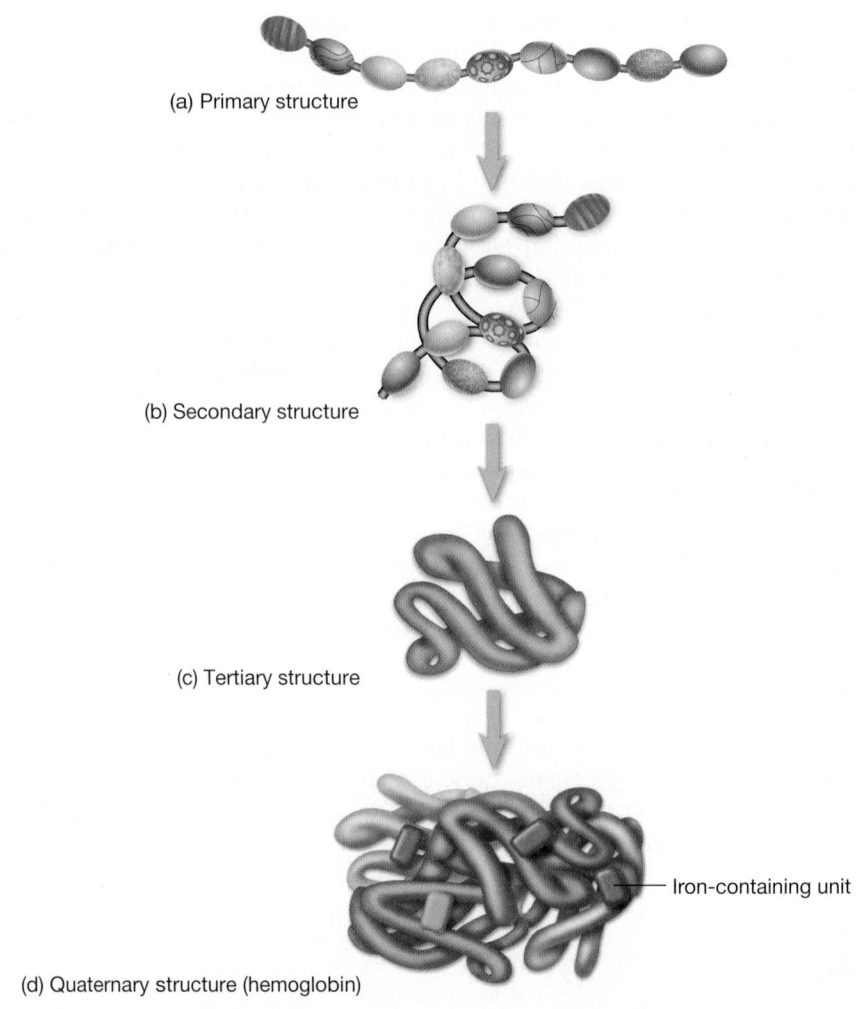

(a) Primary structure

(b) Secondary structure

(c) Tertiary structure

(d) Quaternary structure (hemoglobin)

Iron-containing unit

peptides small chains of amino acids

polypeptides proteins comprised of 50 or more amino acids

primary structure refers to the basic structure of protein; a linear chain of amino acids linked by peptide bonds

secondary structure refers to the coiling of a polypeptide chain

tertiary structure refers to the three-dimensional, twisted structure of a polypeptide chain that includes interactions between various amino acid groups on the chain

quaternary structure refers to the structure of protein that is comprised of two or more polypeptide chains arranged together in a unique manner

sickle cell anemia inherited form of anemia

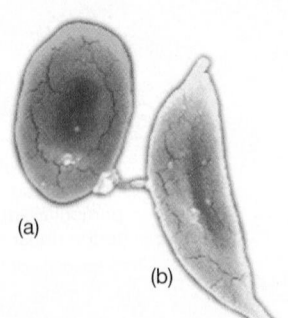

(a)

(b)

FIGURE 7.8 Sickle cell anemia. This microscopic view of red blood cells shows (*a*) normal disk-shaped cells and (*b*) a sickle cell that contains abnormal hemoglobin.

- The **primary structure** of a protein refers to the linear chain of amino acids linked by peptide bonds. As you look at Figure 7.7a, you are looking at the primary structure of that short protein.

- The **secondary structure** of the protein reflects the polypeptide chain's coiling, because of chemical attractions between certain components of the chain's amino acids (Fig. 7.7b).

- The **tertiary structure** refers to the protein's final three—dimensional form (Fig. 7.7c).

- In some proteins, two or more polypeptide chains associate with each other to form large complexes **(quaternary structure)**. For example, *hemoglobin*, a protein in red blood cells, is comprised of an arrangement of four polypeptide chains (Fig. 7.7d).

The shape of a protein is important because it influences the compound's function in the body. Occasionally, an incorrect amino acid is introduced into the amino acid chain during the protein synthesis process. If the DNA code is faulty, however, the wrong amino acid will be inserted into the chain consis—tently, forming an abnormal polypeptide. Such errors often cause genetic defects that have devastating, even deadly, effects. **Sickle cell anemia**, for example, is an inherited condition characterized by abnormal hemoglobin (Fig. 7.8). If the hemoglobin—producing DNA codes for the insertion of a particular wrong amino acid in two of hemoglobin's four polypeptide chains, the resulting protein is defective and does not function correctly. Sickle cell anemia is a common genetic disorder that generally affects people with African, Caribbean, or Mediterranean ancestry. There is no cure for sickle cell anemia.

denaturation altering a protein's natural shape and function by exposing it to conditions such as heat, acids, and physical agitation

Protein Denaturation

A protein undergoes **denaturation** when it is exposed to various conditions that alter its natural folded and coiled shape (Fig. 7.9). Protein—rich foods are often cooked to make them more digestible and safe to eat, but heat also causes the proteins in foods to unfold. The protein in raw egg white, for example, is almost clear and has a jellylike consistency. When the egg white is cooked, it becomes white and firm as its proteins become denatured.

Other treatments often used during food preparation also denature proteins, including whipping or exposing them to alcohol or acid. Wine, for example, is often used in marinades, because the alcohol it contains denatures proteins in meat, helping tenderize it. Adding acidic lemon juice to milk denatures ("cur—dles") the proteins in milk. In your stomach, hydrochloric acid denatures food proteins, making them easier to digest. Denaturation does not "kill" a protein (because proteins are not living), but the process usually permanently alters the protein's shape and functions. Once an egg white has been cooked or milk has curdled, the food cannot return to its original state.

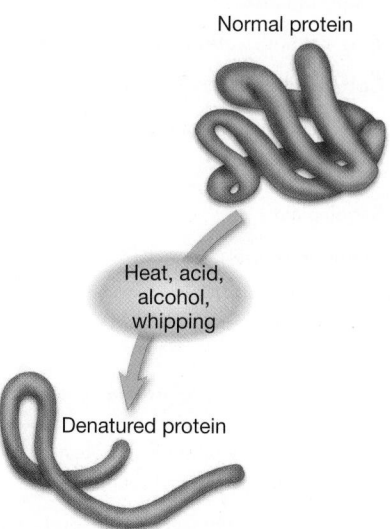

FIGURE 7.9 Denaturation. A protein undergoes denaturation when exposed to various conditions that alter its natural folded shape.

ASSESS YOUR PROGRESS

6 *What is a gene?*

7 *Identify the type of bond that links amino acids in a protein.*

8 *Explain the basic steps involved in protein synthesis.*

9 *Describe the four levels of protein structure from simplest to most complex.*

10 *Explain why an egg white changes its appearance when it is cooked.*

7.4 Proteins in Foods

LEARNING OUTCOMES

1 *Identify foods that are good sources of high-quality proteins and foods that are sources of low-quality proteins.*

2 *Discuss dietary protein recommendations.*

People often associate protein with animal foods, but beans, nuts, seeds, grains, and certain vegetables are good sources of protein, too. Although nearly all foods contain protein, no naturally occurring food is 100% protein. Protein comprises only about 20 to 30% of the weight of a piece of beef; 25% of the weight of drained, water—packed tuna fish; and only 12% of an egg's weight. Animal foods gen—erally provide higher amounts of protein than similar quantities of plant foods. A 3—ounce serving of broiled lean ground beef supplies 23 g of protein; a 3—ounce serving of steamed broccoli or cooked carrots provides only about 1 g of protein. In general, most plant foods provide less than 3 g of protein per ounce. Table 7.3 lists some commonly eaten foods and their approximate protein content per serving.

Certain parts of plants contain more protein than other parts. Seeds, tree nuts, and legumes supply more protein per serving than servings of fruit or the edible leaves, roots, flowers, and stems of vegetables. Tree nuts include walnuts, cashews, and almonds; **legumes** are plants that produce pods that have a single row of

DID **YOU** KNOW?

The sleepiness that often follows a turkey dinner can be, at least in part, attributed to the presence of the essential amino acid tryptophan. Tryptophan is a precursor for serotonin, a regulatory amine that enhances mood and promotes relaxation.[2] However, turkey is not the only food source of tryptophan; other types of poultry, including chicken, are also rich in the essential amino acid.

legumes plants that produce pods with a single row of seeds

TABLE 7.3 Approximate Protein Content of Some Commonly Eaten Foods per Serving

Food	Serving Size	Protein g/Serving	Food	Serving Size	Protein g/Serving
Chicken, breast, roasted, meat only	4 oz	34	Milk, fat-free	1 cup	8
Ham, lean, cooked	4 oz	33	Peanut butter, smooth	2 Tbsp	8
Hamburger, 80% lean, broiled	4 oz	29	Baked beans, vegetarian	½ cup	6
Pepperoni pizza, regular crust, 14" pie	2 slices (200 g)	24	Egg, large, hard cooked	1	6
Tuna, canned, water-packed, drained	4 oz	22	American processed cheese	1 oz	5
Cottage cheese, 2% low-fat	4 oz	13	Vanilla ice cream	1 cup	4
Lasagna with meat sauce	6 oz	12	White rice, cooked	1 cup	4
Tofu, regular	½ cup	10	Peas, green, cooked	½ cup	4
Bagel, plain	1 (3 ½" diam.)	10	Banana, medium	1	1
Almonds, whole	¼ cup	8			

Source: *USDA national nutrient database for standard reference, release 25 2012.*

high-quality (complete) protein protein that contains all essential amino acids in amounts that support the deposition of protein in tissues and the growth of a young person

low-quality (incomplete) protein protein that lacks or has inadequate amounts of one or more of the essential amino acids

limiting amino acid essential amino acid found in the lowest concentration in a protein source

seeds, such as peas, peanuts, lentils, and the many varieties of beans, including soybeans (Fig. 7.10). A 3—ounce serving of almonds, dry—roasted peanuts, or sun—flower seed kernels supplies about 20 g of protein. Many seeds and nuts, however, pack a lot of calories from fat. Snack on just 3 ounces of almonds, dry—roasted peanuts, or sunflower seed kernels, and you will add almost 500 kcal to your diet!

FRESH TIPS

Commercially canned beans often have considerable amounts of salt added to them. Consider rinsing the beans in water to remove the salt, or purchasing canned or frozen beans that have little or no added salt. Dried beans do not have salt added to them, but they take a long time to cook, unless you soak them for several hours before cooking. The soaking process softens the beans, reducing their cooking time, and making them more digestible and less likely to contribute to intestinal gas.

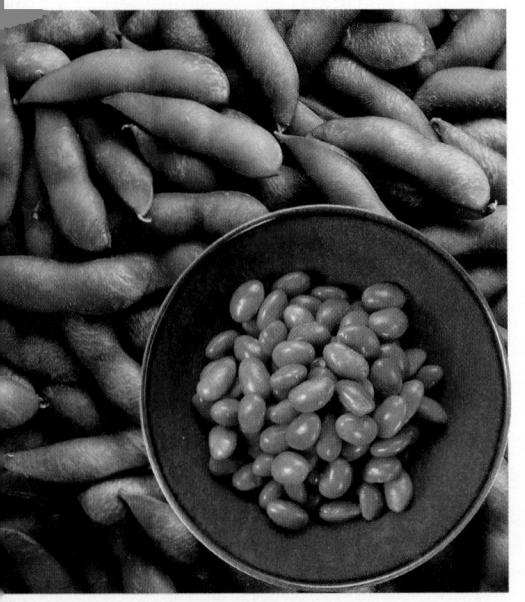

FIGURE 7.10 Legumes. Legumes, such as soybeans, are plants that produce pods that have a single row of seeds.

Protein Quality

Foods differ not only in the amount of protein they contain but also in their pro—tein quality. A **high—quality** or **complete protein** contains all essential amino acids in amounts that support protein deposition in muscles and other tissues, as well as supporting the growth of a young child.[3] High—quality proteins are well digested and absorbed by the body. Meat, fish, poultry, eggs, and milk and milk products contain high—quality proteins. Egg protein generally rates very high for protein quality, because it is easy to digest and has a pattern of essential amino acids that closely resembles that needed by humans.

A **low—quality** or **incomplete protein** lacks or contains inadequate amounts of one or more of the essential amino acids. Furthermore, the human digestive tract does not digest low—quality protein sources as efficiently as foods con—taining high—quality protein. The essential amino acids that are in relatively low amounts are referred to as **limiting amino acids**, because they reduce the protein's ability to support growth, repair, and maintenance of tissues. In most instances, tryptophan, threonine, lysine, and the sulfur—containing amino acids methionine and cysteine are the limiting amino acids in foods.[4]

Most plant foods are not sources of high–quality proteins. Quinoa (*keen'–wa*) and soy protein are exceptions. Quinoa is botanically related to sugar beets and spinach, but the quality and amount of protein in quinoa seeds are superior to those of many cereal grains.[5] Cooked quinoa is often used as a cereal. After being processed, the quality of soy protein is comparable to that of most animal proteins.[6] Processed soybeans are used to make a variety of nutritious foods, including soy milk, infant formula, and meat substitutes. Furthermore, eating foods made from soybeans may reduce the risk of osteo–porosis, cardiovascular disease, and certain cancers.[7] More research, however, is needed to determine the long–term health benefits of eating diets that contain soy products.

Understanding the concept of protein quality is important. Regardless of how much protein is eaten, a child will fail to grow properly if his or her diet lacks essential amino acids. Section 7.11, "Vegetarianism," explains how people can obtain these and other essential nutrients by eating only plant foods.

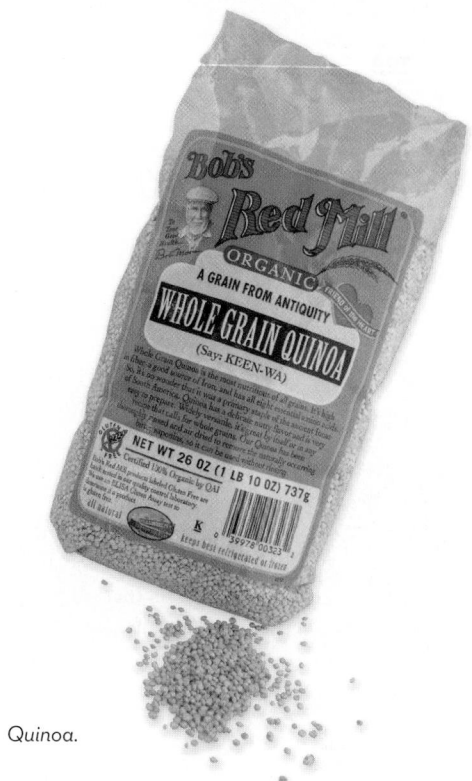

Quinoa.

Measuring Protein Quality

The digestibility and amino acid composition of a protein are the two key factors in determining the quality of that protein. To measure protein quality, these two factors are compared against a **reference protein**, most often egg white protein (*albumin*). There are several tools used to measure protein quality.

- **Biological value (BV)** is a measure of protein quality based on how well and how quickly the body converts food protein into body tissue proteins. Amounts of limiting amino acids in a food determine whether the item has a high or low BV. To calculate BV, food scientists divide grams of nitrogen absorbed by grams of nitrogen retained. The food source with the highest BV, 100%, is egg white protein. Most animal sources of protein, including milk, cheese, and meat, have a high BV, most often between 90 and 100%. In com–parison, the BV of plant sources of protein are highly variable. For example, the BV of whole soybeans is 96%, rice is 83%, tofu is 64%, whole–wheat flour is 64%, and white flour is 41%.

- **Protein digestibility corrected amino acid score (PDCAAS)** is the most commonly used tool used to measure protein quality. Like BV, PDCAAS also takes into consideration the essential amino acid composition of the protein, as well as how well the protein is digested and absorbed. The *amino acid composition score* is a measure of the amount of each essential amino acid in a gram of the food protein divided by the "ideal" amount of each essential amino acid in a reference protein (usually egg white protein). A protein lacking one of the essential amino acids will have an amino acid composition score of 0. The PDCAAS is calculated by multiplying the amino acid composition score of the protein by the protein's digestibility score. Most animal proteins, as well as soy protein, have a PDCAAS of 1.0.

- **Protein efficiency ratio (PER)** is a third measure of protein quality. PER is determined by measuring the weight gain of a growing laboratory animal that consumes a known amount of a specific type of protein. The weight gain of the animal is then compared against weight gain following consumption of a reference protein, most often a milk protein **(casein)**.

Protein: RDA

A healthy adult's RDA for protein is 0.8 g/kg of body weight.[4] Protein needs increase during pregnancy, breastfeeding, periods of rapid growth, and recovery from serious illnesses, blood losses, and burns. The DRI tables at the end of this textbook shows the RDAs for proteins during different stages of the life cycle, including pregnancy and lactation.

reference protein a high-quality protein against which quality of other proteins is measured

biological value (BV) measure of protein quality based on how well and quickly the body converts food protein into body tissue protein

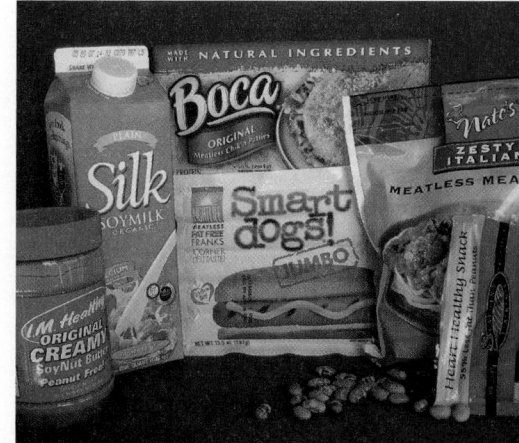

Soy products.

protein digestibility corrected amino acid score (PDCAAS) measure of protein quality based on amino acid composition score and digestibility of a protein food

protein efficiency ratio (PER) measure of protein quality based on the ability of a protein to support weight gain in a laboratory animal

casein high-quality protein found in milk

To determine a person's RDA for protein, multiply his or her weight in kilograms by 0.8 g. If the individual is underweight or overweight, use a healthy weight for the person's height when making this calculation (see the BMI chart in Chapter 13). For example, a healthy man who is 5–feet, 10–inches tall and weighs 75 kg (his weight in pounds divided by 2.2) should consume 60 grams of protein daily (75 kg × 0.8 g) to meet his RDA for the nutrient. The "Personal Dietary Analysis" at the end of this chapter can help you estimate your daily protein intake.

ASSESS YOUR PROGRESS

11 *Explain the difference between a high-quality protein and a low-quality protein.*

12 *Identify at least three dietary sources of high-quality protein and three dietary sources of low-quality protein.*

13 *List three ways to measure protein quality.*

14 *A healthy young woman weighs 136 pounds. Calculate her RDA for protein.*

7.5 Protein Digestion, Absorption, and Transport

LEARNING OUTCOMES

1 *Discuss protein digestion, including enzymes involved in the process.*

2 *Describe how proteins are absorbed by the digestive tract, and identify where they are transported after being absorbed.*

Protein Digestion

Protein digestion begins in the stomach. Hydrochloric acid (HCl) denatures food proteins and activates pepsin from the inactive form of the enzyme, pepsino–gen. Pepsin initiates enzymatic digestion of proteins into smaller polypeptides. Soon after the polypeptides enter the small intestine, the pancreas secretes protein–splitting enzymes, including **trypsin** ($trip'-sin$) and **chymotrypsin** ($ki'-mo-trip'-sin$). Trypsin and chymotrypsin break down polypeptides into shorter peptides and amino acids. Enzymes released by the absorptive cells of the small intestine break down most of the shortened peptides into dipep–tides, tripeptides, and individual amino acids. **Dipeptides** and **tripeptides** are compounds that consist of two and three amino acids, respectively. When the dipeptides and tripeptides contact the microvilli ("the brush border") of villi, enzymes within the microvilli can break down di– and tripeptides into amino acids. Thus, amino acids are the end products of protein digestion.

trypsin protein-splitting enzyme secreted from the pancreas

chymotrypsin protein-splitting enzyme secreted from the pancreas

dipeptides compounds that consist of two amino acids

tripeptides compounds that consist of three amino acids

Protein Absorption and Transport

Following digestion of proteins to amino acids, the amino acids are transported by specific carrier systems into the absorptive cells. After entering the absorptive cell, the amino acids move into the capillary of the villus. Healthy children and adults will have minimal, if any, undigested protein entering the large intestine and being excreted in feces. After being absorbed, the amino acids travel to the liver via the hepatic portal vein. The liver keeps some amino acids for its needs and releases the rest into the general circulation. Figure 7.11 summarizes protein digestion and absorption.

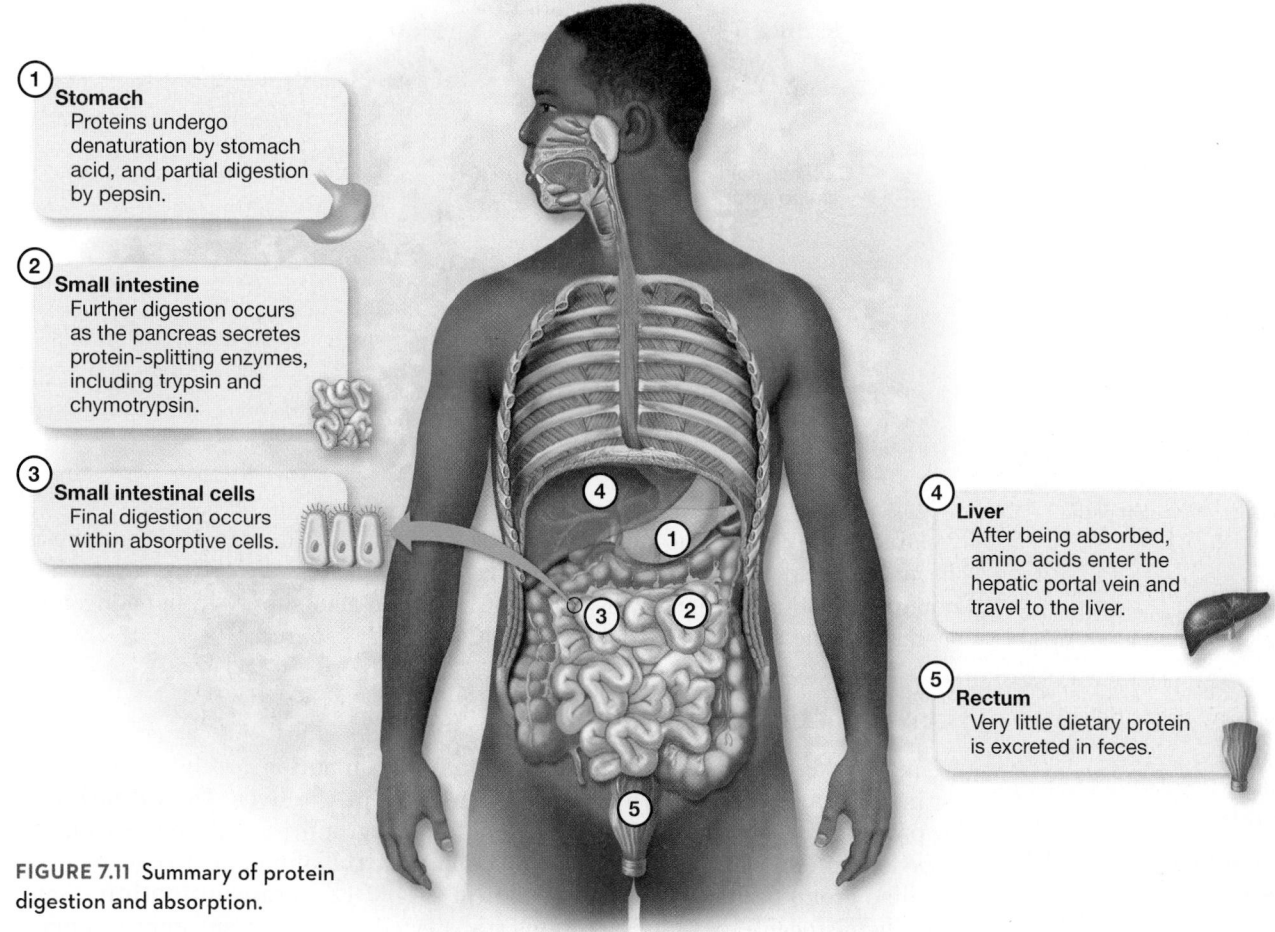

1 Stomach
Proteins undergo denaturation by stomach acid, and partial digestion by pepsin.

2 Small intestine
Further digestion occurs as the pancreas secretes protein-splitting enzymes, including trypsin and chymotrypsin.

3 Small intestinal cells
Final digestion occurs within absorptive cells.

4 Liver
After being absorbed, amino acids enter the hepatic portal vein and travel to the liver.

5 Rectum
Very little dietary protein is excreted in feces.

FIGURE 7.11 Summary of protein digestion and absorption.

ASSESS YOUR PROGRESS

15 *Name two pancreatic enzymes that break down protein in the small intestine.*

16 *Where does the final breakdown step from dipeptides and tripeptides to amino acids take place?*

17 *Describe what happens to the protein in beans after you eat a bowl of chili.*

7.6 Protein Metabolism

LEARNING OUTCOMES

1 *Explain what happens during transamination and deamination.*

2 *Describe common causes of abnormal blood urea nitrogen and urine urea nitrogen levels.*

3 *Discuss nitrogen balance.*

While some amino acids must be consumed in the diet, not all amino acids have to be supplied through dietary sources. **Protein turnover**, the process of breaking down old or unneeded proteins into their component amino acids and recycling them to make new proteins, occurs constantly within cells. Amino acids that are not incorporated into proteins become part of a small amino acid pool, a readily

protein turnover cellular process of breaking down proteins and recycling their amino acids

FIGURE 7.12 Deamination and transamination. In this example, glutamic acid loses its amino group and becomes a carbon skeleton (deamination). Pyruvic acid receives the amino group from glutamic acid, forming alanine, a nonessential amino acid (transamination).

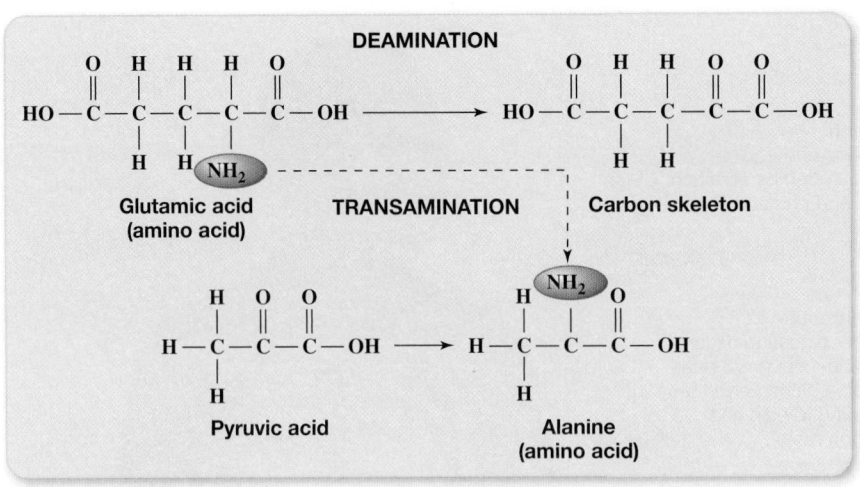

endogenous source of nitrogen from within the body

exogenous source of nitrogen from outside of the body (dietary protein)

deamination removal of the nitrogen-containing group from an amino acid

carbon skeleton remains of an amino acid following deamination and removal of the nitrogen-containing component of the amino acid

transamination transfer of the nitrogen-containing group from an unneeded amino acid to a carbon skeleton to form an amino acid

urea waste product of amino acid metabolism

creatinine nitrogen-containing waste produced by muscles

blood urea nitrogen (BUN) measure of the concentration of urea in blood

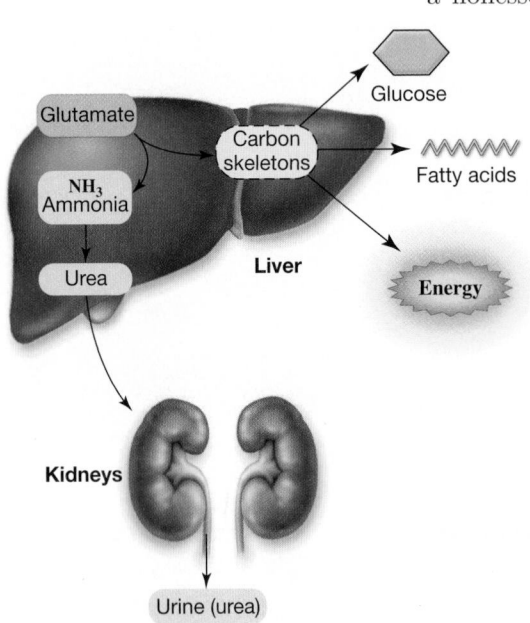

FIGURE 7.13 Urea. The process of deamination results in the production of the highly toxic compound ammonia. In an energy-requiring process, the liver converts ammonia to urea and releases it into the blood. The kidneys pick up urea and other nitrogen-containing wastes and eliminate them in urine.

available supply of amino acids that cells can use for future protein synthesis. The amino acid pool is an **endogenous**, or internal, source of nitrogen. The human body obtains about two–thirds of its amino acid supply from endogenous sources and the remainder from **exogenous** (dietary) sources.

Transamination and Deamination

Chemical reactions called deamination and transamination are involved in the synthesis of amino acids, which occurs primarily in the liver. **Deamination** is the process of removing the nitrogen–containing group (usually NH_2) from an unneeded amino acid. As a result of deamination, the amino acid that gives up its amino group becomes a **carbon skeleton** (Fig. 7.12). **Transamination** occurs when the nitrogen–containing group is transferred to another substance to make a nonessential amino acid. To make the amino acid alanine, for example, liver cells remove the amino group (NH_2) from glutamic acid gluta–mate and transfer it to pyruvic acid (Fig. 7.12). Transamination reactions are reversible.

If a person consumes more protein than he or she needs, what happens to the extra amino acids? The body does not store excess amino acids in muscle or other tissues. The unnecessary amino acids undergo deamination, and some of the excess NH_2 is transported to the liver in glutamate (a form of glutamic acid). Liver cells remove NH_2 from the amine component of glutamate, forming *ammonia* (NH_3), a highly poisonous waste product (Fig. 7.13). The liver can use the ammonia to make **urea**, a metabolic waste product that is released into the bloodstream. The kidneys filter urea, small amounts of ammonia, and **creatinine** (a nitrogen–containing waste produced by muscles) from blood and eliminate the compounds in urine. After an amino acid undergoes deamination, the carbon skeleton that remains can be used for energy or converted to other compounds, such as glucose. Muscle cells can deaminate certain amino acids and use their carbon skeletons for energy (Fig. 7.13).

Blood Urea Nitrogen and Urine Urea Nitrogen

Urea levels in both blood and urine are used as markers of dietary protein intake and chronic disease. **Blood urea nitrogen (BUN)** is a blood test often used to assess kidney function. Normal val–ues for BUN are between 7 and 20 mg/dL. An elevated BUN level occurs when the kidneys are diseased and unable to filter

TABLE 7.4 Blood Urea Nitrogen (BUN)

High BUN (>20 mg/dL) May Indicate:	Low BUN (<7 mg/dL) May Indicate:
Congestive heart failure	Liver failure
Excessive protein intake (generally considered greater than 100 g/day)	Inadequate protein intake
GI bleeding	Malnutrition
Heart attack	Overhydration (too much water in the bloodstream)
Kidney disease, kidney failure, urinary tract obstruction	
Shock	

Source: National Institutes of Health: *Blood urea nitrogen.* http://www.nlm.nih.gov/medlineplus/ency/article/003474.htm Accessed: January 19, 2014.

urea from the blood properly. In such cases, urea accumulates in the blood and causes toxicity. As kidney disease progresses, the amount of urea filtered through the kidneys continues to diminish. Thus, BUN levels continue to increase if the condition is untreated. A person with elevated BUN due to kidney disease is often advised to eat less protein so that his or her kidneys have less work to do. A registered dietitian can counsel patients who have high BUN levels to ensure they are consuming enough protein but not too much.

Kidney disease is not the only cause of elevated BUN levels; heart disease, bleeding in the GI tract, and urinary tract obstructions can contribute to high BUN. Table 7.4 identifies common causes of both high and low BUN levels.

Urine urea nitrogen (UUN) is also evaluated as part of certain patients' health care screening. UUN can be used as a marker of protein intake. The more protein a person consumes, the more amino acids need to undergo deamination, and therefore, urea synthesis will increase. Normal values for UUN measured from a 24-hour urine sample are between 12 and 20 g.

In addition to signaling excessive protein intake, an elevated UUN may indicate excessive breakdown of protein in the body. Thus, low UUN levels are commonly used as an indicator of low protein intake and malnutrition. Table 7.5 identifies factors that often contribute to high and low UUN levels.

Nitrogen Balance

Although the body conserves nitrogen by recycling amino acids, each day some protein and nitrogen are lost. Urinary elimination of urea and creatinine accounts for most of the lost nitrogen.[9] Daily nitrogen losses also occur as nails and hair grow and when the outermost layer of the skin and cells from the intestinal tract are shed. The body uses amino acids from foods to replace the lost nitrogen.

Normally, an adult's body maintains its protein content by maintaining **nitrogen balance** or **nitrogen equilibrium**, that is, balancing nitrogen intake and protein turnover with losses. During certain stages of life or physical conditions, however, nitrogen intake and retention do not equal nitrogen losses.

When the body is in a state of **positive nitrogen balance**, it retains more nitrogen than it loses as proteins are being added to tissues. Positive balance occurs during periods of rapid growth such as pregnancy, infancy, and puberty, and when people are recovering from illness or injury. Hormones such as insulin, growth hormone, and testosterone stimulate positive nitrogen balance. Performing weight (resistance) training also leads to nitrogen retention.[10,11]

When the body is in a state of **negative nitrogen balance**, it loses more nitrogen than it retains. Negative balance occurs during starvation, serious illnesses, and severe injuries. Recovery from the illness or injury involves replacing the protein that was lost (refeeding). Refeeding results in positive nitrogen

TABLE 7.5 Urine Urea Nitrogen (UUN)

High UUN (>20 g) May Indicate:	Low UUN (<12 g) May Indicate:
Excessive intake of protein	Inadequate protein intake, malnutrition
Increased breakdown of protein in the body	Kidney problem

Source: National Institutes of Health: *Urine urea nitrogen.* http://www.nlm.nih.gov/medlineplus/ency/article/003605.htm Accessed: January 19, 2014.

DID YOU KNOW?

Health care practitioners can obtain clues about a patient's health by determining the pH of the person's urine. Results of a study of over 1000 males indicated that low urine pH was associated with an increase in waist circumference, fasting blood glucose, and blood triglycerides.[8] Acidic urine is more common with high-protein diets due to excess urea elimination.

urine urea nitrogen (UUN) measure of the concentration of urea in urine

nitrogen balance (equilibrium) balancing nitrogen intake with nitrogen losses

positive nitrogen balance state in which the body retains more nitrogen than it loses

negative nitrogen balance state in which the body loses more nitrogen than it retains

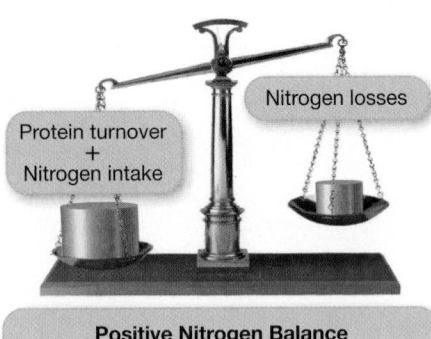
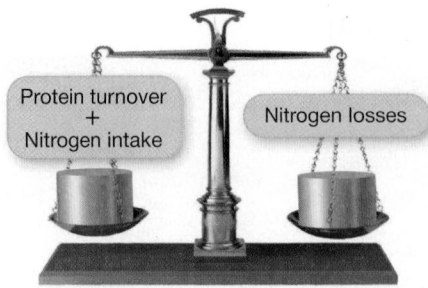
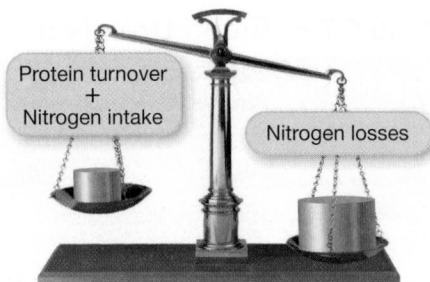

Positive Nitrogen Balance

- Growth
- Pregnancy
- Recovery from illness/injury
- Increased levels of the hormones insulin, testosterone, and growth hormone
- Resistance exercise

Nitrogen Equilibrium

- Healthy adult meets protein and energy needs

Negative Nitrogen Balance

- Inadequate protein intake or digestive tract diseases that interfere with protein absorption
- Increased protein losses resulting from certain kidney diseases or blood loss
- Bed rest, fever, injuries, or burns
- Increased secretion of thyroid hormone or cortisol (a "stress hormone")

FIGURE 7.14 Nitrogen balance. This diagram illustrates the concept of nitrogen balance and lists conditions that result in positive and negative nitrogen balance.

balance until nitrogen equilibrium is restored. Figure 7.14 illustrates the concept of nitrogen balance and lists conditions that result in positive and negative nitrogen balances.

ASSESS YOUR PROGRESS

18 Compare transamination and deamination.

19 Identify two causes each for high BUN and low BUN.

20 Describe two causes each for high UUN and low UUN.

21 Explain conditions that can cause the body to be in positive nitrogen balance and in negative nitrogen balance.

7.7 Meeting Protein Needs

LEARNING OUTCOMES

1 Identify the Acceptable Macronutrient Distribution Range (AMDR) for protein intake in healthy adults.

2 Describe how complementary protein combinations are used in diet planning.

In 2009–2010, protein comprised about 15% of the typical adult American's total energy intake for a day.[12] For healthy adults, this level of consumption is within the Acceptable Macronutrient Distribution Range (AMDR), which is 10 to 35% of energy from protein.[4] A young woman who consumes 15% of her calories from protein on a 2000–kcal diet is eating approximately 75 grams of protein per day, which is the approximate amount of protein in a 10–ounce steak. Animal foods, such as beef, supply almost two–thirds of the protein in the American diet. The following sections discuss ways of reducing consumption of red meat and other animal sources of protein without sacrificing the protein quality of diets.

Combining Complementary Proteins

Although research findings indicate that it is not necessary to consume all essen– tial amino acids during each meal for the body to utilize them for growth, certain plant—based recipes ensure that these compounds are consumed at one time. **Complementary combinations** are mixtures of certain plant foods that provide all essential amino acids without adding animal proteins. To make dishes that contain complementary amino acid combinations, consumers must know (1) which plant foods are good protein sources and (2) which essential amino acids are limiting or low in those plant foods.

Most plant foods are poor sources of one or more essential amino acids, particularly tryptophan, threonine, lysine, and methionine. Green peas, for example, are good sources of lysine, but they contain low amounts of tryptophan and methionine. Cereal grains such as wheat, rice, and corn are good sources of tryptophan and methionine, but they tend to be low in lysine. Wheat germ, however, is a rich source of lysine. Legumes are low in methionine. Seeds such as sesame seeds and sunflower seeds are generally low in lysine. Walnuts, cashews, almonds, and other tree nuts also contain low amounts of lysine. Although most fruits and some kinds of vegetables are poor sources of protein, they add appealing colors and textures as well as vitamins, minerals, and phytochemicals to plant—based meals.

In many cultures, traditional foods already combine complementary proteins. Rice and beans, as one example, contain complementary proteins, as do rice and tofu, a soy product. A peanut butter sandwich also combines two foods that supply complementary plant proteins. Peanuts are a fair source of lysine, while bread provides some methionine but is very low in lysine. Table 7.6 lists some other foods that are examples of complementary protein combinations. When menu planning, people can combine a variety of legumes, grains, tree nuts, and seeds with vegetables to prepare dishes that provide adequate mixtures of the essential amino acids. Figure 7.15 shows three categories of plant proteins (legumes, grains, and

TABLE 7.6 Complementary Protein Dishes

- Red beans and rice
- Peanut or soynut butter on bagel, sprinkled with wheat germ
- Hummus (mashed chickpeas/garbanzo beans) with sesame seeds
- Hummus on whole-grain pita bread
- Black beans and cornmeal tortilla
- Split pea soup with toasted whole-wheat bread
- Meatless kidney bean chili with macaroni
- Cornmeal tortilla with black bean salsa
- Peanut butter on whole-grain crackers, sprinkled with wheat germ
- Green beans with brown rice and cashews

complementary combinations mixing certain plant foods to provide all essential amino acids without adding animal protein

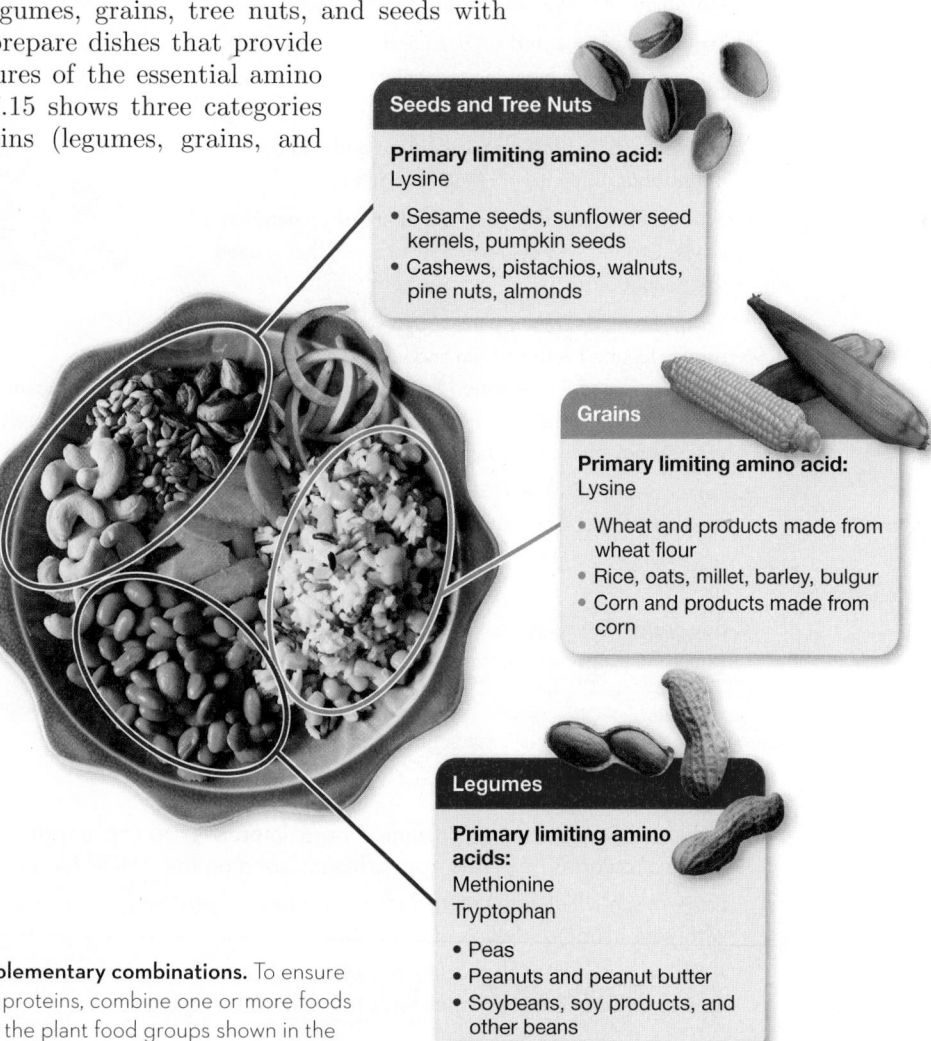

Seeds and Tree Nuts

Primary limiting amino acid:
Lysine

- Sesame seeds, sunflower seed kernels, pumpkin seeds
- Cashews, pistachios, walnuts, pine nuts, almonds

Grains

Primary limiting amino acid:
Lysine

- Wheat and products made from wheat flour
- Rice, oats, millet, barley, bulgur
- Corn and products made from corn

Legumes

Primary limiting amino acids:
Methionine
Tryptophan

- Peas
- Peanuts and peanut butter
- Soybeans, soy products, and other beans

FIGURE 7.15 Complementary combinations. To ensure an adequate mix of proteins, combine one or more foods from at least two of the plant food groups shown in the illustration (legumes, grains, and seeds and tree nuts).

tree nuts and seeds) that make complementary combinations when one or more foods from at least two different groups are mixed together.

Not every mixture of plant foods creates a complementary combination. For example, making a fruit salad by combining apples, grapes, and oranges will not provide a complementary mixture of essential amino acids. Fruits are nutritious foods, but they are generally poor sources of protein. Similarly, combining Boston, iceberg, and romaine varieties of lettuce with carrots and onions makes a tasty salad, but simply mixing leafy greens with other vegetables does not make a complementary combination. However, adding sunflower seeds, kidney or black beans, cashews, and bread cubes to the salad boosts the amount of protein and provides a complete mix of amino acids. To increase the essential amino acid content of the salad even further, add a small amount of hard-cooked egg, shredded cheese, or tofu to it. Processed soybean foods are good sources of essential amino acids. The "Fresh Tips" feature on this page provides information about some of the more popular foods made from soybeans.

FRESH TIPS

The following information describes popular soybean foods and offers tips for how to use them in menu planning.

- Tofu is made from pureed soybeans and has the consistency of thick jelly. Plain tofu has little flavor, so it can be added to a variety of foods, including stir-fried vegetables; with some seasoning, the soybean product can be used as a replacement for scrambled eggs.

- Tempeh is a fermented soybean and grain mixture that can substitute for meat in sandwiches and casseroles.

- Miso is also made from fermented soybeans. Miso can be used to boost the protein content and add flavor to other foods, but it is very high in sodium.

- Soynuts are roasted soybeans that are often eaten as a snack. Ground soynuts form a soft spread that is used like peanut butter.

- Soymilk is made from crushed soybeans. Soymilk is usually fortified with calcium and vitamins A, D, B-12, and riboflavin. Read the Nutrition Facts panel for information about the percent DV of calcium and vitamin D in the milk. Regular soymilk can substitute for cow's milk as a beverage or in recipes. Soy cheeses and yogurt are also available.

- Texturized soy protein (TSP) is made from soybean flour. TSP is often processed to imitate the texture, taste, and appearance of meat or poultry. A TSP product that resembles ground beef can be used to replace half or all of the ground beef in meatloaf, meatball, chili, taco, or meat sauce recipes.

- Soy protein concentrate is a high-protein, high-fiber refined soybean product that is used to boost the protein content of foods.

ASSESS YOUR PROGRESS

22 *Hien is 24 years old and consumes approximately 3200 kcal per day. Calculate the range of calories he needs from protein, based on the AMDR for adult protein intake.*

23 *List ways in which you can reduce your intake of protein from animal foods, starting with your usual food choices.*

24 *A recipe mixes cereals made from wheat, rice, and corn. What plant foods could you add to this combination of cereals to make the recipe a source of high-quality protein?*

7.8 Protein Malnutrition

LEARNING OUTCOMES

1 *Describe health consequences of overconsumption of protein.*

2 *Describe protein-energy malnutrition, including differences between marasmus and kwashiorkor.*

If some protein is necessary for proper growth and good health, can eating extra amounts of the nutrient make a person *extra* healthy or physically fit? Intuitively, the idea of eating more protein to improve one's health seems logical, but protein is no different from other nutrients. If a diet contains adequate amounts of protein, then eating more is not better.

In many parts of the world, the lack of foods containing high–quality proteins is a serious problem, particularly for young children. Protein deficiency interferes with a child's normal growth and development, and contributes to many child–hood deaths. The following sections examine protein malnutrition.

Excessive Protein Intake

Heart disease and cancer are the leading causes of death in developed countries, including the United States. In these nations, the typical Western diet that contains high amounts of animal proteins and saturated fat is associated with increased risk of certain chronic diseases, particularly heart disease,[13–15] colorectal cancer,[16,17] and probably prostate cancer.[18,19] Consumption of red meats and processed meats, such as ham and sausage, is associated with increased risk of pancreatic cancer[20] as well as stomach and esophageal cancer.[21,22] Furthermore, high intakes of red meat may increase the risk of certain breast cancers.[23] More research, however, is needed to clarify the role of high–protein diets and red and processed meats in the risk of certain cancers.

High–protein diets are generally not recommended for healthy individuals. Such diets may lead to higher–than–normal urinary losses of calcium.[24] Urine calcium losses may be more likely to occur when people, particularly women, consume diets that contain more animal than vegetable proteins. Some nutrition experts suspect that diets that supply a lot of animal protein are associated with osteoporosis, a condition characterized by thin bones that fracture easily.[27] Chapter 11 discusses dietary and other factors that may contribute to osteoporosis.

Excess amino acid or protein intake can lead to dehydration, because the kidneys need more water to dilute and eliminate the toxic waste products of amino acid metabolism in urine. Dehydration is a potentially life–threatening condition in which the body's water level is too low. People with liver or kidney diseases may need to avoid protein–rich diets and amino acid supplements because metabolizing the excess amino acids is a burden to their bodies. Chronic intake of a very high–protein diet (over 35% of energy) may also be detrimental to kidney health, particularly in athletes.[28,29] Chapter 15 discusses the protein needs of athletes.

Protein Deficiency

In the United States, protein deficiency is uncommon, but people suffering from alcoholism, anorexia nervosa, or certain intestinal tract disorders are at risk of protein malnutrition. Individuals with low incomes, especially those who are elderly, are also at risk of protein deficiency. Many older adult Americans have limited incomes and must make difficult choices concerning their expenses.

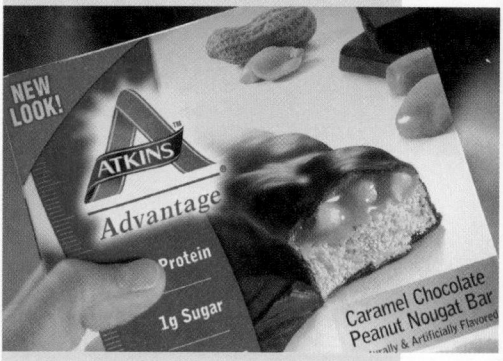

DID **YOU** *KNOW?*

Certain popular weight-loss diets, such as the Atkins, Protein Power, and Sugar Busters® diets, promote high intakes of protein. While following high-protein diets to lose weight, people often report decreased feelings of hunger and increased sense of fullness (satiety) after meals.[25] This response is probably because protein contributes to satiety to a greater extent than fat or carbohydrate.[26]

A person who is 80 years of age and needs to take several medicines daily to treat heart disease, breathing problems, and abnormally high fluid pressure in his or her eyes may think it is more important to purchase costly prescription medications than nutritious foods.

Undernutrition, the lack of food, is often widespread in poor nations in which populations endure frequent famine resulting from crop failures, political unrest, or civil wars. In these countries, **protein–energy malnutrition (PEM)** affects people whose diets lack sufficient protein as well as energy. The failure to consume adequate amounts of protein and energy also results in vitamin and mineral deficiencies.

When food is limited, it is often more difficult for children than for adults to obtain nutritionally adequate diets. Adults may be able to consume enough plant proteins to meet their protein and energy needs, but children have smaller stomachs and higher energy and protein needs per pound of body weight than adults. They are unable to eat enough plant foods to meet their relatively high protein and other nutrient requirements.

According to the World Health Organization, one in every five children in developing countries is underweight due to malnutrition.[30] Impoverished children in Asia and Africa are most likely to develop PEM, and the effects of PEM are especially devastating for the very young. Children with PEM do not grow and are very weak, irritable, and vulnerable to dehydration and infections, such as measles, that can kill them. If these children survive, their growth may be permanently stunted and their intelligence may be lower than normal because malnutrition during early childhood can cause permanent brain damage.

At one time, nutrition experts thought there were only two types of PEM, *kwashiorkor* and *marasmus*. The distinctions between these conditions, however, are often blurred, because protein deficiency is unlikely when a person's energy intake is adequate. Nevertheless, dietitians generally consider *marasmus*, *kwashiorkor*, and *marasmic kwashiorkor* as forms of PEM.

Forms of PEM

Severe PEM causes extreme weight loss and a condition called **marasmus** (*mahraz'–mus*), which is commonly referred to as starvation (Fig. 7.16). Obvious signs of marasmus are weakness and wasting. The body of a starving person loses most of its subcutaneous fat and deeper fat stores. The marasmic person is so thin that his or her ribs, hips, and spinal column are visible through the skin. People suffering from marasmus avoid physical activity to conserve energy, and they are often irritable.

Kwashiorkor (*qwash'–e–or'–kor*) primarily occurs in developing countries where mothers commonly breastfeed their infants until they give birth to another child. The older child, who is usually a toddler, is fairly healthy until abruptly weaned from his or her mother's milk to make way for the younger sibling. Although the toddler may obtain adequate energy by consuming a traditional diet of cereal grains, the diet lacks enough complete protein to meet the youngster's high needs, and he or she soon develops signs of protein deficiency.

Children affected by kwashiorkor have stunted growth; unnaturally blond, sparse, and brittle hair; and patches of skin that have lost their normal coloration. Children with kwashiorkor have some subcutaneous (under the skin) fat, and their swollen cheeks, arms, legs, and bellies make them look well fed, but their appearance is misleading. An important function of certain proteins in blood is to maintain proper fluid balance within cells and blood vessels, as

undernutrition lack of food

protein-energy malnutrition (PEM) occurs when the diet lacks sufficient protein and energy

marasmus form of undernutrition that results from starvation; diet lacks energy and nutrients

kwashiorkor form of undernutrition that results from consuming adequate energy and insufficient high-quality protein

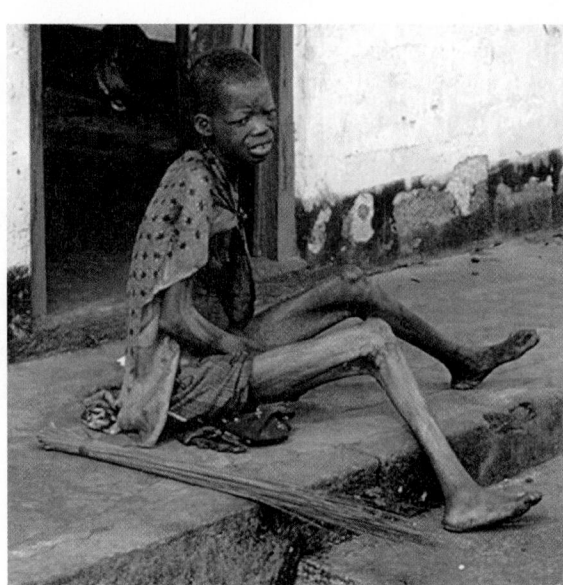

FIGURE 7.16 Severe protein-energy malnutrition. This photo of a Nigerian person suffering from marasmus was taken during the civil war that occurred in the late 1960s.

well as between cells. During starvation, levels of these proteins decline, resulting in edema, which can make the protein–deficient child look plump and overfed instead of thin and undernourished.

In many cases, the child suffering from kwashiorkor does not obtain enough energy and eventually develops **marasmic kwashiorkor**, a condition character– ized by edema and wasting (Fig. 7.17). *Wasting* is the loss of organ and muscle proteins as the body tears down these tissues to obtain amino acids for energy metabolism.

The World Health Organization has guidelines for identifying and treating children with PEM.[31] According to these guidelines, treatments for kwashiorkor, marasmic kwashiorkor, and marasmus are similar. The sickest children need hospitalization, carefully controlled refeedings, and frequent health assessments to recover from PEM.[32,33]

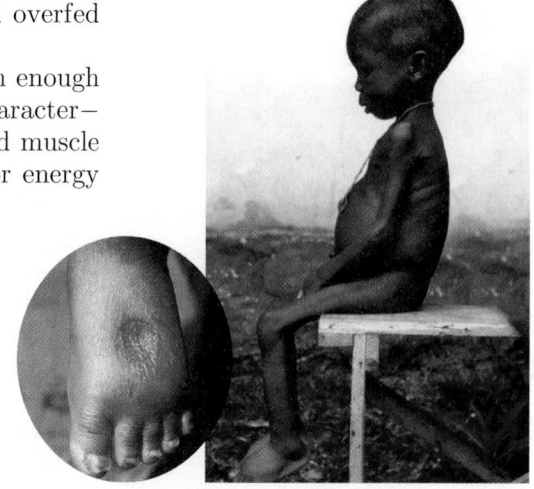

FIGURE 7.17 Mild to moderate protein-energy malnutrition. This Nigerian child is suffering from marasmic kwashiorkor. Note the edema in the child's abdomen, lower legs, and feet. The inset photo shows "pitting" edema: swollen tissues that become deformed when pressed with a finger. These photos were taken during the Nigerian civil war that occurred in the late 1960s.

marasmic kwashiorkor form of undernutrition that results in a child with kwashiorkor who then starts to not consume enough energy; characterized by edema and wasting

ASSESS YOUR PROGRESS

25. *In the United States, which groups of people are most likely to suffer from protein malnutrition?*

26. *Explain why protein-energy malnutrition (PEM) is especially devastating for young children.*

27. *Police bring a 2-year-old child into a clinic; the child is weak and has has arms and upper legs that are so thin, the skin hangs from them. The police report indicates the child was severely neglected by the parents. According to this information, is this child suffering from kwashiorkor, marasmus, or anorexia nervosa? Choose one of these conditions and explain why you selected it.*

7.9 Food Allergies, Food Intolerances, and Phenylketonuria

LEARNING OUTCOMES

1. *Describe the incidence, causes, and treatment of food allergies.*
2. *Explain the difference between a food allergy and a food intolerance, and provide examples of each condition.*
3. *Explain the cause of phenylketonuria (PKU), and discuss diagnosis and treatment of the disorder.*

Although cells need amino acids to function properly, in some cases, certain amino acids or proteins can harm the body and even cause death. The following sections take a closer look at protein–related conditions that affect the lives of millions of Americans: food allergies, food intolerances, and phenylketonuria. By following special diets, people with these conditions can live normal and productive lives.

What Is a Food Allergy?

A food allergy is an inflammatory response that results when the body's immune system reacts inappropriately to one or more harmless substances (*allergens*) in a food. In most cases, the allergen is a protein. In many cases, some protein in a food does not undergo complete digestion, and the small intestine absorbs the

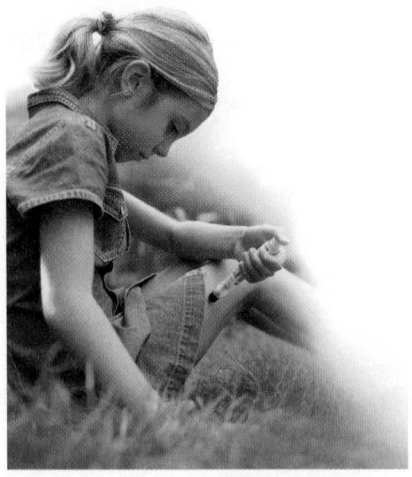

FIGURE 7.18 Treatment for anaphylaxis. Emergency treatment for anaphylaxis involves injecting a medication that prevents or blunts the allergic response.

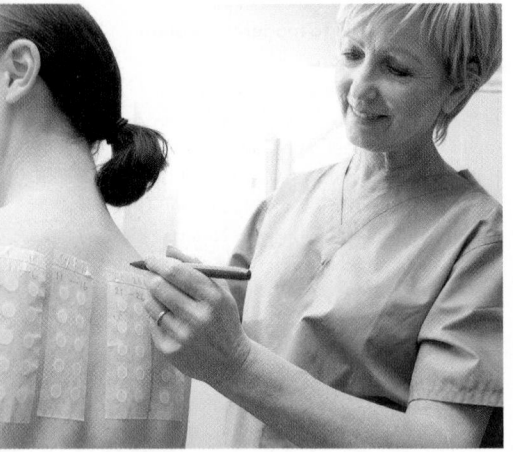

FIGURE 7.19 Skin patch testing for allergies. Skin patch testing involves applying an allergen to a patch, which is then placed on the skin. The skin will become irritated and itch if antibodies to the allergen are present in the body.

TABLE 7.7 Top Food Allergens (United States)

- Milk
- Eggs
- Fish (such as bass, cod, and flounder)
- Crustacean shellfish (such as crab, lobster, and shrimp)
- Tree nuts (such as almonds, cashews, and walnuts)
- Peanuts
- Wheat
- Soybeans

anaphylaxis serious drop in blood pressure that occurs when sensitive people are exposed to food allergens; can be fatal

food intolerances conditions characterized by unpleasant physical reactions following consumption of certain foods

whole molecule. Immune system cells in the small intestine recognize the food protein as a foreign substance and try to protect the body by mounting a defensive response. As a result of the immune response, the individual experiences typical signs and symptoms of food allergy: *hives*, red raised bumps that usually appear on the skin; swollen or itchy lips; a scaly skin rash (eczema); difficulty swallowing; wheezing and difficulty breathing; and abdominal pain, vomiting, and diarrhea.

Allergic reactions generally occur within a few minutes to a couple of hours after eating the offending food. In severe cases, sensitive people who are exposed to food allergens can develop *anaphylactic shock*, a serious drop in blood pressure that affects the whole body. **Anaphylaxis** ($an-a-pha-lax'-is$) can be fatal, unless emergency treatment is provided (Fig. 7.18). Genetics play a major role in the risk of food allergies; people who have family histories of allergies to specific foods or substances in foods are more likely to develop these conditions.

Although any food protein has the potential to cause an allergic reaction in a susceptible person, the most allergenic proteins are in cow's milk, eggs, peanuts and other nuts, wheat, soybeans, fish, and shellfish. In the United States, approximately 8% of young children suffer from food allergies, with 30% of those children having multiple food allergies.[34] In addition, 40% of children with food allergies have experienced a significant allergic reaction.[34] Since 1997, the prevalence of food allergies among children under 18 years of age has been increasing in the United States. Most young children outgrow their food allergies by the time they are 5 years old. Allergies to peanuts, tree nuts, seafood, and wheat, however, usually are not outgrown. According to the American Academy of Allergy, Asthma, and Immunology (www.aaaai.org), 3 to 4% of adults in the United States have one or more food allergies.[34]

Accurate diagnosis of a food allergy should be undertaken by an immunologist, a physician who specializes in the diagnosis and treatment of allergies. Skin testing is a reliable way to identify allergens (Fig. 7.19). Although hair analysis, cytotoxic or electrodermal testing, and kinesiology are promoted by alternative medical practitioners to diagnose allergies, these are unproven diagnostic methods.[35]

Treatment of food allergies involves strict avoidance of the offending foods. Parents or caregivers of young children with food allergies should read food labels carefully to check for allergens listed among ingredients. Additionally, they should educate teachers and other adults who associate with the allergic child about the importance of not exposing the youngster to specific foods. Food manufacturers must identify potentially allergenic ingredients on product labels (Fig. 7.20).[36] The foods and food groups listed in Table 7.7 account for approximately 90% of all food allergies in the United States.[36]

Food Intolerances

Many people experience **food intolerances**, unpleasant physical reactions, including headaches and intestinal discomfort, after they consume nonprotein substances in foods such as lactose, monosodium glutamate (MSG), or *sulfites*. A food intolerance is not the same as a food allergy because the offending substance in the food does not trigger the body's immune response.

Sulfites are a group of sulfur-containing compounds that result from the metabolism of certain amino acids. Sulfites can be naturally in foods, but the compounds are often added to wines, fruits, vegetables, and shellfish to prevent spoilage or preserve flavors.[37] People who suffer from asthma often develop breathing difficulties after consuming food treated with sulfites. Other sulfite-sensitive people report skin flushing (redness and warmth), hives, difficulty swallowing, vomiting, diarrhea, and dizziness after consuming foods that contain the compounds. The U.S. Food and Drug Administration (FDA) requires manufacturers of alcoholic beverages that contain 10 or more mg sulfite/L to include a warning, such as "contains sulfites," on the product's label.[38]

Phenylketonuria

Phenylketonuria ($fen-ul-key-toe-nur'-e-ah$) or PKU is a rare genetic metabolic disorder affects about 1 in every 15,000 infants in the United States.[39] The condition usually occurs when cells are unable to produce the enzyme *phenylalanine hydroxylase* or produce an inactive form of the enzyme. Phenylalanine hydroxylase converts the essential amino acid phenylalanine ($fen-ul-al'-ah-neen$) into the nonessential amino acid tyrosine ($tie'-roe-seen$). As a result, phenylalanine or its toxic by-products build up in tissues and damage cells, including nerve cells in the brain (Fig. 7.21). If PKU is not diagnosed and treated within a few weeks of birth, the affected infant can develop intellectual disability during the first year of life.[39]

To diagnose PKU, physicians generally rely on a simple blood test that is conducted on infants within 48 hours after their birth. In the United States, more than 98% of newborns undergo testing for PKU and several other treatable inherited diseases.[40] Phenylalanine is essential for growth and development; therefore, pediatricians often recommend infants with PKU consume a small amount of the amino acid, which most are able to do without any side effects.[41] Specialized formulas are available for infants with PKU. As the children grow and mature, fruits, vegetables, and special low-protein foods can be added to the formula diet. However, children and adults with the disorder need to avoid foods that are rich sources of phenylalanine, such as nuts, milk products, eggs, meats, and other animal foods. Additionally, people with PKU should not consume diet soft drinks and other foods and beverages containing the alternative sweetener aspartame, because the sweetener is a source of phenylalanine (see Chapter 5 for information about aspartame).

In the past, children with PKU were often allowed to eat regular foods after they were about 6 years of age. However, the importance of continuing the low-phenylalanine diet became evident when many of the children experienced learning and behavioral problems as they matured. Thus, individuals with PKU should follow the phenylalanine-restrictive diet and ensure adequate intake of tyrosine, which becomes conditionally essential in an individual with PKU.

People with the disorder need to undergo frequent blood tests to make sure they are maintaining a healthy concentration of phenylalanine in their bodies. Monitoring blood phenylalanine is especially important during pregnancy. An expectant woman who has PKU must carefully control her phenylalanine level to avoid exposing her embryo/fetus to excessive amounts of the amino acid. If she fails to control the concentration of phenylalanine in her blood, she can give birth to a baby with severe birth defects, including a smaller-than-normal brain. The "Real People, Real Stories" on page 210 features Dallas Clasen, a young adult who has PKU.

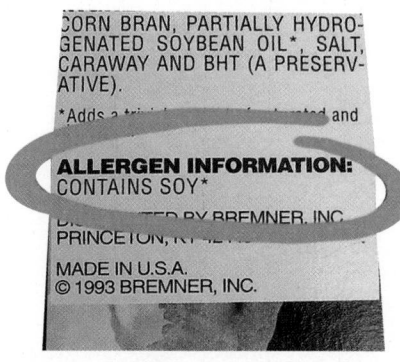

FIGURE 7.20 Allergen labeling. Food manufacturers must identify potentially allergenic ingredients such as soy, milk, and peanuts on product labels.

phenylketonuria (PKU) genetic metabolic disorder characterized by the inability to convert the amino acid phenylalanine into tyrosine, resulting in accumulation of phenylalanine

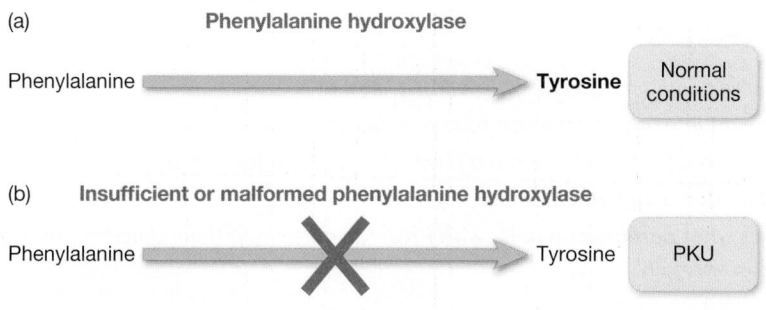

FIGURE 7.21 Phenylalanine metabolism. (*a*) Under normal conditions, the enzyme phenylalanine hydroxylase converts phenylalanine into tyrosine. (*b*) In PKU, the body makes insufficient amounts of phenylalanine hydroxylase. Therefore, the phenylalanine and/or its toxic by-products accumulate in the bloodstream.

REAL People, REAL Stories

Dallas Clasen

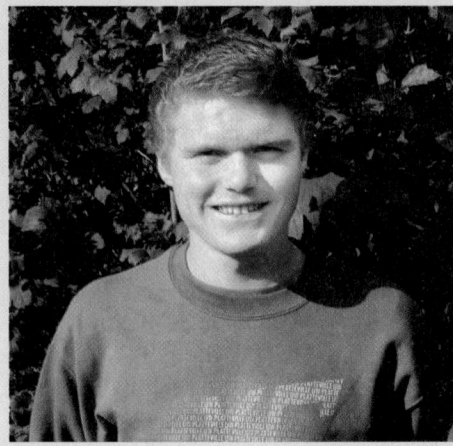

Dallas Clasen is majoring in engineering at the University of Wisconsin–Platteville. In addition to keeping up with his coursework, he runs cross country at school and participates in triathlons. Like most college students, Dallas is very busy, but unlike most students, he has to pay very close attention to his diet. Dallas was born with a rare inherited metabolic disorder called phenylketonuria (PKU).

A few days after birth, Dallas underwent standard newborn blood testing. The results of the test indicated that the level of phenylalanine in his blood was about 40 times higher than the normal amount, a sign of PKU. To avoid developing severe brain damage and other physiological effects of PKU, Dallas received care from a physician who specialized in treating children with the disorder. The primary treatment for PKU is a low-phenylalanine diet.

Most foods that are rich sources of protein, especially high-quality animal proteins, contain more phenylalanine than people with PKU can tolerate. Thus, from the time Dallas was a week old, he has consumed a formula that does not contain the amino acid. In addition to the formula, Dallas can eat limited amounts of grain products and most fruits and vegetables. He also consumes special low-phenylalanine foods that resemble "regular" foods but are not available in supermarkets. As part of Dallas's college meal plan, he has access to the special foods through the university's food service.

Foods that are eaten away from home can present problems for people with PKU. When at a restaurant, Dallas usually orders French fries or "sub" sandwiches that are made with vegetables but do not contain any cheese or meat. Instead of drinking milk, Dallas drinks his special formula or sports drinks that do not contain the nonnutritive sweetener aspartame (see Chapter 5). He is so accustomed to his special diet, he thinks meat looks "gross." In addition to following the special diet, Dallas takes Kuvan®, a prescription medication that stimulates the enzyme that converts phenylalanine to tyrosine. He takes 14 capsules after breakfast with apple juice. The medication does not help everyone with PKU, but it allows Dallas to consume more foods that contain phenylalanine. "I can eat double the amount of the amino acid," Dallas says. To determine whether his special diet and medication are working, each week, Dallas pricks his finger and allows a few drops of blood to soak into a special paper. Then he sends the paper to a laboratory that checks the level of phenylalanine in his blood.

Dallas is aware of the consequences that can occur if he does not limit his phenylalanine intake, and he accepts the need to follow the special diet for the rest of his life. "Being on a strict diet has not only made me disciplined, it has taught me to do whatever is needed to always take good care of myself," Dallas says. "I have learned that we are all different, anyway. So, accept who you are!"

ASSESS YOUR PROGRESS

28 *List three common signs or symptoms of food allergy.*

29 *Identify at least three common food allergens.*

30 *Explain the difference between a food allergy and a food intolerance.*

31 *What causes anaphylactic shock?*

32 *Discuss what parents of infants with PKU can do to help their children grow and develop normally.*

7.10 Celiac Disease and Gluten Sensitivity

LEARNING OUTCOMES

1 *Explain why celiac disease causes malabsorption in the small intestine.*

2 *Identify grains that contain gluten.*

3 *Explain factors that contribute to celiac disease, and discuss the condition's diagnosis and dietary management.*

Celiac (*see'–lee–ak*) **disease** is an autoimmune disorder that results in poor absorption of nutrients (malabsorption) in the small intestine. People with the disease cannot tolerate foods that contain **gluten**, a protein in wheat, barley, and some other cereal grains. Gluten contains the peptide *gliadin*. In cases of celiac disease, gliadin enters the intestinal mucosa and activates the immune system, which inflames or destroys villi. Even though the affected person's food intake may be nutritionally adequate, undernutrition results because his or her intestinal tract lacks healthy villi. Celiac disease is also known as nontropical sprue and gluten–induced or gluten–sensitive enteropathy (*ent–er–op'–a–thee*).

In the United States, about 1 in 133 people has celiac disease.[42] Although the tendency to develop the disease is probably inherited, environmental factors often play a role by triggering the condition. A serious viral infection or severe emotional stress, for example, may activate the disorder in a genetically susceptible person. Infants who consume formula may be more likely to develop the condition than breastfed babies.[42] Also, infants who are fed gluten–containing foods when they are too young (3 months of age, for example) may have a higher risk of developing celiac disease than infants who are not introduced to such foods until they are older.[42]

Diagnosing Celiac Disease

The signs and symptoms of celiac disease vary from person to person but usually include abdominal bloating, chronic diarrhea, and weight loss. Children with this condition also experience poor growth due to nutrient malabsorption and protein malnutrition. Some people have no obvious signs or symptoms of the disease, despite the damage occurring to their small intestines. Serious health problems such as anemia (a blood disorder), osteoporosis (weak bones), liver disease, and intestinal cancer can result from untreated celiac disease.

Blood tests (e.g., transglutaminase antibody test) and intestinal biopsies are often used to diagnose celiac disease. Intestinal biopsy involves removing tiny pieces of tissue from the small intestine. The tissue samples undergo micro–scopic examination to evaluate the condition of the villi. The presence of damaged villi can help confirm the diagnosis of celiac disease.

Treating Celiac Disease

There is no cure for celiac disease, but persons with the condition can achieve and maintain good health by follow–ing a gluten–free diet very carefully. Today, many super–markets carry a variety of gluten–free foods. Table 7.8 lists foods that must be avoided by people with celiac disease, as well as those that are safe for them to consume. Although people with the condition can eat corn, rice, and soy prod–ucts, these foods may be contaminated with gluten if they

celiac disease inherited condition in which the protein gluten cannot be absorbed; results in damage to the small intestine and poor absorption of nutrients

gluten type of protein found in many grains; provides texture and shape to baked products

TABLE 7.8 Gluten in Common Foods

Foods to Avoid		Generally Safe Foods	
Barley	Wheat	Arrowroot	Oats (small
Rye	Wheat-enriched flour	Buckwheat	amounts)
Triticale	Durum flour	Cassava	Quinoa
	Graham flour	Corn	Rice
	Semolina flour	Flax	Sorghum
	Farina	Millet	Soy
	Wheat bran	Nuts	Tapioca
	Wheat germ		
	Cracked wheat		
	Wheat protein		

gluten sensitivity uncomfortable symptoms develop following consumption of gluten, but the individual does not have damage to the small intestine

Every summer, thousands of children head off to summer camp; sports, computer, band, and even health camps are all popular. A recent trend is the "gluten-free" camp. Children with celiac disease who attended a week-long gluten-free camp showed improvement in well-being, self-perception, and emotional outlook. The camp had the greatest positive impact on those children who had been following a gluten-free diet for less than 4 years.[44]

TABLE 7.9 Gluten-Free Flour Substitutes

Substitute 1 cup wheat flour with:
- ⅞ cup rice flour
- ⅝ cup potato starch flour
- 1 cup soy flour plus ¼ cup potato starch flour
- 1 cup corn flour
- 1 cup tapioca flour

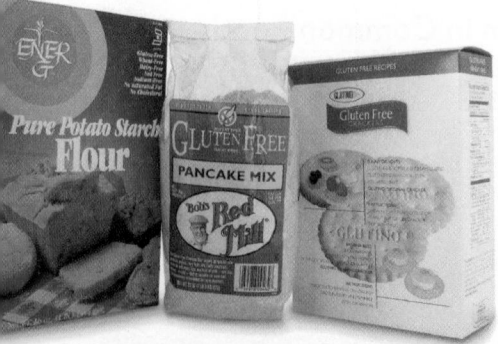

Gluten-free foods are often available in supermarkets.

are processed in factories that also manufacture wheat products. Because gluten may be used to make medications, dietary supplements, and lipsticks, people with celiac disease should read ingredient lists to determine whether such "hidden" sources of gluten are present.

Gluten Sensitivity

In recent years, **gluten sensitivity** has become recognized as a separate condition from celiac disease. Compared to celiac disease, people with gluten sensitivity do not have damage to the small intestine. Individuals who are sensitive to glutens may test negative for celiac disease, yet they report signs and symptoms that are similar to celiac disease after consuming gluten. At this time, clinicians do not have a reliable method of diagnosing gluten sensitivity,[43] so they rely on patient-reported symptoms to identify cases of the condition. Like celiac disease, treatment for gluten sensitivity involves a gluten-free diet.

Planning a Gluten-Free Diet

Eating a gluten-free diet means avoiding all foods, beverages, medications, and supplements that contain gluten (Table 7.8). For many, the most challenging aspect of gluten-free eating is avoiding products made from wheat, one of the most commonly consumed grains in the United States. Table 7.9 identifies commonly used substitutes for wheat flour. When a recipe calls for "flour," it is often best to use a combination of gluten-free flours, including rice flour, potato starch flour, or soy flour.

A food that is gluten-free is not necessarily nutrient dense and a healthy addition to the diet. There are many gluten-free potato chips, cakes, and cookies that are high in simple sugars, fat, and sodium. Consumers choosing gluten-free foods should read nutrition labels carefully.

Gluten-Free Labeling

As of 2013, the FDA has adopted a gluten-free labeling standard.[45] According to the FDA, a product can be labeled as gluten free if it contains less than 20 parts per million (ppm) of gluten, the equivalent of about 6 mg of gluten per serving. Currently available methods and equipment can detect this amount of gluten; equipment to verify lower levels is not available at this time. The following "Fresh Tips" feature provides advice for gluten-free eating.

Katie Adams was diagnosed with celiac disease when she was in college. The "Real People, Real Stories" feature on page 213 introduces Katie and describes how she manages her diet to avoid signs, symptoms, and complications of celiac disease.

FRESH TIPS

- Read all ingredient lists. Gluten-containing ingredients are often "hidden" in processed foods.
- Uncontaminated, pure oats can be used in moderation (less than 1 cup, cooked, per day).
- "Wheat-free" does not always mean gluten-free. Check the ingredient list to be safe.
- Distilled alcoholic beverages and vinegars are gluten-free, but most beers contain the protein. Gluten-free beers and ales are often available at specialty food stores.
- Consult a registered dietitian for more information on planning a gluten-free diet.

REAL People, **REAL** Stories

Katie Adams

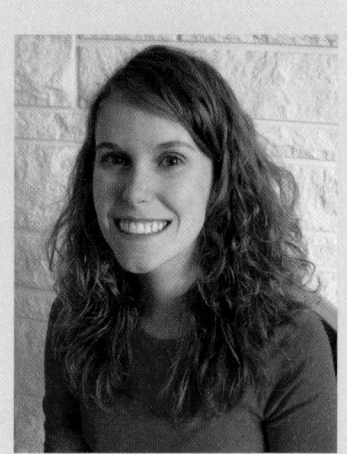

When Katie Adams was an American college student, she had the opportunity to attend England's renowned Cambridge University during her junior year. Within a few months after Katie began her studies in England, she began to experience frequent bouts of abdominal pain not long after eating. Making matters even worse, she suffered from nearly constant diarrhea. Although her weight was at a healthy level when she first went to England, she began to lose pounds despite eating adequate amounts of food.

While at Cambridge, Katie was examined by a physician who thought her signs and symptoms were the result of celiac disease. Katie, however, decided to forgo being tested for the condition until she returned to the United States.

After coming home from England, Katie underwent specialized testing by a gastroenterologist, a physician who diagnoses and treats conditions affecting the intestinal tract. The tests included determining whether certain antibodies were present in her blood. This testing detected the presence of antibodies to proteins in gluten. She also underwent an endoscopic examination of her upper gastrointestinal tract. This exam enabled the gastroenterologist to see the condition of her small intestine and remove a small part of the damaged tissue to view under a microscope. As a result of these definitive tests, Katie was diagnosed with celiac disease. The only treatment for celiac disease is complete avoidance of gluten-containing foods. After a couple of weeks on a gluten-free diet, she began to feel better.

Eating out is especially difficult for people with celiac disease, because of restaurants' widespread inclusion of breads, rolls, pasta, and desserts made from wheat flour in menus. Katie learned how to locate the few restaurants in her community that cater to people with celiac disease by having kitchens that are dedicated to gluten-free food preparation. People with the condition can patronize these eating establishments without worrying about eating any gluten-containing or contaminated foods.

Today, Katie maintains her good health by continuing to avoid gluten. Although her diet is very restrictive, she knows from experience that if she "cheats" by eating even a small amount of food that contains gluten, she'll get sick again. After such occasions, she returns to following a gluten-free diet.

According to Katie, people who are unfamiliar with celiac disease should take the condition seriously and accommodate the special dietary needs of people who have the disease. For example, if you invite someone with celiac disease to share a meal or snack with you, wash your hands after you prepare foods that contain gluten and don't offer those foods to the person. Additionally, prepare some gluten-free foods for your guest who has celiac disease to eat safely. She says, "It's discouraging when people think I'm simply a 'picky eater' and just making life hard for them. The more people who understand celiac disease, the easier my life becomes!"

Diet and Autism Spectrum Disorders

Autism spectrum disorders (ASDs), often simply called **autism**, are neuro—developmental disorders characterized by deficits in social interaction and verbal and nonverbal communication, and by repetitive behaviors or interests.[46] There is great variability in a child's degree of ASD; some children experience very mild symptoms that are only noticeable to parents and close caregivers.

The incidence of diagnosed autism has increased more than 10—fold in the past 20 years.[47] Today, ASDs affect 1 in 110 children in the United States. Boys are four to five times more likely to have autism than girls. Although

autism spectrum disorders (ASDs, autism) neurodevelopmental disorders characterized by deficits in social interaction, verbal and nonverbal communication, and by repetitive behaviors or interests

environmental factors probably play a role in the condition's development, genetic factors are also involved.

At this time, there is no cure for ASD. Many caregivers turn to alternative therapies for the disorders, including special diets that exclude gluten and casein, a protein in milk. A recent dietary intervention study found that a gluten−free/casein−free (GF/CF) diet was beneficial for autistic children.[48] However, other studies have shown no benefits for autistic children who follow GF/CF, casein−free, or gluten−free diets. Some scientists caution that following such diets could cause malnutrition because of the limited food choices.[49] More long−term, well−designed studies are necessary determine whether there is a relationship between a gluten−free or GF/CF diet and ASD.

ASSESS YOUR PROGRESS

33 *What is gluten?*

34 *List four kinds of grains that contain gluten and four that are gluten-free.*

35 *Describe the causes and symptoms of celiac disease and how it can be managed with diet.*

36 *List three strategies people can employ for following a gluten-free diet.*

7.11 Vegetarianism

LEARNING OUTCOMES

1 *Explain the differences between the composition of a Western diet and the compositions of different vegetarian diets.*

2 *Discuss the pros and cons of vegetarian diets.*

vegetarians people who eat plant-based diets

Vegetarians are individuals who rely heavily on plant foods; they may or may not include some animal foods in their diets. About 2.3% of American adults do not eat meat, fish, or poultry, and about 1.4% of adults avoid eating any food from animal sources.[51]

Classifying Vegetarian Diets

semivegetarian ("flexitarian") a person who usually avoids red meat but consumes other animal foods, including fish, poultry, eggs, and dairy products

pescavegetarian vegetarian who consumes fish, milk products, and eggs for animal protein

lactovegetarian vegetarian who consumes milk and milk products for animal protein

ovovegetarian vegetarian who eats eggs for animal protein

lactoovovegetarian vegetarian who consumes milk products and eggs for animal protein

vegan vegetarian who eats only plant foods

There are many different types of plant−based vegetarian diets, including some that contain animal foods. A **semivegetarian ("flexitarian")**, for example, usu−ally avoids red meat but consumes other animal foods, including fish, poultry, eggs, and dairy products. A **pescavegetarian** eats fish, eggs, and dairy products but avoids red meat, poultry, or other animal products. A **lactovegetarian** (*lacto* = milk) obtains animal protein by consuming milk and milk products, including yogurt, cheese, and ice cream. An **ovovegetarian** (*ovo* = egg) eats eggs, and a **lactoovovegetarian** consumes milk products and eggs. A **vegan**, or *total vege−tarian*, eats only plant foods. Table 7.10 lists common types of vegetarian diets.

Is Vegetarianism a Healthy Lifestyle?

Vegetarian diets are often lower in fat and energy than Western diets that contain animal foods, particularly plenty of red meat. Compared to people who eat meat, vegetarians tend to have a lower risk of obesity, type 2 diabetes, hypertension, and certain cancers.[52,53] Furthermore, vegans tend to be leaner than nonvegans.[54] It is difficult, however, to pinpoint diet as being responsible for vegetarians' good health status. Vegetarians often adopt other healthy lifestyle practices, such as

TABLE 7.10 Common Types of Vegetarian Diets

Type of Vegetarian Diet	Animal Foods Included
Pescavegetarian	Milk, milk products, and eggs; fish but no other animal foods
Semivegetarian	All except red meats
Lactovegetarian	Milk and milk products; no animal flesh or eggs
Ovovegetarian	Eggs but no other animal foods
Lactoovovegetarian	Milk and milk products and eggs but no other animal foods
Vegan	No animal foods

exercising regularly; practicing relaxation activities, such as yoga or meditation; and avoiding tobacco products and excess alcohol.

Compared to the typical American diet, vegetarian diets provide more fiber, phytochemicals, folic acid (a B vitamin), vitamins E and C, and the minerals potassium and magnesium.[51] In addition, vegetarian diets often supply less saturated fat than diets that include animal foods.

In general, plant foods have low energy density: they add bulk to the diet without adding a lot of calories. Thus, vegetarians may feel "full" soon after eating a meal of plant foods, and they may not consume as much energy and nutrients as they need. Poorly planned plant-based diets may not contain enough energy; high-quality protein; omega-3 fatty acids; vitamins B-12, D, and riboflavin; and minerals zinc, iron, and calcium to meet a person's nutritional needs.[52,54]

Humans digest animal proteins to a greater extent than plant proteins.[51] Therefore, vegetarians may need to increase their protein intakes by about 10% to compensate. Total vegetarians, including some vegan athletes, can obtain adequate amounts of the essential amino acids by eating processed soybean products and foods that combine complementary plant proteins.[55]

Vegetarians who do not consume seafood may need to obtain omega-3 fatty acids by eating algae or taking algae supplements. Plant foods contain little or no vitamin B-12,[56] and there are few dietary sources of vitamin D other than fortified cow's milk. Furthermore, some mineral nutrients are more available from animal foods than from plant foods. Plants often contain phytochemicals that interfere with the body's absorption of minerals, particularly iron, zinc, and calcium. Vegans have lower calcium intakes and a higher risk of bone fractures than vegetarians who include milk and milk products in their diets.[51]

Vegans can obtain vitamin B-12, vitamin D, iron, zinc, and many other micronutrients by consuming fortified foods such as soy and rice beverages, "Red Star®" vegetarian nutritional yeast, and breakfast cereals. Vegetarians can also take a multiple vitamin/mineral supplement to provide dietary "insurance." Table 7.11 summarizes the nutritional advantages and possible nutritional disadvantages of vegetarian diets.

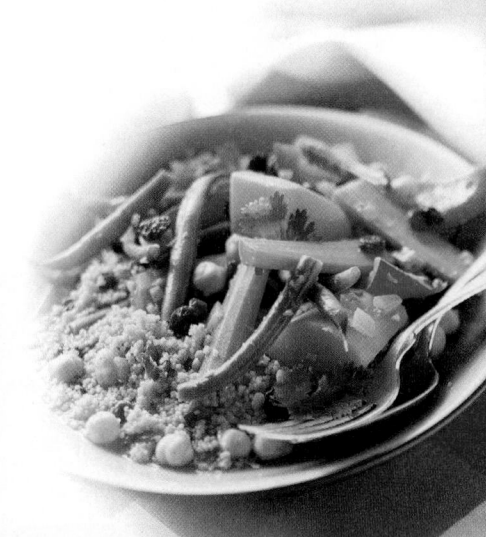

A vegan might enjoy this dish: couscous with vegetables and chickpeas. Couscous is a grain product.

Vegetarianism During Certain Life Stages

Children have higher protein and energy needs per pound of body weight than an adult. Because plant foods add bulk to the diet, vegan children are likely to eat far less food than adult vegans because they become full sooner during meals. Thus, very young vegans may be unable to eat enough plant foods to meet their protein and energy needs. Therefore, it is very important for parents or other caretakers to plan nutritionally adequate diets for vegetarian children and monitor the children's growth rates.[57]

Pregnant vegan women should consult with their physicians about the need to take a vitamin B-12 supplement to reduce the likelihood of having a baby who is deficient in this nutrient. Vegan women who breastfeed their infants

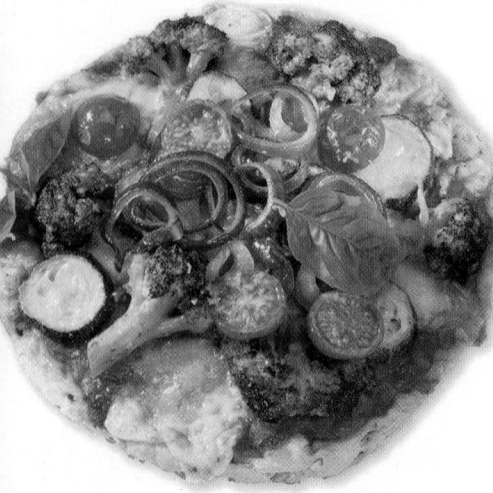

TABLE 7.11 Vegetarian Diets: Nutritional Aspects

Advantages	Possible Disadvantages
High: Vitamins C , E, and folic acid Phytochemicals Fiber Magnesium and potassium	**Low:** Vitamins B-12, D, and riboflavin Zinc, iron, and calcium Omega-3 fatty acids Certain essential amino acids Energy
Low: Fat (saturated)	

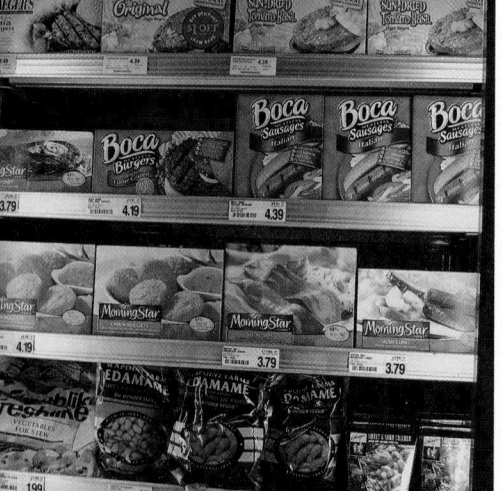

may produce milk that is deficient in vitamin B−12, particularly if the mothers' diets lack the vitamin. Infants of these mothers have a high risk of developing severe developmental delays associated with neurological damage, especially when breast milk is their only source of vitamin B−12.[58]

Many American teenagers and young adults are adopting vegetarian diets. Switching from the typical Western diet to vegetarianism can be a healthy practice for teens; vegetarian youth often eat more fruits and vegetables and less fat than their nonvegetarian peers.[51] However, vegetarian teenagers may have a higher risk of unhealthy weight control practices and eating disorders, such as *anorexia nervosa*, than young people who eat meat. Anorexia nervosa ("anorexia") is a serious psychological disorder that can result in starvation and death. Chapter 14 provides more information about anorexia nervosa and other eating disorders.

Meatless Menu Planning

Many common menu items can be converted into vegetarian foods by removing the meat, fish, or poultry. For example, pizza and lasagna can be prepared without meat and still provide plenty of protein from the cheese as well as the crust or pasta. The following "Fresh Tips" feature presents more meatless menu suggestions.

Commercially prepared vegetarian foods that substitute for meat, fish, and poultry items are often available in the frozen−food section of supermarkets. These vegetarian products can look and taste like their nonvegetarian counterparts, but they may be lower in saturated fat. Such foods include soy−based sausage patties or links, soy hot dogs, "veggie" burgers, and soy "crumbles" that look like bits of cooked ground beef. Restaurants may offer vegetarian menu items, or their cooks can modify menu items by substituting meatless sauces, omitting meat from stir−fries, and adding vegetables or pasta in place of meat.

FRESH TIPS

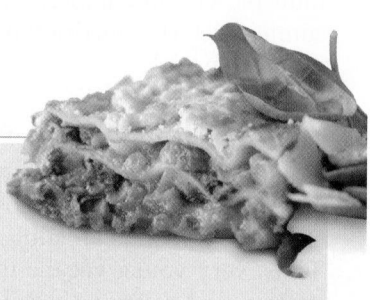

Try one of the following meatless meal menu ideas.

- Cooked pasta with marinara sauce and grated Parmesan or part-skim mozzarella cheese
- Vegetable lasagna with layers of thinly sliced zucchini, mushrooms, and bell peppers
- Vegetable stir-fry with bits of tofu and cheese
- Grilled vegetable kabobs served over cooked rice and black beans
- Black or red bean burritos
- Bean and corn tacos

With careful planning, vegetarians can overcome the nutritional limitations of a plant—based diet and consume adequate nutrients.[51] The MyPlate website also offers suggestions for planning nutritionally adequate meatless meals.

ASSESS YOUR PROGRESS

37 *Compare and contrast the different types of vegetarian diets.*

38 *List potential health benefits of vegetarian diets.*

39 *Identify nutrients that can be low or lacking in a vegan's diet.*

40 *Explain why one must be careful when planning vegan meals for children.*

7.12 Nutritional Genomics

LEARNING OUTCOMES

1 *Distinguish between nutrigenomics and nutrigenetics.*

2 *Explain how genetic testing may be used in dietary recommendations.*

In 1990, scientists began the Human Genome Project, an effort to identify and sequence the approximately 23,000 *genes* that code for protein synthesis in human DNA.[59] As a result of this project, scientists discovered that people's food choices can affect their genes' expression (activity that results in protein syn—thesis). Furthermore, researchers used such information to develop the science of **nutritional genomics** (Fig. 7.22). Nutritional genomics has two components:

- **Nutrigenomics**—the study of how nutrients affect the expression of a person's genome, and

- **Nutrigenetics**—the study of how inherited genetic variations influence the body's responses to specific nutrients and nutrient combinations.[59]

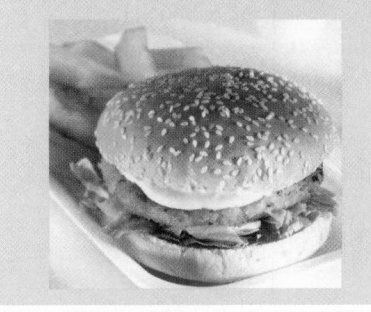
nutritional genomics study of nutrigenomics and nutrigenetics

nutrigenomics study of how nutrients affect the expression of a person's genome

nutrigenetics study of how inherited genetic variations influence the body's responses to specific nutrients and nutrient combinations

Nutrigenetics

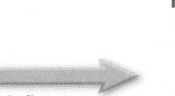

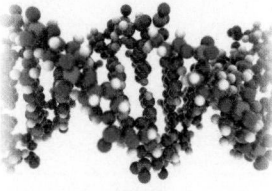

Genes

Influence →

Nutrient Needs
Example: Variation in human nutrient requirements

Metabolism
Examples: Diabetes and obesity development

Nutrigenomics

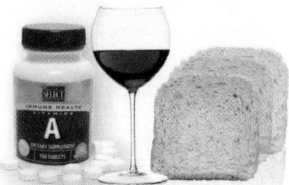

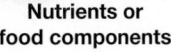

Nutrients or food components

Influence →

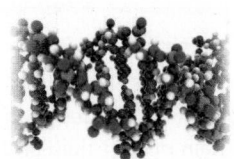

Genetic Expression

Examples:
- Excess vitamin A during pregnancy causes birth defects in embryo
- Alcohol consumption during pregnancy causes birth defects in embryo
- Food allergies and intolerances in vulnerable persons

FIGURE 7.22 Nutritional genomics.

personalized nutrition making dietary choices based on one's genetic makeup

inborn errors of metabolism conditions that occur when genes undergo mutations that disrupt metabolism of specific nutrients

mutation change to the typical sequence of a gene's DNA components

Nutritional genomics may explain why dietary interventions can have different effects on the health of different individuals.[60] For example, a low-fat diet may lower the blood cholesterol level of one person, but the same diet may have no effect on another person's cholesterol level. A young man, for example, may develop kidney stones while taking a daily dietary supplement that contains 1000 mg of vitamin C. However, another man who is the same age and takes the same amount of vitamin C each day does not form kidney stones. Thus, the effectiveness of a specific diet, dietary supplement, medication, or lifestyle intervention may be largely dependent on one's genes. Such differences may need to be considered when prescribing treatments.

Personalized Nutrition

The concept of **personalized nutrition**, making dietary choices based on one's genetic makeup, is based on nutritional genomics. This means that in addition to relying on traditional forms of health assessment, including height, weight, and blood pressure, health care professionals need to consider the influence that an individual's genetic background can have on dietary recommendations.

Personalized nutrition is not a new concept. For decades, medical experts have treated infants who have certain **inborn errors of metabolism** with special diets. An inborn error of metabolism occurs when a gene undergoes a **mutation**, that is, a change in the typical sequence of the gene's DNA components. PKU is an example of an inborn error of amino acid metabolism that is treated with a special diet.

The Future of Nutritional Genomics

Nutritional genomics is a dynamic field, and the results of research in this field can influence the work of health care professionals. Registered dietitians now face the opportunity and challenge to make genetically driven dietary recommendations.[62] The shift away from providing standard dietary advice and toward personalized dietary planning is in an early phase. Students who study dietetics or human nutrition may consider taking courses in genetics, specifically nutritional genomics, to prepare for this emerging trend.

ASSESS YOUR PROGRESS

41 Identify the major outcomes of the Human Genome Project.

42 Explain the effects that nutritional genomics can have on an individual's health.

43 Discuss how personalized nutrition affects the dietetics profession.

SUMMARY

SECTION 7.1 Introducing Proteins

- Proteins are organic compounds that contain nitrogen.
- Proteins have numerous functions in the body, including forming tissues such as muscles and bones, catalyzing chemical reactions, transporting other nutrients, and helping maintain proper fluid and acid-base balance.

SECTION 7.2 Amino Acids

- The chemical structure of an amino acid includes a nitrogen-containing (amine) group, a carboxylic acid group, and an R group.
- The diet must supply nine of the amino acids, the essential amino acids, because the body cannot make them or cannot make enough of them to meet its needs.

SECTION 7.3 **Protein Synthesis and Structure**

- Cells produce proteins by linking amino acids together in specific sequences that are dictated by instructions coded in DNA. Errors in the DNA code can result in the wrong amino acids being inserted into peptide chains.
- Proteins have four levels of structure—primary, secondary, tertiary, and quaternary.

SECTION 7.4 **Proteins in Foods**

- A high-quality, complete protein contains all nine of the essential amino acids in necessary amounts. The quality of a protein is measured against a reference protein, which is usually egg white protein.
- The adult RDA for protein is 0.8 g/kg of body weight daily. Protein requirements increase during pregnancy; breastfeeding; periods of growth; and recovery from serious illnesses, blood losses, and burns.

SECTION 7.5 **Protein Digestion, Absorption, and Transport**

- Protein digestion begins in the stomach, where hydrochloric acid denatures food proteins and pepsin breaks proteins into polypeptides.
- In the small intestine, enzymes secreted by the pancreas and absorptive cells digest polypeptides. The end products of protein digestion, amino acids, travel to the liver. The liver uses the amino acids or releases them into the general circulation.

SECTION 7.6 **Protein Metabolism**

- If an essential amino acid is not available when protein synthesis occurs, protein synthesis stops, and the amino acids in the unfinished peptide are removed and returned to the amino acid pool through deamination.
- Following deamination, the nitrogen-containing group, in the form of ammonia, is converted into urea in the liver and eventually excreted in the urine.
- The more protein a person consumes, the more urea is in his or her urine, leading to an elevated urine urea nitrogen level. Having high blood urea nitrogen may indicate the kidneys are not filtering blood correctly.
- An adult's body maintains its protein content by carefully balancing nitrogen intake and losses.

SECTION 7.7 **Meeting Protein Needs**

- The AMDR for adults is 10 to 35% of energy intake from protein.
- Complementary protein combinations are mixtures of plant foods that provide all essential amino acids without adding animal proteins.

SECTION 7.8 **Protein Malnutrition**

- Protein-energy malnutrition (PEM) affects people whose diets lack sufficient protein as well as energy; children are more likely to be affected by PEM than adults.
- Severely undernourished children do not grow and are very weak, irritable, and vulnerable to dehydration and life-threatening infections.

SECTION 7.9 **Food Allergies, Food Intolerances, and Phenylketonuria**

- A food allergy is an inflammatory response that results when the body's immune system reacts inappropriately to one or more allergens in the food. Anaphylaxis is a serious allergic reaction, resulting in a drastic drop in blood pressure.
- The most common food allergens in the United States are milk, eggs, fish, crustacean shellfish, tree nuts, peanuts, wheat, and soybeans. In the United States, food manufacturers must identify potentially allergenic ingredients on product labeling.
- Phenylketonuria occurs when cells are unable to produce an enzyme that converts the amino acid phenylalanine to other compounds. Individuals with PKU must avoid foods that are rich sources of phenylalanine.

SECTION 7.10 **Celiac Disease and Gluten Sensitivity**

- Celiac disease is an inherited condition that results in an individual not being able to tolerate the protein gluten, leading to malabsorption of nutrients in the small intestine. Common signs of celiac disease include abdominal bloating, chronic diarrhea, and weight loss. Treatment for celiac disease includes avoiding foods that contain gluten.

SECTION 7.11 **Vegetarianism**

- Vegetarian diets are based on plant foods and limit animal foods either partially or completely. If not properly planned, plant-based diets may not contain enough energy; high-quality protein; omega-3 fatty acids; vitamins B-12 and D; and zinc, iron, and calcium to meet a person's nutritional needs, especially children's needs.

SECTION 7.12 **Nutritional Genomics**

- Nutritional genomics may predict how one's diet affects his or her genetic makeup and how one's genetic makeup affects how his or her body responds to food and diet.

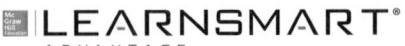 Get the most out of your study of nutrition with McGraw-Hill's innovative suite of adaptive learning products including McGraw-Hill LearnSmart®, SmartBook®, McGraw-Hill LearnSmart Achieve®, and McGraw-Hill LearnSmart Prep®. Visit www.learnsmartadvantage.com.

Critical Thinking

1. Plan a day's meals and snacks for a healthy 132-pound adult female who is not pregnant or breastfeeding and who is following a lactoovovegetarian diet. Your meal plan can range from 1800 to 2200 kcal, and it should follow the recommendations of the MyPlate food guide.

2. Abhi is a freshman in college who weighs 175 pounds. Although his diet supplies an average of 120 g of protein daily, he thinks he needs to consume more meat. What would you tell Abhi about his daily protein intake and whether it is necessary for him to add more meat to his diet?.

3. After having a routine physical exam, John's physician told him to have further testing because his BUN level was 25 mg/dL. Explain what BUN represents, and provide some conditions that would raise a person's BUN to 25 mg/dL.

4. A recipe for bean salad has the following main ingredients:

   1 cup kidney beans   1 ½ cups wine vinegar
   1 cup green beans   ⅓ cup canola oil
   1 cup butter beans   ¼ cup chopped onion
   1 cup black beans

   Explain why this recipe is not a complementary mixture of plant proteins. What plant foods could you add to the recipe to make it a complementary mixture?

5. Chaitra has been experiencing abdominal bloating, cramping, and frequent diarrhea. She reports that the pain and diarrhea is worst after she eats a lot of bread. What may be causing Chiatra's GI symptoms? How should she modify her diet to help alleviate some of the symptoms?

CASE STUDY RESPONSE

MEETING PROTEIN NEEDS

BASED ON MANUEL'S BODY WEIGHT OF 175 POUNDS, he should consume approximately 64 grams of protein per day (0.8 g protein/kg body weight). He currently consumes nearly double this daily protein recommendation.

Manuel does not have to eat only meat to consume high-quality protein and meet his daily protein requirements. He can meet his protein needs by choosing meatless snacks and meal options, such as:

- Hummus on whole-grain pita bread or whole-grain crackers
- Peanut or soynut butter on an apple or banana
- Bean (e.g., pinto or black) burrito or taco
- Vegetarian chili with beans and mixed vegetables
- Homemade trail mix with walnuts, almonds, sunflower seeds, and dried fruit, such as raisins

Like many Americans, Manuel is already exceeding his daily protein requirements. He is currently consuming 1.5 g/kg body weight of protein. Thus, Manuel does not need to consume a protein shake in addition to the protein he currently consumes. Excess may contribute to osteoporosis and dehydration. He should eat a well-balanced diet that includes protein from both animal and plant sources.

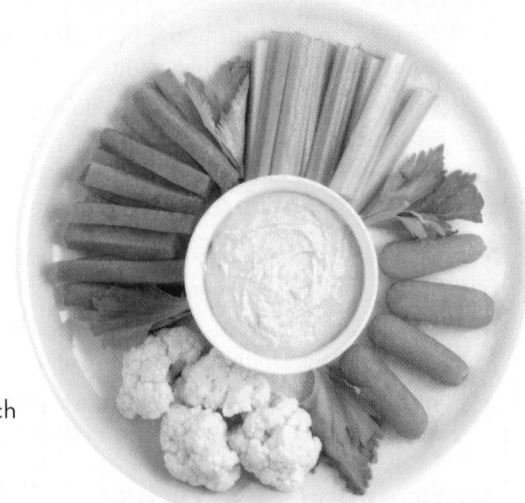

Hummus is made from chickpeas (also called garbanzo beans).

TEST KITCHEN
Modifying Recipes for Healthy Living

Sixteen-year-old Lily recently told her parents that she wants to follow a lactoovovegetarian diet. Lily's parents are concerned because the meals they prepare at home often have beef, chicken, pork, or fish as the main dish. For the family's Fourth of July cookout, Lily's parents usually prepare a dinner menu that includes hamburgers and frankfurters, pork and beans, and corn on the cob. The family would still like to enjoy this dinner, but they want to have vegetarian-friendly options available for Lily. Consider the family's typical complete dinner menu, and provide suggestions for adapting this menu for a lactoovovegetarian.

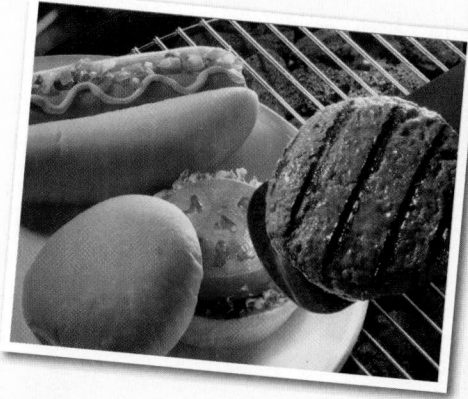

TYPICAL DINNER MENU FOR LILY'S FAMILY COOKOUT

STEP 1 Brainstorm

Examine the menu. What options can Lily choose to eat on her lactoovovegetarian diet? Can these options by themselves constitute a well-balanced meal?

STEP 2 Develop a modified dinner menu for the family

Identify vegetarian-friendly options that could be added to the menu. When planning the new menu, consider recommendations of MyPlate. List the new menu.

STEP 3 Nutritional analysis

Develop a table that compares the number of calories and amounts of total fat, saturated fat, carbohydrates, and protein in a hot dog, a 3- to 4-ounce hamburger, and 3- to 4-ounce commercially available veggie burger. Describe the key nutrient differences.

OPTIONAL ACTIVITIES

STEP 4 Prepare the proposed lactoovovegetarian-friendly menu

Keep notes on any changes you make to the menu.

STEP 5 Reflect on your findings

Was the revised menu satisfying? Did the revised menu provide a well-balanced meal with carbohydrates, fat, and protein?

STEP 6 Add any new recipes to your collection

MENU

Hamburgers and hot dogs on white buns

Pork and beans

Deviled eggs

Corn on the cob

Unsweetened iced tea

PERSONAL Dietary Analysis

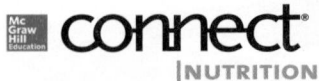

Complete the Personal Dietary Analysis activity online at www.mcgrawhillconnect.com, where you will also find McGraw-Hill LearnSmart®, SmartBook®, NutritionCalc Plus, and many other dynamic learning tools.

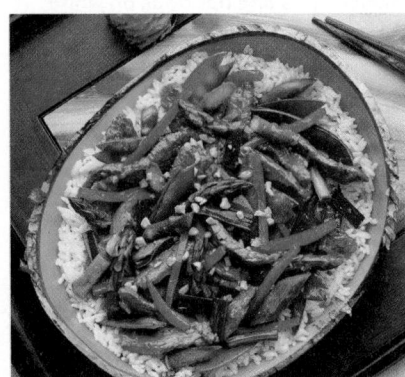

1. Refer to the 3-day food log from the "Personal Dietary Analysis" feature in Chapter 5. Calculate your average protein intake by adding the grams of protein eaten each day, dividing the total by 3, and rounding the figure to the nearest whole number.

Sample Calculation: _____

Day 1   <u>76</u> g

Day 2   <u>55</u> g

Day 3   <u>103</u> g

Total grams   <u>234</u> g ÷ 3 days = <u>78</u> g of protein/day

Your Calculation: _____

Day 1   ___ g

Day 2   ___ g

Day 3   ___ g

Total grams   ___ ÷ 3 days = ___ g/day

My average daily protein intake was ___ g.

2. The RDA for protein is based on body weight. Using the RDA of 0.8 g of protein/kg of body weight, calculate the amount of protein that you need to consume daily to meet the recommendation. To determine your body weight in kilograms, divide your weight (pounds) by 2.2, then multiply this number by 0.8 to obtain your RDA for protein. Then round the figure to the nearest whole number.

My weight in pounds ___ ÷ <u>2.2</u> = ___ kg

My weight in kg ___ × <u>0.8</u> = ___ g

My RDA for protein = ___ g

a. Did your average intake of protein meet or exceed your RDA level that was calculated in step 1? ___ Yes ___ No

b. If your answer to 2a is yes, which foods contributed the most to your protein intake?

Foods: _____

3. Review the log of your 3-day food intake. Calculate the average number of kilocalories that protein contributed to your diet each day during the 3-day period.

a. Each gram of protein provides about 4 kcal; therefore, you must multiply the average number of grams of protein obtained in step 1 by 4 kcal to obtain the average number of kcal from protein.

Sample Calculation: _____

<u>78</u> g/day × <u>4</u> kcal/g = <u>312</u> kcal from protein

Your Calculation: _____

___ g/day × <u>4</u> kcal/g = ___ average number of kcal from protein

4. Determine your average energy intake over the 3-day period by adding the kilocalories for each day and dividing the sum by 3, and round to the nearest whole number.

Sample Calculation:

Day 1   <u>2500</u> kcal

Day 2   <u>3200</u> kcal

Day 3   <u>2750</u> kcal

Total kcal   <u>8450</u> ÷ 3 days = <u>2817</u> kcal/day (average caloric intake)

Your Calculation:

Day 1   ___ kcal

Day 2   ___ kcal

Day 3   ___ kcal

Total kcal   ___ ÷ 3 days = ___ kcal/day (average)

5. Determine the average percentage of energy that protein contributed to your diet by dividing the average kilocalories from protein obtained in step 3 by the average total daily energy intake obtained in step 4. Then round this figure to the nearest one-hundredth. Multiply this value by 100, move the decimal point two places to the right, drop the decimal point, and add a percent symbol.

Sample Calculation:

312 kcal from protein ÷ <u>2817</u> kcal intake = <u>0.11</u> (rounded)

<u>0.11</u> × <u>100</u> = <u>11%</u>

Your Calculation:

___ kcal from protein ÷ ___ kcal intake = ___

___ × 100 = ___ %

6. Did your average intake of protein meet the recommendation of 10 to 35% of total calories? If your average protein intake was below 10%, list at least five foods you could eat that would boost your intake.

Foods: _____

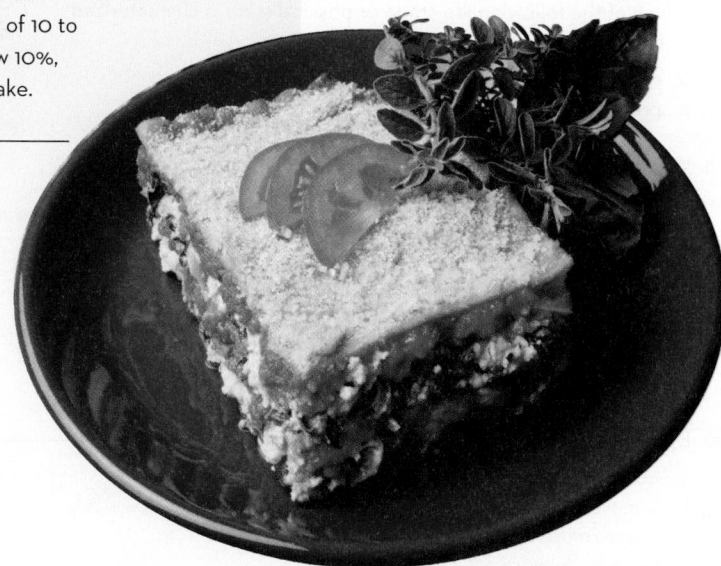

Practice Test

Select the best answer.

1. A protein
   a. is comprised of glucose molecules.
   b. has nitrogen in its chemical structure.
   c. provides more energy per gram than carbohydrate.
   d. is a complex inorganic molecule.

2. Which of the following statements is false?
   a. Certain hormones are proteins.
   b. Nearly all enzymes are proteins.
   c. Proteins are part of triglycerides.
   d. The body uses protein to make antibodies.

3. Which of the following foods is not a source of complete protein?
   a. peanut butter   c. fish
   b. cheese   d. eggs

4. In cells, _____ controls the assembly of amino acids into proteins.
   a. food   c. insulin
   b. DNA   d. AMDR

5. _____ is the process of removing nitrogen from an amino acid.
   a. Transamination
   b. Denaturation
   c. Hydrogenation
   d. Deamination

6. Following the breakdown of an amino acid, the remaining nitrogen is converted into urea in the _____ and then filtered by the _____ for excretion.
   a. kidneys; kidneys
   b. pancreas; large intestine
   c. liver; kidneys
   d. gallbladder; liver

7. Which of the following life stage or physical state is characterized by negative nitrogen balance?
   a. starvation   c. puberty
   b. pregnancy   d. infancy

8. What is the RDA for protein of a healthy adult woman who weighs 62 kg?
   a. 49.6 g   c. 69.6 g
   b. 59.6 g   d. 79.6 g

9. A person following a vegan diet would eat
   a. eggs.   c. nuts.
   b. cheese.   d. fish.

10. By eating more protein than needed, a person can
    a. build bigger muscles.
    b. lose weight.
    c. absorb more calcium.
    d. become dehydrated.

11. People with celiac disease should
    a. take amino acid supplements.
    b. limit their protein intake to 20 g per day.
    c. avoid foods that contain gluten.
    d. eliminate protein from plant sources.

12. Which of the following foods is most likely to cause an allergic reaction?
    a. shellfish   c. apples
    b. corn   d. broccoli

13. When a protein chain begins to coil, its _____ structure forms.
    a. primary   c. tertiary
    b. secondary   d. quaternary

14. Protein digestion begins in the
    a. liver.
    b. small intestine.
    c. mouth.
    d. stomach.

15. A person with PKU should avoid
    a. aspartame.
    b. bread.
    c. corn.
    d. fruit.

1-b; 2-c; 3-a; 4-b; 5-d; 6-c; 7-a; 8-a; 9-c; 10-d; 11-c; 12-a; 13-b; 14-d; 15-a

ANSWERS TO PRACTICE TEST

ANSWERS TO CHAPTER 7 QUIZ Yourself

1. Red meat is the only source of high-quality protein. **False** (pp. 196, 197)
2. Americans typically consume inadequate amounts of protein. **False** (p. 202)
3. Certain hormones and enzymes are proteins. **True** (p. 190)
4. Vegetarian diets are often lower in saturated fat and calories than typical "Western" diets. **True** (p. 214)
5. To maintain good health, individuals with celiac disease should follow a gluten-free diet. **True** (p. 211)

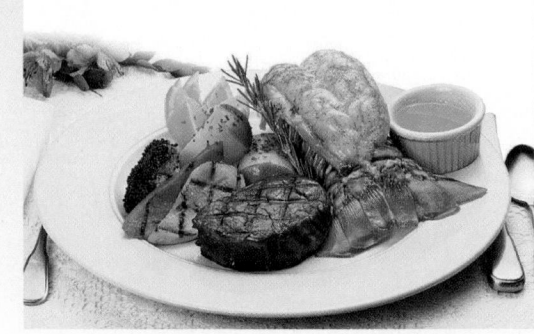

References

1. Saladin KS: *Anatomy & physiology.* 5th ed. Boston: McGraw-Hill Publishing Company, 2010.

2. Qureshi NA, Al-Bedah AM: Mood disorders and complementary and alternative medicine: A literature review. *Journal of Neuropsychiatric Disease and Treatment* 9:639, 2013.

3. Reeds PJ: Dispensable and indispensable amino acids for humans. *Journal of Nutrition* 130:1835S, 2000.

4. Food and Nutrition Board: *Dietary Reference Intakes for energy, carbohydrates, fiber, fat, fatty acids, cholesterol, protein, and amino acids (macronutrients).* Institute of Medicine of the National Academies, Washington, DC: National Academies Press, 2005.

5. Vega-Galvez A and others: Nutrition facts and functional potential of quinoa (Chenopodium quinoa willd.), an ancient Andean grain: A review. *Journal of Science & Food Agriculture* 90(15):2541, 2010.

6. Young VR: Soy protein in relation to human protein and amino acids nutrition. *Journal of the American Dietetic Association* 91(7):828, 1991.

7. Messina M: Insights gained from 20 years of soy research. *Journal of Nutrition* 140(12):2289S, 2010.

8. Otsuki M and others: Association of urine acidification with visceral obesity and the metabolic syndrome. *Endocrinology Journal* 58(5):363, 2011.

9. Tomé D, Bos C: Dietary protein and nitrogen utilization. *Journal of Nutrition* 130(7):1868S, 2000.

10. Hartman JW and others: Resistance training reduces whole-body protein turnover and improves net protein retention in untrained young males. *Applied Physiology, Nutrition, and Metabolism* 31(5):557, 2006.

11. Moore DR and others: Resistance training reduces fasted- and fed-state leucine turnover and increases dietary nitrogen retention in previously untrained young men. *Journal of Nutrition* 137(4):985, 2007.

12. U.S. Department of Agriculture Agricultural Research Service: *What We Eat in America 2009-2010.* http://www.ars.usda.gov/Services/docs.htm?docid=18349 Accessed: January 19, 2014.

13. Preis SR and others: Dietary protein and risk of ischemic heart disease in middle-aged men. *American Journal of Clinical Nutrition* 92(5):1265, 2010.

14. Bernstein AM and others: Major dietary protein sources and risk of coronary heart disease in women. *Circulation* 122(9):876, 2010.

15. Bernstein AM and others: Dietary protein sources and the risk of stroke in men and women. *Stroke* 43(3):637, 2012.

16. Kim E and others: Review of the association between meat consumption and risk of colorectal cancer. *Nutrition Reviews* 33(12):983, 2013.

17. Alexander DD and others: Meta-analysis of prospective studies of red meat consumption and colorectal cancer. *European Journal of Cancer Prevention* 20(4):293, 2011.

18. Salem S and others: Major dietary factors and prostate cancer risk: a prospective case-control study. *Nutrition & Cancer* 63(1):21, 2011.

19. Hori S and others: Prostate cancer and diet: Food for thought? *BJU International* 107(9):1348, 2011.

20. Larsson SC, Wolk A: Red and processed meat consumption and risk of pancreatic cancer: Meta-analysis of prospective studies. *British Journal of Cancer* 106(3):603, 2012.

21. Hu J and others: Salt, processed meat and the risk of cancer. *European Journal of Cancer Prevention* 20(2):132, 2011.

22. Cross AJ and others: Meat consumption and risk of esophageal and gastric cancer in a large prospective study. *American Journal of Gastroenterology* 106(3):432, 2011.

23. DiMaso M and others: Red meat and cancer risk in a network of case-control studies focusing on cooking practices. *Annals of Oncology* 24(12):3107, 2013.

24. Weikert C and others: The relation between dietary protein, calcium, and bone health in women: Results from the EPIC-Potsdam Cohort. *Annals of Nutrition & Metabolism* 49:312, 2005.

25. Busetto L and others: High-protein low-carbohydrate diets: What is the rationale? *Diabetes and Metabolism Research and Reviews* 27(3):230, 2011.

26. Bendtsen LQ and others: Effect of dairy proteins on appetite, energy expenditure, body weight, and composition: A review of the evidence from controlled clinical trials. *Advances in Nutrition* 4(4):418, 2013.

27. Marcason W: What is the effect of a high-protein diet on bone health? *Journal of the American Dietetic Association* 110(5):812, 2010.

28. Wakefield AP and others: A diet with 35% of energy from protein leads to kidney damage in female Sprague-Dawley rats. *British Journal of Nutrition* 106(5):656, 2011.

29. Tipton KD: Efficacy and consequences of very-high-protein diets for athletes and exercisers. *Proceedings of the Nutrition Society* 70(2):205, 2011.

30. World Health Organization: *Data and Statistics.* Updated January 2014. http://www.who.int/research/en/ Accessed: January 19, 2014.

31. World Health Organization: *Management of the child with a serious infection or severe malnutrition.* Department of Child and Adolescent Health and Development. Geneva, Switzerland: WHO, 2000. http://www.who.int/child_adolescent_health/documents/fch_cah_00_1/en/ Accessed: January 19, 2014.

32. Grover Z, Ee LC: Protein energy malnutrition. *Pediatric Clinics of North America* 56(5):1055, 2009.

33. Manary M: Protein source and quality in therapeutic foods affect the immune response, outcome in severe malnutrition. *Food and Nutrition Bulletin* 34(2):256, 2013.

34. American Academy of Allergy, Asthma, and Immunology (AAAAI): *Food Allergy* http://www.aaaai.org/media/statistics/allergy-statistics.asp#foodallergy Accessed: January 19, 2104.

35. Niggemann B, Gruber C: Unproven diagnostic procedures in IgE-mediated allergic diseases. *Allergy* 59(8):806, 2004.

36. U.S. Food and Drug Administration: *Food Allergen Labeling and Consumer Protection Act of 2004 (Public Law 108-282, Title II).* Updated February 2013. http://www.fda.gov/food/guidanceregulation/guidancedocumentsregulatoryinformation/allergens/ucm106187.htm Accessed: January 19, 2014.

37. Vally H and others: Clinical effects of sulphite additives. *Clinical and Experimental Allergy* 39(11):1643, 2009.

38. U.S. Food and Drug Administration: *CRF: Code of Federal Regulations, Title 21 (volume 2), Subpart G, exemptions from food labeling requirements. Section 101.100.* Updated June 2013. http://www.accessdata.fda.gov/scripts/cdrh/cfdocs/cfcfr/CFRSearch.cfm?CFRPart=101&showFR=1&subpartNode=21:2.0.1.1.2.7 Accessed: January 19, 2014.

39. National Institutes of Health, U.S. Department of Health and Human Services, National Human Genome Research Institute: *Learning about phenylketonuria (PKU).* Updated January 2012. http://www.genome.gov/pfv.cfm?pageID=25020037 Accessed: January 19, 2014.

40. Centers for Disease Control and Prevention: Newborn screening can help prevent problems. Updated August 2011. http://www.cdc.gov/Features/NewbornScreening/ Accessed: January 19, 2014.

41. U.S. National Library of Medicine and the National Institutes of Health: *Medical encyclopedia: Phenylketonuria.* Updated June, 2013. http://www.nlm.nih.gov/medlineplus/ency/article/001166.htm Accessed: January 19, 2014.

42. National Institutes of Health, National Digestive Diseases Information Clearinghouse: *Celiac disease.* Last updated January 2012. http://digestive.niddk.nih.gov/ddiseases/pubs/celiac/ Accessed: January 19, 2014.

43. Carroccio A and others: Non-celiac wheat sensitivity is a more appropriate label than non-celiac gluten sensitivity. *Gastroenterology* 146(1):320, 2014.

44. Bongiovanni TR and others: Impact of gluten-free camp on quality of life of children and adolescents with celiac disease. *Pediatrics* 125(3):e525, 2010.

45. Food and Drug Administration. *What is gluten-free? FDA has an answer.* Updated August 2013. http://www.fda.gov/ForConsumers/ConsumerUpdates/ucm363069.htm#gluten-free Accessed: January 19, 2014.

46. National Institute of Mental Health, National Institutes of Health: *Autism spectrum disorders.* http://www.nimh.nih.gov/health/topics/autism-spectrum-disorders-pervasive-developmental-disorders/index.shtml Accessed: January 19, 2014.

47. Centers for Disease Control and Prevention: *Autism spectrum disorders: Data and statistics.* Updated December 2013. http://www.cdc.gov/ncbddd/autism/data.html Accessed: January 19, 2014.

48. Whitely P and others: Gluten- and casein-free dietary intervention for autism spectrum conditions. *Frontiers in Human Neuroscience* 6:344, 2013.

49. Hjiej H and others: Substitutive and dietetic approaches in childhood autistic disorder: Interests and limits. *Encephale* 34(5):496, 2008.

50. Gaesser GA, Angadi SS: Gluten-free diet: Imprudent dietary advice for the general population? *Journal of the Academy of Nutrition and Dietetics* 112(9):1330, 2012.

51. American Dietetic Association: Position of the American Dietetic Association: Vegetarian diets. *Journal of the American Dietetic Association* 109(7):1266, 2009.

52. McEvoy CT and others: Vegetarian diets, low-meat diets and health: A review. *Public Health Nutrition* 15(12):2287, 2012.

53. Kahleova H and others: Vegetarian diet improves insulin resistance and oxidative stress markers more than conventional diet in subjects with Type 2 diabetes. *Diabetic Medicine* 28(5):549, 2011.

54. Craig WJ: Health effects of vegan diets. *American Journal of Clinical Nutrition* 89(5):1627S, 2009.

55. American Dietetic Association: Position of the American Dietetic Association, Dietitians of Canada, and the American College of Sports Medicine: Nutrition and Athletic Performance. *Journal of the American Dietetic Association* 109:509S, 2009.

56. Watanabe F: Vitamin B-12 sources and bioavailability. *Experimental Biology & Medicine* 232:1266, 2007.

57. Chisholm K: Vegetarian diets in children. *Advance for Nurse Practitioners and Physician Assistants* 2(1):39, 2011.

58. Anon: Neurologic impairment in children associated with maternal dietary deficiency of cobalamin—Georgia, 2001. *Morbidity and Mortality Weekly Report* 52(4):61, 2003.

59. Prasad C and others: Introducing nutritional genomics teaching in undergraduate dietetic curricula. *Journal of Nutrigenetics and Nutrigenomics* 4(3):165, 2011.

60 Neeha VS, Kinth P: Nutrigenomics research: A review. *Journal of Food Science and Technology* 50(3):415, 2013.

61. Saukko PM and others: Negotiating the boundary between medicine and consumer culture: Online marketing of nutrigenetic tests. *Social Science and Medicine* 70:744, 2010.

62. Cormier H and others: Nutrigenomics—perspectives from registered dietitians: A report from the Quebec-wide e-consultation on nutrigenomics among registered dietitians. *Journal of Human Nutrition and Dietetics* 27(4): 391, 2014

8 Metabolism

Very-low-carbohydrate diet

TO CONTROL HER WEIGHT, Louisa began following a very-low-carbohydrate diet that supplied, on average, less than 5% of her daily kilocalories from carbohydrates. Louisa, however, did not change her daily caloric intake, which averaged 1600 kcal per day. Compared to her previous diet, her new diet emphasized lean meats and healthy fats. After following the very-low-carbohydrate diet for 4 weeks, Louisa has reported experiencing extreme fatigue. Several of her friends have noted that her breath smells fruity, similar to fingernail polish remover.

- Why has Louisa been experiencing extreme fatigue and fruity breath? Explain why her body needs some glucose. How has Louisa's metabolism changed since she stopped eating her usual mixed-macronutrient diet of approximately 55% carbohydrates, 30% fat, and 15% protein?

The suggested Case Study Response can be found on page 263.

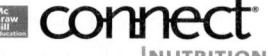 Check out the Connect site at www.mcgrawhillconnect.com to further explore this case study.

QUIZ Yourself

How does the body obtain energy? Can carbohydrates and proteins be converted to and stored as fat? What role do vitamins play in generating energy? Test your knowledge of energy metabolism by taking the following quiz. The answers are provided on page 265.

1. Fats are metabolized by a process called glycolysis. __T __F

2. Many B vitamins are components of coenzymes that work with enzymes in energy metabolism. __T __F

3. Lactate is a molecule that accumulates in tissues when oxygen is not available. __T __F

4. Following an overnight fast, insulin stimulates the liver cells to increase glucose production. __T __F

5. Body size, sex, and age affect an individual's metabolism of alcohol. __T __F

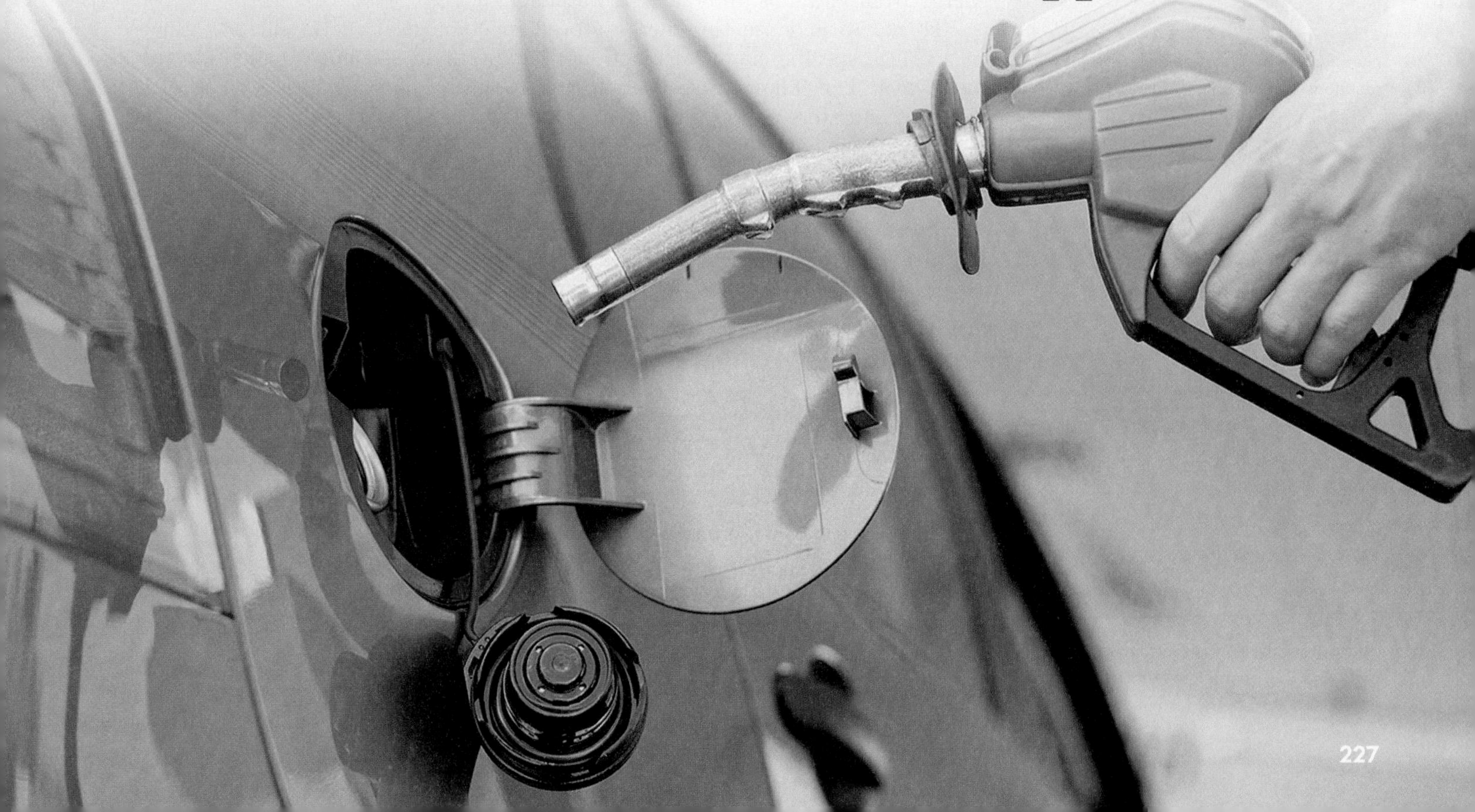

8.1 Fueling the Body

LEARNING OUTCOMES

1 *List at least three forms of energy.*
2 *Identify the sources of energy for the human body.*

What if you were in charge of designing a more efficient car engine—a machine that runs continuously? To run continuously and efficiently, your new gasoline—powered engine will need an unlimited supply of high—quality fuel, which will be stored in the car's gas tank. The tank will need to be refilled when the gas runs out. Finally, your engine has many small parts that must work together precisely and in sequence to keep running. In essence, your body is very much like a car engine; both are complex systems that need to generate energy, store excess energy until needed, and maintain a proper running temperature.

In this chapter, we discuss how the human body obtains the energy it needs by extracting it from macronutrient fuels. We also discuss alcohol and how the body obtains energy from this nonnutrient.

What Is Energy?

energy the capacity to perform work.

Energy is the capacity to perform work. Energy has many forms, includ—ing chemical, mechanical, electrical, heat, solar, and nuclear energy. The total amount of energy in a system is constant; that is, energy can neither be created nor destroyed. However, energy can undergo *transformations*. Chemical energy, for example, can change into heat energy, which explains why a car's engine heats up as it burns gasoline and muscles warm up during exercise.

The cells in the human body release, transfer, and use energy constantly. Human cells obtain energy by releasing the chemical energy that is stored in macronutrients and alcohol. It is important to remember that only carbohy—drates, lipids, proteins, and alcohol can be utilized for energy; cells cannot release energy from vitamins, minerals, or water.

chemical pathways specific chemical reactions that occur in sequences

To access and use the energy stored in "biological fuels" such as glucose, cells utilize specific chemical reactions that occur in sequences called **chemical pathways**. The following sections focus on the primary pathways that release, transfer, and store energy in human cells. We begin by providing a basic over—view about the components of energy metabolism.

ASSESS YOUR PROGRESS

1 *Identify substances that the human body can use as fuel.*
2 *Which form of energy is stored in macronutrients?*

8.2 Energy Metabolism

LEARNING OUTCOMES

1 *Compare and contrast anabolic and catabolic reactions.*
2 *Identify nutrients that act as coenzymes in energy metabolism.*
3 *Discuss ATP, including why it is important, and where it is made.*

energy metabolism involves the chemical pathways that enable the human body to obtain and use energy from macronutrients and alcohol

Metabolism is the sum of all chemical reactions that occur in living cells, including the reactions that release energy from biological fuels, synthesize proteins, and eliminate waste products. **Energy metabolism** involves the chemical pathways that enable the human body to obtain and use energy from macronutrients and alcohol. Metabolic reactions may be catabolic or anabolic.

Catabolism (*cah−ta−bo′−lizm*) refers to metabolic pathways that break down larger molecules into smaller ones (Fig. 8.1). Examples of catabolic reactions include the breakdown of glucose, fatty acid, and amino acid molecules to form carbon dioxide (CO_2) and water (H_2O). Catabolic reactions are considered "downhill," because they result in the release of more energy than is used to initiate the reactions. Heat comprises some of the energy that is released: "Heat of metabolism" helps the body maintain its normal temperature. Cells use the remaining energy to power chemical reactions.

Anabolism (*a−nah−bo′−lizm*) refers to metabolic pathways that build larger molecules from smaller ones (Fig. 8.2). Anabolic reactions include building glycogen from glucose molecules, triglycerides from glycerol and free fatty acids, and proteins from amino acids. Anabolic reactions are "uphill," because they require the input of more energy than is released by the reactions. The newly formed molecules store this extra "input" energy for later use by the body.

The Roles of Enzymes and Coenzymes

Most chemical reactions that occur in living cells require specific enzymes that facilitate (*catalyze*) the reactions, but the enzymes remain unchanged as a result of the process. Reactions involved in metabolic pathways also require the activity of specific enzymes.

Enzymes generally will not catalyze reactions without the help of cofactors. Many vitamins and minerals function as cofactors. **Coenzymes** are a particular group of organic cofactors that often have B vitamins in their chemical structures. Coenzymes that contain the B vitamins thiamin, riboflavin, niacin, pantothenic acid, and vitamin B−6 participate in several of the reactions that release energy from macronutrients. Table 8.1 lists these B vitamins and their coenzymes.

NAD⁺ and FAD

During certain catabolic processes, macronutrient molecules release hydrogen ions (H^+) that contain *high−energy electrons* (e^-). Two different coenzymes accept and transport the ions. These particular coenzymes have forms of the B vitamins niacin or riboflavin in their chemical structures (Table 8.1). Niacin is a component of the coenzyme **nicotinamide adenine dinucleotide** (**NAD⁺**) (*nik′−o−tin′−ah−mide a′−deh−neen di−new′−cle−o−tide*). When NAD⁺ picks up two hydrogen ions and two electrons, the coenzyme becomes *NADH + H⁺* (Fig. 8.3). For simplification, we may use *NADH* for NADH + H⁺. Riboflavin is a component of the coenzyme **flavin adenine dinucleotide (FAD)** (*fla′−vin a′−deh−neen di−new′−cle−o−tide*). FAD can pick up two hydrogen ions along with two electrons. When this reaction occurs, FAD becomes *FADH₂* (Fig. 8.3b). NAD⁺ and FAD shuttle hydrogen ions and electrons to a place within cells where their energy can be extracted.

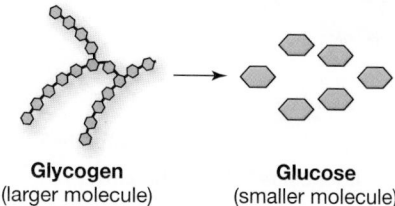

FIGURE 8.1 Catabolic reaction.

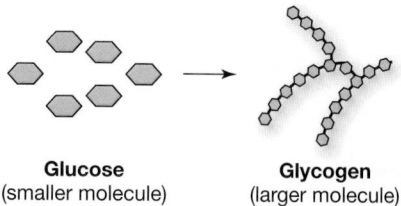

FIGURE 8.2 Anabolic reaction.

catabolism refers to metabolic pathways that break down larger molecules into smaller ones

anabolism refers to metabolic pathways that build larger molecules from smaller ones

coenzymes group of organic cofactors that often have B vitamins in their chemical structures

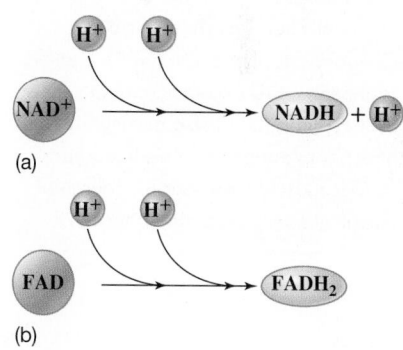

FIGURE 8.3 **NAD⁺ and FAD.** NAD⁺ and FAD shuttle hydrogen ions and electrons to a place within cells where their energy can be extracted.

nicotinamide adenine dinucleotide (NAD⁺) niacin-containing coenzyme

flavin adenine dinucleotide (FAD) riboflavin-containing coenzyme

TABLE 8.1 B Vitamins and Their Coenzymes

B Vitamin	Coenzyme
Thiamin	Thiamin pyrophosphate (TPP)
Riboflavin	Flavin adenine dinucleotide (FAD, FADH₂, FMN)
Niacin	Nicotinamide adenine dinucleotide (NAD⁺, NADH, NADP)
Pantothenic acid	Coenzyme A (CoA)
Vitamin B-6	Pyridoxal phosphate (PLP)

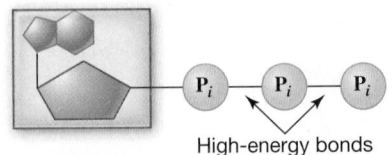

Adenosine Triphosphate (ATP)

FIGURE 8.4 Adenosine triphosphate (ATP).

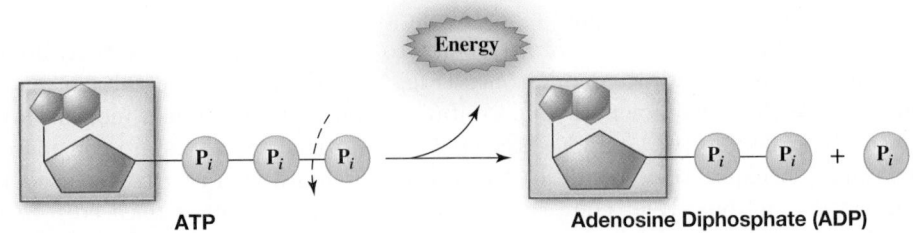

FIGURE 8.5 Forming ADP from ATP. ATP is converted to ADP when the last high-energy bond is cleaved.

ATP (Adenosine Triphosphate)

Most of the energy released by the break down of macronutrients is captured in chemical form as **adenosine triphosphate** ($a-den'-uh-seen\ try-fos'-fate$) **(ATP)**. Figure 8.4 shows that ATP is comprised of adenosine bound to three ($tri-$) inorganic phosphate groups (P_i).

ATP is a high–energy phosphate compound. When an enzyme "cleaves" (breaks) the bond between the last two phosphate groups of ATP, the high–energy molecule loses some of its power. Cells can use the energy released in this reaction for anabolic activities. When ATP loses its terminal phosphate group, it becomes **adenosine *di*phosphate (ADP)** (Fig. 8.5). Note that ADP has adeno–sine bound to two ($di-$) inorganic phosphate groups.

ATP can be re–formed by **phosphorylation**, an anabolic reaction that results in the attachment of a P_i group to ADP (Fig. 8.6). Phosphorylation reactions, however, require the input of some energy. The recycling of ATP from ADP and P_i is essential for meeting the energy demands of cells. The catabolism of macronutrients (and alcohol) supplies energy to produce ATP.

Mitochondria: The Cell's Powerhouses

The chemical pathway that initiates the breakdown of glucose and produces some ATP occurs in the cytoplasm. **Mitochondria** ($my'-toe-con'-dree-ah$; singular: *mitochondrion*) are organelles that synthesize most of the ATP that cells need to function (Fig. 8.7). Mitochondria are the "powerhouses" inside of cells that catabolize macronutrients and transfer the energy released from these molecules to ATP.

adenosine triphosphate (ATP) high-energy phosphate compound

adenosine diphosphate (ADP) molecule that forms when ATP loses its terminal phosphate group

phosphorylation anabolic reaction that results in the attachment of a P_i group to ADP

mitochondria organelles that synthesize most of the ATP that cells need to function

DID **YOU** KNOW?

ATP and ADP are not the only sources of chemical energy that cells use. *Guanosine* triphosphate (GTP), *uridine* triphosphate (UTP), and *cytidine* triphosphate (CTP) also participate in phosphorylation reactions. In addition to ATP, muscles use another source of chemical energy, *creatine phosphate*.

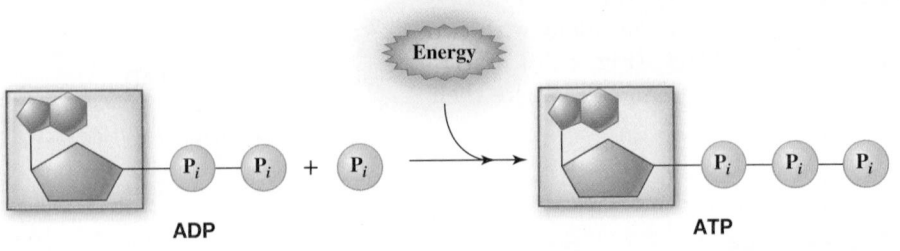

FIGURE 8.6 Forming ATP from ADP. ADP can be converted back to ATP by the addition of a phosphate group.

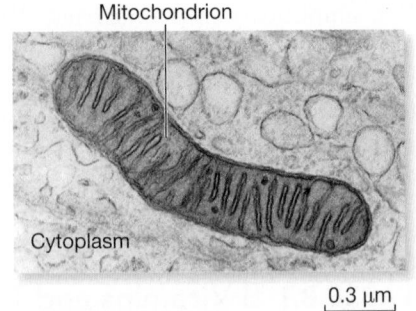

FIGURE 8.7 Mitochondrion.

ASSESS YOUR PROGRESS

3 *Explain the difference between catabolism and anabolism.*

4 *What is a coenzyme?*

5 *What is ATP, and what is its role in living cells?*

8.3 Obtaining Energy from Carbohydrate

LEARNING OUTCOMES

1 *Discuss the main chemical pathways of carbohydrate catabolism.*

2 *Describe the metabolism of carbohydrates under anaerobic and aerobic conditions.*

3 *Explain glycogenolysis and describe how carbohydrates are stored in the human body.*

Have you ever had to run across campus to get to your next class on time? You may be able to run at full speed for only about 30 to 120 seconds. At that point, you are likely to be "out of breath" and unable to continue running so quickly. You have to slow down because the availability of oxygen determines the amount of ATP that can be produced by cells. You are unable to sustain the intense physical activity when your lungs and circulatory system cannot deliver enough oxygen to your muscle cells to support adequate ATP synthesis for running.

When adequate oxygen is present in a cell, mitochondria can make lots of ATP **(aerobic metabolism)**. When the cell's oxygen supply is inadequate to support the functioning of mitochondria, the cell can still obtain ATP by using a pathway that does not require oxygen **(anaerobic metabolism)**. Compared to aerobic metabolism, however, the amount of energy made under low−oxygen conditions is much less.

Carbohydrate Catabolism

Under normal conditions, human cells rely heavily on glucose to function prop−erly. Cells in the central nervous system (CNS) are highly dependent on glucose, rather than fatty acids or amino acids, to meet their energy needs. If glucose is unavailable, however, most cells are resourceful in that they can metabolize more than one fuel for energy. Although we focus on glucose catabolism, cells can also use fructose and galactose to synthesize ATP, particularly in the liver.

Glycolysis: Glucose to Pyruvate

The first phase of glucose catabolism occurs in a series of chemical reac−tions called **glycolysis** (*glyco* = glucose, *lysis* = breakdown). Glycolysis ultimately leads to ATP production from the *oxidation* of glucose. Oxidation involves the loss of electrons during chemical reactions. In many instances, oxygen participates in oxidative reactions by chemically combining with a substance.

Glycolysis is an anaerobic pathway that occurs in the cytoplasm of cells. In a series of chemical reactions, the six−carbon glucose molecule is converted into two three−carbon molecules of **pyruvate** (*pie′−ru−vate*), which is also known as *pyruvic acid* (Fig. 8.8). During this process, two NADH and four ATP molecules form. Several steps in the *glycolytic* pathway can flow in either direction. In most cells, however, pyruvate cannot be used to re−form glucose, because the cells lack the unique set of enzymes that are required for reversing the glycolytic pathway.

A car needs a spark (energy) from the battery to start its engine. In cells, energy from two ATP molecules is the "spark" required to initiate the catabolism of a glucose molecule and crank up our "metabolic engine." Although glycolysis uses two ATP to get started, the process forms four ATP. By subtracting the two ATP needed to spark glycolysis from the four ATP that are formed, the cell gains only two ATP (4 ATP produced − 2 ATP used = 2 ATP gained). Thus, glycolysis does not provide much ATP.

aerobic metabolism ATP production that occurs in the presence of oxygen

anaerobic metabolism metabolic pathways that do not require oxygen

glycolysis first phase of glucose catabolism

pyruvate three-carbon molecule that results from the breakdown of glucose during glycolysis

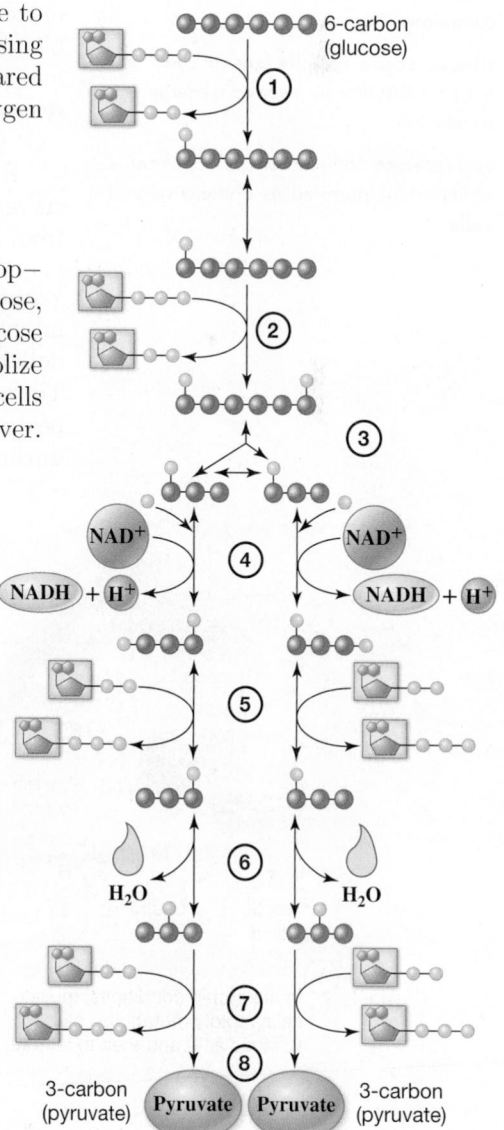

FIGURE 8.8 Glycolysis.

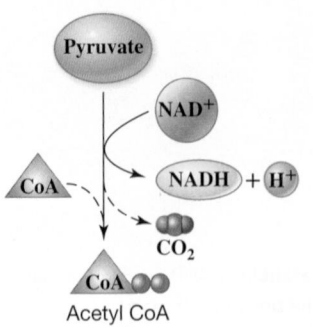

FIGURE 8.9 Conversion of pyruvate to acetyl CoA.

acetyl coenzyme A two-carbon molecule formed from pyruvate

lactic acid three-carbon molecule that forms from pyruvate under anaerobic conditions

citric acid cycle complex series of chemical reactions that that are involved in energy metabolism

oxaloacetate four-carbon molecule that is an important intermediate of the citric acid cycle

Pyruvate's Fate

Human cells use pyruvate in two major ways, depending on the availability of oxygen. When the body has access to plenty of oxygen, the pyruvate molecules enter mitochondria. Within a mitochondrion, pyruvate undergoes conversion into a two−carbon compound, **acetyl coenzyme A** (Fig. 8.9). Acetyl coenzyme A is often referred to simply as "acetyl CoA." Because glycolysis resulted in the formation of two pyruvate molecules, two molecules of acetyl CoA can be formed from one molecule of glucose (see Fig. 8.8).

The coenzymes NAD^+, coenzyme A, and thiamin pyrophosphate ("TPP") are needed to form acetyl CoA from pyruvate. During the formation of acetyl CoA, pyruvate releases a molecule of CO_2 and two hydrogen ions that are picked up by NAD^+. This reaction is irreversible: Acetyl CoA cannot be used to re−form pyruvate. Thus, the formation of acetyl CoA is the "point of no return" for glucose catabolism.

Anaerobic Conditions: Pyruvate to Lactate Under anaerobic conditions, each molecule of pyruvate converts to **lactic acid**, another three−carbon molecule. Lactic acid releases two H^+, forming lactate as a result (Fig. 8.10). Cells, espe−cially vigorously contracting muscles, release lactate into the bloodstream.

What happens to the lactate? Muscle cells lack the enzymes necessary to make glucose from lactate, so the three−carbon compound is released into the bloodstream. Liver cells remove the lactate from the bloodstream and recycle it into glucose, using a pathway called the *Cori cycle* (Fig. 8.10). After the liver releases the newly made glucose into circulation, it is available again as fuel for cells (lactate shuttle).

Recall that glycolysis results in the production of two ATP. The Cori cycle is an energy−requiring pathway in that it requires the energy of six ATP to make glucose from lactate. Therefore, the Cori cycle is too inefficient to continue indefinitely.

What Is "Oxygen Debt"? The body's need for oxygen increases after a bout of intense physical activity, such as sprinting or lifting weights. *Oxygen debt*, a deficiency of oxygen in the body, occurs as a result of the vigorous exercise. To "pay off" the debt, cells needs extra oxygen ("recovery oxygen" or "excess postexercise oxygen consumption") to recycle the lactic acid that accumulated during exercise.[1]

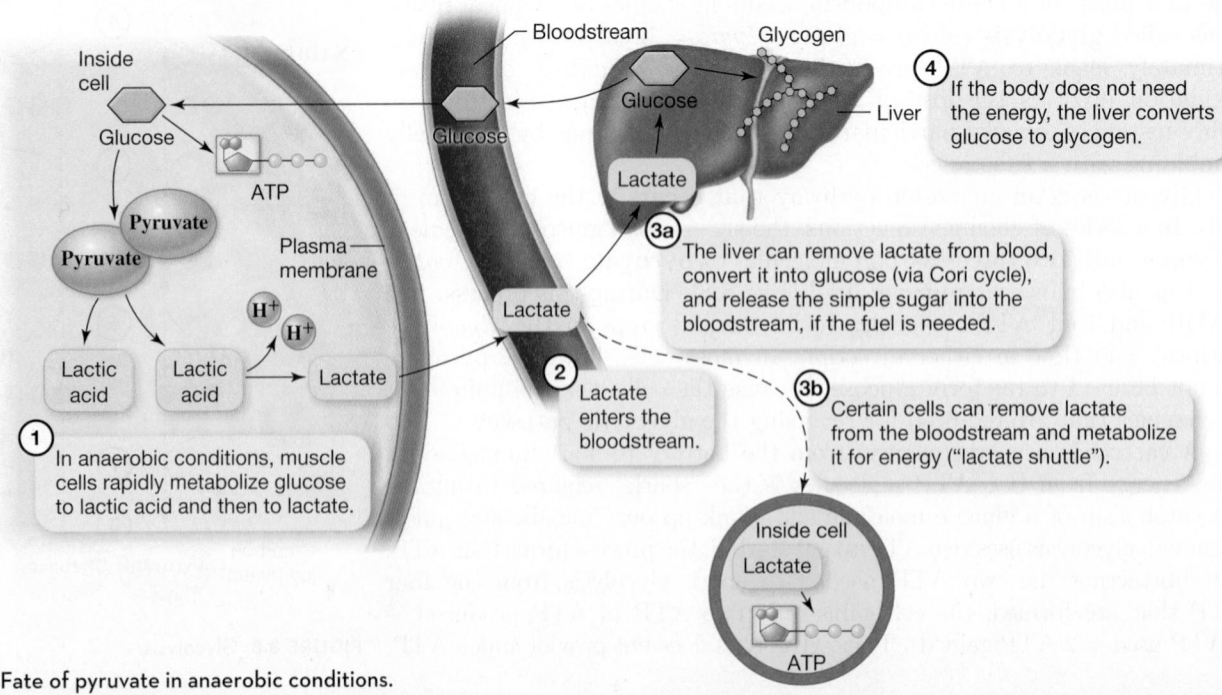

FIGURE 8.10 Fate of pyruvate in anaerobic conditions.

Oxygen debt contributes to fatigue and muscle soreness, and the need for extra oxygen can last several hours after the intense exercise ceases. Athletes, however, can often minimize the effects of oxygen debt by training properly.

Coenzymes: Health and Nutrition Significance

The chemical reactions that oxidize (breakdown) glucose to produce ATP are significant from a nutritional and health standpoint. The water—soluble B vitamins thiamin, pantothenic acid, niacin, and riboflavin are components of coenzymes TPP, coenzyme A (CoA), NAD^+, and FAD, respectively. If a person's diet does not supply adequate amounts of these vitamins, his or her cells will be unable to synthesize the coenzymes necessary for catabolism. When this occurs, cells cannot convert enough pyruvate into acetyl CoA to meet their needs, and the person becomes fatigued.

The lack of acetyl CoA results in decreased ATP formation, and the signs and symptoms of thiamin, pantothenic acid, niacin, and riboflavin deficiency disorders soon become apparent. Common symptoms of these deficiencies include "lack of energy" (fatigue) and weakness, because cells are unable to metabolize macro—nutrients for energy. Chapter 10 discusses these and other B vitamins in depth.

The Citric Acid Cycle

Acetyl CoA is a key molecule in metabolism. The oxidation of acetyl CoA is the second phase of glucose catabolism. When cells need energy, acetyl CoA enters the **citric acid cycle**, which is also known as the *TCA cycle* or *Krebs cycle*. The citric acid cycle is a complex series of chemical reactions that converts the two—carbon acetyl CoA molecules into CO_2 and H_2O molecules. Much of the energy that is released in the process is ultimately captured in ATP. The following steps summarize the major changes that occur to acetyl CoA during the citric acid cycle:

1. The two—carbon acetyl CoA enters the citric acid cycle and binds to **oxaloacetate**, a four—carbon molecule. This initial reaction forms the six—carbon molecule, *citrate* (Fig. 8.11).

2. Citrate is converted to an intermediate compound that undergoes oxidation and loses a carbon atom in the form of CO_2. NAD^+ becomes NADH, and the five—carbon intermediate molecule, *alpha—ketoglutarate*, forms (Fig. 8.12).

3. Alpha—ketoglutarate undergoes oxidation, losing a carbon atom in CO_2. Once again, a NAD^+ molecule picks up hydrogen and becomes NADH (Fig. 8.13). As a result, succinyl—CoA forms.

4. During the next series of reactions, one ATP forms from *GTP* (a related compound), and the four—carbon intermediates (succinate and fumarate) release hydrogen ions that are picked up by FAD and NAD^+ (Fig. 8.14).

5. Eventually, the cycle reaches the "ending point" by re—forming the four—carbon molecule, oxaloacetate (Fig. 8.15). As a result, oxaloacetate binds with acetyl CoA, so the cycle of chemical conversions can repeat itself (see Fig. 8.11).

Each molecule of acetyl CoA goes through one cycle of the citric acid cycle (Fig. 8.16). Under normal conditions, two acetyl CoAs are available from the catabolism of the six—carbon sugar, glucose. Therefore, the citric acid cycle repeats itself once again for each glucose molecule that enters the catabolic pathway.

The most important products of chemical transforma—tion that occur during the citric acid cycle are the coenzymes that are produced. NAD^+ and FAD pick up hydrogen ions and

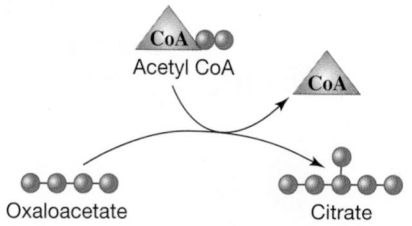

FIGURE 8.11 Citric acid cycle "starting point."

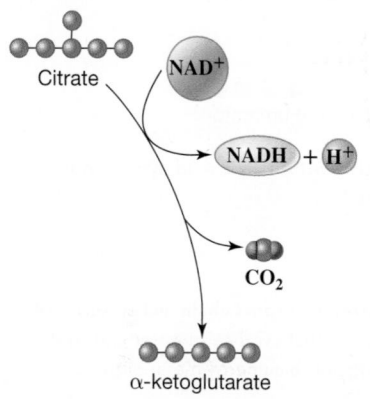

FIGURE 8.12 Forming alpha-ketoglutarate.

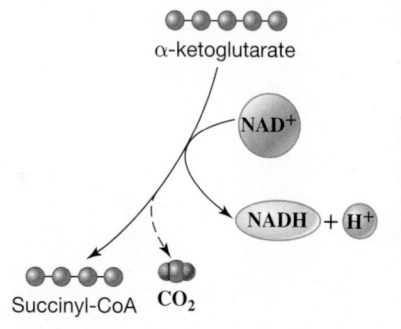

FIGURE 8.13 Alpha-ketoglutarate undergoes oxidation.

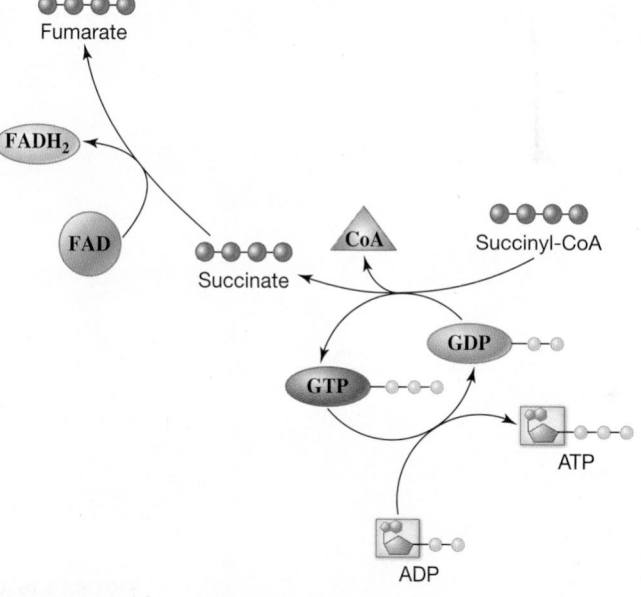

FIGURE 8.14 Succinyl-CoA to fumarate.

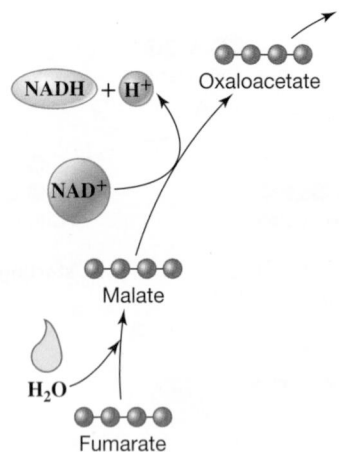

FIGURE 8.15 Citric acid cycle "ending point."

electron transport chain linked series of enzymes that synthesize water and ATP during aerobic energy metabolism

electrons. These high−energy electrons move on to the next phase of glucose catabolism and are responsible for the production of ATP.

The Electron Transport Chain

The coenzymes NADH and $FADH_2$ carry hydrogen ions and their high−energy electrons from the citric acid cycle to a linked series of enzymes called the **electron transport chain** (Fig. 8.17a). This "chain" consists of enzymes within mitochondria. The steps by which the electron transport chain produces water and ATP during aerobic energy metabolism are as follows:

1. Electrons (e^-) from the hydrogen ions are passed through the chain that includes the iron−containing *cytochromes (sigh'−toe−crowns)* (Fig. 8.17b).

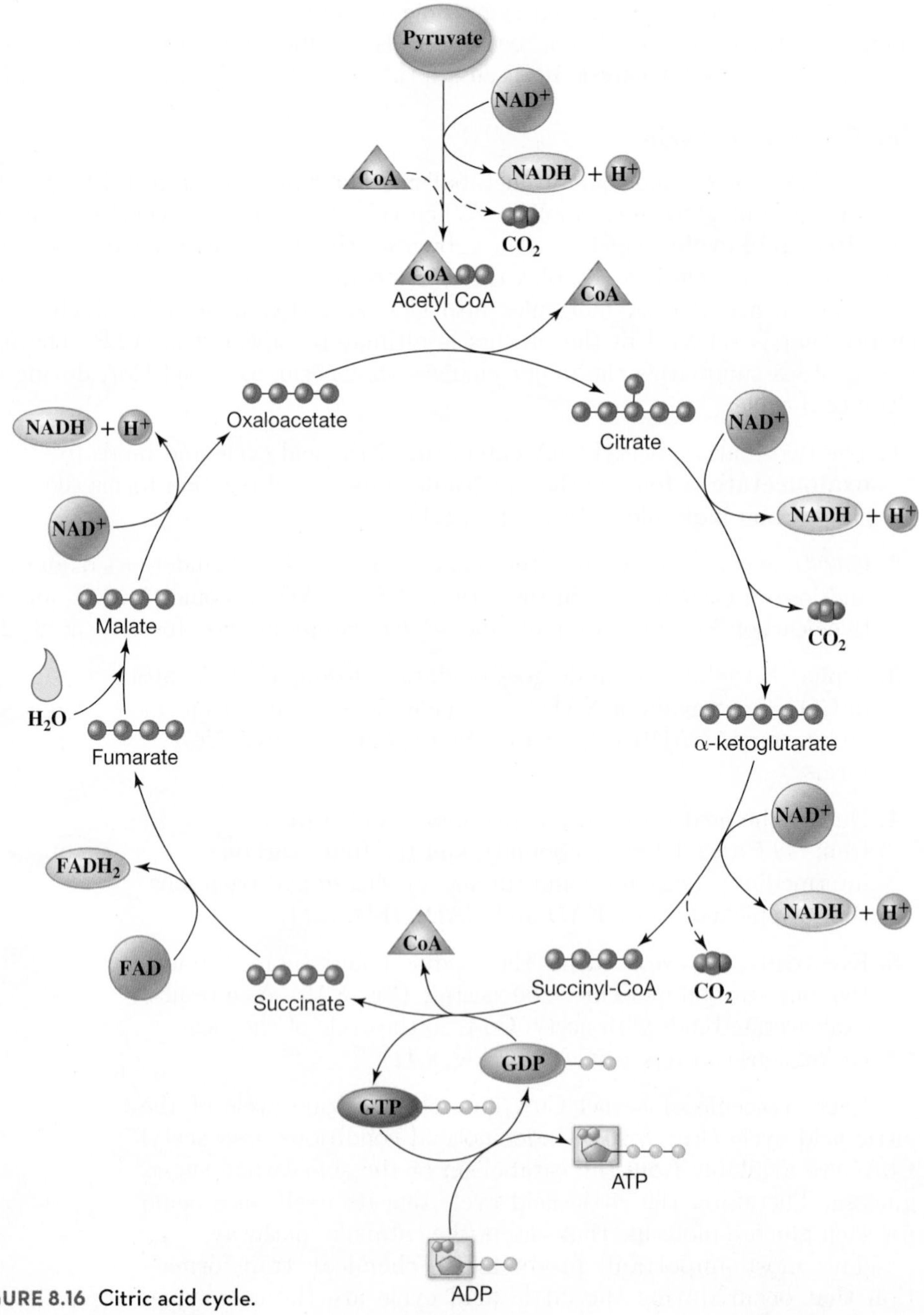

FIGURE 8.16 Citric acid cycle.

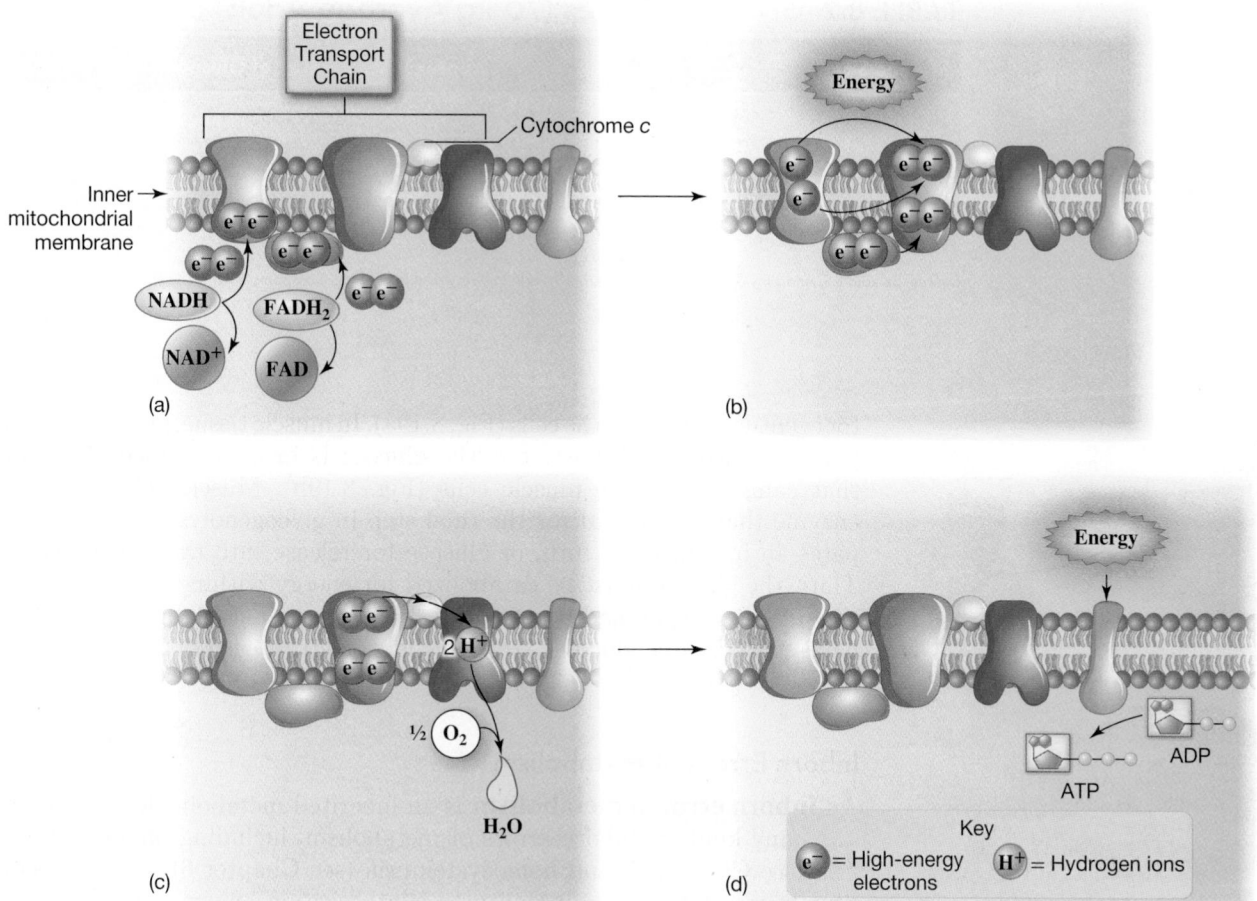

FIGURE 8.17 Electron transport chain.

2. **Cytochrome c** facilitates the bonding of two hydrogen ions (H^+) with an atom of oxygen, forming H_2O as a result (Fig. 8.17c). This H_2O may be referred to as "metabolic water" or the "water of metabolism."

3. Most important, some of the energy released during the electron transfer is used to bind a P_i group to ADP, forming ATP (Fig. 8.17d).

ATP yields for each NADH and each $FADH_2$ that enter the electron transport chain are not precisely known. Biochemists estimate the values to be approximately 2.5 ATP for NADH and 1.5 for $FADH_2$, respectively.[2] The complete catabolism of one glucose molecule yields approximately 30 to 32 molecules of ATP.[2]

Glycogenolysis

When the body needs energy but its cells do not have a direct source of glucose readily available, the cells can obtain the monosaccharide by **glycogenolysis** ($gly'-ko-jen'-ol-eh-sus$), the breakdown of glycogen into glucose molecules (Fig. 8.18). The coenzyme *pyridoxal phosphate* (*PLP*) is needed for the conversion of glycogen to glucose molecules. The liver and muscle tissue are the primary sites for glycogen storage and degradation (Table 8.2).

Liver Versus Muscle Glycogenolysis

In the liver, glycogenolysis occurs when any tissue of the body needs energy. The liver degrades its supply of glycogen and releases glucose into the bloodstream

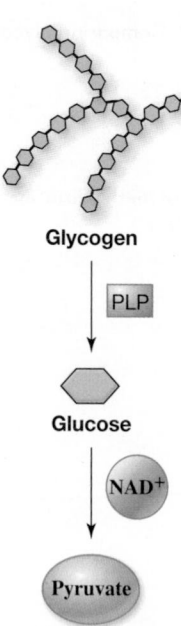

FIGURE 8.18 Glycogenolysis.

cytochrome c component of the electron transport chain

glycogenolysis pathway that breaks down glycogen into glucose molecules

TABLE 8.2 Glycogen Stores (70-kg Average Adult)

Storage Site	Approximate Amount of Glycogen (g)
Skeletal muscles	300–340
Liver	70–100
Cardiac muscle and other tissues	5–10
TOTAL	400–450

Source: Saladin KS: *Anatomy & Physiology.* 5th ed. New York: McGraw-Hill Publishing Company, 2010

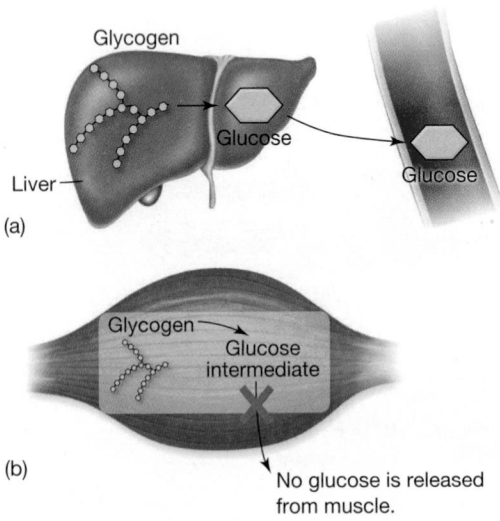

(a)

(b)

No glucose is released from muscle.

FIGURE 8.19 Comparing glycogenolysis in the liver and muscle.

inborn error of metabolism an inherited metabolic defect

gluconeogenesis synthesis of glucose from noncarbohydrate precursors

for eventual uptake by the cells (Fig. 8.19a). In muscle tissue, glycogenolysis releases glucose molecules, but the glucose is in an intermediate form that cannot leave the muscle cells (Fig. 8.19b). Muscle cells lack the enzyme that is required for the final step in glycogenolysis, which prepares an intermediate form of glucose for release into the bloodstream. Thus, the glucose must be catabolized for energy within the muscle cell where the glycogen had been stored. This adaptation enables muscles to have stockpiles of glucose (stored as glycogen) in case of a "fight—or—flight" response.

Inborn Errors of Metabolism

An **inborn error of metabolism** is an inherited metabolic defect. There are many kinds of inborn errors of metabolism, including phenylketonuria (see Chapter 7) and homocysteinuria (see Chapter 6). Such defects usually result from the inability to synthesize an enzyme needed for a chemical pathway to proceed. In some cases, the error has little or no effects on health, but in other instances, the biochemical defect is severe and its effects are *lethal* (deadly). If no effective treatment is available, babies born with severe metabolic errors often die in infancy or early childhood.

Glycogen Storage Diseases Some individuals are born with a form of glycogen storage disease (GSD), an inborn error of metabolism. Each form of GSD results from a defect that relates to an enzyme involved in carbohydrate metabolism. The cells of a person with GSD are unable to synthesize one or more of the enzymes needed to make or degrade glycogen properly. Thus, the person's muscle and/or liver cells may store improperly formed glycogen or abnormal amounts of the polysaccharide, depending on the type of GSD. As a result, abnormal glucose metabolism occurs in all cases of GSD. Signs and symptoms of the disorder include hypoglycemia (low blood glucose), fatigue, irritability, and liver and kidney enlargement.

The "Real People, Real Stories" feature on page 237 is about Andrew Tonkin, a young man who has a mild case of GSD. For more information about GSDs, visit the Association for Glycogen Storage Disease's website at www.agsdus.org.

Alternative Sources of Glucose

Glucose is such an important biological fuel, the body can make the simple sugar, primarily in the liver. **Gluconeogenesis** (*gluco* = glucose, *neo* = new, *genesis* = formation) is the synthesis of glucose from noncarbohydrate precursors that include glycerol, lactate, pyruvate, and most amino acids (Fig. 8.20). Gluconeogenesis is not the reverse of glycolysis, because some steps in the glycolytic pathway flow in only one direction: toward the citric acid cycle.

What About Energy Drinks?

Caffeine powder is available for commercial use as a food additive in soft drinks, but health food stores and Internet dietary supplement outlets also promote the product as a "thermogenic" ("fat–burner") supplement. Caffeine is a stimulant drug, because it increases the activity of the nervous system. The drug, however, can cause unpleasant side effects, including anxiety, restlessness, tremors ("the shakes"), rapid heart rate, and sleep disturbances.

Over the past few years, consumption of energy drinks that contain caffeine has grown in the United States, especially among teens and young adults. In addition to caffeine, energy drinks may contain B vitamins and other dietary supplements, including *taurine*, a derivative of the amino acid cysteine, and *guarana*, an herbal product. Guarana naturally contains caffeine and two chemically related stimulants, *theobromine* and *theophylline*. Can these ingredients actually increase energy and enhance the ability to concentrate on mental tasks?

The benefits of energy drinks do not live up to the marketing hype used to promote the products. Although caffeine increases alertness, the compound does not provide any energy (calories). Simply consuming an energy drink that contains caffeine and other naturally occurring stimulants may reduce feelings of fatigue, but it will not lead to having more energy. The body highly regulates ATP production in response to the body's energy demands and not to consumption of such products. Any beverage that contains digestible carbohydrate, such as sucrose or lactose, provides energy for the body.

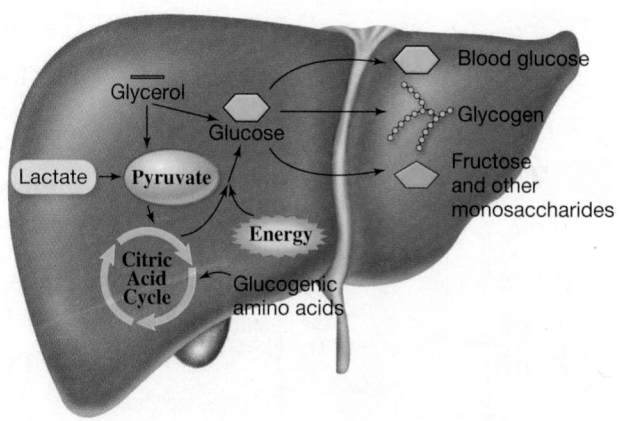

FIGURE 8.20 Gluconeogenesis.

REAL People, **REAL** Stories

Andrew Tonkin

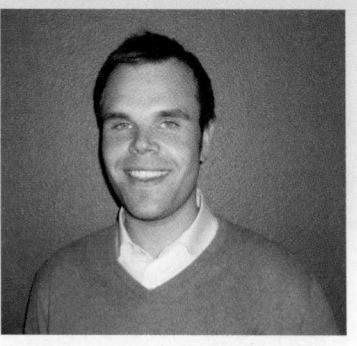

Every 4 hours that he is awake, Andrew Tonkin fixes a mixed drink for himself. Andrew's drink, however, does not contain alcohol. He carefully measures 3 tablespoons of corn starch, stirs the carbohydrate-rich powder into a cup of sugar-free sports drink, and then quickly consumes the solution. Why would someone need to drink such a concoction regularly?

Andrew was born with a form of glycogen storage disease. To maintain normal blood glucose levels throughout the day, he must regularly consume an easily but slowly digested source of glucose that is inexpensive and convenient: cornstarch. In the small intestine, cornstarch is broken down into glucose, and the molecules are absorbed into the blood, without causing a dramatic spike in blood glucose. If Andrew does not consume cornstarch every 4 hours, he begins to show signs and symptoms of low blood glucose (hypoglycemia). "It's hard to describe," he says, "but I start to feel strange—uncomfortable. But soon after I drink the cornstarch mixed with the sports drink, I feel better."

Andrew does not allow his metabolic disorder and his unusual "drinking habit" to interfere with his activities. "I am immensely grateful for the care and attention that the University of Washington's Medical Center have provided," he says. "They have truly saved my life and continue to do so." With continued treatment, Andrew's medical prognosis is excellent. "While a cure would be life-altering and amazing," he says, "what has made me successful in managing my health is accepting the dietary treatment as a way of life."

DID **YOU** KNOW?

In November 2012, the Center for Food Safety and Applied Nutrition of the U.S. Food and Drug Administration (FDA) released a safety alert that linked certain energy drinks to 92 illnesses and 13 deaths. Anyone consuming these drinks should be cautious and not exceed recommended amounts. For more information, visit http://www.fda.gov/food/ recallsoutbreaksemergencies/ safetyalertsadvisories/ucm328536.htm .

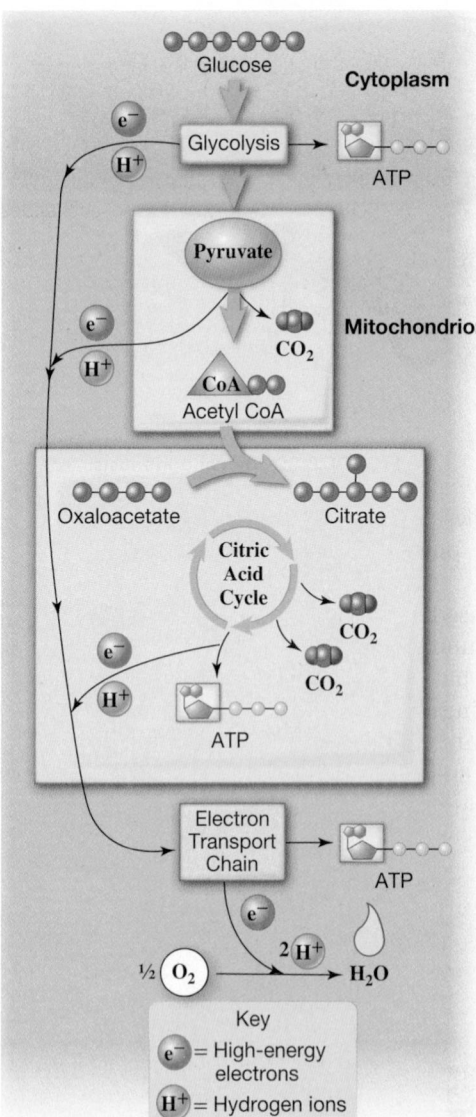

FIGURE 8.21 Catabolism of glucose for energy.

Carbohydrate Catabolism: Putting the Puzzle Together

The following points and Figure 8.21 summarize the three major events that occur in the complete breakdown of glucose that results in the production of CO_2, H_2O, and ATP.

- **Phase 1: Glycolysis**

  Under aerobic conditions, a six-carbon glucose molecule undergoes glycolysis, forming two three-carbon pyruvate molecules in the cytoplasm. Two ATP molecules are utilized, and four ATP molecules are formed in the process, for a net gain of two ATP.

  - **Pyruvate's aerobic conversion to acetyl CoA**

    The two pyruvate molecules enter a mitochondrion, and with the help of coenzyme A, each three-carbon molecule is broken down into acetyl CoA, a two-carbon molecule. During this process, NAD^+ picks up hydrogen ions to form NADH, and carbon dioxide is released.

- **Phase 2: Citric acid cycle**

  The two acetyl CoA molecules formed in the previous step undergo conversion in the citric acid cycle, combining with oxaloacetate. During the cycle, intermediates form: NAD^+ and FAD pick up hydrogen ions and their electrons to become NADH and $FADH_2$, and more CO_2 is released. Each molecule of acetyl CoA that enters the cycle results in one molecule of ATP.

- **Phase 3: Electron transport chain**

  The NADH and $FADH_2$ that were produced in earlier steps shuttle their hydrogen ions to the inner membrane of the mitochondrion, where the electron transport chain is located. The enzymes that comprise the chain pass the electrons along, releasing much of their energy in the process. Some of the energy is captured during the formation of ATP from ADP and P_i. At the end of the chain, an atom of oxygen accepts two hydrogen ions. This final reaction forms water.

ASSESS YOUR PROGRESS

6 *What is the primary advantage of aerobic metabolism over anaerobic metabolism?*

7 *Distinguish between glycolysis and the citric acid cycle, and between the citric acid cycle and the electron transport chain.*

8 *What happens in the catabolism of glucose under anaerobic conditions?*

9 *Describe the functions of NAD^+ and FAD in production of ATP.*

8.4 Obtaining Energy from Fat

LEARNING OUTCOMES

1 *Discuss beta-oxidation.*

2 *Describe how fatty acids are transformed to enter the citric acid cycle.*

3 *Describe ketogenesis, and explain why ketosis occurs in individuals with poorly controlled diabetes.*

Triglycerides are the most energy-dense macronutrient group, and the human body stores more energy in fat cells than in its glycogen stores. (Table 8.3). Fat cells (*adipocytes*) contain the enzyme **hormone sensitive lipase (HSL)**. When cells, especially muscle cells, need to catabolize fatty acids for energy, HSL facilitates *lipolysis* (*lipo* = lipids, *lysis* = breakdown) by removing the three fatty acids from the glycerol backbone of a triglyceride (Fig. 8.22). The glycerol and fatty acid molecules exit adipocytes and enter the bloodstream. The fatty acids bind to *albumin*, a protein that is water soluble and serves as a carrier molecule. Once bound to albumin, the fatty acid circulates to tissues, where it can be picked up and used for energy.

What happens to the glycerol molecules? Glycerol is chemically similar to pyruvate in that it contains three carbons. The liver can remove glycerol from the blood and convert it to pyruvate or glucose (gluconeogenesis). Glycerol catabolism, however, does not produce much ATP. Most of the energy in a triglyceride molecule is stored in its fatty acids.

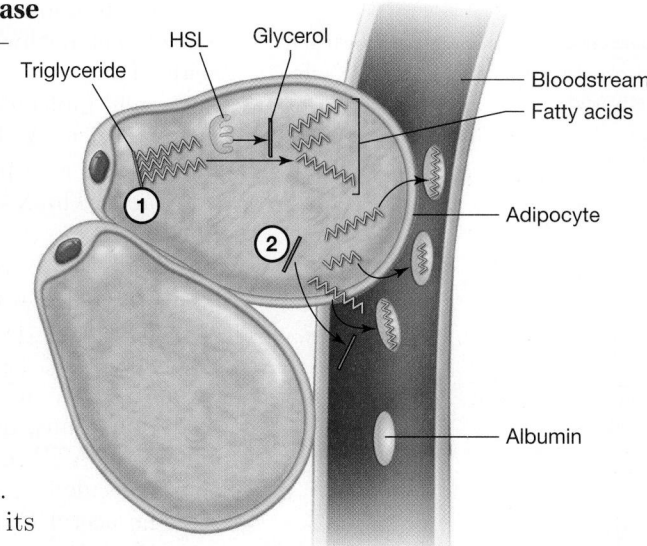

FIGURE 8.22 Lipolysis.

hormone sensitive lipase (HSL) enzyme in fat cells that removes the three fatty acids from a triglyceride

TABLE 8.3 Approximate Macronutrient Fuel Content (70-kg Adult)

Macronutrient	Fuel Content (kcal)	Approximate Percentage of Total Fuel Content
Fat	140,000	78
Protein	38,000	21
Carbohydrate	2000	1

Adapted from: Widmaier EP and others: *Vander's Human Physiology*, 12th ed. New York: McGraw-Hill Publishing Company, 2011.

Beta-Oxidation: Fatty Acids to Acetyl CoA

When certain cells, such as a muscle cell, need ATP, they can take up fatty acids from the bloodstream. Fatty acids undergo catabolism in the mitochondria. While these lipids are still in the cell's cytoplasm, they are prepared for catabolism ("activated") by binding to coenzyme A. The activation process requires energy from two ATP. After activation, fatty acids must pass through the outer and inner mitochondrial membranes with the help of a molecule called **carnitine** (Fig. 8.23).

carnitine molecule that helps fatty acids pass through the outer and inner mitochondrial membranes

FIGURE 8.23 Carnitine activity.

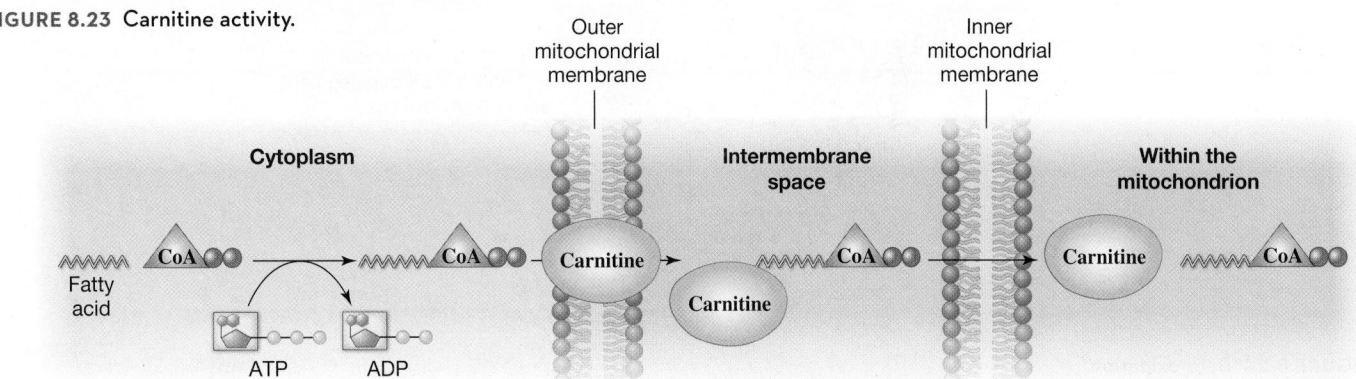

beta-oxidation chemical pathway that is involved in the catabolism of an activated fatty acid

In mitochondria, the catabolism of an activated fatty acid begins with a chemical pathway called **beta–oxidation**. Most naturally occurring fatty acids have an even number of carbon atoms. During beta–oxidation, fatty acid molecules are cleaved into two–carbon segments that are converted into acetyl CoA. Except for the final cleavage reaction, one NADH and one $FADH_2$ are also produced when a two–carbon segment is removed from the fatty acid. The NADH and $FADH_2$ that result from beta–oxidation yield about four ATP.

To illustrate what happens during beta–oxidation, we will use palmitic acid, a saturated fatty acid with 16 carbon atoms. After entering a mitochondrion, enzymes cleave the activated palmitic acid molecule repeatedly into two–carbon segments (Fig. 8.24). The fatty acid molecule yields eight acetyl CoA, seven NADH, and seven $FADH_2$ molecules as a result of undergoing beta–oxidation. Thus, beta–oxidation of palmitic acid produces about 28 ATP. That amount of ATP may not seem to be impressive, but the catabolism of the fatty acid molecule is not complete.

The acetyl CoA molecules that form during beta–oxidation enter the citric acid cycle and are catabolized to produce ATP (Fig. 8.25). Furthermore, the NADH and $FADH_2$ molecules that result from beta–oxidation and the citric acid cycle shuttle energy–containing ions to the electron transport chain to generate even more ATP. The end result: The complete oxidation of a palmitic acid molecule yields a net of 106 ATP. In comparison, the complete catabolism of a glucose molecule yields only about 30 to 32 ATP.

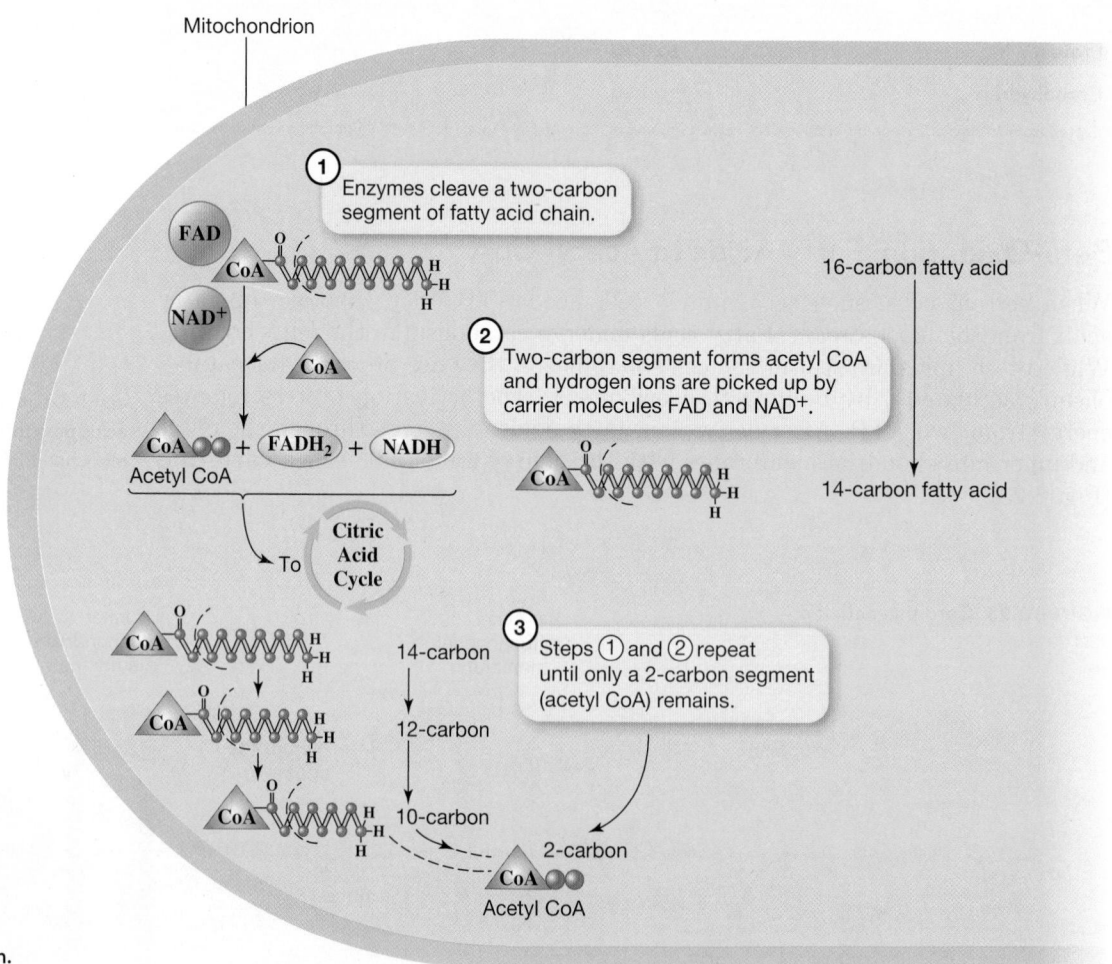

Mitochondrion

① Enzymes cleave a two-carbon segment of fatty acid chain.

FAD

NAD⁺

CoA

CoA ●● + FADH₂ + NADH
Acetyl CoA

To → Citric Acid Cycle

② Two-carbon segment forms acetyl CoA and hydrogen ions are picked up by carrier molecules FAD and NAD⁺.

16-carbon fatty acid

14-carbon fatty acid

14-carbon

12-carbon

10-carbon

③ Steps ① and ② repeat until only a 2-carbon segment (acetyl CoA) remains.

2-carbon

CoA ●●
Acetyl CoA

FIGURE 8.24 Beta-oxidation.

The fatty acids that are typically in foods contain more carbon atoms than the six–carbon glucose molecule, so fatty acids have the potential to form more acetyl CoA, NADH, and FADH$_2$ molecules during their catabolism than glucose. This chemical difference explains why an ounce of pure fat provides more energy than an ounce of pure carbohydrate. Although fatty acids have the potential to yield larger amounts of energy than glucose, human cells cannot metabolize them to make glucose. Having an adequate supply of glucose for energy is important, because red blood cells, the brain, and the nervous system rely predominately on glucose as a fuel source.

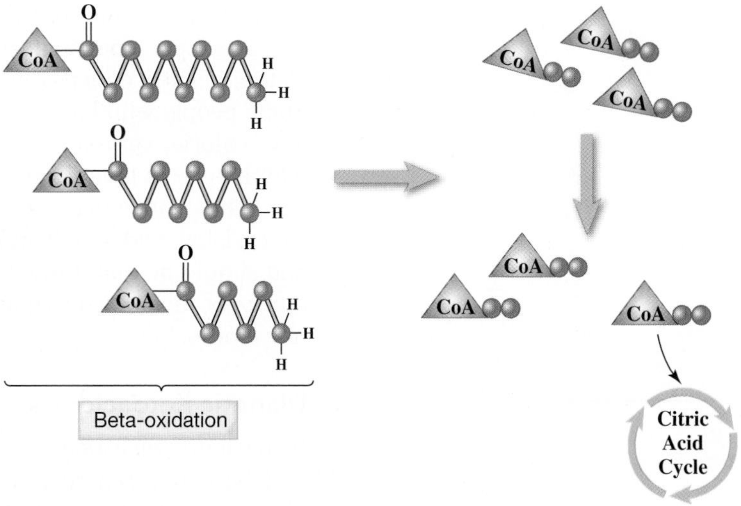

FIGURE 8.25 Fate of acetyl CoA.

"Fat Burns in a Flame of Carbohydrate"

Most cells normally oxidize glucose as their primary fuel. However, if cells do not have enough glucose to "burn" for energy, beta–oxidation of fatty acids increases, which produces excessive amounts of acetyl CoA. When this occurs, the citric acid cycle cannot use the fatty acid molecules efficiently, because the acetyl CoA molecules outnumber the oxaloacetate molecules that are available. Recall that the first step in the citric acid cycle requires acetyl CoA to bind to oxaloacetate, forming citrate (see Fig. 8.11). Normally, cells synthesize oxaloacetate from pyruvate that is derived from glycolysis (see section 8.3). Thus, a "spark" from a carbohydrate "match" helps burn fat for energy. If cells do not have enough pyruvate to make oxaloacetate for the citric acid cycle, acetyl CoA molecules that result from beta–oxidation accumulate.

What Is Ketogenesis?

When excess acetyl CoA production occurs in liver cells, the cells convert the extra molecules to *acetoacetate*, *beta–hydroxybutyrate*, and *acetone* (Fig. 8.26). These compounds, collectively referred to as ketone bodies, are released into the bloodstream. Ketone body formation is called **ketogenesis**.

Acetone is toxic to cells, but the lungs remove the compound by exhaling it. Cells, excluding liver cells, can use acetoacetate and beta–hydroxybutyrate as sources of acetyl CoA. When glucose is unavailable (such as during starvation), most cells, even brain cells, can adapt to the altered metabolic state and catabolize acetoacetate and beta–hydroxybutyrate for energy.

ketogenesis ketone body formation

ketogenic diet high-fat diet

What Is a Ketogenic Diet?

A **ketogenic diet** supplies most of its energy from fat. Such low–carbohydrate diets are often popular with people who want to lose weight. Limiting carbohydrate intake to less than 50 g per day not only rapidly depletes glycogen stores, but it also results in ketosis, the formation of excess ketone bodies. Ketosis usually causes loss of appetite, so people who are trying to lose weight may find this symptom desirable. The long–term health effects of mild ketosis are unknown. To avoid ketosis, the average person needs to consume 100 g of digestible carbohydrates per day.[3]

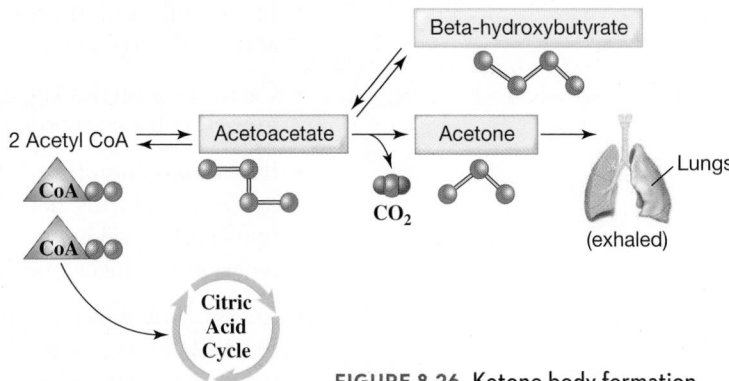

FIGURE 8.26 Ketone body formation.

Physicians may use low–calorie, ketogenic diets to treat children and adults with epilepsy, particularly in cases that do not respond well to medication. Patients with epilepsy have abnormal brain functioning that causes seizures.[4] Some people who have epilepsy are less likely to have seizures when they follow a low–calorie, very–low–carbohydrate diet, but scientists do not fully understand why ketosis is beneficial in these cases.

While following a ketogenic diet, children with epilepsy need close medical supervision and monitoring to determine whether the diet is safe and effective and should be maintained for more than a few months. Side effects of a ketogenic diet may include constipation, dehydration, micronutrient deficiencies, and kidney stones.[5]

Diabetic Ketoacidosis

In patients with poorly controlled diabetes mellitus, glucose cannot enter cells and be converted to pyruvate. Because of the lack of pyruvate, cells catabolize more fat for energy, and acetyl CoA molecules accumulate. Under these conditions, ketogenesis occurs at a rapid pace. Cells soon become overwhelmed with the "flood" of ketone bodies and cannot oxidize them fast enough to maintain normal blood chemistry. High concentrations of acetoacetate and beta–hydroxybutyrate in the bloodstream lower the blood's pH and cause **ketoacidosis**.

Ketoacidosis is a potentially life–threatening condition that requires immediate medical care. Signs and symptoms of ketoacidosis include excessive thirst, frequent urination, and a blood glucose level of more than 250 mg/dL.[6] Individuals with the condition may also have nausea, vomiting, abdominal pain, fatigue, and confusion. The breath of a person with ketoacidosis typically has a "fruity" or acetone odor; acetone is a chemical that is often in fingernail polish remover. If untreated, ketoacidosis can lead to coma (loss of consciousness) and death. Proper management of diabetes, including regular testing of blood glucose levels, is crucial for preventing ketoacidosis.[7]

ketoacidosis condition that occurs when excess acetoacetate and beta-hydroxybutyrate in the bloodstream lower the blood's pH

Fat Catabolism: Putting the Puzzle Together

The following points and Figure 8.27 summarize the major events that occur in the complete oxidation of fatty acids that results in the production of CO_2, H_2O, and ATP:

- Hormone sensitive lipase facilitates the removal of three fatty acids from the glycerol "backbone" of a triglyceride molecule. The free fatty acids enter the bloodstream and bind to albumin for transport to cells, particularly muscle cells.

  - After being transported to muscle tissues, fatty acids are released from albumin and enter the muscle cell.

- In the cell's cytoplasm, a fatty acid binds to coenzyme A, forming an activated fatty acid.

- Carnitine shuttles the activated fatty acid into the region of the mitochondrion where beta–oxidation occurs.

- In the mitochondrion, the activated fatty acid is catabolized by beta–oxidation. During beta–oxidation, the fatty acid molecule is cleaved into two–carbon segments that are converted into acetyl CoA. Each cleavage reaction produces one NADH and one $FADH_2$ molecule.

- Acetyl CoA molecules enter the citric acid cycle and undergo catabolism for ATP production. NADH and $FADH_2$ transfer electrons to the electron transport chain, where, in the final step, the electrons are accepted by oxygen, producing water and releasing energy for the synthesis of ATP.

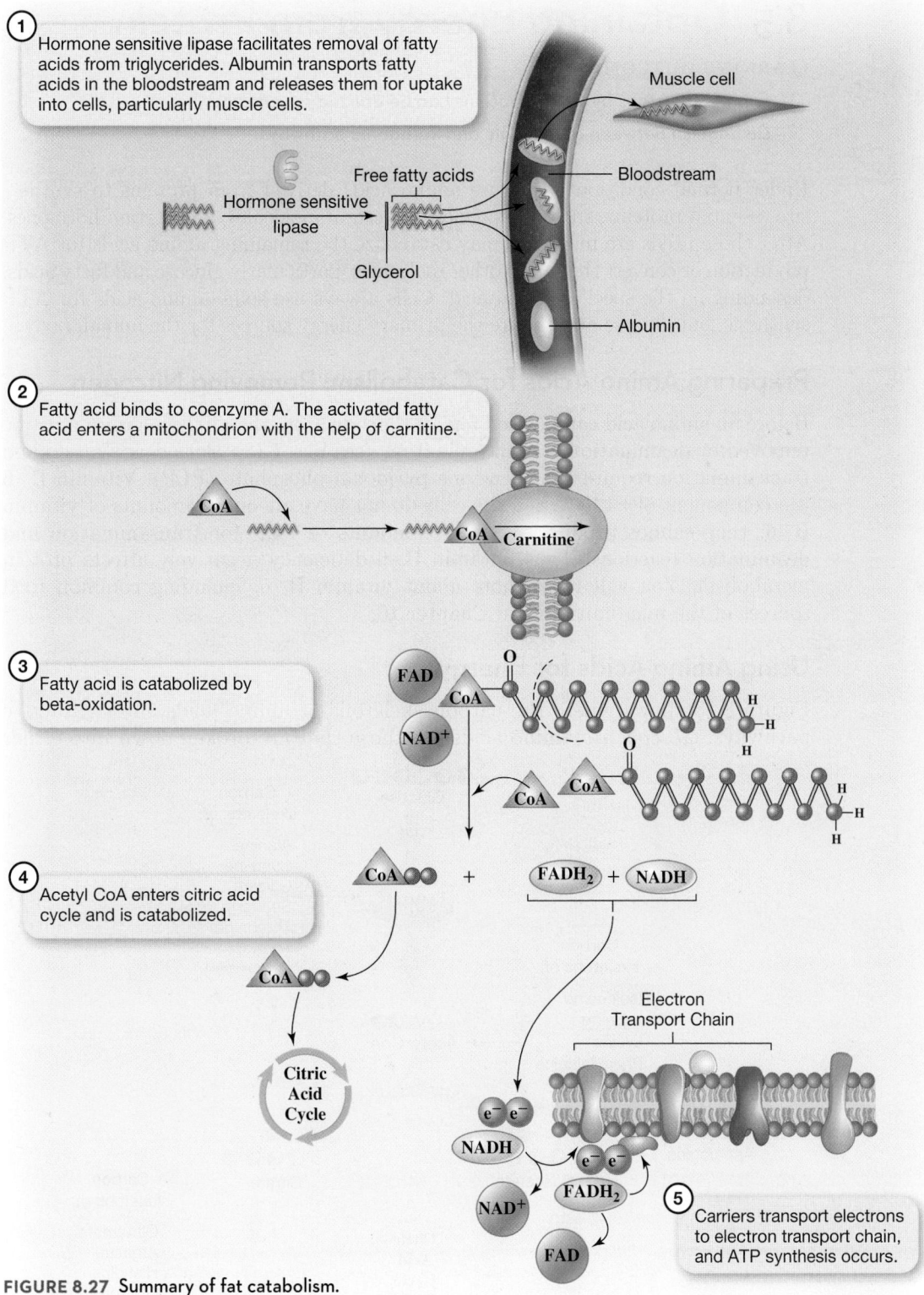

(1) Hormone sensitive lipase facilitates removal of fatty acids from triglycerides. Albumin transports fatty acids in the bloodstream and releases them for uptake into cells, particularly muscle cells.

Muscle cell

Free fatty acids

Hormone sensitive lipase

Bloodstream

Glycerol

Albumin

(2) Fatty acid binds to coenzyme A. The activated fatty acid enters a mitochondrion with the help of carnitine.

CoA

CoA Carnitine

(3) Fatty acid is catabolized by beta-oxidation.

FAD

CoA

NAD$^+$

CoA CoA

(4) Acetyl CoA enters citric acid cycle and is catabolized.

CoA + FADH$_2$ + NADH

CoA

Citric Acid Cycle

Electron Transport Chain

e$^-$ e$^-$

NADH

NAD$^+$

e$^-$ e$^-$

FADH$_2$

FAD

(5) Carriers transport electrons to electron transport chain, and ATP synthesis occurs.

FIGURE 8.27 Summary of fat catabolism.

ASSESS YOUR PROGRESS

10 *What happens to a fatty acid during beta-oxidation?*

11 *Describe how cells utilize fatty acids as a source of energy when glucose is in short supply.*

12 *Explain why ketoacidosis can occur under certain conditions.*

8.5 Obtaining Energy from Protein

LEARNING OUTCOMES

1 *Explain the steps by which proteins can be utilized for energy.*
2 *Distinguish between glucogenic and ketogenic pathways.*

Under normal conditions, cells use amino acids derived from proteins to synthe—size essential proteins, such as enzymes, structural molecules, and certain hormones. After those needs are met, cells may catabolize the remaining amino acids for ATP production or convert them into other molecules, particularly glucose and fatty acids, depending on the specific amino acid. Cells always use some amino acids for ATP synthesis, but glucose and fat are the primary energy sources for the human body.

Preparing Amino Acids for Catabolism: Removing Nitrogen

Before an amino acid can be used for ATP production, the nitrogen group must be removed by deamination or transamination (see Fig. 7.12). Both deamination and transamination require the coenzyme pyridoxal phosphate (PLP). Vitamin B—6 is a component of PLP. When the cells do not have adequate amounts of vitamin B—6, they cannot produce sufficient amounts of PLP for transamination and deamination reactions. Thus, vitamin B—6 deficiency negatively affects protein metabolism. You will learn more about vitamin B—6, including common food sources of the micronutrient, in Chapter 10.

Using Amino Acids for Energy

Figure 8.28 shows where the carbon skeletons of amino acids enter catabolic pathways. *Glucogenic* amino acids are those that are broken down into either

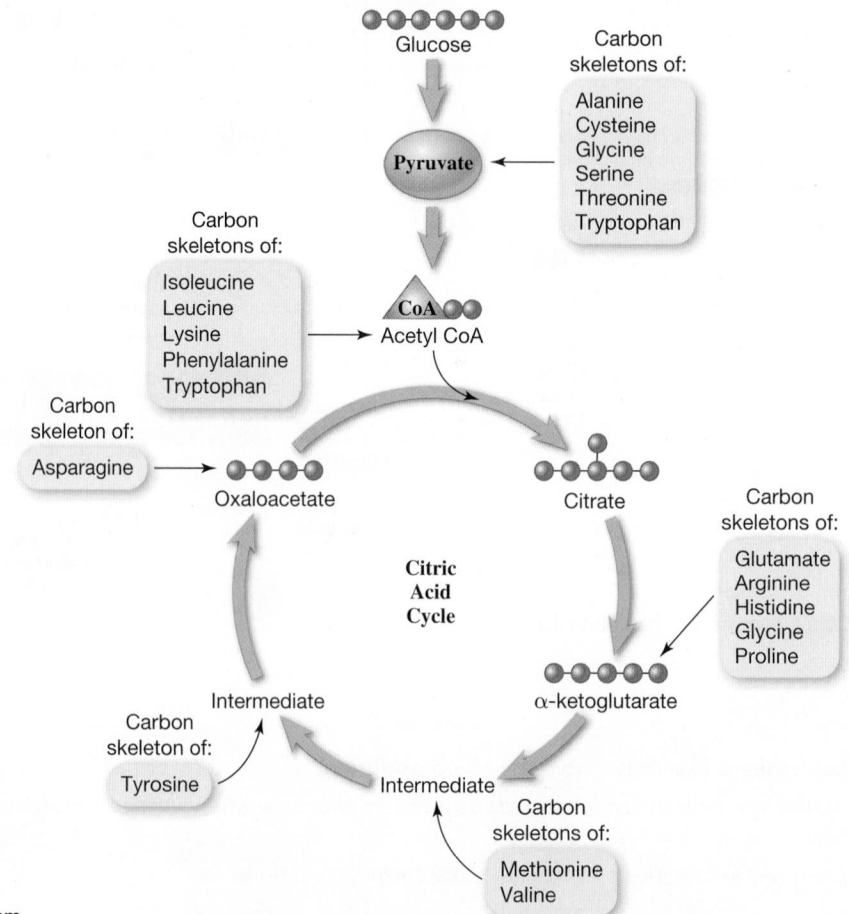

FIGURE 8.28 Amino acids and energy metabolism.

pyruvate or intermediates of the citric acid cycle. Amino acids that enter the catabolic energy pathways as acetyl CoA are *ketogenic*. The amount of ATP formed by the catabolism of a carbon skeleton depends on where it entered into the catabolism pathways. Although cells can use amino acids for producing ATP, amino acid catabolism (alanine, for example) yields less energy than the catabolism of a fatty acid (palmitic acid) or glucose molecule (Table 8.4).

Protein Catabolism: Putting the Puzzle Together

Figure 8.29 summarizes the major events that occur in the complete breakdown of amino acids that results in CO_2, H_2O, and ATP. The amount of ATP formed by the catabolism of an amino acid depends on where its carbon skeleton entered into the catabolic pathways.

ASSESS YOUR PROGRESS

13 *What process must an amino acid undergo before it can be used for energy?*

14 *Explain the differences between the glucogenic and ketogenic pathways for using proteins for energy.*

15 *Which molecule would you expect to produce the most energy: the amino acid lysine, the disaccharide maltose, or the fatty acid linoleic acid? Explain your answer.*

8.6 Energy Storage

LEARNING OUTCOMES

1 *Identify the major sites of energy storage in the body.*

2 *Describe the process by which triglycerides are stored.*

3 *Explain what happens to excess carbohydrate when glycogen stores are full.*

4 *Explain the fate of excess protein or amino acids.*

Fortunately, you do not have to eat continuously to produce ATP when you need energy. When cells have adequate amounts of ATP available and more fuel molecules than necessary to meet their immediate needs, these extra sources of energy are stored, rather than catabolized. Table 8.5 indicates the approximate energy values for glycogen and fat stores in an average healthy adult. These values may vary significantly based on body size, body composition, level of physical fitness, and diet.

What happens metabolically when you are not consuming foods, such as during sleep? Your cells make ATP by breaking down triglycerides stored in adipocytes and the glucose derived primarily from glycogen stored in liver and

TABLE 8.4 ATP Yields

Alanine → 14 ATP	
Palmitic acid → 106 ATP	
Glucose → 30–32 ATP	

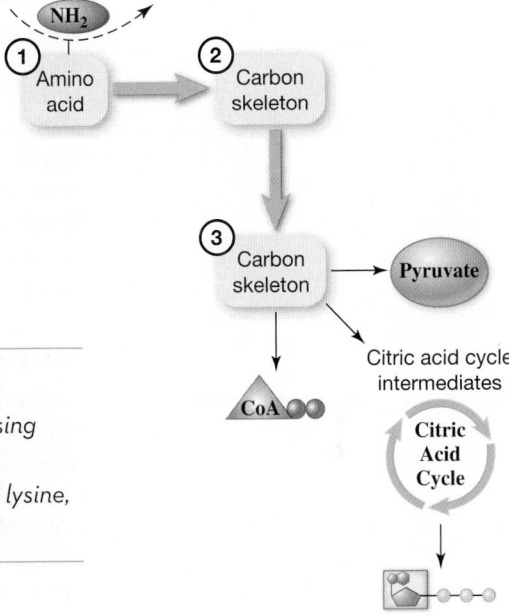

FIGURE 8.29 Summary of using amino acids for energy. (*1*) The nitrogen-containing side group of an amino acid is removed by transamination or deamination. (*2*) As a result of this reaction, a carbon skeleton forms. (*3*) The newly formed carbon skeleton can be converted into pyruvate, acetyl CoA, or an intermediate of the citric acid cycle.

TABLE 8.5 Carbohydrate and Fat: Energy Stores in the Body

Macronutrient	Storage Site and Form	Approximate kcal Stored
Carbohydrate	Liver glycogen	300–400
	Muscle glycogen	1200–1600
Fat	Adipose cell triglycerides	80,000–100,000

Adapted from: Williams MH: *Nutrition for Health, Fitness, & Sport,* 9th ed. New York: McGraw-Hill Publishing Company, 2010.

muscle cells. Although your body's proteins are abundant sources of amino acids, protein—rich tissues are not normally broken down and catabolized for energy.

Synthesizing and Storing Triglycerides

After a fatty meal, the absorption of triglycerides results in an influx of tri—glycerides into the liver. Some of the fat remains in the liver, but a considerable amount of the lipid is incorporated into very—low—density lipoproteins (VLDLs; see Fig. 6.14). After the liver releases VLDL into the bloodstream, adipocytes and other cells can access the lipoproteins' lipid contents, particularly fatty acids, through the action of lipoprotein lipase. This enzyme cleaves the three fatty acids from the glycerol backbone of a triglyceride molecule in lipoproteins. As a result, the free fatty acids and glycerol can enter cells. After entering, three fatty acids can be attached to a glycerol molecule, re—creating a triglyceride molecule. Making triglycerides from fatty acids and glycerol molecules requires very little energy input. Therefore, triglyceride synthesis is the primary route for storing excess fatty acids, especially in adipocytes.

Fatty Acid Synthesis

lipogenesis synthesis of fatty acids

Certain cells can make fatty acids **(lipogenesis)**. The synthesis of a fatty acid requires different enzymes and chemical pathways than the oxidation of a fatty acid. Furthermore, lipogenesis occurs in the cell's cytoplasm, instead of in mito—chondria, and requires the input of energy and the help of the electron carrier mol—ecule NADPH (this molecule is different from NADH because it has a phosphate group). In a series of repeating sequential reactions, two—carbon acetyl CoA units are bound together to form the hydrocarbon chain of the fatty acid. With each addition of an acetyl CoA molecule, the fatty acid elongates and stores energy.

Storing Glucose as Glycogen

When glucose enters cells that need energy, the monosaccharide undergoes gly—colysis and is rapidly catabolized for ATP production. What happens when cells no longer need glucose to synthesize ATP? Under normal conditions, the body does not eliminate the excess glucose by excreting the monosaccharide in urine. Instead, liver and muscle cells can store the glucose as glycogen through a path—way called **glycogenesis**.

glycogenesis pathway that enables certain cells to store glucose as glycogen

The process of glycogenesis involves the help of specific enzymes that bind single glucose molecules together into long branched chains of glycogen (see Fig. 5.6c). As described in section 8.2, when cells require glucose for energy, a different set of enzymes cleaves individual glucose molecules from glycogen (glycogenolysis). The body stores limited amounts of glycogen, and storage sites can fill up quickly. What happens when your cells have no additional space to store glycogen and you continue to eat foods that are sources of glucose?

Excessive Glucose

Cells may use excess dietary glucose molecules to form triglycerides, but the conversion requires more steps and more energy. Thus, only a small percentage of extra dietary glucose is converted to triglycerides and stored in adipocytes.

When a person consumes a surplus of glucose, his or her cells catabolize the monosaccharide molecules for ATP production instead of breaking down fatty acids (Fig. 8.30a). The end result of this metabolic shift is the synthesis and storage of triglycerides in adipocytes (Fig. 8.30b). In a sense, the extra glucose molecules "spare" (conserve) fatty acids by enabling the lipid molecules to be made into triglycerides and stored for ATP production in the future. This process explains why people who eat excess carbohydrates can gain body fat.

When Amino Acids Are in Excess

As mentioned earlier, cells preferentially use amino acids for protein synthesis rather than for energy. What happens if the diet provides an excess of amino acids and cells do not need energy? Under these conditions, the amino acids will be stripped of their nitrogen group and used to make either glucose or fat.

The liver and, to some extent, the kidneys are able to use glucogenic amino acids to make glucose (gluconeogenesis). Liver cells can use the glucose formed by gluconeogenesis to synthesize glycogen or release the simple sugar into the bloodstream for other cells to use (see Fig. 8.20).

Recall that *ketogenic* amino acids, such as leucine and tryptophan, have carbon skeletons that can be converted into acetyl CoA. Ketogenic amino acids cannot be used to make glucose, because the step that converts pyruvate to acetyl CoA is not reversible (see Fig. 8.9). If the acetyl CoA molecules that were derived from these carbon skeletons do not enter the citric acid cycle, they may be used for fatty acid synthesis. Thus, consuming more protein or amino acids than your body needs for protein or ATP synthesis can increase your body fat.

Many people consume protein supplements because they think it will help them gain muscle mass. Obtaining adequate amounts of energy from all macronutrients and exercising muscles is necessary to build muscle size, strength, and endurance. Simply consuming protein or amino acid supplements is likely to result in gaining adipose tissue instead of lean body mass. Table 8.6 reviews the metabolic fates of amino acids, as well as glucose, fatty acids, and alcohol.

As you can see, the human body is an amazing living machine that obtains energy from a variety of sources and extracts the energy in many ways. The body is also able to store excess energy for future use, primarily in two forms (fat and glycogen). The availability of ATP in your cells determines the fate of the macronutrient molecules that you consume in your next meal or snack. In the following section, we consider how hormones regulate the metabolism and availability of nutrients.

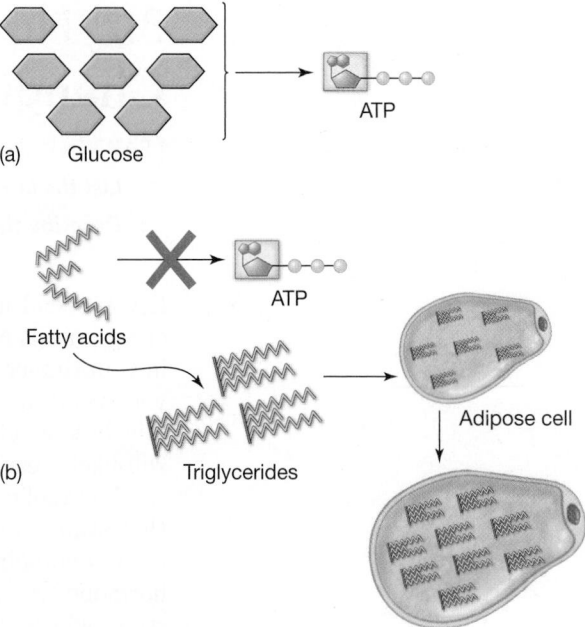

FIGURE 8.30 Excess glucose and fat storage.

TABLE 8.6 Metabolism: The Fates of Macronutrients and Alcohol

Energy Source	Yields Glucose?	Yields Amino Acids?	Yields Fat?
Amino acids	Yes, except for ketogenic amino acids	Yes	Yes
Glucose	Yes	Yes*	Yes
Fatty acids	No	No	Yes
Alcohol	No	No	Yes

*Only nonessential amino acids if nitrogen is available.

ASSESS YOUR PROGRESS

16 *Trace the path of triglycerides from the liver to storage in adipose tissue.*

17 *How does excess carbohydrate consumption increase body fat deposits?*

18 *Which tissues are the primary sites for glycogen synthesis and storage?*

19 *Describe the conversion of excess protein into glucose or fatty acids.*

8.7 Hormonal Responses to Changing Energy Needs

LEARNING OUTCOMES

1 *List the key hormones that direct or regulate metabolic activities.*
2 *Describe the major effects of metabolic hormones.*

If you spend much of the day engaging in vigorous physical activity, your body's energy needs are high. In this situation, your cells will process the macronutrients in your dinner meal by way of ATP—producing, catabolic pathways. In contrast, if you spend most of the day sitting around, your body's energy needs are comparatively low. Therefore, any surplus of food energy provided by your evening meal will likely result in energy storage, because your cells favor anabolic pathways.

Metabolic pathways are coordinated by hormones, "chemical messengers" that stimulate and regulate cellular activities. Key hormones that direct or regulate metabolic activities are insulin, glucagon, cortisol, epinephrine, and thyroid hormone. Actions of each metabolic hormone depend on the body's metabolic state, which can be categorized as either *absorptive* (when the digestive tract is absorbing nutrients) or *postabsorptive* (when the digestive tract is not active). The information in Table 8.7 is a summary of the basic physiological effects of major metabolic hormones.

Insulin: Anabolic Metabolism

We first described insulin in Chapter 5 when we discussed maintaining normal blood glucose levels. Beta cells in the pancreas synthesize insulin, a protein that serves as the primary anabolic hormone. After a carbohydrate—containing meal, the beta cells detect the rise in blood glucose levels (absorptive state) and secrete insulin. The hormone attaches to special receptors on the cell membranes of adipocytes and muscle cells. This attachment results in a signal to glucose transport proteins that are also in the cell membrane (Fig. 8.31). In response to the signal, the glucose transport molecules pass the monosaccharide across the cell membrane and into the cytoplasm. Thus, insulin helps maintain normal blood glucose levels by enabling the entry of glucose into many kinds of cells.

Insulin directs liver and muscle cells to slow down their glycogenolysis rates and increase their rates of glycogenesis. Such actions shift glucose molecules into storage as glycogen. Insulin also increases the fatty acid uptake and triglyceride

TABLE 8.7 Physiological Effects of Major Metabolic Hormones

Hormone	Overall Metabolic Effect	Effects in Liver	Effects in Adipose Tissue	Effects in Muscle
Insulin	Anabolic	Increases glycolysis and glycogenesis	Increases glucose uptake; increases lipogenesis	Increases glucose and amino acid uptake; increases glycogenesis and protein synthesis
Glucagon	Catabolic	Increases glycogenolysis and gluconeogenesis		
Cortisol	Catabolic	Increases glycogenolysis and gluconeogenesis	Increases lipolysis	Increases proteolysis
Epinephrine	Catabolic	Increases glycogenolysis and gluconeogenesis	Increases lipolysis	
Thyroid hormone	Regulates metabolic rate			

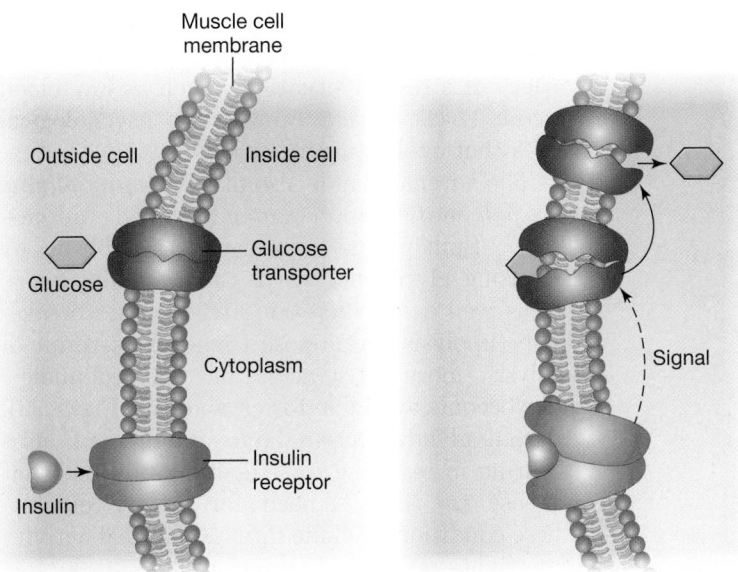

FIGURE 8.31 Transporting glucose across cell membranes.

cortisol catabolic hormone made in the adrenal cortex of the adrenal glands

synthesis of adipocytes. Furthermore, insulin stimulates protein synthesis in cells. To summarize, insulin promotes energy storage (Fig. 8.32).

Glucagon, Cortisol, and Epinephrine: Catabolic Metabolism

Glucagon, cortisol, and epinephrine are hormones that instruct cells to use catabolic rather than anabolic pathways. The cells that synthesize these catabolic hormones release higher amounts of them in response to intense exercise, extreme stress, or starvation. The collective activity of these hormones is to increase fuel mobilization from storage, so sources of energy are available for all of the body's cells (Fig. 8.33).

Glucagon, which we also discussed in Chapter 5, is made by the alpha cells of the pancreas. Alpha cells secrete glucagon in response to blood glucose levels that drop to below normal levels (*postabsorptive* state). The liver is the main target organ for glucagon's action. Glucagon signals liver cells to increase glycogenolysis and gluconeogenesis from glucogenic amino acids. This action enables the liver to produce more glucose for release into the bloodstream (Fig. 8.33). The primary result of glucagon's activity is an increase in blood glucose levels.

Cortisol is a catabolic hormone made in the *adrenal cortex* of the adrenal glands, which are located on top of the kidneys. Cortisol promotes protein catabolism and stimulates the liver to increase its use of amino acids for gluconeogenesis.

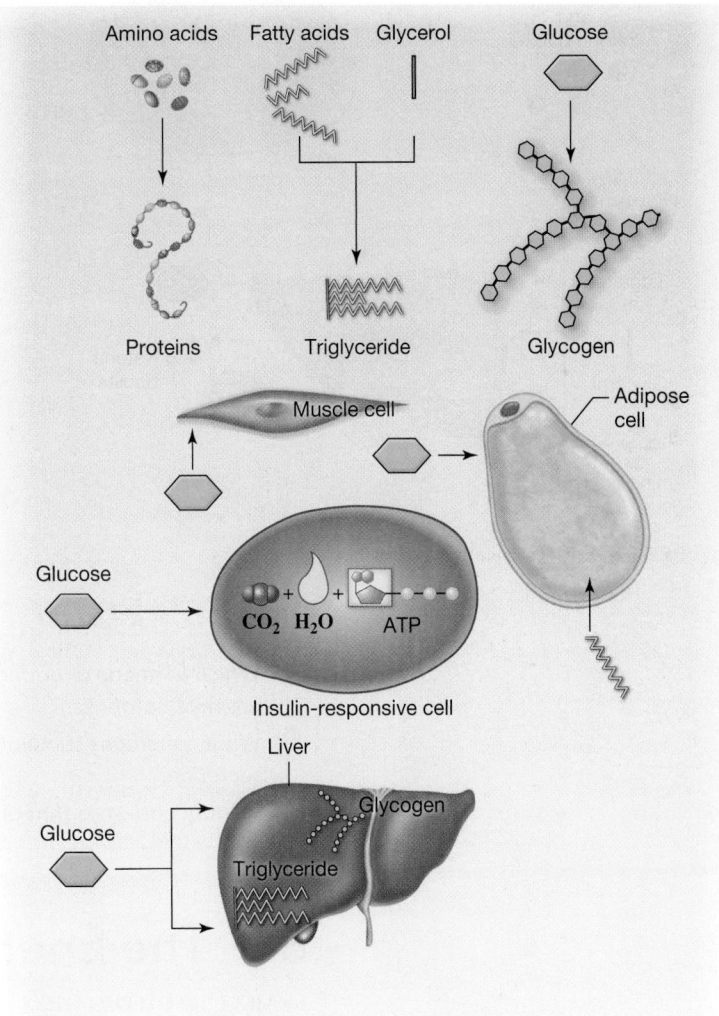

FIGURE 8.32 Insulin action.

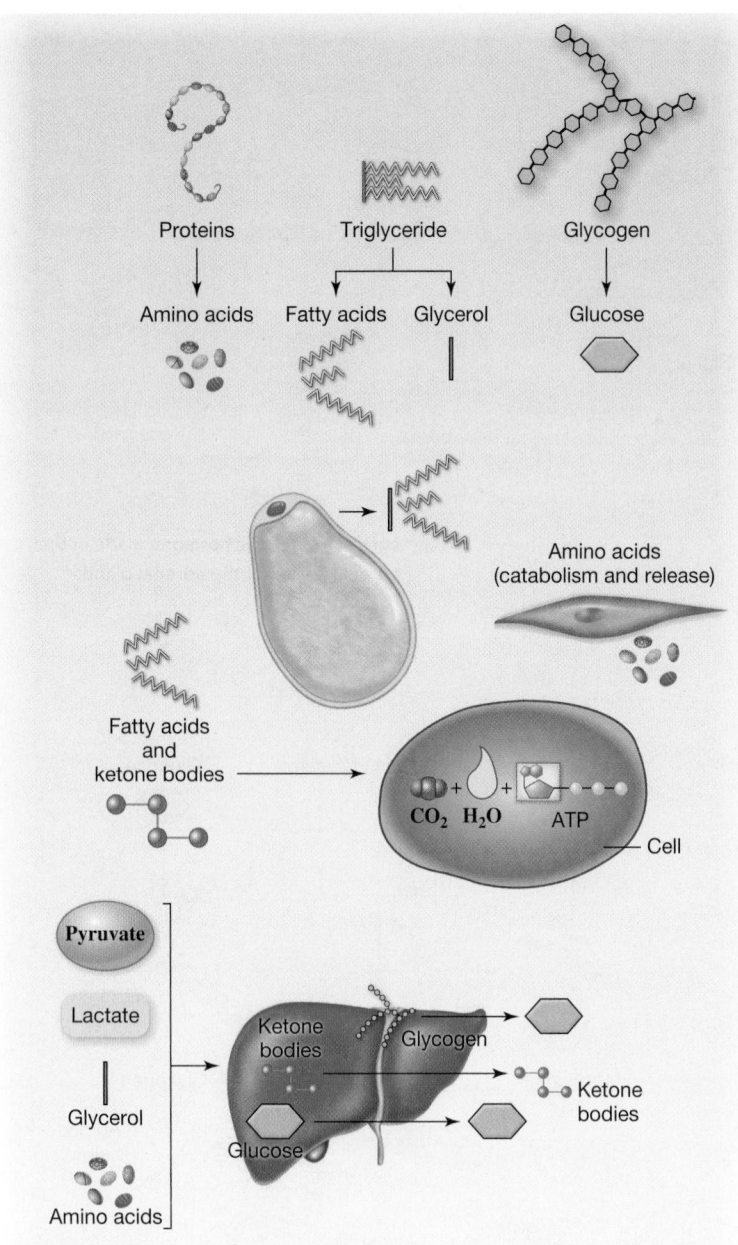

FIGURE 8.33 Effects of catabolic hormones.

Cortisol is often referred to as a "stress hormone," because it is secreted in response to a variety of stressful situations, such as low blood glucose levels, severe injuries, or psychological states that evoke anxiety or fear.

The adrenal glands also produce *epinephrine* (*eh−peh−nef'−rin*), commonly called "adrenaline." Epinephrine stimulates catabolism by increasing glycogenolysis in the liver and muscle, as well as by increasing triglyceride breakdown (lipolysis) in adipose tissue. As a result of lipolysis, more fatty acids and glycerol molecules become available for catabolism (Fig. 8.33). Adrenal glands secrete large amounts of epinephrine in response to stressful conditions that increase the body's need for energy quickly. These conditions include intense physical activity and "fight−or−flight" situations.

Thyroid Hormone: Adaptation to Changing Conditions

The thyroid gland at the base of the throat synthesizes and secretes two hormones that are collectively referred to as thyroid hormone. This hormone helps the body adapt to different situations by increasing or decreasing the rate of metabolism. Therefore, the hormone can have catabolic or anabolic actions. Thyroid hormone increases the rate of glucose catabolism, lipolysis, and protein synthesis. As a result of these actions, cells are able to develop and grow normally. Thus, thyroid hormone levels increase during times of growth and development. When food is not available, such as during periods of starvation, thyroid hormone production decreases. This response is important because it helps conserve the body's fuel stores.

ASSESS YOUR PROGRESS

20 *Which hormone or hormones promote anabolism? Which hormone or hormones promote catabolism?*

21 *What conditions stimulate insulin secretion? What conditions stimulate glucagon secretion?*

22 *Identify pathways that are stimulated by the catabolic hormones.*

8.8 The Energy Balancing Act

LEARNING OUTCOMES

1 *List the metabolic responses to short-term and prolonged fasting.*

2 *Explain the relationship between insulin resistance and metabolic syndrome.*

The anabolic and catabolic hormones that were described in section 8.7 manage your body's fuel supplies and utilization so your body can function normally without the need for you to consume food constantly. How do cells manage their energy supplies during an overnight fast or when food is severely limited?

Metabolic Responses to an Overnight Fast

As blood glucose levels fall during the early part of an overnight fast, the pancreas responds by releasing glucagon. Glucagon instructs liver cells to increase glycogenolysis. This process helps maintain blood glucose levels within normal limits, but the supply of liver glycogen is limited and becomes depleted over the course of about 12 hours.

When the liver's glycogen supply is "on empty," glucagon stimulates liver cells to convert certain amino acids derived from muscle tissue into pyruvate and then glucose (gluconeogenesis). During this time, the liver and muscle tissue use mainly fatty acids for fuel. Once a person "breaks the fast" by eating a carbohydrate—rich meal, the usual insulin response to the influx of glucose into the bloodstream effectively turns the metabolic tide from a catabolic state to an anabolic state. Figure 5.14 illustrates how insulin and glucagon work together to manage blood glucose levels in a healthy individual.

Metabolic Responses to Prolonged Fasting (Starvation)

The body is adapted to survive an extended period without food intake. The same physiological adaptations that occur during an overnight fast also occur as the fast continues. Over a longer period of fasting—*starvation*—the body makes some additional changes to ensure that cells have access to a variety of fuels.

Liver and muscle glycogen stores become depleted with extended fasting. When that situation occurs, muscle cells begin to rely more on fatty acids for energy. Adipose tissue responds to starvation by increasing lipolysis, and as a result, the level of fatty acids increases in the bloodstream. The fatty acids supply some energy for muscle tissue, and they are also taken up by the liver.

Eventually, the rapid influx of fatty acids into the liver becomes too much for the organ's cells to handle. When this occurs, liver cells rely on ketogenesis to convert acetyl CoA into ketone bodies, an alternative fuel source described in section 8.4. During prolonged fasts, even the brain can catabolize ketone bodies for energy.

Under normal conditions, glucose and fatty acids are the body's primary fuels, and they "spare" the body's proteins from being used as a major energy source. During starvation, however, muscle cells experience a severe change: They begin to break down and release amino acids. This degradation process is called proteolysis (*pro′—tee—o—lie′—sus*). The liver can use some of the amino acids for gluconeogenesis (Fig. 8.33). Nevertheless, the body relies more heavily on stored fat than protein for energy during prolonged starvation.

The breakdown of adipose and muscle tissue to provide fuel sources for the starving person contributes to the extreme weight loss, muscle wasting, and weakened condition of the affected individual (see Fig. 7.16). Starvation is a highly catabolic state, characterized by glycogenolysis, lipolysis, proteolysis, and ketogenesis. Although these metabolic responses are necessary for survival, the starving person is in a very dangerous metabolic state and will likely die if the lack of access to nourishing foods continues.

Obesity and Insulin Resistance

Muscle, fat, and liver cells have insulin receptors on their cell membranes.[8] Insulin binds to these receptors, which conveys specific information to the cells. As a result of this binding, these cells allow glucose and fatty acids to enter them, and the cells can store energy (see Fig. 8.31).

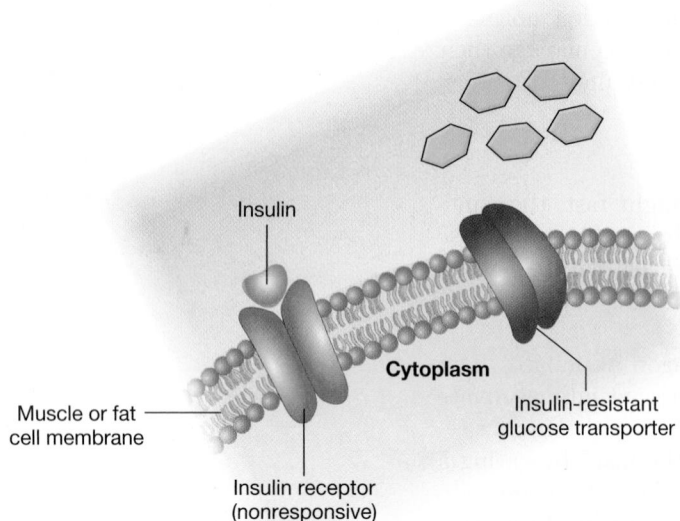

FIGURE 8.34 Insulin resistance.

nonalcoholic fatty liver abnormal accumulation of fat in the liver that is not caused by alcohol consumption

In cases of obesity, the increase in adipose tissue often results in abnormal metabolic changes in fat and muscle cells. These changes make the cells resistant or unresponsive to the effects of insulin. *Insulin resistance* in muscle cells and adipocytes occurs because the insulin receptors no longer function properly (Fig. 8.34). Thus, obesity is highly associated with insulin resistance, a condition that can lead to type 2 diabetes.

Nonalcoholic Fatty Liver

Insulin resistant cells do not take up glucose and fatty acids from the bloodstream and store energy effectively. Thus, blood glucose levels stay abnormally elevated (*hyperglycemia*) long after a meal is consumed. In addition, lipolysis in adipocytes is not restricted, resulting in the release of more fatty acids into the bloodstream. As a result of these metabolic changes, levels of glucose and fatty acids in blood increase dramatically. In the liver, the influx of fatty acids stimulates triglyceride synthesis. The excess fat can accumulate in liver cells and lead to a condition called **nonalcoholic fatty liver**. Regardless of whether the cause of a fatty liver is insulin resistance or excess alcohol intake, the condition is a sign of impending liver damage.

Metabolic Syndrome

When liver cells become insulin resistant, their ability to regulate glycogen synthesis and gluconeogenesis becomes altered. The liver continues to produce glucose and release the monosaccharide into the bloodstream. As the blood glucose level rises even higher, the pancreas secretes more insulin. This vicious cycle results in *metabolic syndrome* (see Chapter 5). Having excess body fat is a major risk factor for developing metabolic syndrome and type 2 diabetes.[9] Thus, people can reduce their risk of both conditions by keeping their weight within a normal range.

ASSESS YOUR PROGRESS

23 *Discuss the metabolic processes that occur during an overnight fast.*

24 *List the major metabolic responses that occur in muscle, adipose tissue, and the liver during starvation.*

25 *Explain why insulin resistance may lead to the development of nonalcoholic fatty liver disease and metabolic syndrome.*

8.9 Putting the Metabolism Puzzle Together

LEARNING OUTCOME

1 *Summarize the catabolic and anabolic pathways and actions of glucose, fat, and amino acids.*

Glucose, fat, and amino acids work together to fuel the body under a variety of physical conditions. Table 8.8 and Figure 8.35 summarize key pathways in the anabolism and catabolism of these energy-supplying nutrients.

TABLE 8.8 Energy Metabolism Summary

Macronutrient	Catabolism	Anabolism
Carbohydrate	Pathways:	Pathways:
	Glycolysis	**Gluconeogenesis**
	Glucose → Pyruvate	Pyruvate → Glucose (certain cells)
	Glycogenolysis	**Glycogenesis**
	Glycogen → Glucose	Glucose → Glycogen
Fat	Pathways:	Pathways:
	Beta-oxidation	**Fatty acid synthesis**
	Fatty acids → Acetyl CoA	Acetyl CoA → Fatty acids
	Lipolysis	**Lipogenesis**
	Triglycerides → Glycerol + Fatty acids	Fatty acids + Glycerol → Triglycerides
Protein	Pathways:	Pathways:
	Proteolysis	**Protein synthesis**
	Proteins → Amino acids	Amino acids → Proteins
	Deamination	
	Amino acids → Carbon skeletons	**Gluconeogenesis**
	Transamination	Amino acids → Glucose
	Amino acids → Carbon skeletons	

Understanding how the pathways and actions of the metabolic hormones (Table 8.8) are interrelated will help you recognize what can happen to the body's nutritional status during disease states. For example, a young male patient with type 1 diabetes who has signs and symptoms of ketosis is under your care. You know that insulin usually enables glucose to enter cells. Therefore, this patient's lack of insulin is causing glucose to accumulate in his bloodstream. By recognizing that ketosis occurs when glucose cannot be utilized as a fuel source, you know that the patient's cells are breaking down fatty acids to form ketone bodies, an alternative fuel source. To treat this patient effectively, you and his other health care providers must address the need to manage his blood pH, as well as his insulin requirements.

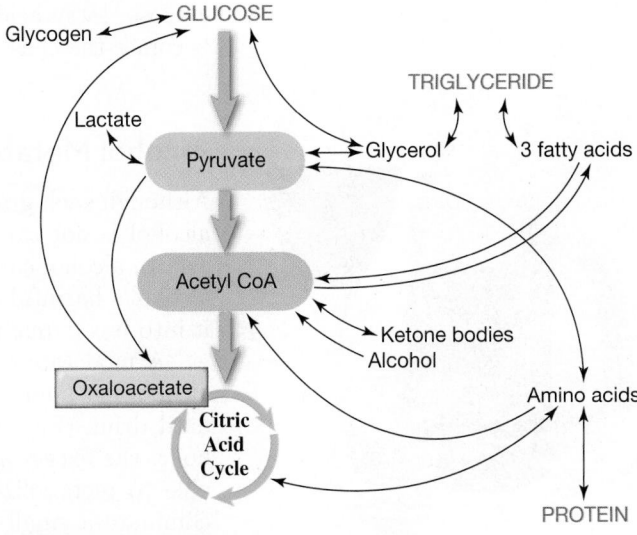

FIGURE 8.35 Summary of energy metabolism.

ASSESS YOUR PROGRESS

26 *Explain the differences between glycogenesis and glycogenolysis, and lipogenesis and lipolysis. Why is gluconeogenesis repeated in Table 8.8?*

8.10 Alcohol as an Energy Source

LEARNING OUTCOMES

1 *Explain how alcohol can be utilized for energy.*

2 *Identify factors that affect alcohol metabolism.*

3 *Discuss alcohol's effects on health.*

$$CH_3 — CH_2 — OH$$

Ethanol

FIGURE 8.36 Ethanol.

ethanol simple two-carbon molecule that is more commonly called "alcohol"

standard drink approximately 12 ounces of beer, 5 ounces of wine, or 1 ½ ounces of liquor

gastric alcohol dehydrogenase enzyme that detoxifies some alcohol while it is in the stomach

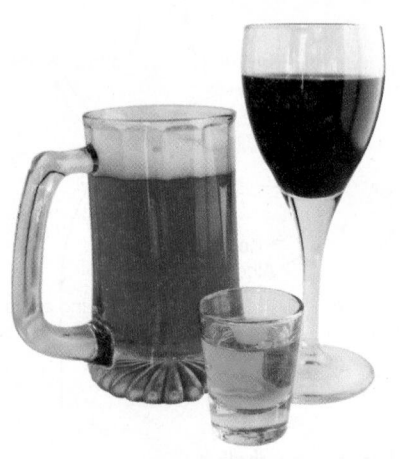

FIGURE 8.37 What is a standard drink?

alcohol dehydrogenase pathway catabolic pathway that metabolizes alcohol in the liver

acetaldehyde highly toxic substance formed during the first step of the alcohol dehydrogenase pathway

aldehyde dehydrogenase enzyme that helps convert acetaldehyde to acetate, a less toxic substance

Another "fuel" that the body can use for energy is **ethanol**, a simple two—carbon molecule that is more commonly called "alcohol" (Fig. 8.36). Alcohol is soluble in water, and alcoholic beverages generally contain a considerable amount of water. Beers are typically 3 to 6% alcohol, and wines contain about 8 to 14% alcohol by volume. Distilled spirits (hard liquors) such as whiskey, bourbon, and vodka are generally 40 to 50% alcohol. Beer and wine contain simple carbohy—drates and small amounts of certain minerals and B vitamins. Distilled spirits have essentially no nutritional value other than water. Mixing distilled spirits with juices, cocktail mixes, or other flavorings increases the alcoholic bever—age's energy content and may add some nutrients, particularly simple sugars, depending on the ingredients in the mixer. A **standard drink** (approximately 12 ounces of beer, 5 ounces of wine, or 1½ ounces of liquor) contains 13 to 14 g of alcohol (Fig. 8.37).

Alcohol Absorption

When a person drinks an alcohol—containing beverage, his or her stomach and small intestine rapidly absorb the drug. When alcohol is consumed with meals, food delays its absorption from the stomach and slows the rate at which sub—stance enters the bloodstream. In contrast, the intestinal tract absorbs alcohol faster when it is in carbonated beverages, such as beer, "sparkling" wines, and drinks made by mixing carbonated soft drinks with liquor.

If alcohol mixes with food in the stomach, some detoxification of the drug occurs by the action of **gastric alcohol dehydrogenase**. The liver, however, is the primary site for metabolizing the alcohol that has been absorbed by the digestive tract. Once alcohol enters liver cells, the normal metabolic processing of glucose, fatty acids, and amino acids slows down, and the catabolism of alcohol becomes the cells' top priority.

Alcohol Metabolism

Although each gram of alcohol can be metabolized for energy and provide 7 kcal, alcohol is not a nutrient; it is a mind—altering, toxic drug. When consumed in excess, alcohol can damage every organ of the body and lead to death. To reduce alcohol's harmful effects, the body *detoxifies* the simple molecule by converting it into less damaging compounds.

A moderate drinker with a healthy liver can metabolize about 12 to 15 g of alcohol per hour.[10] This amount is approximately the alcohol content of a stan—dard drink (Fig. 8.37). If the drinker consumes more than one standard drink/hour, the excess alcohol circulates in his or her bloodstream until liver cells are able to metabolize it. Respiration in the lungs and perspiration from the skin eliminate a small percentage of the alcohol; that is why you can smell alcohol when you are around someone who has been drinking. The kidneys also filter some of the drug from the bloodstream and eliminate it in urine.

Alcohol Dehydrogenase Pathway

When a person drinks low to moderate amounts of alcohol, the liver relies primar—ily on the **alcohol dehydrogenase pathway** to metabolize the drug. In the first step of this process, most of the alcohol is converted to **acetaldehyde**, a highly toxic substance (Fig. 8.38). However, the enzyme **aldehyde dehydrogenase** helps convert acetaldehyde to acetate, a less toxic substance. Acetate can be converted to acetyl CoA (Fig. 8.38). Acetyl CoA may be further metabolized via the citric acid cycle to form CO_2 and H_2O, or the molecule can be used to synthesize fatty acids or ketone bodies.

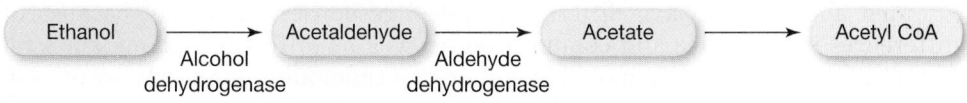

FIGURE 8.38 Alcohol metabolism: Actions of alcohol dehydrogenase and aldehyde dehydrogenase.

Microsomal Ethanol-Oxidizing System

If a person consumes excessive amounts of alcohol in one session, such as during a drinking binge, the liver's ability to metabolize the drug using the alcohol dehydrogenase pathway is overwhelmed. When this occurs, a secondary pathway for processing alcohol, the **microsomal ethanol–oxidizing system (MEOS)**, takes over. Metabolizing alcohol by the MEOS also produces acetaldehyde that must be further processed to yield acetyl CoA. Chronic and excessive alcohol intake leads to increased production of MEOS enzymes. As a result of this adaptation, the liver can metabolize the excess alcohol more rapidly.

microsomal ethanol-oxidizing system (MEOS) secondary pathway for processing alcohol in the liver

Unlike the alcohol dehydrogenase pathway, the MEOS wastes energy in the form of body heat. Thus, alcohol–dependent people (alcoholics) may gain little weight from their energy intake, particularly when alcohol supplies most of their energy. Furthermore, alcoholics are at risk of hypothermia (lower–than–normal body temperature) when exposed to cold. The reason is that to remove the excess heat that results during the metabolism of alcohol, blood vessels relax (*vasodilation*). Vasodilation increases the circulation of blood to the skin, enabling body heat to dissipate into the environment more readily. As a result, alcoholics may "feel" warm and fail to wear proper clothing when in cold conditions. If not recognized and treated promptly, hypothermia can be deadly.

Factors That Influence Alcohol Metabolism

You may have noticed that some of your friends who drink can "hold their liquor" better than others. Several physiological factors account for the variability. Besides the amount and timing of alcohol consumption, personal characteristics such as sex, body size and composition, age, and prior drinking history affect a person's detoxification rate (Fig. 8.39).

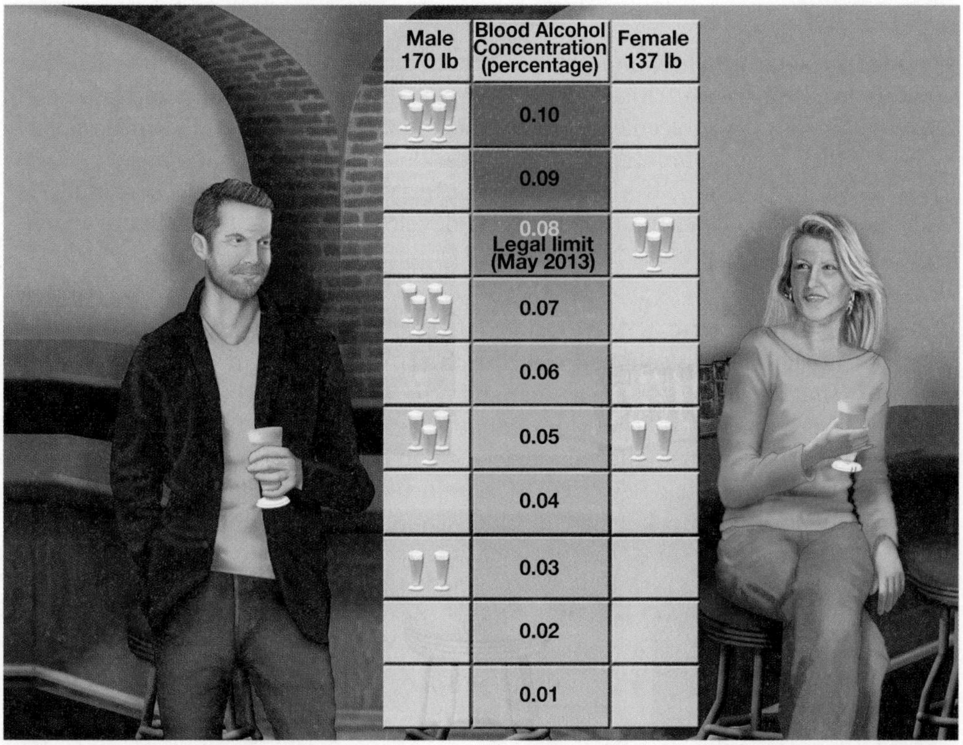

Male 170 lb	Blood Alcohol Concentration (percentage)	Female 137 lb
	0.10	
	0.09	
	0.08 Legal limit (May 2013)	
	0.07	
	0.06	
	0.05	
	0.04	
	0.03	
	0.02	
	0.01	

FIGURE 8.39 Blood alcohol concentration (BAC). The BAC indicates the percentage of alcohol in a person's bloodstream. Increases in the BAC reflect a person's alcohol consumption rate. Furthermore, men and women have different physical responses to alcohol.

DID YOU KNOW?

Excess alcohol intake can interfere with the kidneys' ability to excrete uric acid, a by-product of nucleic acid (DNA and RNA) metabolism. As a result, uric acid accumulates in the bloodstream and can form tiny needlelike crystals in body fluids. These crystals contribute to the signs and symptoms of *gout*, an extremely painful form of arthritis that often causes inflammation in the joints of toes. Thus, people who have gout should avoid drinking excess alcohol because the drug aggravates their condition.

cirrhosis of the liver condition characterized by the accumulation of scar tissue in the liver, which permanently damages the organ

Men and women have different physical responses to alcohol because of differences in body size and composition, as well as differences in metabolism. Larger livers can detoxify more alcohol at one time, and more body water will allow the alcohol to be diluted. In addition, men produce more gastric alcohol dehydrogenase than women.[11] This means that men can metabolize more alcohol before it leaves the stomach, so less is absorbed into the bloodstream from the intestine. These factors help to explain the increased risk of serious health problems faced by women, even if they abuse lower amounts of alcohol than men.[12]

Genetic background is another factor that can influence alcohol metabolism. Many Asian Americans, especially people with Japanese, Chinese, and Korean ancestors, have difficulty metabolizing alcohol because they have inherited genes that result in low activity of aldehyde dehydrogenase.[13] When these individuals consume alcohol, they tend to experience facial flushing, along with other uncomfortable side effects, including nausea, drowsiness, rapid heartbeat, and a subsequent hangover.

Alcohol's Effects on Liver Metabolism Alcohol directly affects the liver by disrupting the normal metabolism of glucose, fatty acids, and amino acids. The two dehydrogenase reactions in the metabolism of alcohol (see Fig. 8.38) each result in the transfer of an electron to the electron carrier molecule NAD^+, producing NADH. As NADH accumulates in liver cells, the amount of NAD^+ becomes depleted (Fig. 8.40a). This change in the ratio of NADH to NAD^+ has the following effects on liver cells' normal metabolic pathways:

- The rate of glycolysis slows, because the glycolytic pathway requires NAD^+ to metabolize glucose molecules. When NADH accumulates in liver cells, more pyruvate is converted to lactic acid (Fig. 8.40b). Because of these changes, ATP production from glucose is impaired.

- The increased ratio of NADH to NAD^+ can lead to hypoglycemia, because not enough NAD^+ is available to maintain the normal rate of gluconeogenesis (Fig. 8.40c).

- Because of the lack of NAD^+, the activity of the citric acid cycle slows (Fig. 8.40d).

- Some of the acetyl CoA molecules enter the citric acid cycle and are catabolized for energy (Fig. 8.40e). However, liver cells use most of the excess acetyl CoA molecules to make fatty acids for triglyceride synthesis (Fig. 8.40f). The accumulation of triglycerides in liver cells can cause "alcoholic fatty liver." If a person with a fatty liver continues to consume alcohol, he or she eventually is likely to develop **cirrhosis of the liver**, which permanently damages the liver (Fig. 8.41).

Blood Alcohol Concentration (BAC)

Increases in the blood alcohol concentration (BAC) reflect an alcohol consumption rate that exceeds the liver's capacity to metabolize the drug. To determine whether someone is legally intoxicated as a result of drinking alcohol, law enforcement officials use special devices to analyze the alcohol in expired air for estimating a person's BAC. BAC is reported as a percentage that indicates the concentration of alcohol in the bloodstream. In the United States, a BAC of 0.08% is the legal limit for intoxication for automobile operators who are 21 years of age or older (see Fig. 8.39). Some states have a lower legal limit, and the national limit for BAC may be reduced to 0.05% in the future.

Alcohol's effects on the central nervous system, especially the brain, appear within a few minutes of having a drink. Alcohol acts as a depressant, slowing the

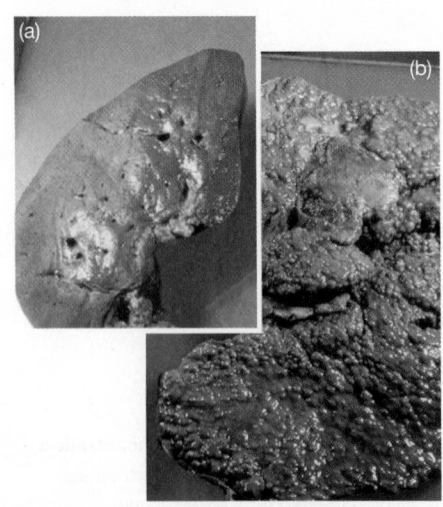

FIGURE 8.41 Cirrhosis of the liver.
(a) Healthy liver; (b) cirrhotic liver.

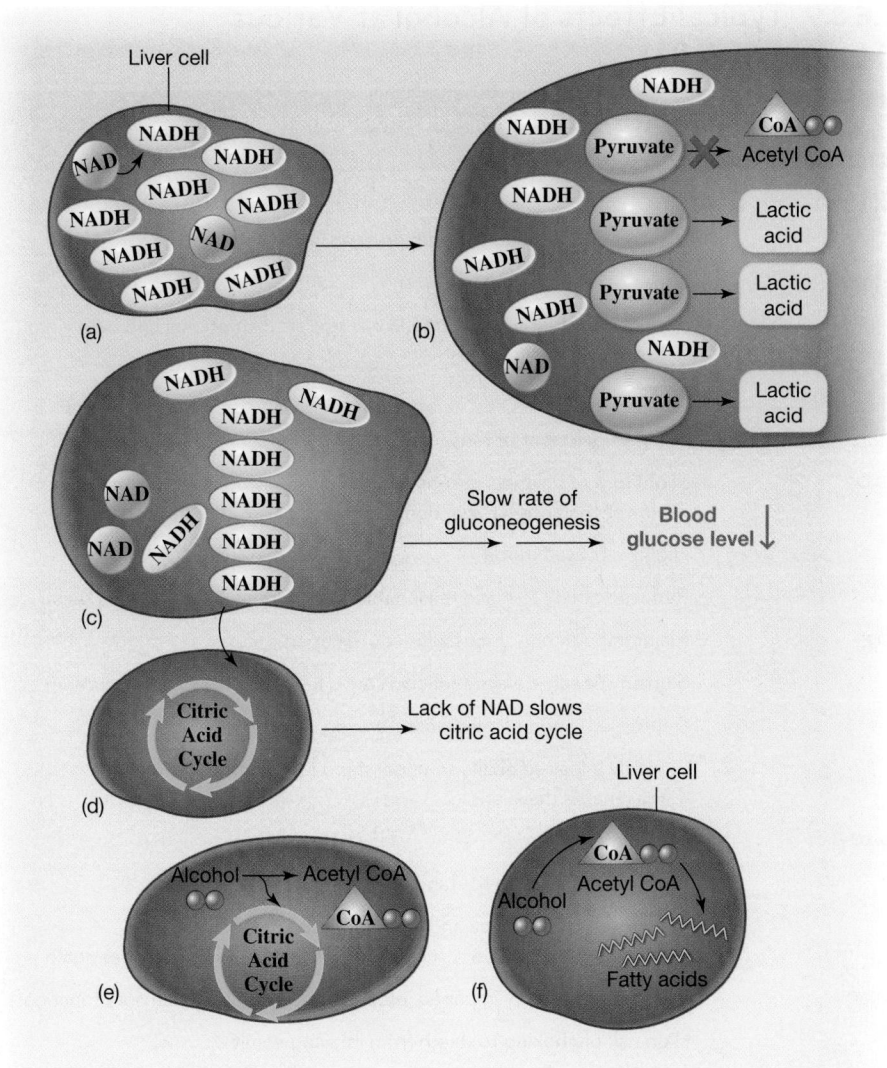

FIGURE 8.40 Effects of alcohol metabolism on the liver. (*a*) NADH accumulates in liver cells, and the amount of NAD$^+$ becomes depleted. (*b*) When NADH accumulates in liver cells, more pyruvate is converted to lactic acid. (*c*) Hypoglycemia occurs as a result of the accumulation of NADH. (*d*) Because of the lack of NAD$^+$, the activity of the citric acid cycle slows. (*e*) Some acetyl CoA is metabolized for energy, but (*f*) liver cells use most of the excess acetyl CoA molecules to make fatty acids for triglyceride synthesis.

transmission of messages between nerve cells. When the drinker's BAC reaches 0.20 to 0.30%, his or her brain is unable to process information. Higher BACs (0.30 to 0.50%) usually result in loss of consciousness (passing out). Moreover, coma and even death can occur as the brain loses control over lung and heart functioning. Table 8.9 lists BAC levels and typical nervous system effects at each level.

Alcohol's Effects on the Body

Anyone who drinks alcohol at a rate that exceeds his or her ability to metabolize the drug may experience a hangover the next day. The headache and nausea, sensitivity to light and noise, fatigue, and thirst associated with a hangover are, in part, explained by the accumulation of the toxic molecule acetaldehyde in various tissues throughout the body. The toxic effects of alcohol on the brain, as well as alcohol's dehydrating and hypoglycemic effects, are also thought to contribute to the discomfort.

Alcohol affects every cell in the body, and when consumed in excess, the drug damages every system in the body, particularly the gastrointestinal, nervous, and cardiovascular systems. Figure 8.42 summarizes major damaging physiological

TABLE 8.9 Typical Effects of Alcohol at Various BAC Levels (Adults)

Blood Alcohol Concentration	Typical Physiological and Psychological Effects
0.02–0.03	Increased sociability, slightly elevated mood, and mild relaxation
	May experience mild light-headed sensation
0.04–0.06	Sense of warmth, well-being, and relaxation
	Reduced inhibitions, resulting in exaggerated emotional and behavioral responses to situations
	Highly elevated mood
	Minor impairment of reasoning
0.07–0.09	Slight loss of balance, may have difficulty carrying on a conversation, slower than normal reaction time
	Highly elevated mood
	Reduced ability to make reasonable decisions and control one's behavior
0.10–0.15	Major impairment of muscular coordination
	Slurred speech, delayed reaction time, hearing and visual impairment
	Depressed mood and increased anxiety
	Severely impaired ability to understand information and make reasonable decisions
0.16–0.20	Disoriented
	May need assistance to stand and walk
	May experience nausea and vomiting; can choke on vomit. May black out, that is, not recall what has occurred when sober again
0.25–0.30	In a stupor (severely impaired intellectual, physical, and sensory functions)
	High risk of choking to death from inhaling vomit
	High risk of accidental injuries
	May pass out
0.35–0.40 and higher	Onset of coma (become unconscious and unable to be awakened for a long period of time)
	Death due to respiratory arrest

Source: Oklahoma University: *Blood alcohol content calculator.* 2009. www.ou.edu/oupd/bac.htm Accessed: August 23, 2013

effects of alcohol. Pregnant women who drink alcohol can cause irreversible damage to their unborn offspring. Chapter 16 discusses the effects that the drug can have on a developing human being.

Alcohol Consumption in the United States

According to results of a national study conducted in 2012, approximately 51% of adults (>18 years of age) in the United States were "current drinkers" of alcohol.[14] A current drinker consumed at least one alcohol–containing drink in the 30 days prior to the survey. Although there are no universally accepted definitions for "light," "moderate," or "heavy" drinking, medical practitioners and alcohol researchers often follow the classification guidelines listed in Table 8.10. In 2012, about 6% of American adults were *heavy* drinkers.[15] Nearly 61% of full–time college students were current drinkers and 13.6% were heavy drinkers in 2011.[16]

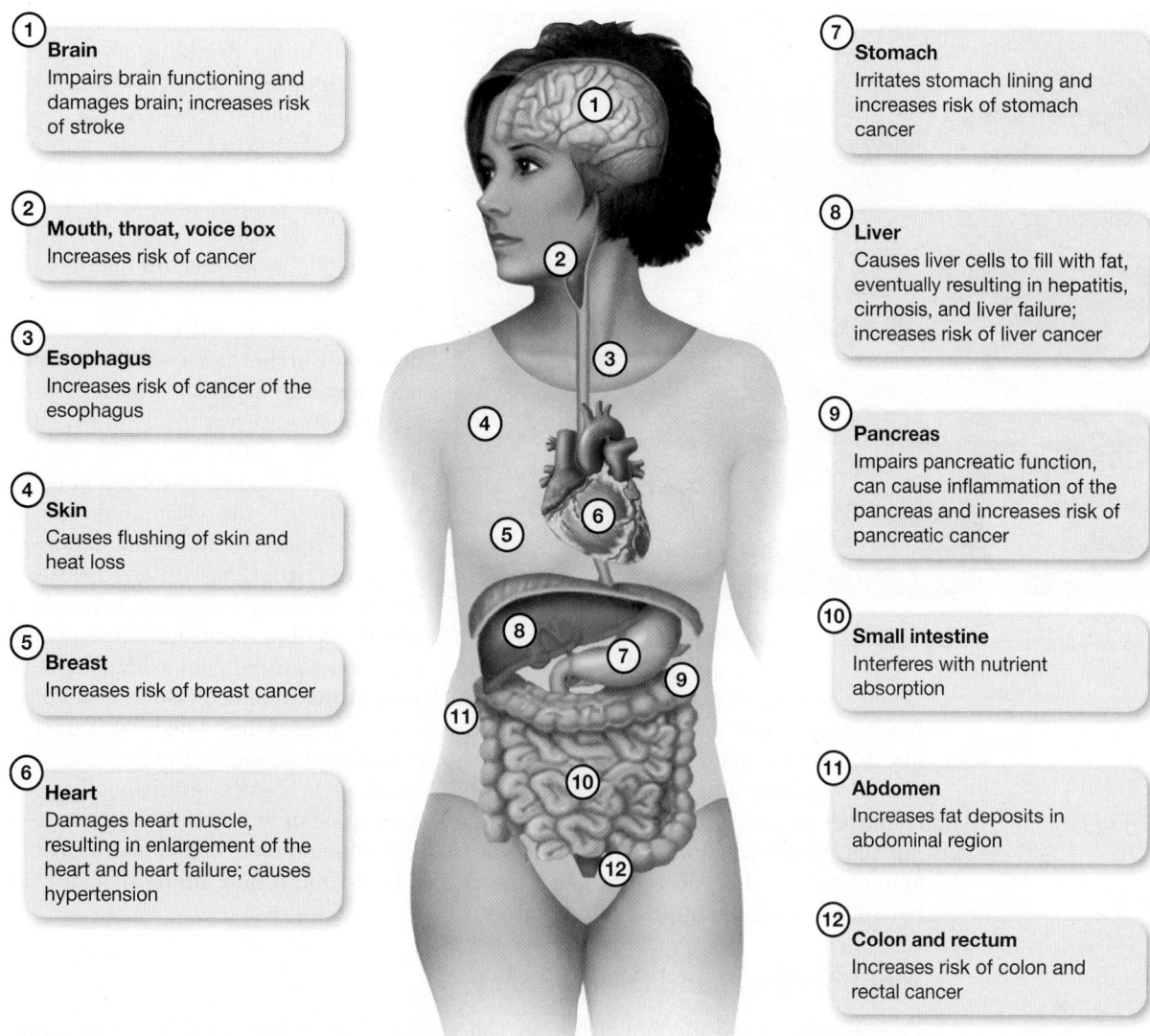

1 Brain
Impairs brain functioning and damages brain; increases risk of stroke

2 Mouth, throat, voice box
Increases risk of cancer

3 Esophagus
Increases risk of cancer of the esophagus

4 Skin
Causes flushing of skin and heat loss

5 Breast
Increases risk of breast cancer

6 Heart
Damages heart muscle, resulting in enlargement of the heart and heart failure; causes hypertension

7 Stomach
Irritates stomach lining and increases risk of stomach cancer

8 Liver
Causes liver cells to fill with fat, eventually resulting in hepatitis, cirrhosis, and liver failure; increases risk of liver cancer

9 Pancreas
Impairs pancreatic function, can cause inflammation of the pancreas and increases risk of pancreatic cancer

10 Small intestine
Interferes with nutrient absorption

11 Abdomen
Increases fat deposits in abdominal region

12 Colon and rectum
Increases risk of colon and rectal cancer

FIGURE 8.42 Alcohol's effects on the body.

Binge Drinking In 2012, about 17% of Americans who were 18 years of age or older reported being binge drinkers during the 30 days prior to the survey.[17] Binge drinking is a form of heavy drinking, but the definition of binge drinking differs according to sex. Binge drinking is defined as having four or more drinks for females and five or more drinks for males per two–hour occasion.[17]

TABLE 8.10 Classifying Drinkers

Level	Amount of Alcohol Consumed (Standard Drinks)
Abstainer	None or fewer than 12 drinks/year
Light	1–13 drinks/month
Moderate	4–14 drinks/week
Heavy	3 or more drinks/day (males); 2 or more drinks/day (females)
Binge drinker	5 or more drinks/about 2 hours (males); 4 or more drinks/about 2 hours (females)

Source: Modified from: Dufour MC: What is moderate drinking? Defining "drinks" and drinking levels. *Alcohol Research & Health*, 23(1):5, 1999.

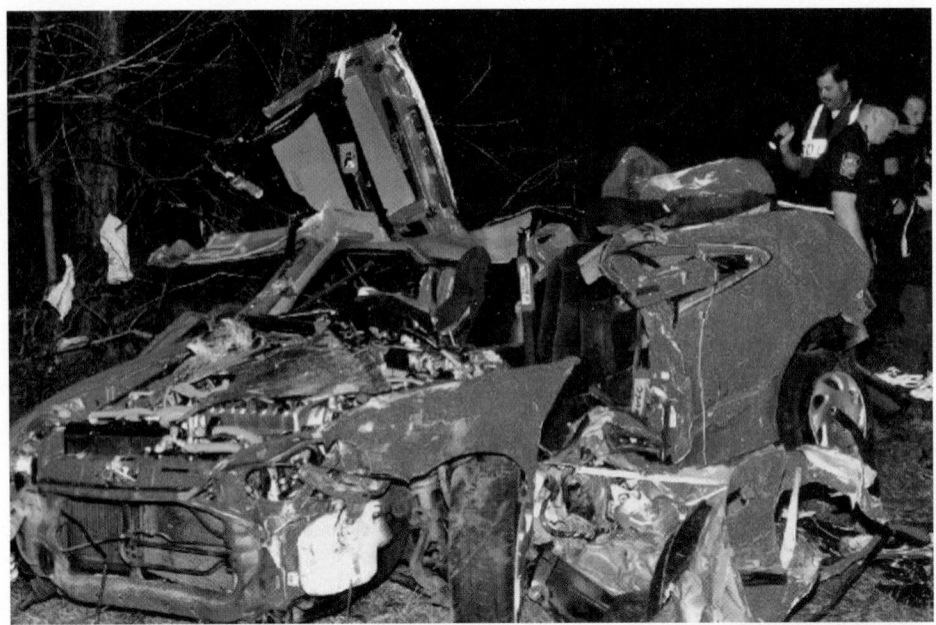

The three teenagers who died in this automobile had consumed alcohol before the accident.

As a college student, you may have observed binge drinking or engaged in the practice; about two in five college students binge drink regularly.[18] According to one survey, binge drinking rates were highest among people who were 18 to 24 years of age.[19] Youthful binge drinking is a serious public health concern because the behavior is often associated with driving while drunk. Furthermore, the practice may increase a person's later risk of alcoholism and can result in death.

During 2001 to 2005, binge drinking was responsible for more than 50% of the estimated 79,000 alcohol-related deaths that occurred annually in the United States.[20] Binge drinking increases a person's blood alcohol concentrations rapidly and to a point at which signs of alcohol poisoning occur. An individual suffering from alcohol poisoning is confused, passes out and cannot be aroused (comatose), breathes slowly and irregularly, and has pale or bluish skin. Alcohol poisoning can cause the heartbeat to slow down and lungs to stop functioning, resulting in death. Additionally, if a comatose person vomits, his or her stomach contents can enter their lungs, causing the person to choke to death. If you suspect someone has consumed a deadly amount of alcohol, do not waste time trying to estimate how many drinks that person has drunk; call 911 immediately.

Alcohol Abuse and Dependency

People who abuse alcohol drink to the extent that it harms their mental and physical health, as well as their interpersonal relationships.[21] Additionally, alcohol abusers place themselves and others in danger by driving or operating heavy machinery while intoxicated. Table 8.11 lists signs of alcohol abuse. According to government estimates, almost 15 million Americans who were 12 years of age and older were dependent on or abused alcohol in 2012.[22]

TABLE 8.11 Signs of Alcohol Abuse

You *might be abusing alcohol if you*
Drink to relax, forget your worries, or improve mood
Lose interest in food as a result of your drinking habits
Binge drink
Lie about your drinking habits or try to hide them
Drink alone
Hurt yourself or someone else while drinking
Were drunk more than three or four times last year
Need to drink more alcohol than you used to drink to get "high"
Feel irritable when you are not drinking
Have medical, social, or financial problems caused by drinking habits
Have been cited for driving while intoxicated (DWI) or driving under the influence of alcohol (DUI)

A person who is dependent on alcohol (an alcoholic) has an uncontrollable need to drink; is unable to limit his or her alcohol consumption; suffers with‐drawal symptoms, such as shakiness and anxiety, when alcohol is unavailable after a period of heavy drinking; and experiences tolerance to the drug. According to government estimates, over 700,000 Americans aged 12 and older were alcohol dependent in 2010.[22]

If you are concerned about your drinking or that of a friend or relative, con‐sider contacting these organizations:

- National Drug and Alcohol Treatment Referral Routing Service, 1‐800‐662‐HELP

- Alcoholics Anonymous, www.aa.org

- Substance Abuse and Mental Health Services Administration (http:samhsa.gov)

- Al‐Anon/Alateen, for families and friends of alcoholics and alcohol abusers, www.al‐anon.alateen.org

FRESH TIPS

Alcohol can be a dangerous drug. The following tips can help you protect yourself when you are in social situations where alcohol is available:

- Consider not drinking alcohol. When attending social occasions, you can bring a nonalcoholic beverage to consume. This allows you to blend in with others at the event by holding a glass that is filled with a beverage.

- Pace yourself. Limit your alcohol consumption to one standard drink per hour and have water or another nonalcoholic beverage in between alcoholic drinks.

- Eat ahead of and during the event. Food slows down alcohol absorption, which gives the liver more time to process it.

- At large parties, do not allow others to make drinks for you or provide an already-opened bottle of an alcohol-containing beverage for you to sample. If you place a drink down and leave it for any length of time, discard it when you get back. In your absence, someone may have added an illegal drug to it.

- Set a "cutoff" time of at least an hour before you plan to leave the party and drive elsewhere. After this time, you will not have any more alcoholic drinks. Consider calling a taxi instead of driving. When you attend parties with friends, take turns being the "designated driver" who refrains from alcohol during the events.

DID **YOU** KNOW?

Caffeinated alcoholic beverages (CABs) are commercially available drinks that are popular among younger drinkers. However, mixing caffeine and alcohol can be a dangerous combination. The person who consumes CABs may be awake, but he or she is still under the influence of alcohol and capable of serious errors of judgment. Furthermore, the caffeine in the beverages does not affect the body's ability to metabolize alcohol.[23] Thus, the person's BAC will not be reduced as a result of drinking CABs.

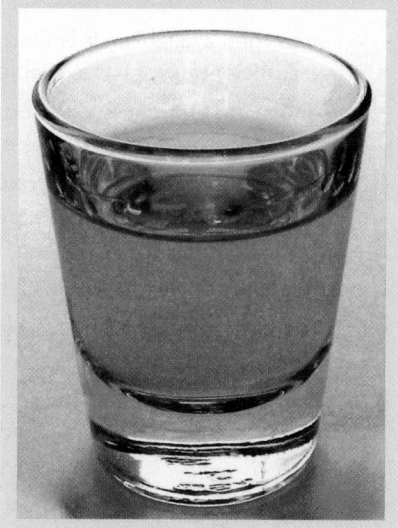

ASSESS YOUR PROGRESS

27 Describe the two pathways that metabolize alcohol.

28 Summarize the effects of alcohol on the liver.

29 What is BAC? What is the legal limit for BAC in the United States?

30 Describe at least two effects of alcohol on the body.

31 Define binge drinking and explain why it can be deadly.

32 Compare alcohol abuse and alcohol dependency.

SUMMARY

SECTION 8.1 Fueling the Body

- The primary fuels for the body are the macronutrients, predominantly carbohydrates and fats.
- Energy is defined as the capacity to do work; the body runs on chemical energy from the metabolism of macronutrients.

SECTION 8.2 Energy Metabolism

- *Metabolism* is defined as all of the chemical processes that take place in living cells. Metabolic pathways can be catabolic (energy releasing) or anabolic (energy requiring).
- Coenzymes are a particular group of organic molecules that participate and facilitate enzyme reactions.
- Cellular energy is held in adenosine triphosphate (ATP) molecules. ATP is a "high-energy" phosphate compound. The energy in ATP can be used to drive metabolic reactions.

SECTION 8.3 Obtaining Energy from Carbohydrate

- When oxygen availability is limited (anaerobic conditions), cells can release very limited amounts of energy in the cytoplasm. When sufficient oxygen is available (aerobic conditions), pathways that occur in mitochondria produce far more ATP.
- Glycolysis, the first phase of carbohydrate catabolism, occurs in the cytoplasm. Glycolysis is an anaerobic process that results in the conversion of glucose to two pyruvate molecules and a net gain of two ATP molecules.
- Under anaerobic conditions, pyruvate is converted to lactic acid. The liver can use lactic acid to remake glucose via the Cori cycle. Under aerobic conditions, pyruvate is converted into acetyl CoA for entry into the citric acid cycle.
- The citric acid cycle is a sequence of chemical reactions that results in the release of CO_2, hydrogen ions, and electrons from intermediates of citrate. Oxaloacetate, the cycle's starting compound, is re-formed in the process.
- The coenzymes FAD and NAD^+ pick up hydrogen ions and electrons that were released during glycolysis and the citric acid cycle and carry them to the electron transport chain, resulting in the production of ATP.
- Glycogenolysis is the utilization of stored glycogen in the liver and in muscles to supply the glucose needed for short-term energy needs. Glycogen storage diseases are hereditary disorders that reduce the availability of glycogen, requiring regular starch supplementation.

SECTION 8.4 Obtaining Energy from Fat

- Fatty acid catabolism occurs in the mitochondria via beta-oxidation. Ketogenesis occurs when acetyl CoA molecules cannot be used efficiently in the citric acid cycle. This condition results when the glucose supply in cells is insufficient and cells must rely on fatty acids as a major fuel. The acetyl CoA molecules that accumulate can be converted to an alternative fuel called ketone bodies. Ketoacidosis results from an excess of ketone bodies in the blood.

SECTION 8.5 Obtaining Energy from Protein

- Amino acids are catabolized after undergoing deamination or transamination. The remaining carbon skeleton may be used to make glucose, fatty acids, or ketone bodies.

SECTION 8.6 Energy Storage

- Energy is stored in the body primarily as glycogen or triglycerides. Liver and muscle cells store most of the glycogen in the body. Adipose tissue is the main storage site for triglycerides.
- Triglyceride synthesis can occur in the liver, muscle cells, and adipocytes. Metabolically, cells easily can convert fatty acids to triglycerides. The body can make triglycerides from excess amino acids, but the process is complicated.
- Human cells cannot form glucose from fatty acids. Normally, most cells rely on glucose as their predominant fuel source. When glucose supplies are adequate, fatty acids and amino acids are "spared" from being used for energy.

SECTION 8.7 Hormonal Responses to Changing Energy Needs

- The enzymes and reactions that facilitate ATP production and energy storage in the body are coordinated and regulated by specific hormones.

- In the absorptive state, insulin promotes anabolic pathways and nutrient storage. In the postabsorptive state, glucagon acts mainly on the liver to stimulate glucose production by increasing glycogenolysis and gluconeogenesis.

SECTION 8.8 **The Energy Balancing Act**

- The metabolic responses to an overnight fast include the use of liver glycogen stores, as well as gluconeogenesis, to maintain adequate blood glucose levels. Glucagon stimulates these pathways. During starvation, multiple catabolic hormones, including glucagon and cortisol, instruct cells to release all fuel sources into the bloodstream.
- Obesity often results in a state of insulin resistance. In this condition, cells do not take up blood glucose, and hyperglycemia occurs.

SECTION 8.9 **Putting the Metabolism Puzzle Together**

- Glucose, fat, and amino acids work together to fuel the body under a variety of physical conditions.

SECTION 8.10 **Alcohol as an Energy Source**

- Ethanol (alcohol) is metabolized primarily in the liver. Once alcohol enters liver cells, the drug becomes the focus of the organ's catabolic activities. Low doses of alcohol are converted to acetyl CoA using alcohol dehydrogenase and aldehyde dehydrogenase enzymes. Alcohol metabolism is influenced by sex, age, body size, frequency of drinking, and genetics.
- Excess alcohol consumption can lead to fatty liver and eventually to cirrhosis of the liver.
- Blood alcohol concentration (BAC) indicates level of alcohol consumption. Binge drinking can be deadly because an individual can drink a toxic amount of alcohol without realizing it.

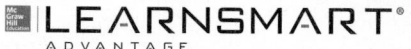

CASE STUDY RESPONSE

VERY-LOW-CARBOHYDRATE DIET

UNDER NORMAL CONDITIONS, LOUISA'S BODY catabolizes primarily carbohydrate and fat for energy. However, she has been consuming a diet that is very low in carbohydrates. Therefore, her body lacks adequate amounts of glucose for normal metabolism. Cells need about 100 g of carbohydrate daily to metabolize fat properly.

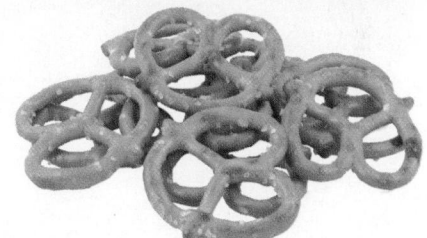

Without adequate carbohydrate, Louisa's cells rely much more heavily on fats as an alternative energy source. The significant increase in fatty acid breakdown results in ketogenesis, which supplies acetoacetate and beta-hydroxybutyrate that can be catabolized in cells of her body. However, ketone body accumulation leads to ketosis and, in severe cases, to ketoacidosis, a potentially dangerous condition characterized by abnormally low blood pH, "fruity breath," and fatigue. Louisa should consider consuming at least 100 g of carbohydrate daily to prevent ketosis and check with her physician to assess her health.

Critical Thinking

1. Explain why gluconeogenesis is an important metabolic activity.
2. Ahmed jogs on a treadmill as part of his workout routine. Although he exercises in an air-conditioned gym and has a fan blowing cool air on him, he feels warm after less than 10 minutes of jogging. Explain why he has trouble keeping cool while exercising.
3. Very-low-fat diets have a history of being popular for weight loss. Explain how a person may still gain body fat on this type of diet.
4. Emma drinks at least six 12-ounce cans of beer daily, and sometimes she consumes whiskey along with the beer. Although she spends most of her income on alcoholic beverages and eats very little, she has gained a lot of fat, especially in the abdominal section of her body. Explain why Emma has gained the fat.
5. Many energy drinks contain very high amounts of B vitamins, such as vitamin B-12 and niacin. Do these B vitamins provide energy? Describe why or why not.

TEST KITCHEN

Modifying Recipes for Healthy Living

For this activity, compare the ingredients in a serving of a commercial energy drink to a serving of a smoothie that you can make at home. Then, answer the following questions.

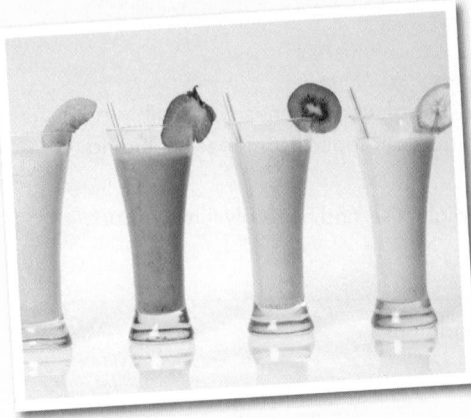

Commercial Energy Drink			High-Caliber Smoothie†		
Ingredients		kcal	Ingredients		kcal
Water	12 oz	0	Nonfat milk	1 cup (8 oz)	80
Sucrose	1 Tbsp	120	Nonfat plain yogurt	¼ cup	35
Glucose	1 tsp	40	Frozen raspberries, unsweetened	¼ cup	30
Caffeine	100 mg		Frozen blueberries, unsweetened	¼ cup	20
B vitamins*			Banana	1 medium	100
Niacin	20 mg				
B-6	1.5 mg				
B-12	2.5 μg				
Pantothenic acid	10 mg				
Total kcal:		160	Total kcal:		265

*All amounts at least 100% of RDA
†To make the smoothie, combine all ingredients and blend until smooth.

1. What are the sources of energy in the two drinks?
2. Not long after the drinks are consumed, blood sugar levels begin to rise. which stimulates the pancreas to release insulin. Assume the person consuming the commercial energy drink does not need the calories from the beverage for energy. In this situation, what effect would the insulin have on the body?
3. Which drink is a healthier source of energy? Explain your choice of drinks.

Practice Test

1. Metabolism is the ___ that occur in living cells.
   a. total of all chemical reactions
   b. sum of all catabolic reactions
   c. sum of all anabolic reactions
   d. difference between anabolic and catabolic reactions

2. Glycolysis
   a. requires oxygen.
   b. results in a net gain of 10 ATP.
   c. occurs in mitochondria.
   d. results in the formation of pyruvate.

3. When oxygen is not available in a working muscle cell, pyruvate will be converted to
   a. acetyl CoA.
   b. oxaloacetate.
   c. lactic acid.
   d. palmitic acid.

4. During beta-oxidation, fatty acids are
   a. anabolized to yield acetyl CoA molecules for conversion to glucose.
   b. converted to triglycerides and stored in adipocytes.
   c. oxidized to yield acetyl CoA molecules for the citric acid cycle.
   d. formed in the cytoplasm and used for amino acid synthesis.

5. Which of the following statements is true?
   a. Ketone bodies are produced from acetyl CoA molecules.
   b. When excess amino acids are consumed, acetyl CoA molecules accumulate in cytoplasm.
   c. Acetyl CoA molecules enter the electron transport chain.
   d. Accumulated acetyl CoA can be converted pyruvate.

6. Which of the following best describes the most likely fate of excess glucose molecules in the body after a meal?
   a. Liver cells convert the excess glucose molecules to glycogen.
   b. Mitochondrial enzymes in the adrenal glands anabolize the excess glucose to amino acids for storage in muscle protein.
   c. The kidneys degrade the excess glucose molecules into urea for elimination in urine.
   d. Intestinal cells use the excess glucose molecules to synthesize ketone bodies.

7. Metabolic postabsorptive responses are mainly under the influence of
   a. glucagon.
   b. cortisol.
   c. progesterone.
   d. insulin.

8. Glucagon instructs liver cells to
   a. synthesize fatty acids.
   b. synthesize glycogen to store glucose.
   c. degrade glycogen to release glucose.
   d. degrade insulin.

9. During prolonged fasting, the following pathways are all active, except
   a. glycogenolysis.
   b. gluconeogenesis.
   c. ketogenesis.
   d. fatty acid synthesis.

10. The cells of an obese person may
    a. become insulin resistant.
    b. increase their catabolism of fatty acids.
    c. become hypermetabolic.
    d. increase their synthesis of glucose from fatty acids.

11. Alcohol metabolism in the liver can result in all of the following, except
    a. production of acetyl CoA.
    b. synthesis of glucose.
    c. synthesis of fatty acids.
    d. production of acetaldehyde.

12. ___ has riboflavin in its chemical structure.
    a. NAD^+
    b. $FADH_2$
    c. PLP
    d. Coenzyme A

13. Which of the following hormones promotes glycogenesis?
    a. insulin
    b. cortisol
    c. glucagon
    d. epinephrine

14. Kenny's BAC is 0.025. At this BAC, you would expect him to be
    a. relaxed.
    b. angry.
    c. in a stupor.
    d. in a coma.

15. Low to moderate amounts of alcohol are metabolized through the
    a. microsomal ethanol-oxidizing system (MEOS).
    b. pyruvate dehydrogenase shuttle.
    c. alcohol dehydrogenase pathway.
    d. beta-oxidation pathway.

ANSWERS TO PRACTICE TEST
1-a; 2-d; 3-c; 4-c; 5-a; 6-a; 7-d; 8-c; 9-d; 10-a; 11-b; 12-b; 13-a; 14-a; 15-c

ANSWERS TO CHAPTER 8 QUIZ Yourself

1. Fats are metabolized by a process called glycolysis. **False** (p. 240)
2. Many B vitamins are components of coenzymes that work with enzymes in energy metabolism. **True** (p. 229)
3. Lactate is a molecule that accumulates in tissues when oxygen is not available. **True** (p. 232)
4. Following an overnight fast, insulin stimulates the liver cells to increase glucose production. **False** (p. 251)
5. Body size, sex, and age affect an individual's metabolism of alcohol. **True** (p. 255)

References

1. LaForgia J and others: Effects of exercise intensity and duration on the excess postexercise oxygen consumption. *Journal of Sports Sciences* 24(12):1247, 2006.

2. Nelson DL, Cox MM: *Lehninger principles of biochemistry.* 5th ed. W.H. Freeman and Company: New York, 2008.

3. Otten JJ and others, eds: *Dietary Reference Intakes: The essential guide to nutrient requirements.* Washington, DC: National Academies Press, 2006.

4. PubMed Health: *Epilepsy.* Reviewed 2012. http://www.ncbi.nlm.nih.gov/pubmedhealth/PMH0001714/ Accessed: August 22, 2013

5. Runyon AM, So T-Y: The use of ketogenic diet in pediatric patients with epilepsy. *ISRN Pediatrics* Article ID 263139, 10 pages, 2012. DOI:10.5402/2012/263139

6. Westerberg DP: Diabetic ketoacidosis: Evaluation and treatment. *American Family Physician* 87(5):337, 2013.

7. Kordella T: Diabetic ketoacidosis. As dangerous as it sounds. Knowing what diabetic ketoacidosis is and how to prevent it can save you a trip to the hospital. *Diabetes Forecast* 58(3):40, 2005.

8. McKinley MP and others: *Anatomy & physiology: An integrative approach.* McGraw-Hill Publishing Company: New York, 2013.

9. National Institutes of Health, National Heart, Lung, and Blood Institute: *What is metabolic syndrome?* 2011. http://www.nhlbi.nih.gov/health/health-topics/topics/ms/ Accessed: February 2, 2014

10. Jones AW. Evidence-based survey of the elimination rates of ethanol from blood with applications in forensic casework. *Forensic Science International.* 200(1-3):1, 2010. DOI: 10.1016/j.forsciint.2010.02.021. Epub March 20, 2010.

11. Greenfield SF and others: Substance abuse in women. *Psychiatric Clinics of North America* 33(2):339, 2010.

12. Ceylan-Isik AF and others: Sex difference in alcoholism: Who is at greater risk for development of alcoholic complication? *Life Sciences* 87(5-6):133, 2010.

13. Yokoyama A and others: Alcohol and aldehyde dehydrogenase polymorphisms and a new strategy for prevention and screening for cancer in the upper aerodigestive tract in East Asians. *Keio Journal of Medicine* 59(4):115, 2010.

14. National Center for Chronic Disease Prevention & Health Promotion. Behavioral Risk Factor Surveillance System: Prevalence and trends data. *Alcohol consumption—2012. Adults who have had at least one drink of alcohol within the past 30 days.* http://www.cdc.gov/brfss/ Accessed: February 2, 2014

15. National Center for Chronic Disease Prevention & Health Promotion. Behavioral Risk Factor Surveillance System: *Prevalence and trends data. Alcohol consumption—2012. Heavy drinkers (adult men having more than two drinks per day and adult women having more than one drink per day).* http://www.cdc.gov/brfss/ Accessed: February 2, 2014

16. Substance Abuse and Mental Health Services Administration: *Results from the 2011 National Survey on Drug Use and Health: Summary of National Findings.* NSDUH Series H-44, HHS Publication No. (SMA) 12-4713. Rockville, MD: Substance Abuse and Mental Health Services Administration, 2012. http://www.samhsa.gov/data/NSDUH/2k11Results/NSDUHresults2011.htm Accessed: February 2, 2014

17. National Center for Chronic Disease Prevention & Health Promotion. Behavioral Risk Factor Surveillance System: *Prevalence and trend data. Alcohol consumption—2012. Binge drinkers (males having five or more drinks on one occasion, females having four or more drinks on one occasion)* http://www.cdc.gov/brfss/ Accessed: February 2, 2014

18. Hingson RW and others: Magnitude of and trends in alcohol-related mortality and morbidity among U.S. college students ages 18-24, 1998–2005. *J. Stud. Alcohol Drugs* Suppl. 16:12-20, 2009.

19. Naimi TS and others: The intensity of binge alcohol consumption among U.S. adults. *American Journal of Preventive Medicine* 38(2):201-207, 2010.

20. Centers for Disease Control and Prevention: Vital signs: Binge drinking among high school students and adults—United States, 2009. *Morbidity and Mortality Weekly Report* 59(39): 1274, 2010. www.cdc.gov/mmwr/preview/mmwrhtml/mm5939a4.htm?s_cid=mm5939a4_ Accessed: February 2, 2014

21. Centers for Disease Control and Prevention: *Alcohol and public health, frequently asked questions.* Updated July 2013. http://www.cdc.gov/alcohol/faqs.htm#alcoholismAbuse Accessed: February 2, 2014

22. U.S. Department of Health and Human Services, Substance Abuse and Mental Health Services Administration: Figure 7.1 Substance dependence or abuse in the past year among persons aged 12 or older: 2002-2012. 2013. *Results from the 2012 National Survey on Drug Use and Health: Summary of National Finding.* http://www.samhsa.gov/data/NSDUH/2012SummNatFindDetTables/Index.aspx Accessed: February 2, 2014

23. Centers for Disease Control and Prevention: *Alcohol and public health: Fact sheets—caffeinated alcoholic beverages.* 2010. http://www.cdc.gov/alcohol/x.fact-sheets/cab.htm Accessed: February 3, 2014

9 Vitamin Overview and Fat-Soluble Vitamins

Vitamin D and bone health

SEVENTY-YEAR-OLD JOSETTE LEARNED at her last physician's appointment that she is 2 inches shorter than she was 5 years ago. Her physician noted that Josette has developed curvature of her upper spine and recommended that she have additional testing to determine the cause. Additional testing revealed that Josette has low blood levels of vitamin D.

Josette has lived in northern Maine her entire life. After spending the past 30 years working outdoors, she has retired and now spends the majority of her day indoors.

- Describe the relationship between vitamin D and developing curvature of the upper spine.

- Explain to Josette how living in northern Maine may be contributing to her low blood levels of vitamin D.

- Recommend at least five vitamin D–rich foods for Josette to include in her diet.

The suggested Case Study Response can be found on page 298.

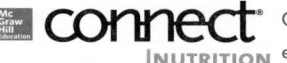

connect NUTRITION   Check out the Connect site at www.mcgrawhillconnect.com to further explore this case study.

QUIZ Yourself

Can vitamins give a person more energy or reduce his or her chances for developing chronic disease? What happens if someone consumes too little or too much of a particular vitamin? Test your knowledge of vitamins by taking the following quiz. The answers are found on page 301.

1. Vitamins are a source of "quick" energy. ___T ___F

2. A deficiency of vitamin A can lead to night blindness. ___T ___F

3. Fruits are a rich dietary source of vitamin D. ___T ___F

4. Vitamin E is an antioxidant. ___T ___F

5. Vitamin K is necessary for blood clotting. ___T ___F

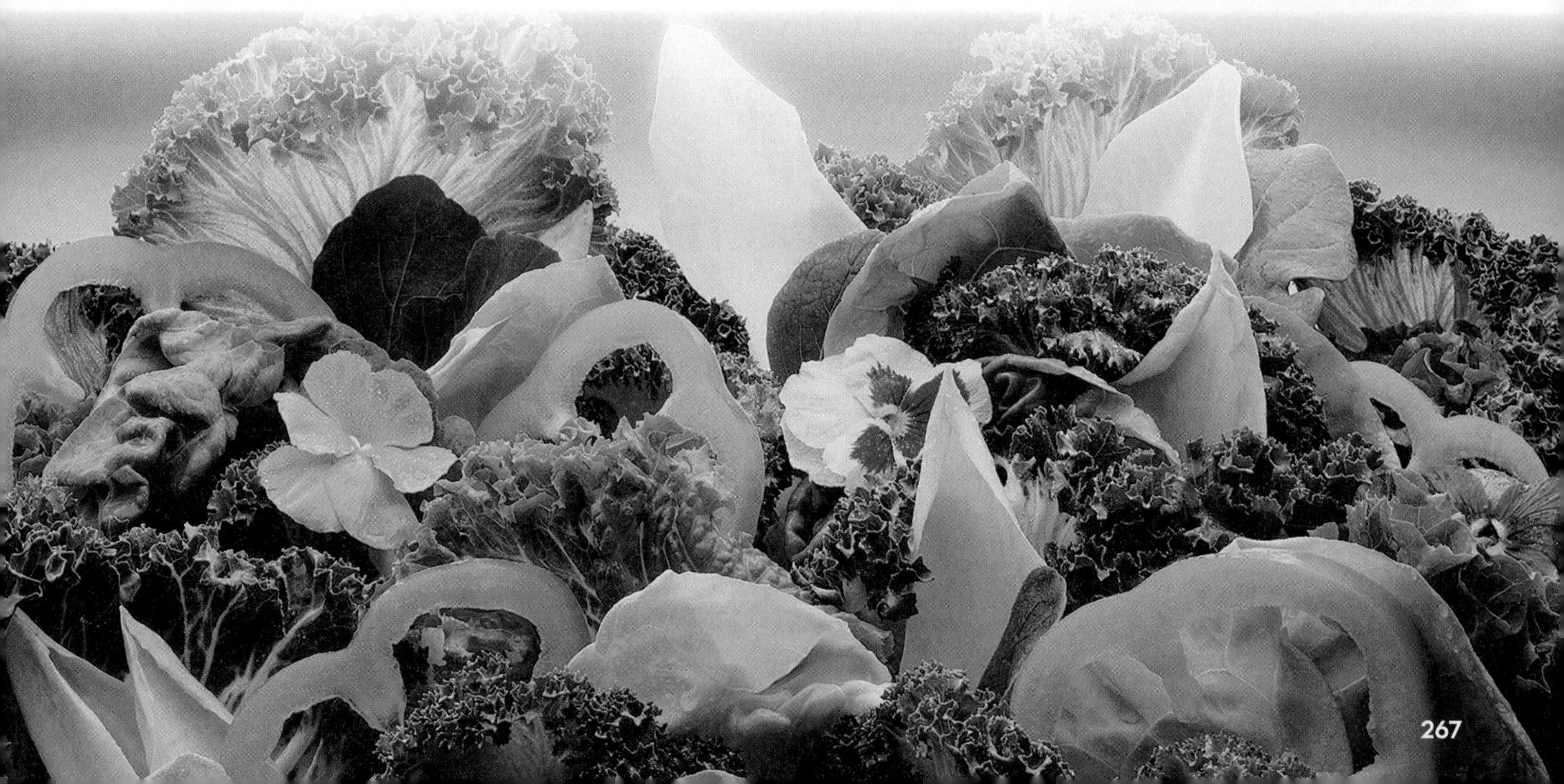

9.1 Introducing Vitamins

LEARNING OUTCOMES

1 *State the meaning of the term* vitamin.

2 *Explain why it is unlikely that any vitamins have yet to be discovered.*

Vitamins were first defined in 1912 when Polish chemist Casimir Funk coined the termed *vitamine* (*vita* = necessary for life; *amine* = a type of nitrogen–containing substance) after discovering a substance, now known as thiamin, in an extract made from rice bran. Dr. Funk thought that this substance would cure the disease beriberi—and he was correct.

The term *vitamine* was later modified to *vitamin* when scientists determined that there were several kinds of these substances in foods and not all were amines. By the end of the twentieth century, scientists had added riboflavin, niacin, biotin, B–6, B–12, pantothenic acid, folate, ascorbic acid, A, D, E, and K to the list of vitamins.

It is unlikely that any vitamins still need to be discovered. Evidence for this conclusion is that babies grow and thrive on infant formulas, synthetic liquid diets containing vitamins and other nutrients known to be essential for health. Additionally, very ill people who cannot eat solid food can be kept alive for years on liquid synthetic feedings that contain all known nutrients, including vitamins. If a vitamin remained undiscovered, infants and people who are unable to consume solid foods would not be able to survive on formula diets.

This chapter and Chapter 10 present information about the 13 vitamins, and the vitamin–like substances choline, inositol, carnitine, taurine, and lipoic acid. By reading these chapters, you will learn what can happen to the body when consumption of certain vitamins is too small or too great. Many Americans take vitamin supplements to prevent disease. This and the next chapter examine current scientific evidence concerning the usefulness of taking megadoses of certain vitamins. In general, a megadose is at least 10 times the recommended amount of the micronutrient.[1]

ASSESS YOUR PROGRESS

1 What is the literal meaning of vitamin?

2 Why is it unlikely that additional vitamins have yet to be discovered?

9.2 Vitamins: The Basics

LEARNING OUTCOMES

1 *List the fat-soluble and water-soluble vitamins.*

2 *Compare and contrast general characteristics of fat- and water-soluble vitamins.*

3 *Describe the activity of antioxidants.*

4 *Identify factors that affect the bioavailability of a vitamin.*

5 *Explain how the vitamin content of a food can be conserved.*

vitamin complex organic molecule that regulates certain metabolic processes

A **vitamin** is a complex organic compound that regulates certain metabolic processes in the body and meets the following criteria:

- The body cannot synthesize the compound or make enough to maintain good health (it is an *essential nutrient*);

- The compound naturally occurs in commonly eaten foods;

- Signs and symptoms of a health problem (*deficiency disorder*) eventually occur when the substance is missing from the diet or is not properly metabolized; and

- Good health is restored if the deficiency disorder is treated early by supplying the missing substance.

Although vitamins are organic molecules in foods, they are distinctly different from car‒bohydrates, fats, and proteins. For example, carbohydrates, fats, and proteins are metab‒olized for energy, but vitamins are not. In addition, foods generally contain much smaller amounts of vitamins than of macronutrients. A slice of whole‒wheat bread, for example, weighs 28 g. Of that weight, only about 0.005% (1.48 mg) is comprised of vitamins; carbo‒hydrate, water, protein, fat, and minerals make up the remaining weight of the bread. Furthermore, the body requires vitamins in milligram or microgram amounts, but it needs grams of macronutrients.

In the past, amounts of most vitamins in foods, particularly fat‒soluble vitamins A, D, and E, were often expressed in *International Units (IUs)*. Today, IUs have largely been replaced by more precise milligram or micro‒gram measures. One microgram of vitamin D, for example, equals 40 IUs of the vitamin. Food composition tables and the information panels on food and sup‒plement labels often still list IU values for fat‒soluble vitamins. Table 9.1 pro‒vides IU conversion values for vitamins A, D, and E.

A slice of bread weighs about 1 ounce (28 g). Vitamins comprise only about 0.005% (1.48 mg) of the weight of the bread.

Classifying Vitamins

Vitamins A, D, E, and K are **fat‒soluble vitamins**. These vitamins are found in the lipid portions of foods and tend to associate with lipids in the body. The fat‒soluble vitamins are digested and absorbed with fats in the GI tract. Therefore, foods rich in fat often contain vitamins A, D, E, and/or K.

fat-soluble vitamins vitamins A, D, E, and K

Thiamin, riboflavin, niacin, vitamin B‒6, pantothenic acid, folate, biotin, vitamin B‒12 (collectively known as the B vitamins), and vitamin C are **water‒soluble vitamins**. The vitamin‒like compounds choline, carnitine, and lipoic acid are also water soluble. Water‒soluble vitamins dissolve in the watery components of food and the body.

water-soluble vitamins thiamin, riboflavin, niacin, vitamin B-6, pantothenic acid, folate, biotin, vitamin B-12, and vitamin C

TABLE 9.1 International Unit (IU) Conversion Values for Vitamins A, D, and E

Vitamin A	Vitamin D	Vitamin E
1 IU vitamin A activity = 0.3 µg retinol = 3.6 µg beta-carotene	**1 IU vitamin D activity** = 0.025 µg cholecalciferol	**1 IU vitamin E activity** = 0.67 mg alpha-tocopherol
1 µg retinol = 3.33 IU vitamin A	**1 µg cholecalciferol** = 40 IU vitamin D	**1 mg alpha-tocopherol** = 1.49 IU vitamin E

TABLE 9.2 Classifying Vitamins

Fat-Soluble Vitamins
A (retinol)
D (cholecalciferol, ergocalciferol)
E (alpha-tocopherol, other tocopherols)
K (phylloquinones, menaquinones)
Water-Soluble Vitamins
Thiamin (thiamine, B-1)
Riboflavin (B-2)
Niacin (B-3, nicotinamide, nicotinic acid)
B-6 (pyridoxine)
B-12 (cobalamin, cobalamine)
Biotin (H)
Pantothenic acid (B-5)
Folate (folic acid)
C (ascorbic acid)
Vitamin-Like
Carnitine
Choline
Inositol
Lipoic acid
Taurine

DID **YOU** KNOW?

Smoking tobacco or being exposed to tobacco smoke causes the production of free radicals. Children exposed to second-hand smoke have lower levels of antioxidants in their body, regardless of their dietary and supplement intake. Blood levels of the antioxidant vitamins A, C, and E are lower in children whose parents smoke.[2] Therefore, parents and other caregivers should be concerned about this additional risk of second-hand smoke in the home.

oxidizing agent or **oxidant** substance that removes electrons from atoms or molecules

free radical substance with an unpaired electron

antioxidant substance that gives up electrons to free radicals to protect cells

Vitamins may have more than one name. Table 9.2 presents the vitamins and provides some other names that may be used to identify them.

Why is it important to know the difference between fat– and water–soluble vitamins? The reason is that the body generally has more difficulty eliminating excess fat–soluble vitamins because these nutrients do not dissolve in watery substances such as urine. As a result, the body stores extra fat–soluble vitamins, primarily in the liver and in adipose tissue. Over time, these vitamins can accumulate and cause toxicity. In contrast, the body stores only limited amounts of most water–soluble vitamins; vitamin B–12 is an exception. Furthermore, kidneys can filter excesses of water–soluble vitamins from the bloodstream and eliminate them in urine. Thus, water–soluble vitamins are generally not as likely to be toxic as fat–soluble vitamins.

Roles of Vitamins

Vitamins play numerous roles in the body, and each of these micronutrients gen–erally has more than one function (Fig. 9.1). Some vitamins, such as vitamin D, act as hormones; other vitamins, such as vitamin C and thiamin, participate in chemical reactions by accepting or donating electrons. In general, vitamins regulate a variety of body processes, including those involved in cell division and development as well as the growth and maintenance of tissues.

Advertisements for vitamin supplements often promote the notion that these micronutrients can "give" you energy. Vitamins, however, are not a source of energy, because cells do not metabolize them for energy. Although not used directly for energy, many vitamins participate in the chemical reactions that release energy from glucose, fatty acids, and certain amino acids. Recall that in Chapter 8, you learned that NAD^+ and $FADH_2$, which are important cofactors in metabolism, are derived from niacin and riboflavin, respectively. Appendix E presents a simplified view of energy metabolism and indicates vitamins that are involved in the various steps of the process.

Most vitamins have more than one chemical form that functions in the body. For example, *retinol*, *retinal*, and *retinoic acid* are chemically related types of vitamin A that have roles in the body. Additionally, some vitamins have precursors (*provitamins*) that do not function as vitamins until the body converts them into active forms. For example, the plant pigment beta–carotene is a provitamin for vitamin A, and the amino acid tryptophan is a precursor for the B–vitamin niacin.

What Is an Antioxidant?

When many biochemical reactions take place, the compounds participating in the reactions lose or gain electrons. An atom or molecule that loses one or more electrons has been *oxidized*. An **oxidizing agent** or **oxidant** is a substance that removes electrons from atoms or molecules. An oxidation reaction can form a **free radical**, a substance with an unpaired electron.

Free radicals are highly reactive, that is, chemically unstable, and they remove electrons from more stable molecules, such as proteins, fatty acids, and DNA (Fig. 9.2). As a result, free radicals can damage or destroy these mole–cules. If the loss of electrons is uncontrolled, a chain reaction can occur in which excessive oxidation takes place and affects many cells. Many medical researchers suspect excess oxidation is responsible for promoting chemical changes in cells that ultimately lead to heart attack, stroke, cancer, Alzheimer's disease, and even the aging process.

Some free radical formation in the body is necessary and provides some benefits.[3] Free radicals, for example, stimulate normal cell growth and division. Additionally, white blood cells generate free radicals as part of their activities in destroying infectious agents. Under normal conditions, cells regulate oxidation reactions by using antioxidants such as vitamin E. **Antioxidants** protect cells by giving up electrons to free radicals. When a chemically unstable substance accepts an electron, it can form a more stable structure that does not pull electrons away

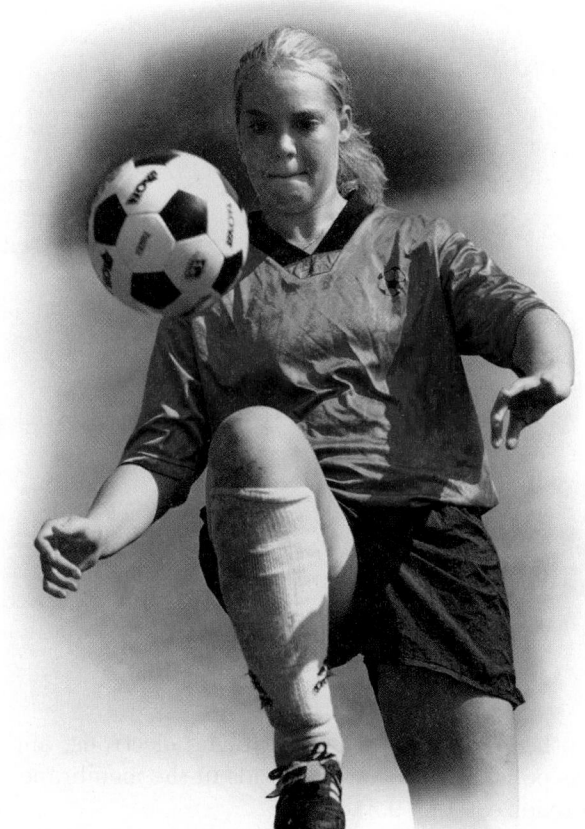

Bone Health

Vitamin A
Vitamin D
Vitamin K
Vitamin C

Energy Metabolism

Thiamin
Riboflavin
Niacin
Pantothenic acid
Biotin
Vitamin B-12
Vitamin B-6

Blood Clotting

Vitamin K

Amino Acid Metabolism

Vitamin B-6
Folate
Vitamin B-12
Vitamin C
Choline

Growth and Development

Vitamin A
Vitamin D
Choline

Red Blood Cell Formation

Vitamin B-6
Vitamin B-12
Folate
Riboflavin (indirect)

Immune Function

Vitamin A
Vitamin C
Vitamin D
Vitamin E

Antioxidant Defense

Vitamin E
Vitamin C (likely)
Certain carotenoids

FIGURE 9.1 Functions of vitamins and related compounds. Groups of vitamins and related compounds (e.g., choline and certain carotenoids) work together to maintain good health.

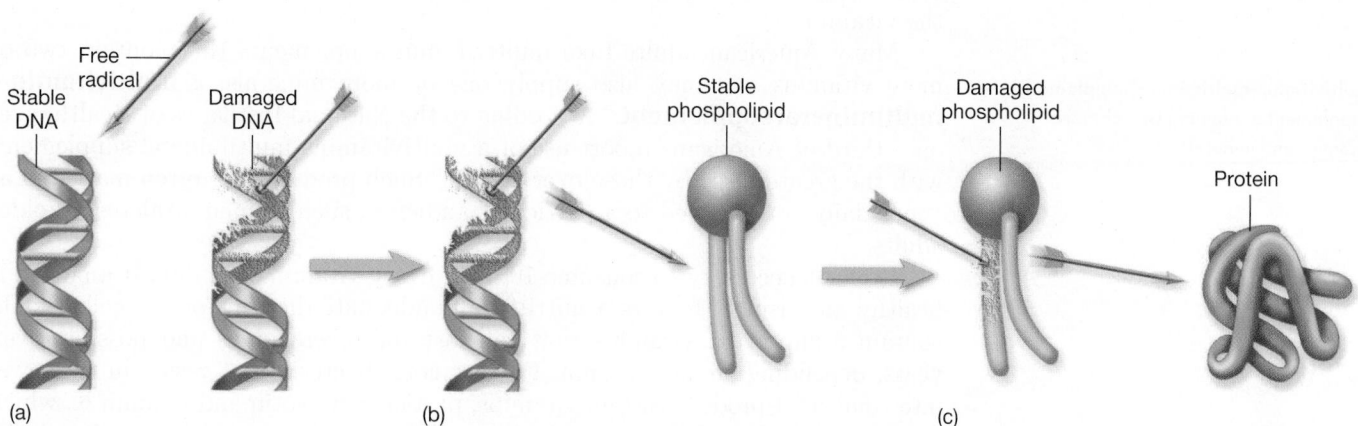

(a)   (b)   (c)

FIGURE 9.2 Free radical activity. (*a*) A free radical acts as an "arrow" by hitting a vulnerable molecule such as DNA. (*b*) The damaged molecule becomes the source of another free radical that "strikes" another vulnerable molecule; in this case, a phospholipid. (*c*) The reaction repeats itself.

FIGURE 9.3 Antioxidant action.
By sacrificing electrons, antioxidants protect molecules such as polyunsaturated fatty acids in the plasma membrane or DNA in the nucleus from being oxidized.

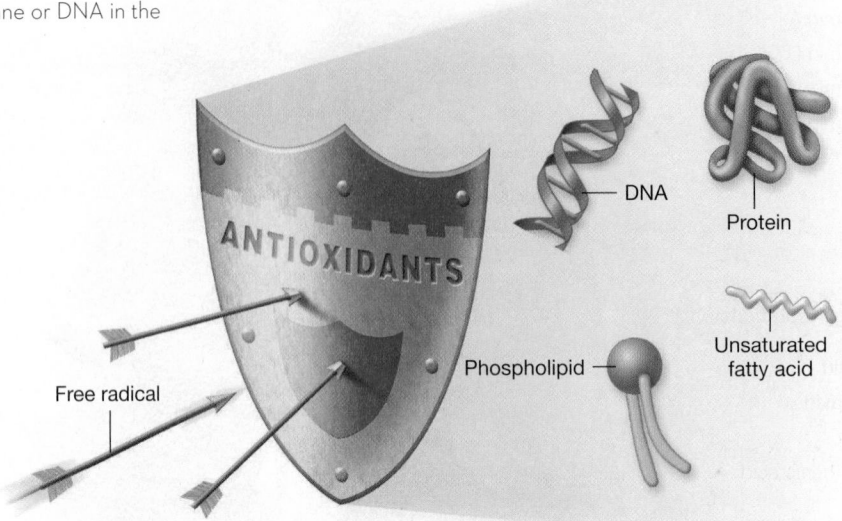

from other compounds. By sacrificing electrons, antioxidants protect molecules such as polyunsaturated fatty acids in the membrane or DNA in the nucleus from being oxidized (Fig. 9.3).

Sources of Vitamins

Plants, animals, fungi, and even bacteria supply natural forms of vitamins in our diets. In addition to foods, vitamin supplements are another source of these micronutrients. Although chemists can synthesize vitamins, certain types of bacteria and algae produce vitamins. These organisms can be grown in laboratory settings for the purpose of "harvesting" their vitamins to use in supplement production.[4]

Regardless of whether a particular vitamin is naturally found in foods or synthesized in a laboratory, it generally has the same chemical structure and works equally well in the body. However, there are exceptions. The natural form of vitamin E has more **biological activity**, that is, it produces more effects in the body, than synthetic vitamin E. In contrast, *synthetic folic acid*, the type of folate that is added to flour and many readytoeat and cooked cereals, has almost twice the biological activity as the natural form of the vitamin.

Many American adults take multivitamin supplements that contain two or more vitamins and may also supply one or more minerals, a **multivitamin–multimineral supplement**.[5] According to the National Institutes of Health, over onethird of Americans report use of a multivitamin–multimineral supplement, with the greatest use by those over age 70.[6] Such products are often marketed as "once daily" or targeted to a particular audience, such as men, athletes, or older adults.

It is not necessary to consume 100% of every vitamin each day. If a person is healthy and usually follows a nutritionally adequate diet, his or her cells should contain a supply of vitamins that can last for several days and possibly even years, depending on the vitamin. Furthermore, bacteria that reside in the lower intestinal tract produce certain vitamins, particularly biotin and vitamin K, which can be absorbed to some extent. Additionally, the body can synthesize vitamin D, niacin, and choline under certain conditions.

biological activity describes vitamin's degree of potency or effects in the body

multivitamin-multimineral supplement supplement containing two or more vitamins and minerals

Bioavailability of Vitamins

Food processing and preparation, as well as digestion and absorption all affect the bioavailability of a vitamin, the amount of that vitamin that is actually available for use by the body. Factors that affect vitamin bioavailability include:

- Changes to the normal GI transit time. When foods move too quickly through the GI tract, such as in cases of frequent diarrhea, vitamin bioavailability is decreased.

- Health conditions that affect absorption of fats also affect fat—soluble vitamin absorption, reducing vitamin bioavailability.

- Food processing and preparation techniques.

- Source of the vitamin. Most vitamins are more bioavailable from natural food sources, but that is not always the case. For example, folate is nearly two times as bioavailable from synthetic sources as from food sources.

When working with a client who has a vitamin deficiency, it is important for the health care provider to evaluate factors that may be negatively affecting the vitamin's bioavailability. Adjustments can be made in the source of the vitamin, food preparation techniques, and overall dietary habits to maximize bioavailability and correct deficiencies.

Vitamin Enrichment and Fortification

In Chapter 3, we discussed nutrient enrichment and fortification. Enrichment helps protect Americans from developing the deficiency diseases associated with the lack of thiamin, riboflavin, niacin, folate, and iron. However, enrichment does not replace the vitamin E, vitamin B—6, magnesium, several other micronutrients, and fiber that were naturally present in the unrefined grains. This is the major reason dietitians and other nutrition experts promote regular consumption of whole—grain products, such as whole—wheat bread and brown rice.

Some food manufacturers add vitamins to (fortify) foods and beverages, particularly flavored drinks, which would otherwise be considered "empty—calorie" items. Many nutrition experts are concerned that by substituting such human—made products for more natural foods and beverages, Americans may consume excessive amounts of a few vitamins while reducing their intake of others.

Vitamin Absorption

The small intestine is the primary site of vitamin absorption. However, the intestine does not absorb 100% of the vitamins in food. Vitamin absorption tends to increase when the body's needs for the micronutrients are also higher than usual. The body's requirements for vitamins generally increase during periods of growth, such as infancy and adolescence, and during pregnancy and breastfeeding.

Fat—soluble vitamins are chemically similar to lipids, and the vitamins are in fatty portions of food. Thus, processes that normally occur during fat digestion facilitate the absorption of fat—soluble vitamins. For example, bile enhances lipid as well as fat—soluble vitamin absorption. In the small intestine, the presence of fat stimulates the secretion of the hormone cholecystokinin (CCK) that causes the gallbladder to release bile. Therefore, adding a small amount of fat to low—fat foods, such as tossing raw vegetables with some salad dressing, adding a teaspoon of soft margarine to steamed carrots, or stir—frying green beans in peanut oil, can enhance the intestinal tract's ability to absorb the fat—soluble vitamins in these foods. To review lipid digestion, see Chapter 6.

Diseases or conditions that affect the GI tract can reduce vitamin absorption and result in deficiencies of these micronutrients. People with the inherited disease *cystic fibrosis* (*sis'—tik fie—broe'—sis*) are unable to digest fat properly.

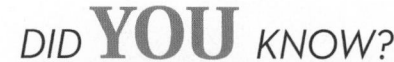

DID **YOU** *KNOW?*

A plant's vitamin content is largely determined by its genetic makeup; by growing conditions, including soil composition and sunlight exposure; and by its maturity when harvested.

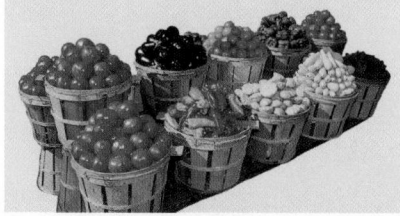

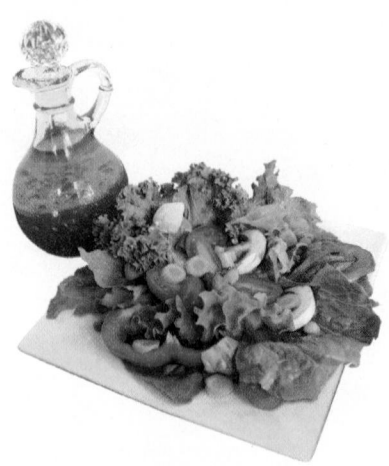

Promote absorption of fat-soluble vitamins by tossing salad with salad dressing, such as an olive oil-based vinaigrette.

Blockages form in ducts that convey pancreatic enzymes to the small intestine, reducing fat absorption. People suffering from the disease often develop deficiencies of fat—soluble vitamins. Section 9.8 provides more information about cystic fibrosis and the problems that can result from malabsorption of fat—soluble vitamins.

People who are unable to absorb vitamins efficiently may need to take large oral doses of vitamin supplements just to enable small amounts of the vitamins to be absorbed. In other cases, injections of vitamins may be needed.

Deficiency and Toxicity of Vitamins

A diet that contains adequate amounts of a wide variety of foods, including min—imally processed fruits, vegetables, and whole—grain breads and cereals, can help supply the vitamin needs of most healthy people. Vitamin deficiency disorders gen—erally result from inadequate diets or conditions that increase the body's require—ments for vitamins, such as reduced intestinal absorption or higher—than—normal excretion of the micronutrients. Today, severe vitamin deficiencies are uncommon in the United States, thanks in part to modern food preservation practices, food enrichment and fortification, and the year—round, widespread availability of fresh fruits and vegetables from other countries. Many Americans, however, consume less than recommended amounts of vitamins A, D, E, and K.[7]

Certain segments of the population are at risk for vitamin deficiencies. These vulnerable people include alcoholics, older adults, and patients who are hospital—ized for lengthy periods. Additionally, people who suffer from the eating disorder anorexia nervosa, have intestinal conditions that interfere with vitamin absorption, or have rare metabolic defects that increase their vitamin requirements are more likely to develop vitamin deficiency disorders than people who do not have these conditions.

A nutritionally adequate diet that occasionally lacks proper vitamin intake is not likely to cause a deficiency disease, because body cells store vitamins to some extent. The likelihood of developing a deficiency disease increases when a diet consistently lacks one or more vitamins. When this happens, the person's body stores or tissue levels of the vitamin become depleted, and the signs and symp—toms of the nutrient's deficiency disease begin to occur.

With vitamins, more is not necessarily better. When cells are saturated with a vitamin, they contain all they need and cannot accept additional amounts of the micronutrient. In this situation, continuing to take the vitamin can produce a toxicity disorder, because exposure to the excess micronutrient or its by—products can damage cells. Liver damage can also occur as a result of the intake of toxic levels of some vitamins.[8]

Most people do not need to be concerned about vitamin toxicity unless they are taking excessive amounts (megadoses) of vitamin supplements or consuming large amounts of vitamin—fortified foods regularly. In their natural states, most commonly eaten foods do not contain toxic levels of vitamins. Taking a "once daily" type of multivitamin supplement regularly is unlikely to cause toxic effects in adults because these products usually contain less than two times the Daily Values of each micronutrient component.

Preserving the Vitamin Content of Foods

Regardless of whether fruits and vegetables are picked fresh from a backyard garden or purchased from a farmers' market or supermarket, many kinds of produce, especially berries and leafy vegetables, are highly perishable. Therefore, these foods should be eaten soon after they are harvested or purchased to ensure maximum vitamin retention.

In many instances, unpackaged ("bulk") fresh fruits or vegetables that are sold in supermarkets do not have dates indicating when they should be used, and consumers have no way of knowing when the produce was harvested. When buying fresh produce, avoid items that are bruised, wilted, or shriveled, or that shows signs of decay, such as mold. Consumers who are uncertain of how to choose ripe fruits and vegetables should ask the person who manages the produce section of the store for advice.

Some vitamins, such as niacin and D, resist destruction by usual food storage conditions or preparation methods. Others—particularly vitamin C, thiamin, and folate—are easily destroyed or lost by improper food storage and cooking methods. Fresh produce retains its natural vitamin content better when stored at temperatures near freezing, in high humidity, and away from air. Most fresh fruits and vegetables should be kept in plastic packaging and chilled until they are used. Tomatoes, bananas, and garlic should be stored at room temperature.

Exposure to excessive heat, alkaline substances (such as baking soda), light, and air can destroy certain vitamins, especially vitamin C. To reduce such losses, wait to trim, peel, and cut raw fruits and vegetables until just before eating or serving them. Keep in mind that the darker leaves of vegetable greens generally contain more vitamins than the paler inner leaves or stems.

Water—soluble vitamins can leach out of food and dissolve in the cooking water, which is often discarded. Cooking vegetables in small amounts of water and reusing that water for soups or sauces helps retain those water—soluble nutrients. Cutting produce into large pieces reduces the amount of surface area exposed to heat, water, and other conditions that can increase vitamin losses. Cooking fruits and vegetables with their skins on helps keep nutrient content, as does consuming edible skins.

Quick cooking methods that involve little contact between produce and water, such as microwaving, steaming, and stir—frying, can conserve much of the vitamin content of the food (Fig. 9.4). According to the Food and Drug Administration (FDA), microwave cooking does not reduce the nutrient content of foods any more than do conventional cooking methods.[9] Microwave cooking may help conserve more vitamins in food because the method cooks quickly and without the need to add much water. Stir—fried vegetables should be cooked briefly to retain their nutrients as well as their appealing textures, flavors, and colors (Fig. 9.5).

Are fresh fruits and raw vegetables better sources of vitamins than canned or frozen versions? Sometimes they are. During the canning process, the heating of food can destroy certain vitamins. However, produce that is frozen immediately after being harvested and then properly stored can be just as nutritious as fresh produce. Frozen fruits and vegetables are often economical alternatives to fresh produce, but they need to be cooked without thawing to conserve much of their vitamin content.

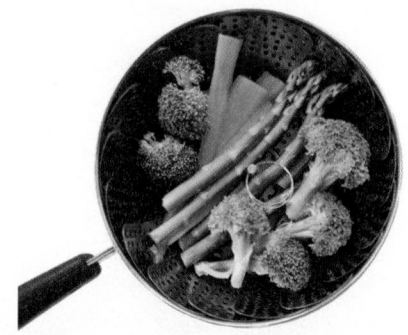

FIGURE 9.4 Conserving vitamins: Steaming. Steaming vegetables can conserve much of the vitamin content of the produce.

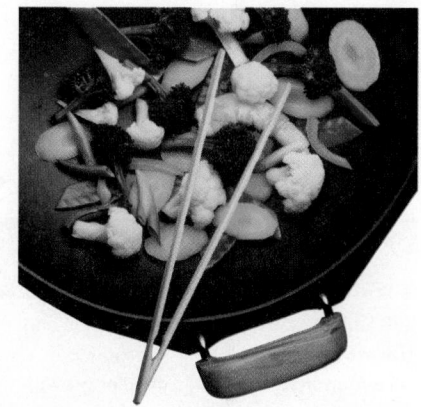

FIGURE 9.5 Conserving vitamins: Stir-frying. Stir-frying conserves vitamins by cooking vegetables quickly without adding water.

DID **YOU** KNOW?

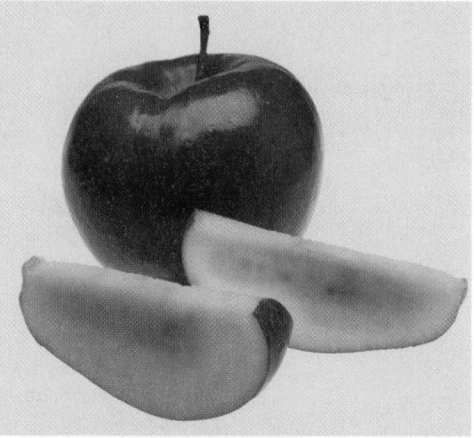

Have you ever wondered why a freshly peeled apple, eggplant, potato, or banana eventually turns brown? Damaged plant cells release an enzyme that results in the production of brown pigments when it is exposed to air. The action of this enzyme can be reduced by sprinkling salt or sugar on cut pieces of raw food; coating the pieces with an acidic solution, such as lemon juice; or covering them with airtight plastic wrap and chilling the food. Because heat destroys this enzyme, the unappetizing discoloring will not occur if you cook the fruit or vegetable immediately after peeling.

ASSESS YOUR PROGRESS

3 *List at least three criteria used to designate a substance as a vitamin.*

4 *Identify the four fat-soluble vitamins and nine water-soluble vitamins.*

5 *Describe how antioxidants protect against free-radical damage.*

6 *List at least three factors that affect the bioavailability of a vitamin.*

7 *Discuss at least five ways to preserve the vitamin content of fruits and vegetables during food preparation and storage.*

9.3 An Overview of Fat-Soluble Vitamins

LEARNING OUTCOMES

1 *Explain why vitamins A, D, E, and K are soluble in fat.*

2 *Summarize the main functions of each of the fat-soluble vitamins.*

The four fat–soluble vitamins are grouped together because of their solubility, and this in turn is related to their structures. All four of the fat–soluble vitamins' structures include a hydrocarbon chain—not unlike the long chains of fatty acids (see Appendix D). This characteristic makes them compatible with, and soluble in, fats. Table 9.3 summarizes the characteristics of fat–soluble vitamins. Figure 9.6 indicates food groups of MyPlate that are good food sources of these vitamins.

TABLE 9.3 Summary of Fat-Soluble Vitamins

Vitamin	Major Functions in the Body	Adult RDA/AI (adult RDA = bold)	Major Dietary Sources	Major Deficiency Signs and Symptoms	Major Toxicity Signs and Symptoms
Vitamin A (preformed and provitamin A)	Normal vision and reproduction, cellular growth, and immune system function	**700–900 µg RAE**	Preformed: liver, milk, fortified cereals Provitamin: yellow-orange and dark green fruits and vegetables	Night blindness, xerophthalmia, poor growth, dry skin, reduced immune system functioning	**Adult Upper Limit (UL) = 3000 µg/day** Nausea and vomiting, headaches, bone pain and fractures, hair loss, liver damage, interference with vitamin K absorption
Vitamin D	Absorption of calcium and phosphorus, maintenance of normal blood calcium, calcification of bone, maintenance of immune function	**15–20 µg**	Vitamin D–fortified milk, fortified cereals, fish oils, fatty fish	Rickets in children, osteomalacia in adults: soft bones, depressed growth, and reduced immune system functioning	**Adult UL = 100 µg/day** Poor growth, calcium deposits in soft tissues
Vitamin E	Antioxidant	**15 mg** (alpha-tocopherol)	Vegetable oils and products made from these oils, certain fruits and vegetables, nuts and seeds, fortified cereals	Loss of muscular coordination, hemolysis of red blood cells resulting in anemia	**Adult UL = 1000 mg/day** Excessive bleeding as a result of interfering with vitamin K metabolism
Vitamin K	Production of active blood-clotting factors	90–120 µg	Green leafy vegetables, canola and soybean oils, and products made from these oils	Excessive bleeding	**Adult UL = undetermined** Unknown

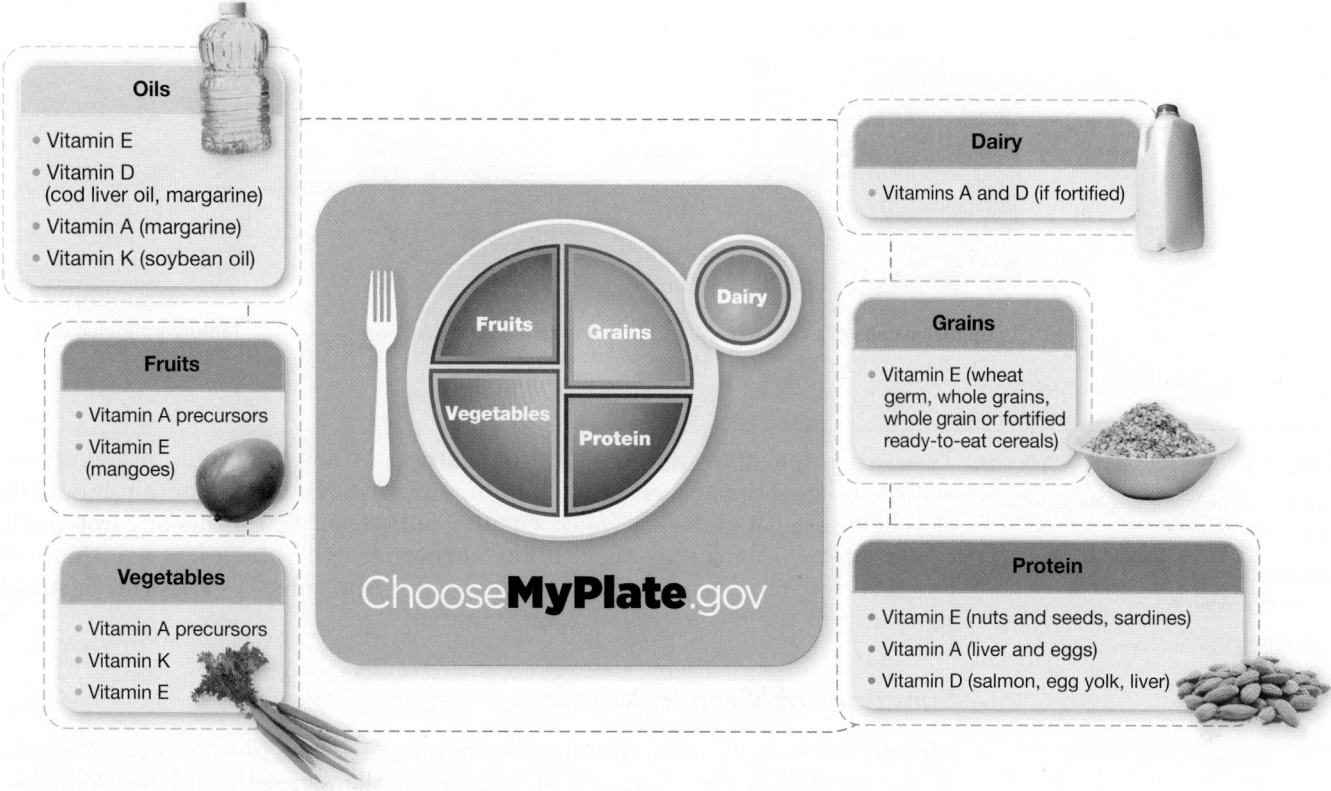

FIGURE 9.6 MyPlate and fat-soluble vitamins. This illustration highlights MyPlate food groups that are generally good sources of fat-soluble vitamins.

In the sections that follow, we discuss each vitamin's major functions in the body and its main sources in foods. Additionally, we describe what can happen when too little or too much of each fat—soluble vitamin is consumed and the role of these vitamins in chronic disease.

ASSESS YOUR PROGRESS

8 *What feature makes vitamins A, D, E, and K soluble in fat?*

9 *List the major functions of each fat-soluble vitamin.*

9.4 Vitamin A

LEARNING OUTCOMES

1 *Identify the different forms of vitamin A.*

2 *Explain the major functions of vitamin A in human health.*

3 *List food sources of vitamin A.*

4 *Discuss vitamin A deficiency and toxicity disorders.*

5 *Describe the relationship between vitamin A and cardiovascular disease, cancer, and age-related macular degeneration.*

Classifying Forms of Vitamin A

Vitamin A is actually a family of compounds that includes *retinol, retinal,* and *retinoic acid,* together called **retinoids (preformed vitamin A)**. **Retinol** is the the alcohol form and most active form of the vitamin in the body.

retinoids (preformed vitamin A) family of compounds commonly called vitamin A (retinol, retinal, retinoic acid)

retinol alcohol form of vitamin A and the most active form of vitamin A in the body

FIGURE 9.7 Vitamin A and epithelial cells. Vitamin A is necessary for immature epithelial cells to mature and function properly.

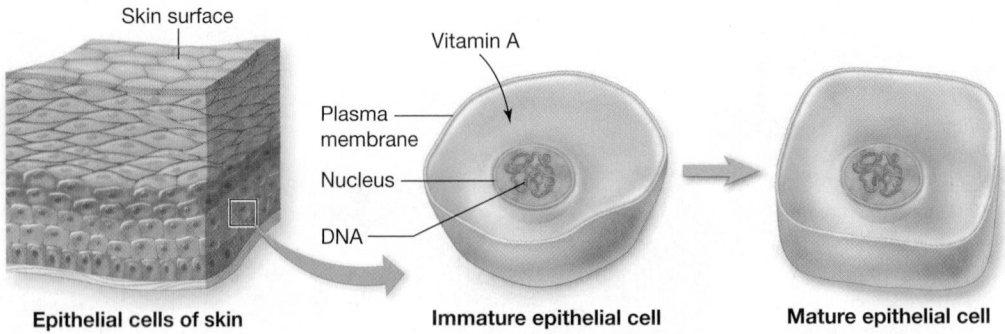

Skin surface

Vitamin A

Plasma membrane

Nucleus

DNA

Epithelial cells of skin

Immature epithelial cell

Mature epithelial cell

retinyl esters storage form of vitamin A

carotenoids yellow-orange pigments in fruits and vegetables

beta-carotene carotenoid that the body can convert to vitamin A

epithelial cells cells that form protective tissues that line the body

The body often stores retinol as **retinyl esters**. Although retinol, retinyl esters, and the other retinoids are only found in animal foods, plants contain hundreds of yellow—orange pigments called **carotenoids**. Over 600 forms of carotenoids exist, but only alpha—carotene, **beta—carotene**, and beta—cryptoxanthin can be converted into a biologically active retinoid. Appendix D shows the chemical structures of the retinoids and beta—carotene.

Functions of Vitamin A

All cells in the body need vitamin A to develop and function properly. Vitamin A participates in the processes of cell production, growth and development, function, and maintenance. As one example, the vitamin is necessary for the production, maturation, and maintenance of **epithelial cells**, cells that form protective tissues that line the body, including skin and linings of the digestive, respiratory, and reproductive tracts (Fig. 9.7). Certain epithelial cells secrete *mucus*, a slippery and sticky fluid that keeps the tissue moist and forms a barrier against many environmental pollutants and infectious agents. When the mucus—secreting epithelial cells do not have vitamin A, they deteriorate and no longer produce mucus. A lack of vitamin A can also reduce fertility, because the vitamin is required for maintaining the epithelial cells that line the female and male reproductive tracts.

Certain white blood cells produce antibodies, which are proteins that participate in the body's immune response. Antibodies help destroy infectious agents such as bacteria. Vitamin A plays a role in the pro—duction and activity of white blood cells.[10] Thus, people deficient in vitamin A are at greater risk of infections than those with adequate levels of the vitamin in their bodies.

Normal bone growth and development also require vitamin A. Although bones do not appear to change their shape, they are con—stantly being remodeled by processes that involve tearing down and rebuilding the tissues to meet the physical demands that are placed on them each day. Vitamin A participates with some other vitamins as well as certain minerals in the bone—remodeling process.

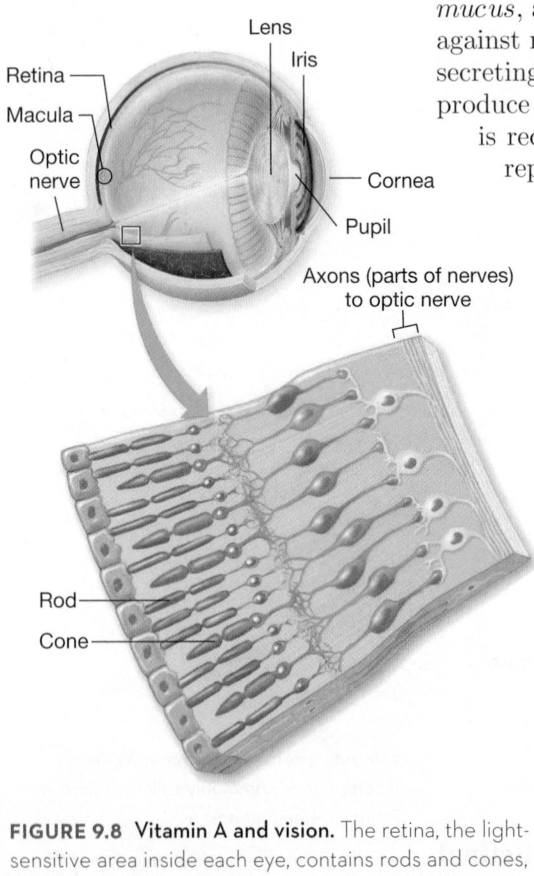

Vitamin A and Vision

The *retina*, the light—sensitive area inside each eye, contains *rods* and *cones*, specialized nerve cells that are essential for vision (Fig. 9.8). Rods enable adaptation to see in poorly lit environments. Cones are responsible for color vision and function in well—lit envi—ronments. Rods and cones both need vitamin A, particularly retinol, to function properly.

Figure 9.9 illustrates the *visual cycle* involving the rods. Rods remove retinol from the bloodstream and convert it to retinal. In

Lens

Iris

Retina

Macula

Optic nerve

Cornea

Pupil

Axons (parts of nerves) to optic nerve

Rod

Cone

FIGURE 9.8 Vitamin A and vision. The retina, the light-sensitive area inside each eye, contains rods and cones, specialized nerve cells that are essential for vision.

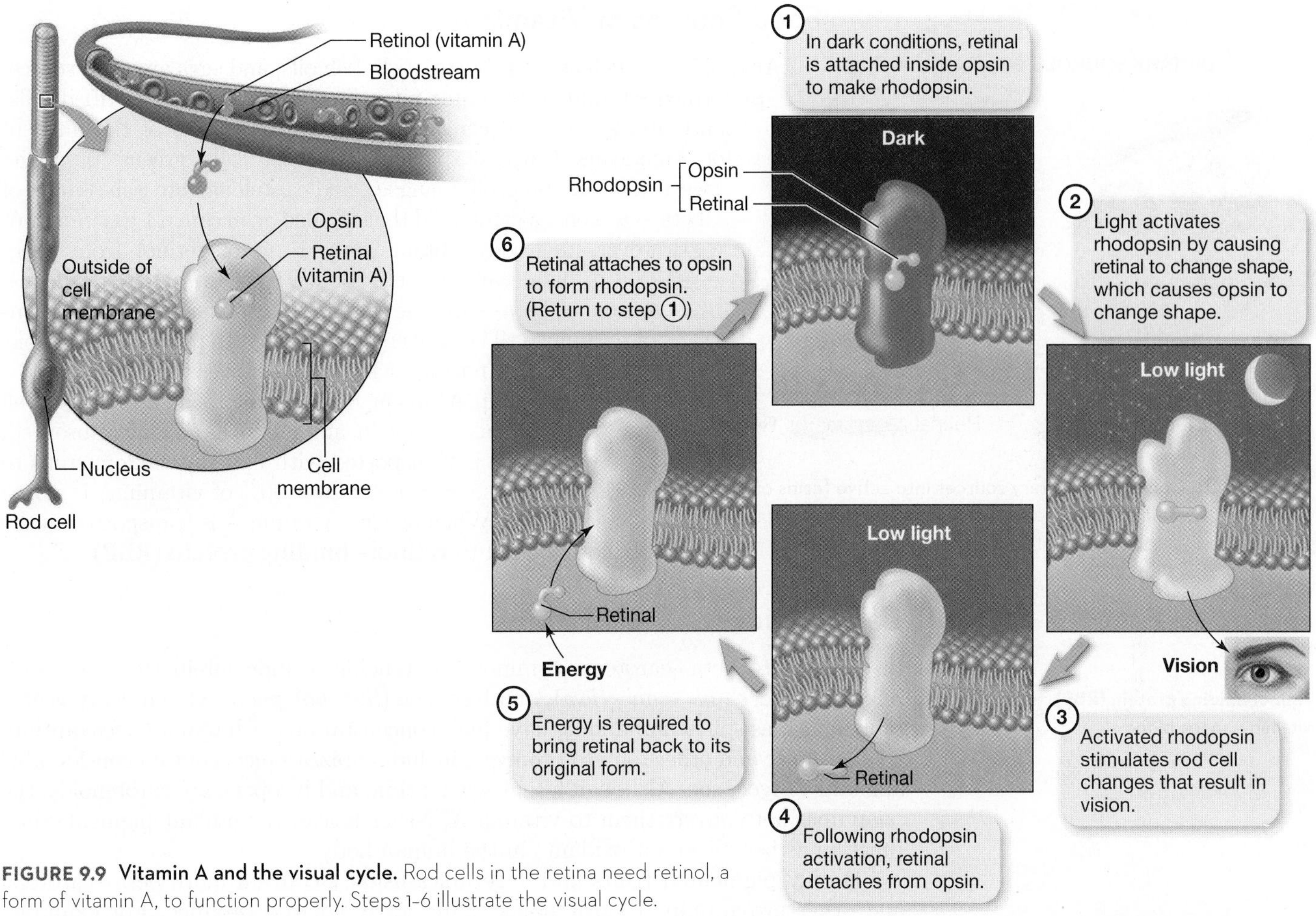

Retinol (vitamin A)
Bloodstream
Outside of cell membrane
Opsin
Retinal (vitamin A)
Nucleus
Cell membrane
Rod cell

Rhodopsin — Opsin / Retinal

① In dark conditions, retinal is attached inside opsin to make rhodopsin.

Dark

② Light activates rhodopsin by causing retinal to change shape, which causes opsin to change shape.

Low light

⑥ Retinal attaches to opsin to form rhodopsin. (Return to step ①)

Retinal

Energy

⑤ Energy is required to bring retinal back to its original form.

Low light

Retinal

④ Following rhodopsin activation, retinal detaches from opsin.

Vision

③ Activated rhodopsin stimulates rod cell changes that result in vision.

FIGURE 9.9 Vitamin A and the visual cycle. Rod cells in the retina need retinol, a form of vitamin A, to function properly. Steps 1-6 illustrate the visual cycle.

dark conditions, retinal binds to a protein called *opsin* to form **rhodopsin** (*visual purple*), which is necessary for vision in dim light. When a person is in a dark environment and exposed to a small amount of light, such as moonlight, the light strikes the rods. This activates rhodopsin, which then alters the shape of the retinal portion of rhodopsin and bleaches the compound. Retinal splits away and opsin is reformed, the final step in the visual cycle. The transformation of rhodopsin to opsin stimulates the rod to send a nervous impulse to the brain that signals the visual processing areas to interpret what is seen. After splitting away from opsin, retinal can bind to the protein, forming rhodopsin again.

What Is Night Blindness?

Have you ever walked from a brightly lit theater lobby into the darkened movie auditorium and felt blinded for a few seconds? This is a normal visual response to the sudden and dramatic reduction in light intensity. It takes a certain amount of time for the rod cells to react to the dim light.

As a result of the visual process shown in Figure 9.9 some retinal that splits away from rod cells is destroyed. To replace the retinal, rods remove some retinol from the bloodstream and convert it to retinal. *Night blindness*, the inability to see in dim light, can occur if retinol is unavailable. Night blindness may be an early sign of vitamin A deficiency.[11,12] Although cone cells also need vitamin A to function, the inability to see certain colors (color blindness) is not the result of a vitamin A deficiency.

rhodopsin vitamin A–containing protein that is needed for vision in dim light

DID **YOU** KNOW?

When preparing salads or meals, don't discard the edible dark green leaves of lettuce, cabbage, or broccoli. These darkly pigmented parts of the plants contribute more provitamin A carotenoids to your diet than the lighter-colored parts. In addition to carotenoids, many fruits and vegetables contain hundreds of other phytochemicals that may benefit your health.

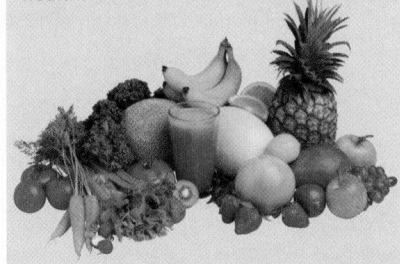

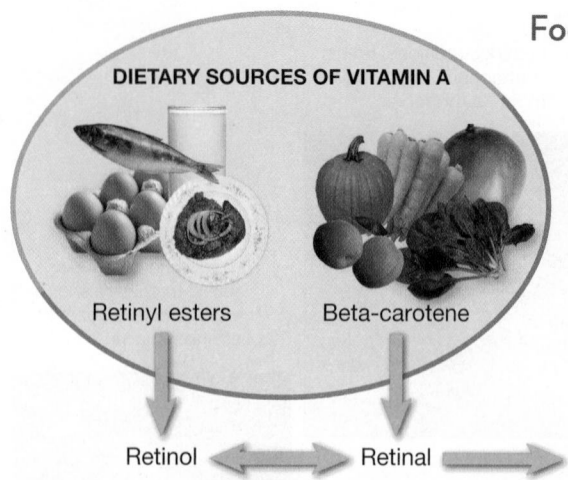

FIGURE 9.10 Converting dietary sources into active forms of vitamin A. Retinyl esters, from animal food sources, and beta-carotene, from plant food sources, are converted into active retinoids.

Food Sources of Vitamin A

Animal foods such as liver, butter, fish, fish oils, and eggs are good sources preformed vitamin A, including retinyl esters. Vitamin A–fortified milk, yogurt, margarine, and cereals are important sources of the nutrient for Americans. Carrots, spinach and other leafy greens, pumpkin, sweet potatoes, broccoli, mangoes, and cantaloupe are rich sources of beta–carotene, a carotenoid that the body can convert to vitamin A. However, the body obtains only 1 μg of retinol from every 12 μg of beta–carotene in a food. Figure 9.10 shows the conversion of beta–carotene and retinyl esters into active forms of vitamin A. The conversion of retinol to retinal is reversible, but retinal to retinoic acid is non–irreversible.

Vitamin A precursors in plant foods are not as well absorbed as retinol in animal foods.[10] Once absorbed, vitamin A is transported with lipids in chylomicrons to tissues for use or storage. Over 90% of vitamin A is stored in the liver. When needed, vitamin A is transported in the blood bound to **retinol–binding protein (RBP)**.

Carotenoids

retinol-binding protein (RBP) transports vitamin A in the blood

In addition to beta–carotene, common carotenoids include lutein (*loo'–tee–en*), zeaxanthin (*zee–ah–zan'–thin*), and lycopene (*lie'–ko–peen*). Green, leafy vegetables, such as spinach and kale, have high concentrations of lutein and zeaxanthin. Tomato juice and other tomato products, including pizza sauce, contain considerable amounts of lycopene. Although lutein, zeaxanthin, and lycopene are carotenoids, the body does not convert them to vitamin A. Nevertheless, these plant pigments may function as beneficial antioxidants in the human body.

Darkly pigmented fruits and vegetables usually contain more beta–carotene and other provitamin A carotenoids than lightly colored produce. For example, carrots, sweet potatoes, and peaches contain more beta–carotene than celery, white potatoes, and bananas. Dark green fruits and vegetables also contain carotenoids, but the green pigment *chlorophyll* hides the yellow–orange pigments. Table 9.4 lists some foods that are sources of vitamin A and its precursors.

TABLE 9.4 Vitamin A Content of Selected Foods

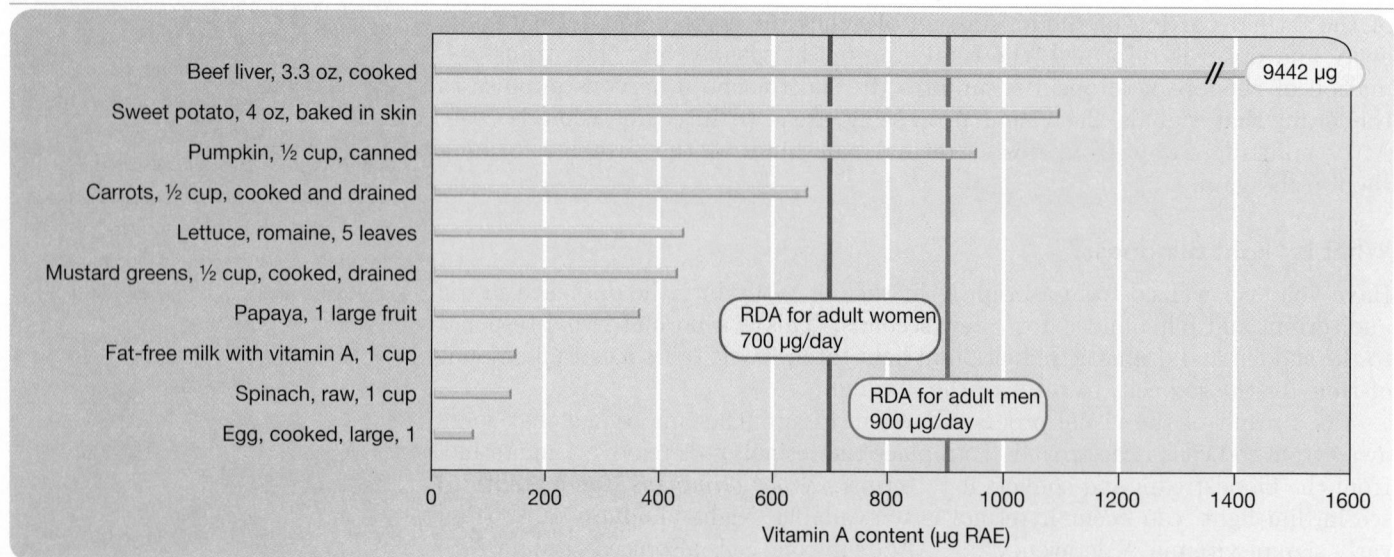

Source: Data from U.S. Department of Agriculture, Agricultural Research Service: *USDA National nutrient database for standard reference*, release 26, 2013.

DID **YOU** KNOW?

Most people associate carrots with the color orange. The next time you are at the market, you may notice carrots that are white, yellow, red, or even purple. All colors of carrots are rich in plant pigments that act as antioxidants in the body. Choose the color that you like the best or that complements the meal that you are preparing.

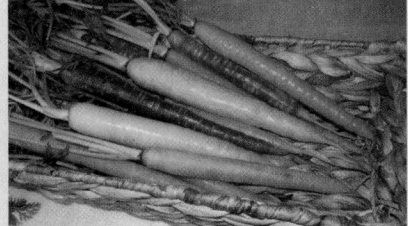

TABLE 9.5 Retinol Activity Equivalents

1 retinal activity equivalent (RAE) is equal to:
1 µg retinol
12 µg beta-carotene
24 µg alpha-carotene or beta-cryptoxanthin

Amounts of vitamin A in food are often reported as micrograms of retinol activity equivalents (RAE). One RAE is approximately 1 µg of retinol, 12 µg beta–carotene, or 24 µg alpha–carotene or beta–cryptoxanthin (Table 9.5). You may still find vitamin A contents identified as IUs (see Table 9.1).

Dietary Adequacy

For adults, the RDA for vitamin A is 700 to 900 µg RAE.[14] The average American diet provides enough vitamin A and its precursors to meet the RDA. Thus, adults generally do not need to take vitamin A supplements. In the United States, pre–school children who do not eat enough vegetables, low–income urban residents, older adults, and people with severe alcoholism, fat malabsorption, or liver diseases are at risk for vitamin A deficiency.

Vitamin A Deficiency

Epithelial cells are among the first to become affected by a deficiency of vitamin A. In skin, vitamin A–deficient epithelial cells produce too much **keratin**, a tough protein found in hair, nails, and the outermost layers of skin. Keratin accumulates within the skin and makes the tissue rough and bumpy. Keratin also forms in tissues that do not normally contain the protein, such as the *cornea*, the clear covering over the iris of the eye (see Fig. 9.8). The cornea enables light to enter the eye. The epithelial cells that line the inner eyelids secrete mucus that helps keep the cornea moist and clean. In a person suffering from chronic vitamin A deficiency, these cells accumulate keratin, become hardened, and stop producing mucus. This condition is called **xerophthalmia** (*zir–op–thal′–me–a*) or "dry eye" (Fig. 9.11). Corneas affected by xerophthalmia can be damaged easily by dirt and bacteria. Unless a person with xerophthalmia receives vitamin A, the condition eventually leads to blindness (Fig. 9.11).

Each year, thousands of children in developing nations, especially in Africa and Southeast Asia, become blind because of severe vitamin A deficiency. Vitamin A deficiency also reduces the effectiveness of the immune system, and many children suffering from vitamin A deficiency die from infections such as measles. Chapter 20 provides more information about global efforts to reduce the prevalence of vitamin A deficiency.

The results of animal studies suggest that women who are vitamin A deficient during pregnancy may give birth to infants with circulatory, urinary, skeletal, and nervous system defects.[15] However, a pregnant woman should not take a vitamin A supplement without consulting her physician. When taken in excess during pregnancy, vitamin A is a **teratogen**, an agent that causes birth defects.

DID **YOU** KNOW?

Tomatoes are a good source of certain carotenoids, particularly beta-carotene and lycopene. Exposure to heat can break down plant cells, and as a result, the cells release carotenoids. Thus, cooking tomatoes can improve the intestinal tract's ability to absorb carotenoids in the food.[13]

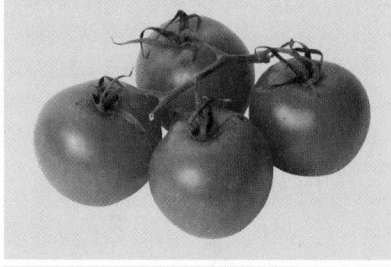

keratin tough protein found in hair, nails, and the outermost layers of skin

xerophthalmia condition affecting the eyes that results from vitamin A deficiency

teratogen an agent that causes birth defects

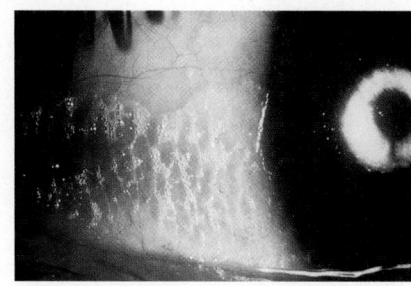

FIGURE 9.11 Early sign of xerophthalmia. Vitamin A deficiency can cause drying of the surface of the eye. The white, foamy areas are signs of such dryness. If untreated, this condition can lead to blindness.

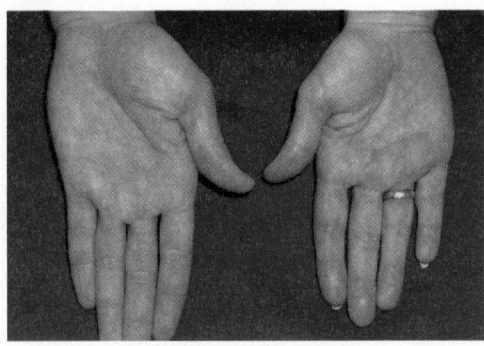

FIGURE 9.12 Carotenemia. Carotenemia results from consuming too much beta-carotene, either from foods or supplements. Notice the slight yellowing of the skin of the woman's hand on the right.

carotenemia yellowing of the skin that results from excess beta-carotene in the body

Vitamin A Toxicity

The UL for vitamin A intake is 3000 μg/day for adults.[14] Excessive consumption of vitamin A can damage the liver, because the organ is the main site for vitamin A storage. Toxicity signs and symptoms include headache, nausea, vomiting, visual disturbances, hair loss, bone pain, and bone fractures.

Carotenemia (*kar′−et−eh−ne′−me−ah*), a condition characterized by yellowing of the skin, can result from eating too much beta−carotene−rich produce or taking too many beta−carotene supplements (Fig. 9.12). This condition occasionally develops in infants who eat a lot of baby foods that contain carrots, apricots, winter squash, or green beans.[16] In most instances, carotenemia is harmless. The skin's natural color eventually returns to normal when the carotenoid−rich foods are no longer eaten.

Because vitamin A has a role in the production of healthy epithelial tissues, physicians may prescribe medications derived from vitamin A, such as isotretinoin (Accutane®) or tretinoin topical (Retin−A®), to treat severe acne and other skin disorders. Although these medications are less toxic than natural vitamin A, ingesting excessive amounts can produce harmful symptoms. Women of childbearing age should avoid pregnancy while using these medications because they can harm the developing fetus.

DID YOU *KNOW?*

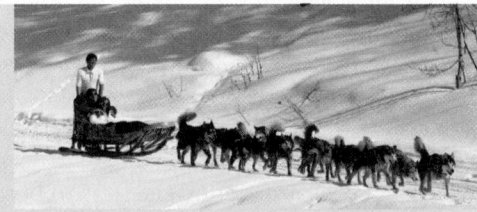

In the early 1900s, teams of explorers raced to discover and explore the North and South Poles. Starvation was a major risk on these expeditions. The Inuits, an Eskimo population of the Arctic, warned the explorers to avoid eating polar bear and seal livers because severe illness and death could result.

Unfortunately, many explorers did not know that their sled dogs' livers were also unsafe to eat. From 1911 to 1913, Douglas Mawson and Xavier Mertz were on an ill-fated expedition near the South Pole. Struggling to reach their winter base camp, the men had no choice but to eat their sled dogs, particularly the animals' livers, to avoid starvation. Both men suffered terrible illness, and Mertz did not survive. Over 50 years later, scientists determined that sled dogs can accumulate large amounts of vitamin A in their livers, and eating just a few ounces of sled dog liver can be toxic for humans.

Vitamin A and Chronic Disease

Findings of observational studies suggest an association between eating diets rich in fruits and vegetables and lower risk of certain cancers, heart disease, and *age−related macular degeneration*, a leading cause of blindness in the United States. Such diets provide plenty of beta−carotene and other antioxidant carotenoids. Scientists have conducted numerous large−scale studies to determine whether carotenoid supplements provide health benefits. The following sections summarize research findings regarding the health effects of taking these supplements.

CVD and Cancer

Results of clinical studies have not provided support for taking vitamin A or beta−carotene supplements to reduce the risk of cardiovascular disease (CVD).[17,18]

Furthermore, the use of beta—carotene supplements does not reduce the risk of cancer.[10] In two major studies, smokers who took beta—carotene supplements were *more* likely to die of lung cancer than smokers who took placebos.[10] Nevertheless, more research is needed to determine whether other carotenoids, such as lycopene and *beta—cryptoxanthin (bay'—ta krip—teh—zan'—thin)*, protect against CVD and cancer.[19,20]

Age-Related Macular Degeneration

In developed countries, **age—related macular degeneration (AMD)** is the leading cause of impaired vision among people over 55 years of age.[21] The disease is associated with changes in the *macula*, the region within the eye that provides the most detailed central vision (see Fig. 9.8). When the macula is damaged, objects appear to be distorted, as shown in Figure 9.13. Major risk factors for AMD are genetics, smoking, and advanced age, but diet also plays a role in the development of the condition.

    The macula contains the carotenoids lutein and zeaxanthin. Diets supplying high amounts of carotenoids (beta—carotene, lutein, and zeaxanthin) may lower the risk of AMD.[21] In the Age—Related Eye Disease Study (AREDS), patients who already had advanced AMD took dietary supplements that contained relatively high amounts of vitamins C and E, beta—carotene, and the mineral zinc.[22] The combination of these substances slowed the progression of vision loss associated with macular degeneration. However, there was no clear scientific evidence that taking antioxidant supplements prevents healthy people from developing AMD. Additionally, the long—term use of these supplements could be harmful.

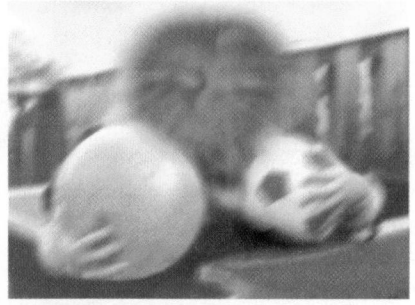

FIGURE 9.13 Visual effect of macular degeneration. Distorted and blurry central vision are signs of age-related macular degeneration (AMD).

age-related macular degeneration (AMD) eye disease resulting in changes in the macula of the eye, causing distorted vision

ASSESS YOUR PROGRESS

10 *Name the three active forms of vitamin A.*

11 *Describe three key functions of vitamin A in the body.*

12 *List at least four good food sources of preformed vitamin A and four good food sources of beta-carotene.*

13 *Explain the role of vitamin A in preventing night blindness.*

14 *What are signs of vitamin A toxicity? What group of people must be especially careful not to exceed recommended vitamin A intake?*

rickets vitamin D-deficiency disorder in children resulting in improper bone growth

9.5 Vitamin D

LEARNING OUTCOMES

1 *Describe the activation of vitamin D from food sources and sunlight exposure.*

2 *Explain the major functions of vitamin D in human health.*

3 *List food sources of vitamin D.*

4 *Discuss vitamin D deficiency and toxicity disorders.*

5 *Describe the relationship between vitamin D and chronic disease.*

By the seventeenth century, some people in parts of northern Europe had learned that exposing children to sunlight or giving the youngsters fish liver oil could prevent or treat **rickets**. Children with rickets have bones that are soft and can become misshapen. Leg bones, for example, bow under the weight of carrying the upper part of the body (Fig. 9.14). Additionally, the affected

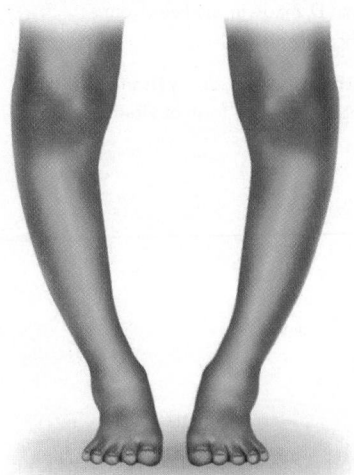

FIGURE 9.14 Typical sign of rickets.

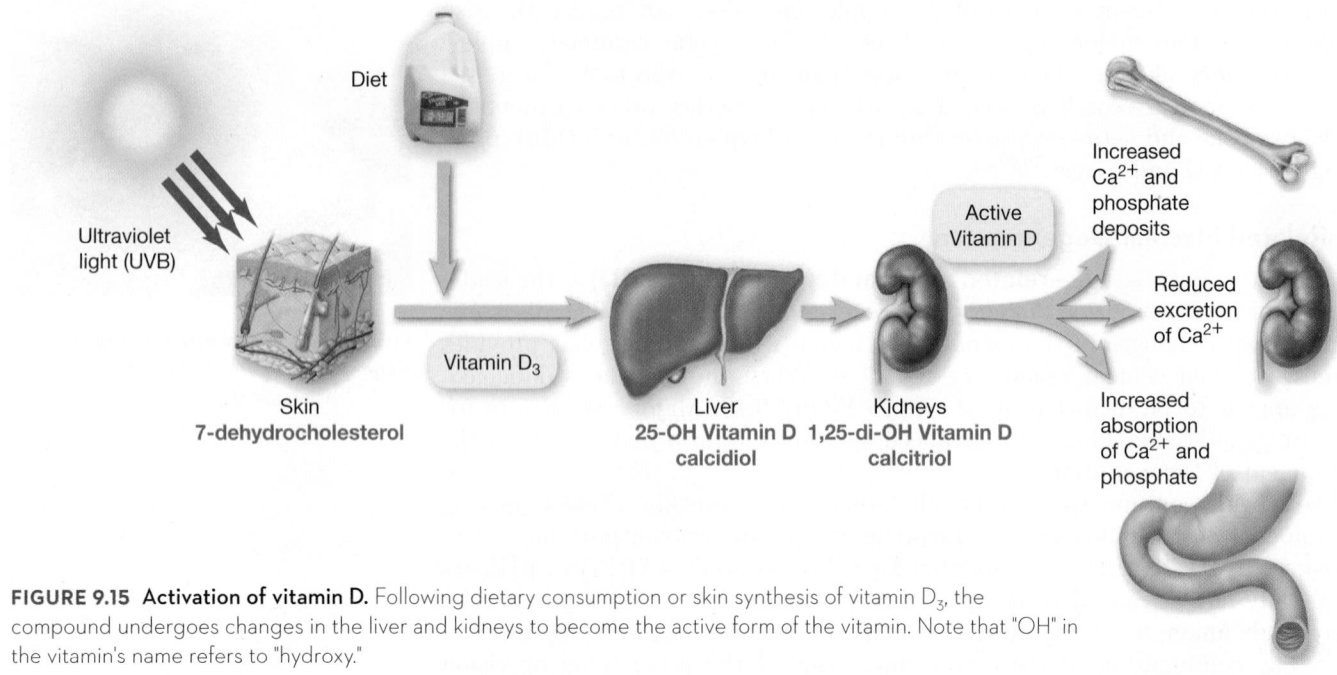

FIGURE 9.15 Activation of vitamin D. Following dietary consumption or skin synthesis of vitamin D_3, the compound undergoes changes in the liver and kidneys to become the active form of the vitamin. Note that "OH" in the vitamin's name refers to "hydroxy."

child's joints, rib cage, and hips (pelvis) become deformed, and the child may complain of muscle pain. By the nineteenth century, scientists learned that rickets can be prevented and treated by taking vitamin D supplements or eating vitamin D–rich foods.

Classifying Forms of Vitamin D

calciferol form of vitamin D found in both plant and animal foods

ergocalciferol (vitamin D_2) form of vitamin D found in plant food sources

cholecalciferol (vitamin D_3) form of vitamin D found in animal food sources

7-dehydrocholesterol precursor for vitamin D found in skin

25-hydroxyvitamin D inactive form of vitamin D, made in the liver from cholecalciferol

calcitriol (1,25-dihydroxyvitamin D) most biologically active form of vitamin D

Vitamin D, **calciferol**, comes from both plant and animal sources. The plant form of vitamin D is called vitamin D_2, or **ergocalciferol** (*er'—go—kal—sif'—er—ol*), whereas the animal form is vitamin D_3, also called **cholecalciferol** (*ko'—lee—kal—sif'—er—ol*). Vitamin D is unique among all other vitamins because it is not considered an essential nutrient. The body can make vitamin D when skin cells are exposed to the sun's ultraviolet radiation, which explains why the nutrient is also considered a hormone and referred to as the "sunshine vitamin."

Ultraviolet radiation converts a substance in skin that is derived from cholesterol, **7—dehydrocholesterol**, into a prohormone, called vitamin D_3. Vitamin D_3 circulates to the liver, where the substance is converted to the inactive compound **25—hydroxyvitamin D** (*calcidiol*). Blood levels of 25—hydroxyvitamin D are used to determine vitamin D status. Eventually, the kidneys convert 25—hydroxyvitamin D into the most biologically active form of vitamin D, **1,25—dihydroxyvitamin D (calcitriol)**. The chemical structures of vitamin D_3 and calcitriol are shown in Appendix D. Full activation of vitamin D requires both a healthy liver and healthy kidneys (Fig. 9.15).

DID YOU KNOW?

Nearly 20 million American adults, 11% of the population, live with chronic kidney disease. As the disease progresses, risk of bone loss and fracture, cardiovascular disease, immune suppression, and death increases.[23] Because the kidneys are not able to convert 25-hydroxyvitamin D into calcitriol, low vitamin D status is common in patients with **chronic renal failure (CRF)**. Higher intake of vitamin D, either through diet or supplements, improves survival rates in patients with chronic kidney disease.[24]

chronic renal failure (CRF) long-term kidney failure

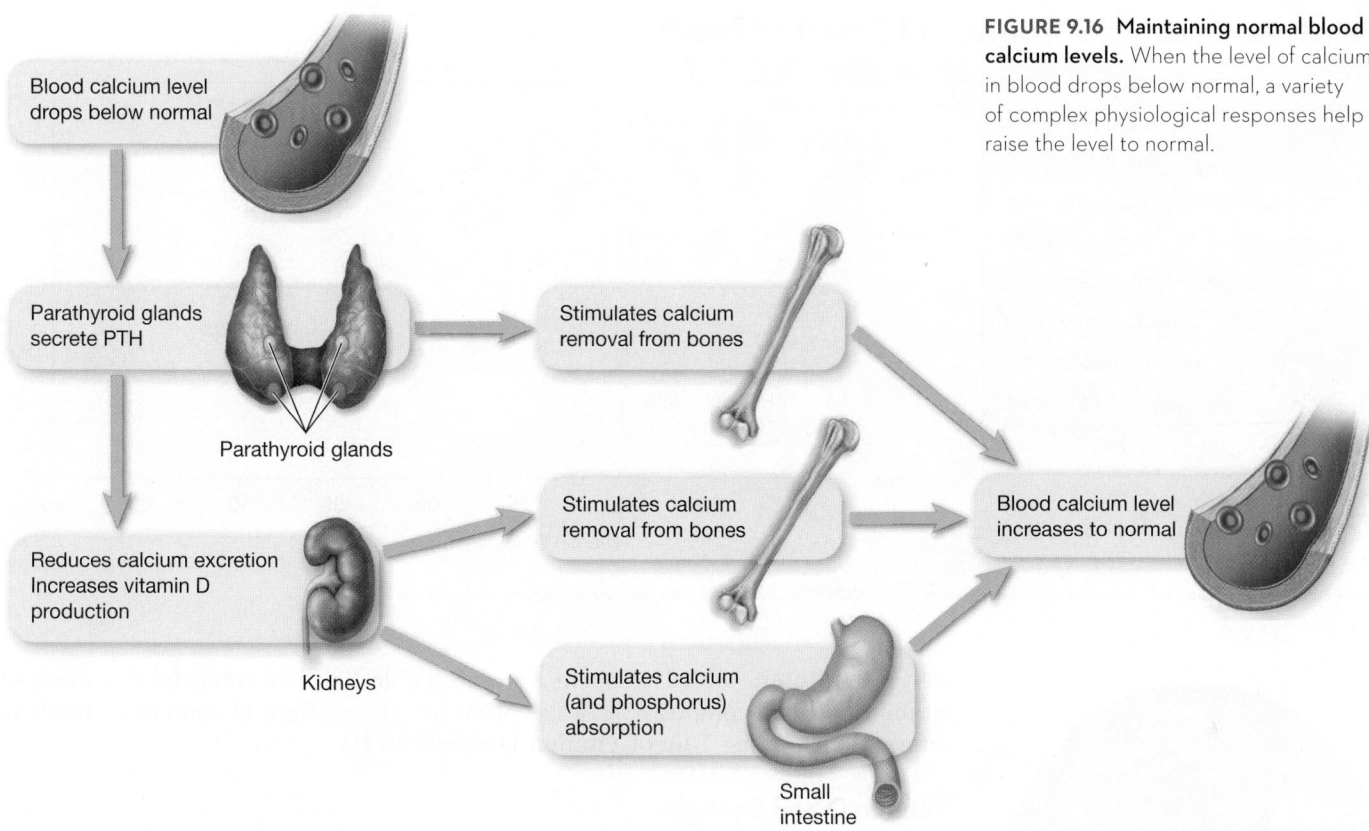

FIGURE 9.16 Maintaining normal blood calcium levels. When the level of calcium in blood drops below normal, a variety of complex physiological responses help raise the level to normal.

Blood calcium level drops below normal

Parathyroid glands secrete PTH

Parathyroid glands

Reduces calcium excretion Increases vitamin D production

Kidneys

Stimulates calcium removal from bones

Stimulates calcium removal from bones

Stimulates calcium (and phosphorus) absorption

Small intestine

Blood calcium level increases to normal

Functions of Vitamin D

Vitamin D is necessary for the metabolism of the minerals calcium and phosphorus, and the production and maintenance of healthy bones. Vitamin D stimulates small–intestine cells to absorb calcium and phosphorus from food. When vitamin D is lacking, the intestine absorbs only 10 to 15% of the calcium in foods; with the vitamin, intestinal absorption of dietary calcium increases to 30 to 80%.[25] Vitamin D also stimulates bone cells to form *calcium phosphate*, the major mineral compound in bone. Without adequate vitamin D, bone cells cannot deposit enough calcium and phosphorus to produce strong bone tissue (Fig. 9.16).

When blood calcium levels drop, vitamin D works with **parathyroid hormone (PTH)** to signal bones to release calcium. PTH also stimulates the kidneys to increase vitamin D production and decrease the elimination of calcium in urine. These actions help raise the level of calcium in blood to normal (Fig. 9.16). Removing too much calcium from bones can weaken them, but calcium is essential for normal heartbeat and other muscle contractions. If bones did not supply calcium for such vital functions, a person could experience serious, even fatal consequences.

Vitamin D has other roles in the body, including regulating neuromuscular and immune function and reducing inflammation.[26] The vitamin may also reduce the risks of heart disease, cancer, diabetes mellitus, multiple sclerosis, asthma, and depression.[27] However, more research is needed to clarify the vitamin's role in chronic disease prevention.

parathyroid hormone (PTH) hormone secreted in response to low blood calcium levels

Food Sources of Vitamin D

Fish liver oils and fatty fish, especially salmon, herring, and catfish, are among the few foods that naturally contain vitamin D. Milk is routinely fortified with vitamin D, and some brands of ready–to–eat cereals, orange juice, and margarine

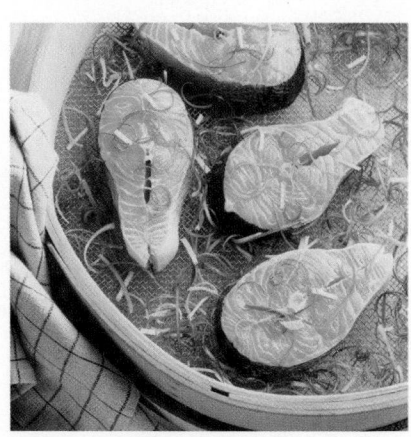

Salmon is a good source of vitamin D.

TABLE 9.6 Vitamin D Content of Selected Foods

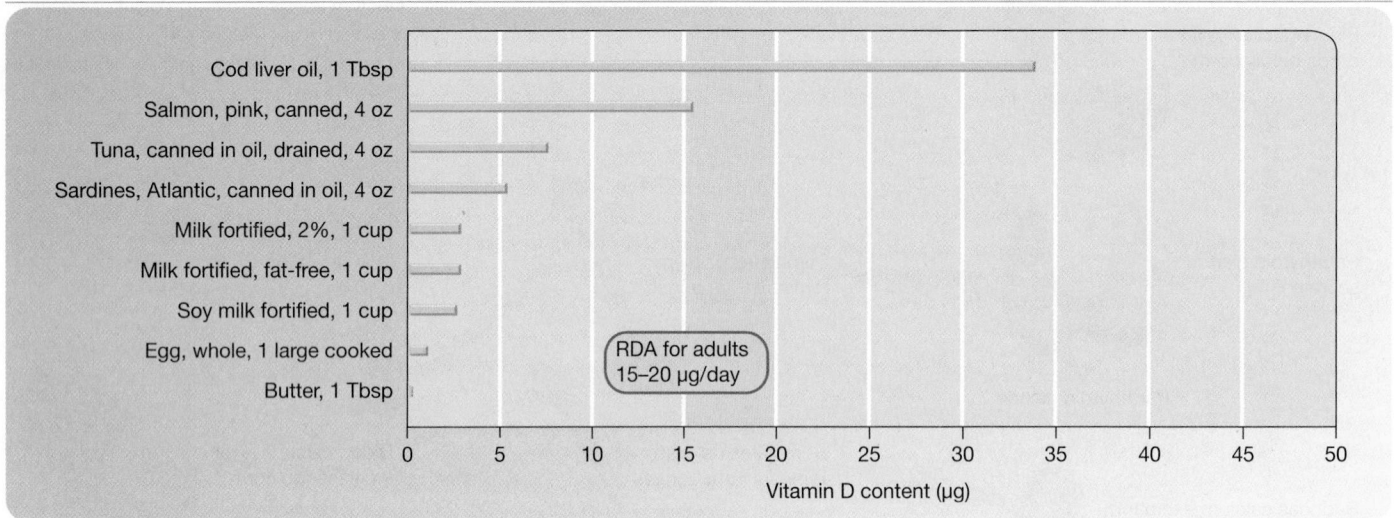

Source: Data from U.S. Department of Agriculture, Agricultural Research Service: *USDA National nutrient database for standard reference, release 26,* 2013.

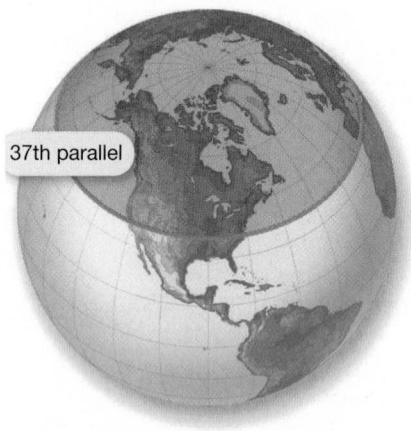

FIGURE 9.17 Latitude and vitamin D status. If you live in North America south of the 37th parallel and are outdoors when sunlight is most intense during the day, you are likely to obtain enough sun exposure to synthesize vitamin D most of the year.

have the vitamin added to them as well. Table 9.6 lists some food sources of vitamin D. Food composition tables often list the vitamin D content of foods in International Units; 1 μg of vitamin D equals 40 IU.

Vitamin D and Sunlight

Vitamin D is not widespread in food; therefore, the body depends on sunlight exposure to synthesize the vitamin. Those living south of the 37th parallel and who are outdoors between 10 A.M. and 3 P.M., when sunlight is most intense, often obtain enough sun exposure to synthesize vitamin D during most of the year. The amount of time one needs to spend in the sun to form adequate amounts of vitamin D depends primarily on his or her location, the time of day and year, age, and skin color.

Earth's atmosphere blocks UV radiation. In North America, the 37th parallel extends from about southern Virginia through southern Missouri to San Francisco, California (Fig. 9.17). For those living north of the 37th parallel, the angle of the winter sun is such that the sun's rays must pass through more of the atmosphere than at other times of the year (Fig. 9.18). As a result, skin cannot make sufficient

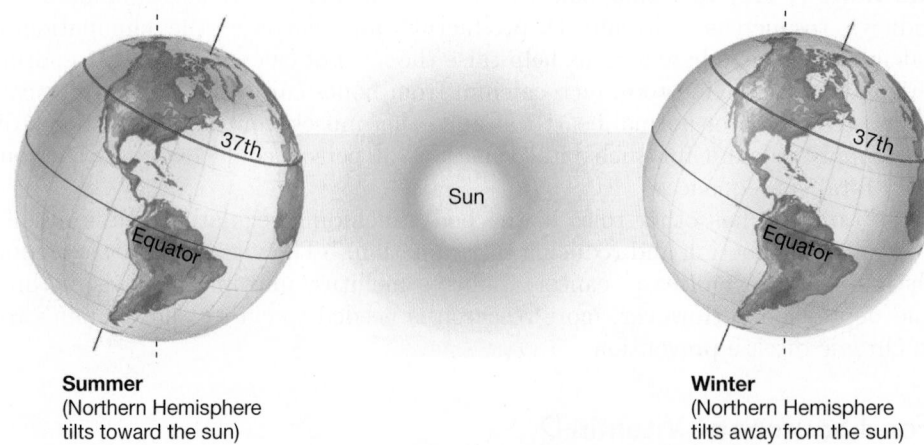

Summer
(Northern Hemisphere tilts toward the sun)

Sun

Winter
(Northern Hemisphere tilts away from the sun)

FIGURE 9.18 Seasonal variation in sunlight intensity. If you live north of the 37th parallel, the angle of the winter sun is such that the sun's rays must pass through more of the atmosphere than at other times of the year. As a result, skin tends to form less prohormone vitamin D in the winter.

amounts of provitamin D during the winter and a person may not have adequate vitamin D stored in his or her body to last until spring.[28] Some individuals need to take a supplement that contains 100% of the adult Daily Value for vitamin D, especially from November through February. Clouds, shade, and air pollution also limit the amount of UV radiation that reaches skin.

Skin contains *melanin*, the brown pigment that can prevent skin from absorbing too much solar radiation and forming toxic amounts of vitamin D. Darker skin contains more melanin than lighter skin. Those who have light skin or a medium degree of pigmentation should expose their skin to sun for at least 15 minutes a day during the summer for adequate synthesis of vitamin D in the body.[28]

Tanning and severe sunburn increase the risk of developing wrinkles and skin cancer. UV radiation is a major risk factor for skin cancer, including melanoma, the most deadly form of skin cancer.[26] Dermatologists often advise people to apply sunscreens consistently before going outdoors. Using a sunscreen, however, may limit the skin's ability to synthesize prohormone vitamin D_3.[29]

Dietary Adequacy

For adults under 70 years of age, the RDA for vitamin D is 15 μg/day (600 IU/day).[30] Many Americans do not consume enough vitamin D to meet the RDA.[7] According to findings of a nationwide survey conducted in 2005–2006, approximately 41% of American adults had low blood levels of vitamin D.[31] Individuals who were female, black, or Mexican−American were more likely to be vitamin D deficient than white, non−Hispanic males.[31] Other factors that were associated with low vitamin D status included having excess body fat; using electronic media or games for more than 4 hours daily; and drinking milk less than once a week. According to the Dietary Guidelines, vitamin D is a "nutrient of public health concern."

Rickets

Although severe rickets is uncommon in the United States, public health officials are concerned about the recent increase in the number of cases reported among infants and toddlers.[32] Breast milk contains insufficient amounts of vitamin D to prevent rickets. Young children who are most likely to develop rickets are breastfed, and they have dark skin, minimal sunlight exposure, and little or no vitamin D intake.[33] Exposing breastfed infants to sunlight reduces their risk of the disease, but medical experts do not know how much sun exposure is necessary. Thus, breastfed infants should consume a supplement containing 400 IU of vitamin D per day soon after birth.[32,34] While infants being formula−fed are at low risk for rickets, health care providers should ensure that the formula is fortified with vitamin D and that the infant is consuming enough formula each day to meet needs.[33] Healthy children should continue to consume at least 400 IU of the vitamin per day through adolescence.[32,35]

Osteomalacia

The adult form of Vitamin D deficiency is called **osteomalacia** (*ahs'−tee−o−mah−lay'−she−a*), or literally, "soft bones." The bones of people with osteomalacia have normal amounts of *collagen*, the protein that provides structure for the skeleton, but their bones contain less−than−normal amounts of calcium. The bones are soft and weak, and bend and break easily as a result. Muscle weakness is also a symptom of osteomalacia.

Adults who are confined indoors or almost fully covered when out−side during the day, such as for religious reasons, are at risk for osteomalacia

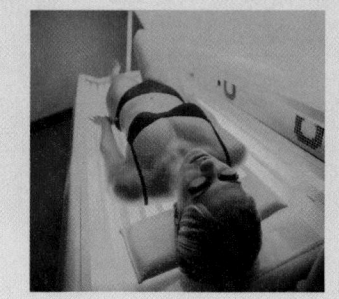
osteomalacia condition characterized by softening of the bones as a result of inadequate vitamin D status in adults

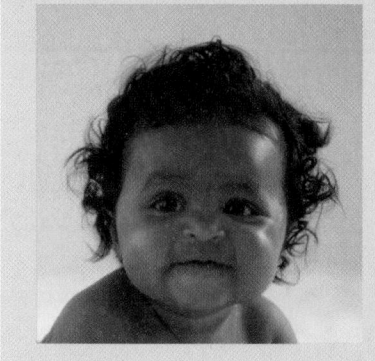

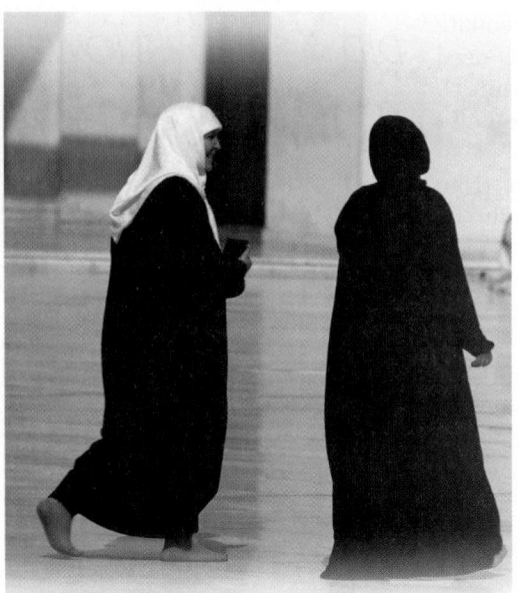

FIGURE 9.19 Clothing and vitamin D status. Adults who are almost fully covered when outside during the day, such as for religious or cultural reasons, are at risk for osteomalacia.

(Fig. 9.19).[37,38] Osteomalacia is a risk for adults who have kidney, liver, or intestinal diseases, because these conditions may reduce both vitamin D production and calcium absorption.

In the United States, mild to moderate cases of vitamin D deficiency among adults may be common. According to results of one national survey, about 42% of African–American women and 4% of white women had low blood levels of vitamin D.[26] Exposing skin to sunlight, eating vitamin D–rich foods, or taking vitamin D supplements can help people avoid vitamin D deficiency and osteomalacia. The "Real People, Real Stories" on this page features Amanda Croker, a college student who learned she is deficient in vitamin D.

As a person ages, production of 7–dehydrocholesterol in skin declines and conversion of the prohormone to active vitamin D in kidneys also decreases. As a result of these age–related changes, older adults are more likely to develop vitamin D deficiency than younger persons.[39] Older adults are also at risk for bone fractures. The bone health of those over 50 years of age may benefit from the use of a daily vitamin D supplement, but more research is needed to determine safe doses.[40]

It is not uncommon for people with osteomalacia to also have *osteoporosis*, a condition characterized by loss of bone mass that usually occurs with aging.[26,41] Although osteoporosis is usually associated with inadequate calcium intakes, a long–term vitamin D deficiency contributes to the condition because calcium absorption is reduced.[26] The calcium section of Chapter 11 provides more information about osteoporosis.

REAL People, **REAL** Stories

Amanda Croker

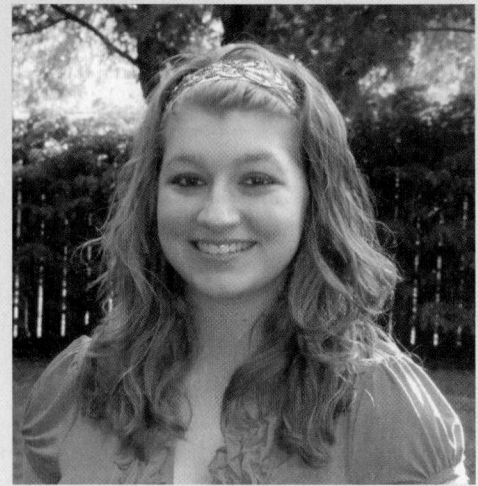

Amanda Croker, a junior majoring in East Asian Language and Culture at the University of Kansas, routinely tried to limit her sun exposure to avoid sunburn and the possibility of skin cancer in the future. "My skin is so light," Amanda says. "I even got a sunburn in Kansas in the middle of October, because I was outside for a couple hours!" She was unaware that her efforts to protect her skin were also limiting her body's ability to make vitamin D, "the sunshine vitamin."

"I'm taking a prescription dose of vitamin D, because my family doctor tested my blood and found out that I didn't have enough of the vitamin in my body," says Amanda. "She told me that people need sunlight to make vitamin D, but she said she wasn't surprised that I'm deficient, since I have red hair. I told her that I try to avoid being out in the sun for more than 30 minutes, because I 'crisp' when I get exposed to sun. Anyway, I don't notice that much of a difference now that I'm on the medication." Although Amanda does not "feel" different now, her bones eventually may have become soft and weak, if her doctor had not discovered that Amanda was vitamin D–deficient. Before the discovery and purification of vitamin D, children were given cod liver oil to prevent rickets, the vitamin's deficiency disease.

As a result of the treatment, Amanda's blood level of vitamin D became normal within a few weeks. Because few foods are good sources of vitamin D, she will need to take a daily supplement of the micronutrient that is available without a prescription for the rest of her life. By taking the supplement, she should be able to maintain a healthy blood level of the fat-soluble vitamin.

Vitamin D Toxicity

The body stores vitamin D, making it a potentially toxic vitamin. Long–term ingestion of high–dose vitamin D supplements that supply 250 to 1250 µg/day (10,000 to 50,000 IU/day) can cause vitamin D to accumulate in the body and produce toxicity.[30] When excess vitamin D is consumed, the small intestine absorbs too much calcium from foods and the mineral is deposited in soft tissues, including the kidneys, heart, and blood vessels. The calcium deposits can inter–fere with cells' ability to function and cause cellular death. Other signs and symptoms of vitamin D toxicity include muscular weakness, loss of appetite, diarrhea, vomiting, and mental confusion. The body does not make toxic lev–els of vitamin D when exposed to sunlight, because skin limits its production of 7–dehydrocholesterol. The Upper Limit (UL) for vitamin D supplementation is 100 µg/day (4000 IU/day).

ASSESS YOUR PROGRESS

15 Sketch a diagram showing how the body makes the most active form of vitamin D, calcitriol, from UV exposure and dietary sources.

16 Explain why vitamin D inadequacy is common in chronic kidney disease.

17 Describe the role of vitamin D when blood calcium levels drop below normal.

18 List at least four good food sources of vitamin D.

19 What groups of people are at the greatest risk for rickets and osteomalacia and why?

9.6 Vitamin E

LEARNING OUTCOMES

1 Compare the sources and biological activities of alpha- and gamma-tocopherol.
2 Explain the major functions of vitamin E in human health.
3 List food sources of vitamin E.
4 Discuss vitamin E deficiency and toxicity disorders.
5 Describe the relationship between vitamin E and cardiovascular disease, cancer, and inflammation.

Vitamin E was first discovered in 1920, when scientists determined that a com–ponent of vegetable oil was necessary for normal reproduction in rats.[42] The researchers called the factor *tocopherol*, derived from the Greek words *toco*, "childbirth," and *pherein*, "to bear." Today, nutrition scientists recognize vita–min E as a potent antioxidant.

Classifying Forms of Vitamin E

Vitamin E exists in one of eight forms; four of the forms are **tocopherols** (*toe–koff'–e–rolls*). Only the **alpha–tocopherol** form of the vitamin is main–tained in plasma and used by the body.[14] Appendix D includes an illustration of the chemical structure of alpha–tocopherol. Alpha–tocopherol is in many foods and vitamin E supplements; **gamma–tocopherol** is also in foods, includ–ing vegetable oil. However, the biological activity of gamma–tocopherol is sig–nificantly lower than that of alpha–tocopherol.

tocopherols group of four structurally similar forms of vitamin E

alpha-tocopherol form of vitamin E used by the body; found in most foods and vitamin E supplements

gamma-tocopherol form of vitamin E that has significantly lower biological activity than alpha-tocopherol

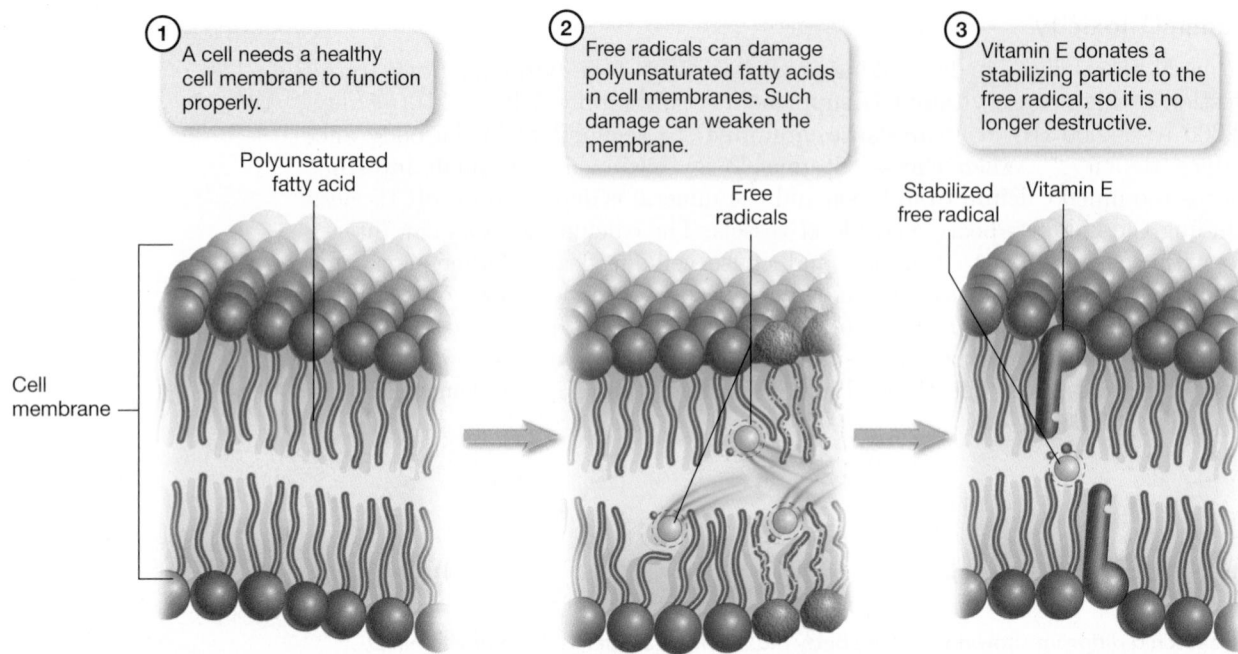

FIGURE 9.20 Vitamin E and the cell membrane.

Functions of Vitamin E

Vitamin E protects polyunsaturated fatty acids in cell membranes from being damaged by free radicals (Fig. 9.20). Such oxidative damage may be associated with the development of atherosclerosis, the process that occurs within arteries and contributes to heart attack and stroke, cancer, and premature cellular aging and death. Other roles for vitamin E include maintaining nervous tissue and immune system function.

Food Sources of Vitamin E

Rich food sources of vitamin E include sunflower seeds, almonds, and plant oils, especially sunflower, safflower, canola, and olive oils. Products made from vitamin E–rich plant oils, such as margarine and salad dressings, also supply the micronutrient. Other important dietary sources of the vitamin include fish, whole grains, nuts, seeds, and certain vegetables. Meats, processed grain products, and dairy products generally do not contain much vitamin E. Table 9.7 lists some common foods that are sources of the micronutrient.

Harvesting, processing, storage, and cooking methods influence the amount of vitamin E retained in food. During the milling process, most of the vitamin E that is in whole grains is lost, and it is not restored by enrichment. Furthermore, vitamin E is highly susceptible to destruction by exposure to oxygen, metals, and light, as well as high temperatures that occur when heating oil for deep–fat frying.

Dietary Adequacy

For adults, the RDA for vitamin E is 15 mg/day of alpha–tocopherol.[14] Although many American adults do not consume recommended amounts of vitamin E, vitamin E deficiency is rare.[43] A healthy body stores the vitamin in body fat, skeletal muscle, and the liver.

TABLE 9.7 Vitamin E Content of Selected Foods

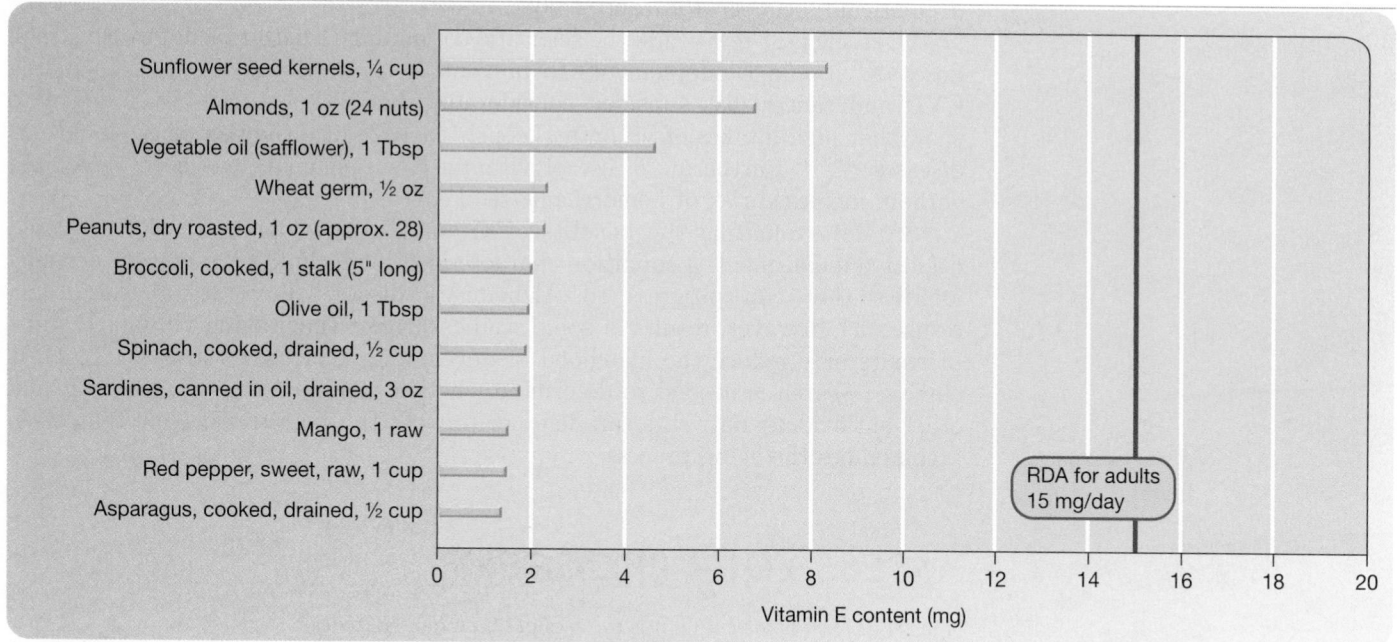

Food	Vitamin E content (mg)

Source: Data from U.S. Department of Agriculture, Agricultural Research Service: *USDA National nutrient database for standard reference,* release 26, 2013.

Amounts of vitamin E may be reported as a number of IUs. One mg of alpha−tocopherol is about 1.5 IU of the natural form of the vitamin. Synthetic vitamin E is used to fortify foods and produce supplements that supply the vitamin. One mg of natural vitamin E is equal to 2.2 IU of the synthetic form of the vitamin.[3]

Vitamin E Deficiency

People who have diseases that interfere with fat absorption may become deficient in vitamin E, because dietary fat enhances intestinal absorption of the micronutrient. Long−term vitamin E deficiency damages the nervous system and results in nerve damage, loss of neuromuscular control, and blindness.[44] Vitamin E deficiency can also reduce the functioning of the immune system.

Vitamin E Toxicity

For healthy adults, the UL for vitamin E is 1000 mg/day of alpha−tocopherol. Consuming high amounts of vitamin E in foods has not been associated with any negative effect on health.[14] However, taking dietary supplements that supply excessive amounts of the vitamin may interfere with vitamin K's role in blood clotting and lead to uncontrolled bleeding (hemorrhage). Therefore, people who are taking medications that interfere with blood clotting ("blood thinners") should check with their physicians before using vitamin E supplements.

Vitamin E and Chronic Disease

In the early 1980s, epidemiological reports indicated that populations who ate vitamin E–rich diets had a lower risk of heart disease than groups who ate diets that did not contain high amounts of the micronutrient. Additionally, results of other studies suggested that vitamin E might reduce the risk of cancer, particularly lung cancer in smokers. Some researchers promoted the use of vitamin E megadoses to slow the decline in mental functioning that is associated with

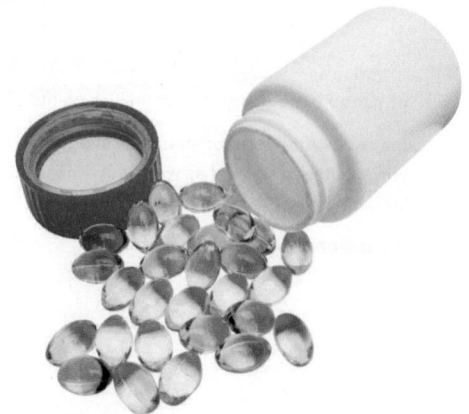

Vitamin E is a popular dietary supplement in the United States.

Alzheimer's disease. Not surprisingly, sales of vitamin E supplements increased dramatically between 1987 and 2000.[45]

Over the past few years, the scientific community's enthusiasm for using high doses of vitamin E supplements to prevent or treat chronic diseases, including CVD and cancer, has subsided considerably. Major long–term trials failed to show that high intakes of vitamin E consistently reduce the risk of these chronic diseases.[43,46–51] Furthermore, use of vitamin E supplements has been associated with an increased risk of hemorrhagic stroke.[52]

Studies evaluating the benefits of vitamin E in people with signs of mild cognitive impairment, a condition characterized by declining thought–processing abilities that can progress to Alzheimer's disease, have found conflicting results.[43,53] However, results of some studies suggest that taking vitamin E supplements may reduce the likelihood of developing Alzheimer's disease.[54,55] More clinical research is needed to determine whether combinations of vitamin E and other antioxidant nutrients can delay or prevent the cognitive decline that often accompanies the aging process.

ASSESS YOUR PROGRESS

20 *What form of vitamin E has the highest biological activity?*

21 *Describe the key functions of vitamin E.*

22 *List four good food sources of vitamin E.*

23 *Explain the consequences of a vitamin E deficiency.*

24 *Summarize the current research findings regarding vitamin E supplements and chronic diseases such as CVD, cancer, and Alzheimer's disease.*

9.7 Vitamin K

LEARNING OUTCOMES

1 *Identify the different forms of vitamin K.*

2 *Explain the major functions of vitamin K in human health.*

3 *List food sources of vitamin K.*

4 *Discuss deficiency and toxicity signs and symptoms of vitamin K.*

5 *Describe vitamin K's relationship to bone health and to metabolic syndrome.*

In the early 1930s, Danish researcher Henrik Dam discovered a factor in alfalfa that played a role in blood clotting (coagulation). Dam named the factor vitamin "K" after *koagulation*, the Danish word for coagulation.

phylloquinone form of vitamin K in plants

menaquinone form of vitamin K in egg yolks, butter, and beef as well as synthesized by bacteria in the large intestine

menadione synthetic form of vitamin K

Vitamin K is a family of compounds that includes **phylloquinone** (*fill–o–kwin'–own*) from plants and **menaquinones** (*men–eh–kwin'–owns*) in egg yolks, butter, and beef. Bacteria that normally live in the large intestine also syn–thesize menaquinones that can be absorbed by the body. Bacterial menaquinone contributes about 10% to the body's vitamin K supply. The biological activity of phylloquinone is greater than that of menaquinone. A synthetic form of vitamin K, **menadione**, can be converted into menaquinone in the body. Appendix D includes the chemical structures of the various forms of vitamin K.

Digestion and Absorption of Vitamin K

The presence of dietary fat, bile, and pancreatic juice enhances vitamin K absorp–tion in the small intestine. Following absorption, some vitamin K is stored in the

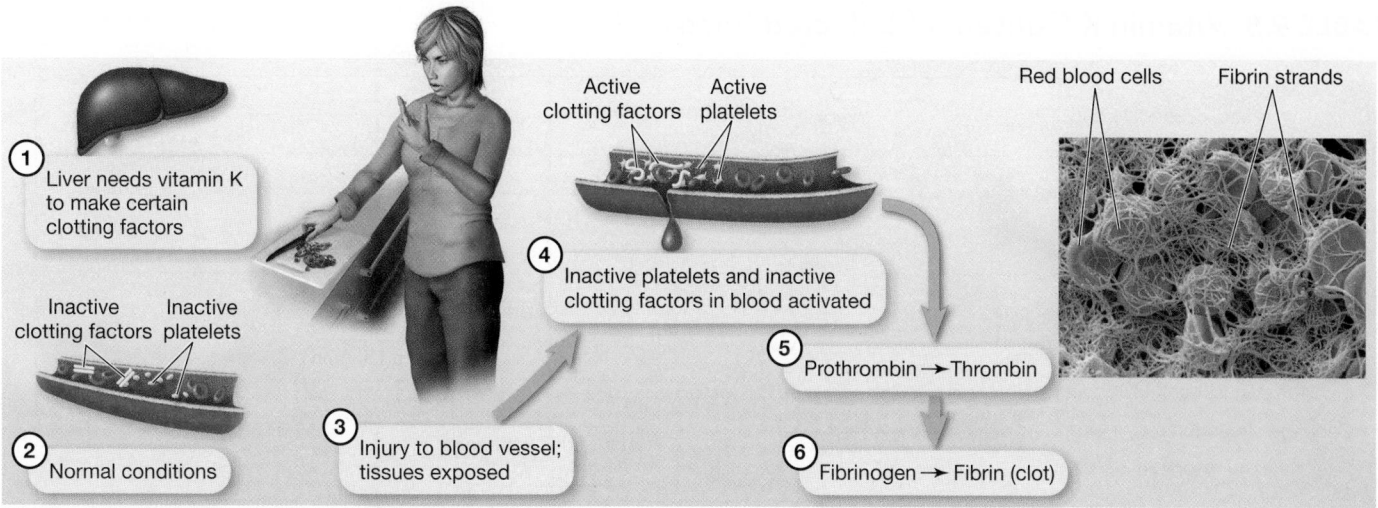

FIGURE 9.21 Vitamin K and blood clotting. When a blood vessel is cut, blood in the injured area undergoes a series of steps to form a clot that stops the bleeding. The liver needs vitamin K to make prothrombin and three other blood-clotting factors.

liver and some is incorporated in lipoproteins for transport in the bloodstream. The liver also breaks down vitamin K and eliminates the vitamin's by—products by adding them to bile.

Functions of Vitamin K

Blood contains inactive clotting factors and cell fragments called *platelets* that are necessary for blood clotting to occur. When a blood vessel is cut, blood in the injured area undergoes a complex series of steps to form a clot that stops the bleed—ing (Fig. 9.21). A clot is comprised of strands of the protein *fibrin* that traps blood cells, forming a mesh. The liver synthesizes several blood—clotting factors, and the organ needs vitamin K to produce four of them, including *prothrombin*, properly.

When vitamin K is unavailable, the blood—clotting factors are inactive, and the blood does not clot effectively. Over 4 million Americans take the prescribed medication warfarin because their blood clots too easily. Vitamin K can inter—fere with warfarin's "blood—thinning" activity, so people who take this medica—tion should not consume vitamin K supplements.[56,57] Additionally, these patients should try to maintain consistent dietary intakes of the vitamin each day.

In addition to vitamin K's role in blood clotting, it is also a cofactor for an enzyme that is essential for bone—building cells to produce *osteocalcin*, a pro—tein needed for normal bone mineralization.[58] Low blood levels of vitamin K are associated with the risk of osteoporosis. However, more research is needed to clarify the vitamin's role in bone health.

Food Sources of Vitamin K

Major food sources of vitamin K are green leafy vegetables such as kale, turnip greens, salad greens, cabbage, and spinach; broccoli; and green beans. Other reli—able sources of the vitamin are soybean and canola oils, and products made from these oils, such as margarine and salad dressing. Table 9.8 lists some foods that are sources of the vitamin.

Dietary Adequacy

No RDAs for vitamin K have been established, but AIs for the vitamin are 120 µg/day for men and 90 µg/day for women. The AIs can be met easily by

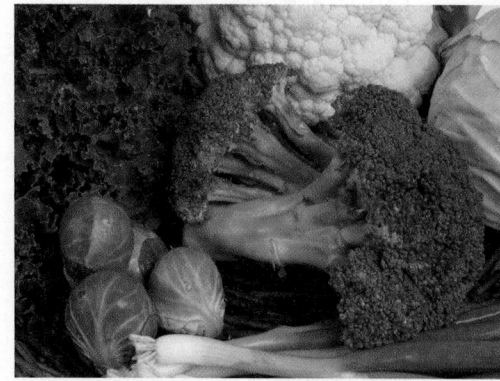

Dark green vegetables, such as broccoli, are a rich source of vitamin K.

TABLE 9.8 Vitamin K Content of Selected Foods

Food	Vitamin K content (µg)
Kale, cooked, ½ cup	530 µg
Beet greens, cooked, ½ cup	349 µg
Turnip greens, cooked, ½ cup	265 µg
Spinach, cooked, ½ cup	444 µg
Brussels sprouts, cooked, 1 cup	219 µg
Spinach, raw, 1 cup	
Broccoli, cooked, 1 cup chopped	
Asparagus, cooked, 1 cup	
Cabbage, shredded raw, 1 cup	
Soybean oil, 1 T	

AI for adult men 120 µg/day

AI for adult women 90 µg/day

Source: Data from U.S. Department of Agriculture, Agricultural Research Service: *USDA National nutrient database for standard reference, Release 26, 2013.*

eating a salad that contains 1 cup of leafy vegetables and 2 tablespoons of salad dressing made with soybean oil. Intake of vitamin K tends to increase with age; middle-aged and older adults eat more green vegetables than young adults.[59]

Vitamin K Deficiency

Although the body stores very little vitamin K, deficiencies among adults rarely occur.[60] Vitamin K deficiency, however, can develop in people who have liver diseases or conditions that impair fat absorption, such as cystic fibrosis. Additionally, long-term antibiotic therapy can reduce the number of bacteria in the colon that synthesize vitamin K and, as a result, contribute to a deficiency of the nutrient. The most reliable sign of vitamin K deficiency is an increase in the time it takes for blood to clot.

Babies are generally born with low vitamin K stores, and a deficiency of the vitamin can occur soon after birth because of the newborn's immature GI tract.[61] Vitamin K–deficient infants are at risk of serious bleeding because their bodies are unable to make certain blood-clotting factors. To prevent vitamin K deficiency from developing during infancy, newborns generally receive a single injection of vitamin K immediately after birth.

Vitamin K Toxicity

Ingesting amounts of vitamin K that exceed the AIs has not been reported to be harmful to humans. Therefore, the Food and Nutrition Board of the National Institutes of Health did not set a UL for the micronutrient. Nevertheless, people should avoid consuming more than the recommended amounts of vitamin K.[14]

Vitamin K and Osteoporosis

Several long-term studies have shown an inverse relationship between vitamin K intake and risk for osteoporosis. The Nurse's Health Study followed over 70,000 nurses for 10 years to evaluate the effects of diet and supplement use on health. They found that participants who consumed the least amount of vitamin K had a 30% higher risk of fracture than women who consumed adequate amounts of vitamin K.[63] However, health care practitioners caution that more research is needed on dosing effects and safety of vitamin K supplementation for bone health.[64]

DID YOU KNOW?

Bone loss is common during and after spaceflight, and some experts speculated that this might be related to vitamin K. The vitamin's status was evaluated in crew members who flew 2 to 6 months on the International Space Station. There was no difference in vitamin K status preflight, in-flight, or postflight. Therefore, it does not appear that vitamin K supplementation is necessary to counteract bone loss during spaceflight.[62]

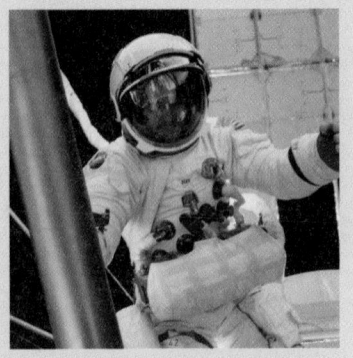

ASSESS YOUR PROGRESS

25 *Identify the three forms of vitamin K and their relationship to each other.*

26 *Describe the role of vitamin K in clotting blood.*

27 *List four good food sources of vitamin K.*

28 *Explain the consequences of vitamin K deficiency and toxicity.*

29 *Discuss the relationship between vitamin K and bone health.*

9.8 Cystic Fibrosis and Fat-Soluble Vitamins

LEARNING OUTCOMES

1 *Describe the cause, signs, and symptoms of cystic fibrosis.*

2 *Summarize general dietary guidelines for cystic fibrosis.*

Millions of Americans suffer from inflammatory bowel disease, pancreatitis, gallbladder disease, and other conditions that negatively affect fat–soluble vitamin digestion and absorption. This section focuses on the inherited disease cystic fibrosis, because the disease interferes with fat–soluble vitamin absorption.

What Is Cystic Fibrosis?

Cystic fibrosis is caused by a defective gene that was first identified in 1989.[65] The presence of this gene leads to the overproduction of thick and sticky mucus that negatively affects the lungs, pancreas, liver, intestines, sinuses, and sex organs. Respiratory and digestive problems are common in cystic fibrosis as the thick mucus builds up, often leading to lung infections. Figure 9.22 shows sticky mucus accumulation in the trachea. Left untreated, children with cystic fibrosis usually experience delayed growth and malnutrition.

Cystic fibrosis is the most common inherited respiratory disease in the Western world with an incidence of 1 per 3000 live births.[65] Individuals whose families have a history of cystic fibrosis can undergo prenatal testing to assess their risk for conceiving a child with cystic fibrosis.

cystic fibrosis inherited respiratory disease caused by a defective gene that leads to overproduction of thick and sticky mucus

Symptoms and Diagnosis

Most children with cystic fibrosis are diagnosed by the time they are 2 years old.[65] People may be diagnosed with the condition when they are teenagers or young adults; however, these individuals have a much milder form of the disease. At this time, most states in the United States conduct newborn screening for cystic fibrosis. A blood sample is sent to a lab for detecting genetic abnormalities that are characteristic in cystic fibrosis. If the blood test comes back positive, a *sweat test* follows. A high level of salt in sweat is a positive sign for cystic fibrosis.

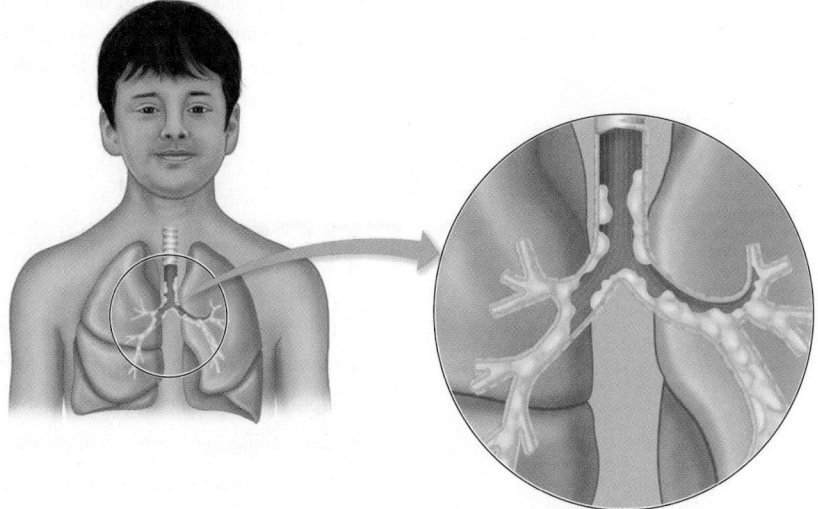

FIGURE 9.22 Mucus accumulation in cystic fibrosis. Overproduction of thick and sticky mucus in cystic fibrosis leads to mucus buildup and lung infections.

TABLE 9.9 Signs and Symptoms of Cystic Fibrosis

- No bowel movements in the first 24 to 48 hours of life
- Failure to gain weight normally during infancy and childhood
- Salty-tasting skin
- Abdominal pain, bloating, gassiness, and severe constipation
- Nausea and loss of appetite
- Foul-smelling feces that contain mucus or float
- Chronic cough with significant mucus accumulation in the sinuses or lungs
- Recurrent fever

Source: National Institutes of Health: *Cystic fibrosis.* Updated May 2012. http://www.ncbi.nlm.nih.gov/pubmedhealth/ PMH0001167/ Accessed: January 25, 2014.

Treatment can be initiated immediately to prevent infection and malnutrition in newborns diagnosed with cystic fibrosis. The most common symptoms of cystic fibrosis are listed in Table 9.9.

Treatment

Treatment for cystic fibrosis includes diet and medications. Nutritional management of cystic fibrosis improves disease management and prevents serious complications of the disease. Such complications include destruction of pancreatic tissue, blockage of the ducts leading to and from the pancreas, and reduced enzymatic activity that can cause nutrient malabsorption. The "Fresh Tips" feature on this page has some basic steps for the dietary management of patients with cystic fibrosis.

Vitamin Malabsorption

As a result of pancreatic enzyme insufficiency and mucus blocking passageways throughout the body, fat–soluble vitamin digestion and absorption is often impaired in cystic fibrosis. Vitamin A is involved in immunity, and poor immune response is a concern of people with cystic fibrosis, because they are already prone to frequent respiratory infections. Although vitamin A supplementation could benefit people with the disease, more research is needed to develop specific guidelines for use of supplemental vitamin A in persons with cystic fibrosis.[66]

Vitamin D deficiency is almost universal in cystic fibrosis patients. Over 20 studies have documented low blood levels of vitamin D in patients with cystic fibrosis, even after supplementation with the micronutrient.[67–69] To conserve bone mass, clinicians routinely supplement such patients with vitamin D. Adequate sun exposure should also be encouraged for those who have cystic fibrosis.[70] However, many cystic fibrosis patients avoid sunlight due to photosensitivity

FRESH TIPS

- A patient taking pancreatic enzyme pills should take those pills with all meals and snacks.
- Patients should eat several small, nutrient-dense meals during the day.
- People who have cystic fibrosis can add calories and protein to their diet by
  - Consuming a nutrient-fortified shake.
  - Topping meals with added cheese and drinking whole milk.
  - Dipping fruits and vegetables in dips or peanut butter.
  - Adding chicken, salmon, eggs, and/or nuts to a vegetable salad.

from antibiotics that are often prescribed to treat frequent lung infections in this population.[67]

Vitamin E deficiency occurs in over one–third of newborn infants with cystic fibrosis.[71] The deficiency can contribute to poor resistance to disease and heart abnormalities.[72,73] Through supplementation, blood levels of alpha–tocopherol can be enhanced in children and adults with cystic fibrosis.[74,75] To maximize absorption, water–soluble forms of vitamin E are often recommended.

Deficiency of vitamin K is common in cystic fibrosis patients who do not take supplements of the micronutrient. However, nutrition experts do not agree on the optimal dosage.

ASSESS YOUR PROGRESS

30 *Describe cystic fibrosis, including common signs and symptoms, and how the disease is diagnosed.*

31 *Explain how cystic fibrosis is treated.*

SUMMARY

SECTION 9.1 Introducing Vitamins

- Vitamins include thiamin, riboflavin, niacin, biotin, pantothenic acid, folate, and vitamins A, B-6, B-12, C, D, E, and K. Choline, carnitine, inositol, lipoic acid, and taurine are vitamin-like nutrients.

SECTION 9.2 Vitamins: The Basics

- Vitamins are organic compounds. Foods generally contain much smaller amounts of vitamins than of macronutrients.
- Vitamins play numerous roles in the body, and each vitamin usually has more than one function. In general, vitamins regulate a variety of body processes, including those involved in cell division and development as well as the growth and maintenance of tissues. Vitamins are not a source of energy.
- Certain vitamins act as antioxidants.
- Vitamins A, D, E, and K are fat-soluble vitamins; thiamin, riboflavin, niacin, vitamin B-6, pantothenic acid, folate, biotin, vitamin B-12, and vitamin C are water-soluble vitamins. The body stores extra fat-soluble vitamins.
- Vitamin deficiency disorders generally result from inadequate diets or conditions that increase the body's requirements for vitamins.
- Most commonly eaten foods do not contain toxic levels of vitamins. Vitamin toxicity is most likely to occur in people who take megadoses of vitamin supplements.
- The bioavailability of a vitamin is dependent on a variety of factors.

SECTION 9.3 An Overview of Fat-Soluble Vitamins

- The fat-soluble vitamins include a hydrocarbon chain as part of their structure.

SECTION 9.4 Vitamin A

- Vitamin A is involved in vision, immune function, and cell development. The vitamin A family includes retinol, retinal, and retinoic acid. The vitamin A precursor, beta-carotene, functions as an antioxidant.
- Dietary sources of preformed vitamin A include liver, fish, and fish oils; provitamin A carotenoids are especially plentiful in dark green and orange fruits and vegetables.
- A deficiency of vitamin A contributes to night blindness and weakened immunity. Excess vitamin A can be toxic and cause birth defects when taken during pregnancy. Eating a diet rich in fruits and vegetables may help prevent chronic diseases, particularly heart disease and cancer.

SECTION 9.5 **Vitamin D**

- Vitamin D is both a hormone and a vitamin. Vitamin D, calciferol, is present in both plant and animal sources; ergocalciferol is present in plant foods, and cholecalciferol is present in animal foods.
- Exposure to sunlight enables human skin to synthesize a precursor of the vitamin from a cholesterol-like substance. The body can convert this substance to the active form of vitamin D.
- Infants and children who do not obtain enough vitamin D may develop rickets, and adults with inadequate amounts of the vitamin in their bodies may develop osteomalacia. Excess intakes of vitamin D can cause the body to deposit calcium in soft tissues.

SECTION 9.6 **Vitamin E**

- Alpha-tocopherol is the most active form of vitamin E. Vitamin E functions primarily as an antioxidant. Plant oils and products made from these oils are generally rich food sources of vitamin E.
- High doses of vitamin E may be detrimental to health.

SECTION 9.7 **Vitamin K**

- Vitamin K is a family of compounds that includes phylloquinone, menaquinone, and menadione. Vitamin K is essential for the blood clotting process and for healthy bone formation.
- Green leafy vegetables, including kale, spinach, and turnip greens, are good dietary sources of vitamin K.
- Inadequate consumption of the vitamin can cause uncontrollable bleeding. Babies are usually born with low vitamin K stores and require an injection of vitamin K soon after birth.

SECTION 9.8 **Cystic Fibrosis and Fat-Soluble Vitamins**

- Cystic fibrosis is a common inherited disease that causes a thick mucus buildup.
- Respiratory and digestive problems are common in cystic fibrosis, with fat and fat-soluble vitamin absorption significantly impaired.
- Mucus buildup reduces the availability of gastrointestinal secretions, contributing to fat malabsorption. Fat-soluble vitamins A, D, E, and K are often deficient in patients with cystic fibrosis. Health care professionals continue to evaluate the potential value of fat-soluble vitamin supplements in treating cystic fibrosis.

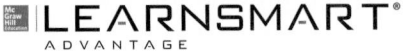 Get the most out of your study of nutrition with McGraw-Hill's innovative suite of adaptive learning products including McGraw-Hill LearnSmart®, SmartBook®, McGraw-Hill LearnSmart Achieve®, and McGraw-Hill LearnSmart Prep®. Visit www.learnsmartadvantage.com.

CASE STUDY RESPONSE

VITAMIN D AND BONE HEALTH

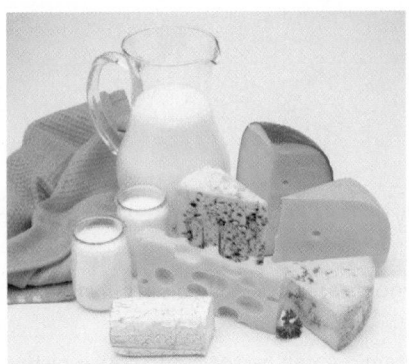

VITAMIN D IS NECESSARY FOR HEALTHY bones, including those of the spine. Vitamin D enhances absorption of phosphorus and calcium in the small intestine, two minerals necessary for bone growth and maintenance. When vitamin D is deficient, bones weaken, leading to osteomalacia. The weakening of the bones in the spine can lead to curvature of the upper spine, which can be identified through monitoring changes in height over time.

Vitamin D is often called the "sunshine vitamin" because the sun can convert a substance in skin, 7-dehydrocholesterol, into active vitamin D. The amount of vitamin D made through sunlight exposure depends on a variety of factors, including where a person lives. Josette lives in northern Maine, a location with long winters. Her low blood vitamin D levels may be a result of her living north of the 37th parallel and spending much of her day indoors.

Dairy foods are generally excellent sources of vitamin D: low- or nonfat milk, yogurt, and cheese are good options. Salmon, tuna, catfish, herring, and sardines are also rich in vitamin D. Some ready-to-eat cereals and breads, orange juice, and margarine have added vitamin D.

TEST KITCHEN
Modifying Recipes for Healthy Living

Adelaine has two young sons, ages 5 and 7, whom she describes as picky eaters. The boys love rice, but they eat very few vegetables. Adelaine is looking for a vegetable-rich chicken and rice dish that incorporates child-friendly vegetables.

CHICKEN AND RICE

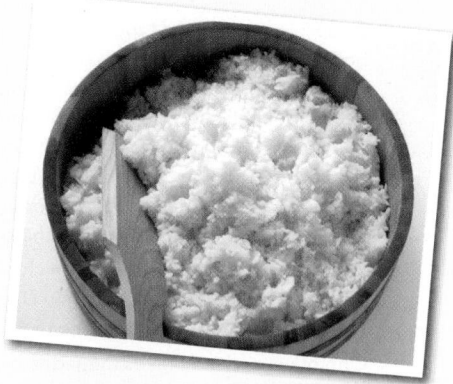

PREPARATION STEPS

1. Preheat oven to 350°F. Grease a shallow baking pan with nonstick cooking spray. Place chicken breasts in pan and add a small amount of water (approximately ¼ cup). Bake chicken for approximately 20 minutes, depending on the thickness of the chicken. Use a meat thermometer to ensure that the internal cooking temperature of the chicken reaches 165°F.

2. While chicken is baking, prepare the rice following package instructions.

3. Drizzle canola oil over the rice and gently stir.

4. Cut chicken into smaller pieces and place over the rice mixture.

5. Serve warm. Serves two.

INGREDIENTS

6 oz boneless, skinless chicken breast

¼ cup water

2 cups uncooked instant whole-grain (brown) rice

3 Tbsp canola oil

STEP 1 Brainstorm

Use diet analysis software to analyze the nutrient and calorie content of the "Chicken and Rice" recipe. List the total calories, carbohydrates, fiber, protein, fat, and vitamin content (vitamins A, D, E, K, thiamin, riboflavin, niacin, pantothenic acid, biotin, B-6, B-12, folate, and C) of the recipe. How do you rate the overall quality of the recipe?

STEP 2 Develop a modified version of this recipe

Develop a modified version of this recipe to increase its vitamin density.

1. List ingredients and amounts.

2. List the preparation steps.

STEP 3 Evaluate the modified recipe

Use diet analysis software to analyze the nutrient and calorie content of the modified "Chicken and Rice" recipe. Develop a table comparing the total calories, carbohydrates, fiber, protein, fat, and individual vitamins in the original and modified recipes. Explain how the rice dishes differ nutritionally.

OPTIONAL ACTIVITIES

STEP 4 Shop for your ingredients

Were the ingredients readily available at the market?
List ingredients that you could not find or that were not available fresh.

STEP 5 Test your new recipe

Keep notes on any changes you make to ingredient amounts as you prepare the chicken and rice.

STEP 6 Reflect on the modified recipe

How does the rice dish look? How does the rice dish taste? Do you think children would enjoy eating this menu item? Explain why they would or would not like it.

STEP 7 Add the recipe to your collection or repeat steps to improve the product

Critical Thinking

1. Choose a vitamin and type the nutrient's name in the search box of an Internet browser. Locate three sites that sell products containing the vitamin. Review the pages of each site, making notes about claims, prices, and the kinds of links provided. Then write a two- to three-page report that describes and compares the information you found at the sites. In your paper, discuss any claims made on behalf of these products that you consider false or misleading. Include the URLs for the sites in your report.

2. Paul was recently diagnosed with chronic kidney disease. Paul's physician recommended a vitamin D and calcium supplement. Describe to Paul the importance of vitamin D in kidney disease.

3. One of your friends takes megadoses of vitamins A and E because she thinks they help her stay healthy. What would you tell her about taking such large doses of these vitamins?

4. Julie's newborn tested positive for cystic fibrosis following screening and a follow-up sweat test. Julie is trying to learn as much as she can about cystic fibrosis and what she can do to ensure her daughter is healthy. Explain to Julie how cystic fibrosis affects blood levels of fat-soluble vitamins. What specific dietary recommendations would you offer Julie?

5. According to MyPlate guidelines, a person who needs 2000 kcal/day should consume 2 cups of fruit and 2.5 cups of vegetables daily. Plan a day's meals and snacks that provide these amounts of fruits and vegetables.

Practice Test

Select the best answer.

1. Megadoses of vitamins are
   a. safe to take, if the vitamins are water soluble.
   b. useful for preventing chronic diseases.
   c. available naturally from a wide variety of foods.
   d. most often consumed from supplements.

2. Vitamins
   a. are metabolized to yield energy.
   b. occur in gram amounts in foods.
   c. are organic molecules.
   d. are macronutrients.

3. People who are unable to absorb fat are likely to develop a ____ deficiency.
   a. vitamin A   c. vitamin B-12
   b. folate   d. riboflavin

4. Enriched grain products have specific amounts of ____ added during processing.
   a. vitamin C   c. vitamin B-12
   b. vitamin A   d. thiamin

5. Which of the following foods is not a rich source of beta-carotene?
   a. beef
   b. carrots
   c. squash
   d. sweet potato

6. A deficiency of vitamin A contributes to
   a. inadequate blood clotting.
   b. night blindness.
   c. sickle cell anemia.
   d. pellagra.

7. The most active form of vitamin A in the body is
   a. retinol.
   b. retinal.
   c. retinoic acid.
   d. cholecalciferol.

8. Children who lack vitamin D can develop
   a. pellagra.
   b. rickets.
   c. beriberi.
   d. scurvy.

9. The most active form of vitamin D is called
   a. cholecalciferol.
   b. calcitriol.
   c. calcidiol.
   d. ergocalciferol.

10. Vitamin D deficiency is most likely in
    a. an infant being breastfed.
    b. a child living in Florida.
    c. a child who drinks fat-free milk.
    d. an infant exposed to sunlight only 30 minutes per day.

11. Vitamin K can be produced by
    a. skin exposure to ultraviolet radiation.
    b. hydrolysis of seawater.
    c. intestinal bacteria.
    d. conversion of lactic acid into lactate.

12. Which of the following vitamins is the most potent antioxidant?
    a. folate
    b. vitamin K
    c. vitamin E
    d. vitamin B-6

13. The form of vitamin K found in spinach and kale is called

    a. menaquinone.
    b. phylloquinone.
    c. menadione.
    d. alpha-tocopherol.

14. ____ may interfere with blood thinning medications, so supplements should generally be avoided.

    a. Vitamin A
    b. Vitamin D
    c. Vitamin E
    d. Vitamin K

15. Which of the following descriptions of cystic fibrosis is false?

    a. A genetic condition affecting the respiratory and digestive systems
    b. A condition leading to excess mucus secretion and buildup
    c. A condition likely to cause a deficiency in fat-soluble vitamins
    d. A condition that can be cured by taking antioxidant supplements

ANSWERS TO PRACTICE TEST

1-d; 2-c; 3-a; 4-d; 5-a; 6-b; 7-a; 8-b; 9-b; 10-a; 11-c; 12-c; 13-b; 14-d; 15-d

ANSWERS TO CHAPTER 9 QUIZ Yourself

1. Vitamins are a source of "quick" energy. **False** (p. 270)
2. A deficiency of vitamin A can lead to night blindness. **True** (p. 279)
3. Fruits are a rich dietary source of vitamin D. **False** (p. 285)
4. Vitamin E is an antioxidant. **True** (p. 289)
5. Vitamin K is necessary for blood clotting. **True** (p. 292)

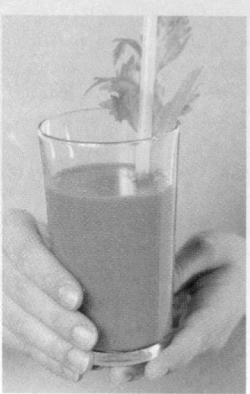

References

1. What is a megadose and why do you recommend against taking megadoses of vitamins? *Johns Hopkins Medical Letter Health After 50*, p. 8, August 2001.
2. Wilson KM and others: Micronutrient levels in children exposed to secondhand tobacco smoke. *Nicotine Tobacco Research* 13(9):800, 2011.
3. Food and Nutrition Board: *Dietary Reference Intakes for vitamin C, vitamin E, selenium, and carotenoids.* Washington, DC: National Academy Press, 2000.
4. Vandamme EJ: Production of vitamins, coenzymes and related biochemicals by biotechnological processes. *Journal of Chemical Technology & Biotechnology* 53(4):313, 1992.
5. Murphy SP and others: Multivitamin-multimineral supplements' effect on total nutrition intake. *American Journal of Clinical Nutrition* 85(Suppl):280S, 2007.
6. National Institutes of Health Office of Dietary Supplements: *Dietary supplement fact sheet: Multivitamin/mineral supplements.* Updated January 2013. http://ods .od.nih.gov/factsheets/MVMS-QuickFacts/ Accessed: January 25, 2014.
7. U.S. Department of Agriculture, Agricultural Research Service: *What we eat in America 2009-2010.* http://www.ars.usda.gov/Services/docs.htm?docid=18349 Accessed: January 19, 2014.
8. Sheth A and others: Potential liver damage associated with over-the-counter vitamin supplements. *Journal of the American Dietetic Association* 108(9):1536, 2008.
9. Food and Drug Administration: *Microwave oven radiation.* Updated October 2014. http://www.fda.gov/Radiation-EmittingProducts/ ResourcesforYouRadiationEmittingProducts/ucm252762.htm Accessed: March 14, 2013.
10. Office of Dietary Supplements: *Dietary supplement fact sheet: Vitamin A and carotenoids.* Updated June 2013. http://ods.od.nih.gov/factsheets/vitamina/ Accessed: January 25, 2104.
11. Lanska DJ: Chapter 29: Historical aspects of the major neurological vitamin deficiency disorders: Overview and fat-soluble vitamin A. *Handbook of Clinical Neurology* 95:435, 2010.
12. Genead MA and others: Fundus white spots and acquired night blindness due to vitamin A deficiency. *Advances in Ophthalmology* 119(3):229, 2009.
13. Fielding JM and others: Increases in plasma lycopene concentration after consumption of tomatoes cooked with olive oil. *Asia Pacific Journal of Clinical Nutrition* 14:131, 2005.
14. Otten JJ and others (eds.): Institute of Medicine: *Dietary Reference Intakes: The essential guide to nutrient requirements.* Washington, DC: National Academies Press, 2006.
15. Zile MH: Function of vitamin A in vertebrate embryonic development. *Journal of Nutrition* 131:705, 2001.
16. Sale TA and Stratman E: Carotenemia associated with green bean ingestion. *Pediatric Dermatology* 21(6):657, 2004.
17. Hak AE and others: Prospective study of plasma carotenoids and tocopherols in relation to risk of ischemic stroke. *Stroke* 35:1584, 2004.
18. Riccioni G and others: Antioxidant vitamin supplementation in cardiovascular diseases. *Annals of Clinical and Laboratory Science* 37(1):89, 2007.
19. Mamede AC and others: The role of vitamins in cancer: A review. *Nutrition & Cancer* 63(4):479, 2011.
20. Mannisto S and others: Dietary carotenoids and risk of lung cancer in a pooled analysis of seven cohort studies. *Cancer Epidemiology, Biomarkers, and Prevention* 13(1):40, 2004.
21. Coleman HR and others: Age-related macular degeneration. *Lancet* 372(9652):1835, 2008.
22. National Eye Institute, National Institutes of Health: *The AREDS formulation and age-related macular degeneration.* Updated November 2011. http://www.nei.nih .gov/amd/summary.asp Accessed: January 25, 2014.
23. Thadhani R and others: Vitamin D therapy and cardiac structure and function in patients with chronic kidney disease: The PRIMO randomized controlled trial. *Journal of the American Medical Association* 307(7):674, 2012.
24. Santoro D and others: Vitamin D status and mortality risk in patients with chronic kidney disease. *Renal Failure* 33(2):184, 2011.
25. Holick MF: Vitamin D deficiency. *New England Journal of Medicine* 357:266, 2007.
26. National Institutes of Health, Office of Dietary Supplements: *Dietary supplement fact sheet: Vitamin D.* Updated June 2011. http://ods.od.nih.gov/factsheets/ vitaminD_pf.asp Accessed: January 25, 2014.
27. Pludowski P and others: Vitamin D effects on musculoskeletal health, immunity, autoimmunity, cardiovascular disease, cancer, fertility, pregnancy, dementia and mortality—a review of recent evidence. *Autoimmunity Reviews* 12(10):967, 2013.

28. Cashman KD and others: Estimation of the dietary requirement for vitamin D in free-living adults ≥ 64 years of age. *American Journal of Clinical Nutrition* 89:1366, 2009.

29. Tsiaris WG, Weinstock MA: Factors influencing Vitamin D status. *Acta-Dermato-venereologica* 91(2):115, 2011.

30. Institute of Medicine Office: *Dietary Reference Intakes for calcium and vitamin D*. Updated November 2010. http://www.iom.edu/~/media/Files/Report%20 Files/2010/Dietary-Reference-Intakes-for-Calcium-and-Vitamin-D/Vitamin%20 D%20and%20Calcium%202010%20Report%20Brief.pdf Accessed: January 25, 2014.

31. Forrest KY, Stuhldreher WL: Prevalence and correlates of vitamin D deficiency in US adults. *Nutrition Research* 31(1):48, 2011.

32. Ozkan B: Nutritional rickets. *Journal of Clinical Research in Pediatric Endocrinology* 2(4):137, 2010.

33. Roth DE: What should I say to parents about vitamin D supplementation from infancy to adolescence? *Paediatric Child Health* 14(9):575, 2009.

34. Bly E and others: Clinical inquiry: What is the best age to start vitamin D supplementation to prevent rickets in breastfed newborns? *Journal of Family Practice* 62(12):755, 2013.

35. Unuvar T, Buyukgebiz A: Nutritional ricks and vitamin D deficiency in infants, children and adolescents. *Pediatric Endocrinology Reviews* 7(3):283, 2010.

36. Godang K and others: Seasonal variation in maternal and umbilical cord 25(OH) vitamin D and their associations with neonatal adiposity. *European Journal of Endocrinology* E-pub: January 22, 2014.

37. Macdonald HM and others: Sunlight and dietary contributions to the seasonal vitamin D status of cohorts of healthy postmenopausal women living at northerly latitudes: A major cause for concern? *Osteoporosis International* 22(9):2461, 2011.

38. Ashwell M and others: UK Food Standards Agency Workshop Report: An investigation of the relative contributions of diet and sunlight to vitamin D status. *British Journal of Nutrition* 104(4):603, 2010.

39. Rizzoli R and others: Vitamin D supplementation in elderly or postmenopausal women: A 2013 update of the 2008 recommendations from the European Society for Clinical and Economic Aspects of Osteoporosis and Osteoarthritis (ESCEO). *Current Medical Research and Opinion* 29(4):305, 2013.

40. Reid IR and others: Effects of vitamin D supplements on bone mineral density: A systemic review. *Lancet* 383(9912):146, 2014.

41. Cardinal RN, Gregory CA: Osteomalacia vitamin D deficiency in a psychiatric rehabilitation unit: Case report and survey. *BMC Research Notes* 2:82, 2009.

42. Wolf G: The discovery of the antioxidant function of vitamin E: The contribution of Henry A. Mattill. *Journal of Nutrition* 135(3):363, 2005.

43. National Institutes of Health, Office of Dietary Supplements: *Dietary supplement fact sheet: Vitamin E*. Updated June 2013. http://ods.od.nih.gov/factsheets/ vitamine/ Accessed: January 25, 2014.

44. Clarke MW, Burnett JR: Vitamin E in human health and disease. *Critical Reviews in Clinical Laboratory Sciences* 45(5):417, 2008.

45. Ford ES and others: Brief communication: The prevalence of high intakes of vitamin E and the use of supplements among U.S. adults. *Annals of Internal Medicine* 143:116, 2005.

46. Mamede AC and others: The role of vitamins in cancer: A review. *Nutrition and Cancer* 63(4):479, 2011.

47. Ledesma MC and others: Selenium and vitamin E for prostate cancer: Post-SELECT (Selenium and Vitamin E Cancer Prevention Trial) status. *Molecular Medicine* 17(1–2):134, 2011.

48. Jiang L and others: Efficacy of antioxidant vitamins and selenium supplement in prostate cancer prevention: A meta-analysis of randomized controlled trials. *Nutrition and Cancer* 62(6):719, 2010.

49. Bjelakovic G and others: Systemic review: Primary and secondary prevention of gastrointestinal cancers with antioxidant supplements. *Aliment Pharmacology and Therapy* 28(6):689, 2008.

50. Fortmann SP and others: Vitamin and mineral supplements in the primary prevention of cardiovascular disease and cancer: An updated systematic evidence review for the U.S. Preventive Services Task Force. *Annals of Internal Medicine* E-pub: November 12, 2013.

51. Pekmezci D: Vitamin E and immunity. *Vitamins and Hormones* 86:179, 2011.

52. Schurks M and others: Effects of vitamin E on stroke subtypes: Meta-analysis of randomized controlled trials. *British Medical Journal* 341:c5702, 2010.

53. Dysken MW and others: Effect of vitamin E and memantine on functional decline in Alzheimer disease: The TEAM-AD VA cooperative randomized trial. *Journal of the American Medical Association* 311(1):33, 2014.

54. Lee HP and others: Antioxidant approaches for the treatment of Alzheimer's disease. *Expert Reviews in Neurotherapeutics* 10(7):1201, 2010.

55. Devore EE and others: Dietary antioxidants and long-term risk of dementia. *Archives of Neurology* 67(7):819, 2010.

56. Chang CH and others: A practical approach to minimize the interaction of vitamin K with warfarin. *Journal of Clinical Pharmacy and Therapeutics* 39(1):56, 2014.

57. Gebuis EP and others: Vitamin K1 supplementation to improve the stability of anticoagulation therapy with vitamin K antagonists: A dose-finding study. *Haematologica* 96(4):583, 2011.

58. Sogabe N and others: Effects of long-term vitamin K(1) (phylloquinone) or vitamin K(2) (menaquinone-4) supplementation on body composition and serum parameters in rats. *Bone* 48(5):1036, 2011.

59. Booth SL and others: Dietary vitamin K intakes are associated with hip fracture but not with bone mineral density in elderly men and women. *American Journal of Clinical Nutrition* 71(5):1201, 2000.

60. Linus Pauling Institute, Oregon State University, Micronutrient Information Center: Vitamin K. Updated December 2011. http://lpi.oregonstate.edu/ infocenter/vitamins/vitaminK/ Accessed: March 14, 2013.

61. Lippi G, Franchini M: Vitamin K in neonates: Facts and myths. *Blood Transfusion* 9(1):4, 2011.

62. Zwart SR and others: Vitamin K status in spaceflight and ground-based models of spaceflight. *Journal of Bone Mineral Research* 26(5):948, 2011.

63. Feskanich D and others: Vitamin K intake and hip fractures in women: A prospective study. *American Journal of Clinical Nutrition* 69(1):74, 1999.

64. Hamidi MS and others: Vitamin K and bone health. *Journal of Clinical Densitometry* 16(4):409, 2013.

65. National Institutes of Health: *Cystic fibrosis*. Updated May 2012. http://www.ncbi .nlm.nih.gov/pubmedhealth/PMH0001167/ Accessed: March 14, 2013.

66. O'Neil C and others: Vitamin A supplementation for cystic fibrosis. *Cochrane Database of Systematic Reviews* Jan 23 (1):CD006751, 2008.

67. Hall WB and others: Vitamin D deficiency in cystic fibrosis. *International Journal of Endocrinology* 2010:218691, 2010.

68. Lark RK and others: Diminished and erratic absorption of ergocalciferol in adult cystic fibrosis patients. *American Journal of Clinical Nutrition* 73(3):602, 2001.

69. Royner AJ and others: Vitamin D insufficiency in children, adolescents, and young adults with cystic fibrosis despite routine oral supplementation. *American Journal of Clinical Nutrition* 86(6):1694, 2007.

70. Robberecht E and others: Sunlight is an important determinant of vitamin D serum concentrations in cystic fibrosis. *European Journal of Clinical Nutrition* 65(5):574, 2011.

71. Sokol RJ and others: Fat-soluble-vitamin status during the first year of life in infants with cystic fibrosis identified by screening of newborns. *American Journal of Clinical Nutrition* 50:1064, 1989.

72. Tanyel MC, Mancano LD: Neurological findings in vitamin E deficiency. *American Journal of Family Physicians* 55:197, 1997.

73. Shamseer L and others: Antioxidant micronutrients for lung disease in cystic fibrosis. *Cochrane Database of Systematic Reviews* Dec 8(12):CD007020, 2010.

74. Sagel SD and others: Effect of an antioxidant-rich multivitamin supplement in cystic fibrosis. *Journal of Cystic Fibrosis* 10(1):31, 2010.

75. Huang SH and others: Vitamin E status in children with cystic fibrosis and pancreatic insufficiency. *Journal of Pediatrics* 148(4):556, 2006.

10 Water-Soluble Vitamins

Vitamin B-12 deficiency in a vegan

DEON HAS BEEN FOLLOWING A VEGAN DIET FOR 7 YEARS. Over the past 6 months, Deon has been experiencing extreme fatigue, headaches, and numbness in his fingers. Following a visit to his health care provider, Deon was diagnosed with *megaloblastic anemia* and a vitamin B-12 deficiency.

Initially, the health care provider recommended Deon take a daily vitamin B-12 pill. However, at follow-up, it was determined that his blood levels of vitamin B-12 were still low after several months of treatment. Therefore, it was recommended he receive monthly vitamin B-12 injections.

- Explain to Deon how his vegan diet may have contributed to the vitamin B-12 deficiency and how this relates to anemia.
- Describe why Deon's health care provider has recommended vitamin B-12 injections.
- Provide dietary advice for Deon to promote increased blood levels of vitamin B-12.
- If Deon chooses to ignore his health care provider's advice to manage the anemia and low blood vitamin B-12, what are additional health consequences he may face from a vitamin B-12 deficiency?

The suggested Case Study Response can be found on page 336.

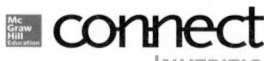 Check out the Connect site at www.mcgrawhillconnect.com to further
|NUTRITION explore this case study.

QUIZ Yourself

Will taking supplements that contain water-soluble vitamins give a person more energy? Does vitamin C prevent the common cold? Can water-soluble vitamins be toxic? Take the following quiz to test your knowledge of the B-vitamins and vitamin C. The answers are found on page 340.

1. Water-soluble vitamins are stored in significant amounts in the human body. ___T ___F

2. High doses of B vitamins are safe to take. ___T ___F

3. Thiamin is necessary to prevent neural tube defects. ___T ___F

4. Vegans are at risk for a vitamin B-12 deficiency. ___T ___F

5. Vitamin C enhances the body's disease-fighting abilities. ___T ___F

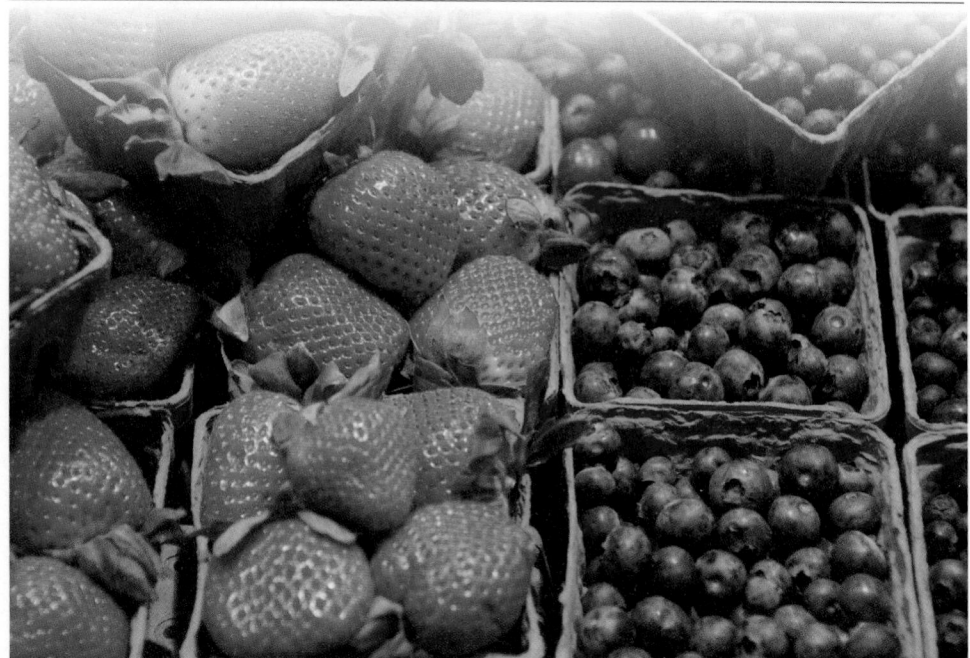

10.1 Introducing Water-Soluble Vitamins

LEARNING OUTCOMES

1 *Describe the fate of excess water-soluble vitamins in the body.*
2 *Identify the water-soluble vitamins.*
3 *Explain the importance of water-soluble vitamins as coenzymes.*

This chapter focuses on vitamin C and the eight B vitamins—thiamin, riboflavin, niacin, biotin, pantothenic acid, vitamin B–6, folate, and vitamin B–12. The physiological roles, major food sources, and consequences of deficiency or toxicity are discussed for each water–soluble vitamin. Additionally, this chapter provides information about the vitamin–like compounds choline, carnitine, inositol, taurine, and lipoic acid.

Water-Soluble Vitamins: Basic Concepts

As discussed in Chapter 9, water–soluble vitamins dissolve in the watery components of food and the body. Compared to fat–soluble vitamins, excesses of most water–soluble vitamins are filtered through the kidneys and eliminated in the urine, rather than stored in large amounts. Therefore, water–soluble vitamins need to be consumed on a regular basis to prevent deficiency.

Table 10.1 provides a summary of the water–soluble vitamins. Unless otherwise noted, RDA/AI values are for adults 19 to 50 years of age, excluding pregnant or breastfeeding women. Figure 10.1 indicates food groups that are good food sources of water–soluble vitamins.

Water-Soluble Vitamins as Coenzymes

In the body, most water–soluble vitamins function as components of specific coenzymes. Many of the chemical reactions involved in the metabolism of carbohydrates, fats, and amino acids involve coenzymes that contain

FIGURE 10.1 MyPlate: Water-soluble vitamins. This illustration highlights MyPlate food groups that generally are good sources of water-soluble vitamins.

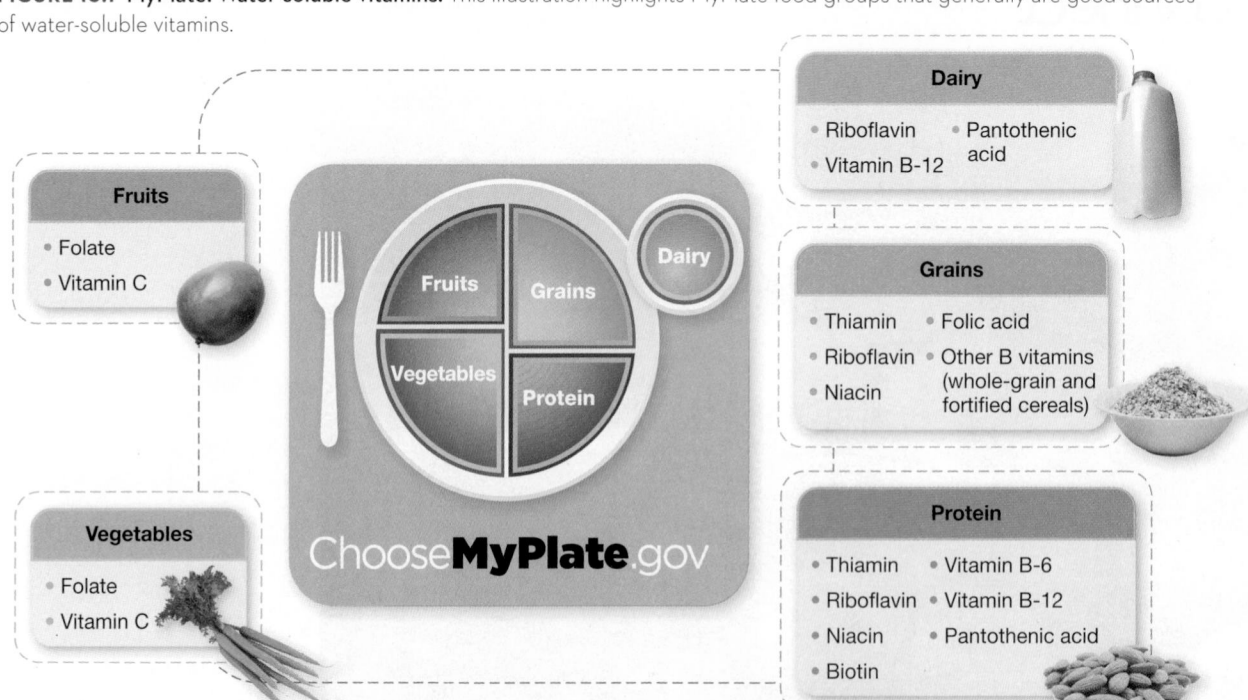

Fruits
- Folate
- Vitamin C

Vegetables
- Folate
- Vitamin C

Dairy
- Riboflavin
- Vitamin B-12
- Pantothenic acid

Grains
- Thiamin
- Riboflavin
- Niacin
- Folic acid
- Other B vitamins (whole-grain and fortified cereals)

Protein
- Thiamin
- Riboflavin
- Niacin
- Biotin
- Vitamin B-6
- Vitamin B-12
- Pantothenic acid

ChooseMyPlate.gov

TABLE 10.1 Summary of Water-Soluble Vitamins

Vitamin	Major Functions in the Body	Adult RDA/AI (adult RDA = bold)	Major Dietary Sources	Major Deficiency Signs and Symptoms	Major Toxicity Signs and Symptoms
Thiamin	Part of TPP, coenzyme needed for carbohydrate metabolism and the metabolism of certain amino acids; may help produce neurotransmitters	1.1–1.2 mg	Pork, wheat germ, enriched breads and cereals, brewer's yeast	Beriberi and Wernicke-Korsakoff syndrome: Weakness, abnormal nervous system functioning	None (upper limit [UL] not determined)
Riboflavin	Part of FMN and FAD, coenzymes needed for carbohydrate, amino acid, and lipid metabolism	1.1–1.3 mg	Milk, yogurt, and other milk products; enriched breads and cereals; liver	Inflammation of the mouth and tongue, eye disorders	None (UL not determined)
Niacin	Part of NAD and NADP, coenzymes needed for energy metabolism	14–16 mg	Enriched breads and cereals, beef, liver, tuna, salmon, poultry, pork, mushrooms	Pellagra • Diarrhea • Dermatitis • Dementia • Death	Adult UL = 35 mg/day Flushing of facial skin, itchy skin, nausea and vomiting, liver damage
Pantothenic acid	Part of coenzyme A that is needed for synthesizing fat and that helps release energy from carbohydrates, fats, and protein	5 mg	Beef and chicken liver, sunflower seeds, mushrooms, yogurt, soy milk, fortified cereals	Rarely occurs	Unknown (UL not determined)
Biotin	Cofactor needed for synthesizing glucose and fatty acids	30 µg	Liver, eggs, peanuts, salmon, pork, mushrooms, sunflower seeds	Rarely occurs: skin rash, hair loss, convulsions, and other neurological disorders; developmental delays in infants	Unknown (UL not determined)
Vitamin B-6	Part of PLP, coenzyme needed for amino acid metabolism, involved in neurotransmitter synthesis and hemoglobin synthesis	1.3–1.7 mg	Meat, fish, and poultry; potatoes, bananas, spinach, sweet red peppers, broccoli	Dermatitis, anemia, depression, confusion, and neurological disorders such as convulsions	Adult UL = 100 mg/day Nerve destruction
Folate	Part of THFA, coenzyme needed for DNA synthesis and conversion of cysteine to methionine, preventing homocysteine accumulation	400 µg	Dark green, leafy vegetables; liver; legumes; asparagus; broccoli; orange juice; enriched breads and cereals (folic acid)	Megaloblastic anemia, diarrhea, neural tube defects in embryos	Adult UL = 1000 µg/day May stimulate cancer cell growth
Vitamin B-12	Part of coenzymes needed for various cellular processes, including folate metabolism; maintenance of myelin sheaths	2.4 µg	Animal foods, fortified cereals, fortified soy milk	Pernicious anemia: megaloblastic anemia and nerve damage resulting in paralysis and death	None (UL not determined)
Ascorbic acid (vitamin C)	Connective tissue synthesis and maintenance, antioxidant, synthesis of neurotransmitters and certain hormones, immune system functioning	75–90 mg (nonsmokers)	Peppers, citrus fruits, papayas, broccoli, cabbage, berries	Scurvy: poor wound healing, pinpoint hemorrhages, bleeding gums, bruises, depression	Adult UL = 2000 mg/day Diarrhea and GI tract discomfort

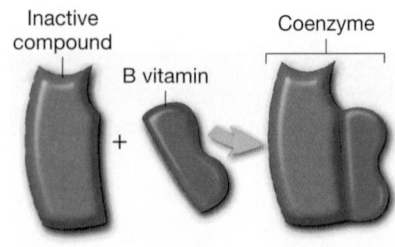

FIGURE 10.2 Coenzyme synthesis.

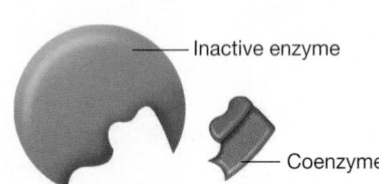

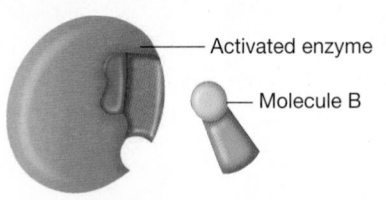

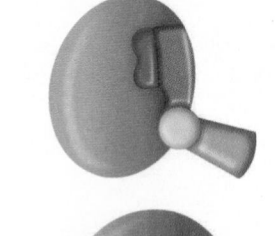

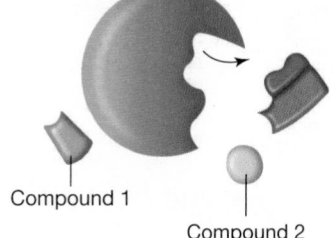

FIGURE 10.3 Coenzyme action. Many enzymes need coenzymes to function. This illustration shows a coenzyme activating an enzyme, which enables it to split a molecule into two parts.

thiamin vitamin B-1; vitamin component of a coenzyme that is important for energy metabolism as part of thiamin pyrophosphate (TPP)

neurotransmitters chemicals produced by nerve cells that enable the cells to communicate with other nerve cells

B vitamins (see Chapter 8). The coenzyme forms of B vitamins are often found in foods; this form of the vitamin undergoes digestion to release the free form of the vitamin. Following absorption, cells combine one of the B vitamins with a nitrogen−containing, nonprotein compound, to synthesize a coenzyme (Fig. 10.2). Upon activation by the coenzyme, the enzyme enables the reaction to occur (Fig. 10.3).

Health−food stores often sell supplements that contain coenzymes; buying these products may be a waste of money. As described above, coenzymes in food or supplements are not absorbed intact in the small intestine. The com−pounds undergo digestion to release their B−vitamin components. The small intestine absorbs many of the B vitamins that are present in foods and sup−plements, and the micronutrients eventually enter the general circulation. As in Chapter 9, the sections that follow present each vitamin's major functions in the body and its main food sources. We also discuss each vitamin's dietary ade−quacy, the symptoms of deficiency, and its toxicity, if applicable. Section 10.12 discusses the role of diet in cancer development; several vitamins may protect against cancer.

ASSESS YOUR PROGRESS

1. *Why do water-soluble vitamins need to be consumed regularly?*
2. *List the water-soluble vitamins.*
3. *Describe how cells use B vitamins to make coenzymes.*

10.2 Thiamin

LEARNING OUTCOMES

1. *Identify the coenzyme form of thiamin.*
2. *Describe dietary sources of thiamin.*
3. *Explain the consequences of a thiamin deficiency or toxicity.*

In the late 1890s, Dutch physician Christiaan Eijkmann observed that chick−ens fed refined (milled) white rice developed a nervous system disease that was similar to *beriberi*, a human disease characterized by severe neurologi−cal problems. Beriberi was common among human populations who ate mostly white rice. When Eijkmann fed the bran and hulls removed from rice during the milling process ("rice polishings") to chickens and humans affected by this nervous system disorder, they recovered. In 1911, Polish chemist Casimir Funk discovered the substance in rice polishings that cured beriberi. Funk called the compound a "vitamine" because of its chemical structure, which contained an amine (a nitrogen−containing substance). We now know this substance as vitamin B−1 or thiamin.

Functions of Thiamin

Thiamin is part of the coenzyme thiamin pyrophosphate (TPP). TPP partic−ipates in chemical reactions that remove a carbon dioxide molecule (CO_2) from a larger compound. This reaction is necessary for the breakdown of carbohy−drates to release energy and for the metabolism of the branched−chain amino acids leucine, isoleucine, and valine. TPP is also necessary for the synthesis of **neurotransmitters**, chemicals produced by nerve cells that enable the cells to communicate with other nerve cells. *Acetylcholine* is a neurotransmitter that requires TPP for synthesis.

Food Sources of Thiamin

Whole–grain and enriched breads and cereals, pork, legumes, and orange juice are good food sources of thiamin. Brewer's yeast is a rich source of thiamin, but most Americans do not eat the product. Table 10.2 lists some common foods that are good sources of thiamin. Overheating food can destroy thiamin.

Thiamin Deficiency and Toxicity

The adult RDA for thiamin is 1.2 mg/day for men and 1.1 mg/day for women.[1] The body stores very little thiamin, so deficiency symptoms can occur within a few days of consuming a thiamin–deficient diet. The thiamin deficiency disease, as noted earlier, is called **beriberi**. People suffering from beriberi are very weak and have poor muscular coordination (Fig. 10.4). The severe lack of thiamin also negatively affects the functioning of their cardiovascular, digestive, and nervous systems.

While rare in the United States, outbreaks of beriberi have occurred in other parts of the world. In 2005, a beriberi outbreak occurred among commercial fishermen on a ship in Thailand.[2] During their 18 months at sea, over half of the men on the ship developed signs of beriberi, including swelling, chest discomfort, and difficulty swallowing. Authorities attribute the outbreak to the fishermen eating only raw seafood and polished rice. Polished rice is a poor source of thiamin, and raw seafood contains *thiaminase*, an enzyme that destroys thiamin. If started immediately, thiamin therapy results in complete recovery from beriberi.

Wernicke–Korsakoff syndrome (*vear'–nih–key kor'–sah–koff*) is a degenerative brain disorder associated with thiamin deficiency. This syndrome occurs primarily in alcoholics in the United States, because alcohol reduces thiamin absorption and increases the vitamin's excretion. Signs of Wernicke–Korsakoff syndrome include abnormal eye movements, staggering gait, and distorted thought processes. Treatment involves eliminating alcohol and obtaining thiamin injections. Without prompt treatment, people with Wernicke–Korsakoff syndrome can become disabled permanently or die.

Toxicity from consuming high amounts of thiamin from food or supplements is rare, probably because the excess vitamin is readily excreted in urine.[3] Thus, no UL has been established for thiamin.

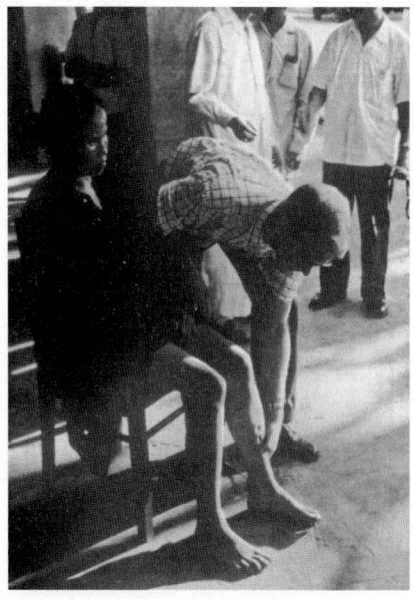

FIGURE 10.4 Beriberi. The woman sitting in the chair has a form of beriberi called "wet beriberi." She suffers from fatigue, nervous system disorders, and abnormalities that result in severe "pitting" edema in her lower legs.

beriberi thiamin deficiency disease characterized by weakness, poor muscular coordination, and abnormal functioning of the cardiovascular, digestive, and nervous systems

Wernicke-Korsakoff syndrome degenerative brain disorder associated with a deficiency of thiamin and most commonly caused by excessive alcohol consumption

TABLE 10.2 Thiamin Content of Selected Foods

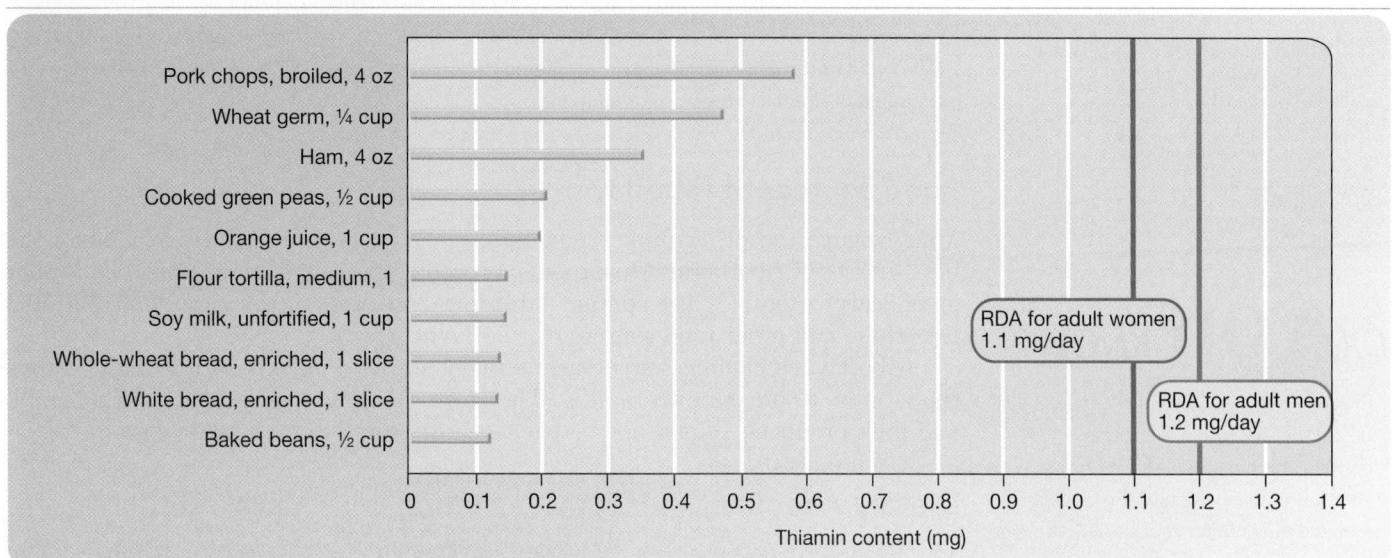

Food	Thiamin content (mg)
Pork chops, broiled, 4 oz	~0.59
Wheat germ, ¼ cup	~0.47
Ham, 4 oz	~0.35
Cooked green peas, ½ cup	~0.20
Orange juice, 1 cup	~0.20
Flour tortilla, medium, 1	~0.14
Soy milk, unfortified, 1 cup	~0.13
Whole-wheat bread, enriched, 1 slice	~0.13
White bread, enriched, 1 slice	~0.12
Baked beans, ½ cup	~0.12

RDA for adult women 1.1 mg/day
RDA for adult men 1.2 mg/day

Source: Data from U.S. Department of Agriculture, Agricultural Research Service: *USDA National nutrient database for standard reference*, release 26, 2013.

DID YOU KNOW?

Large doses of thiamin are used to treat certain inborn errors of metabolism, or metabolic diseases, including *thiamin responsive lactic acidosis*. In this rare condition, lactate accumulates due to abnormal *pyruvate dehydrogenase complex* activity.[4] This enzyme complex is necessary for the conversion of pyruvate into acetyl CoA. When pyruvate is not converted into acetyl CoA, the substance instead accumulates as lactate. Thiamin can increase the activity of pyruvate dehydrogenase, reducing lactate buildup. Early diagnosis and thiamin therapy are necessary to prevent brain damage from thiamin responsive lactic acidosis.[5]

ASSESS YOUR PROGRESS

4 *Name the coenzyme form of thiamin.*

5 *Identify three good food sources of thiamin.*

6 *Discuss the conditions associated with a thiamin deficiency, including signs and symptoms.*

10.3 Riboflavin

LEARNING OUTCOMES

1 *Name the coenzyme forms of riboflavin and discuss the vitamin's primary functions in the body.*

2 *Identify dietary sources of riboflavin.*

3 *List the signs and symptoms of a riboflavin deficiency.*

riboflavin vitamin B-2; important for energy metabolism as part of flavin mononucleotide and flavin adenine dinucleotide

Recall from Chapter 8 that **riboflavin** is a component of flavin mononucleotide (FMN) and flavin adenine dinucleotide (FAD), two coenzymes that play key roles in enzymatic reactions, including those that are critical to energy, fatty acid, and folate metabolism. The liver, kidneys, and heart store small amounts of riboflavin; any excess intake is excreted rapidly in the urine.

DID YOU KNOW?

High doses of riboflavin (200 to 400 mg) may be a low-cost, effective treatment for managing migraines in both children and adults.[6] Several studies have found that supplemental riboflavin reduces the incidence of migraines.[7] However, other studies have shown a significant placebo effect and no benefit with riboflavin supplementation.[8] More research is needed to determine the value of riboflavin therapy for migraines.

Food Sources of Riboflavin

Milk, yogurt and other milk products, enriched cereal, and liver are among the best sources of riboflavin. Mushrooms, broccoli, asparagus, and spinach and other green leafy vegetables also contain substantial amounts of the vitamin. Table 10.3 lists these and other food sources of riboflavin.

Riboflavin's chemical structure is fairly stable, but exposure to light causes the vitamin to break down rapidly. Therefore, riboflavin—rich foods, such as milk and milk products, should not be packaged or stored in clear glass containers.

Dietary Adequacy

The RDA for riboflavin is 1.1 mg/day for women and 1.3 mg/day for men.[1] The typical riboflavin intake of North Americans is about 1.5 mg/day for women and

DID YOU KNOW?

Riboflavin is naturally yellow. If you take a dietary supplement that contains high amounts of riboflavin, your kidneys will excrete the excess, and you may notice your urine has a bright yellow color.

TABLE 10.3 Riboflavin Content of Selected Foods

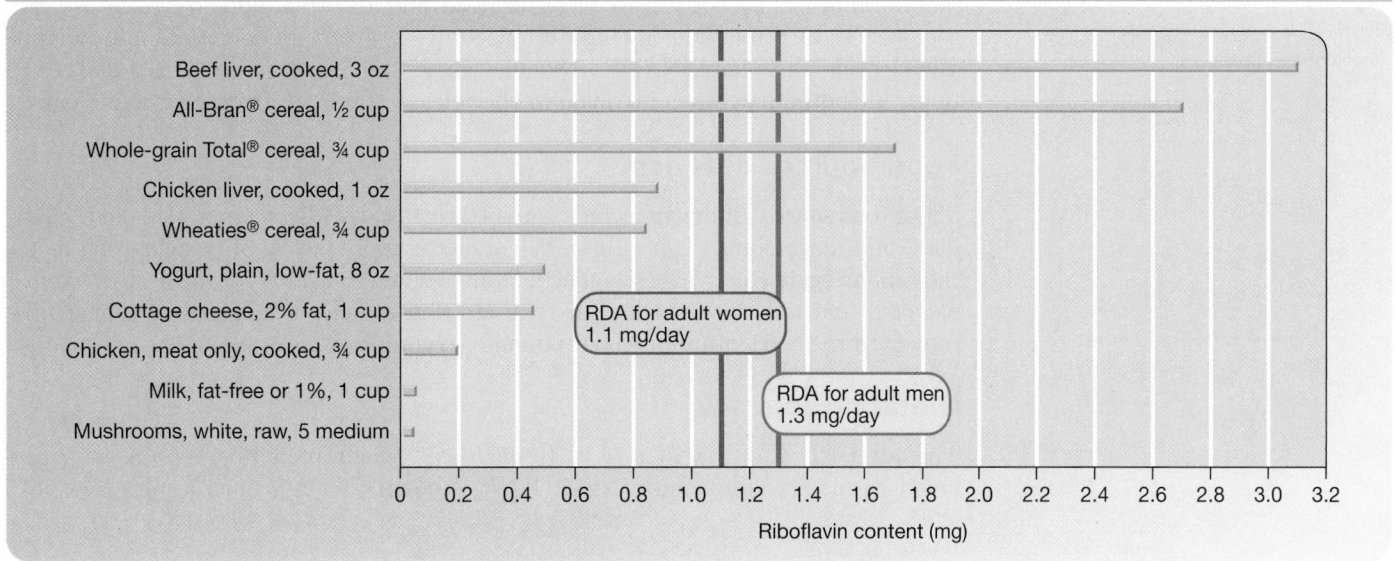

Food	Riboflavin content (mg)

Beef liver, cooked, 3 oz
All-Bran® cereal, ½ cup
Whole-grain Total® cereal, ¾ cup
Chicken liver, cooked, 1 oz
Wheaties® cereal, ¾ cup
Yogurt, plain, low-fat, 8 oz
Cottage cheese, 2% fat, 1 cup
Chicken, meat only, cooked, ¾ cup
Milk, fat-free or 1%, 1 cup
Mushrooms, white, raw, 5 medium

RDA for adult women 1.1 mg/day

RDA for adult men 1.3 mg/day

Riboflavin content (mg): 0 0.2 0.4 0.6 0.8 1.0 1.2 1.4 1.6 1.8 2.0 2.2 2.4 2.6 2.8 3.0 3.2

Source: Data from U.S. Department of Agriculture, Agricultural Research Service: *USDA National nutrient database for standard reference*, release 26, 2013.

2.1 mg/day for men.[3] Riboflavin is rapidly eliminated in urine, so consuming large amounts of the vitamin does not appear to cause side effects. Thus, no UL has been established for riboflavin.

In the United States, the riboflavin deficiency disease **ariboflavinosis** ($a-rie-bo-flay-veh-no'-sis$) rarely occurs, because many commonly eaten foods contain riboflavin. Signs of ariboflavinosis include fatigue, inflammation of the mucous membranes that line the mouth and throat, and **glossitis**, a swollen and sore tongue (Fig. 10.5). The tongue, which also appears lumpy and reddish−purple in color, is called "magenta tongue". Other signs include chapped−appearing lips; **cheilosis** ($key-low'-sis$) scaling and cracking of the skin around the corners of the mouth; a type of dermatitis (inflammation of skin); and eye disorders. Nervous system disorders, such as confusion and headaches, have also been reported. Many signs and symptoms of ariboflavinosis, such as cheilosis and glossitis, are nonspecific and can also occur in other B−vitamin deficiencies. Therefore, specific blood tests may be necessary to determine whether an individual is riboflavin deficient.

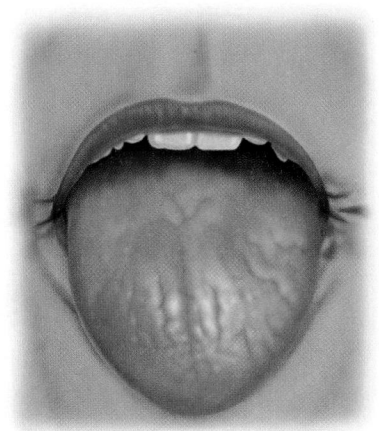

FIGURE 10.5 Glossitis and cheilosis. Glossitis and cheilosis can be symptoms of several medical conditions, including ariboflavinosis. In cases of ariboflavinosis, the tongue is reddish-purple in color.

ASSESS YOUR PROGRESS

7 *Explain the role of riboflavin in energy metabolism.*

8 *List three good food sources of riboflavin.*

9 *Identify two signs or symptoms associated with a riboflavin deficiency.*

10.4 Niacin

LEARNING OUTCOMES

1 *Name the coenzyme forms of niacin and discuss the vitamin's primary functions in the body.*

2 *Identify dietary sources of niacin.*

3 *Explain the signs and symptoms of a niacin deficiency or toxicity.*

4 *Discuss the clinical use of megadoses of niacin.*

ariboflavinosis riboflavin deficiency disease characterized by fatigue, inflammation of the mucous membranes that line the mouth and throat, and glossitis

glossitis swollen and sore tongue

cheilosis scaling and cracking of the skin around the corners of the mouth

niacin vitamin B-3; important for energy metabolism as part of nicotinamide adenine dinucleotide and nicotinamide adenine dinucleotide phosphate

Niacin, vitamin B–3, has two forms: *nicotinic acid* and *nicotinamide* (also called *niacinamide*). The body uses nicotinic acid and nicotinamide to synthesize two coenzymes, nicotinamide adenine dinucleotide (NAD) and nicotinamide adenine dinucleotide phosphate (NADP). Niacin coenzymes participate in at least 200 reactions, including pathways involved in the release of energy from macronutrients.

Food Sources of Niacin

Major food sources of niacin include enriched cereals, beef liver, tuna, salmon, poultry, pork, and mushrooms (Table 10.4). When diets supply plenty of protein–rich foods, the human body can synthesize niacin from the amino acid tryptophan. For example, eggs and milk lack niacin, but they are rich sources of tryptophan that can be converted to the B vitamin. About 60 mg of tryptophan yield about 1 mg of niacin.

Dietary Adequacy

The adult RDA for niacin is 14 to 16 mg/day.[1] Niacin recommendations are provided as niacin equivalents (NEs); 1 NE is equal to 1 mg niacin. NEs take into

DID **YOU** KNOW?

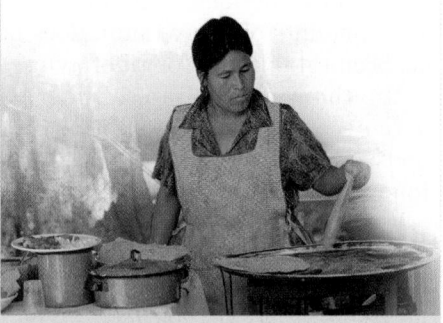

The niacin content of corn is considerably higher than that of most other vegetables, but the B vitamin is tightly bound to a protein that resists digestion. Thus, people who eat corn as their staple food are prone to develop pellagra, the niacin deficiency disease. The traditional Mexican diet is corn-based, but pellagra was not a widespread disease in Mexico, while it was a major health concern in other parts of the world. The Mexican practice of soaking corn kernels in lime water before using them to prepare tortillas helps free the niacin, enhancing its ability to be absorbed. In the United States, corn products such as hominy and grits are sources of niacin because they have been treated with lime before cooking.

TABLE 10.4 Niacin Content of Selected Foods

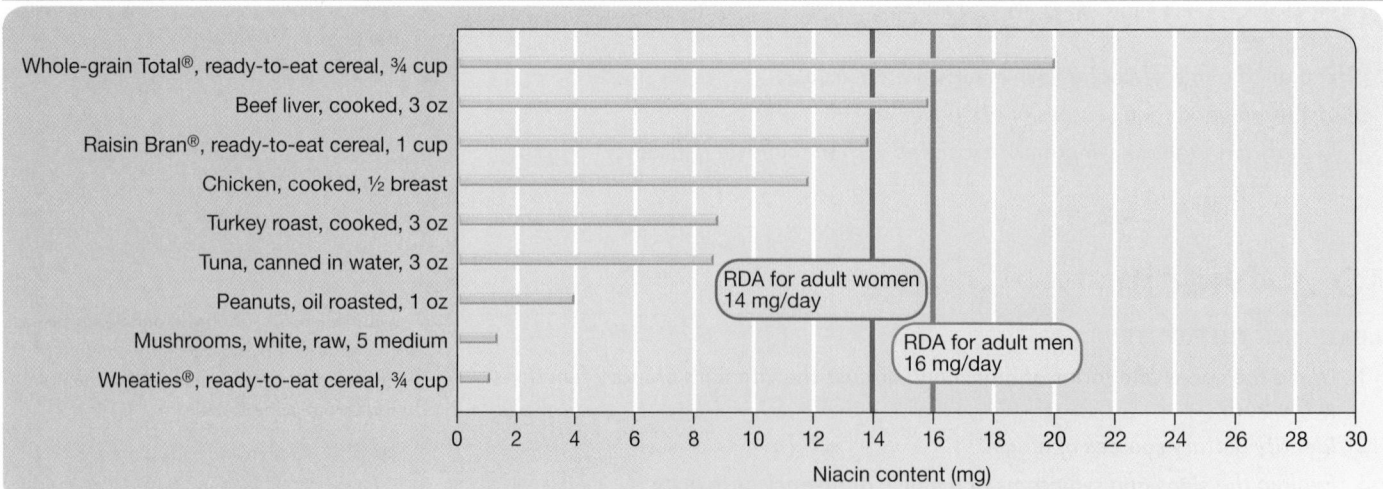

Source: Data from U.S. Department of Agriculture, Agricultural Research Service: *USDA National nutrient database for standard reference*, release 26, 2013.

consideration both the niacin content of a food and the contribution of trypto—phan to niacin. Daily NEs can be estimated from the protein content of the diet.

Step 1: Determine the grams of protein available for niacin synthesis (RDA for protein is 0.8g/kg body weight). The protein available for niacin synthesis is any amount consumed above that amount.

Step 2: Assume that most sources of dietary protein contain approximately 1% tryptophan. Based on this assumption, divide the grams of excess daily protein intake by 100 to obtain the grams of tryptophan. Convert this amount to milligrams (multiply by 1000).

Step 3: Because the body can convert 60 mg of tryptophan into 1 mg of niacin, divide the milligrams of tryptophan from Step 2 by 60. This indicates the NEs available from tryptophan.

Step 4: Add together the amount of food niacin and niacin available from tryptophan (Step 3 above). This amount provides an estimate of dietary niacin.

Niacin Deficiency

In the United States, people with alcoholism, anorexia nervosa (self—starvation), and those with rare disorders that disrupt tryptophan metabolism are generally the only groups at risk of niacin deficiency. Early signs and symptoms of mild niacin deficiency include poor appetite, weight loss, and weakness. Because of the broad, nonspecific symptoms, niacin deficiency is often missed in patients with anorexia nervosa.

If an affected person continues to consume a niacin—deficient diet, the con—dition worsens and **pellagra** (*peh—lah′—gra* or *peh—lay′—gra*) develops. The classic signs and symptoms of pellagra are dermatitis, diarrhea, dementia, and death—the "4 Ds of pellagra" (Fig. 10.6). In the early twentieth century, pellagra was widespread in the southeastern United States. Today, the disease is rare in Western societies, but it still occurs among impoverished populations in devel—oping countries, particularly in regions of Africa, India, and China.

Niacin Toxicity

The adult UL for niacin (nicotinic acid) is 35 mg/day.[1] There have been no reports indicating that the niacin obtained naturally in foods can cause toxicity.[3] However, physicians may prescribe megadoses of niacin supplements containing *nicotinic acid* to reduce elevated LDL cholesterol levels and increase HDL cho—lesterol levels in blood (Fig. 10.7).[9] For patients who cannot tolerate statins (see Chapter 6), taking megadoses of niacin can reduce their risk of stroke and heart attack.[10] Such therapy, however, can have side effects, including flushing of the skin, usually on the face and chest; GI tract upset, such as nausea and vomiting; and liver damage. Using a statin along with a prescribed form of niacin to treat elevated LDL cholesterol levels has not been shown to be safe or effective in reducing risks of stroke and heart attack.[11]

ASSESS YOUR PROGRESS

10 *Identify a coenzyme form of niacin.*

11 *List three food sources of niacin.*

12 *Which amino acid can be a source of niacin?*

13 *Describe the niacin deficiency condition, and list three common symptoms.*

14 *What is the major clinical use of high-dose niacin? What are common signs of niacin toxicity?*

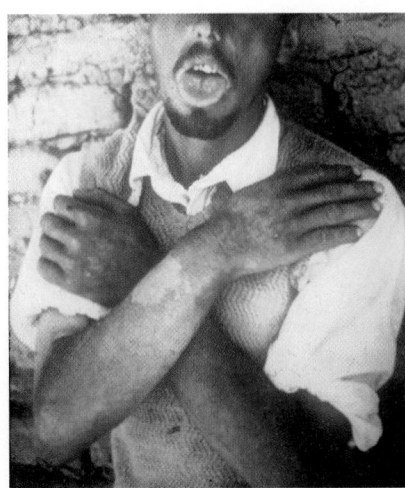

FIGURE 10.6 Pellagra. This man with pellagra shows one of the classic signs of the niacin deficiency disease, dermatitis, particularly on parts of the body exposed to sun.

pellagra niacin deficiency disease characterized by dermatitis, diarrhea, dementia, and death

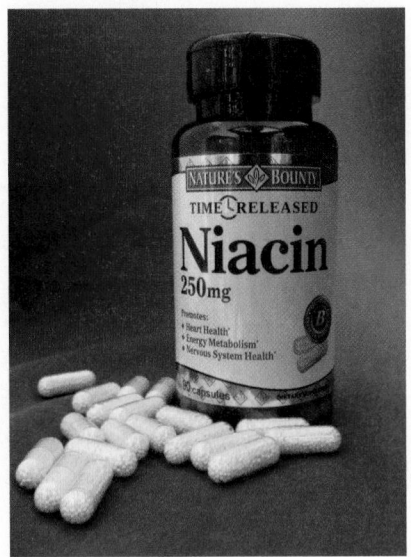

FIGURE 10.7 Niacin as medicine. Megadoses of niacin have been used to treat abnormalities in blood lipids.

10.5 Pantothenic Acid

LEARNING OUTCOMES

1 *Name the coenzyme form of pantothenic acid and discuss the vitamin's primary function in the body.*

2 *Identify dietary sources of pantothenic acid.*

3 *Explain why a pantothenic acid deficiency is rare.*

pantothenic acid vitamin component of coenzyme A (CoA)

coenzyme A pantothenic acid–containing coenzyme that helps release energy from carbohydrates, fat, and protein, and is necessary for fatty acid synthesis

Like the other B vitamins, **pantothenic acid** is a component of a coenzyme; in this case, **coenzyme A**. This coenzyme helps release energy from macronutrients and is needed for fatty acid synthesis.

Food Sources of Pantothenic Acid

In Greek, *pantothen* means "everywhere," which refers to the vitamin's presence in a wide variety of foods. Pantothenic acid, once identified as vitamin B–5, is so widespread in foods that a nutritional deficiency is unlikely to occur among healthy people who eat varied diets. Rich sources of pantothenic acid include cereals that have been fortified with the vitamin, beef and chicken liver, sunflower seeds, mushrooms, peas, and soy milk. Other good sources are meat, cow's milk, and many types of vegetables. Table 10.5 lists these and other common food sources of pantothenic acid.

Dietary Adequacy

The AI for pantothenic acid is 5 mg/day for adults. Most Americans con-sume the AI amount or more daily, and as a result, deficiencies of the vita-min are rare. When scientists experimentally cause pantothenic deficiency to occur in human subjects, they note signs and symptoms that include headache, fatigue, impaired muscle coordination, GI tract disturbances, and *burning feet syndrome*, which causes severe aching in the feet. People who abuse alcohol may develop pantothenic acid and other B–vitamin deficiencies, particularly if their overall diets are nutritionally inadequate. At this time, scientists have not set a UL for the vitamin because there have been no reports of toxicity from taking high doses.

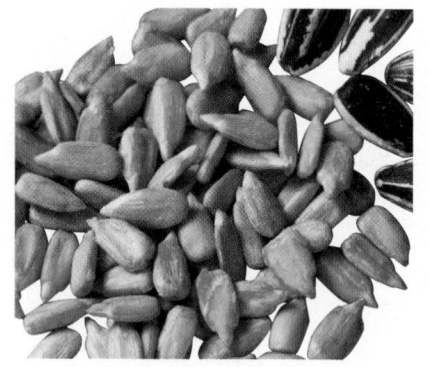

One-quarter of a cup of dry-roasted sunflower seeds provides 2.25 mg of pantothenic acid.

TABLE 10.5 Pantothenic Acid Content of Selected Foods

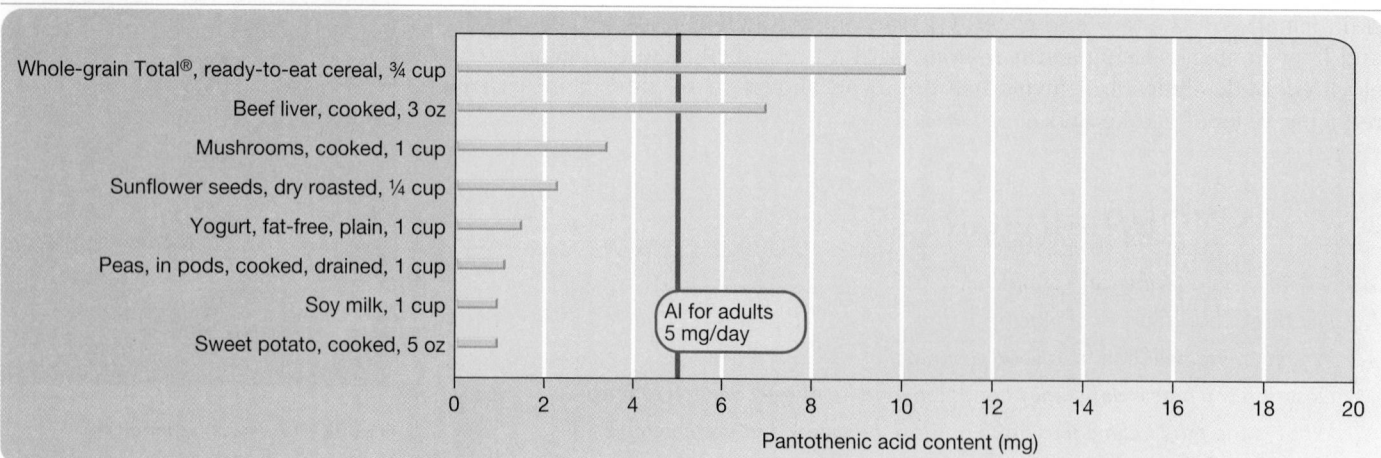

Source: Data from U.S. Department of Agriculture, Agricultural Research Service: *USDA nutrient database for standard reference*, release 26, 2013.

ASSESS YOUR PROGRESS

15 *Explain the role of pantothenic acid in energy metabolism.*

16 *List three food sources of pantothenic acid.*

17 *Which population is at the greatest risk for a pantothenic acid deficiency?*

10.6 **Biotin**

LEARNING OUTCOMES

1 *Summarize the importance of biotin in the body.*

2 *Identify dietary sources of biotin.*

3 *Describe the signs of a biotin deficiency and identify the primary cause of the deficiency.*

In its coenzyme form, **biotin** participates in chemical reactions that add carbon dioxide to other compounds. By doing so, the vitamin promotes the synthesis of glucose and fatty acids and the breakdown of certain amino acids. Biotin as a coenzyme is essential for regenerating oxaloacetate in the TCA cycle (see Fig. 8.16).

Food Sources of Biotin

Table 10.6 provides information about the biotin content of some foods. Liver, eggs, peanuts, salmon, pork, mushrooms, and sunflower seeds are good sources of the vitamin.

Dietary Adequacy

The AI for biotin is 30 µg/day for adults, an amount that is generally met by the typical American adult. Severe deficiencies of biotin rarely occur because intestinal bacteria produce some biotin and the vitamin is found in a wide variety of foods. Signs and symptoms of biotin deficiency include skin rash, hair loss,

biotin vitamin component of a coenzyme that participates in chemical reactions that add carbon dioxide to other compounds

avidin protein found in raw egg whites that binds biotin, thus preventing absorption of the vitamin

DID **YOU** *KNOW?*

Eating raw eggs frequently or in excess can cause a biotin deficiency. A protein in raw egg whites, **avidin**, binds biotin, thus inhibiting absorption. It often takes consumption of 24 or more raw egg whites in a day before biotin absorption is impaired. Consuming cooked eggs is not a cause for concern because heating denatures avidin, as well as kills any potentially dangerous bacteria.

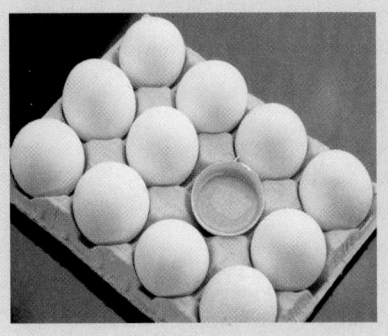

TABLE 10.6 Biotin Content of Selected Foods

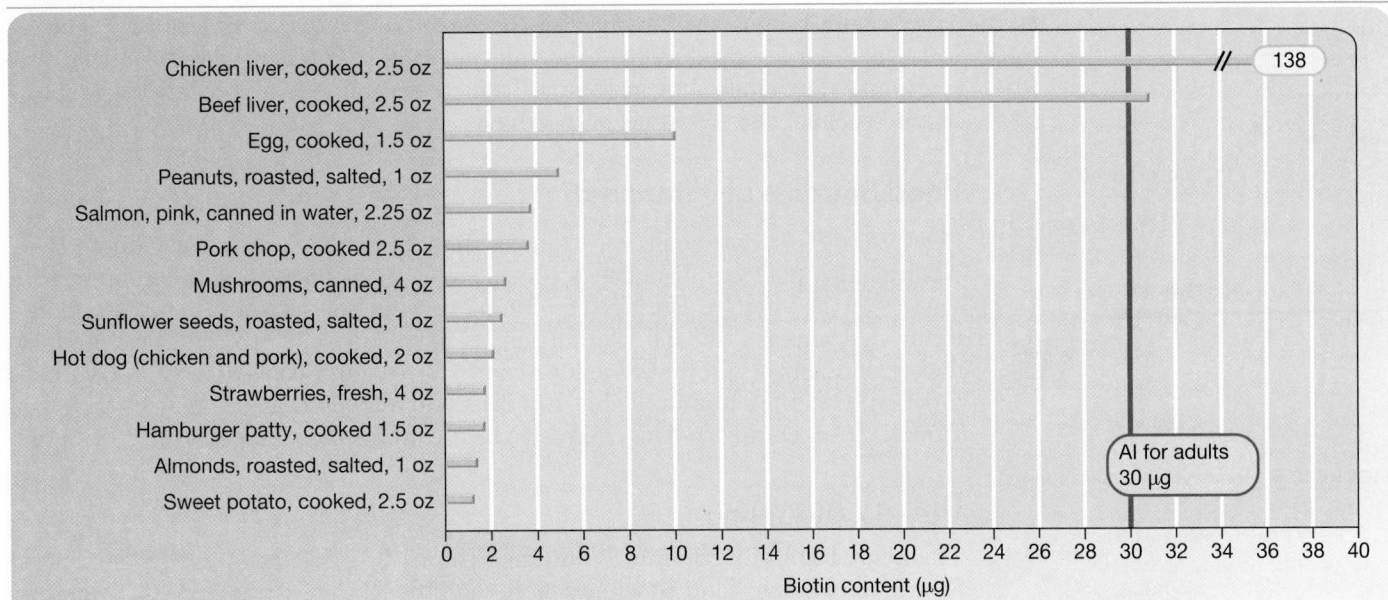

Biotin content (µg)

Chicken liver, cooked, 2.5 oz — 138
Beef liver, cooked, 2.5 oz
Egg, cooked, 1.5 oz
Peanuts, roasted, salted, 1 oz
Salmon, pink, canned in water, 2.25 oz
Pork chop, cooked 2.5 oz
Mushrooms, canned, 4 oz
Sunflower seeds, roasted, salted, 1 oz
Hot dog (chicken and pork), cooked, 2 oz
Strawberries, fresh, 4 oz
Hamburger patty, cooked 1.5 oz
Almonds, roasted, salted, 1 oz
Sweet potato, cooked, 2.5 oz

AI for adults 30 µg

Source: Staggs CG:Determination of the biotin content of select foods using accurate and sensitive HPLC/avidin binding. *Journal of Food Composition and Analysis* 17(6):767, 2004.

convulsions, and other neurological disorders. Infants who are biotin deficient also experience developmental delays. Because biotin appears to be nontoxic, nutrition scientists have not set a UL for the micronutrient.

ASSESS YOUR PROGRESS

18 *What role does biotin play in energy metabolism?*

19 *List three food sources of biotin.*

20 *Why are cases of biotin deficiency uncommon?*

10.7 Vitamin B-6

LEARNING OUTCOMES

1 *Name the coenzyme form of vitamin B-6 and discuss the vitamin's role in the body.*

2 *Identify dietary sources of vitamin B-6.*

3 *Describe the signs and symptoms of a vitamin B-6 deficiency or toxicity.*

vitamin B-6 B vitamin component of the coenzyme pyridoxal phosphate (PLP); important for energy metabolism, particularly protein metabolism, as a part of pyridoxal phosphate (PLP)

Vitamin B−6 is actually a family of three compounds: *pyridoxine* (*pir−ih−doc'−seen*), *pyridoxal* (*peer−ih−doc'−sal*), and *pyridoxamine* (*peer−ih−doc'−sah−mean'*). Cells can convert these forms of the vitamin to the primary B−6 coenzyme, *pyridoxal phosphate* (*PLP*). A major role of PLP is to facilitate enzymatic reactions involved in amino acid metabolism, including the conversion of the amino acid tryptophan to niacin and the transamination reactions that form nonessential amino acids (see Fig. 7.12).

PLP also helps convert a toxic amino acid, homocysteine, to cysteine, a nonessential amino acid. If the body lacks vitamin B−6, homocysteine can accumulate in blood and may contribute to cardiovascular disease (CVD) in some individuals (see Chapter 6). As shown in Figure 10.8, folate and vitamin B−12 are also needed for homocysteine metabolism.

hemoglobin iron-containing protein in red blood cells that transports oxygen

During red blood cell production, PLP participates in the production of heme. Heme is the iron−containing portion of **hemoglobin**, the protein in red blood cells (RBCs) that transports oxygen. If vitamin B−6 is unavailable for heme synthesis, a type of anemia develops.

Vitamin B−6 is also involved in the synthesis of *neurotransmitters*, chemicals that nerves produce to transmit messages. These neurotransmitters are serotonin, dopamine, and histamine from their amino acid precursors, tryptophan, tyrosine, and histidine, respectively.

Food Sources of Vitamin B-6

Liver, meat, fish, and poultry are among the best dietary sources of vitamin B−6. Additionally, potatoes, bananas, spinach, sweet red peppers, and broccoli are good sources of the vitamin. During the refining process, the vitamin B−6 that is naturally in grains is lost, and the nutrient is not added back to the grain products during enrichment. However, many ready−to−eat and cooked cereals have been fortified with the vitamin. Table 10.7 lists some foods that are major sources of vitamin B−6. During cooking, excessive heat can cause major losses of the vitamin.

Dietary Adequacy

The adult RDAs for vitamin B−6 range from 1.3 to 1.7 mg/day.[1] In the United States, the average adult consumes more than the RDA of vitamin B−6. Therefore, cases of vitamin B−6 deficiency are rare, but they can result from alcoholism or genetic conditions that affect vitamin B−6 metabolism. Additionally, patients

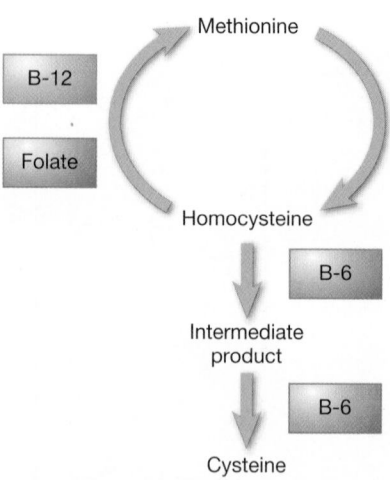

FIGURE 10.8 Homocysteine metabolism. Homocysteine can be converted to cysteine, a nonessential amino acid, in reactions that depend on vitamin B-6-containing enzymes. Methionine can be recycled from homocysteine in reactions that involve vitamin B-12 and folate.

TABLE 10.7 Vitamin B-6 Content of Selected Foods

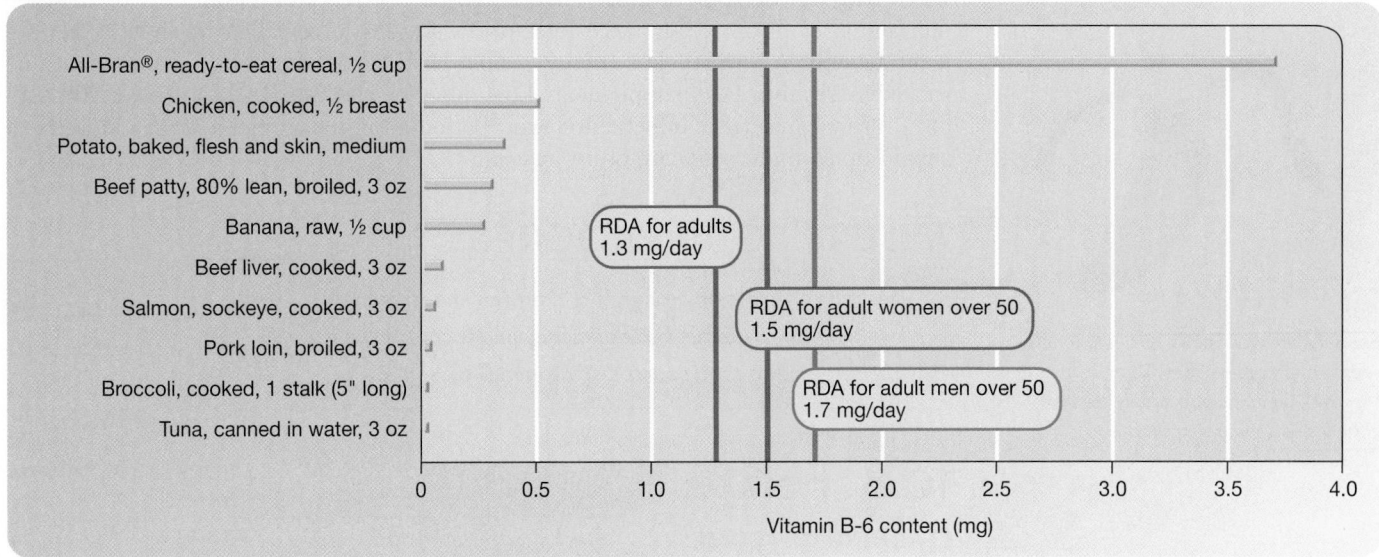

	Vitamin B-6 content (mg)
All-Bran®, ready-to-eat cereal, ½ cup	
Chicken, cooked, ½ breast	
Potato, baked, flesh and skin, medium	
Beef patty, 80% lean, broiled, 3 oz	
Banana, raw, ½ cup	
Beef liver, cooked, 3 oz	
Salmon, sockeye, cooked, 3 oz	
Pork loin, broiled, 3 oz	
Broccoli, cooked, 1 stalk (5" long)	
Tuna, canned in water, 3 oz	

RDA for adults 1.3 mg/day

RDA for adult women over 50 1.5 mg/day

RDA for adult men over 50 1.7 mg/day

Source: Data from U.S. Department of Agriculture, Agricultural Research Service: *USDA National nutrient database for standard reference*, release 26, 2013.

DID YOU KNOW?

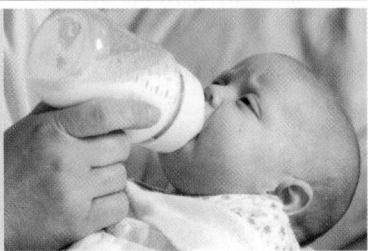

In the early 1950s, some infants became unusually irritable and developed convulsions after being fed a commercial formula. It was determined that the vitamin B-6 in the formula had been destroyed by excessive heating during the manufacturing process. The convulsions may have resulted from a lack of neurotransmitters in the infants' brains. The babies were effectively treated with vitamin B-6.

taking certain medications, particularly those for Parkinson's disease or tuberculosis, may develop vitamin B−6 deficiency because these medications reduce levels of PLP in blood.

Signs and symptoms of vitamin B−6 deficiency include dermatitis, anemia, convulsions, depression, and confusion. Recent evidence suggests that a B−6 deficiency may also contribute to seizures in adults[12,13] and children[14] with epilepsy.

Vitamin B-6 Toxicity

The adult UL for vitamin B−6 is 100 mg/day.[1] Unlike most B vitamins, megadoses of vitamin B−6 are toxic, causing severe sensory nerve damage **(peripheral neuropathy)** when taken in doses that exceed the UL for extended periods.[15] Signs and symptoms of vitamin B−6 toxicity include walking difficulties and numbness of the hands and feet. The nerve damage resolves when affected people stop ingesting megadoses of vitamin B−6.

Popular sources of nutrition information often recommend large doses of vitamin B−6 to treat **premenstrual syndrome (PMS)**, a condition that many women experience a few days before their menstrual period begins. Similarly, vitamin B−6 is a common additive in natural supplements for treatment of nausea and vomiting in early pregnancy, often called *morning sickness*. Chapter 16 mentions the use of a medication that contains a form of vitamin B−6 to treat morning sickness. However, there is not enough scientific evidence to support the use of dietary supplements containing vitamin B−6 for relieving PMS and morning sickness.[16–18] Vitamin B−6 supplementation has also been suggested for the

peripheral neuropathy condition characterized by severe sensory nerve damage

premenstrual syndrome (PMS) condition that many women experience a few days before their menstrual period begins

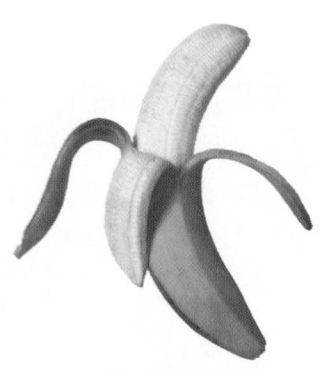

Bananas are well known as being a rich source of potassium (see Chapter 11). However, bananas also supply several vitamins, including vitamin B-6.

treatment of *carpal tunnel syndrome*, a painful nerve disorder that affects the wrist. Results of some studies suggest positive effects of vitamin B–6 in carpal tunnel syndrome, but large long–term studies have failed to show a significant benefit.[19] Nevertheless, many people with carpal tunnel syndrome continue to take a vitamin B–6 supplement. Low doses of vitamin B–6 (less than 200 mg/day) rarely cause toxic effects, however, patients taking supplemental vitamin B–6 should do so under the care of a physician.[20]

ASSESS YOUR PROGRESS

21 *Describe the role of vitamin B-6 in protein metabolism.*

22 *Explain how a vitamin B-6 deficiency might contribute to CVD.*

23 *List three good food sources of vitamin B-6.*

10.8 Folate

LEARNING OUTCOMES

1 *Name the coenzyme form of folate and discuss the vitamin's role in the body.*

2 *Identify sources of folate.*

3 *Compare the absorption of folate from natural and synthetic sources.*

4 *Explain the consequences of a folate deficiency in both pregnant and nonpregnant adults.*

folate B vitamin that is a component of the coenzyme tetrahydrofolic acid (THFA), includes folic acid, and is important for energy metabolism, DNA synthesis, and homocysteine metabolism

Folate is the name for a group of related compounds that includes folic acid. Folic acid refers specifically to the synthetic form of the vitamin found in supplements and added to fortified foods. In the body, cells convert all forms of folate to a group of folate–containing coenzymes collectively called *tetrahydrofolic (tet′–tra–hi′–drow–foe′–lik) acid* or simply *THFA*. THFA accepts a single–carbon group, such as CH_3, from one compound and transfers it to another. As a result, THFA participates in many chemical reactions involved in DNA synthesis and amino acid metabolism. As cells prepare to divide, they need THFA to make DNA.

Certain roles of folate and vitamin B–12 are interrelated. THFA can transfer a CH_3 group to vitamin B–12, which, in turn, transfers the CH_3 group to homocysteine, forming methionine (Fig. 10.9). This process recycles methionine. When vitamin B–12 is unavailable, folate cannot be used, and a deficiency of folate occurs, even though dietary intakes are adequate.

Sources of Folate

Leafy vegetables, liver, legumes, asparagus, broccoli, and orange juice are good natural sources of folate. Enriched grain products and fortified cereals are among the richest sources of folate in the American diet. Foods made with enriched grains supply U.S. adults with about 200 µg folic acid/day—half the RDA.

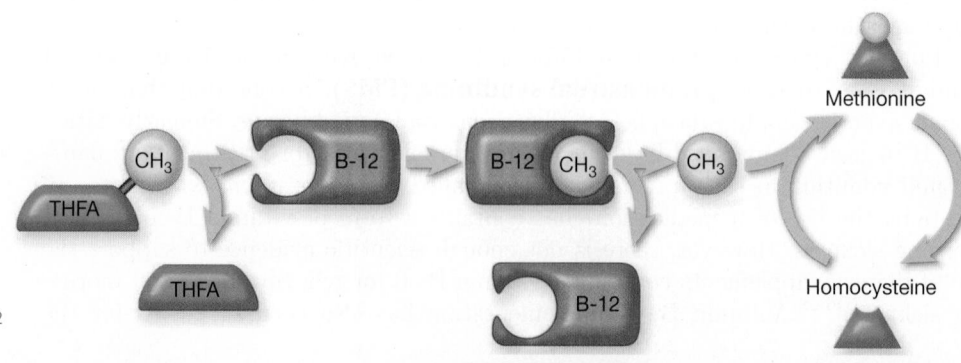

FIGURE 10.9 Folate and vitamin B-12: Working together. This diagram shows how folate (THFA) works with vitamin B-12 to transfer a methyl group (CH_3).

TABLE 10.8 Folate Content of Selected Foods

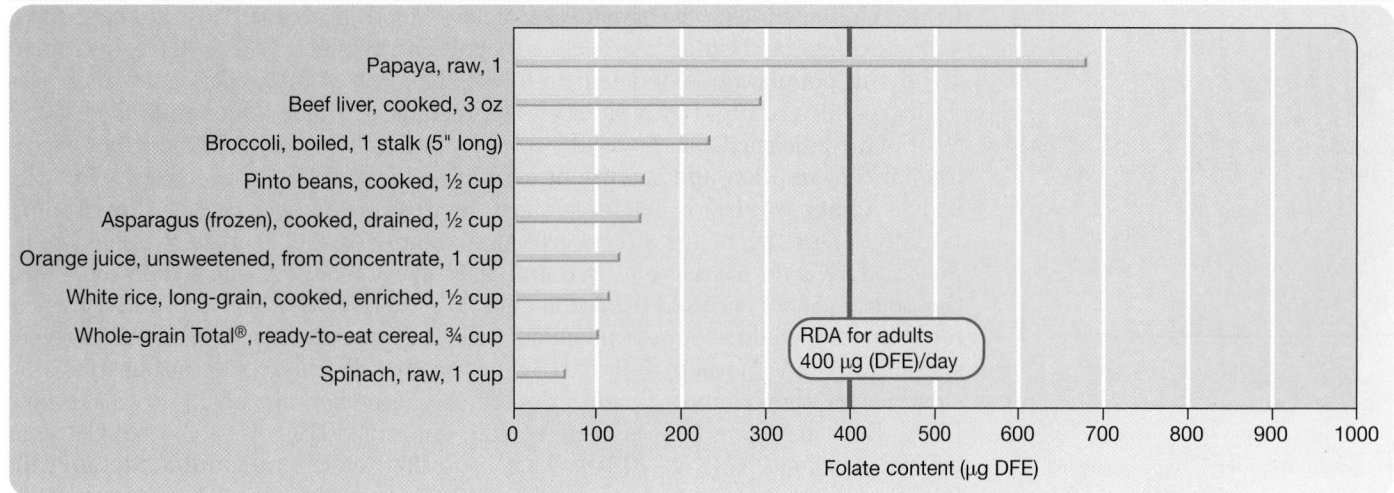

Food	Folate content (µg DFE)
Papaya, raw, 1	~680
Beef liver, cooked, 3 oz	~290
Broccoli, boiled, 1 stalk (5" long)	~230
Pinto beans, cooked, ½ cup	~160
Asparagus (frozen), cooked, drained, ½ cup	~150
Orange juice, unsweetened, from concentrate, 1 cup	~120
White rice, long-grain, cooked, enriched, ½ cup	~110
Whole-grain Total®, ready-to-eat cereal, ¾ cup	~100
Spinach, raw, 1 cup	~60

RDA for adults 400 µg (DFE)/day

Source: Data from U.S. Department of Agriculture, Agricultural Research Service: *USDA National nutrient database for standard reference*, release 26, 2013.

Table 10.8 lists the folate content of selected foods in micrograms of *dietary folate equivalents* (*DFEs*). DFE units account for the difference in absorption of folic acid and that of natural forms of folate.

Folate is easily destroyed by heat, oxidation, and ultraviolet light. Food processing and preparation can destroy 50 to 90% of the folate in food. By eating fresh fruits and raw or lightly cooked vegetables, a person is likely to obtain most of the foods' folate content.

Calculating DFEs

The following equation is used to determine DFEs:

DEF = µg natural food folate + (1.7 × µg folic acid from fortified foods or dietary supplements)

If a person consumes 100 µg of food folate and 200 µg of folic acid from supplements or fortified foods, his or her DFE is:

DFE = 100 µg + (1.7 × 200 µg)

DFE = 100 µg + 340 µg

DFE = 440 µg

Digestion and Absorption of Folate

Folate naturally occurs in foods with a string of glutamates attached to its basic structure (*folate polyglutamate*). Folic acid, the synthetic form of folate that is shown in Appendix D, has a single glutamate molecule bound to folate (*folate monoglutamate*). No enzymatic activity is necessary to digest folic acid. To digest naturally occurring folate, specific intestinal enzymes are necessary to remove all except one of the glutamates, which results in the folic acid form of the vitamin. Because of the additional steps required to remove the glutamates, naturally—occurring folate is not as bioavailable as folic acid.

When folate is in the folic acid form, a three—carbon methyl group (CH_3) is added to the monoglutamate. The folate—CH_3 compound is absorbed in the small intestine. Within the body's cells, folate is activated by removal of the CH_3 group, a process that relies on vitamin B—12.

Dietary Adequacy

The adult RDA for folate is 400 µg (DFE)/day. Needs for the vitamin increase to 600 µg (DFE)/day during pregnancy and 500 µg (DFE)/day in breastfeeding women.[1]

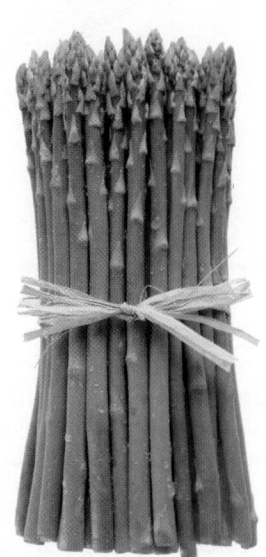

Asparagus is a good source of folate.

Folate Deficiency

In the United States, the prevalence of low blood levels of folate among people 4 years of age and older has declined significantly since 1988–1994.[21] Less than 1% of this population is deficient in folate. The risk of folate deficiency increases during periods of rapid growth, such as pregnancy, infancy, and childhood.[22]

Folate deficiency usually results from nutritionally inadequate diets, but excess alcohol consumption and the use of certain medications can negatively affect the body's ability to absorb and use folate, resulting in deficiencies of the vitamin. Initially, folate deficiency affects cells that rapidly divide, such as red blood cells. Mature RBCs do not have nuclei, and they live for only about 4 months. Thus, the body must replace old or worn—out RBCs constantly. To keep up with their rapid rate of cell division, the precursor cells that mature into RBCs must actively synthesize DNA. Without folate, RBC precursor cells that reside in bone marrow enlarge, but they cannot divide normally, because they are unable to make new DNA. Bone marrow releases some of the abnormal RBCs into the bloodstream before they mature (Fig. 10.10). This condition, called **megaloblastic anemia** (*mega* = large; *blast* = immature cell), is characterized by large, immature RBCs (*megaloblasts*) that still have nuclei and do not carry normal amounts of oxygen.

Because many of folate's metabolic roles are related to those of vitamin B−12, diets that lack either vitamin produce some identical deficiency signs and symptoms. For example, being deficient in folate or vitamin B−12 can cause

megaloblastic anemia type of anemia characterized by large, immature red blood cells; deficiency of folate and/or vitamin B-12 can lead to this form of anemia

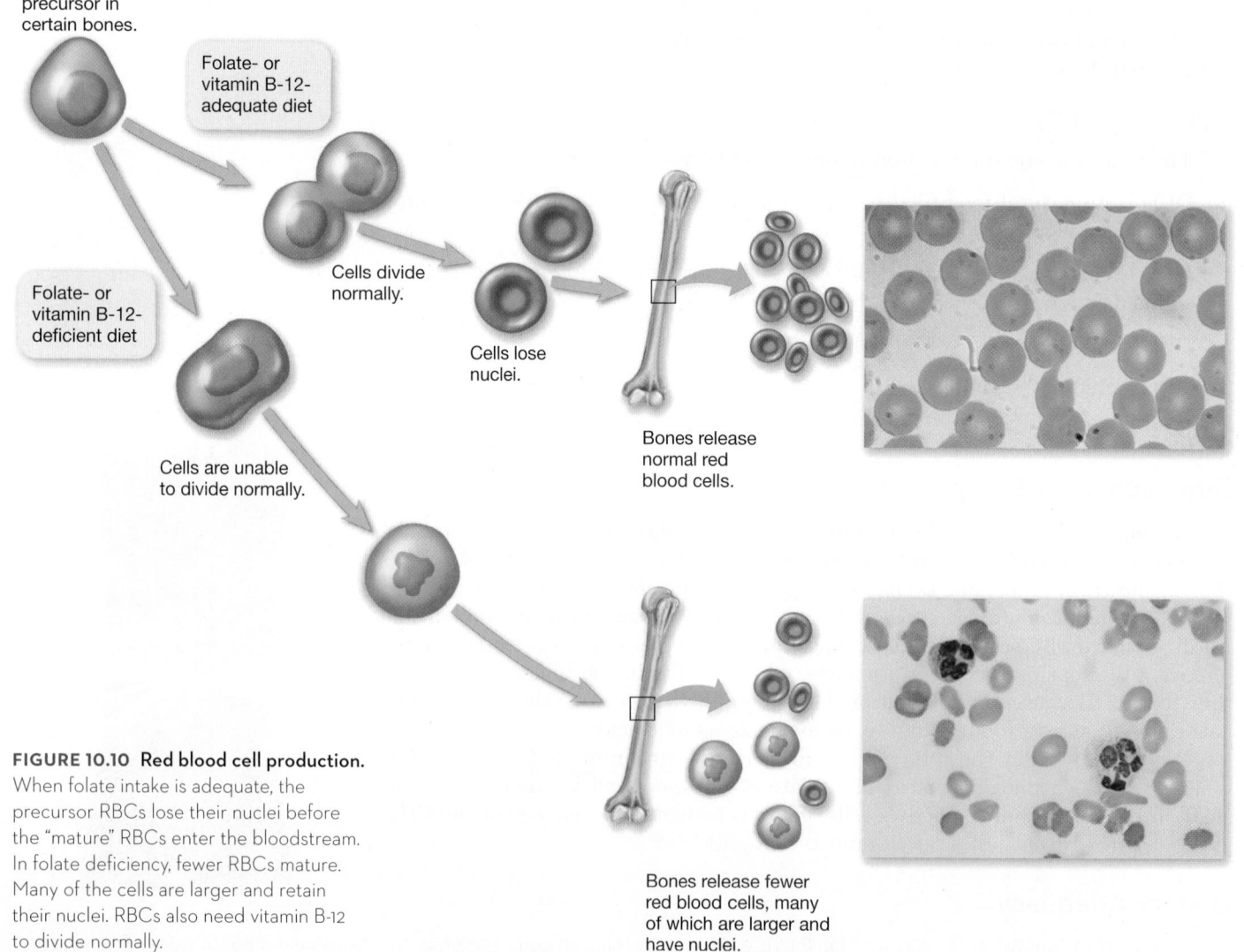

Red blood cell precursor in certain bones.

Folate- or vitamin B-12- adequate diet

Folate- or vitamin B-12- deficient diet

Cells divide normally.

Cells lose nuclei.

Cells are unable to divide normally.

Bones release normal red blood cells.

Bones release fewer red blood cells, many of which are larger and have nuclei.

FIGURE 10.10 Red blood cell production. When folate intake is adequate, the precursor RBCs lose their nuclei before the "mature" RBCs enter the bloodstream. In folate deficiency, fewer RBCs mature. Many of the cells are larger and retain their nuclei. RBCs also need vitamin B-12 to divide normally.

megaloblastic anemia. Therefore, a person with this type of anemia needs further analysis of his or her blood to determine which vitamin is lacking.

Neural Tube Defects A pregnant woman has an increased requirement for folate, because DNA synthesis and cell division take place at a rapid pace during embry—onic development.[23] During the first few weeks after conception, the **neural tube** forms in the human embryo (Fig. 10.11a). This tube eventually develops into the brain and spinal cord. Pregnant women who suffer from folate deficiency have high risk of giving birth to infants with neural tube defects (NTDs). The two most common NTDs are *spina bifida* and *anencephaly*.

Spina bifida (*spy'–na bif'–eh–dah*) occurs when the embryo's spine does not form properly and the bones fail to enclose the spinal cord (Fig. 10.11b). As shown in Figure 10.11c, infants with severe spina bifida have a section of their spinal cord or a sac containing some spinal fluid bulging through an opening in their backs. Often, people with spina bifida are unable to use muscles in the lower part of their bodies, and as a result, they cannot walk independently.

Infants born with **anencephaly** (*an–en–sef'–ah–lee*) have much of their brain malformed or missing, and they usually die shortly after birth. Anencephaly can result from genetic causes as well as from folate deficiency, but folate sup—plementation may lower the risk.

neural tube embryonic structure that eventually develops into the brain and spinal cord

spina bifida type of neural tube defect in which the spine does not form properly before birth and fails to enclose the spinal cord

anencephaly type of neural tube defect in which much of the brain does not form properly or is missing

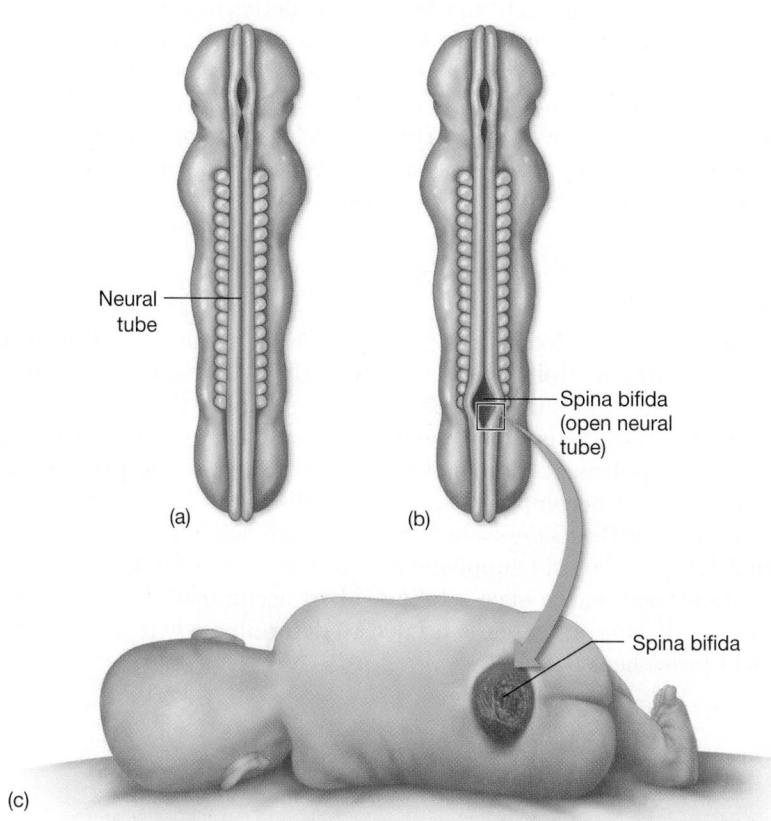

Neural tube

(a)

Spina bifida (open neural tube)

(b)

Spina bifida

(c)

FIGURE 10.11 Neural tube defects. During the first few weeks after conception, the neural tube forms in the human embryo. (*a*) Normal neural tube in an early embryo. (*b*) Spina bifida (abnormal neural tube) in an early embryo. (*c*) Infants born with severe spina bifida have a section of their spinal cord or a sac containing some spinal fluid bulging through their backs.

In 1992, officials with the U.S. Public Health Service recommended that all women capable of becoming pregnant consume 400 μg of folic acid daily to help prevent neural tube defects. This recommendation was followed by the January 1998 guidelines from the FDA requiring the addition of folic acid to enriched flour and cereals. At that time, medical experts estimated that at least half the cases of neural tube defects could be prevented if women consumed sufficient folic acid *before* conception and in early pregnancy.[24,25] For pregnant women, adequate folate status is critical early in pregnancy, because the neural tube begins to form about 21 days after conception.[26] This developmental milestone occurs when many women are not even aware they are pregnant.

Each year, about 1500 babies are born with spina bifida in the United States.[27,28] However, the prevalence of neural tube defects has declined by about 30% since enrichment of foods with folic acid began in 1998.

Folate and Disease Folic acid deficiencies are associated with elevated blood levels of homocysteine. While high levels of blood homocysteine are a marker for heart disease risk, results of research do not provide evidence that lowering homocysteine levels by taking B vitamins reduces the risk of cardiovascular disease.[30] A 2012 meta–analysis of 19 well–controlled studies involving nearly 50,000 subjects concluded that B–vitamin supplementation had no effect on the risk of CVD. However, there was a 12% reduction in stroke risk.[31]

Elevated homocysteine levels may also be a marker or risk factor for Alzheimer's disease (AD). Alzheimer's disease is characterized by a gradual, progressive decline in cognitive functioning, including memory and decision–making skills. The results of one study suggested a relationship between mild cognitive impairment (an early sign of AD) and both folate deficiency and high blood levels of homocysteine.[32] In another study, low intakes of folate, vitamin B–12, and vitamin B–6 were associated with high blood levels of homocysteine and reduced cognitive functioning in aging men.[33] Although taking megadoses of folate can reduce homocysteine levels, such treatment does not improve cognitive functioning.[22] As is often the case, more research is needed to determine whether using folate supplements can reduce the risk of heart disease and stroke, or slow the progression of AD.

Folate Toxicity

Although the folate naturally in foods does not appear to be toxic, the UL for the synthetic form of the vitamin (folic acid) is 1000 μg/day.[1] The UL was established because taking folic acid supplements can cure not only the anemia that occurs in folate deficiency but also the anemia that is a sign of vitamin B–12 deficiency. Folic acid supplementation, however, does not prevent the serious nervous system damage that accompanies the B–12 deficiency. Thus, excess folic acid can "mask" a vitamin B–12 deficiency. Furthermore, some medical experts are concerned that taking folic acid supplements and consuming foods that contain the micronutrient may cause excess folic acid to accumulate in blood and cause health problems.[34] More research is needed to determine whether ingesting too much folic acid poses health risks.

FRESH TIPS

The damage to an embryo due to lack of folic acid occurs early in pregnancy, often before a woman knows she is pregnant. And yet only 30% of women 18 to 24 years of age take an adequate synthetic folic acid supplement.[29] To help guard against neural tube defects, a woman of childbearing potential should track her DFE level to make sure her DFE is above 400 μg. The easiest way to be certain is to take a daily supplement. When pregnancy is discovered, a woman's folic acid intake should be increased to 600 μg per day.

ASSESS YOUR PROGRESS

24 Identify the coenzyme form of folate.

25 Why is folate bioavailability greater from synthetic sources than from natural food sources?

26 Describe the role of folate in red blood cell formation.

27 Why is it important for women who may become pregnant to have adequate folate intake?

10.9 Vitamin B-12

LEARNING OUTCOMES

1 *Identify the functions of vitamin B-12.*
2 *List dietary sources of vitamin B-12.*
3 *Summarize the digestion and absorption of vitamin B-12.*
4 *Discuss the signs and symptoms of a vitamin B-12 deficiency.*
5 *List populations at the greatest risk for a vitamin B-12 deficiency.*

Cells require **vitamin B−12** or **cobalamin**, to make coenzymes that participate in a variety of cellular processes, including the transfer of CH_3 groups in the metabolism of folate. Vitamin B−12 is also needed for homocysteine metabolism and to convert folate to coenzyme forms that are needed for metabolic reactions, including DNA synthesis.

One vital function of vitamin B−12 does not involve folate: maintaining the **myelin sheaths** that wrap around parts of certain nerve cells, insulating them. Myelin enables the nerves to communicate effectively. Without vitamin B−12, segments of myelin sheath gradually undergo destruction that can lead to paralysis. If a person who is vitamin B−12 deficient does not obtain treatment with the vitamin, he or she can die as a result of the deficiency.

vitamin B-12 or **cobalamin** B vitamin that is a component of coenzymes that participate in a variety of cellular processes, including transfer of CH_3 groups in the metabolism of folate

myelin sheath structure that wraps around and insulates a part of certain nerve cells

Food Sources of Vitamin B-12

Only bacteria, fungi (for example, mushrooms and molds), and algae can synthesize vitamin B−12. Plants do not make vitamin B−12; therefore, people rely almost entirely on animal foods to supply the vitamin naturally. Major sources of vitamin B−12 in the typical American diet are meat, milk and milk products, poultry, fish, shellfish, and eggs. Although liver is not a popular food, it is one of the richest sources of vitamin B−12 because the vitamin is stored in the liver. Table 10.9 lists some foods that provide vitamin B−12.

TABLE 10.9 Vitamin B-12 Content of Selected Foods

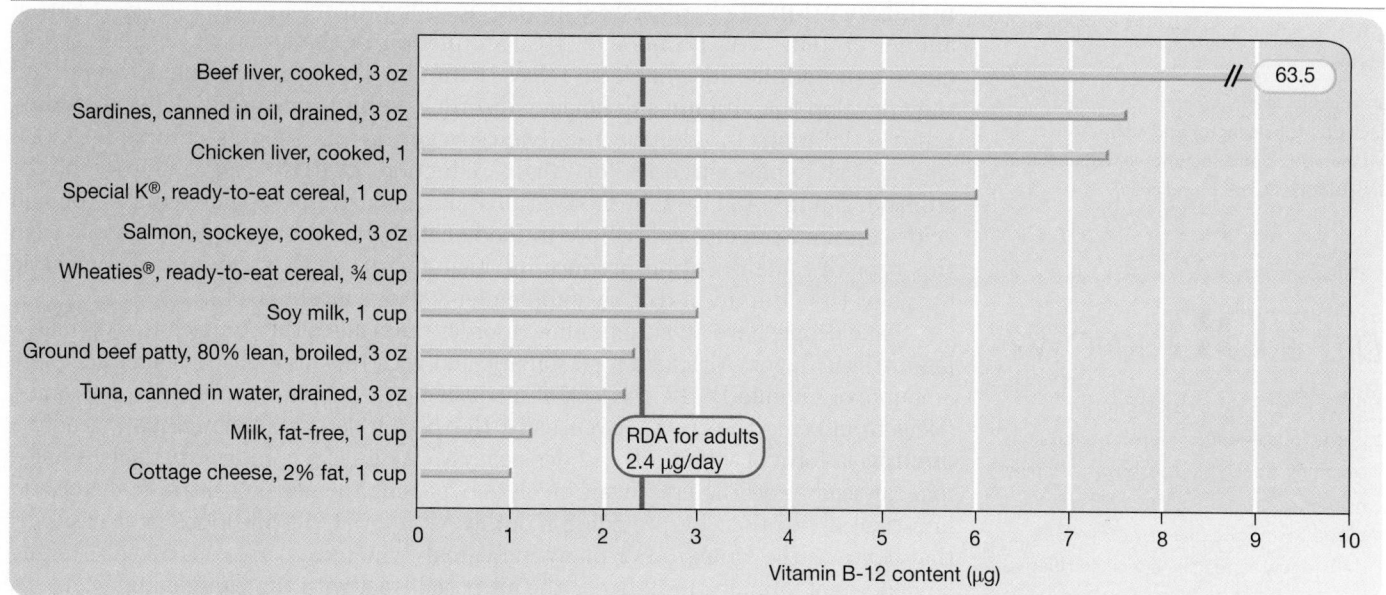

Source: Data from U.S. Department of Agriculture, Agricultural Research Service: *USDA National nutrient database for standard reference*, release 26, 2013.

Digestion and Absorption of Vitamin B-12

Absorbing the vitamin B–12 that is naturally in food requires a complex series of steps (Fig. 10.12). Natural vitamin B–12 is bound to animal protein that prevents its absorption. When the food enters the stomach, the vitamin is released from the protein, primarily by the actions of hydrochloric acid (HCl) in gastric juice. Synthetic vitamin B–12 in dietary supplements or fortified foods is not bound to food protein, so it does not need stomach acid to release the protein. Thus, synthetic vitamin B–12 is more readily absorbed than the natural form of the micronutrient.

In the small intestine, vitamin B–12 binds to intrinsic factor (IF), a compound that is produced by parietal cells of the stomach. Eventually, the vitamin B–12/intrinsic factor complex reaches the ileum of the small intestine, where the vitamin complex is absorbed. Within the absorptive cells, vitamin B–12 is separated from intrinsic factor and attached to transport molecules. The transport molecules enter the bloodstream and travel to the liver via the hepatic portal vein. The liver removes vitamin B–12 from many of the carrier molecules and stores about 50% of the vitamin. A healthy liver has enough vitamin B–12 reserves to last 5 to 10 years.[35] Therefore, a healthy person who decides to follow a diet that completely lacks vitamin B–12 is not likely to experience signs and symptoms of the vitamin's deficiency disorder for as long as 10 years. Even though vitamin B–12 is stored in the liver, no UL has been established for the micronutrient, because no adverse effects have been observed with excess intakes.

Dietary Adequacy

The adult RDA for vitamin B–12 is 2.4 µg/day.[1] Although most Americans who eat animal products consume more than the RDA,[35] some members of the population are at risk of vitamin B–12 deficiency. Vegans, for example, need to be concerned about their intake of vitamin B–12, because plant foods are not sources of the micronutrient (see the "Vegetarianism" section of Chapter 7).

Vitamin B–12 deficiency is characterized by nerve damage and megaloblastic RBCs. Other signs and symptoms of the deficiency include muscle weakness, smooth and shiny tongue, confusion, difficulty walking and maintaining balance, and numbness and tingling sensations, particularly in the hands and feet.

Most cases of vitamin B–12 deficiency result from problems that interfere with intestinal absorption of the vitamin (cobalamin) in foods (*food–cobalamin malabsorption*) and not from inadequate intake.[35] **Food–cobalamin malabsorption** is characterized by the inability to release vitamin B–12 from animal protein.[36] As people age, HCl production in the stomach declines. Thus, many older adults are unable to release vitamin B–12 from animal protein, and they develop the vitamin's deficiency disorder despite consuming diets that contain the vitamin. In addition to advanced age, factors such as chronic alcoholism, gastric bypass surgeries for weight reduction, **gastritis** (inflammation of the stomach lining), and certain medications, particularly those that reduce stomach acid secretion, can also contribute to food–cobalamin malabsorption. People with this type of malabsorption produce intrinsic factor, so they can absorb synthetic forms of the vitamin in dietary supplements that contain B–12.

Some people have an autoimmune disorder that causes the stomach to stop making intrinsic factor. Although a person affected with this disorder consumes adequate amounts of vitamin B–12, the lack of intrinsic factor prevents most of the micronutrient from being absorbed.[37] Eventually, this person develops **pernicious** ("deadly") **anemia** (a form of vitamin B–12 deficiency).[38] As its name implies, pernicious anemia can lead to death. Treatment involves bypassing the need for intrinsic factor and intestinal absorption, by providing monthly vitamin B–12 injections or a nasal gel that contains the vitamin. For many individuals who have pernicious anemia, taking large doses of vitamin B–12 floods the intestinal tract with the vitamin and enables a small amount to be absorbed without the need for intrinsic factor.[39,40]

food-cobalamin malabsorption malabsorption of vitamin B-12 due to the inability to release the vitamin from animal protein during the digestive process

gastritis inflammation of the lining of the stomach

pernicious anemia condition caused by the lack of intrinsic factor and characterized by vitamin B-12 deficiency, nerve damage, and megaloblastic red blood cells

DID **YOU** KNOW?

Family history is a risk factor for pernicious anemia. Therefore, it is recommended that those with a family history of pernicious anemia have blood tests for signs of vitamin B-12 deficiency, especially if a close relative has the condition.

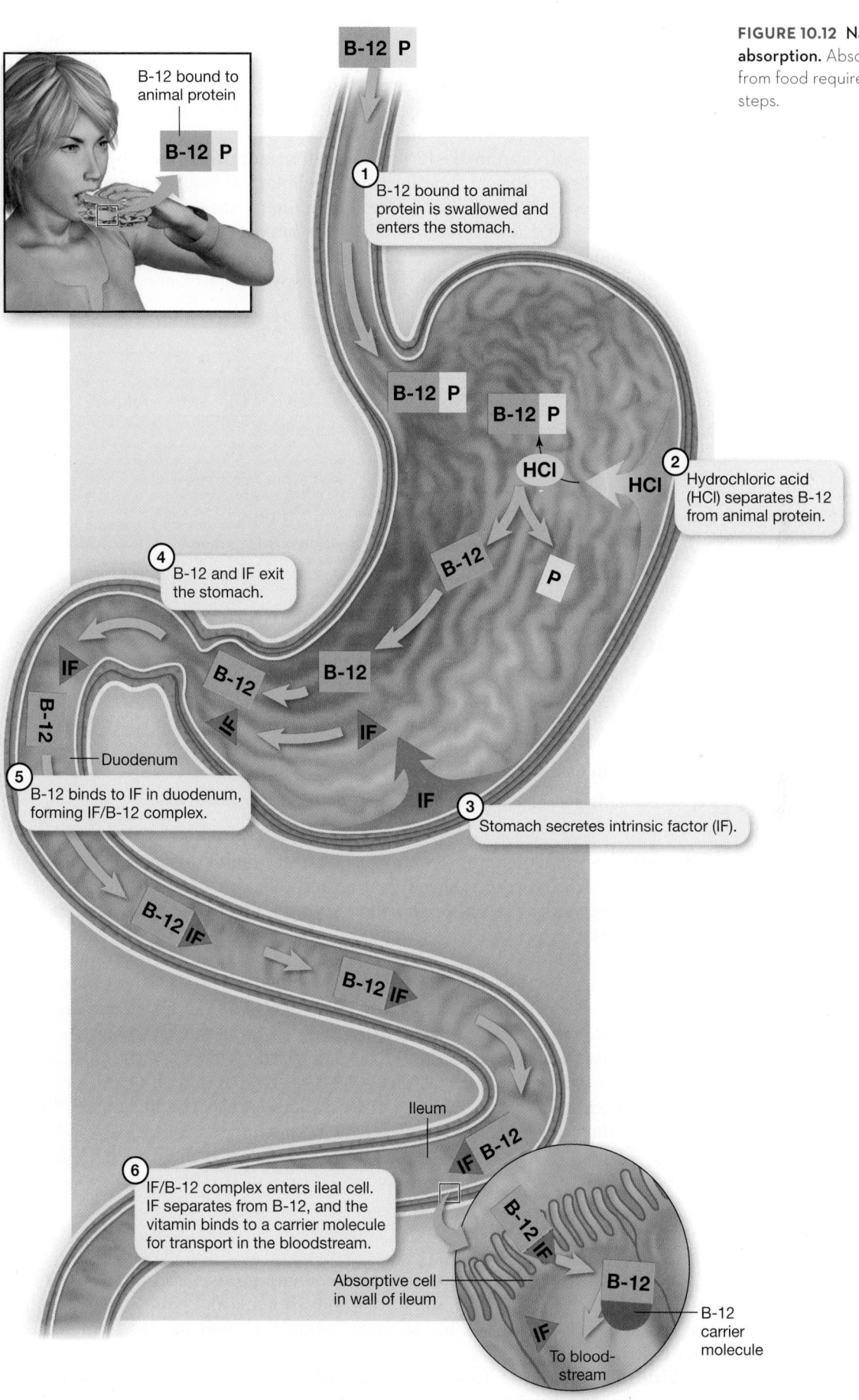

FIGURE 10.12 Natural vitamin B-12 absorption. Absorbing natural vitamin B-12 from food requires a complex series of steps.

B-12 bound to animal protein

B-12 P

① B-12 bound to animal protein is swallowed and enters the stomach.

② Hydrochloric acid (HCl) separates B-12 from animal protein.

④ B-12 and IF exit the stomach.

Duodenum

⑤ B-12 binds to IF in duodenum, forming IF/B-12 complex.

③ Stomach secretes intrinsic factor (IF).

Ileum

⑥ IF/B-12 complex enters ileal cell. IF separates from B-12, and the vitamin binds to a carrier molecule for transport in the bloodstream.

Absorptive cell in wall of ileum

B-12 carrier molecule

To blood-stream

FRESH TIPS

Vegan women who breastfeed their babies need to be aware that their breast milk may contain inadequate amounts of vitamin B-12. Babies fed only vitamin B-12-deficient breast milk are likely to develop megaloblastic anemia and serious nervous system problems. Providing vitamin B-12 to the deficient babies effectively treats the anemia, but some of the damage to the children's nervous systems may be permanent.[41]

Vitamin B-12 Deficiency and Other Health Conditions Like folate, vitamin B−12 may be essential for neural tube development in an embryo. The risk for neural tube defects is two to three times greater in cases of low maternal vitamin B−12 status.[42,43] Thus, nutrition experts often recommend that pregnant women consume foods fortified with vitamin B−12.

Deficiencies of vitamin B−12, folate, and vitamin B−6 have been associated with abnormal neurological function and psychological health, including depression and dementia.[44-46] Evidence from preliminary studies suggests that supplementation with these three vitamins can improve psychological health and cognitive function.[47,48] However, more studies to determine dosing levels and populations most suited for such vitamin therapy are necessary.[47,49]

ASSESS YOUR PROGRESS

28 *What is the one vital function of vitamin B-12 that does not involve folate?*

29 *Describe the digestion and absorption of vitamin B-12.*

30 *List three good food sources of vitamin B-12.*

31 *Identify the symptoms of a vitamin B-12 deficiency.*

32 *Describe gastritis and how it affects vitamin B-12 status.*

33 *Why are vegans at an increased risk for a vitamin B-12 deficiency?*

10.10 Vitamin C

LEARNING OUTCOMES

1 *Describe the role of vitamin C in collagen synthesis, antioxidant activities, iron absorption, and immune function.*

2 *Identify dietary sources of vitamin C.*

3 *Explain the consequences of a vitamin C deficiency or toxicity.*

scurvy vitamin C deficiency disease

For centuries, taking lengthy ocean voyages was a highly dangerous venture, not just because of the threat of severe storms and pillaging pirates, but also because of a terrifying and deadly disease called **scurvy**. At the time, no one knew the cause of scurvy.

In the mid−1700s, British physician James Lind performed a crude experiment on 12 sailors suffering from scurvy. Lind divided the sick sailors into 6 pairs, and each pair received a different treatment. The six treatments were cider, vinegar, sulfuric acid, seawater, nutmeg, or oranges and lemons. According to Lind's observations, the sailors given the citrus fruit were the only ones to recover from scurvy. As a result of his testing, Lind found the cure for scurvy: eating oranges and lemons. Every British sailors earned the nickname "limeys" because at that time, people often referred to citrus fruits collectively as "limes." Today, we know that scurvy results from a deficiency of vitamin C and that citrus fruits are among the richest dietary sources of this vitamin.

Functions of Vitamin C

vitamin C ascorbic acid; cofactor that performs a variety of important cellular functions, primarily by donating electrons to other compounds

Most animals do not need dietary sources of vitamin C (ascorbic acid) because they can synthesize all the vitamin they need. Humans and guinea pigs are among the few species that are unable to make vitamin C, and for these animals, the micronutrient is essential.

Vitamin C does not function as part of a coenzyme as do B vitamins, but instead serves as a nutrient cofactor that facilitates certain chemical reactions. In the body, vitamin C has widespread roles, including collagen synthesis, antioxidant activity, and immune function.

Vitamin C participates in reactions that form and maintain **collagen**, a fibrous protein that gives strength to *connective tissue*. Connective tissues, such as bone, cartilage, and tendons, hold together and support structures in the body. During collagen formation, vitamin C helps create numerous cross—connections between amino acids, which greatly strengthen the connective tissue.

Vitamin C can act as an antioxidant by donating electrons to radicals. Vitamin C also may donate electrons to another antioxidant, vitamin E. Thus, vitamin C recycles vitamin E so it can regain its antioxidant function. Scientists, however, do not know the extent of vitamin C's antioxidant abilities in the human body. Taking excessive amounts of vitamin C may be harmful, because in high doses, the vitamin has **prooxidant** effects. A prooxidant promotes production of free radicals.

White blood cells (WBCs) participate in the body's immune defenses. Compared to other cells, WBCs have a higher concentration of vitamin C. During the immune response to infectious agents, WBCs may generate free radicals. Although this response is intended to kill bacteria, it can also damage the WBCs. The antioxidant activity of vitamin C may limit this self—destruction. Vitamin C may have other roles in immune function that need to be clarified by more research.

Vitamin C is also necessary for the synthesis of bile and certain neurotransmitters; various hormones, including cortisol, the "stress hormone"; aldosterone, a hormone involved in blood pressure regulation; and thyroxin, the thyroid hormone that regulates energy metabolism. Furthermore, the micronutrient enhances the absorption of iron (Fe). Plants are major sources of *nonheme* iron (Fe^{3+}). The small intestine, however, absorbs Fe^{2+} more readily than Fe^{3+}. Vitamin C promotes iron absorption by donating an electron to Fe^{3+}, forming Fe^{2+} as a result. The vitamin may also form a complex with iron that enhances the body's ability to absorb the mineral. Therefore, adding citrus fruits, broccoli, peppers, or other vitamin C–rich foods to meals can increase absorption of nonheme iron.

Food Sources of Vitamin C

Plant foods are the best dietary sources of vitamin C. Peppers, citrus fruit, papaya, broccoli, cabbage, and berries contain relatively high amounts of the micronutrient (Table 10.10). Potatoes and vitamin C–fortified fruit drinks and ready—to—eat cereals also supply vitamin C. Most animal foods are not sources of the micronutrient.

Vitamin C is very unstable in the presence of heat, oxygen, light, alkaline conditions, and the minerals iron and copper. Storing vitamin C–rich foods in cool conditions, such as in the refrigerator, will help preserve the micronutrient. Because vitamin C is easily lost during cooking, eat raw fruits and vegetables whenever possible.

Vitamin C absorption occurs in the small intestine. As intake of the vitamin increases, the rate of absorption decreases. The intestine, for example, absorbs 50% or less of the vitamin when intake totals 1 g or more/day. Additionally, the kidneys increase excretion of the vitamin in response to high intake. Therefore, taking megadoses of vitamin C may be wasteful.

Dietary Adequacy

The adult RDA for vitamin C is 75 mg/day for women and 90 mg/day for men.[1] Cigarette smokers should add an extra 35 mg/day to their RDA, because exposure to tobacco smoke increases radical formation in the lungs.[50] According to MyPlate recommendations, adults should eat 3.5 to 5 cups of fruits and vegetables daily.[51] By choosing vitamin C–rich fruits and vegetables, such as those presented in Table 10.10, healthy people can obtain adequate amounts of vitamin C.

collagen fibrous protein that gives strength to connective tissue such as bone, cartilage, and tendons

prooxidant substance that promotes production of free radicals

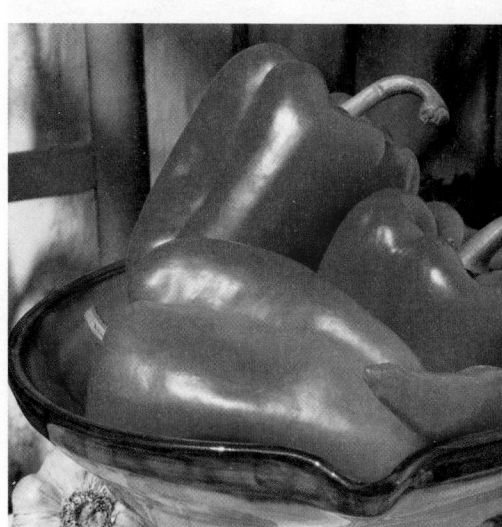

Fresh fruits and vegetables are often excellent sources of vitamin C. This includes red bell peppers, which are readily available in many supermarkets.

TABLE 10.10 Vitamin C Content of Selected Foods

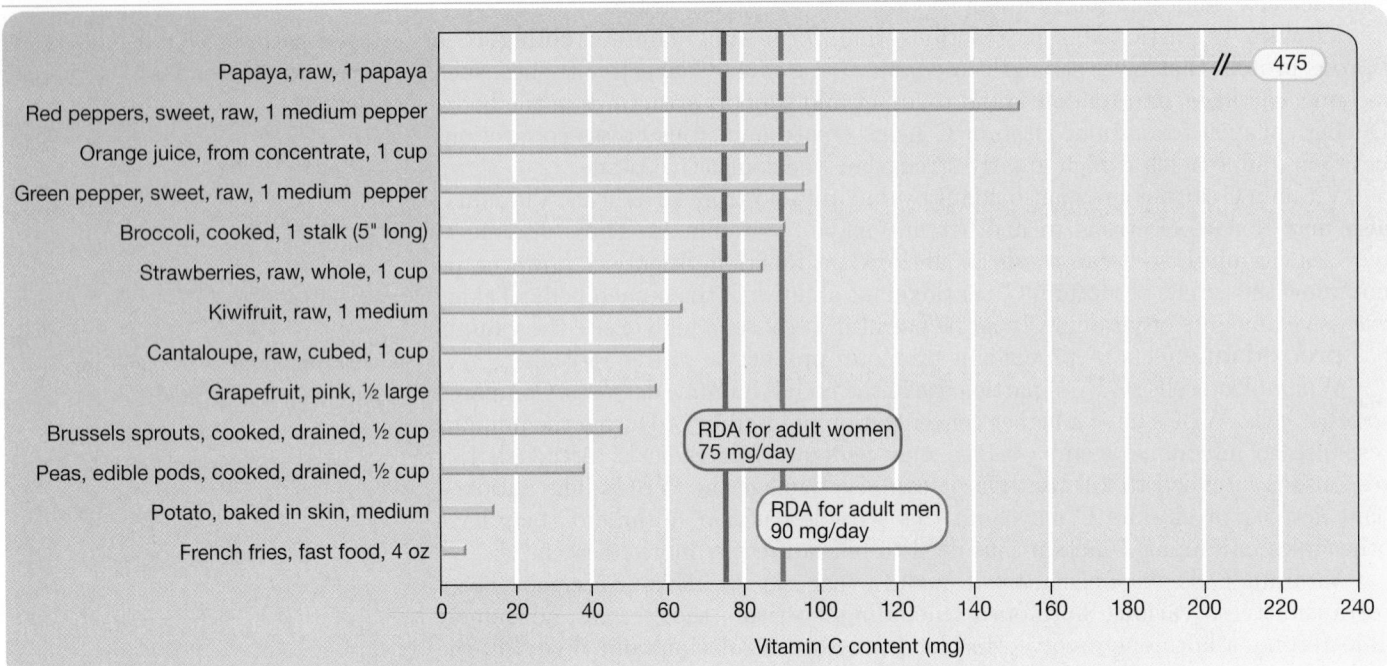

Food	Vitamin C content (mg)
Papaya, raw, 1 papaya	475
Red peppers, sweet, raw, 1 medium pepper	
Orange juice, from concentrate, 1 cup	
Green pepper, sweet, raw, 1 medium pepper	
Broccoli, cooked, 1 stalk (5" long)	
Strawberries, raw, whole, 1 cup	
Kiwifruit, raw, 1 medium	
Cantaloupe, raw, cubed, 1 cup	
Grapefruit, pink, ½ large	
Brussels sprouts, cooked, drained, ½ cup	
Peas, edible pods, cooked, drained, ½ cup	
Potato, baked in skin, medium	
French fries, fast food, 4 oz	

RDA for adult women 75 mg/day

RDA for adult men 90 mg/day

Source: Data from U.S. Department of Agriculture, Agricultural Research Service: *USDA National nutrient database for standard reference*, release 26, 2013.

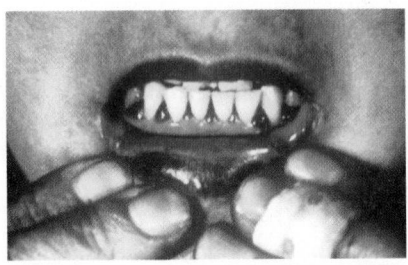

FIGURE 10.13 Scurvy: Swollen gums.
Swollen gums that bleed easily are a sign of scurvy.

Vitamin C Deficiency

Deficiencies in vitamin C are rare; most adults require less than 10 mg of the vitamin daily to prevent scurvy. A 6–ounce serving of fresh orange juice provides about 60 mg of vitamin C—six times the required amount. Additionally, vitamin C is added to many processed foods, including fruit and sports drinks, ready–to–eat cereals, and nutrition or meal replacement bars. Smokers, alcoholics, and people who do not eat fruits and vegetables are most at risk of vitamin C deficiency.

If vitamin C is unavailable, the body forms weak connective tissue and is unable to maintain existing collagen. An early sign of scurvy, pin–point bleeding under the skin (*petechiae*), occur about 20 to 40 days after consuming a vitamin C–deficient diet. The petechiae develop around hair follicles, especially where light pressure has been applied, such as under the elastic bands of clothing. As the dis–ease progresses, the affected person's skin bruises easily; gums become spongy and bleed with the slightest touch (Fig. 10.13); joints swell and ache; and teeth fall out. Without treatment, scurvy victims eventually die, most likely from infection.

Vitamin C Toxicity

The adult UL for vitamin C is 2000 mg/day.[1] When people exceed this amount of the vitamin, gastrointestinal upsets, including diarrhea, often occur.[1] When plasma and circulating cells are saturated with vitamin C (this occurs at approx–imately 400 mg/day), the excess vitamin and *oxalate*, a by–product of breaking

FRESH TIPS

Is there a difference in the vitamin C content of raw orange slices and orange juice? Oranges and orange juice are low in calories and rich sources of vitamin C, but whole oranges contain more dietary fiber (3 g/orange) than orange juice (0.5 g/cup). To meet your vitamin C needs and increase your fiber intake reach for a raw orange.

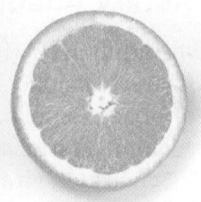

down vitamin C, circulate in the bloodstream.[52] The kidneys filter and eliminate these unnecessary substances in urine, but excess oxalate excretion raises the risk of kidney stones.[53] Therefore, people who are susceptible to develop such stones should avoid consuming megadose vitamin C supplements.

Vitamin C Supplementation and the Common Cold In 1970, Nobel Prize–winning American chemist Dr. Linus Pauling (1901–1994) published *Vitamin C and the Common Cold*. This bestselling book established the popular belief that megadoses of vitamin C could prevent colds. As a result of Pauling's claim, many Americans take large amounts of this micronutrient when they notice the first cold symptoms.

Evidence collected from several scientific studies indicates that routine vitamin C supplementation (200 mg or more of the vitamin daily) does not prevent colds in the general population. However, taking such large doses of the vitamin may reduce the duration of cold symptoms by a day or so.[54] Additionally, vitamin C may reduce the severity of cold symptoms because the micronutrient acts like an antihistamine when taken in very large doses.[55]

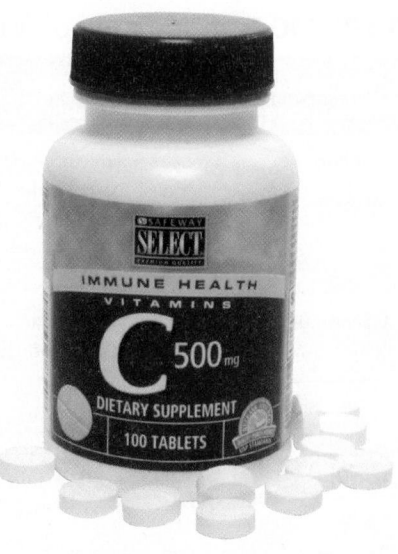

Vitamin C Supplementation: Heart Disease and Alzheimer's Disease As an antioxidant, vitamin C may reduce the oxidation of LDL cholesterol, lowering the risk of CVD. Studies to determine whether vitamin C can help prevent CVD have not provided consistent evidence that the micronutrient reduces the risk of CVD or of dying from the condition.[56] Atherosclerosis takes years and probably decades to result in heart attack, strokes, and other forms of CVD. Thus, more research is needed to determine whether long–term vitamin C supplementation can reduce the risk of this leading killer of Americans.

Results of some observational studies suggest that high intake of vitamin C–rich foods may reduce the risk of Alzheimer's disease.[57] Several studies have examined the benefits of using combinations of antioxidant vitamin supplements, particularly vitamins C and E, to lower the risk of this dreaded disease. In general, the results of these studies were mixed.[58]

ASSESS YOUR PROGRESS

34 *Describe four key functions of vitamin C.*

35 *List three good food sources of vitamin C.*

36 *Identify symptoms of scurvy.*

37 *Would you recommend a vitamin C supplement to a friend with the common cold? Why or why not?*

10.11 Vitamin-Like Compounds

LEARNING OUTCOMES

1 *Describe the difference between vitamins and vitamin-like compounds.*

2 *Explain the importance of choline, carnitine, inositol, taurine, and lipoic acid in human health.*

3 *Identify major dietary sources of each of the vitamin-like compounds.*

Choline, carnitine, inositol, taurine, and lipoic acid are **vitamin–like compounds** necessary to maintain normal metabolism. However, the body synthesizes these vitamin–like compounds; therefore, they are not considered essential nutrients.

The need for vitamin–like compounds generally increases during periods of rapid tissue growth, as occurs in premature infants. The average healthy adult is not at risk of developing deficiencies of vitamin–like compounds. More research is needed to determine whether deficiencies of vitamin–like compounds could

vitamin-like compounds substances that maintain normal metabolism; the body synthesizes these compounds

TABLE 10.11 Summary of Vitamin-Like Compounds

Vitamin-Like Substance	Major Functions in the Body	Adult AI	Major Dietary Sources	Major Deficiency Signs and Symptoms	Major Toxicity Signs and Symptoms
Choline	Neurotransmitter and phospholipid synthesis; methionine metabolism	425–550 mg	Widely distributed in foods; human biosynthesis	Liver damage	**Adult UL = 3500 mg/day** Fishy body odor and reduced blood pressure
Carnitine	Transports long-chain fatty acids for energy metabolism	Not established	Meat, fish, poultry, milk; human biosynthesis	Rarely occurs	No UL established Doses of 3 g/day: nausea, vomiting, diarrhea, abdominal cramps
Inositol	Regulatory role in cells	Not established	Fruits, beans, grains, nuts; human biosynthesis	Unknown	Unknown
Taurine	Vision, antioxidant in white blood cells, insulin action, cell growth and development	Not established	Animal foods; human biosynthesis	Unknown	Unknown
Lipoic acid	Component of metabolic reactions that remove CO_2 from compounds, antioxidant	Not established	Meats, liver, yeast; human biosynthesis	Unknown	Unknown

total parenteral solution liquid mixture that provides nourishment to those who are unable to eat normally; administered intravenously (IV)

occur in certain disease states and whether the compounds should be included in **total parenteral solutions**. A total parenteral solution (TPN) is a liquid mixture that provides nourishment to patients who are unable to eat normally. Such mixtures are administered into a vein (intravenously or IV). Nutrition scientists are also studying whether vitamin–like compounds should be included in infant formulas. At this time, manufacturers of infant formulas often add these vitamin–like compounds to their products.

Table 10.11 summarizes the key vitamin–like compounds. The following sections provide additional information concerning these substances.

Choline

acetylcholine neurotransmitter associated with attention, learning and memory, muscle control, and other nervous system functions

Choline is a part of **acetylcholine**, a neurotransmitter associated with attention, learning and memory, muscle control, and many other nervous system functions. Choline is needed for the production of phospholipids in cell membranes,[59] and the liver uses choline to synthesize part of a lipoprotein that transports lipids. Additionally, the micronutrient participates in the metabolism of the amino acid methionine.

Choline is widely distributed in foods (Table 10.12). Liver, eggs, beef, and pork are among the richest sources of the nutrient. The source of choline in egg yolk is the phospholipid *phosphatidylcholine (foss′–fah–tide′–ull–ko′–lean)*, commonly called **lecithin** *(less′–eh–thin)*. Lecithin is added to certain foods, such as salad dressings and ice cream, during processing for its emulsifying properties. Lecithin helps hold the watery and fatty ingredients together in the product.

lecithin phosphatidylcholine; phospholipid found in egg yolk that acts as an emulsifier in certain foods

The adult AI for choline is 425 to 550 mg/day. The typical American diet provides at least 700 to 1000 mg of choline per day. In addition to food sources of the micronutrient, the body can synthesize choline from serine, an amino acid. It is possible, however, that the body cannot produce enough choline to meet requirements during some life stages.

Choline deficiency has not been reported in healthy persons who eat a variety of foods. To observe the physiological effects of a human choline deficiency, scientists provide choline–free diets to volunteers who are admitted to special research

TABLE 10.12 Choline Content of Selected Foods

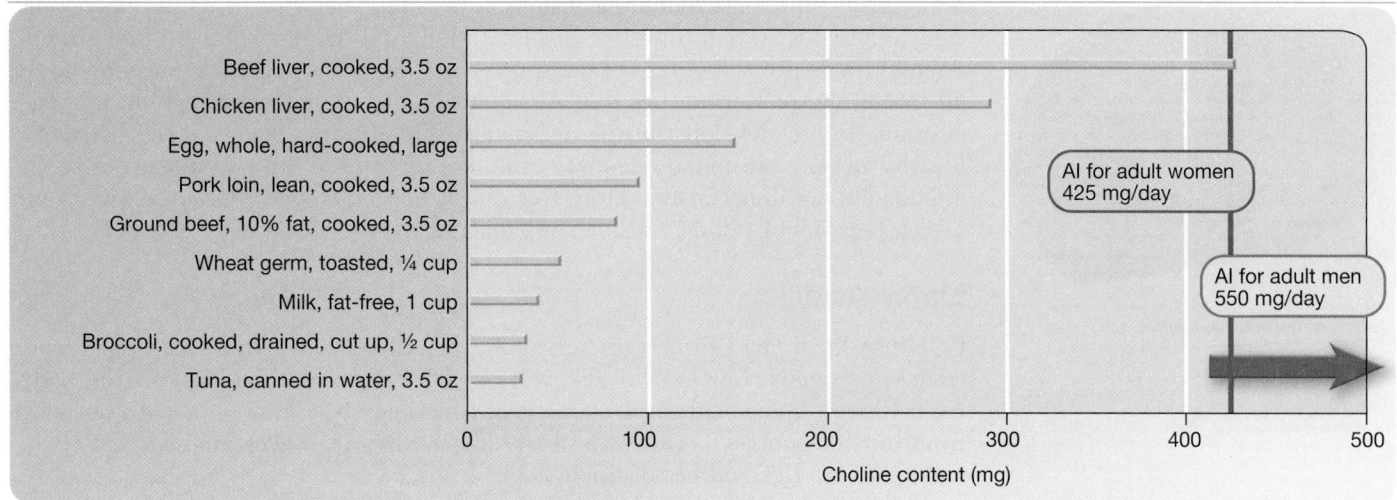

Source: U.S. Department of Agriculture, Agricultural Research Service. *USDA national nutrient database for standard reference*, release 26, 2013. http://www.nal.usda.gov/fnic/foodcomp/search/

clinics. Results of such studies indicate that the amount of fat in the liver increases when the subjects consumed choline–deficient diets. The adult UL for choline is 3.5 g/day. People who consume excessive amounts of the micronutrient often develop a fishy body odor and low blood pressure.

Carnitine

In cells, carnitine transports fatty acids into mitochondria, where the compounds are metabolized for energy. Carnitine also aids mitochondria in removing excess organic acids that are waste products of metabolism. The liver synthesizes carni–tine from the amino acids lysine and methionine. Thus, inadequate supplies of these amino acids can result in abnormal fatty acid metabolism. Human requirements for carnitine are met from biosynthesis and dietary sources, primarily meat and dairy foods. Americans consume about 60 to 180 mg of carnitine/day.[60] Although vegetarian diets are very low in carnitine, healthy vegetarians tend to have nor–mal blood concentrations of carnitine. Thus, medical experts doubt healthy people need dietary sources of carnitine. The vitamin–like compound may be considered a conditionally essential nutrient for premature infants and people recovering from serious diseases or injuries. There is little reliable scientific evidence to support carnitine's use as an aid for exercise or weight loss.[60]

Inositol

Inositol (*ih–noh'–seh–toll*) is in cell membranes and plays important regulatory roles in cells. Inositol–containing phospholipids are precursors of eicosanoids (*eye–ko'–se–noydz*), a family of compounds that have numerous hormone–like actions.

Animal and plant foods are sources of inositol. The average American diet provides about 1 g of inositol per day, and another 4 g/day or more are synthe–sized in the kidneys.

Abnormal inositol metabolism occurs in diabetes, multiple sclerosis, kidney failure, and certain cancers, which may indicate it is an essential compound only under certain conditions. At this time, there is not enough scientific evidence to support the use of inositol supplements for conditions such as cancer and mood disorders—a claim often made by supplement advertisers.[61]

Taurine

The human body synthesizes the amino acid taurine from the sulfur–containing amino acids methionine and cysteine. Muscle, platelets, and nerve tissue are rich

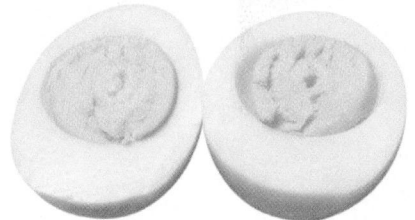

Egg yolks contain choline in the form of phosphatidylcholine, also called lecithin.

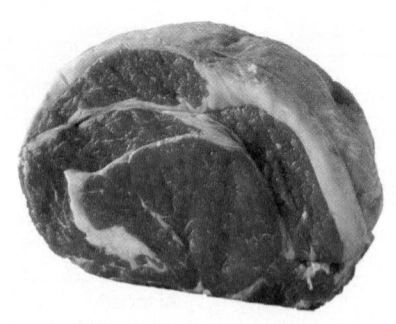

Meat is a rich source of lipoic acid.

in taurine. Additionally, taurine is a component of bile. Taurine is involved in many vital functions, including vision, antioxidant activity in white blood cells, central nervous system function, insulin action, and cell development and growth. Animal foods are the only dietary sources of taurine. Americans consume about 40 to 400 mg of taurine per day Although plants do not contain taurine, veg-etarians do not develop taurine deficiency. This finding suggests the body of a healthy person can make adequate amounts of taurine, and supplements of the amino acid are unnecessary. More research is needed to determine the safety and health benefits of taking taurine supplements.

Lipoic Acid

Cells use lipoic acid in certain metabolic reactions that remove carbon dioxide from compounds. Lipoic acid also works with several antioxidants in the body. Even though lipoic acid serves beneficial functions, it is unnecessary to obtain it from outside sources because the body synthesizes it. Nevertheless, meat, liver, and yeast are rich sources of lipoic acid.

ASSESS YOUR PROGRESS

38 *Identify key functions of the vitamin-like compounds choline, carnitine, inositol, taurine, and lipoic acid.*

39 *List food sources of choline, carnitine, inositol, taurine, and lipoic acid.*

10.12 Diet and Cancer

LEARNING OUTCOMES

1 *Explain cancer development and progression.*
2 *Describe the role of diet in cancer development.*
3 *Summarize the relationship between vitamins and cancer risk.*

According to the American Cancer Society, one in four Americans dies as a result of cancer.[62] Although modern medical technologies have enabled physicians to make great progress in treating many types of cancer successfully, the disease is still the second-leading cause of death in the United States.

In 2014, the three leading sites of new cancer cases (excluding common types of skin cancer) for American men were prostate, lung, and colorectum. The three leading sites of new cancer cases in American women were breast, lung, and col-orectum. As shown in Figure 10.14, lung cancer is responsible for more cancer deaths than prostate (males), breast (females), and colorectal cancers. There is good news: A considerable number of cancer deaths are preventable.

This section focuses on the roles of diet and exercise in the development, pro-gression, and possible prevention of certain cancers. For more information about cancer, including specific forms of cancer, visit the American Cancer Society's web-site at www.cancer.org or the National Cancer Institute's site at www.cancer.gov.

What Is Cancer?

Cancer is the term for a group of chronic diseases characterized by cells that have undergone damage (*mutations*) to certain genes. Genes are portions of DNA that code for the production of specific proteins (see Chapter 7). DNA dictates cellular growth, division, and eventual death. The rate at which healthy cells develop, grow, divide, and die occurs in a controlled fashion.

Cancerous (*malignant*) cells are literally "out of control": They divide repeat-edly and frequently, and they do not die. If genes that regulate cellular growth, division, and death mutate, then abnormal cell development, rapid cell growth,

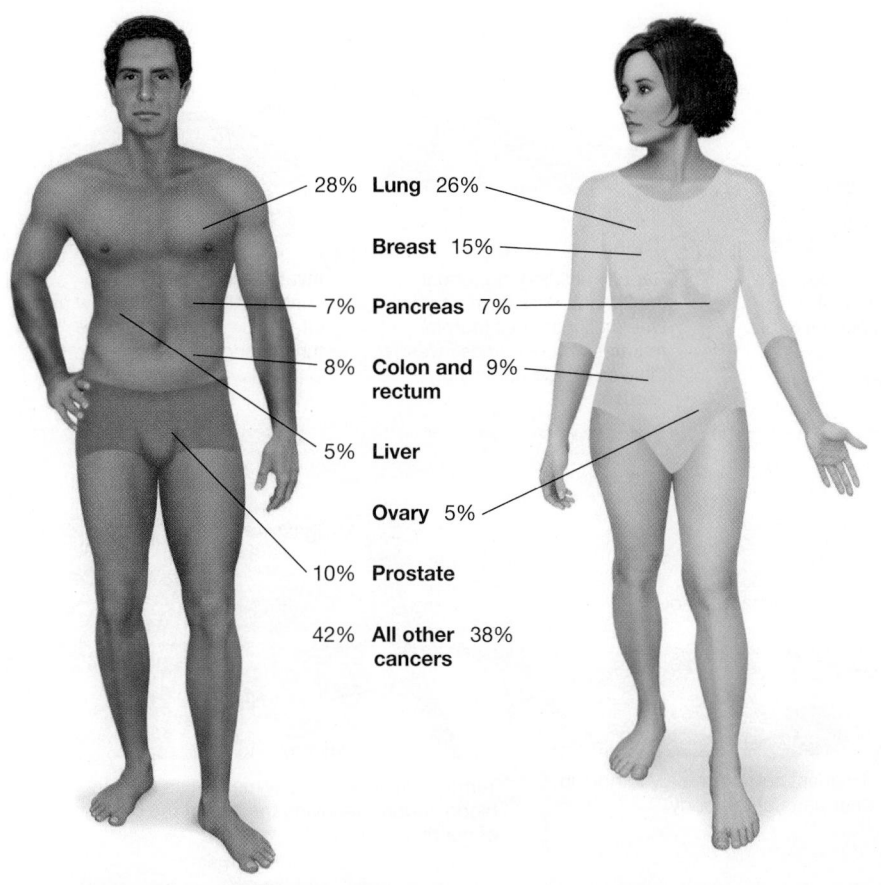

FIGURE 10.14 Leading cancer sites and deaths. This figure indicates leading sites of cancer deaths and percentages of cancer deaths according to 2014 estimates. *Source: American Cancer Society: Cancer facts & figures 2014. www.cancer.org. Accessed: February 1, 2014.*

28% | Lung | 26%

Breast | 15%

7% | Pancreas | 7%

8% | Colon and rectum | 9%

5% | Liver

Ovary | 5%

10% | Prostate

42% | All other cancers | 38%

and unchecked cell division can result. Furthermore, when a cell becomes malignant, it does not perform the specialized functions of the cells from which it was derived. A cancerous liver cell, for example, does not remove toxins from the bloodstream or store nutrients properly.

As a result of their rapid growth rate, many types of cancer cells form masses, called **malignant tumors**. Malignant cells often break away from the tumor. These cells can move to and invade other parts of the body. When cancer spreads to other tissues, the disease is said to have **metastasized** (*meh–tass'–tah–sized*).

Some cells multiply excessively and form **benign** (*bih–nine'*) **masses** or **tumors** as a result. A benign tumor is not cancerous, because the tumor's cells do not destroy nearby tissues or metastasize. Benign tumors are usually harmless. In some cases, however, a benign tumor grows large enough to interfere with the functioning of healthy structures, such as a blood vessel or brain tissue. When this occurs, the tumor needs to be treated to reduce its size or removed.

A **carcinogen** (*car–sin'–o–jin*) is an environmental factor, such as radiation, tobacco smoke, or a virus, that triggers cancer. Some carcinogens damage DNA, causing mutations to genes that control certain cell behaviors. Over time, repeated exposures to carcinogens take their toll on cells, making malignant cells more likely to develop. In fact, it is not unusual for cancerous cells to develop during a person's lifetime. However, a healthy immune system identifies the malignant cells and destroys them before they multiply uncontrollably. Figure 10.15 illustrates major steps in the development and behavior of most cancerous cells.

Because of their rapid growth and frequent cell divisions, malignant cells require more nutrients than normal cells. To supply enough nutrients to meet their needs, cancerous tumors stimulate the body to form blood vessels that divert blood away from healthy cells and into the tumor (Fig. 10.15). Much of the severe body wasting that usually accompanies advanced cases of cancer happens because healthy tissues are unable to obtain adequate supplies of nutrients.

Regular health checkups and a number of screening methods can detect cancer in its early stages, when many forms can be effectively treated. Conventional

malignant tumors masses of cancerous cells

metastasized cancer that has moved from one tissue to other parts of the body

benign masses (tumors) noncancerous tumors that are usually harmless

carcinogen environmental factor, such as radiation, tobacco smoke, or a virus, that triggers cancer

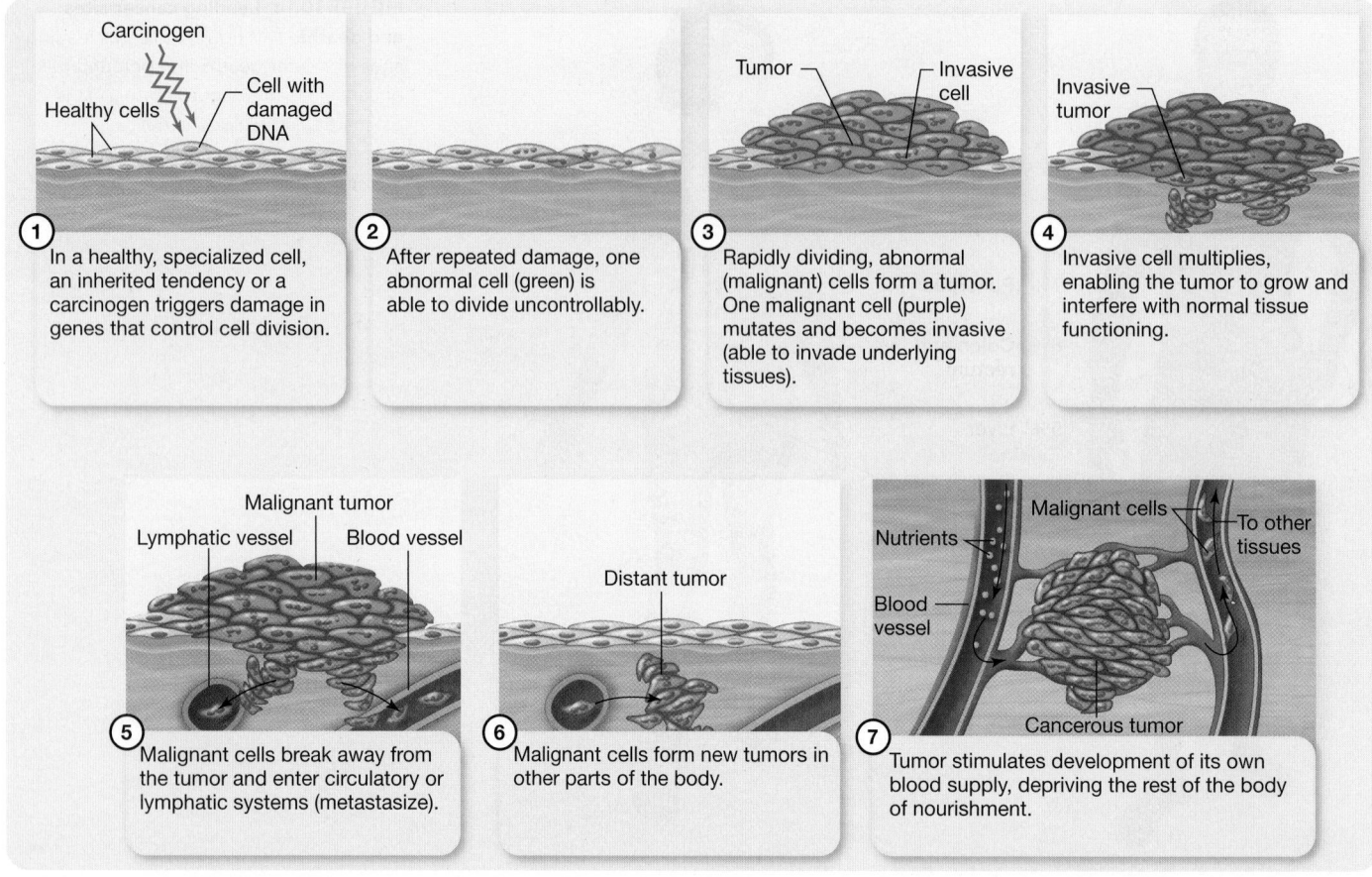

FIGURE 10.15 Cancer development and progression. Several steps are involved as a normal cell progresses into a cancer cell that multiplies out of control.

medical treatments for cancer typically involve surgical removal of cancerous tissue; chemotherapy, the use of medications that are toxic to cancer cells or limit their growth; and radiation therapy that kills cancer cells. Early diagnosis is very important; once cancer metastasizes, it is far more difficult to treat.

What Causes Cells to Become Cancerous?

Medical researchers have discovered several risk factors for many forms of cancer, including the following:

- Aging (most cancers occur in people over 65 years of age)
- Having a family history of cancer
- Using tobacco
- Being exposed to some forms of radiation
- Being exposed to certain environmental substances, such as irritants
- Having certain viral and bacterial infections
- Having elevated levels of certain hormones
- Consuming alcohol and certain foods
- Being physically inactive and having excess body fat[63,64]

People can lower their risk of cancer by avoiding known carcinogens, especially tobacco smoke. Approximately one of every three cancer deaths is associated with smoking tobacco, and nearly 90% of lung cancer deaths are caused by exposure to tobacco smoke.[62] In 2014, experts with the American Cancer Society predicted that over 159,000 Americans would die from lung cancer. Mouth, throat, esophageal, stomach, pancreatic, kidney, and bladder cancers are also associated with tobacco use.

Cancer causation is a complex process. Therefore, it may be impossible to pinpoint a single cause of a patient's cancer. Individuals differ widely in their genetic makeup, lifestyle practices, environmental exposures, and nutritional states. Some forms of the disease are likely to be inherited, but lifestyle factors, including diet, contribute to most cases of cancer.[64]

The Role of Diet in Cancer Development

Rates of specific cancers vary widely among different populations. Men and women living in Asian countries, for example, have lower risks of prostate and breast cancer, respectively, than men and women living in Western countries. After Asian men and women migrate to Western countries, their risks of prostate and breast cancer increase and eventually become similar to the risks of their adopted country's native population. Such findings provide epidemiological evidence of associations between cancer and certain lifestyle choices.

According to results of observational and experimental studies, certain substances in foods and beverages promote cancer development.

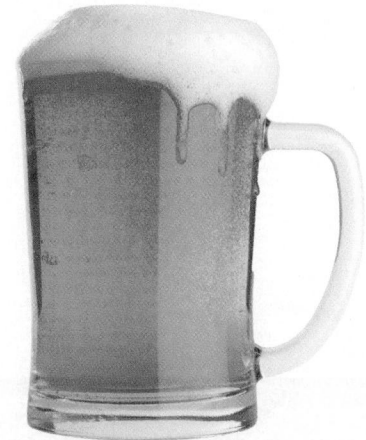

Alcohol is a carcinogen.

- Alcohol is a carcinogen. People who consume two or more alcoholic drinks daily have higher risks of cancers of the mouth, throat, esophagus, larynx, liver, breast, colon, and rectum.[62] The risk increases with amount of alcohol consumed.

- The risk of cancer increases when cigarette smoking is combined with alcohol drinking.

- Certain molds that can grow on nuts or grains produce a chemical called *aflatoxin* (*ah-fla-tox'-in*). Consuming foods that are contaminated with these molds increases the risk of liver cancer. Chapter 19 discusses toxic molds and ways to protect the food supply from them and other food-borne health threats.

- Diets that supply large amounts of processed and/or red meat (defined as beef, pork, and lamb) are associated with increased risk of colon cancer.[62] The sodium nitrate and sodium nitrite added to processed meats ("deli" meats) can form *nitrosamines* (*ni-tros'-ah-menes*), which are carcinogens. Furthermore, eating high amounts of smoked or salt-preserved (cured or pickled) foods may also increase cancer risk, particularly for the stomach and colorectum.[65]

- According to findings of some studies, the risk of colorectal and pancreatic cancer is greater in populations that consume a lot of fried, grilled, or broiled meats. The high temperatures used to cook the meat may cause the formation of a group of carcinogens in the food called *heterocyclic* (*het'-eh-ro-si'-klic*) *amines*. Therefore, risk of certain cancers can be reduced by limiting intake of grilled meats, especially charred areas.

Currently, no scientific evidence indicates that consuming artificial sweeteners, such as aspartame; coffee; fluoridated water; or foods preserved by radiation (*irradiated foods*) causes cancer.[62] However, some dietary practices may *reduce* the risk of cancer.

The charred parts of charcoal-grilled foods may contribute to development of certain types of cancer.

Diet and Cancer Prevention

High intakes of fruits and vegetables reduce the risk of cancer, especially lung, oral, esophageal, stomach, and colon cancers.[62] Fruits and vegetables are rich sources of vitamin C, as well as carotenoids and other phytochemicals that may have antioxidant activity in the body. Antioxidants protect DNA from free-radical damage, preventing potentially cancer-causing mutations from occurring. Although research is ongoing, results of scientific studies generally have not shown that taking dietary supplements containing antioxidants reduces the risk

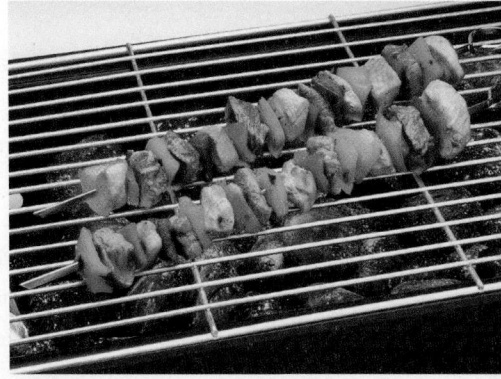

of cancer.[66,67] Some medical experts are concerned that taking antioxidant supplements may *increase* the risk of lung and prostate cancers, especially among smokers and men with family histories of prostate cancer.[68]

Folate, Vitamin C and Vitamin E

Scientists have conducted research to determine whether folate and vitamins C and E intakes are associated with reduced risk of cancer. Some epidemiological studies have found an inverse association between cancer risk and folate status.[22,69] However, results of other studies indicate folate supplementation has no effect or even increases the risk of cancer. Although there is some encouraging scientific evidence that vitamin C may be useful in treating cancer,[70,71] the vitamin may interfere with certain cancer-fighting medications, lowering their effectiveness.[72] Furthermore, taking megadoses of vitamin C can damage DNA, which may increase the likelihood of cancer.[73,74]

The relationship between vitamin E and cancer is unclear. Results of one large study involving over 30,000 subjects found that vitamin E supplementation with alpha-tocopherol increased prostate cancer risk.[75] More research to determine the effects of taking various forms and doses of vitamin E supplements on cancer is necessary.

Reducing the Risk

Although medical researchers are studying the cancer-fighting potential of various chemicals naturally occurring in food, no major breakthroughs have occurred. At this point, the best course of action is to take steps to prevent cancer. According to the American Cancer Society, people can reduce their risk of cancer by:[62]

- Avoiding exposure to tobacco smoke;

- Achieving and maintaining a healthy weight;

- Adopting a physically active lifestyle; and

- Eating a healthy diet that limits intake of red and processed meats and emphasizes plant foods, including fruits, vegetables, and whole grains.

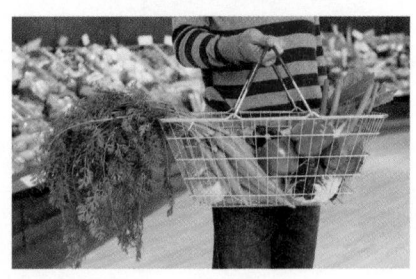
Fresh fruits and vegetables are rich sources of vitamin C.

ASSESS YOUR PROGRESS

40 *List the major steps in cancer development and progress.*

41 *What are the differences between a benign tumor and a malignant tumor?*

42 *Describe how red meat and preparation of red meat may contribute to cancer development.*

43 *Discuss the relationship between folate, vitamin C, and vitamin E and cancer risk.*

SUMMARY

SECTION 10.1 **Introducing Water-Soluble Vitamins**

- Thiamin, riboflavin, niacin, pantothenic acid, biotin, vitamin B-6, folate, vitamin B-12, and vitamin C are water-soluble vitamins. B vitamins function as components of coenzymes necessary for chemical reactions.

SECTION 10.2 **Thiamin**

- Thiamin, a component of thiamin pyrophosphate (TPP), helps cells metabolize carbohydrates, fats, and proteins.

- Enriched grain products, whole grains, pork, legumes, and orange juice are common sources of thiamin.

- Beriberi is the severe thiamin deficiency disease; toxicity from thiamin is very uncommon.

SECTION 10.3 **Riboflavin**

- Riboflavin is a component of flavin mononucleotide (FMN) and flavin adenine dinucleotide (FAD), coenzymes essential to energy metabolism.
- Dairy foods and enriched grains are rich sources of riboflavin.
- A deficiency of riboflavin, ariboflavinosis, is rare; fatigue, glossitis, and cheilosis are common symptoms. Riboflavin is readily excreted in urine.

SECTION 10.4 **Niacin**

- Nicotinic acid and nicotinamide, the two forms of niacin, are components of nicotinamide adenine dinucleotide and nicotinamide adenine dinucleotide phosphate. NAD and NADP participate in over 200 reactions involving carbohydrate, protein, and fatty acid metabolism.
- Enriched grains, liver, fish, poultry, and pork are good sources of niacin. Niacin can also be made from the amino acid tryptophan.
- A niacin deficiency causes pellagra, characterized by dermatitis, diarrhea, dementia, and death—the "4 Ds of pellagra." Physicians may prescribe megadoses of niacin for the treatment of abnormal blood lipid levels. High doses of niacin can cause flushing, itchy skin, nausea, and vomiting.

SECTION 10.5 **Pantothenic Acid**

- Pantothenic acid is a component of coenzyme A, which is essential for energy metabolism.
- Pantothenic acid deficiency is rare, because the vitamin is found in a wide variety of both plant and animal food sources.

SECTION 10.6 **Biotin**

- Biotin participates in chemical reactions that add carbon dioxide to other compounds.
- Biotin is readily consumed in a variety of foods; deficiency is very uncommon.

SECTION 10.7 **Vitamin B-6**

- Vitamin B-6, as pyridoxal phosphate, is involved in protein metabolism.
- Vitamin B-6 may help to relieve morning sickness in pregnancy and premenstrual syndrome, but further research is needed before routine supplementation should be recommended.
- Healthy people can obtain enough vitamin B-6 by eating a varied diet that contains animal foods and rich plant sources of the micronutrient.
- High doses of vitamin B-6 should be avoided because the vitamin can cause nervous system damage.

SECTION 10.8 **Folate**

- Folate plays important roles in DNA synthesis and homocysteine metabolism.
- Rich food sources of folate are leafy vegetables, organ meats, and orange juice.
- Signs of folate deficiency include megaloblastic anemia and neural tube defects in offspring.
- Excess folate in the diet can mask a vitamin B-12 deficiency.

SECTION 10.9 **Vitamin B-12**

- The body needs vitamin B-12 to metabolize folate and homocysteine, and maintain the insulation surrounding nerves.
- Although vitamin B-12 does not occur naturally in plant foods, the vitamin is in animal foods and products that have been fortified with the micronutrient.
- Vitamin B-12 deficiency is more common in older adults due to poor absorption of the vitamin, often a result of gastritis.

- Megaloblastic anemia is an early sign of a vitamin B-12 deficiency. Long-term vitamin B-12 deficiency can result in paralysis.

SECTION 10.10 Vitamin C

- The body uses vitamin C to synthesize and maintain collagen, as an antioxidant, and for normal immune function.
- Fresh fruits and vegetables, especially citrus fruits, are generally good sources of the micronutrient.
- A vitamin C deficiency results in scurvy. Excess vitamin C may cause diarrhea and increase the risk of kidney stones in some people.

SECTION 10.11 Vitamin-Like Compounds

- Choline, carnitine, inositol, taurine, and lipoic acid are examples of vitamin-like compounds. Unlike most vitamins, these compounds can be synthesized by the human body. Deficiencies or toxicities of choline, carnitine, inositol, taurine, or lipoic acid are unlikely.

SECTION 10.12 Diet and Cancer

- Cancer occurs when genes that regulate cellular growth, division, and death mutate, resulting in abnormal cell development, rapid cell growth, and unchecked cell division.
- Research linking specific vitamins to cancer risk is conflicting. Maintaining a healthy body weight, exercising regularly, consuming a diet that supplies plenty of fruits and vegetables, limiting intakes of grilled and processed meats, and avoiding tobacco smoke and excess alcohol may reduce the risk of cancer.

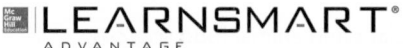

Get the most out of your study of nutrition with McGraw-Hill's innovative suite of adaptive learning products including McGraw-Hill LearnSmart®, SmartBook®, McGraw-Hill LearnSmart Achieve®, and McGraw-Hill LearnSmart Prep®. Visit www.learnsmartadvantage.com.

CASE STUDY RESPONSE

VITAMIN B-12 DEFICIENCY IN A VEGAN

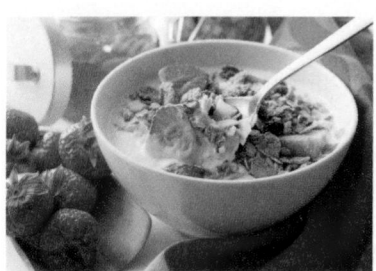

Fortified breakfast cereal served with soy milk provides vitamin B-12 to a vegan's diet.

MAJOR SOURCES OF VITAMIN B-12 in the typical American diet are meat, dairy foods, poultry, fish, shellfish, and eggs. Plants do not make vitamin B-12; therefore, a vegan diet may be deficient in the vitamin.

Absorption of vitamin B-12 requires intrinsic factor. IF binds to vitamin B-12 in the small intestine, allowing for absorption in the ileum. Individuals who lack IF have reduced absorption of vitamin B-12. This eventually leads to deficiency symptoms. Because the daily vitamin B-12 pill that Deon has been taking has not resulted in improved blood levels of vitamin B-12, it is likely that he lacks IF. Therefore, vitamin B-12 injections may be necessary to bypass the need for IF to absorb vitamin B-12 from the small intestine. His doctor may also choose to treat him with monitored megadoses of vitamin B-12.

Deon appears to be vitamin B-12 deficient as a result of both his vegan diet and his impaired IF. As a result, dietary modifications alone are unlikely to correct the anemia and prevent deficiency. However, he should still be encouraged to include vitamin B-12 in his diet, even if only small amounts are being absorbed at this time. Many vegan products are fortified with synthetic vitamin B-12. Deon should consider consuming ready-to-eat cereals and grain products, soy milk, and other dairy-alternatives that contain added vitamin B-12.

A vitamin B-12 deficiency can result in nerve damage, which can lead to paralysis. Long-term deficiency in the vitamin can result in death. With proper treatment, Deon can continue his vegan lifestyle and avoid these negative outcomes.

TEST KITCHEN
Modifying Recipes for Healthy Living

Penny is a 20-year-old college student with a family history of breast cancer. She would like to start incorporating more antioxidant-rich fruits into her diet. Penny's grandmother makes a delicious fruit salad from canned fruits. While Penny enjoys her grandmother's fruit salad, she would like a recipe that incorporates fresh fruits and has less sugar. Develop a healthy "summertime" fruit salad recipe using produce available at a large farmers' market.

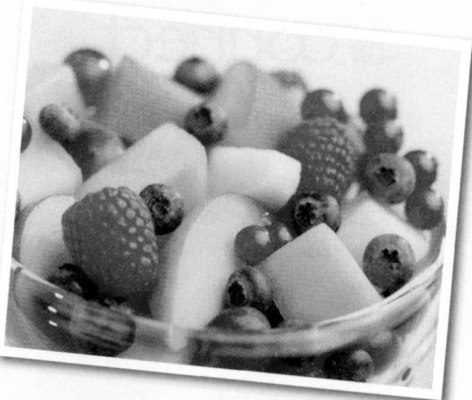

GRANDMOTHER'S PINEAPPLE FRUIT SALAD

PREPARATION STEPS

1. Drain oranges, pineapple, and fruit cocktail.
2. Combine oranges, pineapple, and fruit cocktail in a medium container. Gently mix.
3. Add marshmallows and sugar to fruit mixture.
4. Refrigerate and serve cool.
5. Serves four (½-cup servings).

INGREDIENTS

1 can (8 oz) mandarin oranges
1 can (12 oz) diced pineapple
2 cans (8 oz each) mixed fruit cocktail
1 cup mini-marshmallows
½ cup sugar

STEP 1 Brainstorm

Use diet analysis software to analyze the nutrient and calorie content of the "Grandmother's Pineapple Fruit Salad" recipe. List the total calories, total carbohydrates, sugar, fiber, and vitamin content of the recipe. How do you rate the overall quality of the recipe?

STEP 2 Develop a modified version of this recipe called "Summertime Fruit Salad" that incorporates fresh fruits and less sugar

List the ingredients and amounts of each of them that are needed.
List the preparation steps.

STEP 3 Evaluate the modified recipe

Use diet analysis software to analyze the nutrient and calorie content of the "Summertime Fruit Salad." Develop a table comparing the calories, total carbohydrates, sugar, fiber, and vitamin content in the original and modified recipes. Explain how the fruit salads differ nutritionally.

OPTIONAL ACTIVITIES

STEP 4 Shop for your ingredients

Were the ingredients readily available at your local farmers' market (or supermarket if there is no farmers' market in your area)? List any fruit that you could not find fresh.

STEP 5 Test your new recipe

Keep notes on any changes you make to ingredient amounts as you prepare the "Summertime Fruit Salad."

STEP 6 Reflect on the modified recipe

How does the fruit salad look? How does the fruit salad taste? Would you feel comfortable offering it to friends or family members?

PERSONAL Dietary Analysis

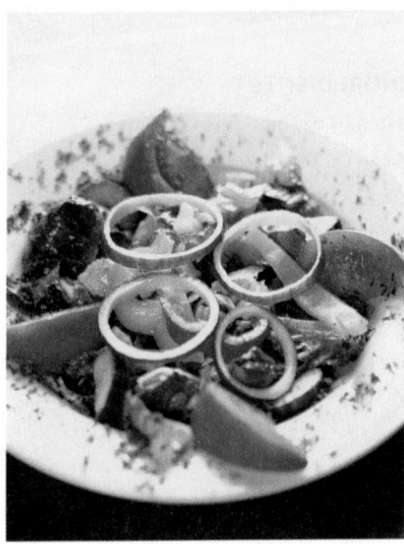

Using the DRIs

1. Refer to your 3-day food log from the "Personal Dietary Analysis" feature in Chapter 5.

   a. Find the RDA values for vitamins under your life stage/sex group category in the DRI tables (see the last pages of this book). Write those values under the "My RDA" column in the table on this page.

   b. Review your personal dietary assessment. Determine your 3-day average intakes of vitamins A, D, E, thiamin, riboflavin, folate, and B-12. Write those values under the "My Average Intake" column of the table.

   c. Calculate the percentage of the RDA you consumed for each vitamin by dividing your intake by the RDA amount and multiplying the figure you obtain by 100. For example, if your average intake of vitamin C were 100 mg/day and your RDA for the vitamin were 75 mg/day, you would divide 100 mg by 75 mg to obtain 1.25. To multiply this figure by 100, simply move the decimal point two places to the right, and replace the decimal point with a percentage sign (125%). Thus, your average daily intake of vitamin C was 125% of the RDA. Place the percentages for each vitamin under the "% of My RDA" column.

   d. Under the ">, <, or =" column, indicate whether your average daily intake was greater than (>), less than (<), or equal to (=) the RDA.

2. Use the information you calculated in the first part of this activity to answer the following questions:

   a. Which of your average vitamin intakes equaled or exceeded the RDA value? _____

   b. Which of your average vitamin intakes was below the RDA value? _____

   c. What foods would you eat to increase your intake of the vitamins that were less than the RDA levels? (Review sources of certain vitamins in this chapter and Chapter 11.)
   _____

   d. Turn in your completed table and answers to your instructor.

Personal Dietary Analysis: Vitamins

Vitamin	My RDA	My Average Intake	% of My RDA	>,<, or =
A				
D				
E				
Thiamin				
Riboflavin				
Niacin				
Folate				
Vitamin B-12				
C				

Critical Thinking

1. Choose three different websites that sell vitamin supplements. Then, choose three different products and compare prices for the same product at the different websites. Then compare prices of the vitamins from these sites with the prices you would pay at a local supermarket, discount department store, or drugstore. Write a one-page report about your findings.

2. Your 70-year-old grandmother complains that she is always tired; her tongue does not "look right," and she is having problems concentrating on tasks and walking. She attributes her health problems to "growing old." Explain why your grandmother may have a vitamin deficiency and how the deficiency is treated.

3. After 10 years as a lactoovovegetarian, Cory recently decided to adopt a vegan diet. What vitamin deficiencies should Cory be most concerned about in his vegan diet? Provide recommendations to Cory to ensure he is meeting his vitamin needs.

4. Two of your roommates have developed common colds in the past week. Your third roommate has started taking an "immune boosting" supplement that contains 500 mg of vitamin C. Do you recommend this supplement? Why or why not?

5. You are a pharmacist technician who routinely dispenses prescribed high doses of niacin. What is the most common reason high-dose niacin is prescribed? What side effects are associated with high-dose niacin?

Practice Test

1. Lack of _____ causes scurvy.
   a. thiamin
   b. riboflavin
   c. vitamin C
   d. vitamin B-12

2. Major food sources of vitamin B-12 include
   a. grain products.
   b. meat and milk products.
   c. fruits and vegetables.
   d. nuts and seeds.

3. Diets that lack niacin can lead to
   a. rickets.
   b. beriberi.
   c. pellagra.
   d. pernicious anemia.

4. To reduce the likelihood of giving birth to babies with neural tube defects, women of childbearing potential should obtain adequate
   a. folate.
   b. biotin.
   c. cellulose.
   d. niacin.

5. _____ is part of pyridoxal phosphate (PLP), the coenzyme necessary for transamination and deamination reactions.
   a. Vitamin B-6
   b. Vitamin B-12
   c. Niacin
   d. Riboflavin

6. Physicians often prescribe therapeutic doses of _____ to treat abnormal blood lipid levels.
   a. vitamin C
   b. vitamin B-12
   c. folate
   d. niacin

7. _____ is a component of coenzyme A.
   a. Vitamin B-6
   b. Riboflavin
   c. Pantothenic acid
   d. Biotin

8. Which of the following statements is false?
   a. Intrinsic factor is needed for vitamin B-12 absorption.
   b. Vitamin B-12 deficiency is common among older adults.
   c. Patients with pernicious anemia are treated with high doses of folic acid.
   d. If untreated, pernicious anemia can be deadly.

9. Which of the following foods is a rich source of vitamin C?
   a. whole milk
   b. egg white
   c. hamburger patty
   d. green pepper

10. Eating large amounts of raw egg whites can cause a _____ deficiency.
    a. folate
    b. biotin
    c. pantothenic acid
    d. riboflavin

11. Deficiency in which of the following vitamins can lead to elevated blood homocysteine?
    a. folate, vitamin B-12, and vitamin B-6
    b. thiamin, niacin, and vitamin B-12
    c. vitamin B-6, folate, and riboflavin
    d. vitamin C, niacin, and vitamin B-12

12. Which of the following practices may reduce your risk of cancer?
    a. eating fruits and vegetables
    b. eating grilled meats regularly
    c. smoking no more than 10 cigarettes daily
    d. consuming 2 to 3 standard alcoholic drinks daily

13. ____ is essential for neurotransmitter and phospholipid synthesis.

    a. Lipoic acid   c. Inositol

    b. Choline   d. Taurine

14. Glossitis and cheilosis are clinical signs of a ____ deficiency.

    a. vitamin B-6   c. riboflavin

    b. pantothenic acid   d. folate

15. ____ can be made from the amino acid tryptophan.

    a. Vitamin B-6   c. Thiamin

    b. Vitamin C   d. Niacin

ANSWERS TO PRACTICE TEST

1-c; 2-b; 3-c; 4-a; 5-a; 6-d; 7-c; 8-c; 9-d; 10-b; 11-a; 12-a; 13-b; 14-c; 15-d

ANSWERS TO CHAPTER 10 QUIZ Yourself

1. Water-soluble vitamins are stored in significant amounts in the human body. **False** (p. 304)
2. High doses of B vitamins are safe to take. **False** (pp. 311, 315, 326)
3. Thiamin is necessary to prevent neural tube defects. **False** (p. 319)
4. Vegans are at risk for a vitamin B-12 deficiency. **True** (p. 322)
5. Vitamin C enhances the body's disease-fighting abilities. **True** (p. 325)

References

1. Otten JJ and others (eds.): Institute of Medicine: *Dietary Reference Intakes: The essential guide to nutrient requirements*. Washington, DC: National Academies Press, 2006.
2. Doung-ngern P and others: Beriberi outbreak among commercial fishermen, Thailand 2005. *Southeast Asian Journal of Tropical Medicine and Public Health* 38(1):130, 2007.
3. Food and Nutrition Board: *Dietary Reference Intakes for thiamin, riboflavin, niacin, vitamin B-6, folate, vitamin B-12, pantothenic acid, biotin, and choline*. Washington DC: National Academy Press, 1998.
4. Naito E and others: Thiamine-responsive lactic acidosis: Role of pyruvate dehydrogenase complex. *European Journal of Pediatrics* 157(8):648, 1998.
5. Toyoshima M and others: Thiamine-responsive congenital lactic acidosis: Clinical and biochemical studies. *Pediatric Neurology* 33(2):98, 2005.
6. Condo M and others: Riboflavin prophylaxis in pediatric and adolescent migraine. *Journal of Headache and Pain* 10(5):361, 2009.
7. U.S. National Library of Medicine, National Institutes of Health: *Riboflavin (vitamin B2)*. Updated November 2012. http://www.nlm.nih.gov/medlineplus/druginfo/natural/957.html Accessed: February 1, 2014.
8. MacLennan SC and others: High-dose riboflavin for migraine prophylaxis in children: A double-blind, randomized, placebo-controlled trial. *Journal of Child Neurology* 23(11):1300, 2008.
9. McKenney J and others: Safety of extended-release niacin/laropiprant in patients with dyslipidemia. *Journal of Clinical Lipidology* 4(2):105, 2010.
10. Keene D and others: Effect of cardiovascular risk of high density lipoprotein targeted drug treatments niacin, fibrates, and CETP inhibitors: meta-analysis of randomized controlled trials including 117 411 patients. *British Medical Journal* 2014;349: g4379 doi:10.1136.bmj.g4379 (published 18 July 2014).
11. The HPS2-THRIVE Collaborative Group: Effects of extended release niacin with Laropiprant in high-risk patients. *New England Journal of Medicine* 371(3):203, 2014.
12. Gerlach AT and others: Vitamin B6 deficiency: A potential cause of refractory seizures in adults. *Journal of Parenteral and Enteral Nutrition* 35(2):272, 2011.
13. Valle-Morales L and others: Epileptic status refractory to conventional treatment caused by vitamin B6 deficiency. *Journal of Perinatology* 29(3):252, 2009.
14. Wang HS and Kuo MF: Vitamin B6 related epilepsy during childhood. *Chang Gung Medical Journal* 30(5):396, 2007.
15. Office of Dietary Supplements, National Institute of Health: *Dietary supplement fact sheet: Vitamin B6*. Updated September 2011. http://ods.od.nih.gov/factsheets/VitaminB6-HealthProfessional/ Accessed: February 1, 2014.
16. Enisiyeh J, Sakineh MA: Comparing ginger and vitamin B6 for the treatment of nausea and vomiting in pregnancy: A randomized controlled trial. *Midwifery* 25(6):649, 2009.
17. Chocano-Bedoya PO and others: Dietary B vitamin intake and incident premenstrual syndrome. *American Journal of Clinical Nutrition* 93(5):1080, 2011.
18. Ebrahimi N and others: Optimal management of nausea and vomiting in pregnancy. *International Journal of Women's Health* 2:241, 2010.
19. Aufiero E and others: Pyridoxine hydrochloride treatment of carpal tunnel syndrome: A review. *Nutrition Reviews* 62(3):96, 2004.
20. Ryan-Harshman M, Aldoori W: Carpal tunnel syndrome and vitamin B6. *Canadian Family Physicians* 53(7):1161, 2007.
21. McDowell MA and others: Blood folate levels: The latest NHANES results. *NCHS Data Brief No. 6*, May 2008.
22. Office of Dietary Supplements, National Institute of Health: *Dietary supplement fact sheet: Folate*. Updated April 2013. http://ods.od.nih.gov/factsheets/Folate-QuickFacts/ Accessed: February 1, 2014.
23. Wilson RD and others: Pre-conceptional vitamin/folic acid supplementation 2007: The use of folic acid in combination with a multivitamin supplement for the prevention of neural tube defects and other congenital anomalies. *Journal of Obstetrics and Gynaecology Canada* 29(12):1003, 2007.
24. Boulet SR and others: Racial/ethnic differences in the birth prevalence of spina bifida—United States, 1995–2005. *Morbidity and Mortality Weekly Report* 57(53):1409, 2009.
25. Houghton LA and others: Long-term effect of low-dose folic acid intake: Potential effect of mandatory fortification on the prevention of neural tube defects. *American Journal of Clinical Nutrition* 94(1):136, 2011.
26. Bramswig S and others: Supplementation with a multivitamin containing 800 micro of folic acid shortens the time to reach the preventive red blood cell folate concentration in healthy women. *International Journal of Vitamin and Nutrition Research* 79(2):61, 2009.
27. Centers for Disease Control and Prevention: *Anencephaly*. Updated July 2013. http://www.cdc.gov/ncbddd/birthdefects/Anencephaly.html Accessed: February 1, 2014.
28. Centers for Disease Control and Prevention: *Spina bifida*. 2013. http://www.cdc.gov/ncbddd/birthdefects/spinabifida.html Accessed: February 1, 2014.
29. Petrini JR and others: Use of supplements containing folic acid among women of childbearing age—United States, 2007. *Morbidity and Mortality Weekly Report* 57(01):5, 2008.
30. Clarke R and others: Effects of lowering homocysteine levels with B vitamins on cardiovascular disease, cancer, and cause-specific mortality: Meta-analysis of 8 randomized trials involving 37,485 individuals. *Archives of Internal Medicine* 170:1622, 2010.
31. Huang T and others: Meta-analysis of B vitamin supplementation on plasma homocysteine, cardiovascular and all-cause mortality. *Clinical Nutrition* 31:448, 2012.
32. Quadri P and others: Homocysteine, folate, and vitamin B-12 in mild cognitive impairment, Alzheimer disease, and vascular dementia. *American Journal of Clinical Nutrition* 80:114, 2004.

33. Tucker KL and others: High homocysteine and low B vitamins predict cognitive decline in aging men: The Veterans Affairs Normative Aging Study. *American Journal of Clinical Nutrition* 82:627, 2005.

34. Mason JB: Folate, cancer risk, and the Greek god, Proteus: A tale of two chameleons. *Nutrition Reviews* 67(4):206, 2009.

35. Dali-Youcef N, Andres R: An update on cobalamin deficiency in adults. *Quarterly Journal of Medicine* 102(1):17, 2008.

36. Office of Dietary Supplements, National Institute of Health: *Dietary supplement fact sheet: Vitamin B12.* Updated June 2011. http://ods.od.nih.gov/factsheets/VitaminB12-QuickFacts/ Accessed: February 1, 2014.

37. Pauling Institute, Micronutrient Information Center, Oregon State University: *Vitamin B-12.* Updated August 2007. http://lpi.oregonstate.edu/infocenter/vitamins/vitaminB12/ Accessed: February 1, 2014.

38. Oh RC and others: Vitamin B12 deficiency. *American Family Physician* 67(5):979, 2003. Grasbeck R and Tanner SM: Juvenile selective vitamin B12 malabsorption: 50 years after its description—10 years of genetic testing. *Pediatric Research* 70(3):222, 2011.

39. Hvas AM and others: The vitamin B12 absorption test, CobaSorb, identifies patients not requiring vitamin B12 injection therapy. *Scandinavian Journal of Clinical and Laboratory Investigation* 71(5):43, 2011.

40. Favrat B and others: Oral vitamin B12 for patients suspected of subtle cobalamin deficiency: A multicentre pragmatic randomized controlled trial. *BMC Family Practice* 13:12, 2011.

41. Codazzi D and others: Coma and respiratory failure in a child with severe vitamin B(12) deficiency. *Pediatric Critical Care Medicine* 6:483, 2005.

42. Wang ZP and others: Low maternal vitamin B(12) is a risk factor for neural tube defects: A meta-analysis. *Journal of Maternal, Fetal, and Neonatal Medicine* 25(4):389, 2011.

43. Ray JG and others: Vitamin B12 and the risk of neural tube defects in a folic-acid-fortified population. *Epidemiology* 18(3):362, 2007.

44. Selhub J and others: B vitamins and the aging brain. *Nutrition Reviews* 68(Suppl 2):S112, 2010.

45. Werder SF: Cobalamin deficiency, hyperhomocysteinemia, and dementia. *Neuropsychiatric Disease Treatment* 6:159, 2010.

46. Morris DW and others: Folate and unipolar depression. *Journal of Alternative and Complementary Medicine* 14(3):277, 2008.

47. Malouf R, Grimley Evans J: Folic acid with or without vitamin B12 for the prevention and treatment of healthy elderly and demented people. *Cochrane Database of Systematic Reviews* October 8 (4):CD004514, 2008.

48. Werder SF: Cobalamin deficiency, hyperhomocysteinemia, and dementia. *Neuropsychiatric Disease Treament* 6:159, 2010.

49. Fava M, Mischoulon D: Folate in depression: Efficacy, safety, differences in formulations, and clinical issues. *Journal of Clinical Psychiatry* 70(Suppl 5):12, 2009.

50. Food and Nutrition Board: *Dietary Reference Intakes for vitamin C, vitamin E, selenium, and carotenoids.* Washington, DC: National Academy Press, 2000.

51. U.S. Department of Agriculture, ChooseMyPlate.gov: *Food groups—Fruits.* Updated 2014. http://www.choosemyplate.gov/food-groups/fruits.html Accessed: February 1, 2014.

52. Levine M and others: A new recommended dietary allowance of vitamin C for healthy young women. *Proceedings of the National Academy of Sciences* 98(17):9842, 2001.

53. Taylor EN and others: Dietary factors and the risk of incident kidney stones in men: New insights after 14 years of follow-up. *Journal of the American Society of Nephrology* 15:3225, 2004.

54. Harvard Health Letter. *What you should know about: Vitamin C.* January 2013. www.health.harvard.edu Accessed: February 1, 2014.

55. Hemila H, Chalker E: Vitamin C for preventing and treating the common cold. *Cochrane Database of Systematic Reviews* 1:CH000980, 2013.

56. Ye Y and others: Effect of antioxidant supplementation on cardiovascular outcomes: A meta-analysis of randomized controlled trials. *PLoS One* 8(2):e56803, 2013.

57. Engelhart MJ and others: Dietary intake of antioxidants and risk of Alzheimer disease. *Journal of the American Medical Association* 287:3223, 2002.

58. Chandrashekhar CD and others: Antioxidants in central nervous system diseases: Preclinical promise and translational challenges. *Journal of Alzheimers Disease* 15(3):473, 2008.

59. Zeisel SH: Nutritional genomics: Defining the dietary requirement and effects of choline. *Journal of Nutrition* 141(3):531, 2011.

60. U.S. National Library of Medicine, National Institutes of Health: *Carnitine.* Updated May 2013. http://ods.od.nih.gov/factsheets/Carnitine-HealthProfessional/ Accessed: February 1, 2014.

61. Sylvia LG and others: Nutrient-based therapies for bipolar disorders—a systemic review. *Psychotherapy and Psychosomatics* 82(1):10, 2013.

62. American Cancer Society: *Cancer facts & figures 2014.* http://www.cancer.org/acs/groups/content/@research/documents/document/acspc-041770.pdf Accessed: February 1, 2014.

63. Harris HR and others: Body fat distribution and risk of premenopausal breast cancer in the Nurses' Health Study II. *Journal of the National Cancer Institute* 103(3):273, 2011.

64. Nahleh Z and others: How to reduce your cancer risk: Mechanisms and myths. *International Journal of General Medicine* 4:277, 2011.

65. Santarelli RL and others: Meat processing and colon carcinogenesis: Cooked, nitrate-treated, and oxidized high-heme cured meat promotes mucin-depleted foci in rats. *Cancer Prevention Research* 3(7):852, 2010.

66. Dolara P and others: Antioxidant vitamins and mineral supplementation, life span expansion and cancer incidence: A critical commentary. *European Journal of Nutrition* 51(7):769, 2012.

67. Han X and others: Antioxidant intake and pancreatic cancer risk: The Vitamins and Lifestyle (VITAL) Study. *Cancer* 119(7):1314, 2013.

68. Lin J and others: Vitamins C and E and beta carotene supplementation and cancer risk: A randomized controlled trial. *Journal of the National Cancer Institute* 101(1):14, 2009.

69. Gibson TM and others: Pre- and post-fortification intake of folate and risk of colorectal cancer in a large prospective cohort study in the United States. *American Journal of Clinical Nutrition* 94:1053, 2011.

70. Ohno S and others: High-dose vitamin C (ascorbic acid) therapy in the treatment of patients with advanced cancer. *Anticancer Research* 29(3):809, 2009.

71. Cabanillas F: Foods, nutrients and the risk of oral and pharyngeal cancer. *British Journal of Cancer* 109(11):2904, 2013.

72. Heaney ML and others: Vitamin C antagonizes the cytotoxic effects of antineoplastic drugs. *Cancer Research* 68(19):8031, 2008.

73. Hoffer LJ and others: Phase I clinical trial of I.V. ascorbic acid in advanced malignancy. *Annals of Oncology* 19(11):1969, 2008.

74. Lee KW and others: Vitamin C and cancer chemoprevention: Reappraisal. *American Journal of Clinical Nutrition* 78:1074, 2003.

75. Klein EA and others: Vitamin E and the risk of prostate cancer: The Selenium and Vitamin E Cancer Prevention Trial (SELECT). *Journal of the American Medical Association* 306(14):1549, 2011.

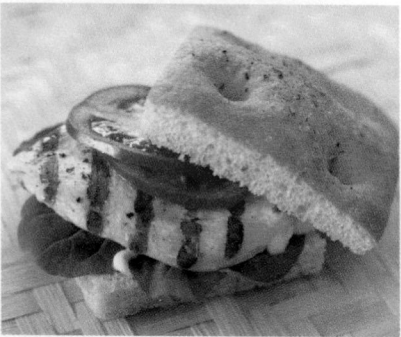

11 Water and Major Minerals

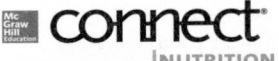
QUIZ Yourself

Can water be toxic when consumed in excess? What is osteoporosis? Test your knowledge of water and major minerals by taking the following quiz. The answers are found on page 381.

1. Cells produce some water as a by-product of metabolism. ___T ___F

2. The kidneys are the major regulator of the body's water content. ___T ___F

3. Consuming too much sodium may contribute to low blood pressure. ___T ___F

4. Weight-bearing exercise can reduce the risk of osteoporosis. ___T ___F

5. Processed foods are rich sources of potassium. ___T ___F

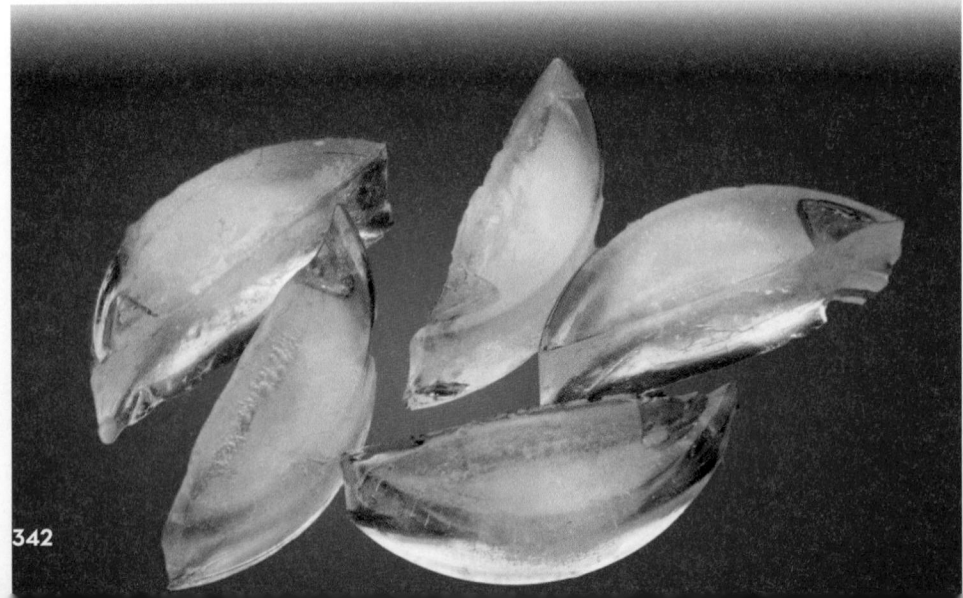

11.1 Water

LEARNING OUTCOMES

1 *Discuss the functions of water in the body.*

2 *Explain differences between intracellular and extracellular water.*

3 *Identify typical sources of water intake and loss.*

Compared to other nutrients, water is so unique, it is in a class by itself. Water is a simple compound (H_2O) that does not need to be digested, and it is easily absorbed by the digestive tract.

We often take water for granted, but this simple molecule is highly essential. You can survive for weeks, even months, if your diet lacks carbohydrates, lipids, proteins, and vitamins. But if you do not have any water, your life will end within a week or two. Fortunately, your body obtains water from beverages and foods, especially fruits, vegetables, and meats. The body also makes some water as a result of metabolism.

Water and Body Composition

Depending on a person's age, sex, and body composition, 50 to 75% of his or her body is water weight (see Fig. 1.1).[1] Lean muscle tissue contains more water (about 73%) than fat tissue (about 20%). On average, young adult men have more lean tissue than young women. Approximately 60% of an average young man's body weight is water; the average young woman's body has more fat and, therefore, slightly less water than an average young man's body. A person's percentage of body weight that is water declines from birth to old age. A newborn's weight may be 75% water, whereas the weight of an older adult's body may be only 45% water.[1]

Functions of Water

Water is a major solvent; many substances, including glucose, dissolve in water. Water often participates directly in chemical reactions, such as those involved in digesting food. Table 11.1 lists these and additional roles of water in the body. Although water has numerous functions in the body, this unique nutrient does not provide energy. The following section discusses details of one of the major functions of water in the body, membrane transport.

Water and Membrane Transport

Water helps transport water–soluble substances within and outside cells. Chapter 4 discussed ways that water and other substance enter cells, including **simple diffusion** (see Figure 4.17a). A **selectively permeable membrane** is a barrier that allows the diffusion of certain substances and prevents the movement of other substances through it. **Osmosis** is the diffusion of a solvent, usually water, through a selectively permeable membrane, such as the plasma membrane of a human cell. The concentration of substances dissolved in the water, such as sodium ions or glucose, influences osmosis. Water moves from a region that has less material dissolved in it (is dilute) to a region that has more material dissolved in it (see Fig. 4.17d). The diffusion stops when the concentrations of the material on either side of the plasma membrane are equal. To survive, a human cell carefully controls the passage of substances through its plasma membrane.

TABLE 11.1 Functions of Water in the Body

Water:
• Is a solvent
• Is a major component of blood, saliva, sweat, tears, mucus, and joint fluid
• Removes wastes
• Helps transport substances
• Lubricates tissues
• Regulates body temperature
• Helps digest foods
• Participates in many chemical reactions
• Helps maintain proper blood pH

simple diffusion molecular movement from a region of higher to lower concentration

selectively permeable membrane barrier that allows the passage of certain substances and prevents the movement of other substances

osmosis movement of a solvent, usually water, through a selectively permeable membrane

FIGURE 11.1 Fluid compartments in the body. Intracellular water is inside cells; extracellular water surrounds cells (tissue or *interstitial* fluid) or is the fluid in blood (*plasma*). Water is exchanged between plasma and interstitial fluids (green arrows), as well as between tissue and intracellular fluids (black arrows).

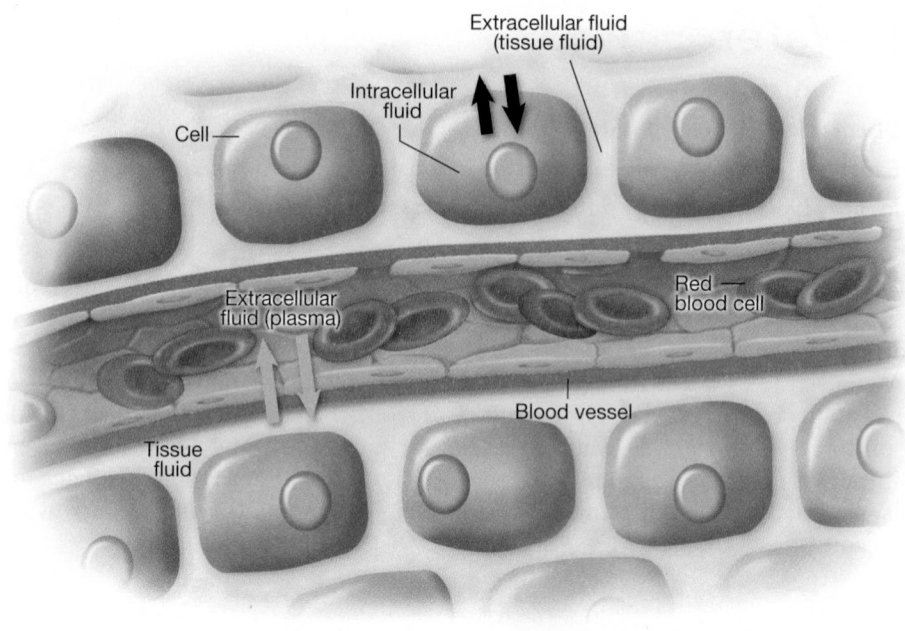

intracellular water water that is inside cells

extracellular water water that surrounds cells or is in the fluid portion of blood

ions elements or small molecules that have electrical charges

Water Distribution: Intracellular and Extracellular Water

The body has two major fluid compartments: intracellular water and extra—cellular water (Fig. 11.1). **Intracellular water** is inside cells. **Extracellular water** surrounds cells (tissue or *interstitial* fluid) or is the fluid portion of blood (*plasma*). About two—thirds of the body's water is in the intracellular compartment.

The body maintains the balance of compartmental fluids primarily by con—trolling concentrations of ions in each compartment. **Ions** are mineral elements or small molecules that have electrical charges, such as sodium, potassium, phos—phate, and chloride ions. These ions are also called *electrolytes*.

Maintenance of intracellular water volume depends to a large extent on the intracellular concentration of potassium and phosphate ions. In contrast, maintenance of extracellular water volume depends primarily on the extracellular concentration of sodium and chloride ions. Changes in the normal concentrations of these ions can cause water to shift out of one compartment and move into the other. For example, extracellular fluid that has fewer—than—normal sodium ions can cause water to move from the extracellular compartment into cells. When this occurs, the cells swell and can burst (Fig. 11.2a).

In the opposite situation, extracellular fluid that has an excess of sodium ions can cause water to move out of cells. As a result, the cells shrink and die because they lack enough intracellular fluid to function (Fig. 11.2b). Recall from Chapter 7 that edema occurs when an excessive amount of water moves into the space surrounding cells (see Fig. 7.1). To function normally, the body must maintain intracellular and extracellular water volumes within certain limits.

Sources of Water

How much water is necessary to drink for good health? Contrary to popular belief, there is no "rule of thumb" recommendation that specifies how many glasses of water to consume each day.[2] Factors such as environmental tem—peratures, health conditions, physical activities, and dietary choices influ—ence individual water requirements. Thus, total water intake varies widely.[3]

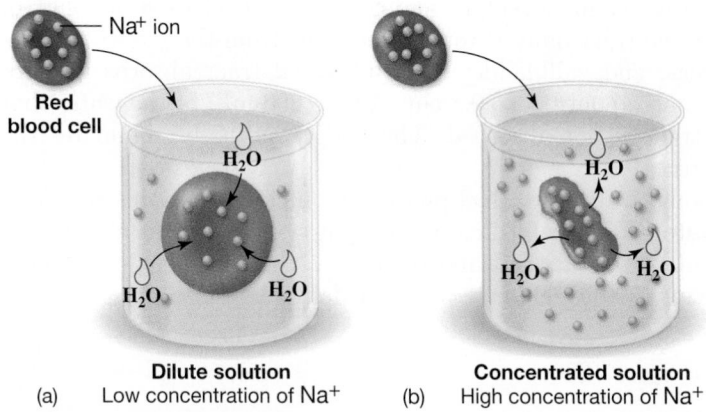

(a) Dilute solution
Low concentration of Na$^+$

(b) Concentrated solution
High concentration of Na$^+$

FIGURE 11.2 Maintaining proper hydration. Cells need to maintain their fluid balance. Changes in the normal concentrations of ions can cause water to shift out of one compartment and move into the other. (a) A red blood cell is placed into a solution containing fewer sodium ions (Na$^+$) than are present inside the cell. As a result, water flows into the cell, which swells and may burst. (b) A red blood cell is placed into a solution containing more sodium ions than are present inside the cell. In this case, water flows out of the cell, which shrivels.

Total water intake refers to water ingested by consuming beverages, including drinking water, and foods.

The Adequate Intake (AI) for total water intake is approximately 11 cups (2.7 L) for young women and approximately 15.5 cups (3.7 L) for young men.[4] Other sources of water include fruit juice, milk, soup, coffee, tea, soft drinks, and flavored bottled water. Most foods also contain some water. Fruits and vegetables appear to be solid, but they generally contain 60 to 95% water weight. Table 11.2 lists some commonly consumed foods and their water content by weight. About 80% of our total water intake is from water and other beverages; food supplies the remaining amount of an American's water intake.[4]

total water intake water ingested by consuming beverages, including drinking water, and foods

TABLE 11.2 Water Content of Selected Foods and Beverages

Food	Water % by Weight
Lettuce	95
Tomato	95
Watermelon	91
Milk, 1% fat	90
Apple, with skin	86
Avocado (Florida)	79
Potato, white, baked with skin	75
Banana	75
Chicken, white meat, roasted	65
Ground beef, 80% lean, broiled	56
Bread, whole wheat	39
Margarine, stick	16
Crackers, saltines	5
Vegetable oil	0

Source: Data from U.S. Department of Agriculture, Agricultural Research Service, USDA Nutrient Data Laboratory: *USDA national nutrient database for standard reference*, release 26, 2013.

DID **YOU** KNOW?

The average adult in the United States consumes 10 to 11 cups of fluids per day, primarily as plain water, soft drinks, coffee, tea, milk, and alcoholic beverages.[5] When comparing tap and bottled water, tap water accounts for about two-thirds of water consumed at home, but only one-half of water consumed away from the home.[6]

metabolic water water formed by cells as a metabolic by-product

In addition to the water in beverages and foods, a considerable amount of water enters the digestive tract daily through secretions from the mouth, stomach, intestine, pancreas, and gallbladder. The intestinal tract absorbs most of this water. Each day, only about 0.4 to 0.8 cup (100 to 200 mL) of the water that enters the digestive tract is not absorbed. The body eventually eliminates the unabsorbed water in feces.

Cells also form some water as a by-product of metabolism; this source is termed **metabolic water**. Physically inactive people typically form about 1 to 1.5 cups (250 to 350 mL) of metabolic water per day; very active people can produce about 2 to 2.5 cups (500 to 600 mL) of water daily.[4]

FRESH TIPS

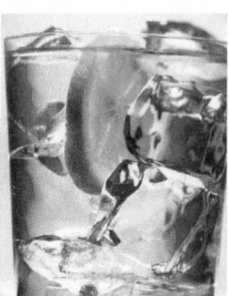

Do you find the taste of plain water bland? Try drinking water ice-cold and flavored with your favorite fruit. Add lemon slices, lime slices, blueberries, raspberries, or strawberries to a pitcher of water and refrigerate for several hours. Serve the fruit-flavored water over ice for a refreshing, healthy, and tasty beverage.

ASSESS YOUR PROGRESS

1. *Identify at least five different functions of water in the body.*
2. *Compare and contrast intracellular and extracellular water.*
3. *Explain the process of osmosis.*

Perspiring helps maintain normal body temperature because water can hold a lot of heat. As sweat evaporates from skin, it takes some heat along with it, cooling the body.

11.2 Water Balance and Hydration

LEARNING OUTCOMES

1 *Discuss how the body maintains its water balance.*
2 *Describe dehydration and water intoxication.*

Water balance is critical to survival, and the body has a number of mechanisms to help maintain a state of proper water balance. **Hydration** is another term for the body's water status. If hydration becomes altered, such as in **dehydration** (body water depletion), an individual can suffer serious consequences.

Water Balance

An average healthy adult consumes and produces approximately 2.5 quarts (2500 mL) of water daily (Fig. 11.3).[1] The body eliminates about 2.5 quarts of water in urine, exhaled air, feces, and perspiration (Fig. 11.3). Thus, a healthy person's average daily water input equals his or her average daily losses (output). A number of factors influence a person's fluid input and output. Environmental conditions such as temperature, humidity, and altitude can affect body water losses. Physiological conditions, especially fever, vomiting, and diarrhea, as well as lifestyle practices such as exercise habits and sodium and alcohol intake, can also alter the body's fluid balance.

hydration water status

dehydration body water depletion

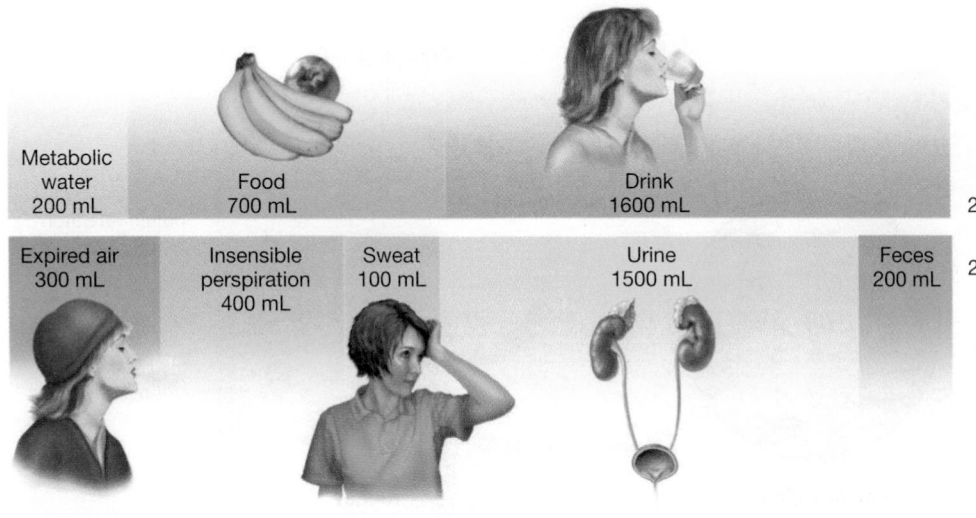

Metabolic water 200 mL
Food 700 mL
Drink 1600 mL

Expired air 300 mL
Insensible perspiration 400 mL
Sweat 100 mL
Urine 1500 mL
Feces 200 mL

Intake 2500 mL/day
Output 2500 mL/day

FIGURE 11.3 Daily water balance. An average healthy adult consumes and produces approximately 2500 mL of water and eliminates about 2500 mL of water daily. A healthy person's average daily water input equals his or her average daily losses.

Kidneys and Water Balance

The kidneys are the major regulator of the body's water content and ion concentrations. In a healthy person, the kidneys maintain proper hydration by filtering excess ions from blood as it flows through the kidneys. When the kidneys remove ions such as sodium, water follows and becomes the main component of urine. If more watery fluids are consumed than the body needs, the kidneys excrete the excess water in urine.

The amount of urine a person produces is determined primarily by his or her total water intake. A healthy person produces about 1 to 2 quarts (1 to 2 L) of urine per day.[1] Healthy kidneys can form more urine, but they become less efficient at urine production when fluid intakes are less than about 2 cups (500 mL) per day.

Kidneys also remove waste products, such as urea, from the bloodstream. Sometimes, minerals and waste products collect into crystals that enlarge and form a hard mass called a kidney stone (Fig. 11.4). As a kidney stone moves out of the kidney and enters the tube leading to the bladder, it can cause considerable pain and bloody urine until it passes out of the body. Pain management and hydration are important in the treatment of kidney stones. However, a kidney stone that is large enough to block the urinary tract requires emergency treatment to remove or break it down. For more information on kidney stones, visit the National Institute of Diabetes and Digestive and Kidney Diseases website at www.kidney.niddk.nih.org.

Hormones, Enzymes, and Water Balance

Antidiuretic hormone (ADH) and **aldosterone** (*al–dahs′–te–rown*) are two hormones that participate in the body's efforts to maintain fluid balance. In response to dehydration, the posterior pituitary gland in the brain releases antidiuretic hormone. Antidiuretic hormone stimulates the kidneys to conserve water. Additionally, the adrenal glands secrete aldosterone. Aldosterone signals the kidneys to reduce the elimination of sodium in urine, and as a result, the kidneys return this mineral to the general circulation. Because water follows sodium, it is conserved as well. Figure 11.5 summarizes the effects of antidiuretic hormone and aldosterone on the kidneys.

The *renin–angiotensin system* also regulates blood volume and blood pressure (Fig. 11.6). The kidneys secrete the enzyme **renin** in response to low blood volume and falling blood pressure. Renin then activates the conversion of a protein synthesized in the liver, angiotensinogen, to angiotensin I. Angiotensin I is inactive and must be converted to angiotensin II, a reaction that primarily occurs in the lungs through the action of *angiotensin–converting enzyme* (*ACE*). **Angiotensin II** (1) stimulates the release of aldosterone from the adrenal glands

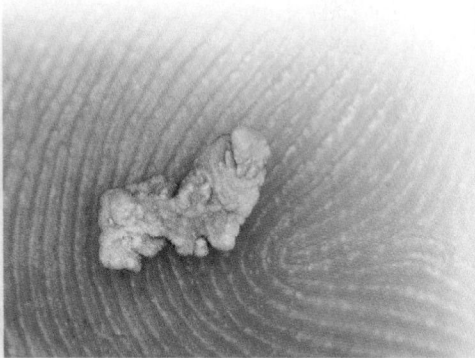

FIGURE 11.4 Kidney stones. Kidney stones typically are tiny crystals of a calcium-containing compound.

antidiuretic hormone (ADH) hormone secreted from pituitary glands in response to dehydration; stimulates kidneys to conserve water

aldosterone hormone secreted from adrenal glands in response to dehydration; stimulates kidneys to conserve sodium and water

renin enzyme secreted in response to low blood volume and falling blood pressure

angiotensin II protein secreted in response to low blood volume and falling blood pressure

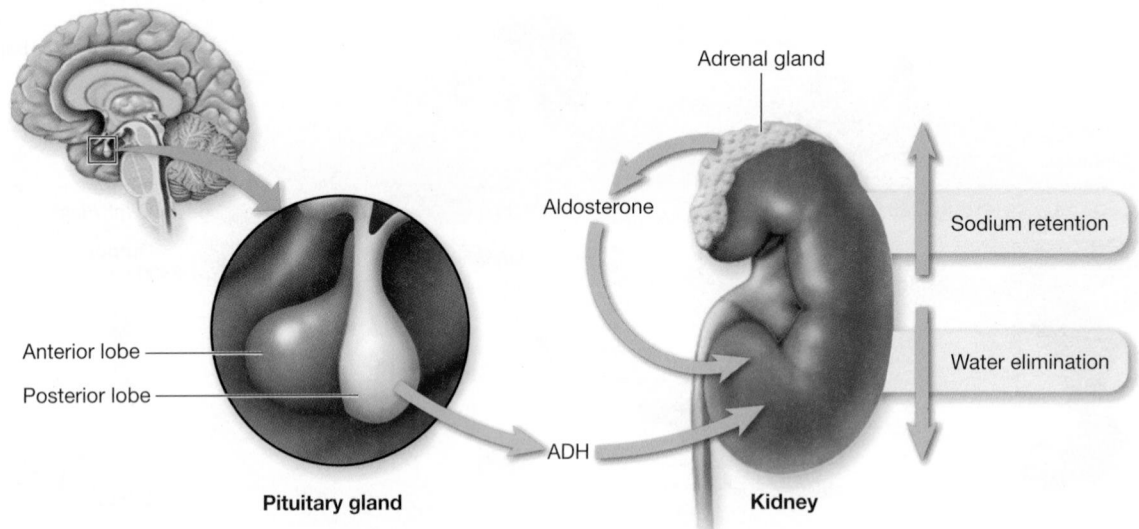

FIGURE 11.5 Effects of antidiuretic hormone and aldosterone on kidneys. In response to dehydration, the posterior pituitary gland in the brain secretes antidiuretic hormone (ADH), which signals the kidneys to conserve water. Additionally, the adrenal glands secrete the hormone aldosterone. Aldosterone reduces urinary excretion of sodium. When the kidneys retain sodium, they return the mineral and water to the general circulation.

vasoconstrictor substance that contributes to the constriction of blood vessels

(Fig. 11.6) and (2) acts as a **vasoconstrictor**, a substance that contributes to the constriction of blood vessels, which causes an increase in blood pressure.

Hydration Status

The simplest way to determine if an individual is consuming enough water is to observe the volume of his or her urine. When fluid intake is adequate, the kidneys produce enough urine to maintain fluid balance. If fluid consumption is more than needed, the kidneys eliminate the excess, and the body produces plenty of urine. If fluid intake is limited or the body loses high amounts of fluid, such as through heavy perspiration, the kidneys produce only small amounts of urine.

In addition to urine volume, the color of urine may be a useful indicator of hydration status. Straw–colored (light yellow) urine can indicate adequate hydration, whereas dark–colored urine may be a sign of dehydration. However, the color of urine is not always a reliable guide for judging a person's hydration status.[8] It is important to recognize that having a urinary tract infection or ingesting certain medications, foods, and dietary supplements, especially those containing the B vitamin riboflavin, can alter urine's color.

FIGURE 11.6 Renin-angiotensin system. The enzyme renin is secreted by the kidneys in response to low blood volume and falling blood pressure.

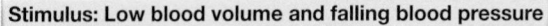

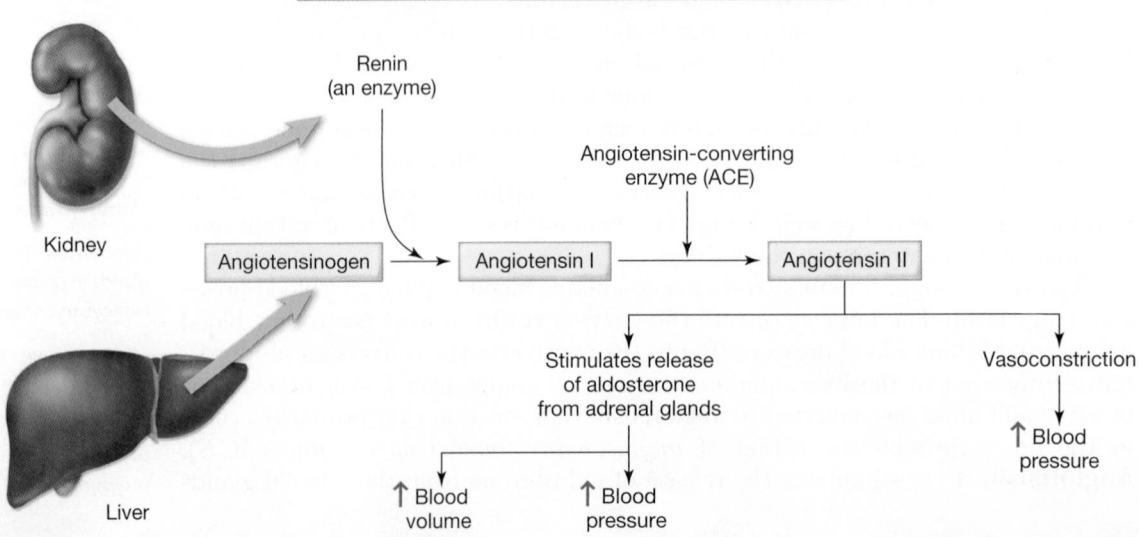

Dehydration

Despite the body's mechanisms to balance its water content, some fluid is constantly being lost, primarily via the skin and lungs. If a person does not consume enough fluids to replace that water, dehydration can occur. Table 11.3 summarizes the most common signs of dehydration.

Rapid weight loss is one of the primary and initial signs of dehydration. Every 16 ounces (about 0.5 L) of water that the body loses represents a pound of body weight. When an individual loses 1 to 2% of his or her usual body weight in fluids, the person feels fatigued and thirsty. For example, if a woman weighs 150 pounds and her weight drops 3 pounds after exercising in hot conditions, she has lost 2% of her body weight, primarily as water weight.

As the loss of body water approaches 4% of body weight, muscles lose considerable amounts of strength and endurance. By the time body weight is reduced by 7 to 10% as a result of body fluid losses, severe weakness results. At a 20% reduction of body weight, coma and death are likely.

Thirst is the primary regulator of fluid intake in most people.[1] The thirst response alerts the person to replenish water that was lost by sweating and other means, before severe dehydration occurs. The majority of healthy people meet their AI for water by letting thirst be their guide.[4] However, people who are dehydrated and older than 60 years of age do not sense thirst as accurately as younger adults.[9] Furthermore, older adults may be more susceptible to developing dehydration than younger persons, because as kidneys age, they become less able to conserve water when fluid intakes are low.[10] Therefore, it may be necessary to remind older adults to drink more fluids, especially when they are physically active or in warm conditions.[11] Nevertheless, healthy older adults are generally able to maintain adequate hydration.[9]

Athletes and other people who work or exercise outdoors, especially in hot conditions, also need to stay properly hydrated to avoid dehydration and heat-related illnesses such as heat exhaustion. These individuals should not rely on thirst alone as a regulator for fluid intake. Rather, regular consumption of fluids before, during, and after exercise is necessary to prevent dehydration. Chapter 15 provides information about heat-related illnesses.

Treating Dehydration People who are sick, especially children with fever, vomiting, diarrhea, and increased perspiration, may need to be given specially prepared solutions of water and electrolytes, called **oral rehydration therapy**, to prevent dehydration. More serious cases of dehydration require intravenous (IV) fluids.[12] The immediate goals of both oral rehydration therapy and IV fluids are to restore blood volume, correct tissue fluid balance, and maintain rehydration.[13]

Diuretics and Dehydration Caffeine is a **diuretic**, a substance that increases urine production. Coffee, tea, "energy" drinks, and soft drinks often contain caffeine or caffeine-related compounds. However, the water consumed in caffeinated beverages is not completely lost in urine, so drinking these fluids can still contribute to meeting a person's water needs.[3]

Alcohol is also a diuretic. Normally, ADH signals the kidneys to conserve water. Alcohol, however, inhibits ADH secretion from the pituitary gland in the brain, enabling the kidneys to eliminate more urine than normal.[3] Alcohol consumption actually results in urinary water losses that are greater than the volume of fluid consumed. Therefore, alcohol contributes to dehydration.

Water Intoxication

There is no Upper Limit (UL) for water.[4] **Water intoxication**, however, can occur when an excessive amount of water is consumed in a short time period or the kidneys have difficulty filtering water from blood. The excess water dilutes the sodium concentration of blood, disrupting water balance and resulting in

TABLE 11.3 Common Signs of Dehydration

Rapid weight loss
Dry or sticky mouth
Low or no urine output
Dark urine
No tears
Sunken eyes
Vomiting and/or diarrhea

oral rehydration therapy specially prepared solutions of water and electrolytes used to prevent and treat dehydration

diuretic substance that increases urine production

water intoxication condition that occurs when too much water is consumed in a short time period or kidneys have difficulty filtering water from blood

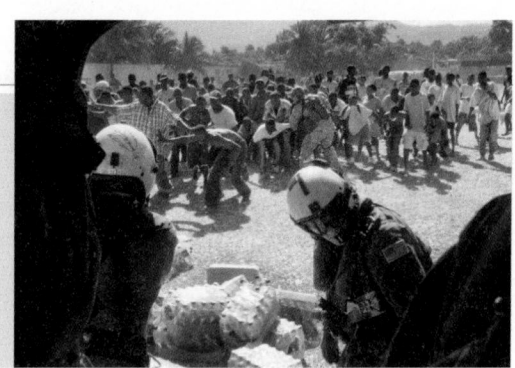

hyponatremia low blood sodium

major minerals essential mineral elements required in amounts of 100 mg or more per day

trace minerals essential mineral elements required in amounts that are less than 100 mg per day

hyponatremia (low blood sodium). As a result of the imbalance, too much water moves into cells, including brain cells. Signs and symptoms of water intoxication may include dizziness, headache, confusion, inability to coordinate muscular movements, bizarre behavior, and seizures.[15] If the condition is not detected early and treated effectively, coma and death can result.

Healthy people rarely drink enough water to become intoxicated. However, water intoxication can develop in people with disorders that interfere with the kidney's ability to excrete water normally. Marathon runners who consume large amounts of plain water in an effort to keep hydrated during competition may be at risk of water intoxication. Chapter 15 discusses the importance of proper hydration and electrolyte balance for athletes.

ASSESS YOUR PROGRESS

4 *Discuss the ways the body loses water.*

5 *Describe how antidiuretic hormone, aldosterone, and the renin-angiotensin system help maintain fluid balance in the body.*

6 *How much water do healthy young men and women need to consume daily (AI values)?*

7 *Identify at least three signs of dehydration.*

8 *Describe treatment options for dehydration in children.*

9 *Why does alcohol act as a diuretic?*

10 *Identify at least three signs of water intoxication.*

11.3 Minerals: The Basics

LEARNING OUTCOMES

1 *Explain the difference between major and trace minerals.*

2 *Classify mineral nutrients as major, trace, or possible essential nutrients.*

3 *Describe key roles of minerals in the human body.*

4 *List good food sources of minerals.*

About 15 mineral elements have known functions in the body and are necessary for human health. The body requires these particular micronutrients in milligram or microgram amounts. The essential minerals are classified into two groups: **major minerals** and **trace minerals** (Table 11.4). If the average adult needs 100 mg or more of a mineral per day, the mineral is classified as a major mineral;

TABLE 11.4 Minerals with Known or Possible Roles in the Body*

Major Minerals	Trace Minerals	Possible Essential Minerals
Calcium (Ca)	Chromium (Cr)	Arsenic (As)
Chloride (Cl⁻)	Fluoride (F⁻)†	Boron (B)
Magnesium (Mg)	Copper (Cu)	Lithium (Li)
Phosphorus (P)	Iodine (I)	Nickel (Ni)
Potassium (K)	Iron (Fe)	Silicon (Si)
Sodium (Na)	Manganese (Mn)	Vanadium (V)
Sulfur (S)	Molybdenum (Mo)	
	Selenium (Se)	
	Zinc (Zn)	

*Chemical symbol is shown in parentheses next to mineral's name.

†Although fluoride is not essential, the mineral plays an important role in strengthening teeth and bones.

otherwise, the micronutrient is a trace mineral. The body also contains very small amounts of other minerals, such as nickel and arsenic. The essential nature of this particular group of minerals has not been fully determined.

Several minerals, including lead and mercury, are often found in the human body, but they are environmental contaminants that have no known function and can cause toxicity. Unlike vitamins, minerals are indestructible. Because minerals cannot be destroyed, heating a food or exposing it to most other environmental conditions does not affect the food's mineral content. However, minerals are water soluble, and they can leach out of a food and into cooking water. By using the cooking water to make soups or sauces, minerals from the food can be retained that would otherwise be discarded.

Functions of Minerals

Essential minerals have many roles in the body (Fig. 11.7). Some minerals form inorganic structural components of tissues, such as calcium and phosphorus in bones and teeth. Minerals may also function as inorganic ions, substances that have negative or positive charges (see Appendix B). For example, calcium ions (Ca^{2+}) participate in blood clotting, and sodium ions (Na^+) help maintain fluid balance. Some ions, such as magnesium (Mg^{2+}) and copper (Cu^{2+}), are cofactors. A **cofactor** is an ion or small molecule that an enzyme requires to function. Many minerals are components of enzymes, hormones, or other organic molecules, such as cobalt in vitamin B−12 and iron in hemoglobin. Although cells cannot metabolize minerals for energy, certain minerals are involved in the chemical reactions that release energy from macronutrients.

In some instances, a person consumes more minerals than his or her body needs, but the excess is excreted, primarily in urine or feces. In other instances, the person's body stores the extra minerals in the liver, bones, or other tissues. Toxicity signs and symptoms occur when excess minerals accumulate in the body to such an extent that they interfere with the functioning of cells. Under normal conditions, the human body does not store large quantities of most minerals, and it loses small amounts of these essential nutrients every day.

cofactor ion or small molecule that an enzyme requires to function

Sources of Minerals

Most foods contain small amounts of minerals; Figure 11.8 (on page 353) indicates food groups from MyPlate that are generally rich sources of various minerals. The digestive tract, however, does not absorb 100% of the minerals in foods or

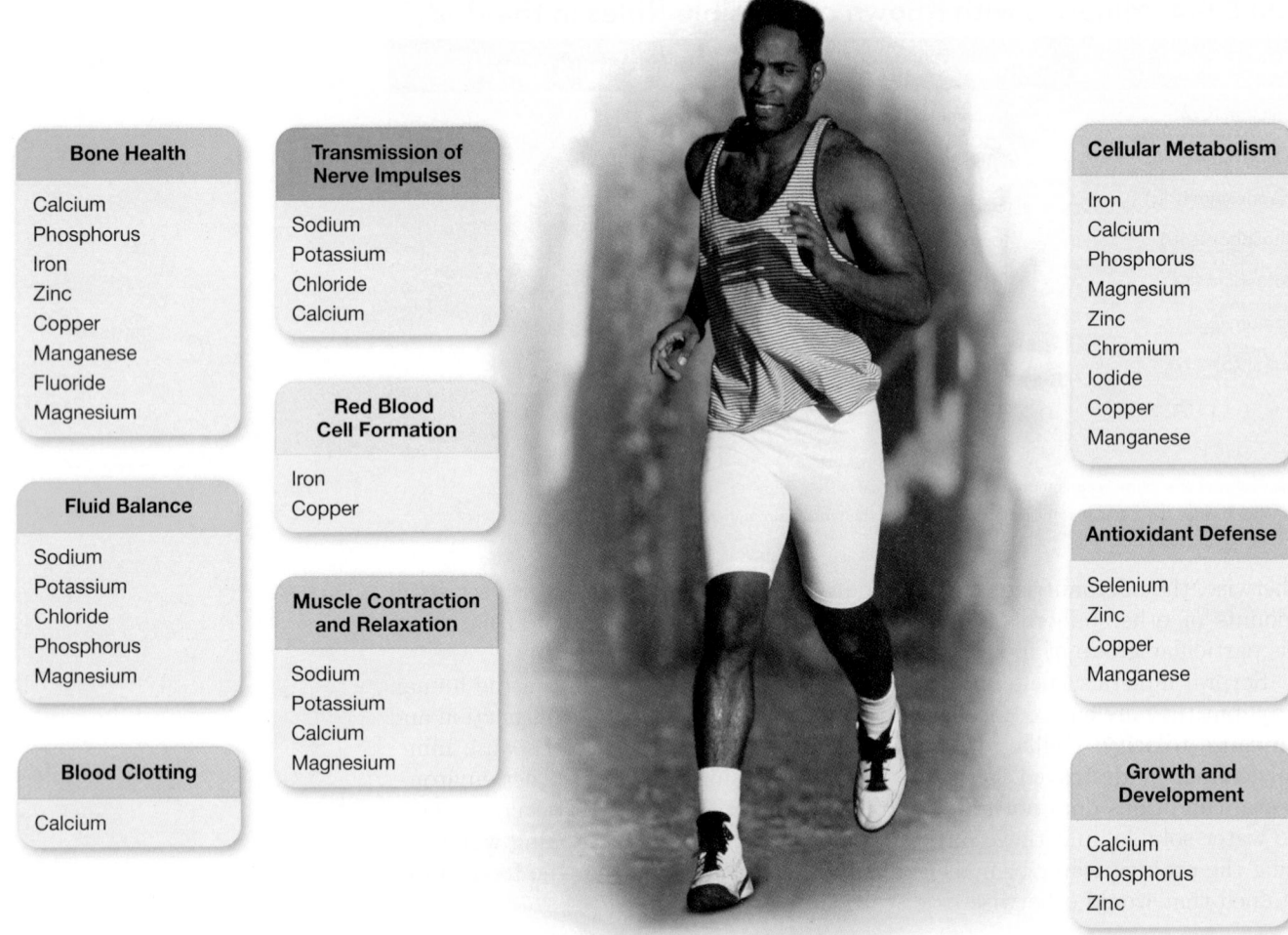

Bone Health

Calcium
Phosphorus
Iron
Zinc
Copper
Manganese
Fluoride
Magnesium

Fluid Balance

Sodium
Potassium
Chloride
Phosphorus
Magnesium

Blood Clotting

Calcium

Transmission of Nerve Impulses

Sodium
Potassium
Chloride
Calcium

Red Blood Cell Formation

Iron
Copper

Muscle Contraction and Relaxation

Sodium
Potassium
Calcium
Magnesium

Cellular Metabolism

Iron
Calcium
Phosphorus
Magnesium
Zinc
Chromium
Iodide
Copper
Manganese

Antioxidant Defense

Selenium
Zinc
Copper
Manganese

Growth and Development

Calcium
Phosphorus
Zinc

FIGURE 11.7 Minerals and their functions. Groups of minerals work together to maintain good health.

dietary supplements. Bioavailability, the body's ability to absorb and use minerals, depends on many factors. A major factor is the body's need for the mineral. In general, a mineral's bioavailability increases during periods of growth, such as infancy and puberty, and during pregnancy and breastfeeding.

Compared to plant foods, animal foods tend to be more reliable sources of minerals, such as iron and calcium. Why? Animal products often have higher concentrations of these minerals, with the exception of magnesium and manganese. Although plants foods may contain minerals, these foods may often contain **phytic** (*fite′−ik*) **acid** or **oxalic** (*awk−sal′−ik*) **acid**, naturally occurring substances that interfere with mineral absorption. Phytic acid is a compound in whole grains and in certain seeds and beans. Spinach, collard greens, and sweet potatoes have high amounts of oxalic acid. In fact, rhubarb leaves are toxic because they contain such high amounts of this chemical.

In general, the more processing a plant food undergoes, the lower its natural mineral content. Cereal grains, for example, naturally contain selenium, zinc, copper, and some other minerals, but these micronutrients are lost during refining. Iron is the only mineral added to grains during enrichment. To obtain a variety of minerals, people should follow MyPlate recommendations (see Chapter 3).

Other Sources of Minerals

The tap water in many communities may be a source of minerals that people may overlook. "Hard" water naturally contains a variety of minerals, including

phytic acid compound found in grains, seeds, and beans that interferes with mineral absorption

oxalic acid substance found in spinach, collard greens, and sweet potatoes that interferes with mineral absorption

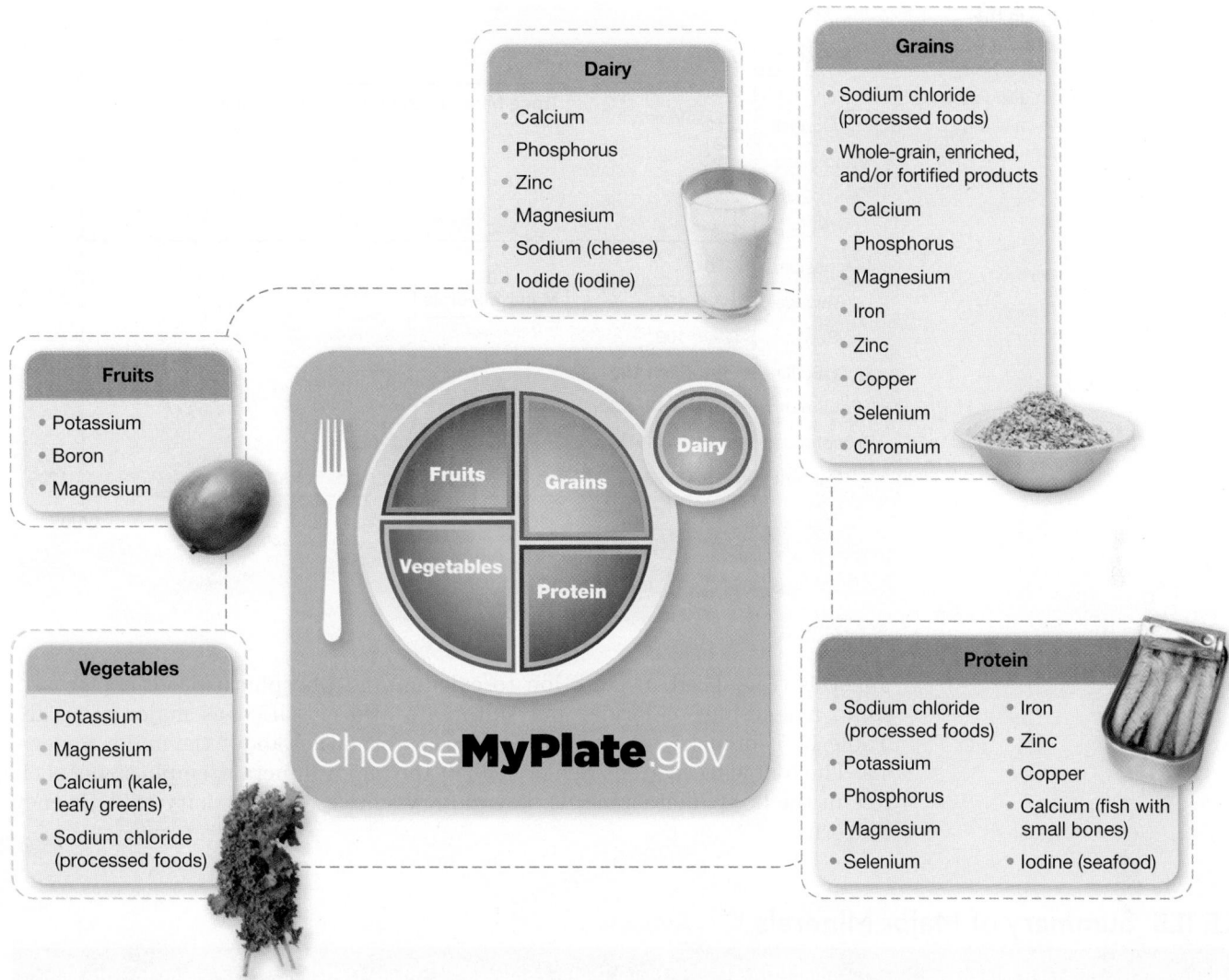

FIGURE 11.8 MyPlate: Food sources of minerals. Each MyPlate food group contributes minerals to the diet.

calcium, magnesium, sulfur, iron, and zinc. Water with high mineral content often tastes and smells unpleasant. Many people drink bottled water as a substitute for tap water because they think bottled water tastes better and is safer. More information on bottled water is available in Chapter 19.

Dietary supplements are another source of minerals. A daily multiple vitamin and mineral supplement is generally safe for healthy people, because a dose of this type of supplement does not provide high amounts of minerals. However, people need to be careful when taking dietary supplements that contain individual minerals, such as iron or selenium. Single-mineral supplements are usually unnecessary unless they are medically prescribed to treat a specific condition, including iron deficiency. An excess of one mineral can also interfere with the absorption or metabolism of other minerals. For example, a large amount of zinc can decrease copper absorption in the intestinal tract.

Major Minerals

Major minerals are called "major" not because of their relative importance to health, but because they are needed in greater amounts in the diet and are stored in larger quantities in the body than are trace minerals. The human body has higher concentrations of calcium and phosphorus than other

FIGURE 11.9 Mineral storage in the body. Major minerals are stored in a higher concentration in the adult body than trace minerals. The most abundant mineral in the human body is calcium, followed by phosphorus, both of which are predominately stored in the skeleton.

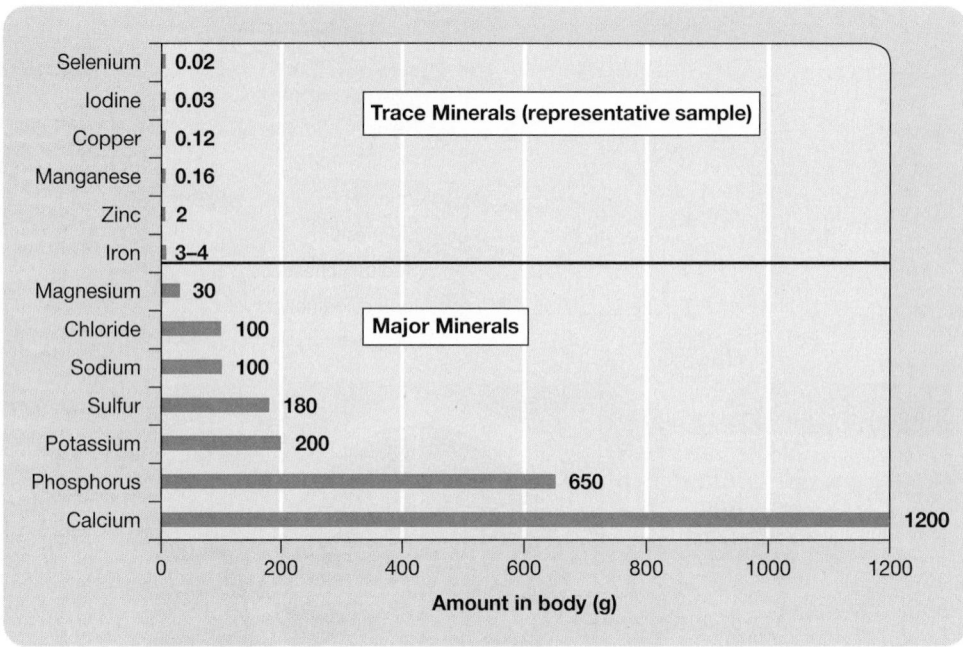

minerals (Fig. 11.9). In addition to calcium and phosphorus, sodium, potassium, magnesium, chloride, and sulfur are also classified as major minerals. Table 11.5 summarizes nutrition-related information about the major minerals. The following sections review each of the major minerals, emphasizing their role in the body, dietary needs, key dietary sources, and toxicity or deficiency concerns.

TABLE 11.5 Summary of Major Minerals

Mineral	Major Functions in the Body	Adult RDA/AI (adult RDA = bold)	Major Dietary Sources	Major Deficiency Signs and Symptoms	Major Toxicity Signs and Symptoms
Calcium (Ca)	• Structural component of bones and teeth • Blood clotting • Transmission of nerve impulses • Muscle contraction • Regulation of metabolism	**1000–1200 mg**	Milk and milk products, canned fish, tofu made with calcium sulfate, leafy vegetables, calcium-fortified foods such as orange juice	• Increased risk of osteoporosis • May increase risk of hypertension	UL = 2.0 to 2.5 g/day • Intakes > 2.5 g/day may cause kidney stones and interfere with absorption of other minerals.
Sodium (Na)	• Maintenance of proper fluid balance • Transmission of nerve impulses • Muscle contraction • Transport of certain substances into cells	1500 mg (19–50 years of age)	Table salt; luncheon meats; processed foods; pretzels, chips, and other snack foods; condiments; sauces	• Muscle cramps	UL = 2300 mg/day • Contributes to hypertension in susceptible individuals • Increases urinary calcium losses
Potassium (K)	• Maintenance of proper fluid balance • Transmission of nerve impulses • Maintenance of acid-base balance	4700 mg	Fruits, vegetables, milk, meat, legumes, whole grains	• Irregular heartbeat • Muscle cramps	No UL has been determined. • Slowing of heart rate that can result in death

Continued

Mineral	Major Functions in the Body	Adult RDA/AI (adult RDA = bold)	Major Dietary Sources	Major Deficiency Signs and Symptoms	Major Toxicity Signs and Symptoms
Magnesium (Mg)	• Strengthens bone • Cofactor for certain enzymes • Heart and nerve functioning	Men: **400–420 mg** Women: **310–320 mg**	Wheat bran, green vegetables, nuts, chocolate, legumes	• Muscle weakness and pain • Poor heart function	UL = 350 mg/day medication-related • Diarrhea
Phosphorus (P)	• Structural component of bones and teeth • Maintenance of acid-base balance • Component of DNA, phospholipids, and other organic compounds	**700 mg**	Dairy products, processed foods, soft drinks, fish, baked goods, meat	• None reported	UL = 4 g/day • Poor bone mineralization
Chloride (Cl)	• Maintenance of proper fluid balance • Production of stomach acid • Transmission of nerve impulses • Maintenance of acid-base balance	2300 mg (19–50 years of age)	Processed foods, salty snacks, table salt	• Convulsions (observed in infants)	UL = 3600 mg/day • Hypertension (because of the association with sodium in sodium chloride [table salt])
Sulfur (S)	• Component of organic compounds such as certain amino acids and vitamins	None	Protein-rich foods	• None reported	• Unlikely from dietary sources

ASSESS YOUR PROGRESS

11 *What is the primary difference between a major mineral and a trace mineral?*

12 *List the seven major minerals.*

13 *Name at least three different functions of minerals in the body, and provide an example of a mineral that performs each function.*

14 *Discuss factors that influence mineral bioavailability.*

11.4 Calcium

LEARNING OUTCOMES

1 *Explain the major functions of calcium in the human body.*

2 *Describe the roles of hormones in maintaining blood calcium homeostasis.*

3 *List the major food sources of calcium.*

4 *Discuss calcium deficiency and toxicity signs and symptoms.*

5 *Explain the relationship between calcium and certain chronic diseases.*

Calcium is the most plentiful mineral element in the human body. Although the body needs calcium to form bones and teeth, the mineral is also involved in muscle contraction, blood clot formation, nerve impulse transmission, and cell

FIGURE 11.10 Thyroid and parathyroid glands. The thyroid gland has the four parathyroid glands embedded in the back (posterior) of the organ. Hormones secreted by the thyroid and parathyroid glands help regulate blood calcium levels.

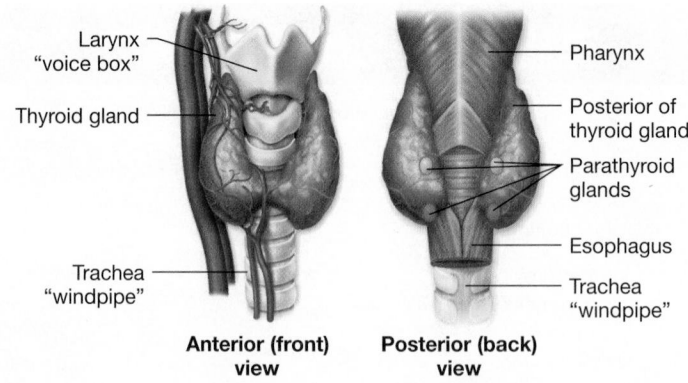

Larynx "voice box"

Thyroid gland

Trachea "windpipe"

Pharynx

Posterior of thyroid gland

Parathyroid glands

Esophagus

Trachea "windpipe"

Anterior (front) view

Posterior (back) view

metabolism. Additionally, calcium may play important roles in maintaining a healthy blood pressure and immune system.

Maintaining Normal Blood Calcium Levels

The body has complex hormonal systems that maintain calcium homeostasis. The thyroid and parathyroid glands secrete certain hormones that help regulate blood calcium levels (Fig. 11.10). In response to falling blood calcium levels, the parathyroid glands secrete parathyroid hormone (PTH), which signals special bone cells called **osteoclasts** to tear down bone tissue. This process releases calcium from bones so the mineral can enter the bloodstream. PTH also works with vitamin D to increase intestinal calcium absorption and reduce calcium excretion in urine (Fig. 11.11).

When the level of calcium in blood is too high, the thyroid gland secretes the hormone **calcitonin** (*cal′−sih−toe−nin*). As shown in Figure 11.11, calcitonin signals another type of bone cell **(osteoblasts)** to remove excess calcium from blood and build bone tissue. Bone formation involves the incorporation of a crystalline structure that contains calcium and phosphorus, called **hydroxyapatite**, on the framework of bone tissue. As this process of **bone mineralization** continues, bone tissue gains strength and rigidity.

osteoclasts bone cells that tear down bone tissue

calcitonin hormone secreted by the thyroid gland when blood calcium levels are too high

osteoblasts bone cells that add bone to where the tissue is needed

hydroxyapatite crystalline structure that forms on the collagen protein complex as bone is made

bone mineralization process by which bone tissue gains strength and rigidity

Sources of Calcium

Table 11.6 lists some foods that are among the richest sources of calcium. Milk products, such as fluid milk, yogurt, and cheese, provide about 75% of the calcium in American diets.[16] Moreover, the calcium in milk products is well absorbed and used by the body. Not all products made from milk are rich sources of calcium. Milk loses about half of its calcium content when it is processed to make cottage cheese, for example (Table 11.6). Although butter, sour cream, and cream cheese are made from whole milk, people generally do not eat enough of these high−fat foods to contribute much calcium to their diets.

Good plant sources of calcium include broccoli and leafy greens, especially kale, collard, turnip, bok choy, and mustard greens. Nevertheless, the calcium in plant foods is generally not as bioavailable as the calcium in milk and milk products. For example, 1 cup of fat−free milk supplies almost 300 mg of calcium, and about 30% of the calcium in milk is bioavailable.[18] A cup of raw spinach supplies 30 mg of calcium, but only about 13% of that amount is bioavailable. Figure 11.12 shows how much spinach, broccoli, and kale a person would need to eat to obtain about the same amount of calcium that is in 1 cup of fat−free milk.

Calcium is added to a variety of foods, including fortified orange juice, margarine, soy milk, cereals, and breakfast bars. Another source of calcium is

Bone remodeling occurs throughout life, and as a result of this process, most of your skeleton is replaced about every 10 years.[17]

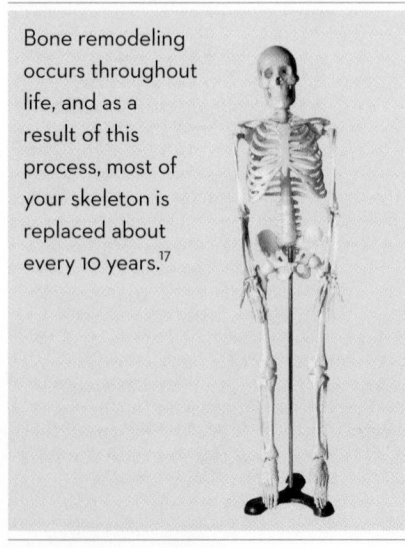

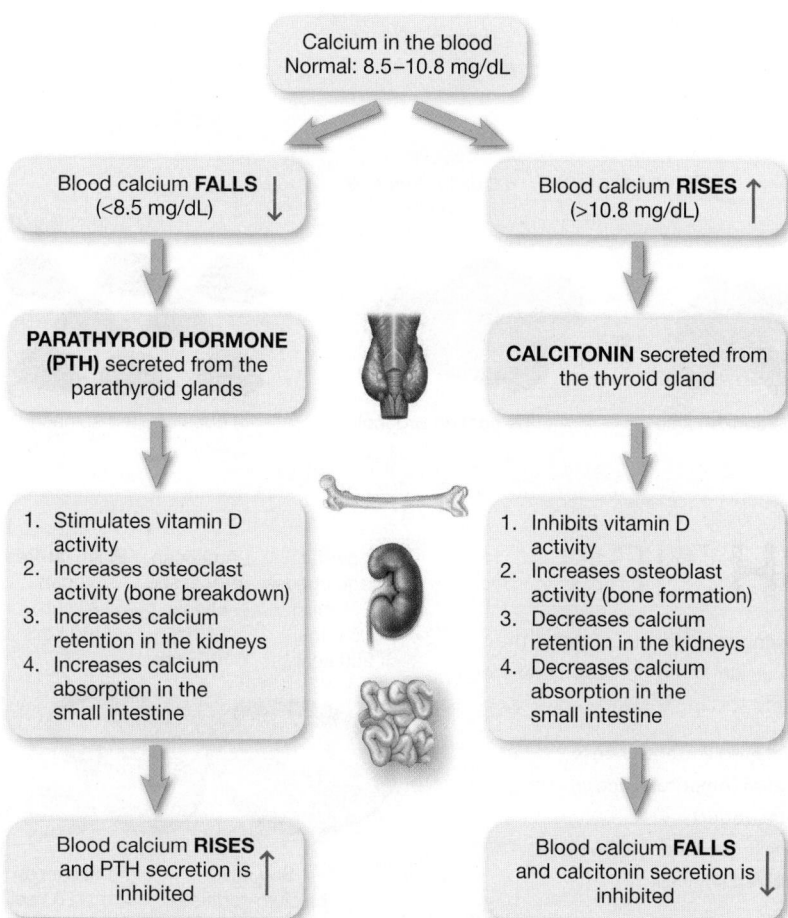

Calcium in the blood
Normal: 8.5–10.8 mg/dL

Blood calcium **FALLS** ↓
(<8.5 mg/dL)

Blood calcium **RISES** ↑
(>10.8 mg/dL)

**PARATHYROID HORMONE
(PTH)** secreted from the
parathyroid glands

CALCITONIN secreted from
the thyroid gland

1. Stimulates vitamin D
   activity
2. Increases osteoclast
   activity (bone breakdown)
3. Increases calcium
   retention in the kidneys
4. Increases calcium
   absorption in the
   small intestine

1. Inhibits vitamin D
   activity
2. Increases osteoblast
   activity (bone formation)
3. Decreases calcium
   retention in the kidneys
4. Decreases calcium
   absorption in the
   small intestine

Blood calcium **RISES** ↑
and PTH secretion is
inhibited

Blood calcium **FALLS** ↓
and calcitonin secretion is
inhibited

FIGURE 11.11 Effects of parathyroid hormone and calcitonin on blood calcium levels. Parathyroid hormone (PTH) and calcitonin work together to maintain blood calcium homeostasis. When blood calcium levels fall, the parathyroid gland secretes PTH. PTH stimulates vitamin D activity and increases osteoclast activity, calcium retention in the kidneys, and calcium absorption in the small intestine. When blood calcium levels rise, calcitonin is secreted from the thyroid gland. Calcitonin inhibits vitamin D, increases osteoblast activity, and decreases calcium retention in the kidneys and calcium absorption in the small intestine.

TABLE 11.6 Calcium Content of Selected Foods

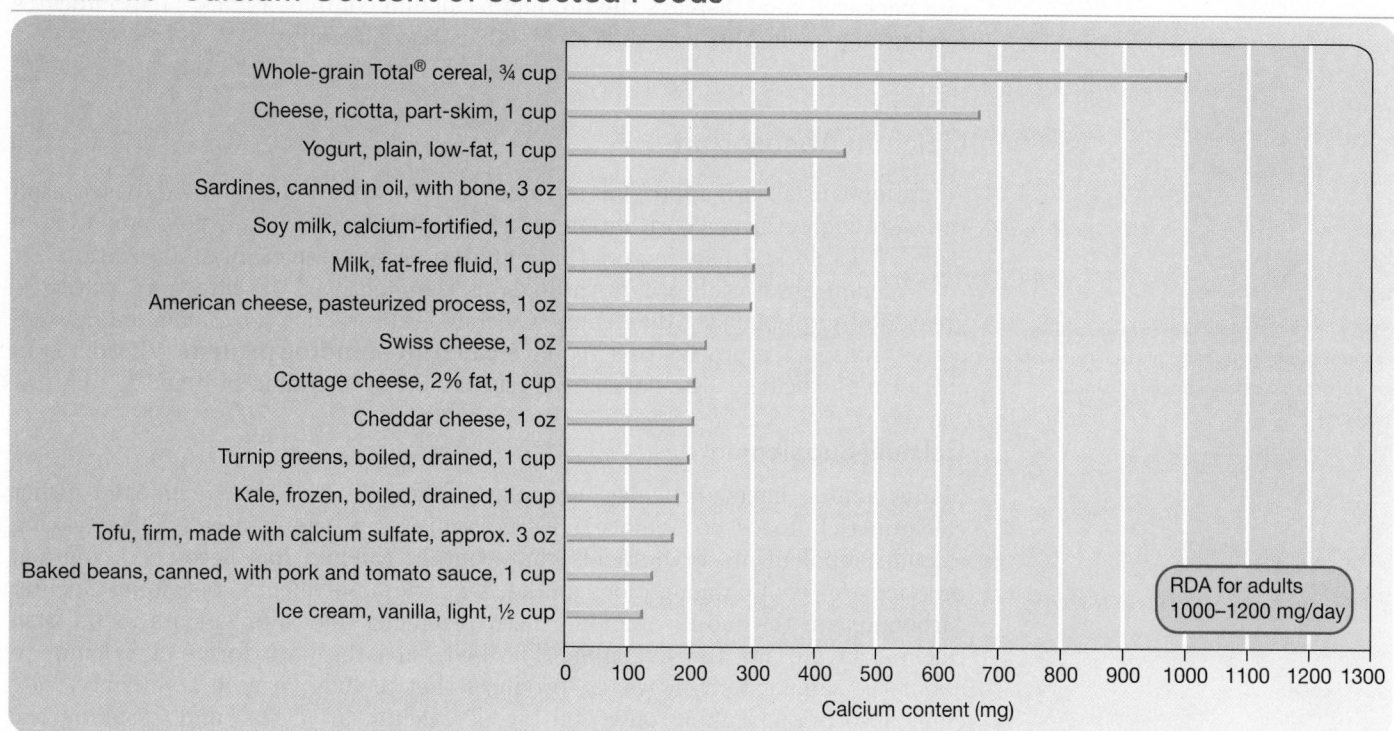

RDA for adults
1000–1200 mg/day

Calcium content (mg)

Source: Data from U.S. Department of Agriculture, Agricultural Research Service: *USDA national nutrient database for standard reference*, release 26, 2013.

FIGURE 11.12 Calcium bioavailability of various foods. To obtain approximately the same amount of calcium that is in 8 fluid ounces of fat-free milk, an individual would need to consume the amounts of the foods shown.

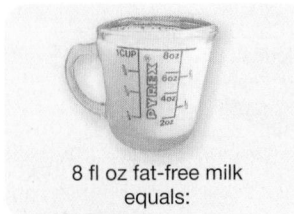

8 fl oz fat-free milk equals:

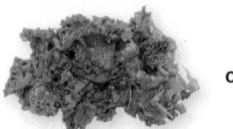   or   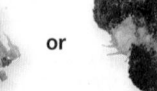   or   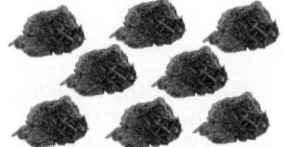

1 ½ cups cooked kale   2 ¼ cups cooked broccoli   8 cups cooked spinach

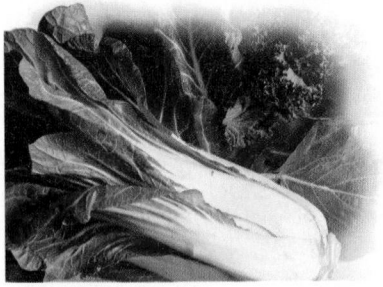

Certain leafy vegetables, such as bok choy and collard greens, contain calcium that is bioavailable.

FRESH TIPS

Each of the following foods contains about the same amount of calcium that is in 1 cup of fat-free milk (approximately 300 mg):

1.5 cups low-fat (2% milk) cottage cheese
1 oz processed cheese (American cheese)
⅔ cup plain, low-fat yogurt
1.5 oz natural cheese (e.g., cheddar or Swiss)
1 cup calcium-fortified soy milk

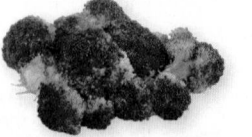

Low-fat cottage cheese (2% milk) 1.5 cups, 200 kcal

American processed cheese 1 oz, 100 kcal

Plain, fat-free yogurt ⅔ cup, 100 kcal

Soy milk, calcium-fortified 1 cup, 80 kcal

Natural cheese 1.5 oz, 170 kcal

---

soybean curd (tofu) that is made with calcium sulfate. The Nutrition Facts panel of a packaged food displays the product's calcium content. Figure 11.13 indicates food groups from MyPlate that are good sources of calcium.

Calcium Absorption

Adult humans absorb approximately one-third of the calcium in food. Absorption rates are higher in newborn infants (55%), children (50%), and pregnant women (65%).[18] Table 11.7 lists factors that enhance or decrease calcium absorption.

Calcium absorption occurs throughout the length of the intestines, with the greatest absorption in the duodenum. Calcium is absorbed in the duodenum through active transport, a process that requires **calcium–binding protein**. Vitamin D in the form of calcitriol stimulates synthesis of calcium–binding protein.

Calcium Supplements

Many adults have difficulty consuming enough milk products and other calcium–rich foods to achieve adequate intake of the mineral. Thus, taking calcium supplements or antacids that contain calcium has become a common practice, especially among older adults. Dietary supplements containing calcium carbonate are the most commonly used products, and supplements made with calcium citrate are also available. The body absorbs both forms of calcium to about the same extent, however, products that include vitamin D enhance cal–cium absorption. Taking only 500 mg of calcium at a time and ingesting the supplement with meals also improves the mineral's absorption.

calcium-binding protein protein necessary for absorption of calcium in the small intestine

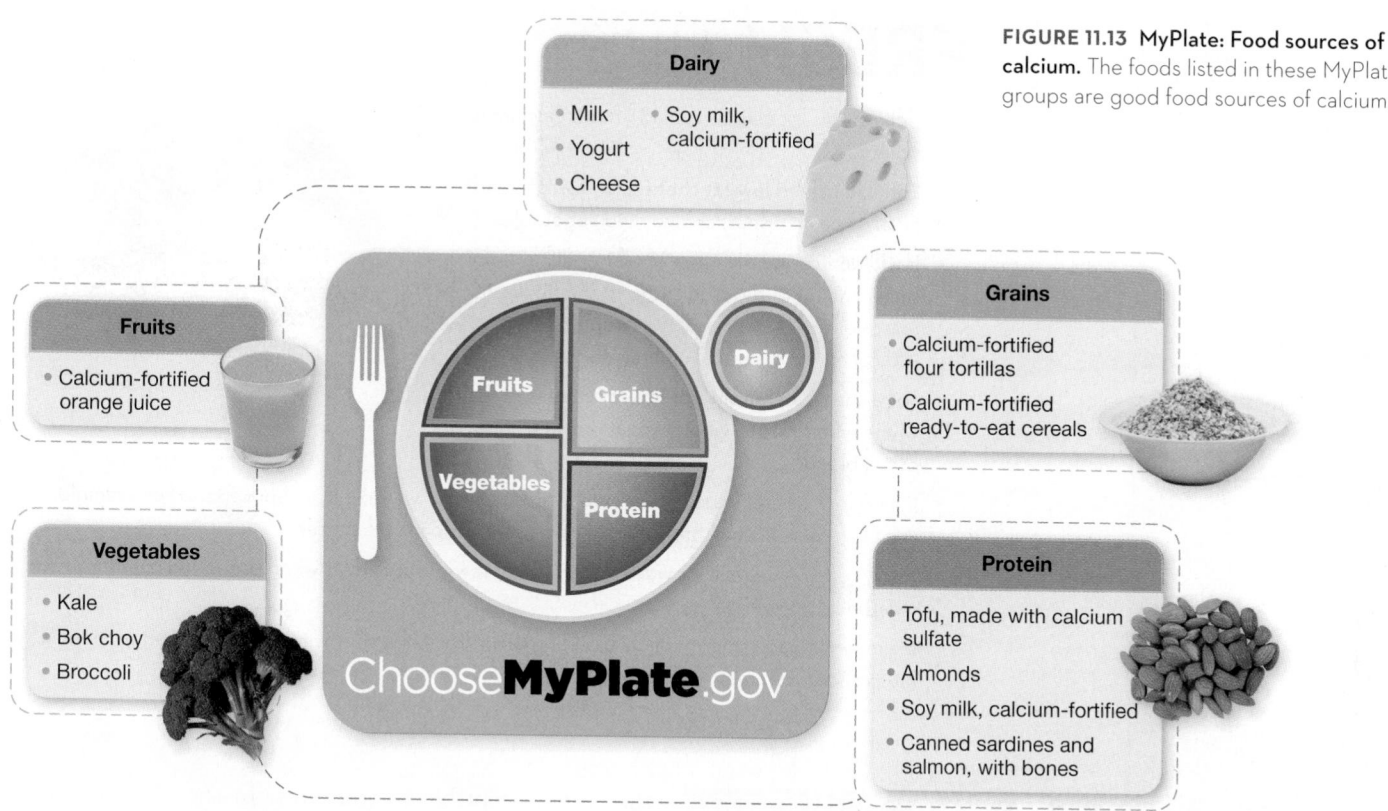

FIGURE 11.13 MyPlate: Food sources of calcium. The foods listed in these MyPlate groups are good food sources of calcium.

Dietary Adequacy

The adult RDA for calcium ranges from 1000 to 1200 mg/day.[19] For children and adolescents between the ages of 9 and 18, the RDA is higher (1300 mg/day) to allow for increases in bone mass during growth and development. In the United States, average calcium intakes were approximately 1116 mg/day for men and 868 mg/day for women in 2011–2012.[20] According to the Dietary Guidelines, calcium is a "nutrient of public health concern." Total vegetarians (vegans) and people who are lactose intolerant are at risk of calcium deficiency, because they often avoid consuming milk and milk products, which are the most reliable dietary sources of calcium.[18]

Calcium Deficiency

Osteoporosis is a chronic disease characterized by low bone mass and reduced bone structure (Fig. 11.14).[20] People with osteoporosis have **osteopenia**, weak bones

TABLE 11.7 Factors That Influence Calcium Absorption

Enhances Calcium Absorption	Decreases Calcium Absorption
Vitamin D (calcitrol)	Vitamin D deficiency
Stomach acid	Reduced stomach acid secretion
Lactose (only in infants)	Phytic and oxalic acid intake
	High fiber intake
	High phosphorus intake
	Chronic diarrhea
	Fat malabsorption

DID **YOU** KNOW?

Many brands of antacids contain calcium carbonate. An antacid pill that contains 750 mg of calcium carbonate provides 300 mg of elemental calcium. Consumers should avoid taking too many antacids or other calcium supplements because of the potential risk of toxicity.

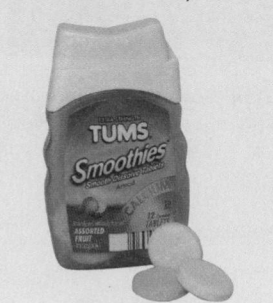

osteoporosis chronic disease characterized by bones with low mass and reduced structure

osteopenia condition in which a person has weak bones that are susceptible to fracture

FRESH TIPS

The following suggestions can add more calcium to your diet:

- Sprinkle grated low-fat cheeses on top of salads, bean or pasta dishes, and cooked vegetables.

- If you do not like the taste of plain milk, try adding a small amount of flavored syrup to the beverage. Two teaspoons of "lite" chocolate syrup add 50 kcal and some trace minerals to the milk.

- For a snack, melt a slice of low-fat cheese on half a whole-wheat bagel, whole-wheat crackers, or a slice of rye bread.

- If a recipe calls for water, substitute fat-free milk for water, if it is appropriate. For example, use fat-free milk when making cooked oatmeal or pancake batter.

- Add ¼ cup nonfat milk powder to 1 pound of raw ground meat when preparing hamburgers, meatballs, or meatloaf.

- Make homemade smoothies by blending plain, low-fat yogurt with fresh or frozen fruit and fat-reduced ice cream or sherbet.

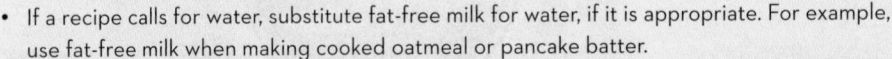

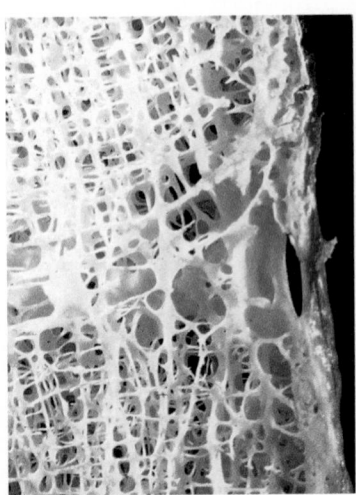 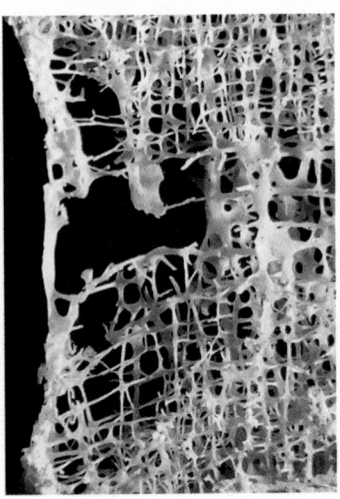

FIGURE 11.14 Bone tissue. Normal spine tissue is on the left; the spine tissue on the right is from a person with osteoporosis.

that are susceptible to fractures. In the United States, osteoporosis is a major public health problem. As many as 10 million Americans who are 50 years of age or older have osteoporosis, and another 34 million are at risk of the disease because they have low bone mass.[21] Most people with osteoporosis are older adult women.

Each year, an estimated 1.5 million Americans experience an osteoporosis–related fracture. Half of women and one–fourth of men who are over 50 years of age will have such a fracture at some point.[21] Many people do not realize that they are developing osteoporosis and their bones are becoming weaker, until they experience a fracture. People with osteoporosis may break a bone by falling, or they may experience spontaneous fractures, in which a fragile bone gives way for no apparent reason. Osteoporosis–related fractures often involve the vertebrae, hip, wrist, or ankle bones. In severe cases, bones in the upper spine fracture and then heal in an abnormally curved position, giving the obvious "widow's hump" appearance associated with osteoporosis (Fig. 11.15).

Fractures, especially hip fractures, can be devastating events for older adults. Only about 15% of older people who break their hip can walk without assistance 6 months after the fracture occurred.[21] Moreover, about 25% of older Americans who experience a broken hip die within 1 year of the injury. Most deaths result from complications after surgery to repair the broken hip.

Causes of Osteoporosis Several factors contribute to bone loss and osteoporosis. Family history of osteoporosis, cigarette smoking, and excessive alcohol consumption are associated with increased risk of the disease. Table 11.8 lists these and other risk factors for osteoporosis. The interactive osteoporosis risk test at the International Osteoporosis Foundation's website (http://www.iofbonehealth.org/iof–one–minute–osteoporosis–risk–test) can help you determine whether you or someone you know is at risk for the disease.

TABLE 11.8 Risk Factors for Osteoporosis

Non-modifiable Risk Factors	Modifiable Risk Factors
Female	Having anorexia nervosa
Growing older	Having low estrogen levels (women) or low testosterone levels (men)
Having white or Asian ancestry	Following diets that contain inadequate amounts of calcium and vitamin D
Having a family history of osteoporosis	Using medications such as steroids or some types of anticonvulsants (antiseizure drugs)
Having a small, thin-boned body frame	Being physically inactive
	Smoking cigarettes
	Consuming excessive alcohol

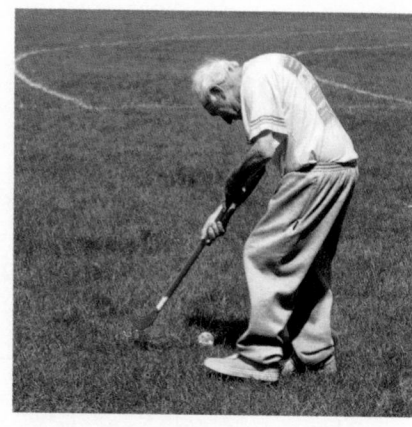

FIGURE 11.15 Osteoporosis. In many people with severe osteoporosis, bones in the upper spine fracture and then heal in an abnormally curved position.

By 20 years of age, healthy young men and women have acquired 85 to 90% of their adult bone mass **(peak bone mass)**.[21] Loss of bone mass begins in mid-adulthood as levels of testosterone and estrogen ("sex hormones"), which are needed for normal bone development and maintenance, begin to decline. In women, however, the rate of bone loss increases significantly after *menopause*; that is, after menstrual cycles have ceased. At this time of life, women have the highest risk of osteoporosis. After menopause, a woman's ovaries produce less estrogen, and as a result, her rate of bone loss exceeds the rate of bone replacement. A simple way to monitor bone mass is by tracking height. Losing an inch or more of adult height may be the first sign that a person has experienced tiny fractures of the spine due to osteoporosis.[21] If osteoporosis is suspected, a person can undergo painless x-ray bone testing to determine the extent of bone loss. People who are at high risk or who already have osteoporosis may require prescription medication to reduce their rate of bone loss.

peak bone mass present when bones have their maximum strength

hypercalcemia high blood calcium

Reducing the Risk of Osteoporosis Efforts to reduce the risk of osteoporosis should begin early to maximize peak bone mass. Proper diet and regular exercise are especially important from early childhood through late adolescence, because the body actively builds bone during these life stages. Exposing skin to sunlight can stimulate the body's ability to form vitamin D, but some people will need to take calcium and vitamin D supplements. Exercise training, especially performing weight-bearing activities, increases bone mass, because contracting muscles keep tension on bones, which stimulates bone-building activity.[22] Table 11.9 lists examples of weight-bearing and non-weight-bearing activities.

These older adults are performing t'ai chi, a weight-bearing activity that can improve balance and may reduce the likelihood of falling.

Calcium Toxicity

The UL for calcium is 2000 to 2500 mg/day for adults.[19] Normally, the small intestine prevents too much calcium from being absorbed. However, taking too many calcium-containing antacids or supplements or drinking too much vitamin D–fortified milk can result in excessive calcium absorption and hypercalcemia. **Hypercalcemia** (*hyper* = excess; *calcemia* = calcium in the blood) is a condition characterized by a higher-than-normal concentration of calcium in blood. Signs and symptoms of hypercalcemia include kidney stones, bone pain, muscle weakness, fatigue, and hypertension.[23] Treatment for hypercalcemia may include avoiding vitamin D and calcium supplements to reduce calcium absorption.

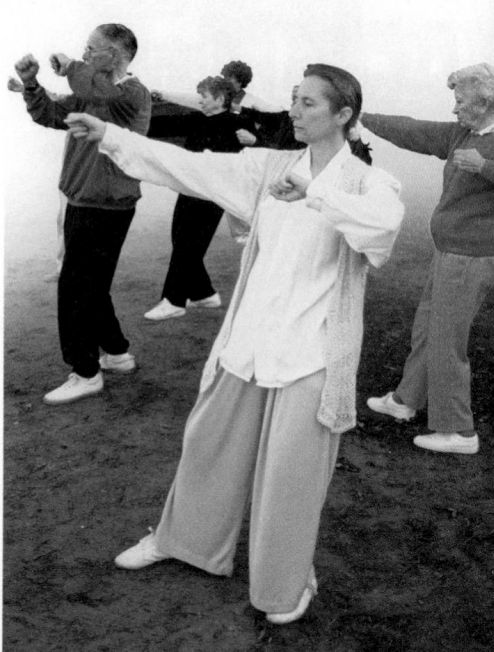

TABLE 11.9 Examples of Weight-Bearing and Non-Weight-Bearing Activities

Weight-bearing	Non-weight-bearing
Low-impact aerobics	Lying in bed
Basketball	Swimming
Running or jogging	Water aerobics
Walking	Cycling
Jumping rope	Traveling in reduced-gravity situations (e.g., space flight)
Dancing	
Hiking	
Stair climbing	
Strength training with weights	
Tennis and other racket sports	

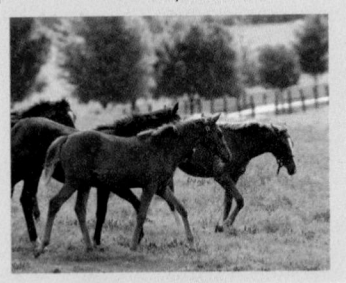

Calcium, Heart Disease, and Weight Control

Calcium—rich diets have beneficial effects on heart disease risk factors, including hypertension, insulin resistance, chronic inflammation, and abnormal blood lipid levels.[24,25] Although dietary calcium may protect against heart disease, calcium supplements have actually been associated with an increased risk of cardiovascular disease (CVD).[26]

Dietary sources of calcium may also be associated with successful weight loss and improved body composition. A high—calcium diet may increase fat breakdown, accelerating fat loss.[27] However, more research is needed to clarify whether calcium intake can reduce the risk of heart disease and aid weight loss efforts.

ASSESS YOUR PROGRESS

15 *Describe at least two key functions of calcium in the human body.*

16 *Compare the specific actions of parathyroid hormone and calcitonin on calcium metabolism.*

17 *List food sources of bioavailable calcium.*

18 *Identify risk factors, symptoms, and treatment for osteoporosis.*

11.5 Phosphorus

LEARNING OUTCOMES

1 *Explain major functions of phosphorus in the human body.*

2 *List rich food sources of phosphorus.*

3 *Discuss phosphorus deficiency and toxicity signs and symptoms.*

Phosphorus is the second most abundant mineral in the body, making up about 1% of a person's total body weight. Approximately 85% of phosphorus is found in combination with calcium as part of bones and teeth. Although phosphorus is concentrated in the skeleton, the mineral is essential for every cell in the human body. Phosphorus is needed to:

- Synthesize adenosine triphosphate (ATP) and creatine phosphate, substances that are essential for energy production;
- Synthesize phospholipids, DNA, and RNA;
- Regulate acid–base balance; and
- Activate many enzymes and hormones necessary for energy metabolism.

Food Sources of Phosphorus

Dairy foods, meat, and cereal grains are the primary sources of phosphorus in the typical American diet. Table 11.10 lists some foods that are good sources of phosphorus. Notice that fruits and vegetables are generally poor sources of the mineral. Figure 11.16 shows food groups that are naturally good sources of phosphorus.

The bioavailability of phosphorus is dependent on whether the nutrient is from plant or animal foods and if it is present in the organic or inorganic form. Plant foods, such as seeds and beans, generally contain organic phosphorus, including phytate. Phytate inhibits the absorption of phosphorus from such foods. Inorganic phosphorus, which is predominately in animal foods, is more bioavailable than the organic forms.[27]

Dietary Adequacy

The Recommended Dietary Allowance (RDA) for phosphorus for both adult males and females is 700 mg/day. The average American consumes well above the RDA, approximately 1400 mg/day.[5] Individuals who eat high amounts of protein–rich foods tend to consume the most phosphorus. Phosphorus deficiencies

TABLE 11.10 Phosphorus Content of Selected Foods

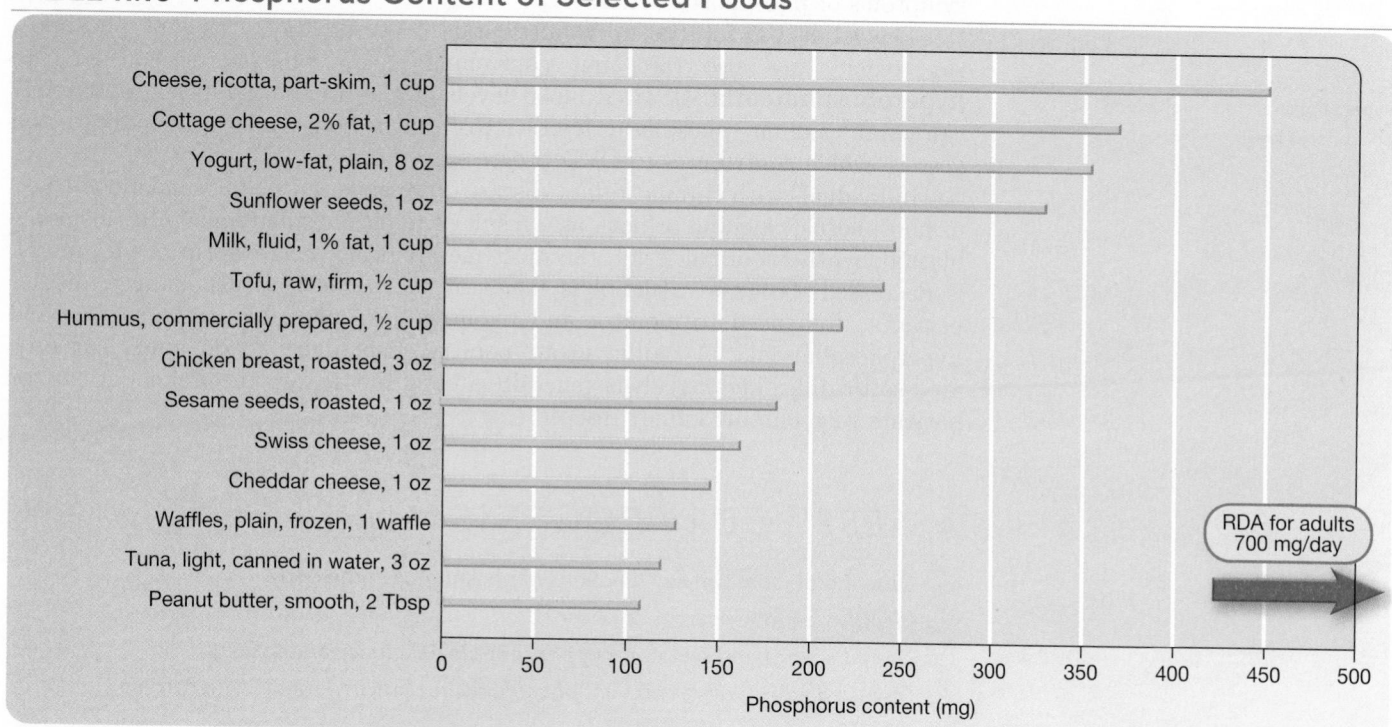

Source: U.S. Department of Agriculture, Agricultural Research Service, USDA Nutrient Data Laboratory: *USDA national nutrient database for standard reference*, release 26, 2013.

FIGURE 11.16 MyPlate: Food sources of phosphorus. The foods listed in these MyPlate groups are good food sources of phosphorus

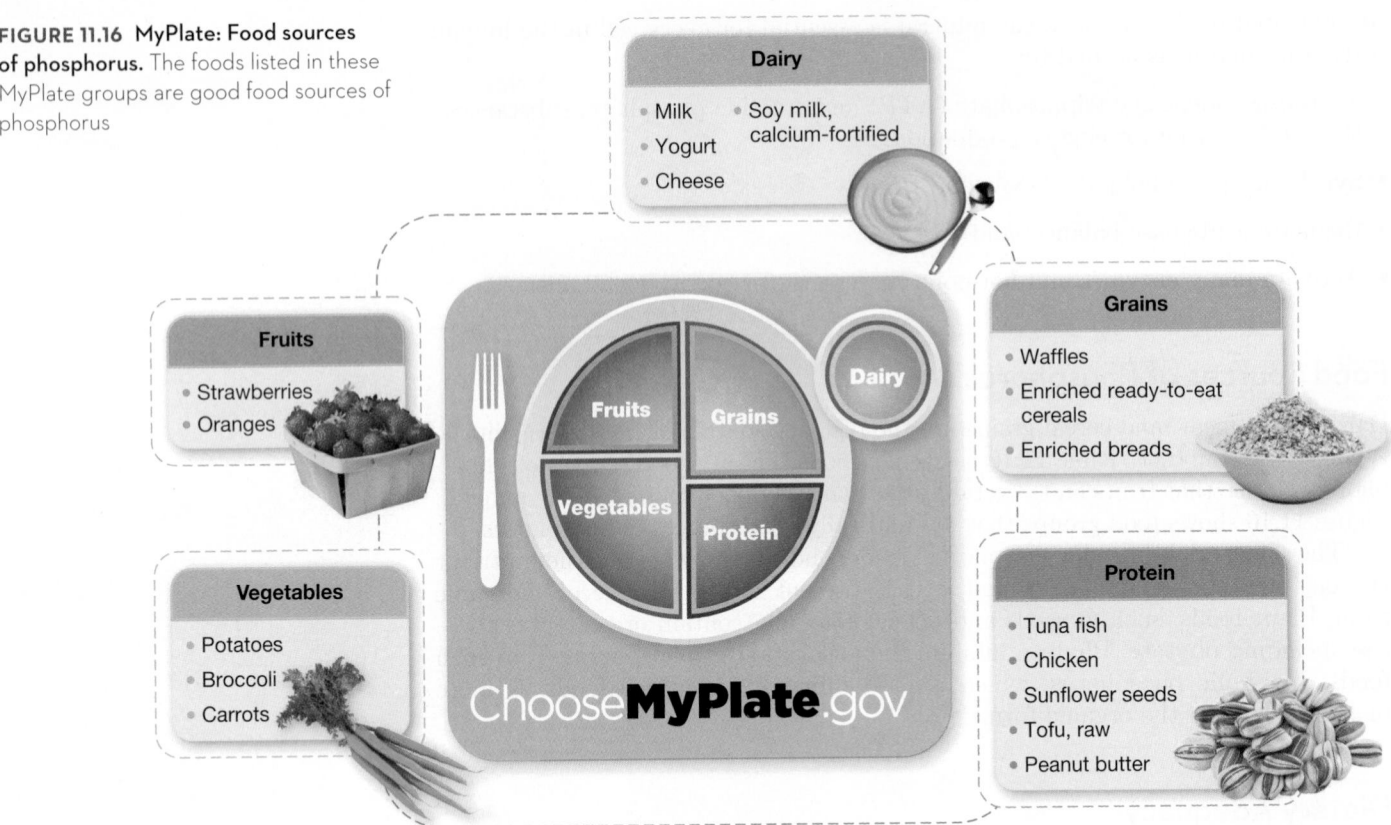

Dairy
- Milk
- Yogurt
- Cheese
- Soy milk, calcium-fortified

Fruits
- Strawberries
- Oranges

Vegetables
- Potatoes
- Broccoli
- Carrots

Grains
- Waffles
- Enriched ready-to-eat cereals
- Enriched breads

Protein
- Tuna fish
- Chicken
- Sunflower seeds
- Tofu, raw
- Peanut butter

are rare. However, when present, a phosphorus deficiency leads to bone loss and decreased bone mineralization and strength. Children who are deficient in phosphorus experience symptoms of rickets. Poor appetite, weight loss, fatigue, muscle pain, weakened immune system, and bone pain are also typical signs and symptoms of phosphorus deficiency.

The adult UL for the micronutrient is 4000 mg/day. Cases of phosphorus toxicity are also rare, but consuming excess phosphorus can lead to **hyperphosphatemia**, elevated blood levels of the mineral. Hyperphosphatemia can cause calcium–phosphate deposits to form in body tissues, including blood vessels, which contributes to CVD progression.[29]

Individuals with chronic kidney disease often experience abnormal blood levels of phosphorus, calcium, or both as a result of hyperphosphatemia.[30] In this population, synthesis of calcitriol, the most metabolically active form of vitamin D, is decreased, because calcitriol is made in the kidneys. Thus, kidney–disease patients often need to monitor and regulate their phosphorus intake to avoid hyperphosphatemia. Avoiding meat, poultry, fish, dairy foods, nuts, carbonated soft drinks, and cereals is generally among the dietary recommendations for patients with chronic kidney disease.

hyperphosphatemia high blood phosphorus level

ASSESS YOUR PROGRESS

19 *Describe at least two key functions of phosphorus in the body.*

20 *Identify rich food sources of phosphorus.*

21 *Describe signs and symptoms of phosphorus deficiency and toxicity.*

22 *Discuss dietary ways to prevent phosphorus toxicity in patients with chronic kidney disease.*

11.6 Sodium

LEARNING OUTCOMES

1 *Explain the major functions of sodium in the human body.*
2 *List rich food sources of sodium.*
3 *Discuss common causes and typical treatment of hyponatremia.*
4 *Describe hypertension, including symptoms, risk factors, prevention, and treatment.*

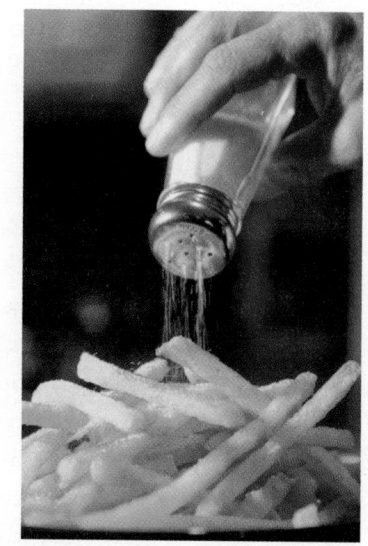

Salt is the primary source of sodium in American diets. The chemical commonly called "table salt" or simply "salt" is actually sodium chloride, a compound comprised of two minerals, sodium and chloride. A teaspoon of table salt supplies 2325 mg of sodium. The human digestive tract absorbs almost all of the sodium that is in foods and beverages. Unless otherwise noted, we refer to sodium chloride simply as "salt" or "table salt."

As mentioned in the "Water" section of this chapter, sodium plays a major role in maintaining normal fluid balance. This mineral is also necessary for the transmitting impulses by nerves, normal functioning of muscles, and transporting small substances such as glucose and amino acids into cells.

Food Sources of Sodium

Most uncooked vegetables, raw meats, and grain products are naturally low in sodium. Thus, most of the sodium Americans consume is from the salt that is added to food during processing, during preparation, or at the table. As a food additive, salt enhances flavors and can prevent the growth of microorganisms responsible for food spoilage. Other common sodium–containing food additives include sodium nitrate, sodium citrate, and *monosodium glutamate (MSG)*, a seasoning that may be added to foods served in Chinese restaurants. Salted snack foods, French fries, canned and dried soups, sauces and gravies, hot dogs and "deli" meats, cheeses, and pickled foods are high in sodium (Table 11.11). Frequent consumption of these foods often leads to higher–than–recommended intakes of sodium. Although sodium is an essential mineral, diets that contain high amounts of sodium are associated with increased risk of hypertension. The American Heart Association, in collaboration with federal agencies, has led efforts to reduce the amount of sodium in the food supply. Several food manufacturers and restaurants have been proactive and voluntarily lowered the sodium content of their products and menu items.[31]

DID **YOU** KNOW?

Between 2005 and 2011, the sodium content of processed foods declined by approximately 3.5%. In some of these products, the sodium content was reduced by over 30%. However, the sodium content of fast-food restaurant foods increased by 2.6% during this same time period.[32]

Dietary Adequacy

Humans require only about 180 mg of sodium per day, but the AI for adults under 51 years of age is 1500 mg/day. The AI for sodium does not apply for people who perspire heavily, such as marathon runners, or people who work in extremely hot conditions.[4] Sweat contains small amounts of sodium, chloride, and some other minerals. Thus, people who perspire heavily can lose large amounts of these minerals in their sweat.

Sodium Deficiency

The typical North American diet supplies far more sodium than the AI amount, and as a result, the average person is unlikely to develop hyponatremia. Although a healthy body is able to regulate its sodium concentration effectively, hypo–natremia can occur in certain situations. While engaging in endurance phys-ical activities, athletes may need to consume sports drinks containing sodium and other electrolytes to avoid dehydration and sodium depletion. Hyponatremia can also result from severe diarrhea or vomiting, and infants are especially at

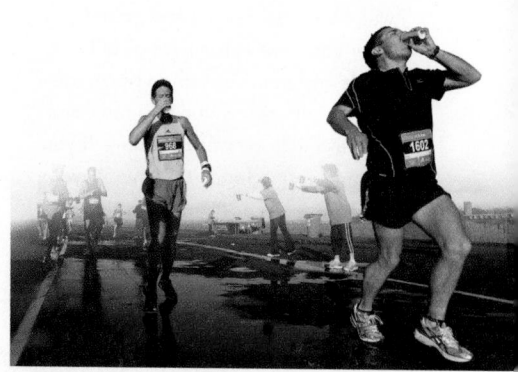

TABLE 11.11 Sodium Content of Selected Foods

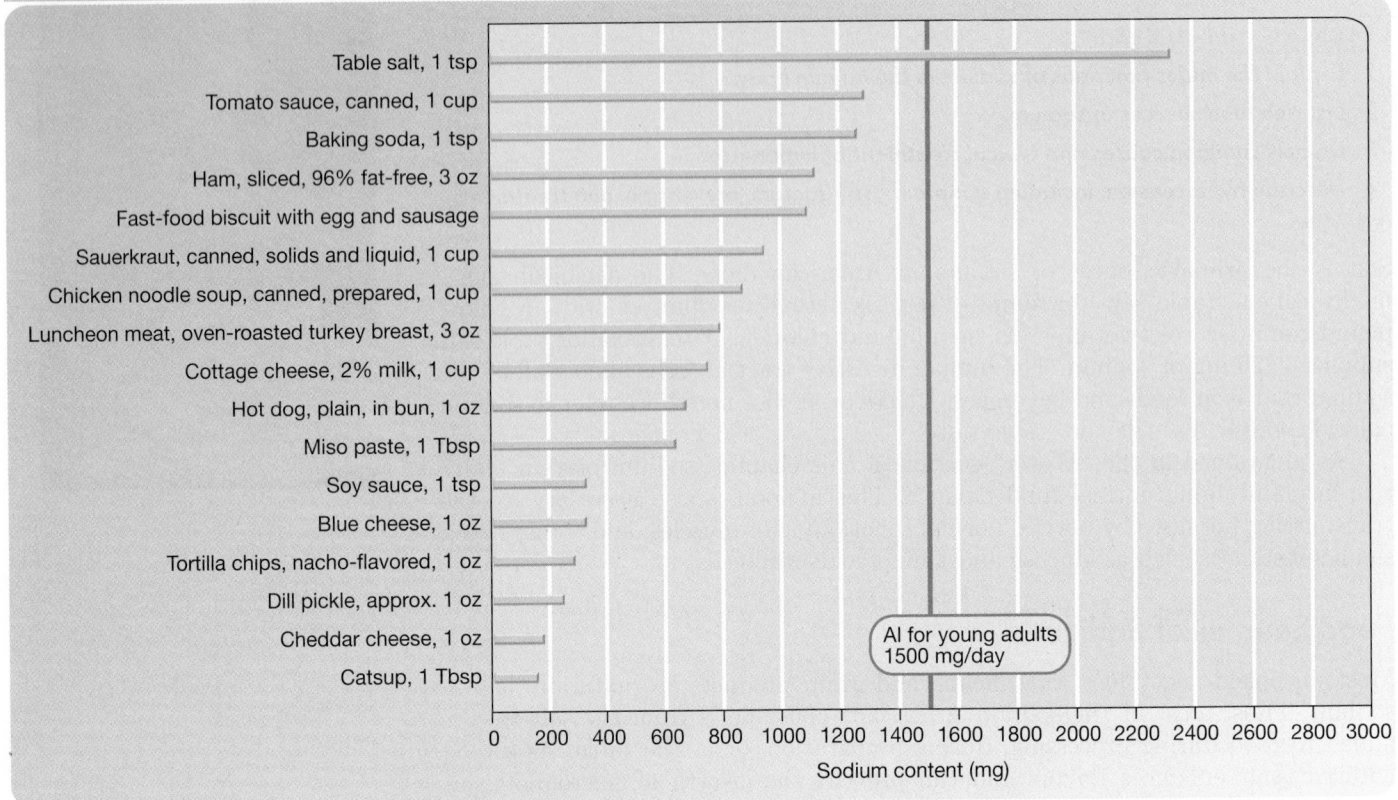

Source: Data from U.S. Department of Agriculture, Agricultural Research Service: *USDA national nutrient database for standard reference,* release 26, 2013.

risk. Symptoms of mild to moderate hyponatremia include weight loss, headache, nausea, vomiting, diarrhea, fatigue, and muscle cramping. Serious hyponatremia can result in seizures, coma, and death if untreated. In such cases, prompt medical care is required to replace lost fluids and electrolytes. Chapter 15 provides additional details about sodium deficiency during physical activity.

Sodium Toxicity

The adult UL for sodium is 2300 mg/day. Americans on average consumed more than 3450 mg of sodium per day in 2011–2012.[20] Most of the typical American's sodium intake comes from food bought in grocery stores, convenience stores, and restaurants. Only 10% of Americans' sodium intake is from salt added at home during food preparation and consumption.[31] A high–sodium diet is associated with increased risk of hypertension, and in some cases, such diets can be a cause of hypertension.[33] A person who is **sodium sensitive** is more likely to develop hypertension as a result of consuming a high–sodium diet than an individual who lacks this sensitivity. The kidneys of a sodium–sensitive person may be unable to eliminate excess sodium as effectively as the kidneys of a healthy person. The excess sodium causes the body to retain water, and blood volume and pressure increase as a result.

Sodium and Hypertension

Hypertension, a condition characterized by persistently elevated blood pressure, is a serious public health problem in the United States. Compared to people with normal blood pressure, hypertensive individuals have greater risk of CVD, especially heart disease and stroke, as well as kidney failure and damage to other organs.[33] Approximately 30% of adult Americans have hypertension.[34] Children

sodium sensitive individual who may develop hypertension as a result of consuming a high-sodium diet

DID YOU KNOW?

Have you ever noticed that your weight increases by a few pounds after you have eaten a lot of salty foods and then consumed beverages? The weight gain is due to a temporary increase in body water volume. If you resume eating foods that supply your usual intake of sodium, your kidneys will eliminate the excess sodium and water in urine within a day. As your body regains its normal fluid balance, your weight also returns to normal.

TABLE 11.12 Categories for Blood Pressure Levels in Adults (Ages 18 years and Older)

	Blood Pressure Levels (Adults)		
	Systolic (mm Hg)		Diastolic (mm Hg)
Normal	< 120	and	< 80
Prehypertension	120–139	or	80–89
Hypertension	≥ 140	or	≥ 90

Source: National Heart, Lung, and Blood Institute: *Your guide to lowering high blood pressure: Categories for blood pressure levels in adults.* ND. http://www.nhlbi.nih.gov/hbp/detect/categ.htm. Accessed: February 2, 2014.

can also develop hypertension; among U.S. adolescents, 22% of boys and 10% of girls have high blood pressure.[35] Justin Steinbruegge, the college student featured in the "Real People, Real Stories" feature on page 369, was 18 when he found out he had hypertension.

Hypertension is often called the "silent killer," because high blood pressure generally does not cause symptoms until the affected person's organs and blood vessels have been damaged. The Centers for Disease Control and Prevention estimates that 20% of adults are not aware that they have hypertension.[34] The best way to detect hypertension is to have regular blood pressure screenings. Because children can develop hypertension, their blood pressure should also be checked regularly, beginning at 3 years of age.

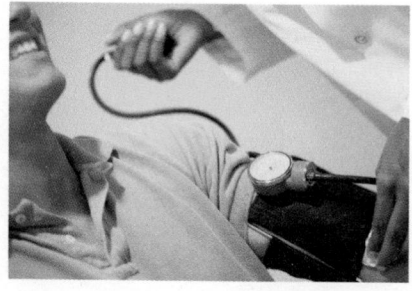

The best way to detect hypertension is to have regular blood pressure screenings.

Blood Pressure Values

When a person's blood pressure is tested, two measurements are taken. The first measurement is the **systolic pressure**, which is the maximum blood pressure within an artery. This value occurs when the ventricles, the heart's pumping chambers, contract. The second measurement is the **diastolic pressure**, which measures the pressure in an artery when the ventricles relax between contractions. The systolic value is always higher than the diastolic value. For adults, healthy blood pressure readings are less than 120/80 millimeters of mercury (mm Hg). Table 11.12 presents categories for blood pressure levels in adults. Systolic and diastolic readings should be recorded and tracked.

Persistent systolic blood pressure readings of 120 mm Hg to 139 mm Hg and diastolic readings of 80 mm Hg to 89 mm Hg are signs of **prehypertension**. People with prehypertension are more likely to develop hypertension than people with normal blood pressure. A person has hypertension when his or her blood pressure persists at systolic values that are greater than or equal to (≥) 140 mm Hg and diastolic values that are ≥ 90 mm Hg (Table 11.12).

Causes of Hypertension

Most cases of hypertension do not have simple causes, but advanced age, African–American ancestry, obesity, physical inactivity, smoking cigarettes, and excessive use of alcohol, and high sodium intake are among the major risk factors for the condition (Table 11.13). Blood pressure usually increases as a person ages, probably in part because of stiffening (*arteriosclerosis*) of the blood vessels. Healthy arteries are flexible tubes that expand with each heartbeat and recoil in between beats. Arteriosclerotic arteries are less flexible and cannot expand as much as healthy arteries. As a result, the heart must work harder to pump blood, and blood pressure becomes chronically elevated.

Health experts generally recommend that Americans limit their sodium consumption. For example, the Dietary Guidelines, recommends less than 2300 mg of sodium daily.[36] That is the amount of sodium in 6 g (about 1 teaspoon)

systolic pressure maximum blood pressure within an artery that occurs when the ventricles contract

diastolic pressure pressure in an artery that occurs when the ventricles relax between contractions

prehypertension persistent systolic blood pressure readings of 120 mm Hg to 139 mm Hg and diastolic readings of 80 mm Hg to 89 mm Hg

TABLE 11.13 Major Risk Factors for Hypertension

Family history
Advanced age
African-American ancestry
Obesity
Physical inactivity
Consuming excess sodium
Cigarette smoking
Consuming excess alcohol
Type 2 diabetes

FRESH TIPS

To reduce sodium intake, consider taking these actions:

- Prepare homemade meals and snacks as much as possible so you have control over your salt intake.

- Do not add salt while preparing foods, even though instructions tell you to "add salt."

- Taste your food before salting it. Adjust to eating foods with less salt in them.

- Do not keep a salt shaker on your table.

- Flavor foods with garlic, citrus juice, and herbs and spices instead of adding salt.

- Use garlic powder and onion powder to flavor foods, instead of "garlic salt" or "onion salt."

- Read the Nutrition Facts panels before purchasing packaged foods to determine sodium contents of the items.

- When ordering items in restaurants, request that no salt be added to your food while it is being prepared.

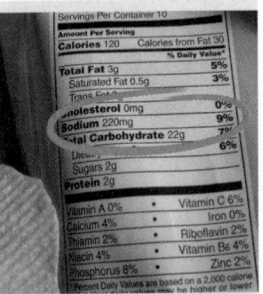

By reading the label, consumers can find foods that have high amounts of added sodium. A serving of these chips provides about 10% of the maximum recommended amount of sodium per day.

of table salt. However, a recent report raised concerns that consuming too little sodium may adversely affect blood lipids and insulin resistance, two risk factors for heart disease.[37] More research is needed to determine ideal sodium intakes for healthy persons. The "Fresh Tips" feature on this page provides some suggestions for reducing salt intake.

Treatment of Hypertension

Treatment for hypertension usually includes following dietary modifications; making some other lifestyle changes, such as managing stress; and taking prescription medications. In the United States, three in four individuals with hypertension are treated with prescription medications, and in many cases, patients require a combination of multiple medications. Such combination therapies have been shown to help hypertensive individuals meet their blood pressure goals.[38]

The *Dietary Approaches to Stop Hypertension (DASH)* diet is low in sodium, total fat, saturated fat, and cholesterol, and high in fruits, vegetables, and low—fat dairy products. Research indicates that people can lower their blood pressure and reduce their risk of CVD by following the DASH diet, losing excess body fat, and increasing their physical activity level.[39] To obtain more information about this diet and some low—sodium recipes, visit the National Heart, Lung, and Blood Institute's website at http://www.nhlbi.nih.gov/files/docs/public/heart/hbp_low.pdf.

Resistant Hypertension Approximately 13% of adults with high blood pressure suffer from **resistant hypertension**.[40] People with resistant hypertension have blood pressure that remains uncontrolled while taking three medications or is controlled only through the continued use of four or more medications. African—Americans, non—black Hispanics, males, obese individuals, and older adults are more likely to develop resistant hypertension than other persons.[40] Individuals with resistant hypertension have a higher—than—average risk of experiencing heart and kidney complications such as coronary artery disease and kidney damage. Regular screening and early treatment are recommended to minimize the risk of such serious complications.

resistant hypertension blood pressure that remains uncontrolled while taking three medications or is controlled only through continued use of four or more medications

REAL People, **REAL** Stories

Justin Steinbruegge

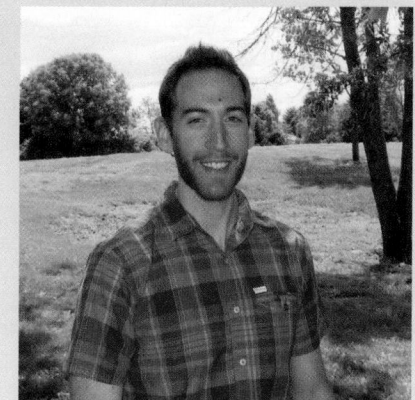

In the spring of his senior year of high school, Justin Steinbruegge was surprised to learn that he had hypertension. "It was a huge shock. I had no signs or symptoms of hypertension. I didn't even know what hypertension was," says Justin. To manage his high blood pressure, he took medication prescribed by his physician, but he had difficulty controlling his sodium intake. "Eating pizzas and salty snacks seemed to keep my blood pressure on a never-ending roller coaster ride," he says.

"When I was 23, I enrolled in a police academy. Four months prior to entering the academy, I started an exercise program, and by the time classes began, I was running 35 or more miles a week. I thought I was in fantastic shape," says Justin, "but I was training too much, and my diet was horrible—loaded with too many processed foods and not enough fresh fruits, vegetables, and meats. I was ignorant about the importance of proper nutrition to good health."

After finishing at the top of his class at the police academy, Justin focused on improving his health. "I developed a healthy combination of diet and exercise that I continue to follow," he says. "I avoid eating out, and I try to cook everything myself. I eat mainly fresh meats, cheeses, nuts, fruits, and vegetables. I drink only water—no juice, soda, or alcohol.

"Exercise is also a necessary part of my health lifestyle. . . . I work out 6 days a week, and I include lifting free weights, rowing, light running, and yoga in my exercise routine. I am able to maintain my weight between 165 and 175 pounds, and my body fat never goes above 13%," says Justin, who is 6-feet, 1-inch tall. "My journey to achieving good health has become a rewarding experience. Now, I don't need to take blood pressure medicine."

ASSESS YOUR PROGRESS

23. *Describe at least two key functions of sodium in the body.*
24. *Identify rich food sources of sodium.*
25. *Describe signs and symptoms of hyponatremia.*
26. *Discuss the relationship between sodium intake and the risk of developing hypertension.*
27. *Describe how hypertension can be managed by making lifestyle modifications.*

11.7 Potassium

LEARNING OUTCOMES

1 *Explain the major functions of potassium in the human body.*
2 *List rich food sources of potassium.*
3 *Discuss potassium deficiency and toxicity signs and symptoms.*

Potassium is the primary positively charged ion in the intracellular fluid. Most of the body's potassium is in cells. All cells need potassium, but nerve and muscle cells contain high amounts of the mineral. Like sodium, potassium plays a key role in maintaining proper fluid balance. Unlike sodium, potassium is associated with lower, rather than higher, blood pressure values. Potassium is also necessary for transmitting nerve impulses, contracting muscles, and maintaining normal kidney function.

TABLE 11.14 Potassium Content of Selected Foods

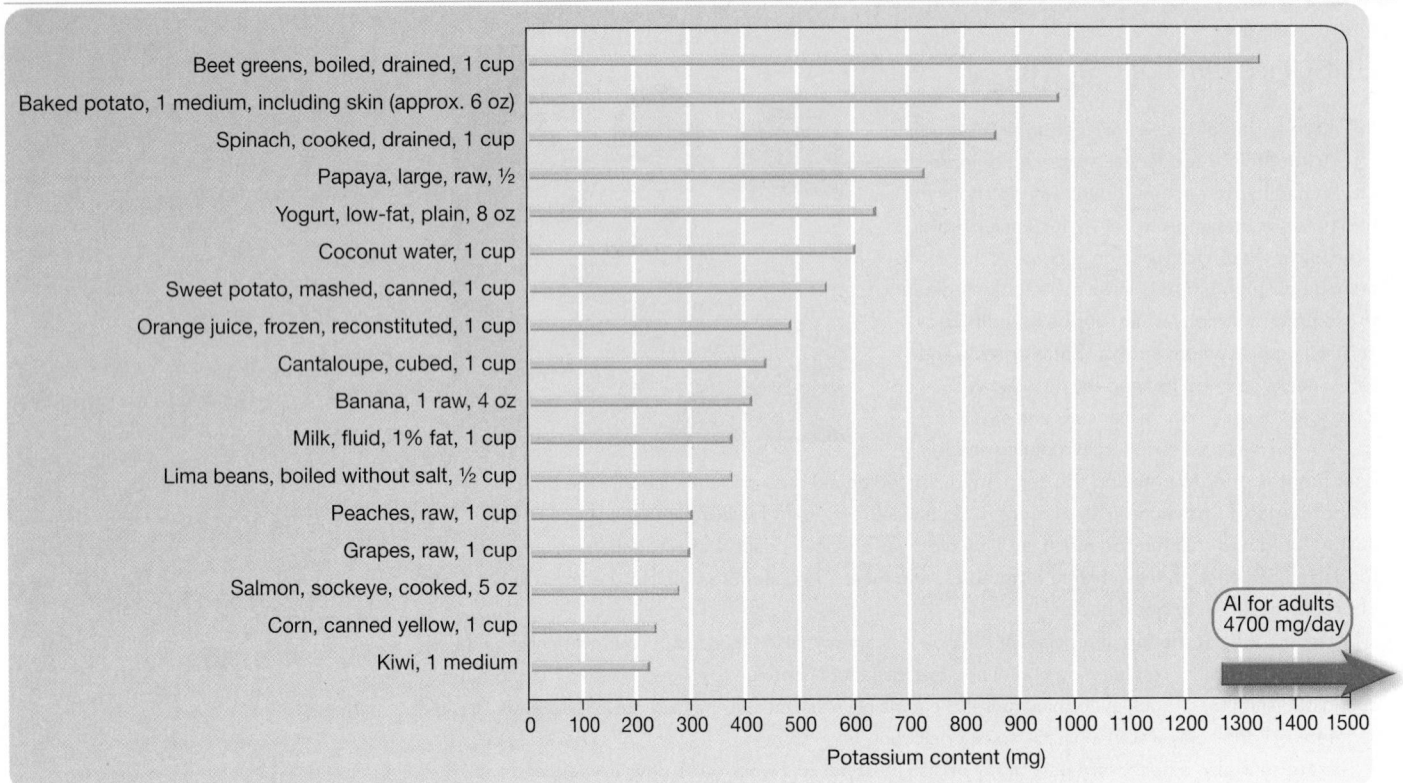

Source: Data from U.S. Department of Agriculture, Agricultural Research Service: *USDA National nutrient database for standard reference,* release 26, 2013.

DID **YOU** KNOW?

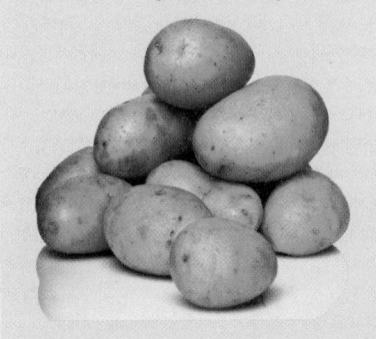

Fresh, white potatoes are one of the richest food sources of potassium. To maximize the mineral content of the cooked potato, consumers can boil, bake, roast, or microwave whole potatoes. Kidney disease patients and people who must reduce their potassium intake should boil small pieces of potato in water. Potassium levels can be reduced by 50 to 75% using this cooking method.[41]

Sources of Potassium

Overall, fresh fruits, fruit juice, and vegetables are good dietary sources of potassium. Milk, whole grains, dried beans, and meats are also major contributors of potassium to American diets. Table 11.14 lists foods that are among the richest sources of this mineral. Figure 11.17 indicates food groups that are naturally good sources of potassium. While processed foods are often concentrated sources of sodium, most processed foods are poor sources of potassium. Potassium is also found as a part of the salt substitute potassium chloride and the artificial sweetener acesulfame–K.

Dietary Adequacy

The adult AI for potassium is 4700 mg per day. On average, Americans con– sume only about 2670 mg of potassium per day.[20] According to the Dietary Guidelines, potassium is a "nutrient of public health concern."[36] People can raise their potassium intakes by increasing their consumption of fruits, vegetables, whole–grain breads and cereals, and low–fat and fat–free milk and milk prod– ucts. Potassium–rich diets, such as the DASH diet, may lower blood pressure, reduce the risk of developing kidney stones, and possibly decrease bone loss.[33]

Potassium Deficiency

The body is unable to conserve potassium as well as it does sodium; therefore, the risk of potassium deficiency is greater than that of sodium deficiency. Individuals suffering from excessive sweating, vomiting, diarrhea, or kidney diseases that increase potassium excretion are at risk for potassium depletion (**hypokalemia**). Signs and symptoms of hypokalemia generally include loss of appetite, muscle cramps, confusion, constipation, and increased urinary calcium excretion. The condition is life–threatening, and treatment should be initiated immediately to prevent serious complications, including death.

hypokalemia low blood potassium

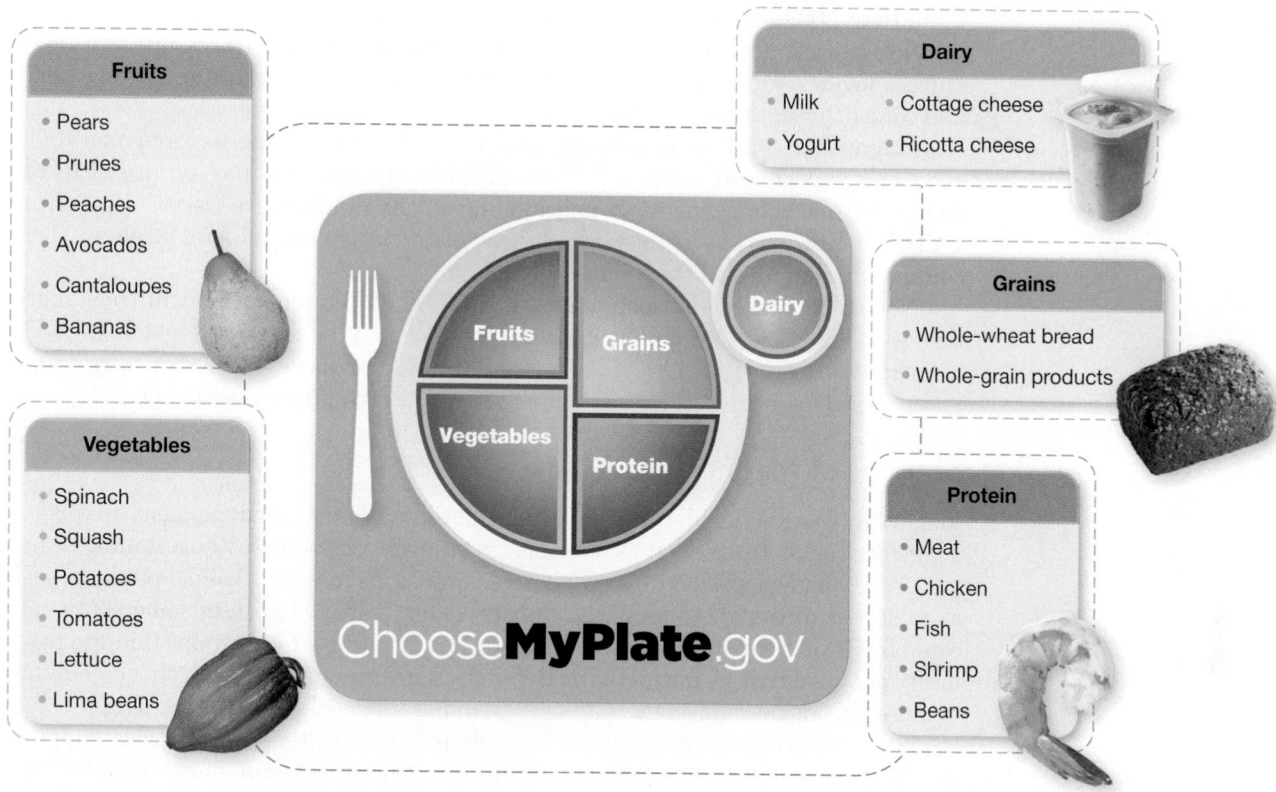

FIGURE 11.17 MyPlate: Food sources of potassium. The foods listed in these MyPlate groups are good food sources of potassium.

Potassium Toxicity

Food consumption of potassium does not lead to potassium toxicity; therefore, there is no UL for the mineral. However, taking potassium supplements can lead to high blood potassium levels, a toxic condition known as **hyperkalemia**. If a person's kidneys are not able to eliminate the excess potassium from the supplements, the mineral accumulates in his or her blood and can cause the heart to stop beating. To avoid toxicity, individuals should not take potassium supplements unless they are under a physician's care.

hyperkalemia high blood potassium

ASSESS YOUR PROGRESS

28 Describe at least two key functions of potassium in the body.

29 Identify rich food sources of potassium.

30 Explain the influence of potassium on blood pressure.

31 Contrast the causes and effects of hypokalemia and hyperkalemia.

11.8 Magnesium

LEARNING OUTCOMES

1 Explain the major functions of magnesium in the human body.

2 List rich food sources of magnesium.

3 Discuss magnesium deficiency and toxicity signs and symptoms.

Magnesium plays an essential role in many important metabolic and physiological activities, including contraction and relaxation of muscles, enzyme function, energy production, and DNA and protein synthesis.[42] Magnesium participates in more than 300 chemical reactions in the body.[42] This essential mineral also helps regulate normal muscle and nerve function, as well as blood pressure and blood glucose levels. Additionally, the body needs magnesium to maintain strong bones and a healthy immune system.

Magnesium may help prevent and treat diabetes, hypertension, metabolic syndrome, CVD, and asthma.[43–45] In addition, magnesium may be useful in the treatment and management of migraine headaches and reduce risk of death from CVD.[46,47] However, more research is needed to clarify the mineral's role in these common chronic health problems.

Normally, humans absorb about 40 to 60% of the magnesium in their diets, but as much as 80% of the magnesium in food may be absorbed when the body is lacking the mineral. The kidneys regulate blood concentrations of magnesium and can reduce urinary losses when the body's magnesium level is low.

Sources of Magnesium

Magnesium is a critical component in chlorophyll, the green pigment in plants. Therefore, plant foods such as spinach, green leafy vegetables, whole grains, beans, nuts, seeds, and chocolate are the richest sources of magnesium. Animal products such as milk and meats also supply some magnesium. Table 11.15 lists some commonly eaten foods that supply magnesium. Figure 11.18 indicates food groups that are nat—urally good sources of magnesium. Refined grains are generally low in magnesium, because the magnesium—rich bran and germ are removed during processing.

Other sources of magnesium are "hard" tap water and dietary supple—ments. However, amounts of magnesium in tap water can vary considerably. Furthermore, the body does not absorb *magnesium oxide*, the form typically found in multivitamin/mineral supplements, very well. Nevertheless, hard water and magnesium supplements can still contribute to a person's magnesium needs.

Dietary Adequacy

Adult RDAs for magnesium range from 310 to 420 mg/day. Many people in the United States do not consume recommended amounts of magnesium; daily

TABLE 11.15 Magnesium Content of Selected Foods

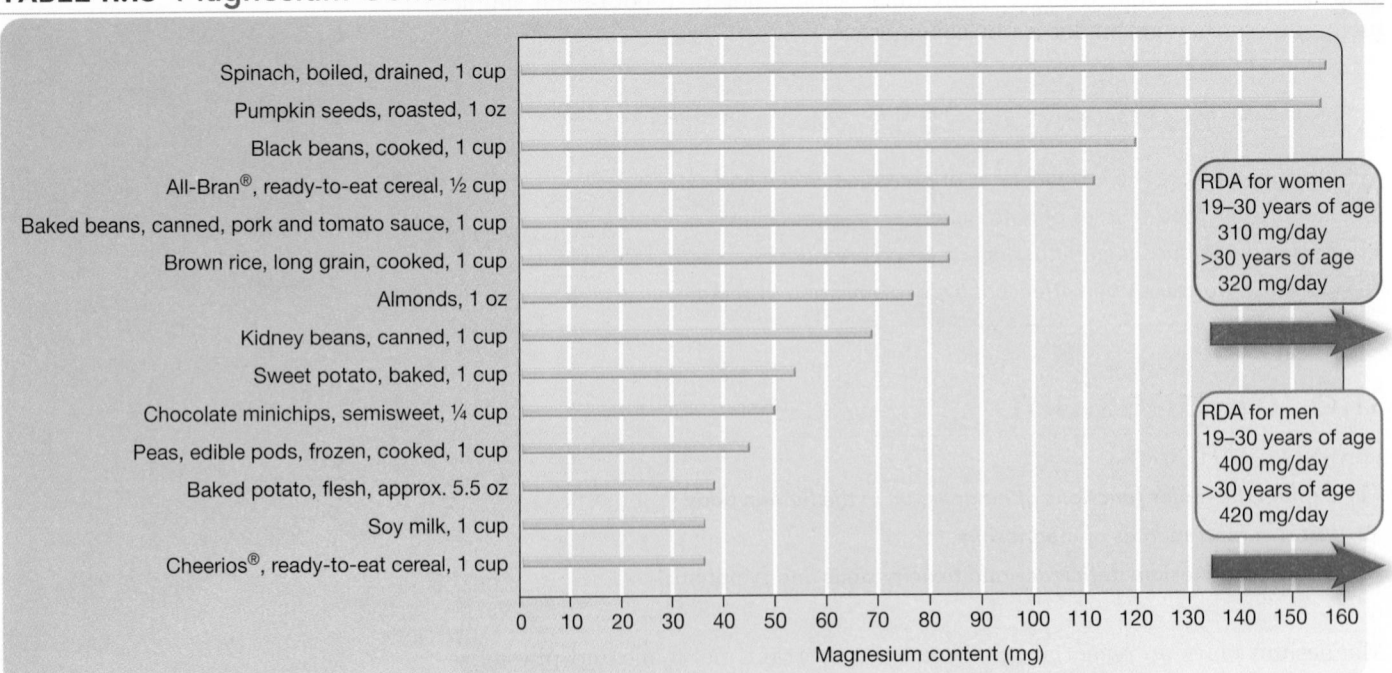

Source: Data from U.S. Department of Agriculture, Agricultural Research Service: *USDA national nutrient database for standard reference*, release 26, 2013.

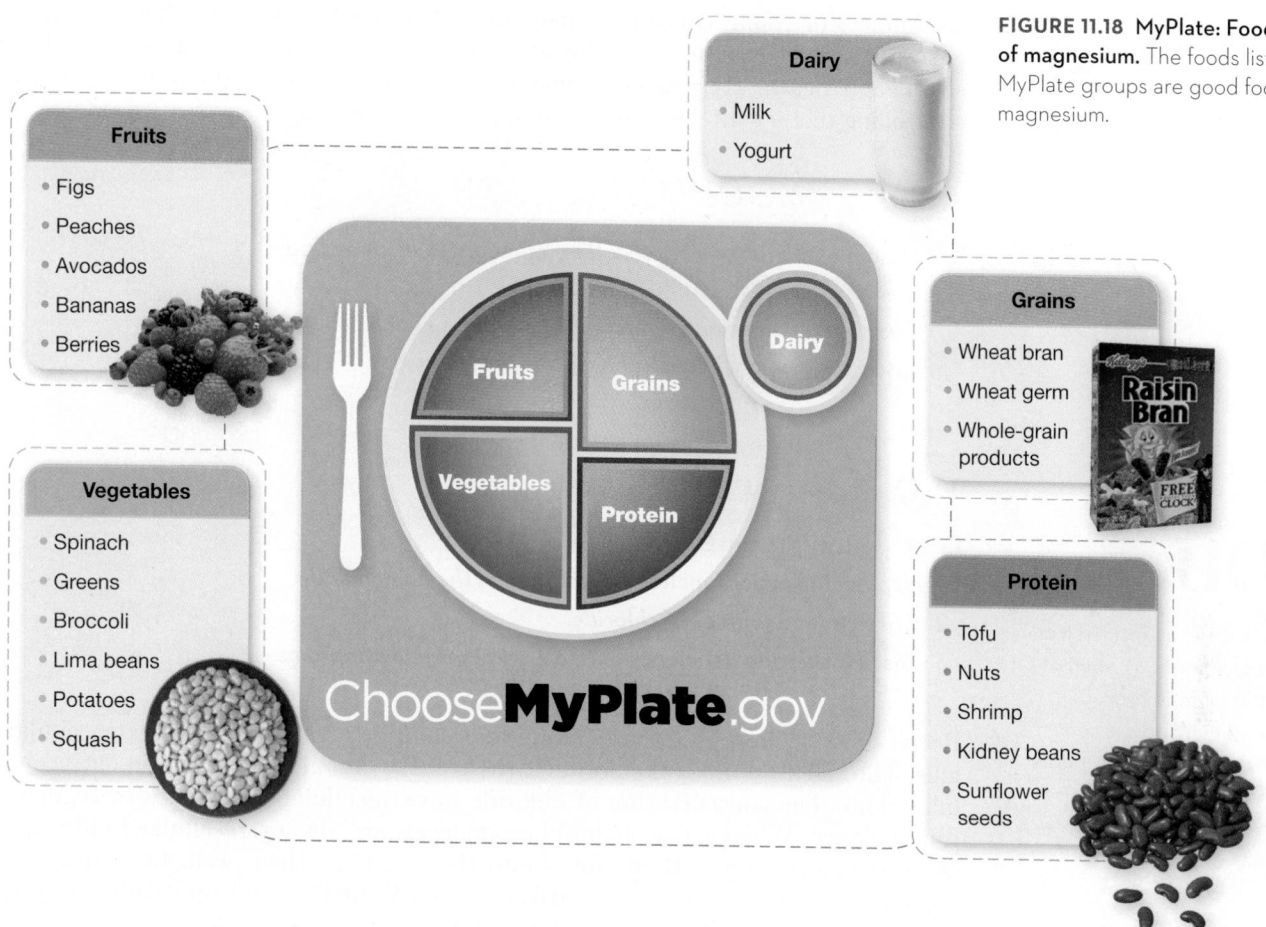

FIGURE 11.18 MyPlate: Food sources of magnesium. The foods listed in these MyPlate groups are good food sources of magnesium.

consumption averages approximately 300 mg.[20] Males tend to consume more magnesium (333 mg/day) than females (261 mg).[20] In the United States, magnesium intake is lower among older adults regardless of their racial and ethnic group.

Although many Americans consume less than recommended amounts of magnesium, cases of magnesium deficiency rarely occur among healthy members of the population.[42] Alcoholics, people with poorly controlled diabetes, or persons who use certain medications (such as diuretics) that increase urinary excretion of magnesium have higher risk of magnesium deficiency. Older adults are also at risk of magnesium deficiency because their bodies absorb less of the mineral and urinary losses increase with advancing age.

In humans, mild magnesium deficiency can cause irritability, weakness, loss of appetite, and muscle twitching. Signs and symptoms of severe magnesium deficiency often include rapid heartbeat, inability to relax muscles, disorientation, and hallucinations. Chronic magnesium deficiency may increase the risk of osteoporosis, because the deficiency lowers the level of calcium in blood.

Magnesium Toxicity

Magnesium toxicity, **hypermagnesemia**, rarely occurs from eating too much magnesium–rich food.[42] The toxicity is more likely to occur from ingesting excessive magnesium from laxatives, antacids, or dietary supplements that contain the mineral. Thus, the UL for the micronutrient (350 mg/day) is for magnesium–containing medications and not food sources. A person who ingests too much magnesium often develops diarrhea as a result.

Patients suffering from kidney failure and older adults have a high risk of magnesium toxicity, because their kidneys do not excrete the mineral as effectively as

hypermagnesemia high blood magnesium

the kidneys of younger, healthier individuals.[48] In cases of kidney failure, the high concentration of magnesium in blood causes weakness, nausea, slowed breathing, coma, and death. Hypermagnesemia in kidney disease patients is managed by controlling dietary intake of magnesium.

ASSESS YOUR PROGRESS

32 Describe at least two key functions of magnesium in the body.

33 Identify rich food sources of magnesium.

34 Describe the signs and symptoms of magnesium deficiency.

35 Discuss the primary cause of hypermagnesemia.

11.9 Chloride

LEARNING OUTCOMES

1 Explain the major functions of chloride in the human body.

2 List rich food sources of chloride.

3 Discuss chloride deficiency and toxicity signs and symptoms.

Recall from Section 11.1 that sodium and chloride are the primary extracellular ions. The essential mineral chloride is the primary anion (Cl^-) found in extracellular fluid. The concentration of chloride in extracellular fluid helps to regulate fluid balance. When extracellular chloride levels are low, extracellular fluid concentrations decrease as fluid moves into the cell. Cells then swell. In addition to regulating fluid balance, the negatively charged chloride and positively charged sodium ion provide electrolytic balance in the extracellular fluid.

Chloride is also important for:

- Hydrochloric acid production (stomach);
- Regulation of acid–base balance;
- Transmission of nerve impulses; and
- Immune fighting response of the white blood cells.

Food Sources of Chloride

The majority of chloride consumed in the typical American diet is in table or sea salt (sodium chloride). Most salt substitutes are comprised of potassium chloride. Many vegetables also contain chloride. Seaweed, rye, tomatoes, celery, and olives are considered excellent sources of the mineral.

Dietary Adequacy

Sodium chloride is composed of approximately 40% sodium and 60% chloride by weight. A teaspoon of table salt supplies 3700 mg of chloride. Dietary recommendations for chloride are based on the amounts of chloride and sodium in table salt. The AI for chloride is 2300 mg.[4]

A chloride deficiency disorder is unlikely because of the excessive intake of table salt by most Americans. However, deficiencies may be seen in cases of extreme vomiting, diarrhea, and/or sweating, as well as with diuretic use. Prolonged vomiting causes increased loss of HCl in gastric juice, resulting in an acid–base and fluid imbalance. Fatigue and loss of appetite are common symptoms of chloride deficiency.

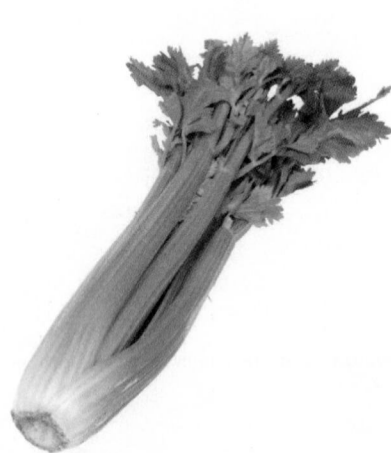

While most chloride in the diet is supplied by table salt (i.e., sodium chloride), several vegetables, including celery, are also rich sources of the mineral.

The UL for chloride is 3600 mg/day.[4] Elevated blood chloride levels may result from excessive table salt intake. As in cases of excess sodium ingestion, consuming too much chloride can contribute to hypertension. In addition, severe dehydration can lead to abnormally elevated blood chloride levels. Replenishing fluids and avoiding foods that contain salt, such as processed foods, can normalize blood chloride levels.

ASSESS YOUR PROGRESS

36 Describe at least two key functions of chloride in the body.

37 Identify the primary food source of chloride.

38 List the two main causes of chloride toxicity.

11.10 Sulfur

LEARNING OUTCOMES

1 Explain the major functions of sulfur in the human body.

2 Describe the relationship between sulfur and the amino acids cysteine and methionine.

Sulfur is a component of several organic compounds, including the amino acids methionine and cysteine, the vitamins biotin and thiamin, and the vitamin-like substance lipoic acid. Some foods and beverages, such as white wine, contain inorganic forms of sulfur (e.g., sulfites), which have been added to preserve the items.

Sulfur is essential to the activity of many enzymes and as part of antioxidant molecules, including **glutathione**, a major antioxidant in the body. Because of their chemical structure, proteins comprised of numerous sulfur-containing amino acids tend to be some of the most rigid in the body. Two such proteins are keratin and collagen, which provide strength to hair, skin, and nails.

Protein-rich foods, including meat, poultry, fish, eggs, milk, cheese, legumes, and nuts, provide ample sulfur to diets. Deficiencies are rare and occur only with severe protein deficiency, which is uncommon in the United States. Sulfur toxicity is unlikely from dietary sources. Thus, there is no AI, RDA, or UL established for sulfur.

glutathione sulfur-containing antioxidant molecule

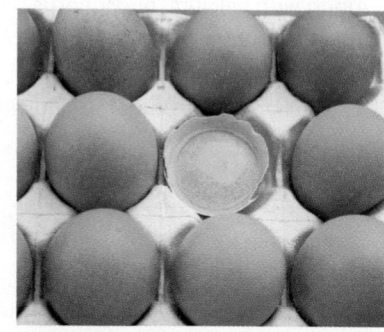

The sulfur-containing amino acids methionine and cysteine are found in both plant and animal food sources. Eggs are an example of a protein-rich food that supplies sulfur.

ASSESS YOUR PROGRESS

39 Describe at least two key functions of sulfur in the body.

40 Identify the two sulfur-containing amino acids.

SUMMARY

SECTION 11.1 Water

- Water has several important roles in the body, including removing waste products, lubricating tissues, regulating body temperature, and maintaining acid-base balance. Water is a major component of blood, saliva, sweat, tears, mucus, and the fluid between joints.

- Water can be found inside of cells (intracellular water) and surrounding cells (extracellular water). Water needs depend on environmental temperatures, health conditions, physical activities, and dietary choices.

SECTION 11.2 **Water Balance and Hydration**

- The kidneys are the body's major regulator of water balance. Antidiuretic hormone (ADH), aldosterone, and the renin-angiotensin system control water balance, primarily through regulation of urine output.
- Dehydration results when water losses are greater than fluid intake. Some cases of dehydration can be treated with oral rehydration therapy, but others require intravenous (IV) fluids. Water intoxication is not as common as dehydration but can result in hyponatremia, low blood sodium.

SECTION 11.3 **Minerals: The Basics**

- Major minerals are those required by the average human adult in excess of 100 mg/day. Those minerals required in lesser amounts are identified as trace minerals.
- The major minerals include calcium, chloride, magnesium, phosphorus, potassium, sodium, and sulfur. Plant foods often contain phytic acid or oxalic acid, substances that reduce the bioavailability of minerals.

SECTION 11.4 **Calcium**

- Calcium is essential for bone and teeth formation, muscle contraction, blood clot formation, nerve transmission, and cell metabolism.
- Parathyroid hormone (PTH) is secreted in response to low blood calcium levels and calcitonin in response to high blood calcium levels. The human skeleton is constantly being remodeled through the activity of osteoblasts and osteoclasts.
- Dairy products, including fluid milk, yogurt, and cheese, are the primary sources of calcium in the typical American's diet.
- A deficiency in calcium results in osteoporosis. Excessive calcium intake results in hypercalcemia.

SECTION 11.5 **Phosphorus**

- Along with calcium, phosphorus is involved in the formation of bones and teeth. Dairy foods, meat, and cereal grains are the primary sources of phosphorus in the typical American diet.
- Phosphorus deficiencies are rare because of the wide variety of foods that supply the nutrient. A deficiency in phosphorus can lead to hyperphosphatemia. Individuals with kidney disease are at an increased risk for phosphorus toxicity.

SECTION 11.6 **Sodium**

- Sodium plays a major role in maintaining normal fluid balance, transmission of nerve impulses, transporting substance into cells, and muscle function.
- Sodium chloride is the primary source of sodium in American diets. Processed foods are high in sodium, whereas uncooked fruits and vegetables are low in sodium.
- While rare, a sodium deficiency leads to hyponatremia. High sodium intakes are associated with hypertension. Hypertension is a risk factor for cardiovascular disease, including heart disease and stroke.

SECTION 11.7 **Potassium**

- As the primary positively charged ion in the intracellular fluid, potassium helps maintain proper fluid and electrolyte balance.
- Fruits and vegetables are excellent sources of potassium. Processed foods are poor sources of potassium.
- A potassium deficiency leads to hypokalemia. People taking potassium supplements may develop hyperkalemia. Both conditions can be fatal.

SECTION 11.8 **Magnesium**

- Magnesium is important for contraction and relaxation of muscles, enzyme function, energy production, and protein synthesis. Adequate magnesium intake may also contribute to the prevention and/or treatment of serious chronic diseases including diabetes and cardiovascular disease.
- Green leafy vegetables, whole grains, beans, nuts, seeds, and chocolate are among the richest sources of magnesium.

- Magnesium deficiency is uncommon among healthy children and adults. Alcoholics, older adults, people with poorly controlled diabetes, and persons taking diuretic medications are at the greatest risk for magnesium deficiency. Hypermagnesemia most often occurs from overuse of laxatives, antacids, and dietary supplements that contain magnesium. People with poor kidney function have a high risk of magnesium toxicity.

SECTION 11.9 Chloride

- Chloride is essential for maintaining proper fluid and electrolyte balance as the primary anion in extracellular fluid. Chlorine is also found in gastric juice as a component HCl.

- For the typical American, the major dietary source of chloride is sodium chloride. Chloride deficiency is unlikely, but excessive chloride intake can contribute to hypertension.

SECTION 11.10 Sulfur

- Sulfur is a component of the sulfur-containing amino acids methionine and cysteine. Therefore, diets rich in protein provide adequate amounts of sulfur. Sulfur is essential for the activity of several enzymes and as part of antioxidant systems. There is no AI, RDA, or UL established for sulfur.

Get the most out of your study of nutrition with McGraw-Hill's innovative suite of adaptive learning products including McGraw-Hill LearnSmart®, SmartBook®, McGraw-Hill LearnSmart Achieve®, and McGraw-Hill LearnSmart Prep®. Visit www.learnsmartadvantage.com.

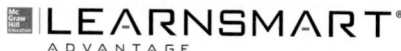

CASE STUDY RESPONSE

MINERALS AND OSTEOPOROSIS

AFTER FRACTURING HER WRIST, Sheryl was told that she is at high risk for osteoporosis. Osteoporosis is a chronic disease characterized by low bone mass and reduced bone structure. The weakening of the bones makes them more susceptible to fractures, particularly of the hip, upper spine, and wrist. Osteoporosis is most common in older woman, those of white or Asian ancestry, those having a smaller body frame, and those with a family history of osteoporosis.

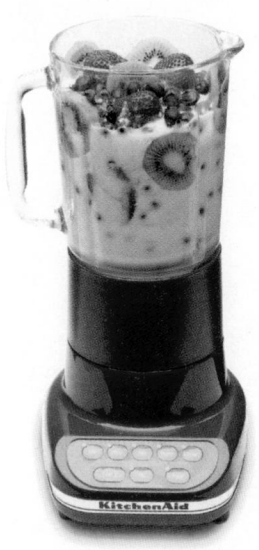

The minerals calcium and phosphorus are most essential to bone health. The formation of bone starts with a collagen protein complex. Then, calcium and phosphorus begin the process of bone mineralization by forming a crystalline structure, called hydroxyapatite, on the collagen complex. The mineralization of bone provides strength and rigidity to the bone.

Lifestyle factors that contribute to osteoporosis include:

- Diets that contain inadequate amounts of calcium, phosphorus, and vitamin D;
- Use of medications, including steroids;
- Lack of physical activity;
- Smoking cigarettes;
- Consuming excessive alcohol; and
- Consuming excess protein, sodium, and/or caffeine.

Dietary recommendations for Sheryl to enhance her calcium intake include:

- Snacking on low-fat yogurt or low-fat cheese sticks at work;
- Drinking a glass of low-fat milk with dinner. Flavor the milk with a small amount of chocolate or strawberry syrup, if necessary;
- Preparing a homemade smoothie from low-fat yogurt and fresh or frozen fruit for an on-the-go breakfast; and
- Drinking calcium-fortified orange juice.

Modifying Recipes for Healthy Living

Tristan, a 30-year-old salesman, leads a stressful life. At his last visit with his physician, he was diagnosed with high blood pressure. A registered dietitian met with Tristan and encouraged him to reduce his salt intake. As football season approaches, Tristan is trying to lower the amount of sodium in his traditional tailgating recipes. He likes to serve his friends a hot spinach dip with store-bought pita chips. Using Tristan's traditional "Hot Spinach Dip" as a guide, develop a lower-sodium version of his hot spinach dip.

HOT SPINACH DIP

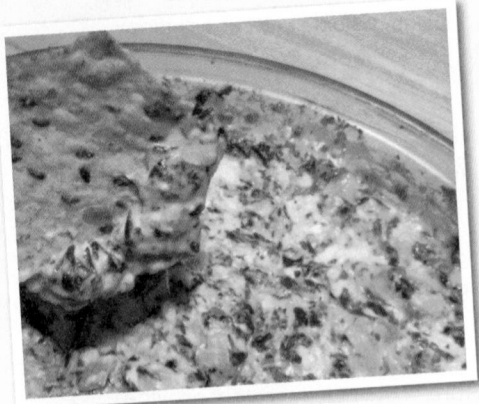

PREPARATION STEPS

1. Defrost spinach (microwave suggested) until tender. Drain and discard liquid.
2. Drain and chop artichoke hearts.
3. Combine spinach and artichoke hearts. Stir in cream cheese, sour cream, mayonnaise, shredded cheese, garlic salt, and red pepper flakes.
4. Bake at 325°F for 15 to 20 minutes. Serve hot with store-bought pita chips.
5. Serves twelve (¼-cup servings).

INGREDIENTS

1 cup frozen spinach

1 cup canned artichoke hearts, chopped

6 oz cream cheese

¼ cup sour cream

¼ cup mayonnaise

¾ cup shredded cheese (Colby Jack, cheddar, or parmesan)

½ tsp garlic salt

¼ tsp red pepper flakes

STEP 1 Brainstorm

Use diet analysis software to analyze the nutrient and calorie content of the "Hot Spinach Dip" recipe. List the total calories, fat, calcium, sodium, potassium, magnesium, phosphorus, chloride, and sulfur content of the recipe. How do you rate the overall taste of the recipe?

STEP 2 Develop a modified version of this recipe

Develop a lower-sodium version of this recipe.

1. List ingredients and amounts of each of them that are needed.
2. List the preparation steps.

What lower-sodium options could you serve with the dip instead of store-bought pita chips?

STEP 3 Evaluate the modified recipe

Use diet analysis software to analyze the total calories, fat, calcium, sodium, potassium, magnesium, phosphorus, chloride, and sulfur content of the modified "Hot Spinach Dip." Develop a table comparing the total calories, fat, calcium, sodium, potassium, magnesium, and phosphorus content in the original and modified recipes. Explain how the two versions of the spinach dip differ nutritionally.

OPTIONAL ACTIVITIES

STEP 4 Shop for your ingredients

Were the ingredients readily available?

STEP 5 Test your new recipe

Keep notes on any changes you make to ingredient amounts as you prepare the "Hot Spinach Dip."

STEP 6 Reflect on the modified recipe

How does the hot spinach dip taste? How does it look? Can you tell that the modified version is lower in sodium than the original recipe?

STEP 7 Add the recipe to your collection or repeat steps to improve the product

PERSONAL Dietary Analysis

Using the DRIs

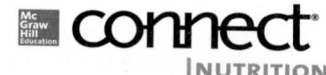

Complete the Personal Dietary Analysis activity online at www.mcgrawhillconnect.com, where you will also find McGraw-Hill LearnSmart®, SmartBook®, NutritionCalc Plus, and many other dynamic learning tools.

1. Refer to your 3-day food log from the "Personal Dietary Analysis" feature in Chapter 5.

   a. Find the RDA/AI values for major minerals under your life stage/sex group category in the DRI tables (see the last pages of this book). Write those values under the "My RDA/ AI" column in the table below.

   b. Review your personal dietary assessment. Find your 3-day average intakes of calcium, phosphorus, sodium, potassium, and magnesium. Write those values under the "My Average Intake" column of the table.

   c. Calculate the percentage of the RDA/AI you consumed for each mineral by dividing your intake by the RDA/AI amount and multiplying the figure you obtain by 100. For example, if your average intake of calcium was 500 mg/day, and your RDA for the mineral is 1000 mg/day, you would divide 1000 mg by 500 mg to obtain .50. To multiply this figure by 100, simply move the decimal point two places to the right, and replace the decimal point with a percentage sign (50%). Thus, your average daily intake of calcium was 50% of the RDA. Place the percentages for each mineral under the "% of My RDA/AI" column.

   d. Under the ">, <, or =" column, indicate whether your average daily intake was greater than (>), less than (<), or equal to (=) the RDA/AI.

2. Use the information you calculated in the first part of this activity to answer the following questions:

   a. Which of your average major mineral intakes equaled or exceeded the RDA/AI?_____

   b. Which of your average major mineral intakes was below the RDA/AI?_____

   c. What foods would you eat to increase your intake of the minerals that were less than the RDA/AI levels? (Review sources of the minerals in this chapter.)

   _____

   d. Turn in your completed table and answers to your instructor.

Personal Dietary Analysis: Minerals

Mineral	My RDA/AI	My Average Intake	% of My RDA/AI	>,<, or =
Calcium				
Phosphorus				
Sodium				
Potassium				
Magnesium				

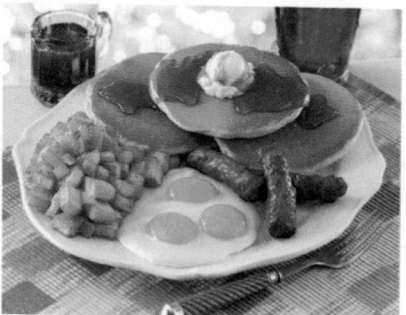

Critical Thinking

1. A friend of yours works for a landscaping company during the summer. He often spends 8 to 10 hours per day working in the heat and humidity. Your friend is concerned that he is becoming dehydrated during the day. Explain to him how to determine if he is dehydrated.

2. Consider your family history and lifestyle to determine whether you are at risk of hypertension. If you are at risk, what steps can you take at this point in your life to reduce your chances of developing this disease?

3. Explain why eating excessive amounts of spinach, collard greens, beans, and/or rhubarb may contribute to a mineral deficiency.

4. What advice would you give Sylvia, a total vegetarian (vegan), concerning her need for calcium, phosphorus, potassium, and magnesium?

5. Stephanie's father has a condition in which his parathyroid glands secrete too much parathyroid hormone. Based on this information, what health complications is he likely to experience as a result of the excess hormone secretion?

Practice Test

Select the best answer.

1. Which of the following statements is false?
   a. Lean tissue contains more water than fat tissue.
   b. Water is a major solvent.
   c. Generally, young women have more body water than young men.
   d. Water does not provide energy.

2. If the extracellular fluid has an excess of sodium ions,
   a. sodium ions move into cells.
   b. intracellular fluid moves to the outside of cells.
   c. phosphate and calcium ions are eliminated in feces.
   d. blood levels of arsenic and oxalate increase.

3. Which of the following foods has the lowest percentage of water?
   a. tomatoes
   b. oranges
   c. whole-grain bread
   d. vegetable oil

4. Which of the following statements concerning antidiuretic hormone is false?
   a. ADH is secreted in response to dehydration.
   b. ADH is secreted from the pancreas.
   c. ADH stimulates reabsorption of water from the kidneys.
   d. ADH maintains normal fluid balance.

5. Water intoxication
   a. develops over several days.
   b. results in high blood sodium levels.
   c. causes dizziness, headache, and confusion.
   d. is more common than dehydration.

6. Major minerals
   a. are more important to human health than trace minerals.
   b. are required in quantities of greater than 100 mg daily.
   c. include calcium, iron, zinc, and iodine.
   d. may be nonessential nutrients.

7. Which of the following foods is not a good source of calcium?
   a. butter
   b. American cheese
   c. canned sardines
   d. kale

8. Calcitonin
   a. is secreted in response to low blood calcium levels.
   b. stimulates activity of osteoblast cells.
   c. inhibits calcium excretion from the kidneys.
   d. is secreted from the parathyroid glands.

9. Henry is concerned about his risk of osteoporosis. Which of the following characteristics is a modifiable risk factor for this chronic condition?
   a. family history
   b. racial/ethnic background
   c. physical activity level
   d. age

10. A phosphorus toxicity is most common in
    a. children.
    b. athletes.
    c. vegetarians.
    d. kidney disease patients.

11. The primary source of sodium in the typical American's diet is
    a. bottled water.
    b. unprocessed food.
    c. fruit.
    d. salt.

12. Which of the following populations has the greatest risk of hypertension?
    a. people with African-American ancestry
    b. young, physically active Asian men
    c. Hispanic women who do not drink alcohol
    d. young adults who consume high amounts of fruits

13. Which of the following statements concerning potassium is false?
    a. High intake is associated with hypertension.
    b. Fruits and vegetables are rich dietary sources.
    c. It is the primary positively charged ion in the intracellular fluid.
    d. Deficiency may result from severe and prolonged vomiting.

14. The mineral found in chlorophyll, the green pigment in plants, is

    a. phosphorus.
    b. chloride.
    c. sulfur.
    d. magnesium.

15. Which mineral is a component of the amino acids cysteine and methionine?

    a. phosphorus
    b. chloride
    c. sulfur
    d. magnesium

ANSWERS TO PRACTICE TEST
1-c; 2-b; 3-d; 4-b; 5-c; 6-b; 7-a; 8-b; 9-c; 10-d; 11-d; 12-a; 13-a; 14-d; 15-c

ANSWERS TO CHAPTER 11 QUIZ Yourself

1. Cells produce some water as a by-product of metabolism. **True** (p. 343)
2. The kidneys are the major regulator of the body's water content. **True** (p. 347)
3. Consuming too much sodium may contribute to low blood pressure. **False** (p. 366)
4. Weight-bearing exercise can reduce the risk of osteoporosis. **True** (p. 361)
5. Processed foods are rich sources of potassium. **False** (p. 370)

References

1. Saladin KS: *Anatomy & Physiology.* 7th ed. Boston: McGraw-Hill Publishing Company, 2015.

2. Negoianu D, Goldfarb S: Just add water. *Journal of the American Society of Nephrology* 19(6):1041, 2008.

3. Campbell SM: Hydration needs throughout the lifespan. *Journal of the American College of Nutrition* 26(Suppl 5):585S, 2007.

4. Food and Nutrition Board, Institute of Medicine. *Dietary reference intakes for water, potassium, sodium, chloride, and sulfate.* Washington, DC: National Academy Press, 2004.

5. Drewnowksi A and others: Water and beverage consumption among adults in the United States: cross-sectional study using data from NHANES 2005–2010. *BMC Public Health* 13:1068, 2013. doi:10.1186/1471-2458-13-1068

6. Sebastian RS and others: *Drinking water intake in the U.S.: What we eat in America, NHANES 2005–2008.* Food Surveys Research Group dietary data brief no. 7, September 2011. www.ars.usda.gov/Services/docs.htm?docid=19476. Accessed: February 20, 2014.

7. National Institute of Diabetes and Digestive and Kidney Disorders, National Institutes of Health: *Kidney stones in adults.* Updated January 2013. http://kidney.niddk.nih.gov/kudiseases/pubs/stonesadults/#who Accessed: February 20, 2014.

8. Valtrin H: "Drink at least eight glasses of water a day." Really? Is there evidence for "8x8"? *American Journal of Physiological Regulation and Integrative Comparative Physiology* 283:R993, 2002.

9. Casa DJ and others: American College of Sports Medicine roundtable on hydration and physical activity: Consensus statements. *Current Sports Medicine Reports* 4:115, 2005.

10. Mentes J: Oral hydration in older adults: Greater awareness is needed in preventing, recognizing, and treating dehydration. *American Journal of Nursing* 106(6):40, 2006.

11. Schols JM and others: Preventing and treating dehydration in the elderly during periods of illness and warm weather. *Journal of Nutrition and Healthy Aging* 13(2):150, 2009.

12. Colletti JE and others: The management of children with gastroenteritis and dehydration in the emergency department. *Journal of Emergency Medicine* 38(5):686, 2010.

13. Canavan A, Arant BS: Diagnosis and management of dehydration in children. *American Family Physician* 80(7):692, 2009.

14. Wober C, Wober-Bingol C: Triggers of migraine and tension-type headache. *Handbook of Clinical Neurology* 97:161, 2010.

15. Yeates KE and others: Salt and water: A simple approach to hyponatremia. *Canadian Medical Association Journal* 170:365, 2004.

16. Montgomery H and others: Finding whole grains and calcium rich food sources on supermarket shelves. *Forum for Family and Consumer Issues* 9: SSN 1540 5273, 2004. http://www.ncsu.edu/ffci/publications/2004/v9-n2-2004-october/ar-2-finding.php Accessed: February 20, 2014.

17. U.S. Department of Health and Human Services: *Bone health and osteoporosis: A report of the surgeon general.* Rockville, MD: U.S. Department of Health and Human Services, Office of the Surgeon General, 2004. http://www.ncbi.nlm.nih.gov/books/NBK45513/ Accessed: February 20, 2014.

18. Office of Dietary Supplements, National Institutes of Health: *Dietary supplement fact sheet: Calcium.* Updated March 2013. http://ods.od.nih.gov/factsheets/Calcium-QuickFacts/ Accessed: February 20, 2014.

19. Food and Nutrition Board, Institute of Medicine: *Dietary reference Intakes for calcium and vitamin D.* Washington, DC: National Academy Press, 2010.

20. United States Department of Agriculture, Agricultural Research Service: *What we eat in America 2011-2012.* Last modified October 2014. http://www.ars.usda.gov/Services/docs.htm?docid=18349 Accessed: November 1, 2014.

21. National Institutes of Health, National Institute of Arthritis and Musculoskeletal and Skin Diseases: *Osteoporosis: Symptoms and diagnosis.* Updated March 2013. http://nihseniorhealth.gov/osteoporosis Accessed: February 20, 2014.

22. Kelley GA and others: Effects of ground and joint reaction force exercise on lumbar spine and femoral neck bone mineral density in postmenopausal women: A meta-analysis of randomized controlled trials. *BMC Musculoskeletal Disorders* 13:177, 2012.

23. Carroll MF, Schade DS: A practical approach to hypercalcemia. *American Family Physician* 67(9):1959, 2003.

24. Torres MR, Sanjuliani AF: Does calcium intake affect cardiovascular risk factors and/or events? *Clinics* 67(7):839, 2012.

25. Nguyen H and others: A review of nutritional factors in hypertension management. *International Journal of Hypertension* E-pub: April 10, 2013.

26. Bolland MJ and others: Effect of calcium supplements on risk of myocardial infarction and cardiovascular events: Meta-analysis. *British Medical Journal* 341:c3691, 2010.

27. Murphy KJ others: Dairy foods and dairy protein consumption is inversely related to markers of adiposity in obese men and women. *Nutrients* 5(11):4665, 2013.

28. Kalantar-Zadeh K and others: Understanding sources of dietary phosphorus in the treatment of patients with chronic kidney disease. *Clinical Journal of the American Society of Nephrology* 5(3):519, 2010.

29. Palit S, Kendrick J: Vascular calcification in chronic kidney disease: Role of disordered mineral metabolism. *Current Pharmaceutical Design* 20(37):5829, 2014.

30. National Institutes of Health, National Kidney Disease Education Program: *Chronic kidney disease.* Updated February 2013. http://nkdep.nih.gov/identify-manage/manage-patients/complications.shtml Accessed: February 20, 2014.

31. American Heart Association: *Sodium (salt or sodium chloride).* Updated February 2014. www.heart.org/HEARTORG/GettingHealthy/NutritionCenter/HealthyDietGoals/Sodium-Salt-or-Sodium-Chloride_UCM_303290_Article.jsp Accessed: February 20, 2014.

32. Jacobson MF and others: Changes in sodium levels in processed and restaurant foods, 2005 to 2011. *Journal of the American Medical Association Internal Medicine* 173(14):1285, 2013.

33. Koliaki C, Katsilambros N: Dietary sodium, potassium, and alcohol: Key players in pathophysiology, prevention, and treatment of human hypertension. *Nutrition Reviews* 71(6):402, 2013.

34. Centers for Disease Control and Prevention: *NCHS Data Brief: Hypertension among adults in the United States, 2009-2010.* No. 107, October 2012. http://www.cdc.gov/nchs/data/databriefs/db107.htm Accessed: February 20, 2014.

35. Shay CM and others: Status of cardiovascular health in US adolescents: Prevalence estimates from the National Health and Nutrition Examination Surveys (NHANES) 2005-2010. *Circulation* 127(13):1369, 2013.

36. U.S. Departments of Health and Human Services and Agriculture: *2015-2020 Dietary Guidelines for Americans.* 2015. http://health.gov/dietaryguidelines/2015/guidelines/ Accessed: January 25, 2016.

37. Institute of Medicine. *Sodium intake in populations: Assessment of evidence.* 2013. http://www.nap.edu/catalog.php?record_id=18311 Accessed: February 20, 2014.

38. Gu Q and others: Trends in antihypertensive medication use and blood pressure control among United States adults with hypertension: The National Health and Nutrition Examination Survey, 2001 to 2010. *Circulation* 126(17):2105, 2012.

39. *National Heart, Lung, and Blood Institute: Explore DASH eating plan.* 2015. http://www.nhlbi.nih.gov/health/health-topics/topics/dash Accessed: January 24, 2016

40. Judd E, Calhoun DA: Apparent and true resistant hypertension: Definition, prevalence and outcomes. *Journal of Human Hypertension* 28(8):463, 2014.

41. Bethke PC, Jansky SH: The effects of boiling and leaching on the content of potassium and other minerals in potatoes. *Journal of Food Science* 73(5):H80, 2008.

42. U.S. National Library of Medicine, National Institutes of Health: *Magnesium in diet.* Updated February 2013. http://www.nlm.nih.gov/medlineplus/ency/article/002423.htm Accessed: February 20, 2014.

43. Kazaks AG and others: Effect of oral magnesium supplementation on measures of airway resistance and subjective assessment of asthma control and quality of life in men and women with mild to moderate asthma: A randomized placebo controlled trial. *Journal of Asthma* 47(1):83, 2010.

44. Wang J and others: Dietary magnesium intake improves insulin resistance among non-diabetic individuals with metabolic syndrome participating in a dietary trial. *Nutrients* 5(10):3910, 2013.

45. Del Gobbo LC and others: Circulating and dietary magnesium and risk of cardiovascular disease: A systematic review of prospective studies. *American Journal of Clinical Nutrition* 98(1):160, 2013.

46. Holland S and others: Evidence-based guideline update: NSAIDs and other complementary treatments for episodic migraine prevention in adults: Report of the Quality Standards Subcommittee of the American Academy of Neurology and the American Headache Society. *Neurology* 78(17):1346, 2012.

47. Reffelmann T and others: Low serum magnesium concentrations predict cardiovascular and all-cause mortality. *Atherosclerosis* 219(1):280, 2011.

48. Kanbay M and others: Magnesium in chronic kidney disease: Challenges and opportunities. *Blood Purification* 29(3):280, 2010.

12 Trace Minerals

CASE STUDY

Selenium toxicity

CARLOS RECENTLY LEARNED THAT HIS 45-YEAR-OLD uncle is undergoing treatment for prostate cancer. Last year, Carlos's 38-year-old brother became the third member of his family to be diagnosed with the disease. At the age of 25, Carlos wants to do whatever he can to avoid prostate cancer.

By recording his typical dietary habits, Carlos estimated that he consumed about 130 μg of selenium per day. After researching information about prostate cancer on the Internet, he became concerned that his selenium intake from foods was too low. Now, he takes a dietary supplement that contains 200 μg of selenium once a day. While investigating food sources of selenium, Carlos discovered that Brazil nuts are a rich source of the trace mineral, so he also eats a handful (about 1 ounce) of Brazil nuts every day.

- What is Carlos's Recommended Dietary Allowance (RDA) for selenium? What is the Upper Limit (UL) for selenium?

- What are the signs and symptoms of selenium toxicity?

- What would you recommend to Carlos regarding the use of a daily selenium supplement as a measure to prevent prostate cancer?

The suggested Case Study Response can be found on page 411.

Connect |NUTRITION Check out the Connect site at www.mcgrawhillconnect.com to further explore this case study.

QUIZ Yourself

Are supplements necessary to provide adequate amounts of trace minerals? Can taking zinc lozenges prevent the common cold? Test your knowledge of trace minerals by taking the following quiz. The answers are found on page 414.

1. In the United States, young men are more likely to be iron deficient than young women. ___T ___F

2. To prevent iodine deficiency, people can use table salt that is fortified with the mineral. ___T ___F

3. Trace minerals are not as important for human health as the major minerals. ___T ___F

4. Symptoms of zinc deficiency include the inability to sense the taste of food. ___T ___F

5. In the United States, copper deficiency is the most common nutritional deficiency. ___T ___F

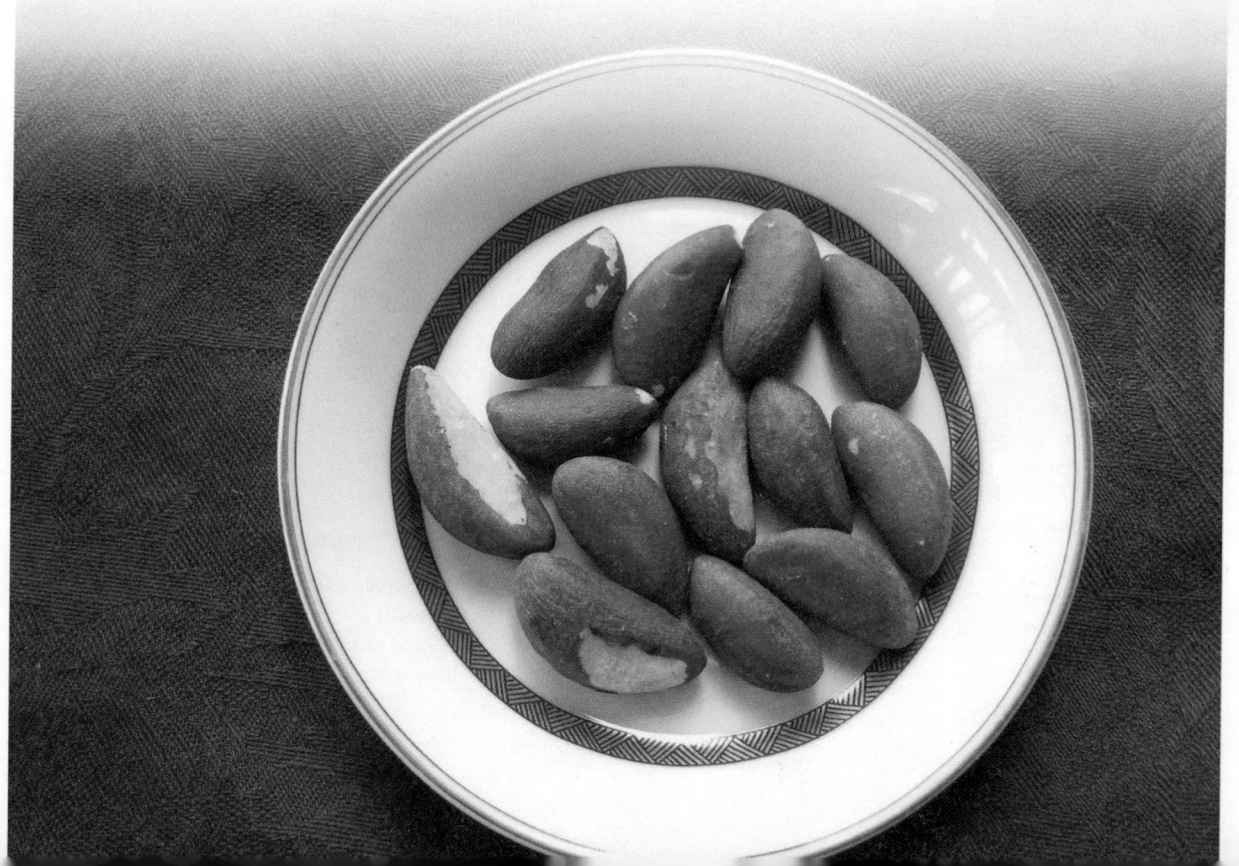

12.1 What Is a Trace Mineral?

1 *Explain the difference between a trace mineral and a major mineral.*

2 *Name the trace minerals.*

In Chapter 11, we discussed major minerals. Recall that the human body needs at least 100 mg/day of each major mineral. In this chapter, we provide information about another group of essential mineral nutrients, the trace minerals. Basic details concerning other trace minerals that may be essential are also provided. Although the body requires each trace mineral in very small amounts (generally less than 100 mg/day), these minerals perform vital roles in the body, and obtaining adequate amounts of them from food can be difficult. Table 12.1 summarizes nutrition–related information concerning the trace minerals. Unless otherwise noted, Dietary Reference Intake (DRI) values are for adults, excluding pregnant or breastfeeding women.

TABLE 12.1 Summary of Trace Minerals

Mineral	Major Functions in the Body	Adult RDA/AI* (adult RDA = bold)	Major Dietary Sources	Major Deficiency Signs and Symptoms	Major Toxicity Signs and Symptoms
Iron (Fe)	• Component of hemoglobin and myoglobin that carries oxygen • Energy generation • Immune system function	Women: **18 mg** Men: **8 mg**	Meat and other animal foods, except milk; whole-grain and enriched breads and cereals; fortified cereals	• Fatigue upon exertion • Small, pale red blood cells • Low hemoglobin levels • Poor immune system function • Growth and developmental retardation in infants	UL = 45 mg/day • Intestinal upset • Organ damage • Death
Zinc (Zn)	• Component of numerous enzymes	Women: **8 mg** Men: **11 mg**	Seafood, meat, whole grains	• Skin rash • Diarrhea • Depressed sense of taste and smell • Hair loss • Poor growth and physical development	UL = 40 mg/day • Intestinal upset • Depressed immune system function • Supplement use can reduce copper absorption.
Copper (Cu)	• Promotes iron metabolism • Component of antioxidant enzymes • Component of enzymes involved in connective tissue synthesis	**0.9 mg**	Liver, cocoa, legumes, whole grains, shellfish	• Anemia • Reduced immune system function • Poor growth and development	UL = 10 mg/day • Vomiting • Abnormal nervous system function • Liver damage
Selenium (Se)	• Component of an antioxidant system	**55 µg**	Meat, eggs, fish, seafood, whole grains	• Muscle pain and weakness • Form of heart disease	UL = 400 µg/day • Nausea • Vomiting • Hair loss • Weakness • Liver damage

Continued

Mineral	Major Functions in the Body	Adult RDA/AI* (adult RDA = bold)	Major Dietary Sources	Major Deficiency Signs and Symptoms	Major Toxicity Signs and Symptoms
Iodine (I)	• Component of thyroid hormones	**150 µg**	Iodized salt, saltwater fish, dairy products	• Goiter • Cretinism (intellectual impairment and poor growth in infants of women who were iodine deficient during pregnancy)	UL = 1100 µg/day • Reduced thyroid gland function
Fluoride (F⁻)	• Increases resistance of tooth enamel to cavity formation • Stimulates bone formation	Men: 4 mg Women: 3 mg	Fluoridated water, tea, seaweed	• No true deficiency, but increased risk of tooth decay	UL = 10 mg/day • Stomach upset • Staining of teeth during development • Bone deterioration
Chromium (Cr)	• Enhances insulin action	Men: 30–35 µg Women: 20–25 µg	Egg yolks, whole grains, pork, nuts, mushrooms	• Blood glucose level remains elevated after meals	• Unknown but currently under scientific investigation • May interact with certain medications
Manganese (Mn)	• Cofactor for certain enzymes, including some involved in carbohydrate metabolism	Men: 2.3 mg Women: 1.8 mg	Nuts, oats, beans, tea	• None in humans	UL = 11 mg/day • Abnormal nervous system function
Molybdenum (Mo)	• Component of certain coenzymes	**45 µg**	Liver, peas, beans, cereal products, leafy vegetables, low-fat milk	• None in healthy humans	UL = 2000 µg/day • Rarely occurs from usual dietary sources • Overdoses of dietary supplements containing molybdenum may cause joint pain and swelling of feet or lower legs

* Values are for adults, excluding pregnant or breastfeeding women.

ASSESS YOUR PROGRESS

1. List at least three trace minerals that are essential nutrients.
2. What distinguishes a trace mineral from a major mineral?

12.2 Iron

LEARNING OUTCOMES

1. *Explain the major functions of iron in the human body.*
2. *List foods that are good sources of iron.*
3. *Discuss factors that affect iron bioavailability.*
4. *Discuss iron deficiency and iron toxicity.*

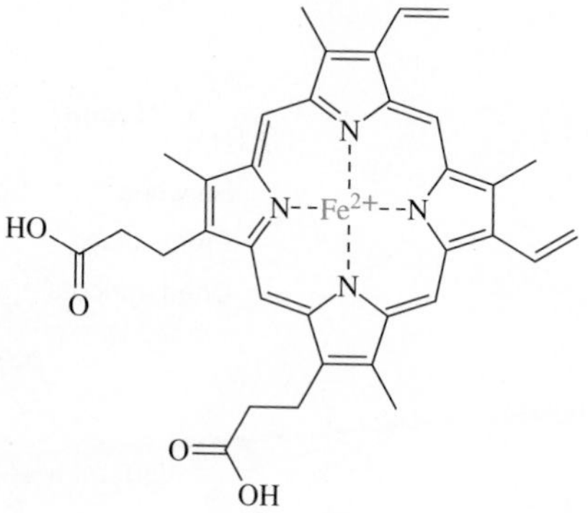

Heme

FIGURE 12.1 Heme.

Iron is necessary for energy metabolism, growth, reproduction, wound healing, and immune function. Table 12.2 lists these and other functions of iron in the body.

Heme is the iron—containing structure in two very important proteins, hemoglobin and myoglobin. In red blood cells (RBCs), hemoglobin enables oxy— gen uptake and transport (Fig. 12.1). **Myoglobin** (*my'—o—glow—bin*) in muscle

heme iron-containing component of hemoglobin and myoglobin

TABLE 12.2 Roles of Iron in the Body

Body Function or System	Role
Oxygen transport and energy metabolism	Needed for production of hemoglobin (red blood cells), myoglobin (muscle cells), and cytochromes (most body cells)
Cell division	Required by an enzyme needed for DNA production
Immune system	Needed for production of lymphocytes (a type of white blood cell) Enables neutrophils (another type of white blood cell) to destroy bacteria
Nervous system	Needed to help maintain the myelin sheath that covers parts of certain nerve cells Needed for the production of neurotransmitters (e.g., dopamine, epinephrine, and norepinephrine) that regulate brain and muscular activity

myoglobin iron-containing protein in muscle cells that controls oxygen uptake from red blood cells

cytochromes group of proteins necessary for certain chemical reactions involved in the release of energy from macronutrients

heme iron form of iron found in meat that is absorbed efficiently

nonheme iron form of iron that is not absorbed as efficiently as heme iron; found in meat, vegetables, grains, supplements, and fortified or enriched foods

cells helps oxygen enter the cells. The oxygen carried by hemoglobin and myoglobin is critical for energy metabolism.

Cells also contain iron in **cytochromes** (*sigh'—toe—crowms*), a group of proteins that are necessary for certain chemical reactions involved in the release of energy from macronutrients (see Chapter 8). If the body does not have enough iron to make hemoglobin, myoglobin, and the cytochromes, cells cannot obtain the energy they need to perform work. Thus, fatigue is a major symptom of iron deficiency.

Food Sources of Iron

Because meat contains hemoglobin and myoglobin, beef, fish, and poultry contain more iron **(heme iron)** than most plant foods. The remaining iron in meat, as well as all the iron in vegetables, grains, dietary supplements, and fortified or enriched foods, is **nonheme iron**. More heme iron than nonheme iron is absorbed in the intestinal tract.[1] Absorption of heme iron ranges from 15 to 35%, whereas absorption of nonheme iron ranges from 2 to 20%.[2]

Products made from enriched cereal grains are other important dietary sources of iron. However, the small intestine absorbs only about 5% of the iron salts that have been added to grain products, because iron salts are not as bioavailable as heme iron.[1,3] Dairy products are poor sources of iron. Table 12.3 lists the iron content of various foods. Figure 12.2 shows some foods of MyPlate food groups that are good sources of iron.

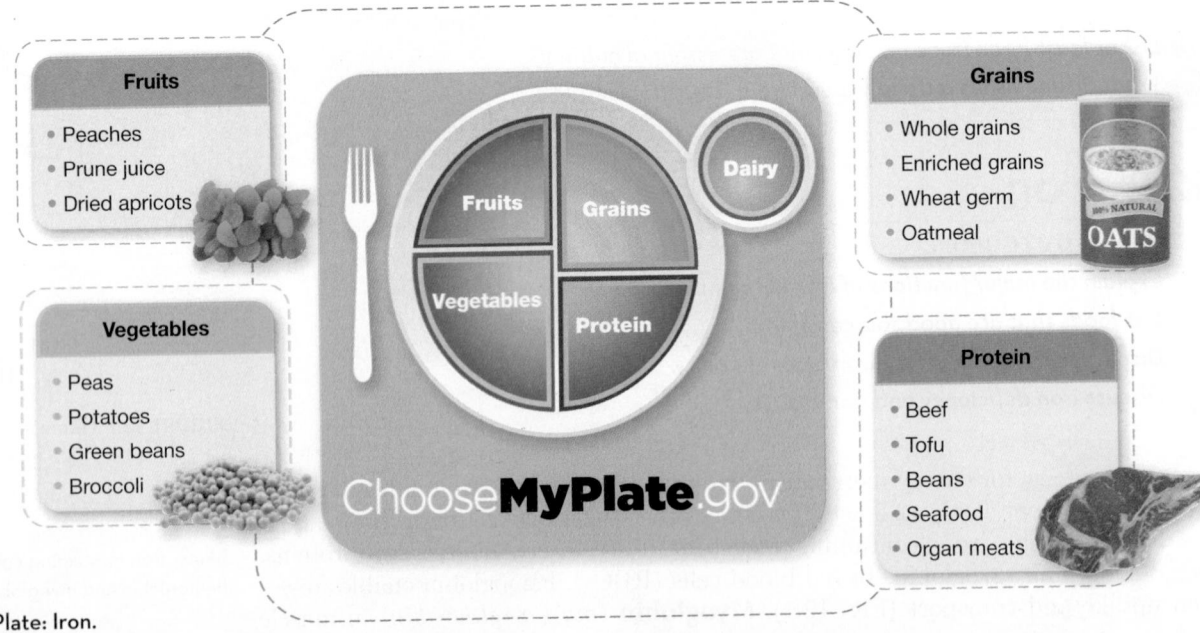

FIGURE 12.2 MyPlate: Iron.

TABLE 12.3 Iron Content of Selected Foods

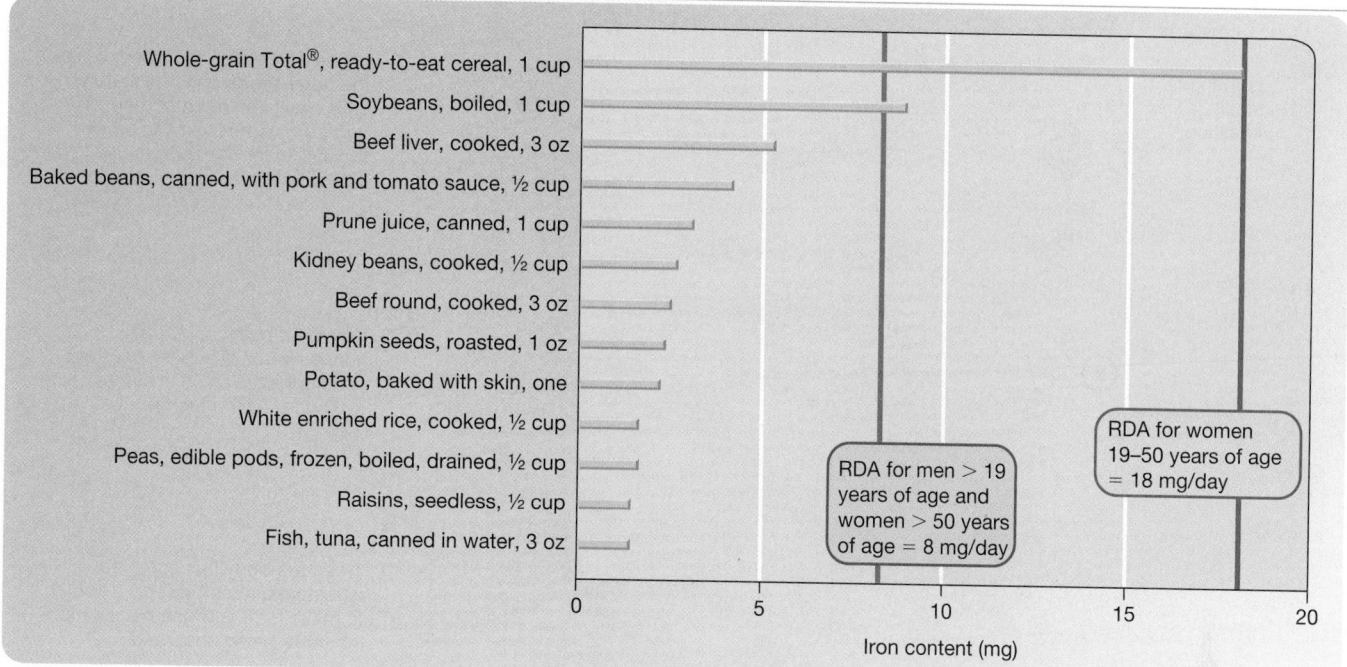

Source: Data from U.S. Department of Agriculture, Agricultural Research Service, USDA Nutrient Data Laboratory: Iron, Fe (mg) content of selected foods per common measure, sorted by nutrient content. *USDA national nutrient database for standard reference,* release 26. Last modified August 2013.

Iron Absorption, Storage, and Transport

A healthy body carefully regulates its iron status to avoid obtaining excessive amounts of the trace mineral. The body uses iron to make **ferritin** (*fer′–ih–tin*), the major storage form of iron. The liver, spleen, and bone marrow are the main sites for iron storage.

In the absorptive cells of the small intestine, ferritin helps regulate iron absorption (Fig. 12.3). When the body has adequate iron stores, the absorptive cells make ferritin, which blocks more iron from being absorbed. If the body lacks iron, ferritin levels drop. When the absorptive cells lack ferritin, they allow more iron to enter the bloodstream. Intestinal cells are constantly being shed into the lumen, and as a result, any ferritin that is stored in the absorptive cells is also shed. Thus, some iron is always needed by the body to replace that which is lost.

Transferrin is a protein in blood that transports iron (Fig. 12.3). When transferrin reaches cells, the protein binds to a receptor on the cell membrane called the **transferrin receptor**. If a cell needs more iron, it increases the number of transferrin receptors on its membrane. A version of transferrin receptor is in the bloodstream in an amount that is proportional to number of membrane–bound receptors. The level of transferrin receptors in the bloodstream increases when the body's iron stores become low.

Iron Absorption

Under normal conditions, the body closely regulates iron absorption and conservation. The digestive system of healthy people absorbs only 5 to 8% of the iron that is in a typical diet.[5] However, the intestinal tract can absorb more iron when the body's need for the trace mineral increases. For example, absorption of non-heme iron can be as high as 23% in women who are iron deficient.[5]

The intestinal tract absorbs the *ferrous* (Fe^{2+}) form of iron more efficiently than the *ferric* (Fe^{3+}) form (Fig. 12.3). Under acidic conditions, ferric iron can be converted to ferrous iron. Thus, medications that decrease stomach acidity,

DID **YOU** KNOW?

Frozen vegetables may lose up to half of their iron content due to processing and cooking.[4] In contrast, fresh vegetables that have been boiled may retain as much as 65% of their iron content, depending on the type of vegetable. To achieve a healthy iron intake, people should consider eating a variety of vegetables, including raw, frozen, and canned forms.

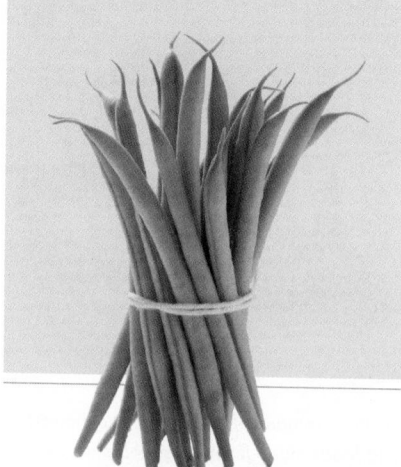

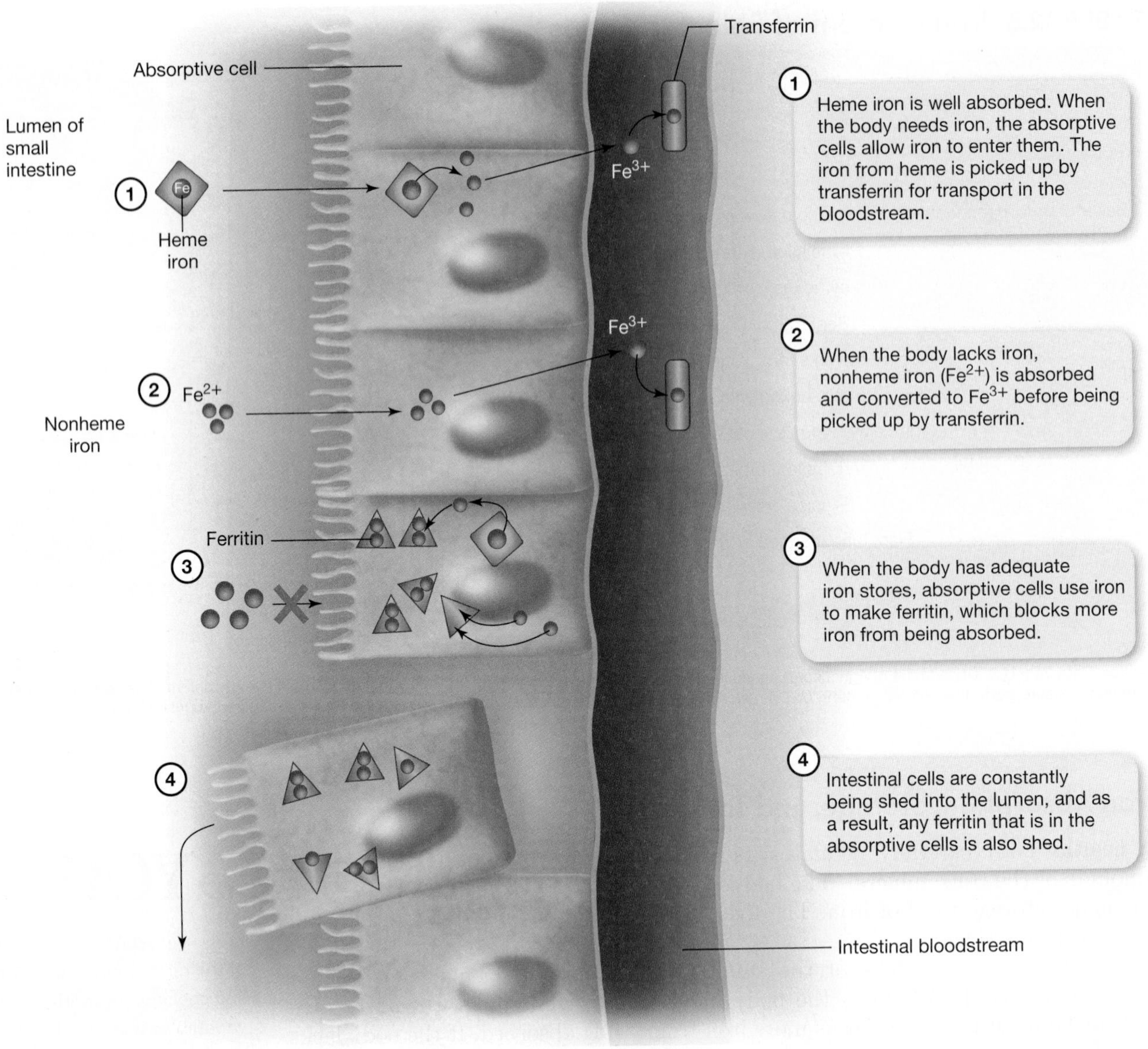

Transferrin

Absorptive cell

Lumen of small intestine

① Fe

Heme iron

Fe³⁺

① Heme iron is well absorbed. When the body needs iron, the absorptive cells allow iron to enter them. The iron from heme is picked up by transferrin for transport in the bloodstream.

② Fe²⁺

Nonheme iron

Fe³⁺

② When the body lacks iron, nonheme iron (Fe²⁺) is absorbed and converted to Fe³⁺ before being picked up by transferrin.

Ferritin

③

③ When the body has adequate iron stores, absorptive cells use iron to make ferritin, which blocks more iron from being absorbed.

④

④ Intestinal cells are constantly being shed into the lumen, and as a result, any ferritin that is in the absorptive cells is also shed.

Intestinal bloodstream

FIGURE 12.3 Intestinal regulation of iron absorption.

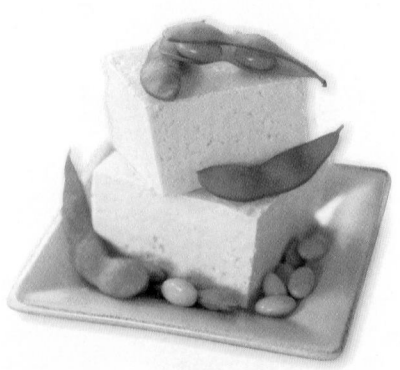

Eating edamame (lightly boiled soybeans) and foods made from soybeans, such as tofu, may inhibit iron absorption.

such as antacids, may reduce iron absorption.[1] Calcium and iron compete for absorption in the small intestine, so a meal with high calcium content can inhibit iron absorption. Therefore, people should consume a variety of food sources of iron throughout the day.

Some plant foods, such as spinach, contain nonheme iron, but *oxalic acid* in spinach binds to the mineral, reducing its absorption. Other naturally occurring compounds that reduce iron absorption include polyphenols, phytic acid (or phytates), and soy protein. Polyphenols are present in tea, coffee, wine, and some fruits and vegetables. Phytates are in several foods, including whole grains, rice, and legumes. Absorption of iron from phytate–containing legumes, such as soybeans, black beans, lentils, and split peas, may be as little as 2%.[1] Soy protein, including the kind used to make tofu, also reduces iron absorption.

Certain dietary factors can enhance iron absorption, especially of nonheme iron. Foods that are high in vitamin C increase intestinal absorption of the trace mineral. Adding a source of vitamin C to meals can increase the absorption of nonheme iron by 20%.[5] People can also increase their absorption of nonheme iron by combining a small amount of heme iron (from meat) with foods that contain nonheme iron. In addition to heme iron, meat, fish, and poultry contain a factor (sometimes called "MFP factor") that enhances the intestinal tract's

TABLE 12.4 Factors That Influence Iron Bioavailability

Enhance	Inhibit
Vitamin C	High intake of calcium with iron-containing food
Heme iron	Medications that reduce stomach acidity
Leavening of bread	Oxalic acid from foods such as spinach
Fermentation	Phytic acid from foods such as whole grains
Soaking beans or grains	Soy protein such as tofu
	Polyphenols from foods and beverages, such as tea

ability to absorb nonheme iron.[3] Table 12.4 lists major factors that enhance or inhibit iron bioavailability.

Dietary Adequacy

For adult men, the RDA for iron is 8 mg/day; for adult women between 19 and 50 years of age, the RDA for iron is 18 mg/day. The average daily intake for American men is about 18 mg, whereas the average daily intake for American women is about 13.6 mg.[6] Thus, women between 19 and 50 years of age are more likely than men to have inadequate iron intake.

Determining Iron Status

A person's iron status reflects his or her iron stores and concentrations of iron in transferrin and plasma (circulating iron), as well as the iron that is in RBCs and tissues involved in RBC production. Blood levels of transferrin receptor are a good indication of a person's iron status, because the level increases when iron stores become depleted. However, measuring blood (serum) ferritin concentration (saturation) is the most commonly used method to assess a person's iron status.[7] **Total body iron** is the ratio of blood transferrin receptor to ferritin. Determining a person's total body iron is the best method of assessing iron status.[7] Figure 12.4 illustrates the continuum of iron status from excess iron (iron overload) to iron deficiency states.

ferritin major storage form of iron; serum concentrations are used to assess iron status

transferrin transport protein for iron in the bloodstream

transferrin receptor membrane-bound receptor that attaches to iron; used to measure iron status

total body iron method of assessing iron status; the ratio of blood transferrin receptor to ferritin

FIGURE 12.4 Indications of iron status.

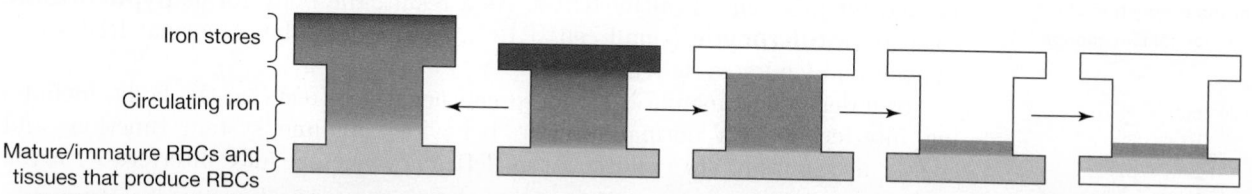

Physiological Feature	Iron Overload	Normal	Iron Depletion	Iron Deficiency	Iron-Deficiency Anemia
Plasma ferritin (µg/L)	>300	100 ± 60	20	10	<10
Iron absorption (%)	>15	5–10	10–15	10–20	10–20
Transferrin saturation (%)	>60	35 ± 15	30	<15	<15
Red blood cells (size and color)	Normal	Normal	Normal	Normal	Small and pale colored

Stage 1: Iron depletion

No apparent health problems

Stage 2: Iron deficiency without anemia (early or mild iron deficiency)

Reduced cognitive functioning in children

Reduced ferritin level

Elevated level of transferrin receptors

Stage 3: Iron deficiency anemia

Microcytic, hypochromic red blood cells

Very high level of transferrin receptors

Signs and symptoms of iron deficiency anemia, poor pregnancy outcomes, heart failure

FIGURE 12.5 Stages of iron depletion.

Iron Deficiency

After RBCs die, the body breaks them down and conserves most of the iron that was in hemoglobin. By doing so, the body can recycle the trace mineral to make hemoglobin for new RBCs. Despite the body's efforts to maintain iron, some of the trace mineral is lost each day via the gastrointestinal tract, urine, and skin. Any form of bleeding, including menstruation, also contributes to iron losses. If such losses are excessive and the affected person is unable to replace the iron, iron deficiency occurs.

Iron deficiency is a condition characterized by abnormally low iron levels in the body. The deficiency usually results from losing blood, consuming diets that lack iron, or being unable to absorb adequate amounts of dietary iron. Anemia is a condition in which the body does not have enough healthy RBCs and oxygen transport in blood is impaired. Over 30% of the world's population has anemia, and many cases of the condition are due to iron deficiency.[8] Iron deficiency can be divided into three stages, which are shown in Figure 12.5.[1]

In the first two stages of iron deficiency, the body's iron stores are lower than normal. A drop in the body's ferritin level is a sign that iron stores are becoming depleted. In the second stage, RBC production is reduced, but the reduction is not enough to be considered anemia. The third stage, **iron deficiency anemia**, is a condition that occurs when the body lacks enough iron to make the hemoglobin needed for producing healthy RBCs. As a result, the body forms **hypochromic** (pale red), **microcytic** (small cell) RBCs. Figure 12.6 shows normal RBCs and hypochromic, microcytic RBCs.

Iron deficiency anemia has widespread negative effects on the body, includ—ing interfering with normal growth, behavior, immune system function, and energy metabolism.[1] In children, iron deficiency anemia may interfere with the

iron deficiency low iron stores in the body

iron deficiency anemia third stage of iron deficiency characterized by a lack of red blood cells or the production of red blood cells that do not contain enough hemoglobin

hypochromic pale color

microcytic small cell

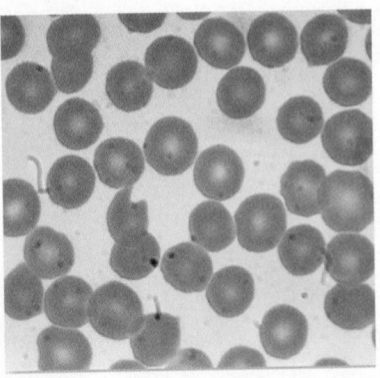
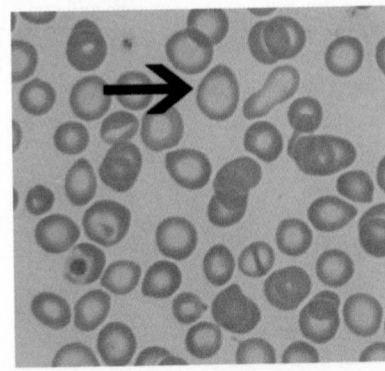

FIGURE 12.6 Iron-deficient red blood cells. (a) Normal red blood cells. (b) Hypochromic, microcytic red blood cells. The arrow points to one abnormal cell.

(a)

(b)

TABLE 12.5 Signs and Symptoms of Iron Deficiency Anemia

- Pale skin and pale mucous membranes (e.g., the membrane under an eyelid)
- Fatigue and weakness
- Irritability
- Shortness of breath
- Brittle, cupped nails
- Decreased appetite (especially in children)
- Difficulty concentrating
- Headache

Source: U.S. Library of Medicine (Medline), National Institutes of Health: Iron deficiency anemia. *Medline plus.* www.nlm.nih.gov/medlineplus/ency/article/000584.htm. Updated February 7, 2012. Accessed: July 16, 2013.

development of cognitive (thought processes) functioning.[7] The following section discusses iron deficiency anemia.

Iron Deficiency Anemia In cases of iron deficiency anemia, not enough RBCs are available to carry oxygen efficiently, or the RBCs do not contain enough hemoglobin. When oxygen is lacking, the body's cells cannot release considerable amounts of energy from macronutrients. This leads to symptoms of anemia, including lack of energy and difficulty concentrating on mental activities. Furthermore, the heart of a person with anemia has to work harder to circulate oxygen-poor blood throughout the body. Over time, anemia can cause rapid or irregular heartbeat, chest pain, an enlarged heart, and even heart failure. Table 12.5 lists common signs and symptoms of iron deficiency anemia.

Iron Deficiency: High-Risk Populations

In the United States, iron deficiency is the most common nutritional deficiency and the leading cause of anemia.[9] According to a 2012 report, 10 to 19% of American females between the ages of 12 to 49 years are iron deficient in contrast to only 1% of males in that age group.[7] Children are also at risk for iron deficiency.

Many factors contribute to iron deficiency. Substantial blood loss that results from severe injuries and serious intestinal conditions, such as colon cancer, is a common cause of iron deficiency anemia. Additionally, women with heavy menstrual blood losses are especially prone to iron deficiency anemia. Young women are also at risk for iron deficiency and iron deficiency anemia, because they may exclude meat and enriched bread and cereal products from their diets.

Iron needs increase during pregnancy and periods of rapid growth. A pregnant woman's need for iron increases as her blood supply expands and new tissues are added to both her body and that of her fetus. Pregnant women who suffer from iron deficiency anemia have a higher risk of dying during pregnancy than healthy pregnant women. Anemic pregnant women are also more likely to give birth to premature or low-birth-weight infants, which are more likely to die during their first year of life. According to the Dietary Guidelines, iron is a "nutrient of public health concern" for pregnant females (see Chapter 3).

Because of their rapid growth rates, infants and toddlers have higher needs for iron than older children. Furthermore, iron appears to be necessary for normal nervous system functioning, including proper brain development. Iron-deficient infants can experience delays in the development of normal motor and mental functions.[9]

Consuming too much milk may play a role in the development of iron deficiency in children. Milk is a poor source of iron, and the calcium that is in milk interferes with iron absorption when the beverage is consumed with foods that contain the trace mineral.[1] To reduce the risk of iron deficiency, children should be encouraged to eat more iron-rich foods, such as lean meats and iron-fortified cereals.

Rapid growth that occurs during puberty increases an adolescent's iron needs.[1] In young females, this growth spurt occurs around the age when menstruation begins. The combination of increased iron needs to support growth, iron losses due to menstruation, and poor dietary choices that are typical of many female teenagers often leads to iron deficiency.

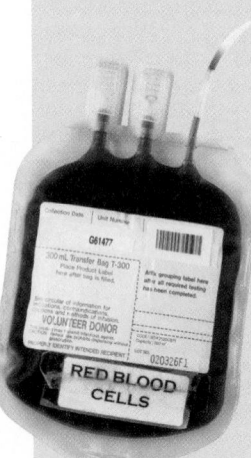

Donating 1 pint (approximately 0.5 L) of blood represents a loss of 200 to 250 mg of iron. Even when a person consumes adequate amounts of iron, his or her body generally needs several weeks to replace the iron that was in the donated blood. According to the American Red Cross, healthy people can give whole blood every 56 days. Young women, however, may need to donate blood less often, especially if they have heavy menstrual losses of blood.

Others at Risk for Iron Deficiency Vegetarians have a higher risk of iron deficiency than people who eat meat, because meat provides heme iron. To avoid iron deficiency and iron deficiency anemia, vegetarians need almost twice as much iron as people who eat meat, up to 14 mg/day for men and 32 mg/day for premenopausal women.[10] Vegetarians should be aware of dietary factors that can enhance or inhibit iron absorption from plant sources. The "Real People, Real Stories" on page 393 features a young woman who became iron deficient while following a vegan diet.

Athletes who regularly perform long-distance running may lose iron during the high-impact activity.[10] The iron in hemoglobin can be lost when RBCs rupture in feet as they pound the pavement. Also, runners experience increased blood loss in the gastrointestinal tract due to the jarring the body undergoes during running. Therefore, long-distance runners may need 30% more iron than people who are not as vigorously active (see Chapter 15).

Treating Iron Deficiency

Treatment for iron deficiency anemia generally includes iron supplements and the addition of iron-rich foods to the diet. The "Fresh Tips" feature on this page suggests practical ways to increase one's intake of dietary sources of iron. It is also important to find and treat nondietary factors that may be causing the deficiency, such as intestinal bleeding.

Iron Supplementation Treatment for iron deficiency may include use of iron supplements. Because of the risk of iron toxicity, an iron supplement should only be taken if it has been recommended by a physician. If men and postmenopausal women take a multivitamin/multimineral supplement, they should choose one with a maximum of 10 mg of iron.[10] Iron supplements can cause gastrointestinal distress, including stomach irritation, nausea, vomiting, diarrhea, or constipation.[1] Taking the iron supplement before or during a meal may be helpful in preventing the gastrointestinal problems.

People should avoid taking an iron supplement at the same time as a calcium or zinc supplement, because these three minerals compete for absorption sites. An acidic environment is ideal for maximizing iron absorption because acid conditions modify the chemical state of iron, making the mineral more bioavailable. Therefore, antacids or other medications that lower stomach acidity should not be taken with an iron supplement.

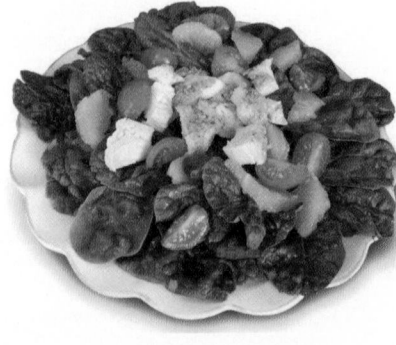

Adding cooked chicken and a source of vitamin C, such as orange segments, to a spinach salad can improve the iron bioavailability of the spinach.

FRESH TIPS

The following suggestions can add iron to your diet and increase its absorption:

- Eat lean meat, poultry, or fish with plant sources of iron.
- Combine soybeans with tomatoes or tomato sauce.
- Sprinkle lemon or lime juice on cooked beans, or serve the beans with salsa.
- Add orange segments, strawberries, or chopped tomatoes to spinach salads or cooked spinach.
- Add chopped onions and green peppers to peas or beans.
- Add lemon or lime juice to salad dressing.
- Serve sweet potatoes with fresh orange segments or dried apricots.
- Add raspberries, strawberries, raisins, or dried apricots to cereal.
- Drink orange juice when eating sandwiches made with nut butter.
- Consume watermelon, dried plums, dried apricots, or raisins for snacks.

Some forms of anemia, such as the anemia that results from having the *thalassemia trait*, are the result of genetic defects and not dietary deficiencies. In these cases, providing supplemental iron does not improve the person's iron status and may be harmful. Blood testing can determine the type of anemia so that the person's condition can be treated properly.

Iron Toxicity

The UL for iron is 45 mg/day. **Iron overload** occurs when toxic amounts of iron supplements are ingested, but toxicity also results from certain genetic conditions. Excess iron in the blood acts as an oxidant. **Oxidants** are free radicals that damage cell membranes, proteins, and DNA (see Chapter 9).

People with **hereditary hemochromatosis** (*he'—mo—crow'—ma—toe'—sis*) **(HH)** absorb too much iron. The body has no way to eliminate the excess iron, so the mineral accumulates in tissues and can cause joint pain; abnormal bronze skin color; and damage to the liver, heart, adrenal glands, and pancreas. The organ damage that results from HH can lead to cirrhosis, liver cancer, diabetes, or *cardiac arrhythmias* (irregular heartbeats).

Common signs and symptoms of HH include fatigue, lack of energy, abdominal pain, loss of sex drive, and heart problems. Even though people with HH begin accumulating iron early in life, they often do not report any signs and symptoms of the disease until they are over 30 years of age. If the disease is not detected early and treated effectively, the organ damage resulting from the condition can be deadly. Treatment usually includes visiting a clinic periodically to have blood removed. This process stimulates the tissues that produce RBCs to use stored iron for hemoglobin production.

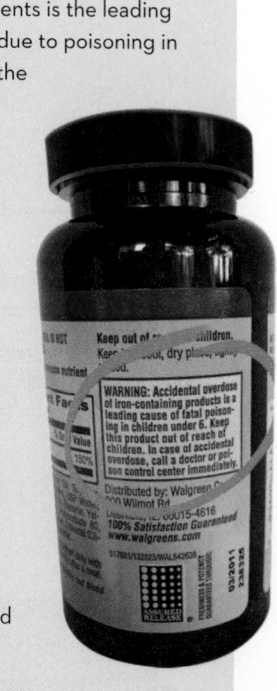

iron overload ingestion of toxic amounts of iron

oxidants free radicals that damage cell membranes, proteins, and DNA

hereditary hemochromatosis (HH) inherited genetic defect that causes people to absorb too much iron

REAL People, **REAL** Stories

Ali Ritto

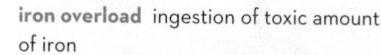

Ali Ritto teaches English at California State University–Long Beach. She's also a part-time yoga instructor. Ali grew up as a lactoovovegetarian, because her parents were lactoovovegetarians. When she was 17 years of age, she decided to become a vegan. She researched information about how to meet all of her nutritional needs by following a vegan diet.

After a year of following the vegan diet, Ali started college. "During my freshman year, I was very busy going to classes and working part-time," Ali says, "so I didn't focus on my nutritional needs, and my diet became unbalanced." When Ali noticed that she didn't have as much energy as in the past, she went to see a physician. According to her doctor, the young woman had a borderline case of iron deficiency. "I was given iron supplements, so I took the supplements daily for about a year. I continued following the vegan diet, but I also started eating better, and my health improved, Now, I pay more attention to my nutrient needs. I eat more broccoli and leafy kale to get enough iron, and I make smoothies with soy milk that's fortified with B-12," says Ali.

"When people find out that I'm a vegan, most of them ask, 'Isn't the diet hard or impossible to follow?' My response is, 'Yes, it's not easy, but it's not impossible.' I recommend that people who are interested in veganism learn as much as possible about the lifestyle before attempting it."

HH is the most common genetic defect among people of northern European descent. Approximately one of every 200 to 250 people in the United States has this inherited defect.[10] Testing is available to determine whether a person has the genes that are responsible for the disease.

ASSESS YOUR PROGRESS

3 *Describe at least three functions of iron in the body.*

4 *Identify two sources of heme iron and two sources of nonheme iron.*

5 *How is iron status assessed? Describe ways of measuring a person's iron status.*

6 *Explain the stages of iron deficiency. Who is at risk for iron deficiency?*

7 *Discuss the physiological effects of iron overload.*

iodide form of iodine that the body absorbs and uses

goiter enlargement of the thyroid gland that is not the result of cancer

thyroid hormone hormones that control the rate of cell metabolism and are dependent on iodine for production

12.3 Iodine (Iodide)

LEARNING OUTCOMES

1 *Explain the major functions of iodine in the human body.*

2 *List rich food sources of iodine.*

3 *Discuss iodine deficiency and toxicity.*

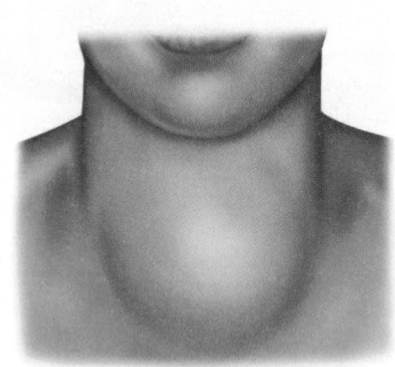

FIGURE 12.7 Goiter.

Elemental iodine (I_2) is a poison, but the iodine in foods is in the form of compounds and salts containing the trace mineral. In the body, the compounds and salts break apart and release the **iodide** ion (I^-), which is the form of iodine that the body absorbs and uses. Most of the iodide in an adult's body is located in the thyroid gland (see Fig. 11.10).

During World War I, physicians noted that men drafted into the U.S. military from the Great Lakes region were far more likely to have a *goiter* than men from some other areas of the country. **Goiter** (*goy'–ter*) is an enlargement of the thyroid gland that is not the result of cancer (Fig. 12.7). Goiters often occur among populations living in areas that lack the mineral iodine in locally produced foods. In general, these regions are inland and far from an ocean. If people in these communities limit their diets to locally produced foods, they might not have enough iodine in their diets.

From 1917 to 1922, researchers in Ohio conducted an experiment on a group of girls in which one group of the children received doses of iodine, while the other group (the control group) did not receive the trace mineral. The results of the study indicated iodine was nearly 100% effective in preventing goiter in the healthy children. Moreover, the majority of the girls who already had goiters when they received the iodine experienced a reduction in the size of their thyroid glands by the end of the study.[11] In 1924, American food manufacturers began adding iodide to table salt, and as a result, cases of goiter caused by iodine deficiency rarely occur in this country. Today, use of iodized salt is the major method of preventing iodine deficiencies in developed nations, but inadequate iodine intake and goiters are still common in central Asia and central Africa.

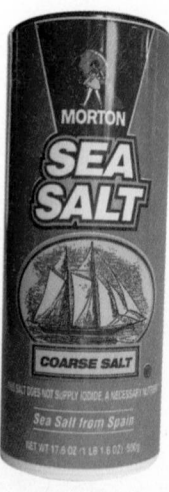

Sea salt is generally not a good source of iodine.

Function of Iodine

People require iodine for normal thyroid function and for the production of different thyroid hormones, which are collectively referred to as **thyroid hormone**. Thyroid hormone controls the rate of cellular metabolism, that is, the rate at which cells use energy. If iodine intake is too low, the thyroid gland enlarges in an attempt to remove as much iodide as possible from the bloodstream. However, an enlarged thyroid gland can also be a sign of certain diseases and conditions that are not related to iodine intake, such as *Graves' disease*. In cases of Graves' disease, the thyroid gland produces and secretes too much thyroid hormone, causing **hyperthyroidism**. Signs and symptoms of hyperthyroidism include rapid heart rate, sweating, anxiety, and weight loss despite increased appetite. In some cases of the disease, the person's eyeballs bulge out of their normal position. Treatment may involve removal of part or all of the thyroid gland, as well as medications that reduce thyroid hormone production.

Sources of Iodine

Major sources of iodine include saltwater fish; seafood; seaweed; some plants, especially the leaves of plants grown near oceans; milk; eggs; and iodized salt. A half teaspoon of iodide–fortified salt supplies the adult RDA for iodine. Adding iodide to salt is voluntary in the United States, so not all salt has the trace mineral added to it.

About 50 to 60% of Americans choose iodized salt.[7] Specialty salts, such as kosher salt and sea salt in particular, are not usually iodized. Other dietary sources of iodine include food additives that contain the mineral, such as certain dough conditioners and food dyes. Table 12.6 lists some foods that are good sources of iodine. The most common food sources of iodine in the United States are dairy products and bread.[12] Many Americans also obtain iodine from multivitamin and mineral supplements.

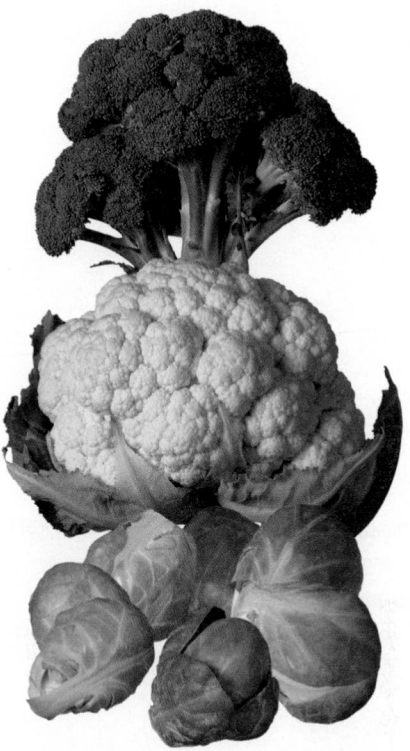
Sources of goitrogens.

Iodine Absorption

The body absorbs nearly all (85 to 90%) of the iodine that is in food. Some plant foods such as cassava, turnips, cabbage, Brussels sprouts, cauliflower, and broccoli, contain **goitrogens**. These compounds inhibit iodide metabolism by the thyroid gland and, as a result, reduce thyroid hormone production. Soy products also contain a compound that inhibits thyroid hormone production. People do not need to be concerned about eating these foods unless they are iodide deficient or they routinely eat large amounts of the vegetables that contain goitrogens or soy products.[12]

hyperthyroidism abnormally high blood levels of thyroid hormone

goitrogens compounds in food that inhibit iodide metabolism by the thyroid gland

TABLE 12.6 Iodine Content of Selected Foods

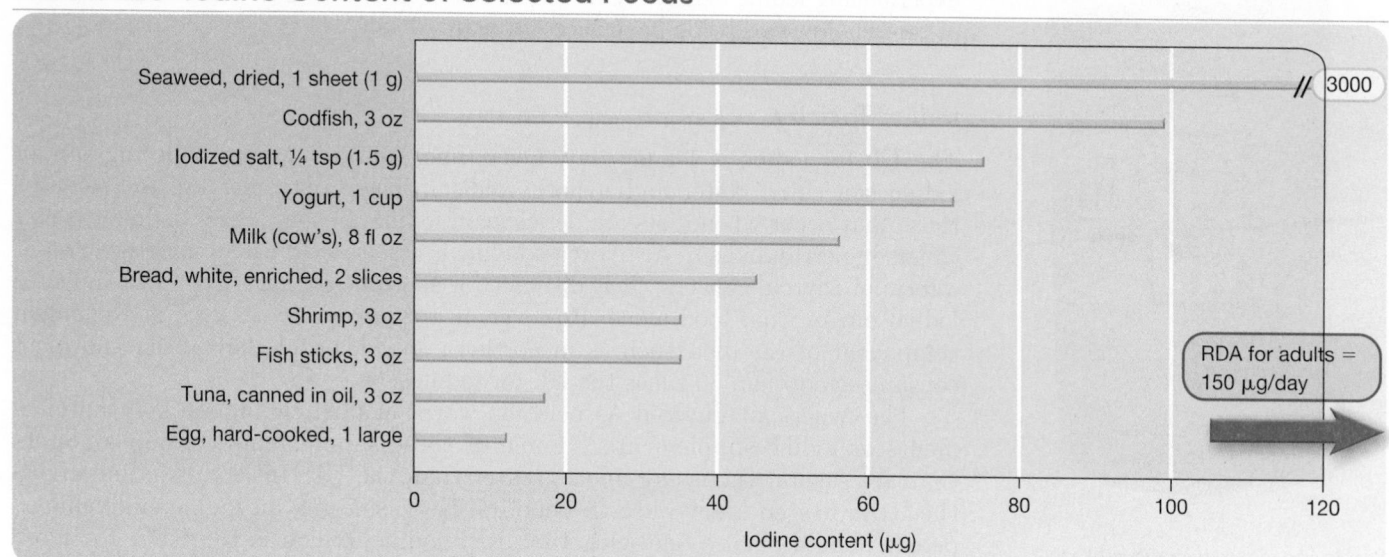

Source: Data from Office of Dietary Supplements, National Institutes of Health: *Dietary supplement fact sheet: Iodine.* Updated June 2011. http://ods.od.nih.gov/factsheets/Iodine-HealthProfessional/ Accessed: April 23, 2014.

Dietary Adequacy

The adult RDA for iodine is 150 µg/day. Although most Americans have adequate iodine intakes,[12] many young, American women have iodine intakes that are marginally adequate.[7] Because iodine needs increase during pregnancy and lactation (milk production), some medical experts recommend that young women take a multivitamin and mineral supplement that provides 150 µg of iodine daily before pregnancy and during pregnancy and lactation.[13] As many Americans, particularly older adults, use less salt to manage their hypertension, this particular population's iodine intake may decline to marginal or inadequate levels.

Iodine Deficiency

Throughout the world, millions of people are at risk of iodine deficiency. Goiter is often the first sign of iodine deficiency. Iodine–deficient people develop **hypothyroidism**, which is characterized by low blood levels of thyroid hormone. Other signs or symptoms of hypothyroidism include reduced metabolic rate, elevated blood cholesterol level, fatigue, difficulty concentrating on mental tasks, weight gain, constipation, and dry skin.

Adequate iodine status is extremely important during pregnancy. Pregnant women who are iodine deficient have higher risk of *stillbirths* (giving birth to a dead infant) or having low–birth–weight babies. During fetal life, thyroid hormone is crucial for normal brain development. Thus, the fetus of an iodine–deficient woman is likely to be born with a condition called **cretinism** (*kre'–tin–ih–zim*). Babies with cretinism have permanent brain damage, reduced intellectual functioning, and growth retardation. Worldwide, iodine deficiency is the most common cause of preventable intellectual disability.[12] Pregnant women can reduce the risk of giving birth to infants with cretinism by consuming adequate amounts of iodine throughout pregnancy.

Iodine deficiency is a serious threat to health in places where soils are iodine deficient and commonly eaten foods are not fortified with the trace mineral. Approximately 35% of the world's population is at risk for iodine deficiency, including people living in regions of Latin America, India, Southeast Asia, and Africa.[14] Currently, international health organizations are engaging in efforts to eliminate iodine deficiency, primarily by promoting the use of iodized salt or iodide–fortified vegetable oils. In the past 10 years, the number of countries experiencing iodine deficiency has been cut in half. It is now estimated that 66% of households worldwide have access to iodized salt.[14]

Iodine Toxicity

The UL for iodine is 1.1 mg/day. Over time, consuming very high amounts of iodine can cause goiter and hypothyroidism. These outcomes are the same as those that occur when diets are deficient in iodine. In some cases, iodine toxicity causes hyperthyroidism. Also, excess iodine is associated with an increased risk of a form of thyroid cancer.[12] It is difficult for someone to reach the upper limit for iodine intake from food alone. However, in regions where seaweed is a common component of the diet, such as in northern Japan, people have been known to consume more than 50 times the UL for iodine.[15]

The American Thyroid Association warns against taking sea kelp supplements or iodine supplements.[16] Some of these supplements contain amounts that are several thousand times greater than the UL. Intake of iodine above the RDA has no known health benefits. If considering an iodine supplement, people should choose one with 150 µg of iodine, which is the RDA for most adults, and should avoid any products with more than 500 µg of iodine per serving.

hypothyroidism low blood levels of thyroid hormone

cretinism condition in infants who are born to iodine-deficient women; the infants have permanent brain damage and growth retardation

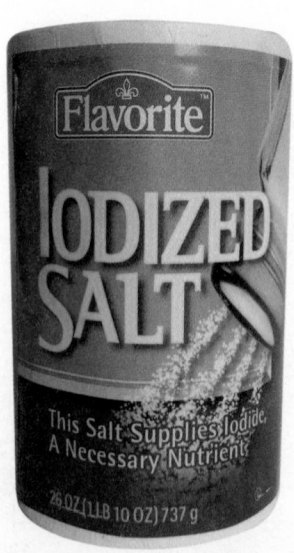

People who reduce their salt intake to manage hypertension may become iodine deficient.

ASSESS YOUR PROGRESS

8 *Identify the main function of iodine in the body.*

9 *List at least three rich dietary sources of iodine.*

10 *What food factors can alter iodine absorption?*

11 *Explain the outcomes of a diet that is too high or too low in iodine.*

12.4 Zinc

LEARNING OUTCOMES

1 *Explain the major functions of zinc in the body.*

2 *List rich food sources of zinc and describe factors that affect the mineral's bioavailability.*

3 *Discuss zinc deficiency and toxicity.*

Over 50 years ago, physician Ananda S. Prasad was working in Iran when he examined a 21-year-old man with dwarfism, intellectual disability, iron deficiency anemia, and underdeveloped sexual organs.[17] Prasad noted that the young man ate unleavened ("flat") bread almost exclusively. When Prasad examined other patients in Iran and Egypt with similar health problems and dietary practices, he hypothesized that diet was responsible for the condition. Eventually, medical researchers determined that Prasad's patients had severe zinc deficiencies. After these patients were given zinc supplements, they began to grow and develop normally.

In the regions where the zinc-deficient people lived, the typical diet was comprised primarily of unleavened whole-wheat bread and little animal protein. Unleavened whole-wheat bread is naturally high in phytic acid and fiber, substances that decrease zinc bioavailability. In places where people use yeast to leaven (raise) bread dough, severe zinc deficiency is less likely to occur. Yeast reduces the binding effects of phytic acid and fiber, making zinc more bioavailable.

Functions of Zinc

Zinc is important for the functioning of over 300 enzymes.[18] The trace mineral is necessary for growth and development, wound healing, the sense of taste and smell, DNA synthesis, and proper functioning of the nervous and immune systems.[18,19]

Sources of Zinc

Zinc is widespread in foods (Table 12.7). Figure 12.8 indicates MyPlate food groups that have foods that are good sources of zinc. Red meat and poultry products supply most of the zinc in the typical American diet.

The bioavailability of zinc is enhanced when foods that contain the mineral are eaten with proteins, especially those with sulfur-containing amino acids.[18] Other factors that influence the bioavailability of zinc include the body's need for the mineral and the presence of large amounts of certain other metals. During times when a healthy body needs zinc, such as during pregnancy, the small intestine absorbs more. However, the presence of excess copper or iron in the small intestine interferes with zinc absorption. Thus, iron supplements should be taken between meals instead of with them to avoid suppressing zinc absorption.[19] People can also obtain zinc from nondietary sources, including denture creams and some over-the-counter products marketed as cold remedies.

TABLE 12.7 Zinc Content of Selected Foods

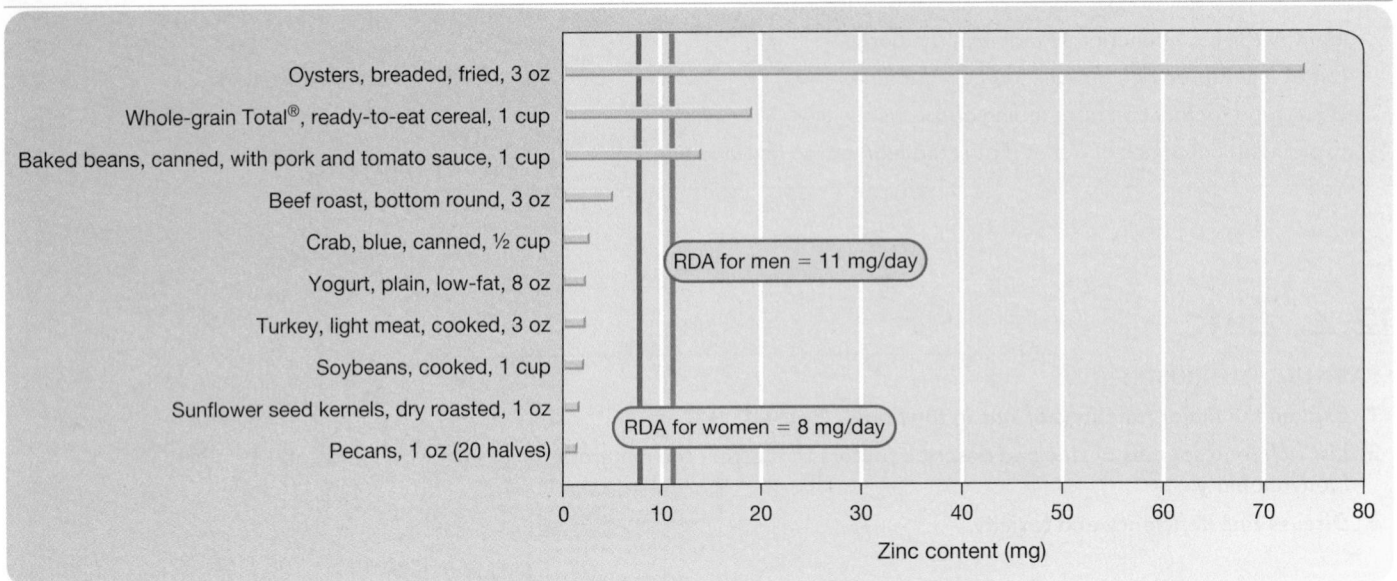

Source: Data from U.S. Department of Agriculture, Agricultural Research Service, USDA Nutrient Data Laboratory: Zinc, Zn (mg)
content of selected foods per common measure, sorted by nutrient content. *USDA national nutrient database for standard reference,* release 26, 2013.

Dietary Adequacy

Currently, there is no established method for assessing zinc status in the body. Humans do not store zinc, so the trace mineral needs to be consumed daily.[19] Adult RDAs for zinc range from 8 mg to 11 mg/day. In the United States, the average intake of zinc is 9.5 mg/day for women and 13.7 mg/day for men.[6] Thus, zinc deficiency is not a widespread problem in the United States. However, alcoholics have high risk of zinc deficiency, because alcohol reduces zinc absorption and increases excretion of the mineral in urine. Furthermore, many people

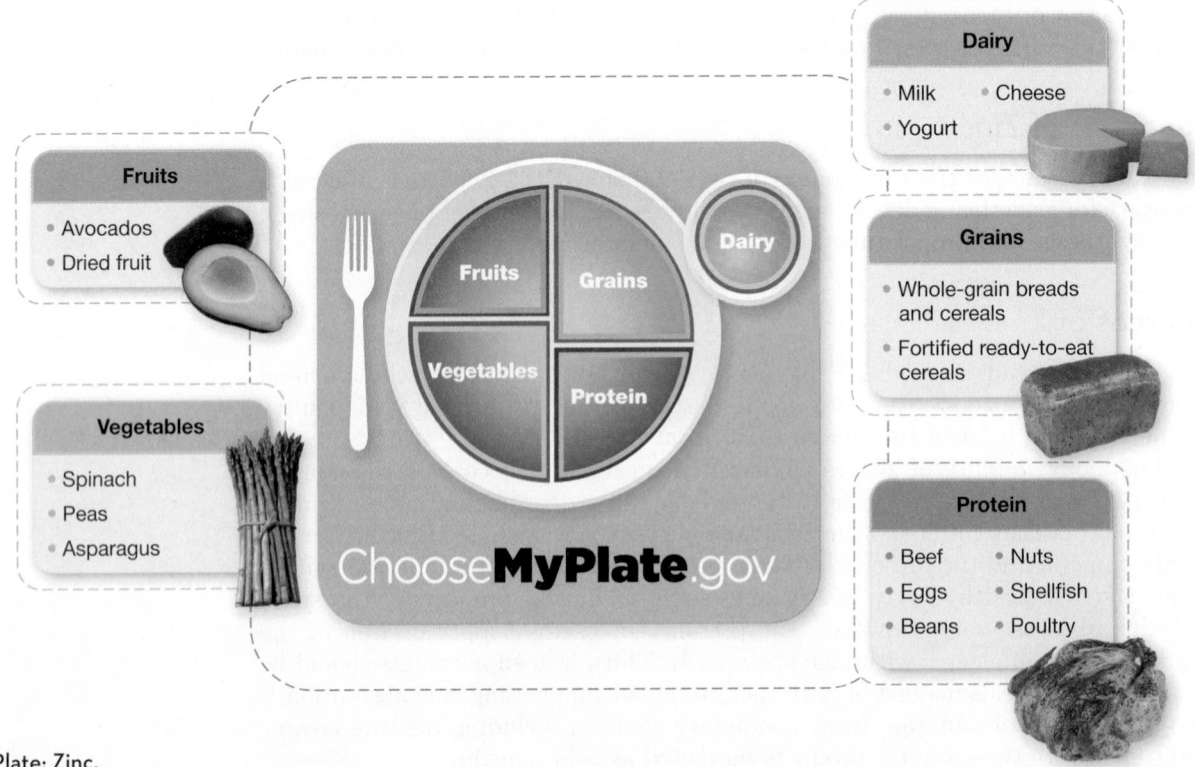

FIGURE 12.8 MyPlate: Zinc.

who suffer from alcoholism do not consume nutritious diets. People with chronic diarrhea or digestive tract diseases can also develop zinc deficiency.

Due to the high phytic acid content of their diet, vegetarians may need up to 50% more zinc than people who eat a "mixed" diet.[18] To optimize zinc absorption, seeds, grains, and legumes can be soaked in water and allowed to sprout before eating to reduce the effects of phytic acid.[20] Also, vegans can eat whole-grain breads made with yeast (leavened bread) instead of unleavened breads.

Zinc Deficiency

Worldwide, approximately 2 billion people have a zinc deficiency.[18] Signs and symptoms of zinc deficiency include loss of appetite, diarrhea, hair loss, skin rash, poor wound healing, impaired sense of taste, and mental slowness.[19] In severe cases, zinc deficiency stunts a child's growth, leading to dwarfism and failure of sexual maturation.

Zinc deficiency during pregnancy can cause serious complications, including premature birth and delivery of a low-birth-weight baby. Breastfed babies may be at risk of developing zinc deficiency. Although breast milk contains zinc, the milk does not supply enough of the trace mineral for infants who are older than 6 months of age. To increase the likelihood that their diets contain enough zinc, breastfed babies who are between 6 and 12 months of age need to consume foods that contain the trace mineral, such as meat and zinc-fortified infant cereal.

The immune system depends on zinc to work properly. A diet that lacks zinc contributes to a weakened immune system, which increases the risk of contracting infections that are often deadly. In developing nations, zinc deficiency contributes to more than 4% of childhood deaths.[18]

Older adults are also at risk of zinc deficiency. In the United States, an estimated 20 to 25% of adults over 60 years of age have zinc intakes that are below the Estimated Average Requirement.[19] One reason for such low intakes may be that older adults on fixed incomes try to save money by not purchasing meat, which is a rich source of bioavailable zinc.

Zinc Toxicity

The UL for zinc is 40 mg/day. Zinc intakes that exceed the UL can reduce beneficial HDL cholesterol levels. Ingesting more than 100 mg of zinc per day can also result in diarrhea, cramps, nausea, vomiting, and depressed immune system function. Additionally, megadoses of zinc may interfere with copper absorption and metabolism. Therefore, people should avoid high zinc supplementation unless they are under a physician's supervision.

Zinc Lozenges and the Common Cold Zinc lozenges or gels may inhibit multiplication of the common cold virus in the nasal or oral cavity and thereby reduce the severity or duration of colds.[19] However, results of studies examining the potential for zinc to reduce the severity or duration of colds are inconsistent. Such inconsistencies may be due to the dose or type of zinc used. Also, benefits may only be experienced if the zinc products are taken within 24 hours of the onset of cold symptoms and continue every 2 to 3 hours while the person is awake. By following these instructions, however, consumers ingest levels of zinc that are higher than the UL. Side effects of such supplementation often include nausea and a metallic taste in the mouth.[18]

In 2009, the Food and Drug Administration (FDA) warned the public about using two *intranasal* ("within the nose") forms of Zicam®, a nonprescription, zinc-containing product marketed for the common cold. The agency had received several reports that this alternative-medicine treatment for the common cold may cause anosmia.[19] Anosmia is the loss of sense of smell, which, in the case of intranasal zinc use, was not always reversible. In response to FDA actions, the manufacturer of Zicam voluntarily recalled the products, removing them from the marketplace.

DID **YOU** *KNOW?*

Having adequate zinc status may prevent the development of age-related macular degeneration, which is a major cause of blindness in older adults.[19] In addition, supplemental doses of zinc along with antioxidants may delay progression of macular degeneration after it occurs.[21] Because of the risk of zinc toxicity, however, consumers should consult their health care provider before considering zinc supplementation.

ASSESS YOUR PROGRESS

12 List at least three major functions of zinc in the body.

13 Identify at least three rich food sources of zinc.

14 List factors that can inhibit zinc absorption.

15 Who is at risk for zinc deficiency?

16 What can happen when someone consumes megadoses of zinc?

12.5 Selenium

LEARNING OUTCOMES

1 Explain the major functions of selenium in the human body.

2 List rich food sources of selenium.

3 Discuss selenium deficiency and toxicity.

Selenium is widespread in Earth's crust, but soils can vary widely in their content of the trace mineral. Areas of the western United States, including parts of Colorado and South Dakota, have unusually high concentrations of selenium in the soil. Certain types of plants that grow in these places accumulate toxic levels of the mineral. Livestock that graze on the selenium–rich plants often ingest poisonous amounts of selenium. In horses and cattle, selenium toxicity can cause hair and weight loss, malformed hooves that can separate from the animals' feet, muscle weakness, loss of muscular function (*paralysis*), and death. Figure 12.9 is a map of the United States that shows the distribution of selenium in soil.

selenoproteins several proteins that require selenium to function; often serve as antioxidants

glutathione peroxidase family of selenoproteins that have antioxidant function.

Functions of Selenium

In the body, selenium functions as a component of several enzymes referred to as **selenoproteins** (*sell'–in–oh–pro'–teens*). **Glutathione peroxidase** is a family

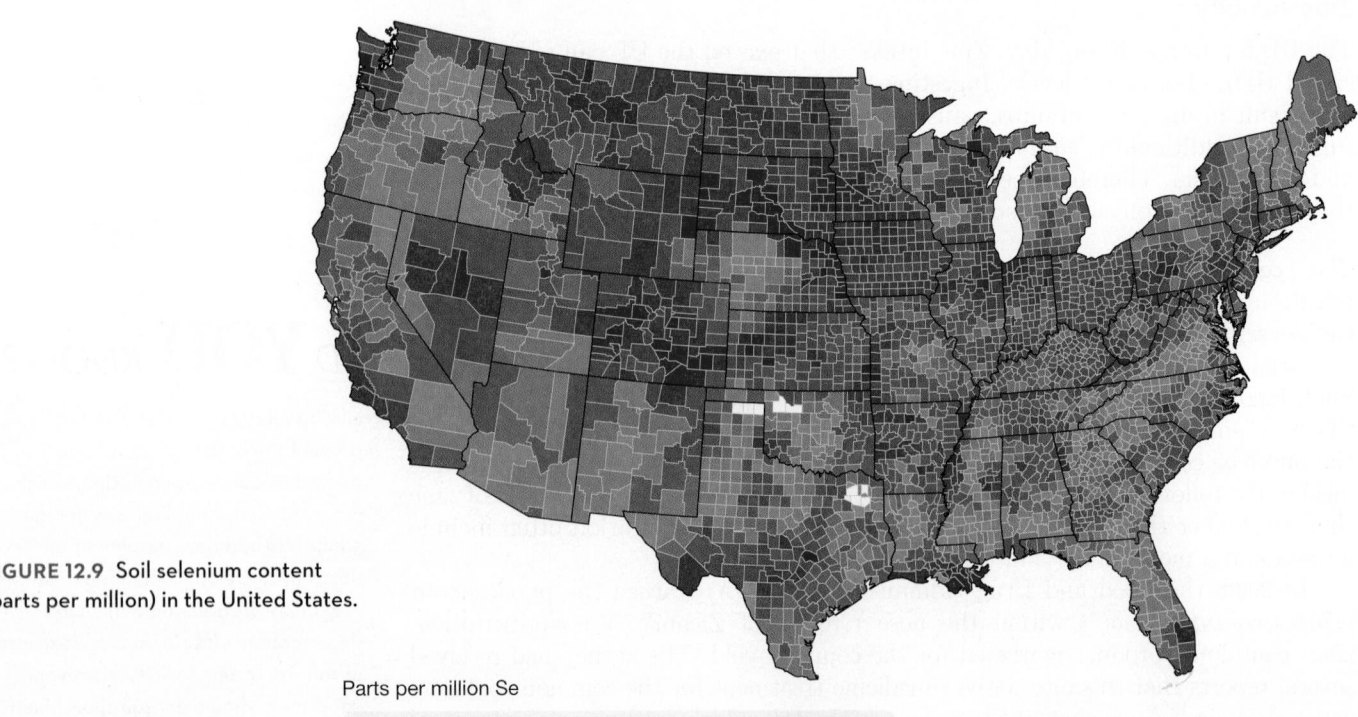

FIGURE 12.9 Soil selenium content (parts per million) in the United States.

Parts per million Se

☐ 0.1–0.22   ■ 0.22–0.38   ■ 0.38–5.32   ☐ No data

Source: U.S. Geological Survey

TABLE 12.8 Selenium Content of Selected Foods

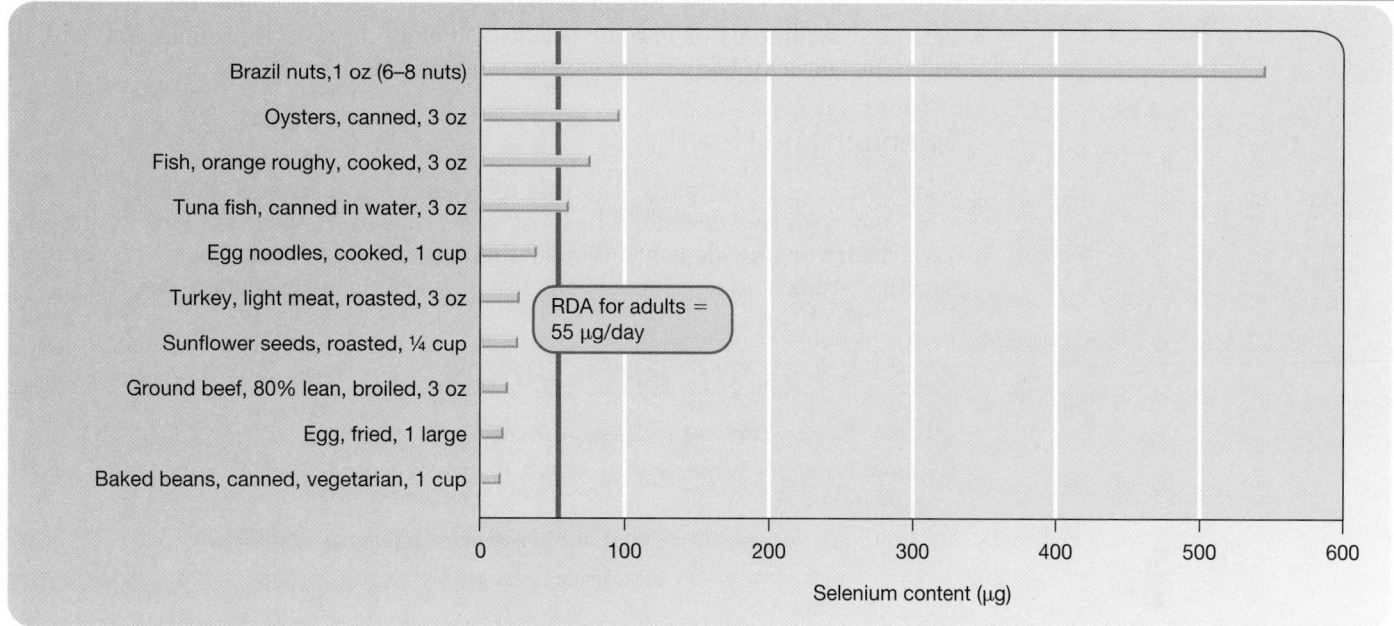

Brazil nuts, 1 oz (6–8 nuts)
Oysters, canned, 3 oz
Fish, orange roughy, cooked, 3 oz
Tuna fish, canned in water, 3 oz
Egg noodles, cooked, 1 cup
Turkey, light meat, roasted, 3 oz
Sunflower seeds, roasted, ¼ cup
Ground beef, 80% lean, broiled, 3 oz
Egg, fried, 1 large
Baked beans, canned, vegetarian, 1 cup

RDA for adults = 55 µg/day

0 100 200 300 400 500 600
Selenium content (µg)

Source: Data from U.S. Department of Agriculture, Agricultural Research Service, USDA Nutrient Data Laboratory: *USDA national nutrient database for standard reference,* release 26, 2013.

of selenoproteins that act as antioxidants, protecting the body from free–radical damage. Other selenoproteins are necessary for the normal functioning of thyroid hormone and the immune system. In addition, selenium is important for reproduction and DNA synthesis.

Sources of Selenium

Rich food sources of selenium include seafood and organ meats, such as liver and kidneys.[22] In the United States, meat, poultry, fish, eggs, nuts, and whole grains are the primary dietary sources of selenium (Table 12.8).[22] As with iodine, the selenium content of crops depends largely on where and how the plants are grown. The body absorbs between 50 to 90% of selenium that is consumed.

Dietary Adequacy

Most Americans consume more than the RDA for selenium (55 µg/day for adults).[6] Thus, selenium deficiency is uncommon in the United States, but the condition may occur in people who have serious digestive tract conditions that interfere with the mineral's absorption. Selenium deficiency reduces thyroid gland activity, which can worsen an iodine deficiency and lead to goiter or cause cretinism. The deficiency also causes male infertility, depresses immune system function, and may contribute to the development of specific forms of heart disease and cancer.

In parts of China where the soil lacks selenium and the population consumes only locally produced foods, diets are typically inadequate in selenium. **Keshan disease**, a *cardiomyopathy* (disease of the heart muscle), was common in selenium–deficient regions of China before food in the area was fortified with selenium. In areas of China, Tibet, Siberia, and North Korea, a form of osteoarthritis called **Kashin–Beck disease** develops as a result of selenium deficiency.[23] Kashin–Beck disease is a degeneration of the cartilage between joints, which leads to deformity and dwarfism.

The UL for selenium is 400 µg/day. In the United States, selenium toxicity **(selenosis)** (*sell'–in–o–sis*) is rare.[22] Chronic selenosis, however, can occur

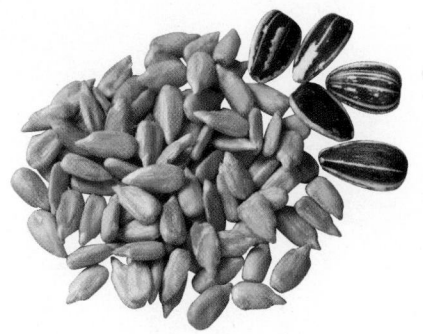

Sunflower seeds are a good source of selenium.

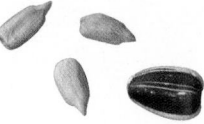

Keshan disease disease of the heart muscle associated with selenium deficiency

Kashin-Beck disease form of osteoarthritis caused by selenium deficiency; leads to joint deformity and dwarfism

selenosis selenium toxicity

from drinking well water that contains naturally high levels of selenium. Selenium toxicity can develop by taking megadoses of dietary supplements. In humans, signs and symptoms of chronic selenosis include brittle fingernails, loss of hair and nails, garlicky body odor, nausea, vomiting, and fatigue.

Selenium and Health

Scientists have investigated the role of selenium in cancer, cardiovascular disease, and cognitive decline.[22] In most cases, however, the results of studies are inconclusive or provide contradictory findings.[22,24] At present, the results of most scientific studies do not support the use of selenium supplementation.

ASSESS YOUR PROGRESS

17 Describe the functions of selenium in the body.

18 Identify rich food sources of selenium. What can cause the selenium content of food to vary widely?

19 What are the signs and symptoms of selenium deficiency and toxicity?

12.6 Fluoride

LEARNING OUTCOMES

1 Explain the role of fluoride in human health.

2 List common sources of fluoride.

3 Discuss the consequences of low and high fluoride consumption.

Fluoride (F^-) is not considered an essential nutrient, because it is not required for growth or to sustain life. However, regular fluoride intake helps mineralize teeth and bones, and can prevent tooth decay. The average adult has about 2.6 g of fluoride in his or her body; 99% of the trace mineral is located in calcified tissue such as bones and teeth.[25]

Functions of Fluoride

Dental erosion can lead to tooth decay (*dental caries* or cavities), but fluoride can remineralize the tooth surface and prevent cavities from developing. In children under 12 years of age, dietary fluoride helps the body build teeth that are resistant to decay. For people with fully formed teeth, fluoride from the diet becomes incorporated in the saliva, which further protects against tooth decay as it bathes the teeth.

In the United States, dental caries are the most prevalent chronic disease in children, but people of all ages can develop tooth decay. Tooth decay often causes jaw pain and tooth loss, altering the ability to eat. As a result, people with tooth decay may reduce their intake of raw or chewy foods, which can negatively affect their nutritional status.

Fluoride also encourages bone development, and the mineral becomes incorporated into bone tissue. Thus, adequate intake of fluoride is important for optimal bone health. For more information about minerals and bone health, see Chapter 11.

Sources of Fluoride

Fluids such as fluoridated water, coffee, tea, soft drinks, beer, and juice are Americans' main dietary sources of fluoride (Table 12.9). In addition, fish and shellfish such as crab, shrimp, and clams are a good source of fluoride. Nonfood sources of fluoride include toothpaste, mouthwash, and dental treatments.

TABLE 12.9 Fluoride Content of Selected Beverages (8 fl oz)

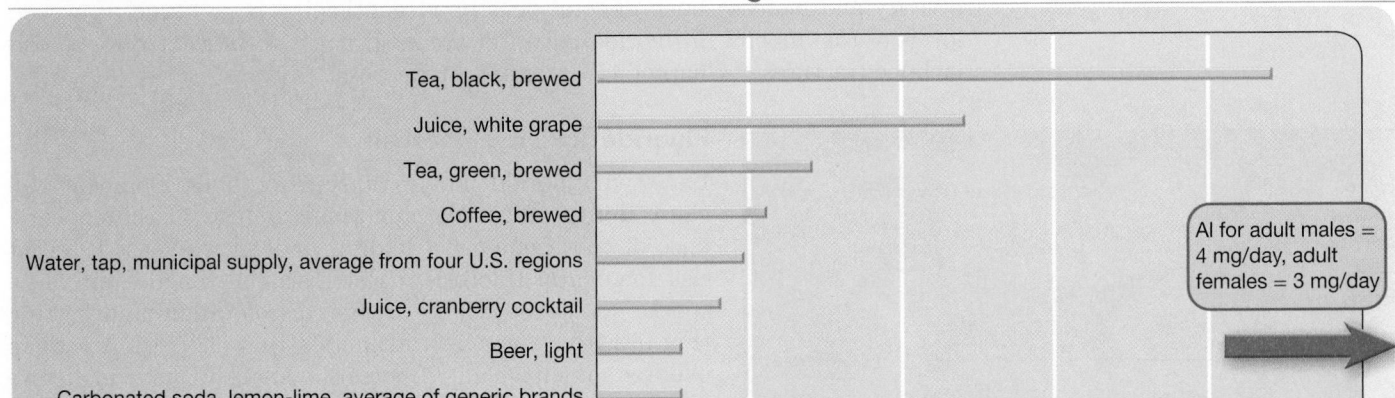

Source: U.S. Department of Agriculture Nutrient Data Laboratory, *USDA national fluoride database of selected foods, release 2.* Last modified August 23, 2011. http://www.ars.usda.gov/Services/docs.htm?docid = 6312 2013.

Fluoridation of Public Water Supplies

In the last 60 years, numerous municipalities in the United States have added healthful amounts of fluoride to the public water supply (fluoridation). In 2012, about 75% of the U.S. population had access to drinking water that contained optimal fluoride levels.[26] A goal of *Healthy People 2020* is to have 80% of Americans drinking fluoridated tap water by 2020.[27] Consumers can obtain information about the fluoride content of their water supply at http://apps.nccd .cdc.gov/MWF/Index.asp.

Most natural sources of water contain fluoride; however, for optimal dental health, many municipalities adjust the amount of fluoride added to the local water supply to achieve a fluoride content of 0.7 to 1.2 mg/L.[28] This concentration of fluoride in water can safely prevent dental caries. Consuming fluoridated water over a lifetime may reduce a person's likelihood of tooth decay by 25%.[29]

In recent years, many Americans have begun to drink bottled water. Relying on bottled water for fluid sources may decrease fluoride intake, because most bottled waters do not contain the mineral. Water filtration systems designed for household use may also reduce the fluoride content of tap water. Consumers can check with the manufacturers of such water filtering systems to determine whether fluoride remains in the filtered tap water.

Despite the scientific evidence concerning the benefits of drinking fluoridated water, some Americans oppose fluoridation for a variety of reasons, including the belief that the practice is a form of involuntary medication. Other people oppose fluoridation because they are concerned about long-term risks of drinking the treated water. For more information about fluoridation, visit www.cdc.gov/Fluoridation/.

Dietary Adequacy

There is not enough information concerning human fluoride requirements to set an RDA for the trace mineral. The Food and Nutrition Board, however, set the Adequate Intake (AI) at 4 mg/day and 3 mg/day for adult men and women, respectively. Because fluoride is not an essential nutrient, it is unlikely that negative consequences will occur from having a low intake of this trace mineral. Nevertheless, people in communities with fluoridated water have 15 to 40% fewer dental caries than fluoride-deficient populations.[30]

At therapeutic doses, fluoride can stimulate osteoblast (bone—building cell) activity and increase bone mineral density, strengthening bone tissue. However, levels of the mineral in fluoridated water are insufficient to prevent osteoporosis or bone fractures.[28] Chapter 11 discusses osteoporosis.

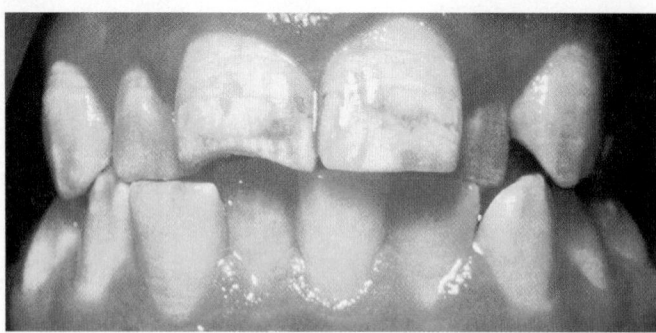

FIGURE 12.10 Dental fluorosis.

Fluoride Toxicity: Fluorosis

Excessive fluoride intakes during tooth development can cause **dental fluorosis**, abnormal changes in the appear—ance of tooth enamel. Children under the age of 8 are at risk for dental fluorosis.[28] Fluorosis can range from white specks on the teeth to severe discoloration and pitting (Fig. 12.10). The CDC estimates that 32% of American children may have mild fluorosis, while 2.5% have moderate to severe forms. Mild cases occur in children who consume fluoride at levels two to three times the AI, and severe dental fluorosis occurs at intakes that are five times the AI.

Dental fluorosis can occur in children who routinely swallow toothpaste and dental rinses. To reduce young children's exposure to excess fluoride, adults should teach youngsters how to use a "pea—sized" amount of toothpaste on their brush, rinse with water, and spit out the excess fluid. Additionally, dental prod—ucts containing fluoride should be kept out of reach of children.

Long—term consumption of high amounts of fluoride can lead to **skeletal fluorosis**, a condition characterized by excess fluoride buildup in bones. Skeletal fluorosis changes bone structure, causing joint stiffness and bone pain. The con—dition also increases the risk of bone fractures. Because of these consequences, fluoride supplements should be used with caution and only under the supervision of a dentist or physician. Skeletal fluorosis rarely occurs in the United States.[25]

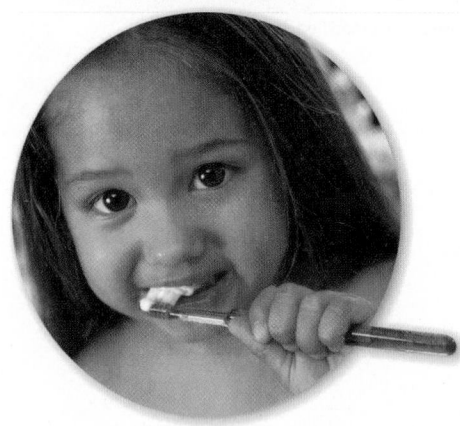

To reduce the risk of fluorosis, young children should use a "pea-sized" amount of toothpaste.

ASSESS YOUR PROGRESS

20 *Describe the role of fluoride in human health.*
21 *Identify common sources of fluoride.*
22 *List two consequences of fluoride toxicity.*

dental fluorosis abnormal change in the appearance of tooth enamel due to chronically high fluoride exposure while the teeth are developing

skeletal fluorosis excess fluoride intake that changes bone structure, causing joint stiffness, bone pain, and increasing risk for bone fractures

12.7 Chromium

LEARNING OUTCOMES

1 *Explain the role of chromium in human health.*
2 *List rich food sources of chromium.*
3 *Discuss chromium deficiency and toxicity.*

The results of scientific studies suggest that chromium plays an important role in maintaining proper carbohydrate and lipid metabolism. The human digestive tract absorbs only about 0.4 to 2.5% of the chromium in foods; the remainder is excreted in the feces.[31] Thus, the concentration of chromium in human tissues is generally low.

Function of Chromium

Chromium enhances the effect of insulin. Recall that cells require insulin to obtain glucose from the bloodstream. Chromium may enhance insulin's action on cell membranes and, in a way, help to "hold the door open" for glucose to enter

DID YOU KNOW?

The form of chromium in food and used by the body is *trivalent chromium (chromium III)*.[31] Trivalent chromium should not be confused with *hexavalent chromium (chromium VI)*, an industrial waste product that contributes to pollution. When inhaled or consumed, hexavalent chromium increases the risk of cancer. Several years ago, the people of Hinkley, California, won a multimillion dollar lawsuit against a gas and electric company for allowing the dangerous mineral to leak into their water supply. The pollution was thought to contribute to high cancer rates for people living in their neighborhood. This story was dramatized in the 2002 movie *Erin Brockovich*.

cells. Chromium is also important for carbohydrate, fat, and protein metabolism and storage. For people who are trying to lose weight, chromium supplementation may contribute to a small amount of weight loss.[32]

Can people who have diabetes experience better blood glucose regulation by taking chromium supplements? Supplementation with chromium improves blood glucose control in people who have diabetes. Additionally, chromium supplementation may improve blood triglyceride and HDL levels in those with diabetes.[33]

Sources of Chromium

Although chromium is widely distributed in foods, most foods contain less than 2 μg of the mineral per serving.[31] Information regarding the chromium content of various foods is difficult to find, because most reliable food composition tables do not include this trace mineral. In general, meat, whole–grain products, yeast, spices, fruits, and vegetables are good sources of chromium. As with selenium, the amount of chromium in plant foods reflects the chromium content of soils where the crops are grown. Table 12.10 lists chromium contents of some foods.

Dietary Adequacy

The adult AIs for chromium are 25 μg for young women and 35 μg for young men. Well–balanced diets typically contain these amounts of chromium. On average, American adults consume diets that meet or exceed their AIs for chromium.[31]

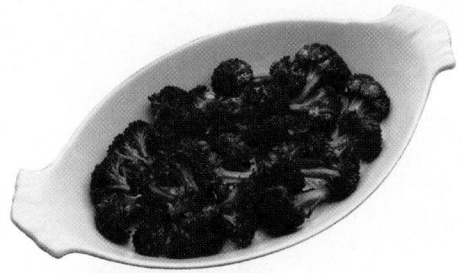

Broccoli is a rich source of chromium.

TABLE 12.10 Chromium Content of Selected Foods

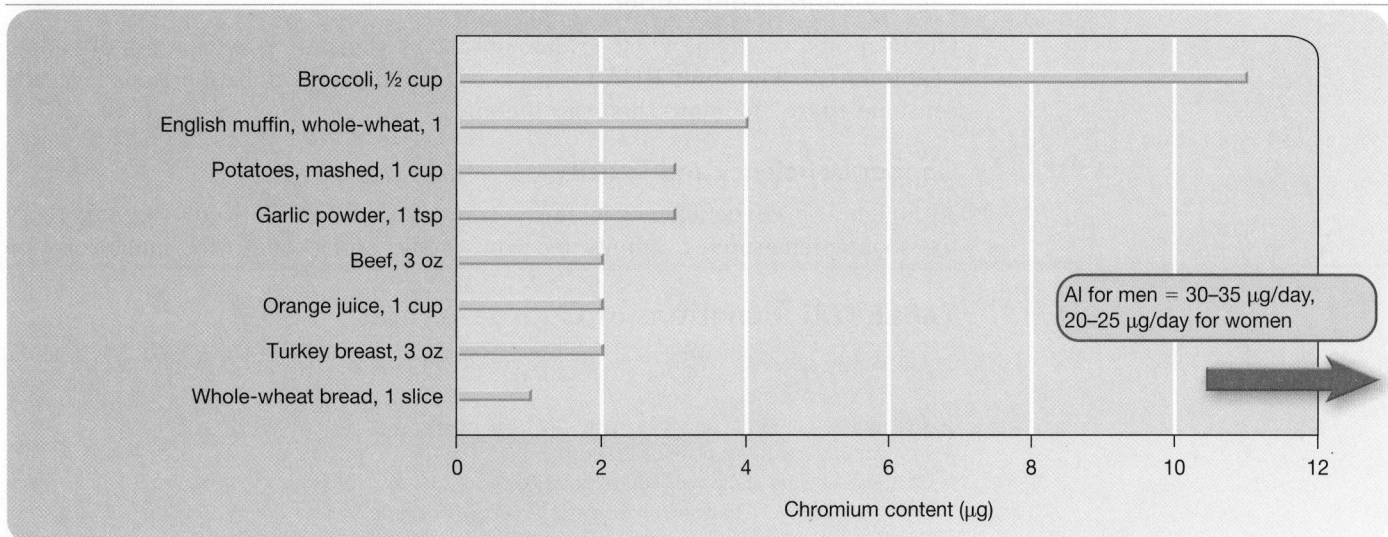

AI for men = 30–35 μg/day, 20–25 μg/day for women

Source: Data from Office of Dietary Supplements, National Institutes of Health: *Dietary supplement fact sheet: Chromium.* Last reviewed: 2013. http://ods.od.nih.gov/factsheets/Chromium-HealthProfessional/

Chromium deficiency can lead to impaired glucose tolerance, which often pre—cedes the development of type 2 diabetes. In addition, elevated blood choles—terol and triglyceride levels can occur with a chromium deficiency. The mechanism by which chromium influences cholesterol metabolism is not known, but it may involve enzymes that control the body's cholesterol production. Cases of chromium deficiency have been reported in people maintained on special—formula diets that did not contain the trace mineral, as well as in severely malnourished children.

The form of chromium that is naturally in foods has not been shown to produce toxicity, so no UL has been set for the trace mineral. The long—term safety of taking various chromium supplements is unknown and requires further scientific investigation.[33]

ASSESS YOUR PROGRESS

 What is the role of chromium in blood glucose regulation?

 What are possible health outcomes of taking chromium supplements?

12.8 Copper, Manganese, and Molybdenum

LEARNING OUTCOMES

1 *Explain the roles of copper, manganese, and molybdenum in human health.*

2 *List rich food sources of copper, manganese, and molybdenum.*

3 *Discuss copper, manganese, and molybdenum deficiencies and toxicities.*

Copper and manganese are components of several enzymes, and molybdenum is necessary for another group of enzymes to function. The following sections pro—vide information about these trace minerals and their roles in health.

Copper

cuproenzymes group of enzymes that require copper to function

Cuproenzymes are a group of enzymes that contain copper. Copper, for example, is a component of *ceruloplasmin*, a protein that is needed for copper transport and iron metabolism. Table 12.11 lists functions of copper—containing enzymes.

Dietary Sources of Copper

Organ meats, shellfish, whole grains, nuts, and seeds are good sources of copper (Table 12.12). The adult RDA for copper is 0.9 mg/day, and Americans typically consume 10 to 70% more than this amount.[6]

Copper Deficiency and Toxicity

Although copper deficiency is fairly rare in the United States, infants born too soon (prematurely), infants fed cow's milk, and people with malabsorption

TABLE 12.11 Functions of Cuproenzymes

- Antioxidant activity
- Energy metabolism
- Collagen formation (connective tissue and bone health)
- Iron storage and transportation
- Synthesis and metabolism of neurotransmitters
- Formation of myelin that surrounds parts of certain nerve cells
- Synthesis of *melanin*, the pigment in hair, skin, and eyes
- Gene expression

TABLE 12.12 Copper Content of Selected Foods

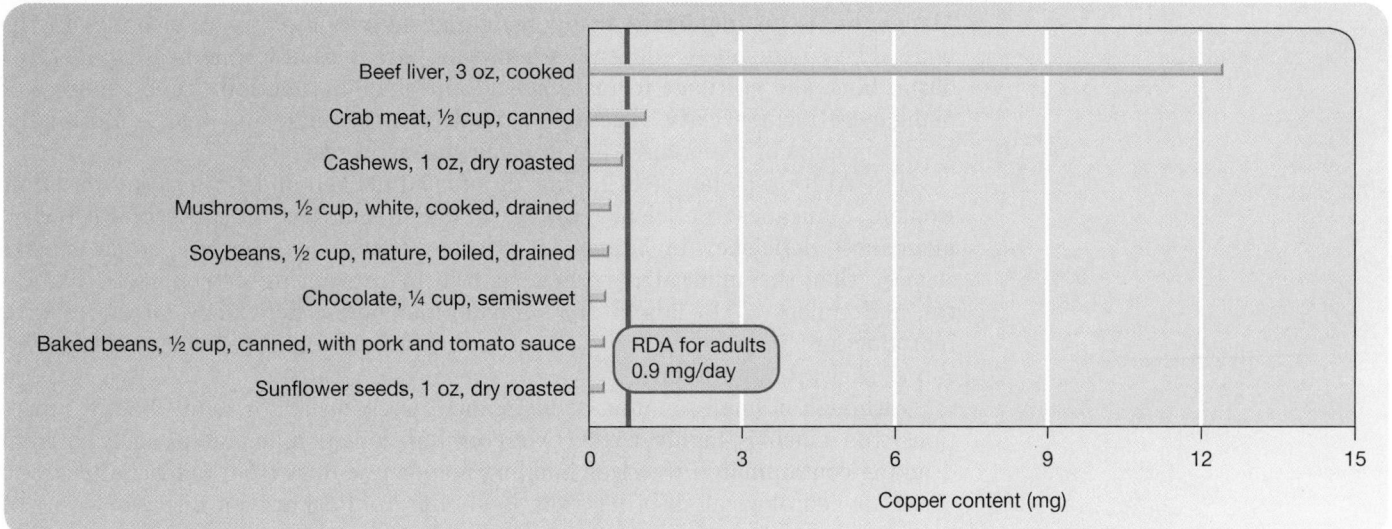

Beef liver, 3 oz, cooked
Crab meat, ½ cup, canned
Cashews, 1 oz, dry roasted
Mushrooms, ½ cup, white, cooked, drained
Soybeans, ½ cup, mature, boiled, drained
Chocolate, ¼ cup, semisweet
Baked beans, ½ cup, canned, with pork and tomato sauce
Sunflower seeds, 1 oz, dry roasted

RDA for adults
0.9 mg/day

0   3   6   9   12   15
Copper content (mg)

Source: Data from U.S. Department of Agriculture, Agricultural Research Service: Copper, Cu (mg) content of selected foods per common measure. *USDA national nutrient database for standard reference,* release 25, 2012.

disorders may be at risk of developing the condition.[34] As a result of this defect, the person's body does not synthesize enough ceruloplasmin, so anemia develops. Poor bone health, abnormal skin pigmentation, impaired neurological and immune system functioning, and poor growth also result from copper deficiency.

Infants who have *Menkes syndrome*, a rare inherited metabolic disorder, can absorb copper, but their cells are unable to metabolize the trace mineral properly. Babies with the syndrome have a variety of physical signs, including brittle, kinky hair; bone defects; and plump, rosy cheeks. Children with Menkes syndrome do not live for more than a few years.

Wilson Disease **Wilson disease** is a rare inherited disorder characterized by the accumulation of toxic amounts of copper in the body, especially in the liver, brain, kidneys, and eyes. Normally, the liver removes excess copper from the bloodstream, stores the trace mineral, or adds it to bile for elimination. In cases of Wilson disease, the liver does not make enough ceruloplasmin, a protein that transports copper in the bloodstream. As a result, the liver's ability to remove copper from storage is severely impaired, so the mineral accumulates in the organ, causing damage. Eventually, the liver releases excess copper into the circulation, and the trace mineral is picked up by other organs.

People with Wilson disease usually develop signs of chronic liver disease, including yellowing of the skin and whites of the eyes (*jaundice*), fluid accumulation in the abdominal region, and enlargement of the liver. Patients may also develop signs and symptoms of nervous system damage, such as impaired muscular coordination and behavioral changes. Physicians can diagnose the disease by measuring copper and ceruloplasmin levels in the blood, and by noting copper deposits in the eyes called **Kayser–Fleischer** rings (Fig. 12.11). A Kayser–Fleischer ring is a greenish–brown or rusty–brown ring that forms around the edge of each iris (the pigmented part of the eye), where it meets the cornea (the clear outer membrane of the eye).

Patients with Wilson disease can take medications that help eliminate copper from their body. Additionally, people who have the disease may need to follow a low–copper diet that excludes liver, crab, cashews, and sunflower seeds (Table 12.12). Furthermore, dietary supplements that contain copper should be avoided. There is no cure for Wilson disease, so people with the condition must continue treatment for the rest of their lives.

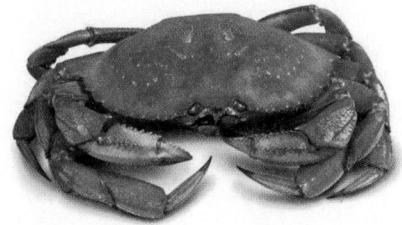

Crabmeat is a good source of copper.

Wilson disease a rare inherited disorder characterized by accumulation of toxic amounts of copper in the body

Kayser-Fleischer rings copper deposits in the eyes that are a sign of Wilson disease

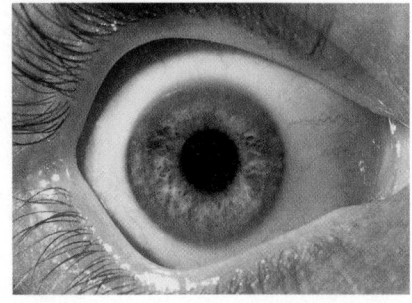

FIGURE 12.11 Kayser-Fleischer ring.

Manganese

Manganese is an important component and activator of many enzymes in the body. These manganese–dependent enzymes play roles in wound healing, metabolism, bone and cartilage formation, and antioxidant function.[35] Food sources of manganese include leafy vegetables, whole grains, nuts, and tea. Additionally, small amounts of manganese are in natural sources of water.

The AI for manganese is 2.3 mg/day for adult men and 1.8 mg/day for adult women. Manganese deficiency rarely occurs in humans. Because of its rarity, manganese deficiency in humans is poorly understood; however, some experts suspect that the mineral may have a role in preventing osteoporosis, diabetes, and epilepsy.[35] In laboratory animals, manganese deficiency interferes with reproduction, impairs growth, alters carbohydrate and lipid metabolism, and causes skeletal abnormalities.[35]

Although a small amount of manganese is essential for many bodily functions, too much is highly toxic. Overconsumption of manganese, such as from drinking contaminated water or inhaling manganese dust from industrial sources, causes a neurological disorder that is similar to Parkinson's disease. Cases of manganese toxicity from food consumption have not been reported.[35]

Molybdenum

Molybdenum is a trace mineral required by all life forms. This essential mineral is a cofactor of four enzymes in humans, including sulfite oxidase and xanthine oxidase.

Legumes such as beans, lentils, and peas are high in molybdenum, and grains and nuts are also good sources. The adult RDA for this mineral is 45 µg/day, and most Americans consume plentiful amounts of this essential mineral.[36] A deficiency of molybdenum has not been reported in healthy individuals, and there is limited evidence of molybdenum toxicity in people who are healthy.[36]

ASSESS YOUR PROGRESS

25 *What do copper, manganese, and molybdenum all have in common regarding their roles in human health?*

26 *What is the likelihood of a person developing deficiencies of copper, manganese, and molybdenum?*

27 *What are the health consequences of copper and manganese toxicities?*

12.9 Possible Essential Minerals

LEARNING OUTCOMES

1 *Identify other minerals that may possibly be essential for human health.*

2 *Discuss practical ways to reduce a person's intake of inorganic forms of arsenic.*

Some minerals, including arsenic, boron, lithium, nickel, silicon, and vanadium, are found in small amounts in the body, but their roles in health are unclear. At present, this group of minerals is not classified as essential nutrients. Table 12.13 summarizes the possible functions, Tolerable Upper Intake Level, and food sources of minerals that may be essential to humans. Although there are reports of severe illness and deaths resulting from environmental exposure to high amounts of

TABLE 12.13 Summary of Other Possible Essential Minerals

Mineral	Possible Functions	Tolerable Upper Intake Level (UL)	Dietary Sources
Arsenic (As)	No clear biological function in humans but may play a role in methionine metabolism, growth, and reproduction (animal studies)	No UL has been established; however, arsenic is highly toxic.	Fish, grains, cereals
Boron (B)	No clear biological function in humans but may be involved in steroid hormone metabolism	20 mg/day	Fruit, leafy vegetables, peanuts, beans, wine
Lithium (Li)	Reproduction Maintenance of appropriate mood	No UL has been established.	Water supply, grains, vegetables
Nickel (Ni)	Amino acid and fatty acid metabolism	1 mg/day	Chocolate, nuts, beans, whole grains
Silicon (Si)	Connective tissue, including bone formation	No UL has been established.	Root vegetables, whole grains
Vanadium (V)	Glucose metabolism Tooth and bone mineralization	1.8 mg/day	Shellfish, mushrooms, black pepper, parsley, dill

Sources: Data from Food and Nutrition Board, Institute of Medicine: *Dietary reference intakes for vitamin A, vitamin K, arsenic, boron, chromium, copper, iodine, iron, manganese, molybdenum, nickel, silicon, vanadium, and zinc.* Washington, DC: Standing Committee on the Scientific Evaluation of Dietary Reference Intakes, National Academy Press, 2006; Schrauzer, GN: Lithium: Occurrence, dietary intakes, nutritional essentiality. *Journal of the American College of Nutrition* 21(1):14, 2002.

these minerals, foods generally do not contain toxic amounts. However, the presence of arsenic in certain commonly eaten foods is a cause for concern.

Arsenic in Food

Arsenic in food can occur in two forms, organic and inorganic. Food crops can be sources of organic arsenic as the plants acquire the mineral naturally from soil deposits, volcanic eruptions, and normal erosion. Seafood is also a source of organic arsenic, because ocean water is a natural source of the mineral. Organic arsenic may be safe as long as dietary intake remains low. However, consuming high amounts of the inorganic form of arsenic can cause health problems, including several forms of cancer.

In some instances, the content of arsenic in soil may increase due to industrial use of inorganic arsenic and previous use of insecticides made with the inorganic form. Use of arsenic–containing insecticides was banned in the United States in 1980. The mineral, however, remains in the soil and may continue to contaminate drinking water and food. The FDA monitors the arsenic content in many foods.

In 2012 and 2013, scientists determined that some brands of apple juice and rice may contain unsafe levels of arsenic.[37] The inorganic arsenic content of rice is of particular concern, because rice cereal and other rice products are often the first foods fed to infants. Furthermore, many children also consume a lot of apple juice and could have elevated inorganic arsenic exposure as a result. Because of their relatively low body weights, infants and children are at greater risk of health consequences due to arsenic intake than adults. Consumers can help lower their intake of dietary sources of inorganic arsenic by:

- Rinsing rice grains before cooking;

- Cooking rice using 6 cups of water for every 1 cup of rice and draining the remaining fluid, once the rice is cooked;

- Limiting apple juice consumption to 4 to 6 ounces/day for children under 6 years of age and 8 to 12 ounces/day for everyone else; and

- Consuming a variety of grains such as wheat, oats, quinoa, and millet.

The FDA continues to monitor amounts of arsenic in rice as well as other foods and beverages. According to officials of the FDA, consumers, including pregnant women, infants, and children, should eat a varied nutritious diet to minimize the possible risks of consuming excessive amounts of arsenic from any one food.[38]

ASSESS YOUR PROGRESS

28 List other possible trace minerals that may be essential for optimal health.

29 Identify commonly eaten foods that may contain high levels of inorganic arsenic.

SUMMARY

SECTION 12.1 What Is a Trace Mineral?

- Trace minerals are essential nutrients required in very small amounts, generally less than 100 mg/day. Trace minerals include iron, iodine, zinc, selenium, fluoride, chromium, copper, manganese, molybdenum and possibly, some other minerals.

SECTION 12.2 Iron

- Iron plays a critical role in oxygen delivery for energy metabolism as part of hemoglobin and myoglobin.
- Dietary iron can be found in two forms, heme and nonheme. The intestinal tract absorbs more of the heme iron than nonheme iron in foods. Naturally occurring components of plant foods, such as phytates and polyphenols, reduce iron absorption.
- Serum ferritin concentrations are the most common method of assessing iron status. Total body iron can be measured by calculating the ratio of blood transferrin receptor to ferritin.
- Iron deficiency occurs in three stages. Iron deficiency anemia has widespread negative effects on the body. Excess iron in the blood acts as an oxidant and causes damage to cell membranes, proteins, and DNA. Iron overload occurs when toxic amounts of iron supplements are ingested, but the condition also results from certain genetic conditions.

SECTION 12.3 Iodine (Iodide)

- Adequate iodine is essential to form thyroid hormone. Major dietary sources of iodine include saltwater fish, seafood, seaweed, and iodized salt.
- Most Americans have adequate iodine intakes. Needs for iodine increase for pregnant and lactating women. Both deficiency and toxicity in iodine causes goiter and hypothyroidism. Infants of iodine-deficient women are likely to be born with cretinism.

SECTION 12.4 Zinc

- Zinc is important for the function of over 300 enzymes. The trace mineral is necessary for growth and development, wound healing, the sense of taste and smell, DNA synthesis, and proper functioning of the immune system.
- Zinc is widespread in foods. Phytic acid and fiber decrease zinc bioavailability.
- Signs and symptoms of zinc deficiency include stunted growth, delayed sexual maturation, poor wound healing, impaired sense of taste, and mental slowness.

SECTION 12.5 Selenium

- Selenium functions as a component of selenoproteins, many of which are antioxidants.
- Foods with the greatest amounts of selenium are seafood and organ meats.
- In the United States, selenium deficiency is uncommon, but the condition may occur in people who have serious digestive tract conditions.

SECTION 12.6 Fluoride

- Fluoride is not considered an essential nutrient, but the trace mineral helps mineralize teeth and bones, and protects against tooth decay.
- Fluoridated drinking water provides 80% of fluoride intake. Nonfood sources of fluoride include toothpaste, mouthwash, and dental treatments. Fluoride toxicity negatively affects bones and teeth.

SECTION 12.7 Chromium

- Chromium enhances the effect of the hormone insulin. Chromium insufficiency may contribute to the development of type 2 diabetes. Signs of chromium deficiency are impaired glucose tolerance and elevated blood cholesterol and triglyceride levels.

SECTION 12.8 Copper, Manganese, and Molybdenum

- Copper is required for the function of a group of enzymes called cuproenzymes. Organ meats, shellfish, whole grains, nuts, and seeds are good sources of copper.
- Manganese is an important component and activator of enzymes in the body. Manganese-dependent enzymes play a role in wound healing, metabolism, bone and cartilage formation, and antioxidant function.
- Molybdenum is a cofactor for four enzymes in humans.

SECTION 12.9 Possible Essential Minerals

- Some minerals, particularly arsenic, boron, lithium, nickel, silicon, and vanadium, are found in small amounts in the body, but their roles in the body are unclear. Arsenic can be toxic, especially inorganic arsenic.

Get the most out of your study of nutrition with McGraw-Hill's innovative suite of adaptive learning products including McGraw-Hill LearnSmart®, SmartBook®, McGraw-Hill LearnSmart Achieve®, and McGraw-Hill LearnSmart Prep®. Visit www.learnsmartadvantage.com.

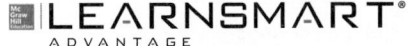

CASE STUDY RESPONSE

SELENIUM TOXICITY

THE RDA FOR SELENIUM (MEN) IS 55 μg; the UL for selenium is 400 μg. The signs and symptoms of selenosis include brittle fingernails, loss of hair and nails, garlicky body odor, nausea, vomiting, and fatigue.

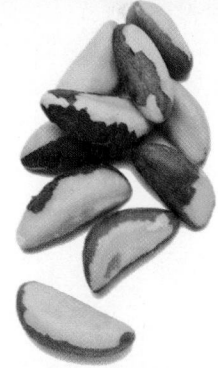

Carlos's usual dietary intake of 130 μg/day and his daily practice of taking the dietary supplement of 200 μg and eating 1 ounce of Brazil nuts (544 μg/day) make his selenium intake well above the UL. While selenosis is rare, it is possible to reach toxic levels, particularly by overuse of selenium-containing supplements. At this dose, Carlos is probably safe taking the dietary supplement but not while consuming Brazil nuts daily. He should focus on eating a healthy diet that supplies sufficient amounts of selenium. Research does not support claims that people can prevent cancer by supplementing a varied, well-balance diet with selenium.

Critical Thinking

1. Bonita is iron deficient. She likes to drink hot or iced tea with her meals and snacks. Based on this information, explain to Bonita why she should consider altering her beverage consumption.

2. Develop a table that lists food sources of heme and nonheme iron. Describe how the difference between the bioavailability of heme and nonheme iron influences a person's risk for iron deficiency.

3. Compare and contrast the outcomes of a zinc and iodine deficiency. Are any of the deficiency consequences similar? How so?

Which outcomes are different? What does this tell us about the functions of zinc and iodine?

4. Why is fluoride an important dietary component, even though it is not an essential nutrient?

5. After reading an article in the newspaper, your sister has decided to stop eating rice and drinking apple juice because she is terrified about the arsenic content in these foods. What are the consequences of consuming too much arsenic? Explain why you support or do not support your sister's avoidance of these foods.

Modifying Recipes for Healthy Living

Ali is a vegan who would like your advice concerning how to modify her favorite Italian dish, pasta primavera, to improve the bioavailability of its iron content. Examine Ali's recipe (below) and suggest ways to change the recipe by adding foods that she will eat and that will enhance the bioavailability of the iron in the ingredients.

PASTA PRIMAVERA

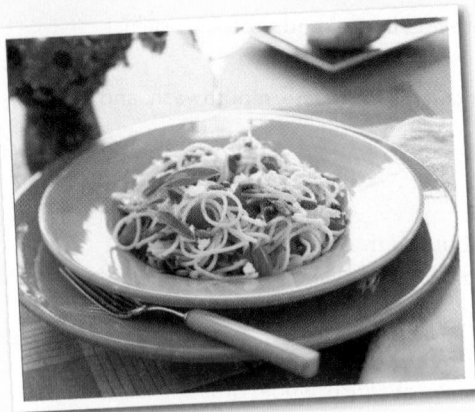

INGREDIENTS

8-oz package of mixed frozen peas and carrots

16 oz pasta (enriched spaghetti or penne forms are recommended)

15 cherry tomatoes

¼ cup olive oil

1 Tbsp dried Italian herbs

Salt and pepper to taste

Yield: 6 servings

PREPARATION STEPS

1. Cook the pasta in a large pan of boiling water until tender. Drain thoroughly.
2. Cook the frozen vegetables in a pan of boiling water. Drain and rinse under cold water.
3. Cut the cherry tomatoes in halves.
4. Gently mix the pasta, vegetables, oil, and herbs in a large bowl.
5. Season with salt and pepper to taste.

STEP 1 Brainstorm

Review information in Section 12.2, including Tables 12.3 and 12.4.

1. What foods could be added to this recipe to increase its iron content?
2. What are some ways to modify this recipe to increase the bioavailability of iron?

STEP 2 Revise the recipe

3. List ingredients and amounts needed.
4. List the preparation steps.

STEP 3 Evaluate the nutrients in the original and modified recipe

5. Use the food composition tables in Appendix I or at the U.S. Department of Agriculture's National Nutrient Database for Standard Reference http://www.ars.usda.gov/Services/docs.htm?docid=8964 to evaluate the nutrient content of the original and modified recipes.
6. Develop a table to compare the amount of iron, calories, carbohydrates, protein, fat, and vitamin C in each recipe.
7. Did your modification(s) improve the iron composition of the meal? Describe these changes.

OPTIONAL ACTIVITIES

STEP 4 Test your new recipe

Keep notes on any changes you make to ingredient amounts as you prepare the pasta dish.

STEP 5 Reflect on your findings

How did the pasta primavera look and taste?

STEP 6 Add the recipe to your collection or repeat steps to improve the product

PERSONAL Dietary Analysis

1. Refer to your 3-day food log from the "Personal Dietary Analysis" feature in Chapter 5.

   a. Find the RDA/AI values for minerals under your life stage/sex group category in the DRI tables (see the last pages of this book). Write those values under the "My RDA/AI" column in the table below.

   b. Review your personal dietary assessment. Find your 3-day average intakes of iron, iodine, zinc, selenium, fluoride, and chromium. Write those values under the "My Average Intake" column of the table.

   c. Calculate the percentage of the RDA/AI you consumed for each mineral by dividing your intake by the RDA/AI amount and multiplying the figure you obtain by 100. For example, if your average intake of iron was 9 mg/day and your RDA for the mineral is 18 mg, you would divide 18 mg by 9 mg to obtain .50. To multiply this figure by 100, simply move the decimal point two places to the right, and replace the decimal point with a percentage sign (50%). Thus, your average daily intake of iron was 50% of the RDA. Place the percentages for each mineral under the "% of My RDA/AI" column.

   d. Under the ">, <, or =" column, indicate whether your average daily intake was greater than (>), less than (<), or equal to (=) the RDA/AI.

2. Use the information you calculated in the first part of this activity to answer the following questions:

   a. Which of your average trace mineral intakes equaled or exceeded the RDA/AI? If one or more were above the RDA/AI, what is a possible consequence of the overconsumption?
   _____

   b. Which of your average trace mineral intakes was below the RDA/AI?_____

   c. What foods would you eat to increase your intake of the minerals that was less than the RDA/AI levels? (Review sources of the minerals in this chapter.)_____

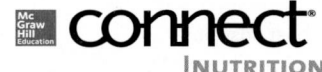

Complete the Personal Dietary Analysis activity online at www.mcgrawhillconnect.com, where you will also find McGraw-Hill LearnSmart®, SmartBook®, NutritionCalc Plus, and many other dynamic learning tools.

Personal Dietary Analysis: Trace Minerals

Mineral	My RDA/AI	My Average Intake	% of My RDA/AI	>, <, or =
Iron				
Iodine				
Zinc				
Selenium				
Fluoride				
Chromium				

Practice Test

Select the best answer.

1. Which of the following lists includes only trace minerals?

   a. selenium, sodium, zinc, and iodide
   b. iron, iodide, selenium, and chromium
   c. calcium, copper, chromium, and phosphorus
   d. magnesium, molybdenum, potassium, and iron

2. Sources of heme iron include

   a. fortified breakfast cereal.
   b. roast beef.
   c. fresh spinach.
   d. raw orange segments.

3. Iron absorption can be increased by

   a. consuming unleavened bread with the source of iron.
   b. drinking tea with the source of iron.
   c. adding a food that contains vitamin C to the meal.
   d. taking a calcium supplement with the meal.

4. Worldwide, which of the following nutrient deficiencies is the most common cause of preventable intellectual disability?

   a. chromium   c. iron
   b. iodine   d. zinc

5. Which of the following statements is false?

   a. In the United States, milk is usually fortified with iodide.
   b. Iodine is necessary for normal thyroid function.
   c. Having too much iodine in the diet can cause a goiter.
   d. Saltwater fish and other seafood are dietary sources of iodine.

6. Which of the following statements is false?

   a. Zinc is important for the proper functioning of over 300 enzymes.
   b. Zinc deficiency can stunt growth and lead to dwarfism.
   c. Zinc deficiency can cause a lack of appetite and impaired sense of taste.
   d. Zinc intake is critical during pregnancy for preventing cretinism.

7. Selenium deficiency can lead to

   a. Wilson disease.
   b. selenosis.
   c. microcytic anemia.
   d. Kashin-Beck disease.

8. Which nutrient can remineralize the tooth surface and prevent cavities?

   a. chromium   c. iron
   b. fluoride   d. iodide

9. Chromium is important for

   a. maintaining proper carbohydrate and lipid metabolism.
   b. synthesizing hemoglobin and myoglobin.
   c. supporting normal thyroid function.
   d. developing healthy teeth.

10. The presence of ___ in a food decreases zinc bioavailability.

    a. phytic acid
    b. glutamic acid
    c. ascorbic acid
    d. lactic acid

11. Garlicky body odor is a sign of

    a. iron deficiency.
    b. hemochromatosis.
    c. selenosis.
    d. iodine toxicity.

12. Which of the following enzymes contains molybdenum?

    a. alcohol dehydrogenase
    b. sucrase
    c. lactase
    d. sulfite oxidase

13. Antoine's eyes have Kayser-Fleischer rings. Based on this information, Antoine has

    a. iron depletion disease.
    b. Wilson disease.
    c. Kashan-Beck disease.
    d. Keshan disease.

14. People who have hereditary hemochromatosis absorb too much

    a. iron.
    b. copper.
    c. zinc.
    d. vanadium.

15. In the United States, table salt is often fortified with

    a. iron.
    b. selenium.
    c. zinc.
    d. iodide.

ANSWERS TO PRACTICE TEST
1-b; 2-b; 3-c; 4-b; 5-a; 6-d; 7-d; 8-b; 9-a; 10-a; 11-c; 12-d; 13-b; 14-a; 15-d

ANSWERS TO CHAPTER 12 QUIZ Yourself

1. In the United States, young men are more likely to be iron deficient than young women. **False** (p. 391)
2. To prevent iodine deficiency, people can use table salt that is fortified with the mineral. **True** (p. 395)
3. Trace minerals are not as important for human health as the major minerals. **False** (p. 384)
4. Symptoms of zinc deficiency include the inability to sense the taste of food. **True** (p. 399)
5. In the United States, copper deficiency is the most common nutritional deficiency. **False** (p. 391)

References

1. Linus Pauling Institute Micronutrient Information Center: *Iron*. Last modified April 2009. http://lpi.oregonstate.edu/infocenter/minerals/iron/ Accessed: February 12, 2014.

2. Office of Dietary Supplements, National Institutes of Health: *Dietary supplement fact sheet: Iron*. Updated August 2007. http://ods.od.nih.gov/factsheets/Iron-HealthProfessional/ Accessed: February 12, 2014.

3. Food and Nutrition Board: *Dietary Reference Intakes for vitamin A, vitamin K, arsenic, boron, chromium, copper, iodine, iron, manganese, molybdenum, nickel, silicon, vanadium, and zinc*. Washington, DC: National Academy Press, 2000.

4. Korus A and others: Effect of different technological and culinary treatments on iron retention, nutritional density and recommended dietary intake in fourteen vegetable species. *International Journal of Food Science and Technology* 47:1882, 2012

5. Collings R and others: The absorption of iron from whole diets: A systematic review. *American Journal of Clinical Nutrition* 98:65, 2013.

6. U.S. Department of Agriculture, Agricultural Research Service: Nutrient intakes from food and beverages: Mean amounts consumed per individual, by gender and age, in the United States, *2011–2012*, 2014. http://www.ars.usda.gov/Services/docs.htm?docid=18349. Accessed: November 4, 2014.

7. Centers for Disease Control and Prevention: *Second national report on biochemical indicators of diet and nutrition in the U.S. population*, 2012. http://www.cdc.gov/nutritionreport/ Accessed: February 12, 2014.

8. World Health Organization: *Micronutrient deficiencies: Iron deficiency anemia*. ND. www.who.int/nutrition/topics/ida/en/ Accessed: February 12, 2014

9. Centers for Disease Control and Prevention: *Iron deficiency*. Last updated February 2011. http://www.cdc.gov/nutrition/everyone/basics/vitamins/iron.html Accessed: February 12, 2014.

10. Schardt D: Heavy metal: Are we getting too much iron? *Nutrition Action Healthletter*, p. 9, January/February, 2012.

11. Carpenter KJ: David Marine and the problem of goiter. *Journal of Nutrition* 135:675, 2005.

12. Office of Dietary Supplements, National Institutes of Health: *Dietary supplement fact sheet: Iodine*. Updated June 2011. http://ods.od.nih.gov/factsheets/Iodine-HealthProfessional/ Accessed: February 12, 2014.

13. American Thyroid Association: *Iodine deficiency*. June 4, 2012. http://thyroid.org/iodine-deficiency/ Accessed: February 12, 2014.

14. World Health Organization: *Micronutrient deficiencies: Iodine deficiency disorder*. ND. www.who.int/nutrition/topics/ida/en/ Accessed: February 12, 2014.

15. Linus Pauling Institute Micronutrient Information Center: *Iodine*. Last updated March 2010. http://lpi.oregonstate.edu/infocenter/minerals/iodine/ Accessed: February 12, 2014.

16. American Thyroid Association: *ATA statement on the potential risks of excess iodine ingestion and exposure*. June 5, 2013. http://www.thyroid.org/ata-statement-on-the-potential-risks-of-excess-iodine-ingestion-and-exposure/ Accessed: February 12, 2014

17. Prasad A: Discovery of human zinc deficiency: 50 years later. *Journal of Trace Elements in Medicine and Biology* 26:66, 2012.

18. Linus Pauling Institute Micronutrient Information Center: *Zinc*. Last updated June 2013. http://lpi.oregonstate.edu/infocenter/minerals/zinc/ Accessed: February 12, 2014.

19. Office of Dietary Supplements, National Institutes of Health: *Dietary supplement fact sheet: Zinc*. Reviewed June 2013. http://ods.od.nih.gov/factsheets/Zinc-HealthProfessional/Accessed: February 12, 2014.

20. Craig WJ, Mangels AR: Position of the American dietetic association: Vegetarian diets. *Journal of the American Dietetic Association* 109(7):1266, 2009.

21. Evans JR, Lawrenson JG: Antioxidant vitamin and mineral supplements for preventing age-related macular degeneration. *Cochrane Database System Reviews* 6:1, 2012.

22. Office of Dietary Supplements, National Institutes of Health: *Selenium*. Updated July 2013. http://ods.od.nih.gov/factsheets/Selenium-HealthProfessional/ Accessed: February 12, 2014.

23. Linus Pauling Institute Micronutrient Information Center: *Selenium*. Last updated January 2009. http://lpi.oregonstate.edu/infocenter/minerals/selenium/ Accessed: February 12, 2014.

24. Berr C and others: Selenium and cognitive impairment: A brief review based on results from the EVA study. *Biofactors* 38(2):139, 2012.

25. Linus Pauling Institute Micronutrient Information Center: *Fluoride*. Last reviewed January 2014. http://lpi.oregonstate.edu/infocenter/minerals/fluoride/ Accessed: February 12, 2014.

26. Centers for Disease Control and Prevention: *2012 water fluoridation statistics*. 2013. http://www.cdc.gov/fluoridation/statistics/2012stats.htm Accessed: April 20, 2014.

27. U.S. Department of Health and Human Services: *Healthy people 2020: Nutrition and weight status*. Last updated 2013. http://www.healthypeople.gov/2020/topicsobjectives2020/objectiveslist.aspx?topicId=29 Accessed: February 12, 2014.

28. Palmer CA, Gilbert JA: Position of the Academy of Nutrition and Dietetics: The impact of fluoride on health. *Journal of the Academy of Nutrition and Dietetics* 112(9):1443, 2012.

29. Centers for Disease Control and Prevention: *Fluoride basics*. Last modified July 2013. http://www.cdc.gov/fluoridation/basics/index.htm Accessed: February 12, 2014.

30. Oral Health in America: A Report of the Surgeon General. *Community and other approaches to promote oral health and prevent oral disease*. 2000. http://www2.nidcr.nih.gov/sgr/sgrohweb/chap7.htm Accessed: February 12, 2014.

31. Office of Dietary Supplements, National Institutes of Health: *Chromium*. Last reviewed 2013. http://ods.od.nih.gov/factsheets/Chromium-HealthProfessional/ Accessed: February 12, 2014.

32. Onakpoya I and others: Chromium supplementation in overweight and obesity: A systematic review and meta-analysis of randomized clinical trials. *Obesity Reviews* 14(6):496, 2013.

33. Suksomboon N and others: Systematic review and meta-analysis of the efficacy and safety of chromium supplementation in diabetes. *Journal of Clinical Pharmacy and Therapeutics* 39(3):292, 2014.

34. Linus Pauling Institute Micronutrient Information Center: *Copper*. Last updated December 2013. http://lpi.oregonstate.edu/infocenter/minerals/copper/ Accessed: February 12, 2014.

35. Linus Pauling Institute Micronutrient Information Center: *Manganese*. Last updated March 2010. http://lpi.oregonstate.edu/infocenter/minerals/manganese/ Accessed: February 12, 2014.

36. Linus Pauling Institute Micronutrient Information Center: *Molybdenum*. Last updated June 2013. http://lpi.oregonstate.edu/infocenter/minerals/molybdenum/ Accessed: February 12, 2014.

37. Anon: Arsenic in your food: Our findings show a real need for federal standards for this toxin. *Consumer Reports Magazine*, November 2012. http://www.consumerreports.org/cro/magazine/2012/11/arsenic-in-your-food/index.htm Accessed: February 12, 2014.

38. Food and Drug Administration: *FDA proposes action level for arsenic in apple juice*. Last updated July 12, 2013. http://www.fda.gov/NewsEvents/Newsroom/PressAnnouncements/ucm360466.htm Accessed: February 12, 2014.

13 Obesity, Energy Balance, and Weight Management

CASE STUDY

Weight loss

TONY IS A 29-YEAR-OLD COMPUTER PROGRAMMER who is 6 feet tall and weighs 245 pounds. His waist circumference is 42 inches. When he was in college, he was the same height, but he weighed 175 pounds, had a waist circumference of 36 inches, and jogged or played basketball for about an hour almost daily. Now, he is so tired after coming home from work, he has little time or energy to do much except watch his favorite teams on TV and then go to bed.

Because Tony has to be at work at 7 A.M., he often skips breakfast. At his workplace, the break room that is next door to his office has several vending machines that are well-stocked with soft drinks, chips, cookies, and candy bars. When Tony feels hungry at work, he often goes to the break room to buy sugar-sweetened soft drinks, chocolate candy bars, and spicy tortilla chips to relieve his hunger.

- What is Tony's body mass index? What information does his BMI provide about his health?

- Explain why Tony should be concerned about his waist circumference.

- What environmental influences are probably contributing to Tony's excess body weight?

- What behavioral modifications would you recommend to help Tony lose weight?

The suggested Case Study Response can be found on page 454.

McGraw Hill Education **connect** | NUTRITION   Check out the Connect site at www.mcgrawhillconnect.com to further explore this case study.

QUIZ Yourself

What is the difference between overweight and obesity? Are there any dietary supplements that help people lose weight safely? Test your knowledge of energy balance, obesity, and weight management by taking the following quiz. The answers are found on page 457.

1. People can determine whether they have an unhealthy amount of body fat by measuring their waistline. ___T ___F

2. The best way to lose weight and keep it off is to follow a low-carbohydrate, high-fat diet, such as the Atkins diet. ___T ___F

3. Dietary supplements that contain ephedra can safely help a person lose 30 pounds in 30 days. ___T ___F

4. When a person consumes more carbohydrates than needed, the excess may be converted to fat and stored in fat cells. ___T___F

5. Liposuction is an easy and safe way to eliminate excess body fat. ___T ___F

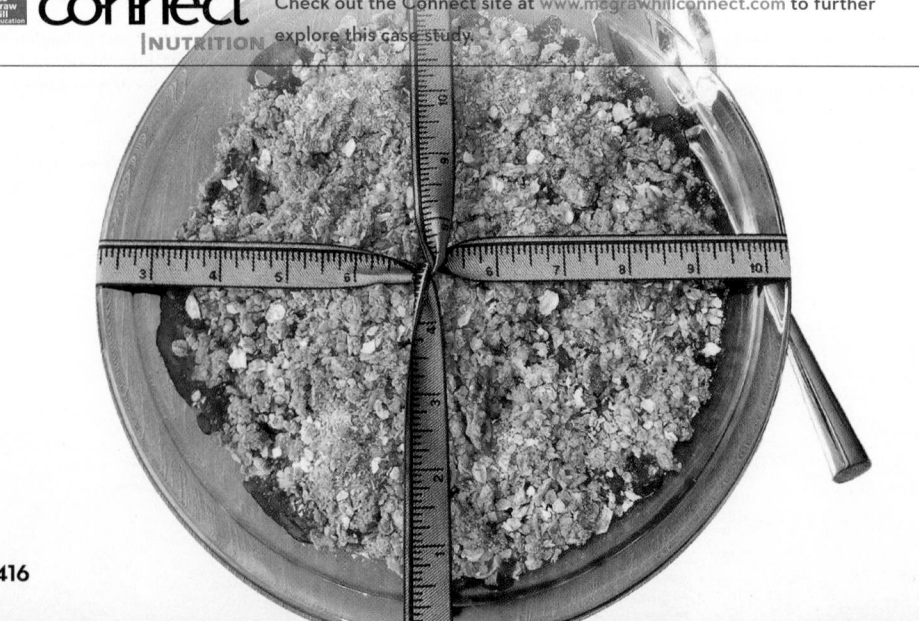

416

13.1 Overweight and Obesity

LEARNING OUTCOMES

1 *Describe recent statistical trends for obesity and overweight in the United States and globally.*

2 *Identify health and economic consequences of obesity.*

In the United States, overweight and obesity are widespread nutritional problems that have reached epidemic proportions (Fig. 13.1). An **overweight** person has extra body weight that is contributed by bone, muscle, body fat, and/or body water.[1] A professional basketball player, for example, may be "overweight" because of his muscular body build—but he has a healthy amount of body fat. **Obesity**, however, is a condition characterized by excessive and unhealthy amounts of body fat. Some body fat is essential for good health, but people who are overweight or obese ("overfat") have a greater risk for serious, chronic health conditions and diseases.

overweight having extra weight from bone, muscle, body fat, and/or body water

obesity condition characterized by excessive and unhealthy amounts of body fat

Prevalence of Overweight and Obesity

According to data collected from a national survey, almost 69% of American adults over the age of 20 were either overweight or obese in 2011–2012.[2] One–third of Americans were overweight, and more than one–third of them were obese. As shown in Table 13.1, the percent of obese adults increased by approximately 50% between 1988–1994 and 2011–2012.[2] People who are classified as being obese can be further categorized into a subgroup of individuals who are "extremely obese." In 2011–2012, over 6% of Americans were classified as being extremely obese. This percentage more than doubled since 1988–1994. The most recent data, however, indicate that the increase in cases of obesity among American adults may be slowing or leveling off.

Compared to non–Hispanic white adults, overweight and obesity are more common among non–Hispanic black and Mexican–American adults.[3] According to experts at the Centers for Disease Control and Prevention (CDC), cultural, behavioral, and environmental factors may be largely responsible for racial/ethnic differences in obesity rates. For example, non–Hispanic black and Mexican–American adults may have more positive attitudes toward overfat body shapes than non–Hispanic white adults. Environmental factors that influence body weight include living in urban areas that lack access to safe outdoor activities or have a high density of fast food outlets.

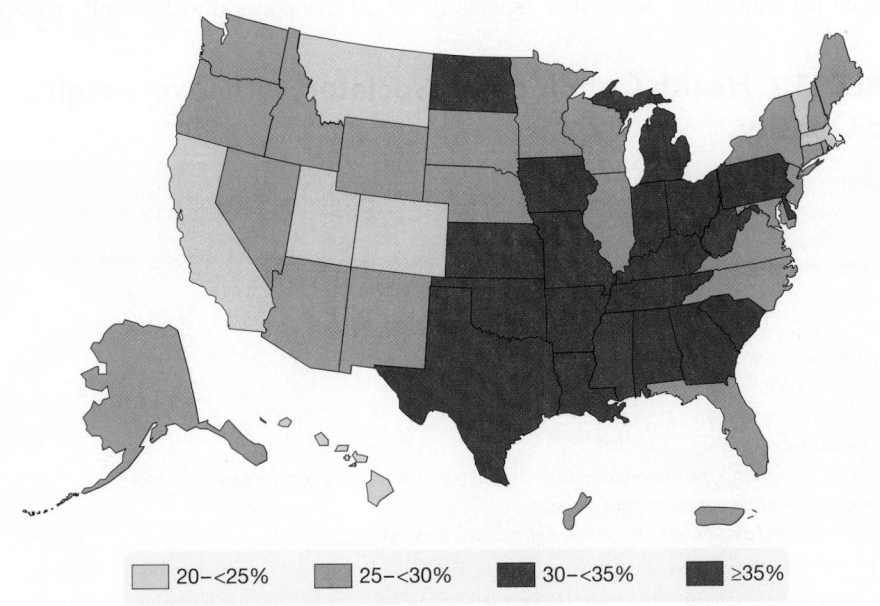

□ 20–<25% ■ 25–<30% ■ 30–<35% ■ ≥35%

Percent of adult population

FIGURE 13.1 Prevalence of self-reported obesity among U.S. adults, 2013.

TABLE 13.1 Age-Adjusted Prevalence of Overweight, Obesity, and Extreme Obesity Among U.S. Adults Aged 20 and Over

Weight Status	1988–1994	2011–2012
Overweight	33.1%	33.6%
Obese	22.9%	34.9%
• Extremely obese	3.0%	6.4%

Source of data: Centers for Disease Control and Prevention: *Obesity and overweight: Data, maps, and trends.* Last updated September 9, 2014. http://www.cdc.gov/obesity/data/databases.html Accessed: October 1, 2014

The prevalence of obesity among American children and adolescents (17%) has also risen sharply over the past two decades.[4] However, the most recent data comparing the prevalence of childhood and adolescent obesity from 2007–2008 to 2009–2010 showed no change.[5] Public health experts are very concerned about the high rate of obesity among children, because these youngsters are more likely to mature into obese adults than children who are not obese. See Chapter 17 for a discussion of childhood obesity.

Globally, overweight and obesity rates are also rising rapidly ("globesity"). In 2008, the World Health Organization estimated that worldwide, 1 *billion* adults were overweight and 500 million adults were obese.[6] Throughout the world, overweight and obesity are responsible for more deaths than underweight.[6]

Health Consequences of Obesity

There are many undesirable chronic health conditions associated with having excess body fat (Table 13.2). Obesity increases risks of type 2 diabetes, coronary artery disease, stroke, and certain cancers. Each year, these chronic diseases are responsible for thousands of deaths among American adults.

Although Table 13.2 does not list social or psychological consequences of obesity, the results of research show that overweight and obesity can be associated with discrimination and stigmatization. Such discrimination may occur when the obese person seeks employment, health care, and relationships.[7] Many people in Western societies think having a healthy body weight is a personal responsibility and simply a matter of exerting some will power or self-control. As a result of this emotionally unsupportive environment, obese people are also likely to have psychological problems, especially mood disorders and low self-esteem.[8]

TABLE 13.2 Health Conditions Associated with Overweight and Obesity

- Coronary artery disease
- Dyslipidemia (high LDL cholesterol, low HDL cholesterol, and/or high levels of triglycerides in the blood)
- Gallbladder disease
- Gout
- Infertility
- Hypertension and stroke
- Low back pain
- Metabolic syndrome
- Osteoarthritis
- *Polycystic ovarian syndrome* (condition that can cause fertility problems for women)
- Sleep apnea and respiratory problems
- Some cancers (particularly, endometrial, breast, and colon cancers)
- Type 2 diabetes

Source: World Health Organization International Obesity Task Force: *Redefining obesity and its treatment.* 2000. http://www.who.int/nutrition/publications/obesity/09577082_1_1/en/index.html Accessed: February 15, 2014.

Furthermore, coping strategies used to deal with psychological stress may include physical inactivity and unhealthy eating behaviors.[7] Chapter 14 provides information concerning such eating practices.

Economic Consequences of Obesity

Treating obesity and dealing with its consequences are costly. Obese individuals often have greater medical care costs than people with healthy body weights.[10] The most costly conditions associated with obesity include arthritis, coronary artery disease, and type 2 diabetes. About half of the costs of treating these conditions are incurred by individuals who are 65 years of age and older and have health insurance covered by tax–supported programs such as Medicare.[11] In 2008, the estimated expenses for taking care of obese patients and related economic costs (e.g., absenteeism and loss of worker productivity) were about $147 billion in the United States.[12] Unless the prevalence of obesity can be reduced, these costs are likely to continue spiraling upward, adding stress to the American health care system and economy as a result.

ASSESS YOUR PROGRESS

1 *In the United States, how has the percent of overweight and obese children and adults changed since 1988?*

2 *List at least three psychological and three physical consequences of being overweight or obese.*

3 *In the United States, what are the economic costs of obesity to the society?*

13.2 Body Mass Index

LEARNING OUTCOMES

1 *Explain how to calculate a person's body mass index (BMI).*

2 *Identify ranges of BMIs that are used to classify people as underweight, healthy weight, overweight, and obese.*

3 *Discuss limitations of using the BMI.*

To determine whether a person's weight is underweight, healthy, overweight, or obese, medical experts generally use the **body mass index (BMI)**. The BMI is a numerical value based on the relationship between body weight and height, and it can be a first step in evaluating a person's risk of chronic health problems associated with excess body fat.[6] BMI is calculated by dividing weight in kg by height in meters, squared.

body mass index (BMI) numerical value of relationship between body weight and risk of chronic health problems associated with excess body fat calculated by dividing weight in kg by height in meters, squared

$$\frac{\text{Weight (kg)}}{\text{Height (m)}^2}$$

To estimate a person's BMI, you can also use the following formula:

$$\frac{\text{Weight (lb)}}{\text{Height (inches)}^2} \times 703$$

For example, a person who weighs 140 pounds and is 5–feet, 3–inches (63–in.) tall has a BMI of approximately 24.8. Calculation:

$$(140 \div [63]^2) \times 703$$

$$(140 \div 3969) \times 703 =$$

$$0.03527 \times 703 = 24.8$$

Health care practitioners can use a BMI calculator, such as the one available at http://www.nhlbi.nih.gov/health/educational/lose_wt/BMI/bmicalc.htm, or consult a BMI chart such as the one shown in Figure 13.2 to determine a range of weight that is healthy for a patient's height without shoes (BMIs of 18.5 to 24.9). According to this chart, an adult whose height is 5—feet, 5—inches has a healthy weight range of about 111 to 149 pounds. Table 13.3 displays classifications according to BMI for adults ages 20 and older.

BMI: Limitations

The BMI can be a reliable indicator of body fatness. However, the usefulness of the BMI may be limited when assessing the health of highly muscular individuals,

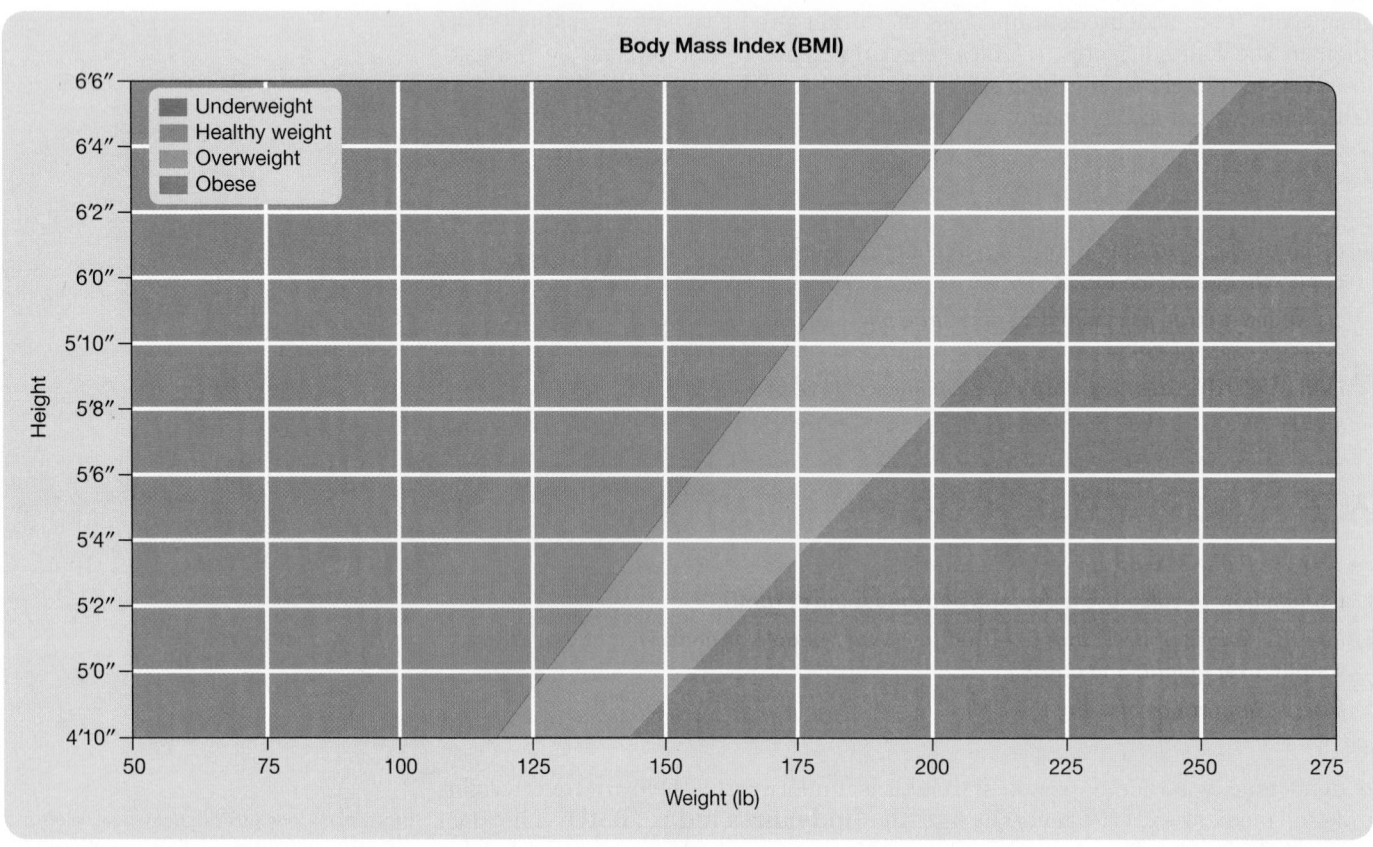

FIGURE 13.2 BMI range chart. To determine your BMI range, locate your height in the left-most column with your left index finger, then locate your weight along the bottom line of the graph with your right index finger. Read across the row with your left finger and up from the bottom with your right finger, until your fingers meet. The chart's color at the point where your fingers meet indicates your body weight classification, according to BMI.

TABLE 13.3 BMI Classifications for Adults

BMI	Classification
< 18.5	Underweight
18.5–24.9	Normal (Healthy)
25.0–29.9	Overweight
30.0–34.9	Obese class I
35.0–39.9	Obese class II
≥ 40.0	Obese class III

Source: World Health Organization International Obesity Task Force: Redefining obesity and its treatment. 2000. http://www .who.int/nutrition/publications/obesity/09577082_1_1/en/index.html Accessed: February 15, 2014.

older adults, or chronically ill persons. Someone with a high degree of muscular—ity may have an elevated BMI but low percent body fat. Thus, a muscular person with a BMI of 25.0 is more likely to be healthy than a sedentary person who also has a BMI of 25.0. Furthermore, BMI may underestimate body fat in people who have lost muscle tissue as a result of illness or aging.[13]

Among older adults, BMI does not reflect excess fat reliably, because peo—ple typically lose weight, especially lean mass, as they age.[14] For example, a 50—year—old woman with a BMI of 23.8 may have a healthy amount of body fat, while an 80—year—old woman with a BMI of 23.8 may have excess fat. However, people with BMIs of 30 or higher generally have excess body fat.

Another limitation of using BMI to assess health is that it does not take a person's sex or race into account. A healthy woman has more body fat than a healthy man who is the same age, weight, and height. BMI tables may not be useful for assessing the health of people with Asian ancestry. Asians, especially Asian women, can have healthy BMIs and unhealthy amounts of body fat.[15]

Normal Weight Obesity

It is possible for a person with low muscularity and a physically inactive life—style to have a normal ("healthy") BMI and also have a high percentage of body fat. This condition is referred to as **normal weight obesity (NWO)**. Scientists estimate that approximately 30 million Americans have NWO, and the condi—tion is associated with increased risk of insulin resistance, diabetes, and coronary artery disease.[16]

NWO becomes more prevalent as a population ages and is most common among Americans between 65 and 75 years of age.[17] NWO is more prevalent in women, regardless of age, and the condition increases risk for cardiovascular *mortality* (death) in women but not men.[16,18] Therefore, having a normal BMI does not nec—essarily protect a person from the health consequences of obesity.

normal weight obesity (NWO) normal body weight as measured by BMI but elevated percent body fat

ASSESS YOUR PROGRESS

④ *Calculate the BMI of someone whose height is 5-feet, 11-inches and whose weight is 190 pounds.*

⑤ *What are the body weight classifications of four 22-year-old individuals who have BMIs of 17, 23, 28, and 34?*

13.3 Body Composition and Fat Distribution

LEARNING OUTCOMES

1 *Identify the components of body composition.*
2 *Explain methods of estimating percent body fat.*
3 *Discuss how waist circumference is used to assess health.*

Health care practitioners can obtain information about the components that make up a patient's body by measuring body composition. **Body composition** is often expressed in percent fat, that is, the percent of the entire body that is **adipose tissue** ("fat cells"). **Total body fat** includes both adipose tissue, which is important for storing energy, and **essential fat**, which is vital for survival and is found in cell membranes, certain bones, and nervous tissue.

Monitoring body composition is important, because it is a component of physical fitness and can indicate risk for certain health conditions. Commonly

body composition measurement of body tissues, usually expressed as percent body fat

adipose tissue fat cells

total body fat adipose tissue and essential fat

essential fat fat that is vital for survival; found in cell membranes, certain bones, and nervous tissue

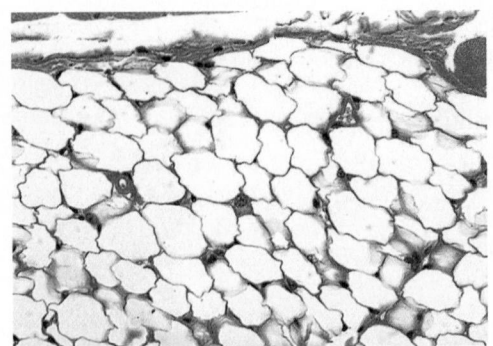

FIGURE 13.3 Microscopic view of adipose tissue.

two-component model method of measuring body composition that divides the body into two compartments: fat mass and fat-free mass

fat-free mass weight of the body that includes body water, bones, teeth, muscles, and organs

subcutaneous fat accumulation of adipose cells in the tissue under the skin

visceral fat large deposit of adipose tissue under the abdominal muscles and over the digestive organs

used approaches to measuring body composition divide the body into two components: fat mass and fat—free mass. This approach is often called the **two—component model** because the entire body is classified as either fat or fat—free mass. **Fat—free mass** includes body water; mineral—rich tis—sues, such as bones and teeth; and protein—rich tissues, including muscles and organs. Some other methods of measuring body composition use three or four components and separately measure body water, bone mineral, or protein from fat mass.

Adipose Tissue: Subcutaneous and Visceral Fat

Subcutaneous (*sub* = under; *cu—ta—ne—ous* [*cue—tay'—nee—us*] = skin) tissue holds skin in place over underlying tissues such as muscles. Subcutaneous tissue also contains adipose cells (Fig. 13.3). When subcutaneous tissue has more adipose cells than other kinds of cells, it is referred to as **subcutaneous fat**.[19] Subcutaneous fat helps insulate the body against cold temperatures and protects muscles and bones from bumps and bruises. Subcutaneous fat is unevenly distrib—uted. This layer of fat is thicker in certain regions of men's and women's bodies, especially in the abdominal area, thighs, and buttocks (Fig. 13.4).

A second type of fat tissue is **visceral** (*viss'—eh—rol*) **fat**. Visceral fat forms a protective structure that is under the abdominal muscles and lies internally over the stomach and intestines (Fig. 13.5). Although there are some gender dif—ferences, women generally have more subcutaneous fat than men, whereas men tend to have more visceral fat than women. Excessive amounts of visceral fat, subcutaneous abdominal fat, or both result in what is commonly called a "beer belly" or the "middle—age spread."

In addition to storing energy, adipose tissue has hormonal functions. Fat cells produce *adipokines*, a group of peptide hormones that alter energy metabolism and feeding behavior. We will discuss two adipokines, *leptin* and *adiponectin*, in section 13.7.

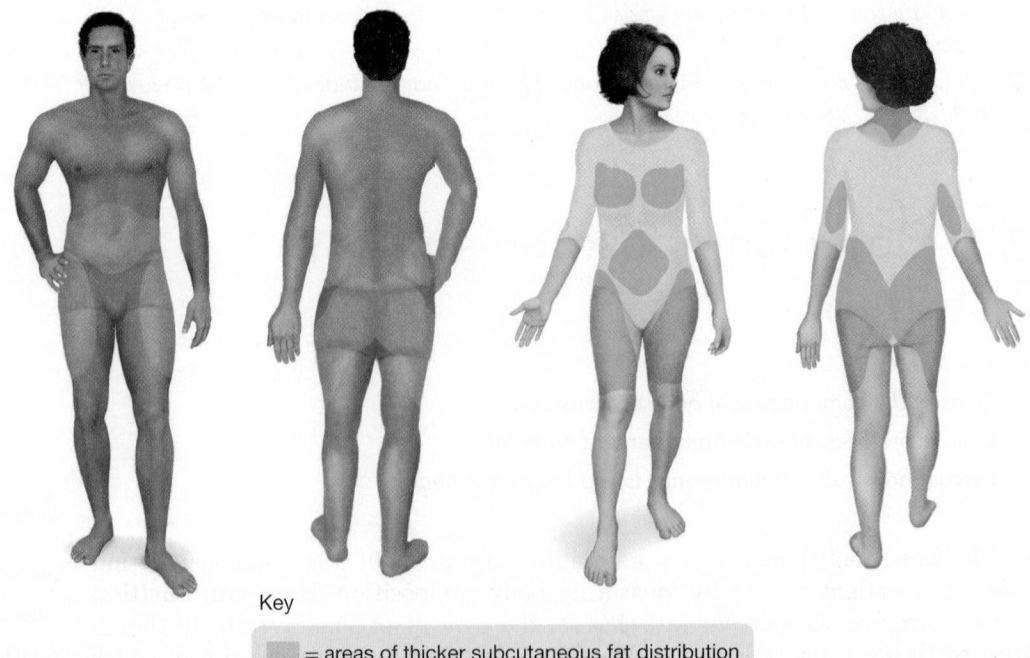

Key

    = areas of thicker subcutaneous fat distribution

FIGURE 13.4 Uneven subcutaneous fat distribution in men and women. Subcutaneous fat is unevenly distributed. Thicker deposits occur in various regions of men's and women's bodies, especially in the abdomen, thighs, and buttocks.

DID YOU *KNOW?*

Cellulite, the lumpy-appearing skin on thighs and buttocks of many adults, especially women, is not a unique type of fat. Scientists have no clear understanding of why cellulite occurs, but it may simply be normal subcutaneous fat held in place by irregular bands of connective tissue. Despite claims by cosmetic manufacturers that their products eliminate cellulite, there are no effective ways to smooth the skin's dimpled appearance.[20]

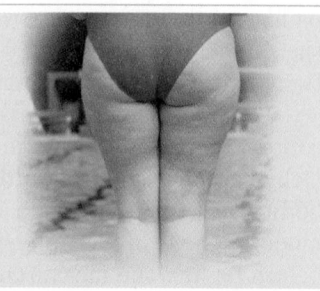

underwater weighing technique of estimating body composition that involves comparing weight on land to weight when completely submerged in a tank of water

air displacement method of estimating body composition by determining body volume

dual-energy x-ray absorptiometry (DXA) technique of estimating body composition that involves scanning the body with two low-energy x-rays

bioelectrical impedance analysis (BIA) technique of estimating body composition in which a device measures the conduction of a weak electrical current through body water

Estimating Percent Body Fat

There is no precise way to measure a living person's percent body fat. Scientists, however, use a variety of methods that indirectly estimate the percentage. The following sections provide information about several of these assessment techniques.

Underwater Weighing

Underwater weighing, also called hydrostatic weighing, involves comparing a person's weight "on land" to his or her weight when completely submerged in a tank of water (Fig. 13.6). Lean tissue is denser than water; fat tissue is not as dense as water. Thus, a person who has more body fat will weigh less when under water than a person who has more lean tissue. The underwater weighing method can be an accurate way of assessing body composition. However, the method is not a convenient, easy, inexpensive, or practical way to estimate percent body fat, because it requires special testing facilities.

Air Displacement

The **air displacement** method assesses the volume of a person's body, which can be used to calculate his or her body composition. After being weighed on a very precise scale, the subject sits in the chamber of a device called the BOD POD (Fig. 13.7). This device measures the volume of air in the chamber while a person is sitting in it and compares it with the volume of air that was in the chamber when it was unoccupied. The person's volume is equal to the amount of air that was displaced after the subject entered the chamber. Air displacement measurements provide highly accurate estimates of body fat content, but the measuring device is expensive and not practical for most consumers to use.

Dual-Energy X-Ray Absorptiometry

Dual–energy x–ray absorptiometry (DXA) involves the use of two low–energy x–rays to scan the entire body. The two levels of x–rays help to differentiate among the densities of adipose, muscle, and bone tissues. The method provides a detailed "picture" of internal structures, including fat deposits (Fig. 13.8). During the scanning process, the equipment emits a dose of radiation that is much lower than that used for a chest x–ray. Although DXA is a highly accurate way to estimate body fat content, the equipment is very expensive and not widely available outside of clinical settings.

Bioelectrical Impedance Analysis

Bioelectrical impedance analysis (BIA) is a quick way to estimate body fat content. This method is based on the principle that water and electrolytes conduct

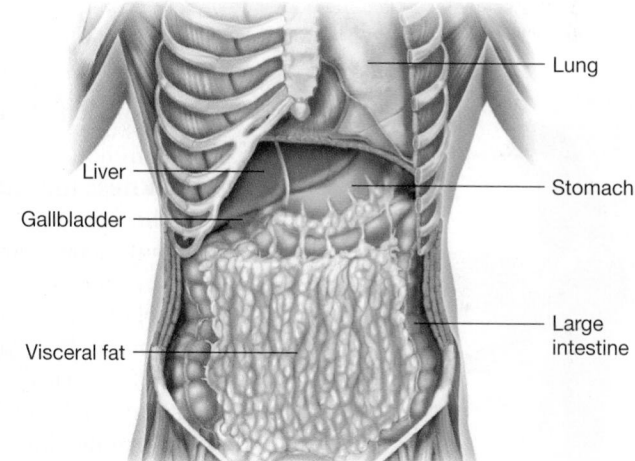

FIGURE 13.5 Visceral fat.

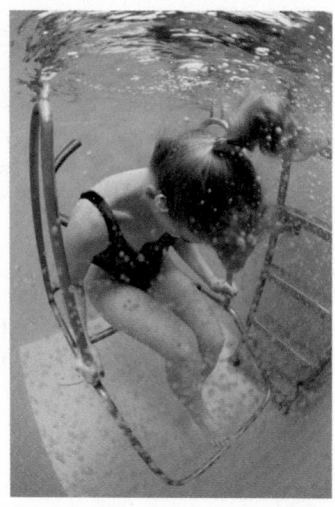

FIGURE 13.6 Underwater weighing.

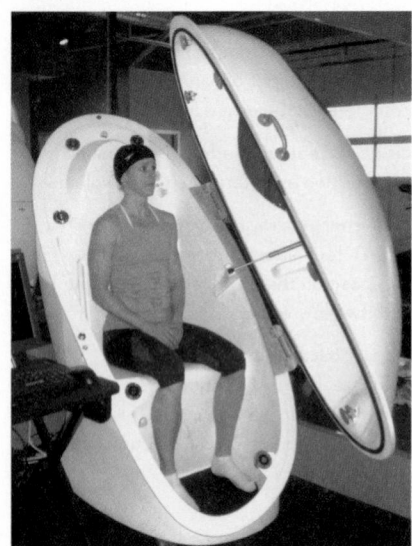

FIGURE 13.7 Air displacement. The BOD POD device estimates a person's body volume.

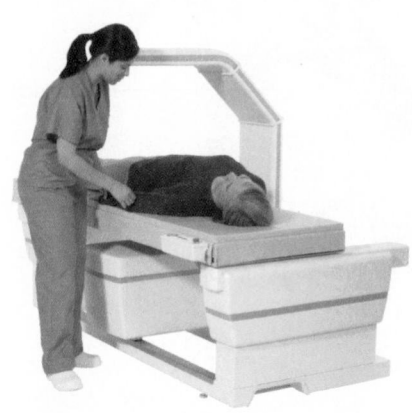

FIGURE 13.8 Dual-energy x-ray absorptiometry. DXA is a highly accurate way to estimate body fat content.

skinfold thickness measurements technique of estimating body composition in which calipers are used to measure the thickness of skinfolds at multiple body sites

electricity. Body fat resists the flow of electricity, because fat tissue contains less water and electrolytes than lean tissue. The bioelectrical impedance device sends a painless, low–energy electrical current through electrodes that are in contact with the subject's skin (Fig. 13.9). Within a few seconds, the device converts information about the body's electrical resistance into an estimate of body fat percentage.

The accuracy and reliability of BIA results heavily depend on body water content. To obtain the most accurate results, proper hydration is necessary. Dehydration results in an overestimation of body fat. Thus, anything that alters body water content, such as consuming food, caffeine, or alcohol; engaging in moderate–to–intense physical activity; and excessive sweating should be avoided before having the measurement taken.

Consumers can purchase a bioelectrical impedance device that resembles a bathroom scale, but research shows that models including hand and foot electrodes are more accurate than devices with only two foot electrodes.[21] The conversion of data concerning electrical resistance to percent body fat requires the use of a population–specific equation. Therefore, many BIA devices that are marketed to consumers are not appropriate for use with diverse populations.[22] Even when used properly, consumer BIA devices may have about ± 7% error in comparison to a "gold standard" method such as air displacement.[23] This means that if a person's body is 20% fat, according to the BIA method of assessment, it is very likely that the subject's true body fat content is between 13 and 27%.

Skinfold Thickness

A common technique for estimating total body fat involves taking **skinfold thickness measurements** at multiple body sites, such as over the triceps muscle of the arm (Fig. 13.10). The thickness of a skinfold indicates the depth of the subcutaneous fat at that site. To perform the measurements, a trained person pinches a section of the subject's skin, gently pulls it away from underlying muscle tissue, and uses specialized calipers to measure the thickness of the subcutaneous fat. After taking the measurements, the values are incorporated into a mathematical formula that provides a fairly accurate estimate of the subject's amount of body fat. Formulas are established for men and women that involve performing skinfold measurement at either three or seven sites.

Skinfold thickness measurements are relatively easy and inexpensive to perform, but the method's accuracy largely depends on the skill of the person performing the measurements. Therefore, a practitioner who wishes to use this measurement technique should be trained by a skilled technician.[24] Practitioners

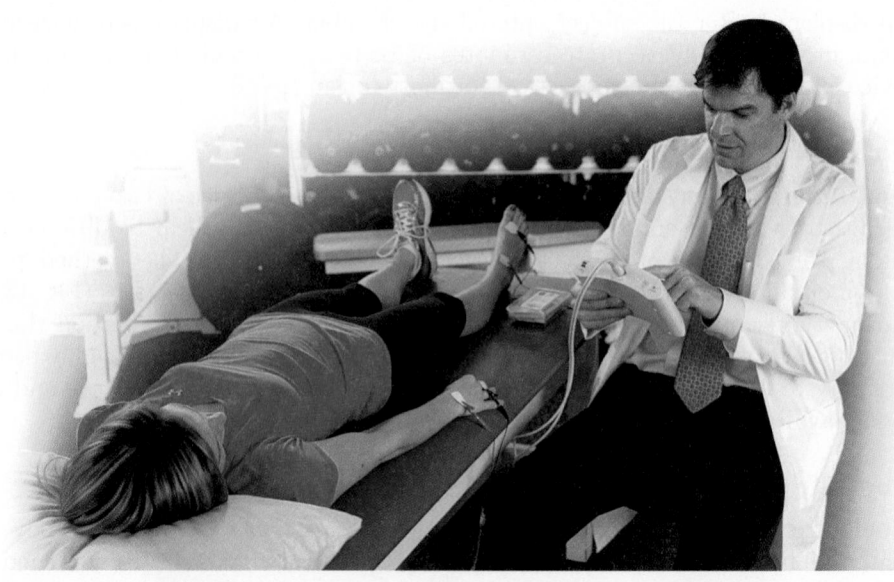

FIGURE 13.9 Bioelectrical impedance.

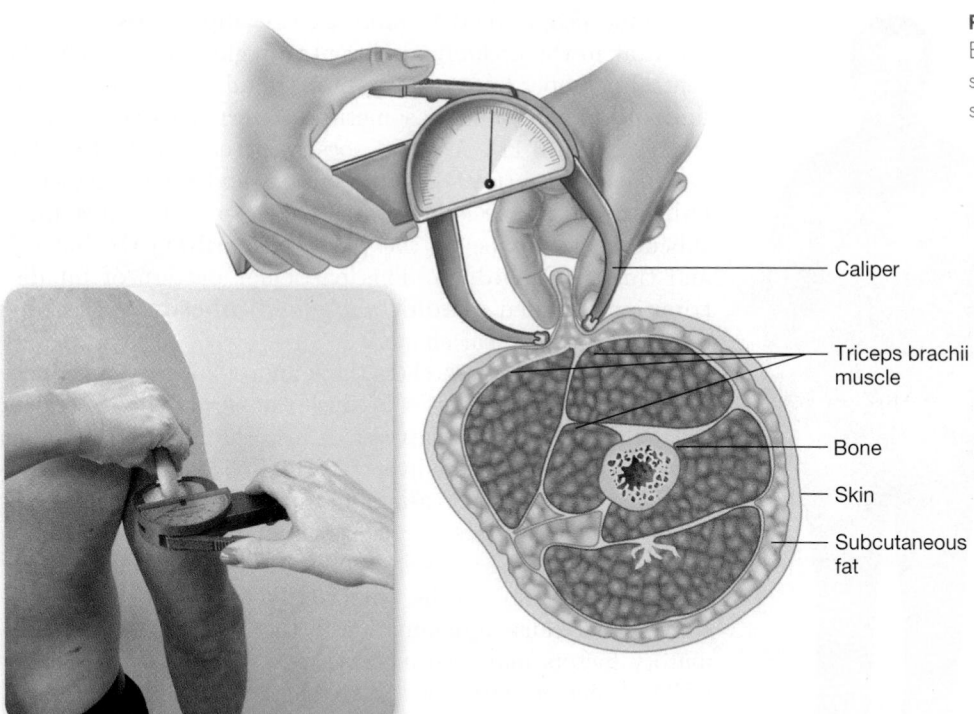

FIGURE 13.10 Measuring skinfolds.
Body fat can be estimated by measuring skinfold thicknesses at multiple body sites, such as over the triceps muscle of the arm.

Caliper

Triceps brachii muscle

Bone

Skin

Subcutaneous fat

can improve the accuracy and precision of their skinfold measurement skills by watching videos that demonstrate proper technique, participating in training workshops, and gaining experience in a supervised environment.

Under ideal testing conditions, the accuracy of predicting percent fat from skinfolds is ± 3.5%.[24] This means if a practitioner uses skinfold assessments to determine that a client is 25% fat, it is very likely that the subject's actual per-cent body fat is between 21.5 and 28.5%.

How Much Body Fat Is Healthy?

Table 13.4 classifies people into weight categories according to their percentage of body fat. A man is overweight when his body is 22 to 25% fat; a woman is over-weight when her body is 32 to 37% fat.[25] A man is obese when fat comprises 26% or more of his body; a woman is obese when fat makes up 38% or more of her body.

Body Fat Distribution

The distribution of excess body fat may be more highly associated with risks of obesity–related diseases than percentage of total body fat. Therefore, the World Health Organization states that BMI and body fat distribution are important for assessing risk of health conditions associated with obesity.[26]

FRESH TIPS

Larger universities with human nutrition and kinesiology departments may have facilities that offer body composition testing, such as bioelectrical impedance, underwater weighing, and air displacement. Check with these departments for more information, including any fees for the testing.

TABLE 13.4 Adult Body Weight Classification by Percentage of Body Fat

Classification	Men Body Fat (%)	Women Body Fat (%)
Healthy	13–21%	23–31%
Overweight	22–25%	32–37%
Obese	26–31%	38–42%
Extremely obese	32% or more	43% or more

Adapted from: Food and Nutrition Board: *Dietary reference intakes for energy, carbohydrate, fiber, fat, fatty acids, cholesterol, protein, and amino acids (macronutrients).* Table 5.5, page 126, 2005. www.nap.edu/openbook/0309085373/html/126.html

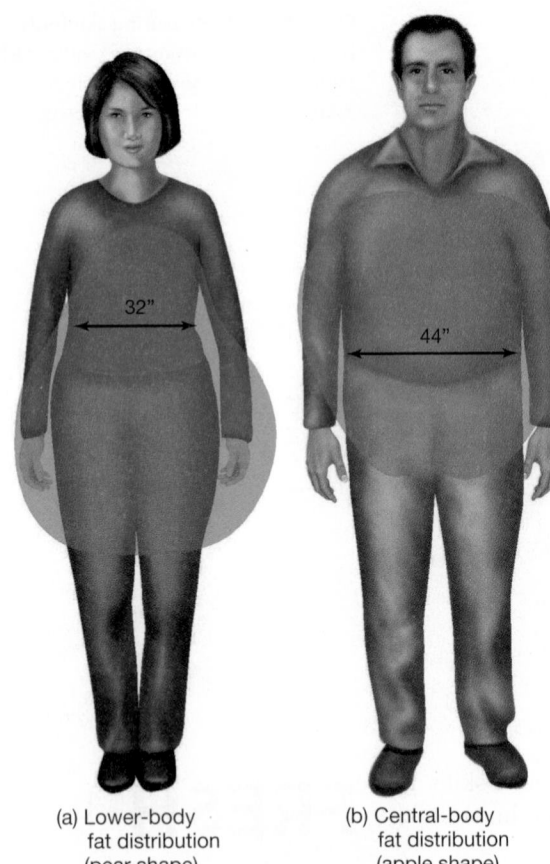

(a) Lower-body
fat distribution
(pear shape)

(b) Central-body
fat distribution
(apple shape)

FIGURE 13.11 Body fat distribution. (a) Lower-body fat distribution (gynoid obesity). (b) Central-body fat distribution (android obesity).

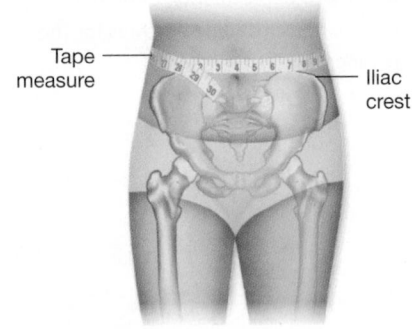

Tape
measure

Iliac
crest

FIGURE 13.12 A method of measuring waist circumference.

android obesity storage of excess body fat in the upper body or abdominal region, leading to an "apple shape"

gynoid obesity storage of excess body fat in the buttocks and thighs, leading to a "pear shape"

Some people tend to store excess adipose tissue as visceral fat in the abdominal or central region of the body. The central or upper body storage of extra adipose tissue is called **android obesity** and is sometimes referred to as an "apple shape" (Fig. 13.11). Android obesity increases risk of cardiovascular disease (CVD), hypertension, and type 2 diabetes.[27] Other people, especially women, tend to store extra fat as subcutaneous fat below the waist, primarily in the buttocks and thighs (Fig. 13.11). This particular pattern of fat distribution is called **gynoid** (*guy'−noid*) **obesity** and is often referred to as a "pear shape."

Many medical researchers think android obesity contributes to certain chronic diseases because the surplus of visceral fat cells releases too many fatty acids into the hepatic portal vein that leads directly to the liver.[28] When flooded with fatty acids, the liver has difficulty using the lipids to make lipoproteins. When this occurs, the fatty acids circulate in the bloodstream, possibly disrupting muscle and liver glucose metabolism.[28] Furthermore, adipose cells, particularly visceral fat, make substances that cause inflammation in the body.[29] These inflammatory factors may also increase risks of type 2 diabetes and CVD. A person with android obesity can have increased risk of type 2 diabetes, hypertension, coronary artery disease, and metabolic syndrome, even if he or she has a normal BMI.

Waist Circumference

A quick and easy method of assessing android obesity and its risk for related disorders is to measure waist circumference. Waist circumference can be measured by placing a cloth measuring tape around the waist, so the tape is at the top of the iliac crest. It is important to use a measuring tape that does not stretch. Figure 13.12 shows a recommended tape measure placement for determining waist circumference.

In people with BMIs that are greater than 25, a waist circumference that is greater than 40 inches for men or 35 inches for women is associated with increased risks of developing type 2 diabetes, abnormal blood lipid levels, hypertension, and CVD.[30] Table 13.5 classifies these risks according to BMI and waist circumference.

TABLE 13.5 Disease Risk for Type 2 Diabetes, Hypertension, and Cardiovascular Disease, Relative to BMI and Waist Circumference

BMI Category	Waist Circumference < 40" for Men or 35" for Women	Waist Circumference > 40" for Men or 35" for Women
Underweight		
Healthy weight		
Overweight	Increased	High
Obesity class I	High	Very high
Obesity class II	Very high	Very high
Obesity class III	Extremely high	Extremely high

Source: National Institutes of Health, National Heart Lung and Blood Institute: *Classification of overweight and obesity by BMI, waist circumference, and associated disease risks.* ND. http://www.nhlbi.nih.gov/health/public/heart/obesity/lose_wt/bmi_dis.htm Accessed: February 15, 2014.

DID **YOU** *KNOW?*

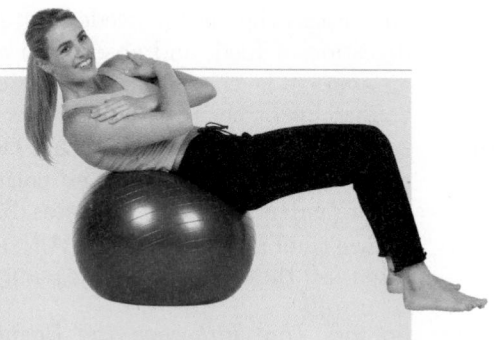

Regular exercise, such as walking, can shrink body fat, but it is not possible to "spot-reduce" by intensely exercising a targeted body region, such as the abdomen.[31] Exercise, however, increases energy expenditure, which can lead to weight loss over time. Regularly exercising specific body parts can improve muscle tone, so that the subcutaneous fat in that part of the body appears less "flabby."

ASSESS YOUR PROGRESS

6 *List the components of body composition.*

7 *Describe three methods of estimating body fat, and identify a drawback of each.*

8 *Identify the health consequences of android obesity.*

9 *What does a person's waist circumference indicate about his or her health?*

13.4 Energy Intake and Expenditures

LEARNING OUTCOMES

1 *Identify the components of total energy expenditure and use formulas to estimate TEE.*

2 *Describe methods of calculating basal metabolic rate, and name factors that alter its value.*

energy intake calories from foods and beverages that contain macronutrients and alcohol

energy output calories cells use to carry out their activities

total energy expenditure (TEE) amount of energy needed for all bodily functions throughout the day

basal metabolism minimum number of calories the body uses for vital physiological activities after fasting and resting for 12 hours

basal metabolic rate (BMR) measurement of basal metabolism

For humans, biological fuels are foods and beverages that contain carbohydrate, protein, and/or fat. Alcohol also provides energy for people who consume the nonnutrient. The amount of calories consumed from these sources is a person's **energy intake**.

Energy output (energy expenditure) refers to the calories cells use to carry out their activities. For example, muscle cells need energy to contract, liver cells use energy to convert toxic compounds to safer substances, and intestinal cells require energy to absorb certain nutrients. In the following sections, we discuss the major ways the body expends food energy. Chapter 8 includes a detailed discussion of energy metabolism.

Energy Expenditures

Total energy expenditure (TEE) is the amount of energy a person needs to carry out all bodily functions throughout an entire day. The components of TEE are basal or resting metabolism, physical activity, thermic effect of food, and non-exercise activity thermogenesis.

Basal and Resting Metabolism

As described in Chapter 8, metabolism is the sum of all chemical reactions that occur in living cells. **Basal metabolism** is the minimum number of calories the body uses for vital physiological activities after fasting and resting for 12 hours. Measuring the rate at which a person uses energy for basal metabolism (**basal metabolic rate** or **BMR**) requires the subject to lie motionless, in a comfortable environment for the duration of the testing (Fig. 13.13).

Basal metabolic processes include breathing, circulating blood, and maintaining constant liver, brain, and kidney functions. Basal metabolism does not

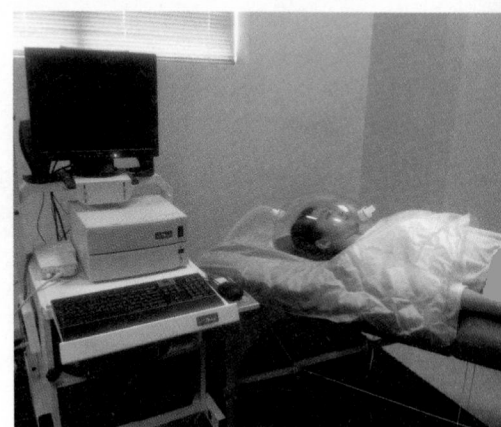

FIGURE 13.13 Indirect calorimetry. This method of measuring energy expenditure quantifies oxygen consumption and carbon dioxide production to estimate caloric expenditure.

resting metabolic rate (RMR) body's rate of energy use a few hours after resting and eating

encompass the energy needed for skeletal muscle movements (physical activity), digestion of food, and absorption and processing of nutrients. For a person with an average level of physical activity, basal metabolism accounts for about 60 to 75% of his or her body's total energy use.[31]

The **resting metabolic rate (RMR)** refers to the body's rate of energy use a few hours after resting and eating. The strict conditions for measuring BMR often lead researchers to assess RMR instead. A person's RMR is about 10% higher than his or her BMR. Although BMR and RMR are different, researchers often use the terms interchangeably in their publications.

Factors That Influence the Basal Metabolic Rate The BMR varies among individuals. Factors that account for this variation include:

- *Body composition:* Lean body mass is the major factor that influences the metabolic rate.[25] Muscle tissue, a component of lean body mass, is more metabolically active than fat tissue. In general, a person who has more muscle mass has a higher BMR than someone with less muscle mass.

- *Sex:* Males generally have higher metabolic rates than females, which may be due to greater lean body mass, on average, in males.

- *Body surface area:* The body constantly loses energy in the form of heat that moves to the skin's surface and then into the environment. Because a taller person has more body surface area than a shorter person, the taller individual loses more body heat.

- *Age:* Basal metabolism declines as one grows older, primarily due to the loss of lean tissues such as muscle. An average adult needs about 150 fewer kilocalories per day for every decade after 20 years of age.[32] Regular exercise helps build and preserve lean body mass.

- *Thyroid hormone:* Thyroid hormone regulates metabolism (Fig. 11.13). Excess thyroid hormone elevates the BMR, while insufficient amounts of the hormone reduce the BMR.

- *Caloric intake:* The body conserves energy use when calorie intake is very low or absent. Very–low–calorie diets reduce the metabolic rate. Therefore, such diets are not generally recommended for weight loss, because a lower metabolic rate can slow the rate of loss.

Although a person's BMR is fairly constant from day to day, a number of factors can influence his or her metabolic rate. Table 13.6 lists several factors that increase or decrease the metabolic rate.

DID **YOU** KNOW?

As many adults grow older, they think their muscles have "turned into" fat. A muscle cell, however, cannot transform itself into a fat cell. During the aging process, lean tissue mass shrinks, as cells in muscle, bone, and organs die and are not replaced. The loss of muscle tissue is called **sarcopenia** (*sar'-koe-pe'-nee-a*).

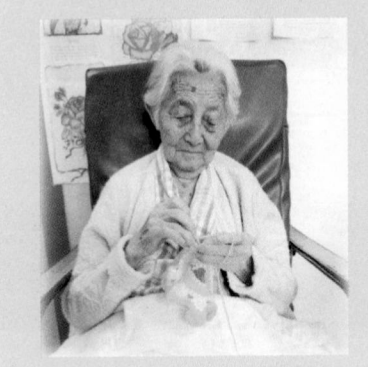

sarcopenia condition characterized by the loss of muscle tissue

TABLE 13.6 Factors That Influence a Person's BMR

Factors That Increase BMR ↑	Factors That Decrease BMR ↓
Body temperature (Fever increases metabolism.)	Starvation or very-low-calorie diets
Excess thyroid hormone	Insufficient thyroid hormone
Periods of growth (i.e., pregnancy, infancy, adolescence)	Aging
Greater body surface area (tall height)	Less body surface area (short height)
Lactation (milk production for breastfeeding)	
Exercise	
Stimulant drugs (e.g., caffeine and amphetamines)	
HIV infection	
Stress	

Calculating Basal Metabolic Rate A person's BMR can be estimated by using three different calculations. The easiest method for healthy young adults to use is a simple rule−of−thumb formula:

$$\text{Factor for men} = 1.0 \text{ kcal/kg of body weight/hr}$$

$$\text{Factor for women} = 0.9 \text{ kcal/kg of body weight/hr}$$

To estimate the number of kilocalories someone needs for basal metabolism, first convert the person's weight in pounds to kilograms by dividing the weight in pounds by 2.2. Then, multiply the weight in kg by the appropriate factor for men or women and fill in the blanks. For example, to estimate the BMR of a woman who weighs 141 pounds, first convert her weight into kilograms by dividing her weight in pounds by 2.2. Then plug her weight into the rule−of−thumb formula for women:

$$141 \text{ lb} \div 2.2 = 64 \text{ kg (rounded up)}$$

$$0.9 \text{ kcal/64 kg/hr} = 57.6 \text{ kcal/hr}$$

The result is the number of kilocalories a woman who weighs 64 kg burns in 1 hour. Multiply this figure by 24 hours to estimate the kilocalories this person metabolizes in an entire day.

$$57.6 \text{ kcal/hr} \times 24 \text{ hr} = \text{approximately } 1382 \text{ kcal/day}$$

The **Harris−Benedict equation** is a scientific formula for estimating the basal metabolic rate. This equation uses age, height, and weight to calculate approximate daily basal metabolic caloric needs for adults. The formula requires information about the person's weight in kg (pounds divided by 2.2), height in centimeters (inches times 2.54), and age in years.

Harris-Benedict equation formula commonly used to estimate basal metabolic rate

Equation for men: $66.47 + (13.75 \times \text{weight}) + (5 \times \text{height}) - (6.76 \times \text{age})$

Equation for women: $655.1 + (9.56 \times \text{weight}) + (1.85 \times \text{height}) - (4.68 \times \text{age})$

For example, to estimate the daily basal metabolic rate of a 25−year−old man whose weight is 165 pounds and height is 5−feet, 10−inches (70 in.), first determine his weight in kg (75 kg) and height in cm (about 178 cm). Then use these values and his age to fill in the blanks of the formula for men:

$66.47 + (13.75 \times 75) + (5 \times 178) - (6.76 \times 25) = \text{approximately } 1819 \text{ kcal/day}$

The **Mifflin−St. Jeor equation** can predict basal calorie needs of people who have excess body fat. This equation also uses weight in kg, height in cm (inches times 2.54), and age in years.

Mifflin-St. Jeor equation method of predicting basal calorie needs of individuals who have excess body fat

Males: $(10 \times \text{weight}) + (6.25 \times \text{height}) - (5 \times \text{age}) + 5$

Females: $(10 \times \text{weight}) + (6.25 \times \text{height}) - (5 \times \text{age}) - 161$

These three different methods of calculating the BMR only provide an esti−mate of a person's daily basal metabolic needs. To estimate a person's *total* energy requirement for a 24−hour period, the other components of total energy expenditure, such as kilocalories used for exercise and other physical activities, need to be added to the BMR value.

Physical Activity

Physical activity resulting from voluntary skeletal muscle movement increases energy expenditure above basal energy needs. *Voluntary* muscles are muscles that are under conscious control; for example, the neuromuscular control of the fingers that is needed to text a message. Energy expended during physical activity is the component of total energy expenditure that varies the most among individuals. The number of kilocalories a particular physical activity burns depends largely on the type of activity, how long it is performed (duration), the degree of effort (intensity) used while performing the activity, and the weight of the person. A heavy person expends more kilocalories when performing the same activity for the same duration and at the same intensity than a lighter person. The reason for this difference is that the muscles of the heavier person must work harder to move the larger body.

Table 13.7 lists various physical activities and the approximate number of kilocalories an individual who weighs 150 pounds expends while performing each activity for a minute. For example, a 150—pound person who walks for 30 minutes (3.5 mph) burns approximately 153 kcal during the walk (30×5.1). To estimate energy needs for a physical activity or to estimate how much is expended on a typical day, visit https://www.supertracker.usda.gov/default.aspx and click on "Physical Activity Tracker."

Thermic Effect of Food

The body needs a relatively small amount of energy to digest foods and bev—erages, as well as to absorb and further process the macronutrients. The energy used for these tasks, generally 5 to 10% of total caloric intake, is referred to as the **thermic effect of food (TEF)**. For a person whose energy intake is 3000 kcal/day, TEF would account for 150 to 300 kcal of that amount of energy.

Nonexercise Activity Thermogenesis

Nonexercise activity thermogenesis (*thermo* = heat; *genesis* = production) or **NEAT** refers to *involuntary* skeletal muscle activity, that is, physical activity that a person does not consciously control. NEAT activities include shivering, fidgeting, maintaining muscle tone, and maintaining body posture when not lying down. Studies have shown that people vary in the amount of energy they use

thermic effect of food (TEF) energy used to digest foods and beverages as well as absorb and further process the macronutrients

nonexercise activity thermogenesis (NEAT) energy expended during involuntary skeletal muscular activities such as fidgeting

TABLE 13.7 Approximate Energy Expenditures of Selected Physical Activities (150-Pound Person)

Physical Activity	Approximate kcal/min
Sitting and playing cards	1.9
Bowling	4.1
Walking (3.5 mph)	5.1
Bicycling (10 mph)	6.4
Canoeing (4 mph)	6.7
Dancing (active)	6.8
Hiking (with pack, 3 mph)	6.8
Walking (4.5 mph)	7.1
Tennis (singles, recreational)	7.5
Weight training	7.8
Touch football (vigorous)	8.3
Aerobic dancing	9.0
Swimming (vigorous breaststroke)	9.6
Running/jogging, steady pace (5.5 mph)	10.0
Bicycling (15 mph)	10.9
Karate	12.8

Source: Williams MH: *Nutrition for health, fitness, and sport.* 10th ed. New York: McGraw-Hill Publishing Company, 2012.

TABLE 13.8 Physical Activity (PA) Level Estimates

Activity Level	PA (Males)	PA (Females)
Sedentary (no exercise)	1.00	1.00
Low activity (e.g., walking the equivalent of 2 miles/day at 3-4 mph)	1.11	1.12
Active (e.g., walking 7 miles/day at 3-4 mph or jogging for 40-45 minutes/day)	1.25	1.27
Very active (e.g., walking 17 miles/day at 3-4 mph or jogging for 1.5 hours/day)	1.48	1.45

Adapted from: Food and Nutrition Board, National Institute of Medicine: *Dietary reference intakes for energy, carbohydrate, fiber, fat, fatty acids, cholesterol, protein, and amino acids (macronutrients)*. Washington, DC: National Academies Press, 2005.

for NEAT, but the expenditure may be more than 800 kcal daily.[33] It is possible that some individuals resist weight gain from overeating because they have higher−than−average energy expenditures for NEAT. Nevertheless, the contribution of NEAT to overall calorie needs is fairly small for most people.

Estimating Total Energy Expenditure

To estimate an individual's daily TEE, it is necessary to add the kilocalories used for basal metabolism, physical activity, TEF, and NEAT in a single day. Alternatively, an easier method is to use one of the formulas published by the Food and Nutrition Board of the Institute of Medicine.[25] The following formulas are for men and women who are 19 years of age or older. The variables are age in years, weight in kilograms (pounds divided by 2.2), height in *meters* (inches divided by 39.4), and the physical activity estimate (PA) (Table 13.8).

Males: $662 - (9.53 \times \text{age}) + (\text{PA} \times [\{15.91 \times \text{weight}\} + \{539.6 \times \text{height}\}])$

Females: $354 - (6.91 \times \text{age}) + (\text{PA} \times [\{9.36 \times \text{weight}\} + \{726 \times \text{height}\}])$

For a 150-pound person, performing karate for 30 minutes burns approximately 384 kcal.

ASSESS YOUR PROGRESS

10 List the four components of total energy expenditure (TEE).

11 Calculate your basal metabolic rate using one of the equations presented in this section.

12 Discuss at least five factors that influence basal metabolic rate.

13.5 Measuring Energy Expenditure

LEARNING OUTCOMES

1 *Discuss direct and indirect measures of energy expenditure.*

In section 13.4, we presented mathematical formulas that can be used to estimate total energy expenditure. In this section, we discuss direct and indirect methods of estimating energy expenditure. When compared to direct methods of measurement, indirect methods may provide different results. Direct methods, however, are complex and require sophisticated laboratory tools, whereas indirect methods are relatively inexpensive, involve minimal equipment, and can be completed outside the laboratory.

calorimetry measurement of heat energy

direct calorimetry measure of the amount of heat produced by someone inside a specialized chamber

indirect calorimetry determination of the amount of heat someone produces by measuring the amount of oxygen consumed and the amount of carbon dioxide produced

Calorimetry

Calorimetry is a measurement of heat energy. The amount of heat, or energy, the body expends can be measured via direct and indirect methods. Scientists use this information to estimate basal, resting, and total energy expenditures.

Direct Calorimetry

Direct calorimetry measures the body's heat of metabolism. This method requires use of a calorimetric ("metabolic") chamber, a special airtight laboratory room that is surrounded by water (Fig. 13.14). When someone is in the chamber, his or her body's metabolic activity releases heat that warms the air and water surrounding the chamber. Researchers can then use the change in temperature to calculate the energy expended by the person's body. To accurately measure basal metabolic rate, direct calorimetry would require someone to be inside the chamber for 24 hours. Thus, direct calorimetry is impractical and expensive, so the method is rarely used.

Indirect Calorimetry

Instead of measuring body heat, **indirect calorimetry** measures a person's oxygen consumption and carbon dioxide production. The use and production of these gases are directly related to energy metabolism and can be used to calculate an individual's caloric expenditure. For every 1 L of oxygen cells consume, the body expends 4.82 kcal of energy. Indirect calorimetry requires a subject to breathe through a mouthpiece or mask that is connected to special equipment that records the volume of oxygen consumed and carbon dioxide produced (see Fig. 13.13). Some versions of the equipment are portable and allow for assessment to take place in the laboratory, at a patient's bedside, and even when a person is exercising outdoors.

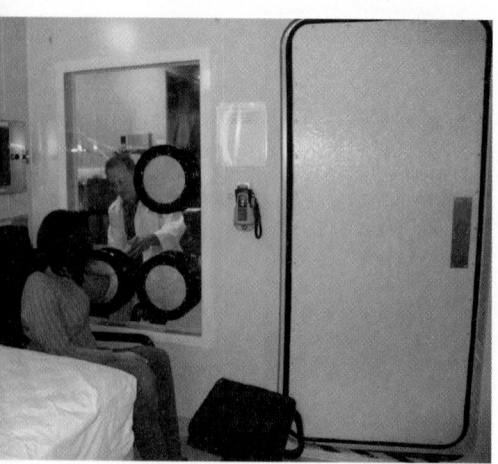

FIGURE 13.14 Calorimetric chamber for direct calorimetry. This direct calorimetry chamber is located at the University of North Carolina-Chapel Hill.

Other Methods of Estimating TEE

Other methods of predicting TEE involve techniques, such as heart rate monitors and accelerometers, that do not involve measuring the amount of heat generated by the body or gas exchange. These methods can often be used with free–living subjects and without the need for expensive equipment.

Heart rate monitors are useful in estimating energy expenditure during exercise of low to moderate intensity (Fig. 13.15). A linear relationship exists between oxygen consumption and heart rate; that is, as heart rate increases, so does energy expenditure. Assessing heart rate during exercise reflects the amount of oxygen consumed and, therefore, the number of calories burned. Compared to the other methods of assessing TEE that are discussed in this section, heart rate monitoring is less complicated. Furthermore, the monitors allow for assessment outside of a laboratory setting. Their major drawback, however, is decreased accuracy.

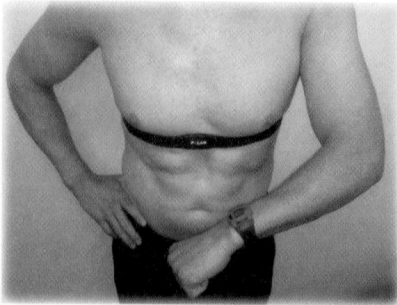

FIGURE 13.15 Heart rate monitor. Heart rate monitors are helpful in estimating energy expenditure.

DID **YOU** KNOW?

The *doubly labeled water* method of estimating TEE involves having the subject drink water that contains two stable isotopes (^2H of hydrogen and ^{18}O of oxygen). These isotopes are heavier than the more common isotopes of elemental hydrogen and oxygen, and they can be measured in urine. The difference in the excretion rates of the two isotopes can be used to calculate the subject's energy expenditure. A major advantage of the doubly labeled water method of measuring TEE is that it is an objective measurement. However, the isotopes are expensive, and measuring their excretion in urine requires sophisticated equipment and expertise.

Accelerometry is the measurement of acceleration, which is a change in speed or direction. An accelerometer is a small device that is worn to record all acceleration made by the body over specific periods of time (Fig. 13.16). During exercise, the body frequently changes direction and speed, both of which can be recorded by the accelerometer. The acceleration record can later be downloaded to calculate calories expended. Use of accelerometer devices is a convenient, objective, and easy method of estimating energy expenditure in free–living environments.

Accelerometry is an accurate method of estimating energy expenditure due to physical activity. However, how the device is used can influence results. For example, wearing the accelerometer at the wrist versus at the waist will lead to different results. Also, the equations used to convert acceleration into energy expenditure will influence the accuracy of the measurement.

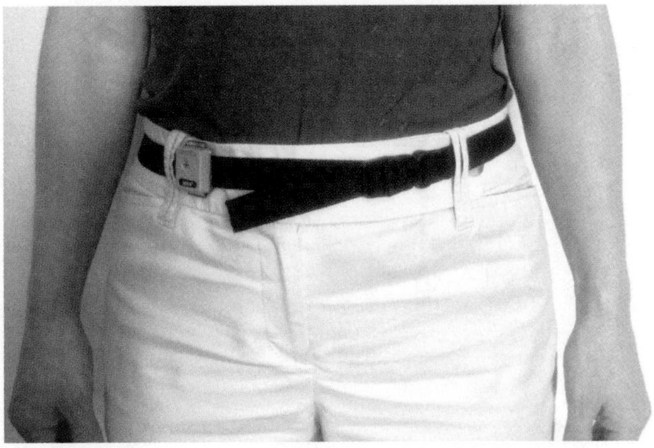

FIGURE 13.16 Accelerometer. This small device can be worn on a belt.

accelerometry method of measuring calorie expenditure during physical activity based on changes in speed and direction

Physical Activity Questionnaires

The information obtained in questionnaires can be used to estimate a person's energy use during physical activity. These questionnaires often require an individual to recall normal activity patterns during a specific period of time and record his or her typical activities, including details about each activity's duration, speed, intensity, and distance. When this information is used along with body weight, a person can estimate the number of calories expended during daily activities. Using the "Physical Activity Tracker" at https://www.supertracker.usda.gov/default.aspx is an easy method to monitor the number of kilocalories expended in physical activity.

ASSESS YOUR PROGRESS

13 *Explain differences between direct and indirect calorimetry.*

14 *Describe how heart rate monitors and accelerometers are used to estimate energy expenditure.*

13.6 The Body's Energy States

LEARNING OUTCOMES

1 *Explain the role of energy balance in weight management.*

2 *Describe factors that create the physiological states of energy balance.*

3 *Use a formula to predict weight changes over time.*

Understanding energy balance is critical to being able to explain why people gain, lose, or maintain weight. The body is in a state of *energy equilibrium* and "balanced" when calorie intake from food and beverages equals calorie output (Fig. 13.17a). Maintenance of **energy balance**—matching calorie intake to calorie output over the long term—is critical for achieving and controlling a healthy body weight.

If the calorie intake from macronutrients (and alcohol) is greater than calorie output, this situation creates a **positive energy balance** (Fig. 13.17b). In this state, the body stores excess dietary fat in adipose cells. Additionally, the body converts surplus dietary carbohydrate, protein, and alcohol to triglycerides to store in adipose cells. Weight gain results from long–term positive energy status.

energy balance matching calorie intake to calorie output over the long term

positive energy balance calorie intake is greater than calorie output

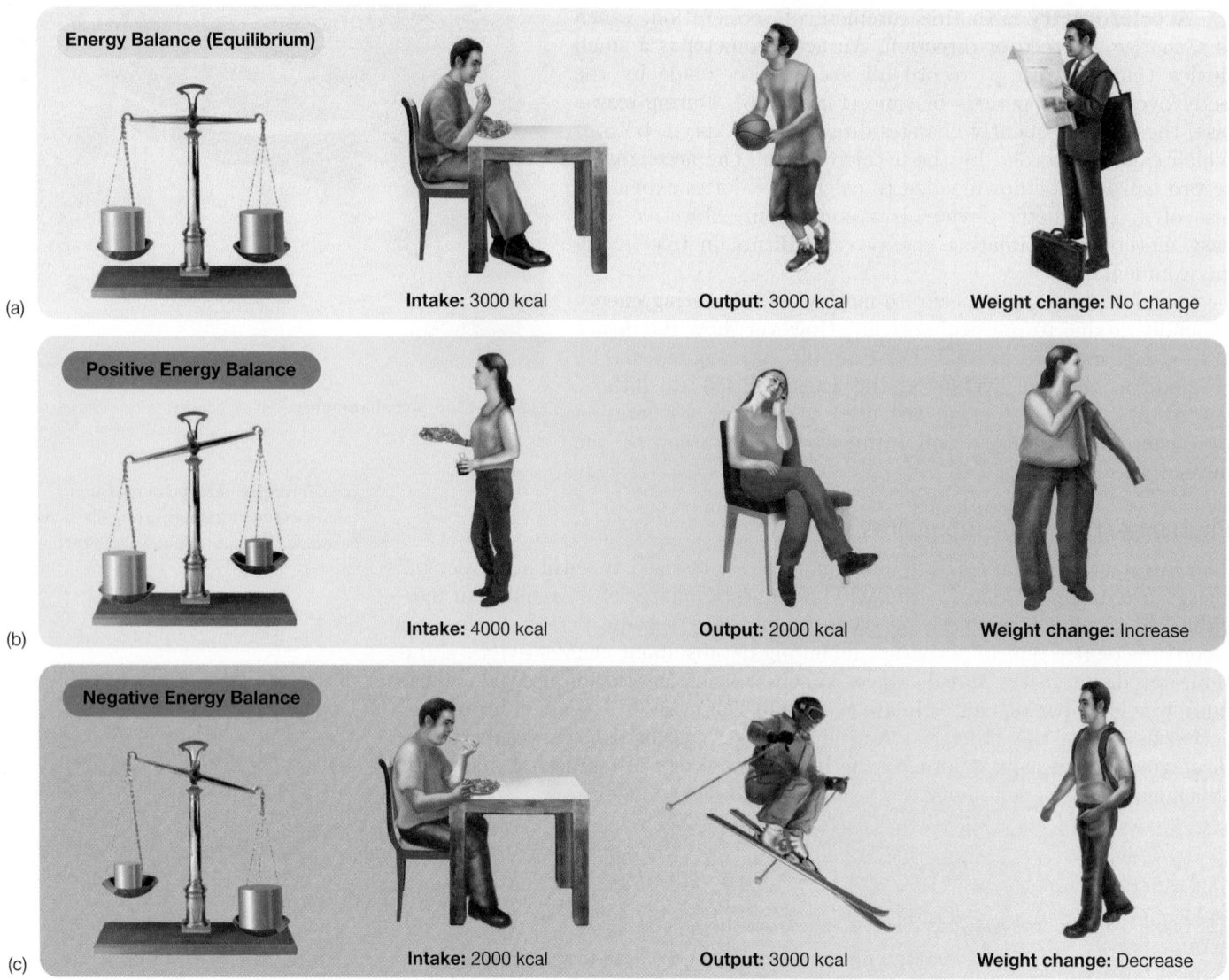

FIGURE 13.17 States of energy balance.

Positive energy balance is necessary for pregnant women, because extra calories are needed to add new tissues that support the pregnancy (anabolism). Positive energy balance also occurs during periods of growth, such as during fetal development, infancy, childhood, and adolescence. However, gaining excessive and unhealthy amounts of body fat is the result of long−term positive energy balance.

If calorie intake is lower than calorie output, **negative energy balance** occurs. In this state, the body needs more calories to carry out its activities than the diet supplies. Therefore, the body metabolizes stored fat, ketone bodies, and some amino acids for energy (see Chapter 8). As indicated in Figure 13.17c, weight loss results when a person is in a negative energy state for an extended period. The following section describes factors that influence energy balance.

negative energy balance calorie intake is less than calorie output

Predicting Weight Change over Time

One pound of body fat contains about 3500 kcal. In the past, this fact was used to estimate how changes in caloric intakes and expenditures could predict weight changes. According to the 3500 kcal rule−of−thumb, a person should lose or gain approximately one pound of fat in a year for every 10 kcal/day reduction or increase in his or her caloric intake (10 kcal/day × 365 days = 3650 kcal). For example, to lose 25 pounds in a year, you should consume 250 fewer kcal/day than your body needs.

Scientists, however, have challenged the reliability of using the 3500–kcal rule for predicting weight change over the long term. According to their new formula, cutting your caloric intake by 250 kcal/day would enable you to lose only about 12.5 pounds in one year.[34] Furthermore, it would take over 3 years of following the calorie–reduced diet for you to lose about 25 pounds. At that point, your body reaches a *weight plateau* (state of energy equilibrium), and no further weight would be lost. This new formula helps explain why people who reduce their usual calorie intakes do not lose as much weight as they expect over time and eventually their weight plateaus. To estimate your daily caloric intake to achieve weight change by using this formula, visit http://bwsimulator .niddk.nih.gov.

ASSESS YOUR PROGRESS

15 What happens to body weight when calorie intake is greater than calorie output?

16 What happens to the body weight when calorie intake is less than calorie output?

17 Use the new weight change formula to predict how much weight you would lose in a year if you reduced your usual caloric intake by 20 kcal/day and made no other changes to your lifestyle.

13.7 Factors That Influence Body Weight

LEARNING OUTCOMES

1 Explain how various physiological factors can influence body weight.

2 Describe the influence of food composition, hormones, and environment on eating behavior.

3 Identify how physical activity and other factors influence body weight.

Many factors can influence a person's body weight. Some of these factors are physiological and not under one's control, while others are related to lifestyle choices and the person's environment. Although people cannot easily change their physiology, they can modify their lifestyles and environments. This section dis–cusses major factors that influence body weight.

Genetic Factors

Genetic factors play an important role in the development of obesity. Most physical characteristics are inherited, including metabolic rate, hormone produc–tion, body frame size, and pattern of fat distribution. All of these characteristics affect body weight.

The results of scientific studies support the hypothesis that obesity is pri–marily an inherited trait. Children are more likely to become overweight or obese if their mothers were overfat prior to becoming pregnant.[35] Infants of overweight mothers tend to have more body fat than infants of lean mothers.[36] Nevertheless, genes do not control everything about a person's health, including his or her weight. Environmental and other factors can modify the expression of genes. For example, children whose mothers are obese may have inherited genes that increase the risk for obesity. However, these children may avoid becoming obese if they adopt a physically active lifestyle and do not overeat.

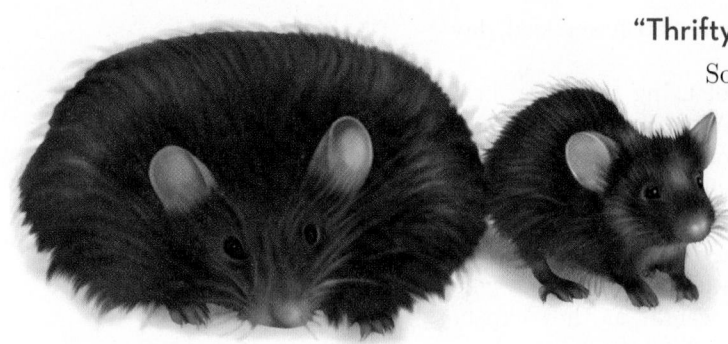

The genetically engineered mouse on the left became obese because it lacked genes to make a hormone that inhibits fat storage.

DID **YOU** KNOW?

Prader-Willi syndrome is a rare condition that results from a particular gene's lack of activity. People with this incurable condition have skeletal deformities, delayed motor development, decreased intellectual functioning, food cravings, and insatiable appetites. If their access to food is not restricted, people with Prader-Willi syndrome eat constantly and become obese.

set-point theory scientific notion that the body's fat content and body weight is genetically predetermined

weight cycling repeated bouts of losing and gaining significant amounts of weight

hunger uncomfortable physiological sensation that drives a person to consume food

appetite desire to eat appealing food

satiety sense that enough food or beverages have been consumed to satisfy hunger

"Thrifty" Genes and Set Points

Some rats and mice are genetically predisposed to become obese because they have inherited a "thrifty gene" for a conservative metabolism. Rodents with the thrifty gene are more efficient at storing excess energy as fat than rodents who do not have the same genetic predisposition. It is possible that humans who gain weight easily have genes that code for thrifty metabolisms as well. Throughout history, there have been times when certain populations did not have access to adequate amounts of food or the availability of food was unpredictable. People had to eat as much as they could when food was plentiful. When there was enough food to eat, individuals with "thrifty metabolisms" stored more excess food energy as body fat than persons who did not have such efficient metabolisms. The people who lacked thrifty metabolisms expended the excess food energy as body heat. Thus, people with thrifty metabolisms may have been more likely to survive periods of starvation than people who did not have the thrifty genetic makeup.

In many modern societies, high-calorie food is available 24 hours a day and starvation is unlikely. As a result, having a thrifty metabolism is no longer beneficial because depositing excess body fat often results in serious health problems.

The majority of people who intentionally lose weight regain the weight over time. According to the **set-point theory**, the body's fat content (and therefore, body weight) is genetically predetermined. The set point acts like a home thermostat, except that it regulates body weight instead of temperature. For example, a person infected with an intestinal virus tends to lose a little weight because he or she has no interest in eating for several days. During and after recovery, the person generally regains the lost weight. This observation provides support for the set-point theory.

Biochemical and metabolic studies also support the set-point theory. When calorie intake is reduced, blood levels of thyroid hormone decline, depressing the normal basal metabolic rate. Additionally, the caloric cost of performing weight-bearing activities decreases when a person loses weight. As a result, an activity that required 100 kcal before weight loss may burn only 80 kcal after weight loss. Furthermore, weight loss seems to make the body become more efficient at storing calories from macronutrients as fat.

When a person gains weight and stays at that weight for a while, his or her body tends to establish a new and higher set point. According to the theory, all these changes protect the body from losing weight and explain why weight loss is so difficult to achieve and perhaps even harder to maintain. Furthermore, the set point theory may help explain **weight cycling** or "yo-yo dieting." Weight cycling occurs when someone loses a lot of weight but then regains the weight and then repeats the cycle again. A genetic set-point could be limiting this person's ability to maintain the weight loss.

Opponents of the set-point theory argue that weight does not remain constant throughout adulthood. Most adults gain weight slowly, at least until they reach old age. Thus, body weight may result more from lifestyle practices and environmental influences than predetermined biological controls such as a set point.

Physiological Factors: Regulation of Eating Behavior

From a physiological standpoint, eating behavior is complex and largely involves interactions among the nervous, endocrine, and digestive systems as well as fat tissue. *Hunger* and *satiety* are key sensations that regulate eating behavior. **Hunger** is an uncomfortable physiological sensation that drives a person to consume food. Hunger differs from **appetite**, which is the desire to eat appealing food. **Satiety** is the sense that enough food or beverages have been consumed to satisfy hunger.

Physical Sensations

The stomach helps regulate eating behavior by:

- ***Producing certain physical sensations.*** As the time between meals increases, the stomach signals "it's time to eat" by contracting, causing hunger pangs. As the contractions become stronger, the person feels compelled to eat or drink something to relieve the discomfort.

- ***Expanding.*** During meals, the stomach stretches as it fills. The sensation that the stomach has reached its capacity can make a person stop eating. Nevertheless, many overfat persons do not recognize the sensation of stomach fullness, and as a result, they may continue to eat even when their stomachs are full.

Food Composition Factors

During the past few decades, easy access to high–calorie foods and the reduction in energy–expending activities have led to an **obesogenic environment** (an environment that promotes excessive weight gain) in the United States. Dietary factors, particularly amounts of fat and certain carbohydrates in the diet, can influence body fat production and appetite. Fatty foods are more energy dense than foods that contain mostly carbohydrate, protein, and water.[37] Thus, high–fat diets are associated with excess calorie intakes and rising obesity rates.[38] Eating a diet based on foods with low calorie density can aid in weight maintenance, weight loss, and even maintenance of weight loss.[39–41]

Starting a meal with a low–calorie–dense soup, salad, or piece of fruit increases satiety and contributes to eating fewer calories.[39] Also, high–protein meals and snacks can delay hunger and lead to less snacking.[42,43] When low–calorie–density foods replace other foods in the diet, weight loss can occur. Calorie density of favorite recipes can be lowered by adding vegetables or fruit, which are heavy due to their water content but still low in calories. Refer to Chapter 1 for a discussion of energy density.

obesogenic environment external conditions that promote excessive weight gain

Hormonal Influences

An area of the **hypothalamus**, a structure in the brain, controls hunger and satiety (Fig. 13.18). Scientists think this region functions as a "hunger/satiety center." The stomach, small intestine, pancreas, and fat tissue produce hormones and proteins that stimulate nerve cells involved in the regulation of hunger and satiety. These hormones and proteins act as chemical messengers, signaling the brain when to eat or when to stop eating. Dozens of hormones affect hunger and satiety, including the ones discussed in the following sections.

Ghrelin **Ghrelin** (*grel′—in*), a hormone secreted mainly by the stomach, stimulates eating behavior and promotes energy storage. Some scientists think that reducing ghrelin production or activity is the key to helping people lose or maintain weight. A person with Prader–Willi syndrome (see the "Did You Know?" feature on page 436) has ghrelin levels that are three to four times greater than normal, which explains why people with this syndrome have an appetite that is difficult to control.[44]

Hormones of the Intestines The small and large intestines release **peptide YY**, a protein hormone that signals the stomach to reduce ghrelin secretion. The small intestine also releases cholecystokinin (CCK), a hormone that stimulates the gallbladder to contract and the pancreas to release digestive enzymes (see Chapter 4). Additionally, CCK stimulates the brain and other nervous tissue, suppressing appetite as a result.

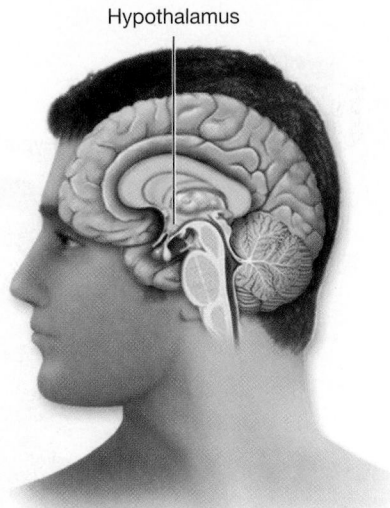

Hypothalamus

FIGURE 13.18 Hypothalamus.

hypothalamus structure in the brain that controls hunger and satiety

ghrelin hormone secreted by the stomach and other tissues that stimulates eating

peptide YY protein hormone that signals the stomach to reduce ghrelin secretion

amylin hormone secreted by the pancreas that slows gastric emptying and reduces hunger

leptin hormone secreted by the adipose tissue to signal the brain when enough energy has been stored

adiponectin hormone produced by adipose tissue that increases muscle cells' uptake of fatty acids from the bloodstream and metabolism of the fatty acids for energy

Pancreatic Hormones The pancreas secretes insulin, glucagon, and amylin, which are hormones that regulate blood glucose and influence appetite.[45] Chapter 5 describes the actions of insulin and glucagon in regulating blood glucose. **Amylin** is a hormone that is secreted by the beta cells of the pancreas at the same time as insulin. Amylin slows the digestion process by delaying gastric emptying and signaling the hypothalamus to reduce hunger.[45]

Fat Tissue Hormones In addition to storing excess energy and providing shape for the body, fat tissue helps regulate hunger and satiety. As mentioned in sec—tion 13.3, fat cells secrete a group of hormones called adipokines. **Leptin** is an adipokine that reduces hunger and inhibits fat storage in the body. A person's blood leptin level is directly proportional to his or her amount of body fat.[19] The brain obtains information about the status of body fat stores by monitoring the level of leptin in blood. When researchers administer leptin to genetically modified mice that cannot synthesize the hormone, the rodents lose weight, because the hormone reduces the animals' interest in eating and increases their rate of fat metabolism.[46] Studies involving humans, however, generally find that obese people produce high amounts of leptin, but their bodies resist the hor—mone's hunger—suppressing action, and they consume more calories as a result.[47] Figure 13.19 illustrates the complex effects of ghrelin, peptide YY, CCK, amylin, and leptin on hunger and satiety.

Adiponectin is an adipokine that increases muscle cells' uptake of fatty acids from the bloodstream and metabolism of the fatty acids for energy. High

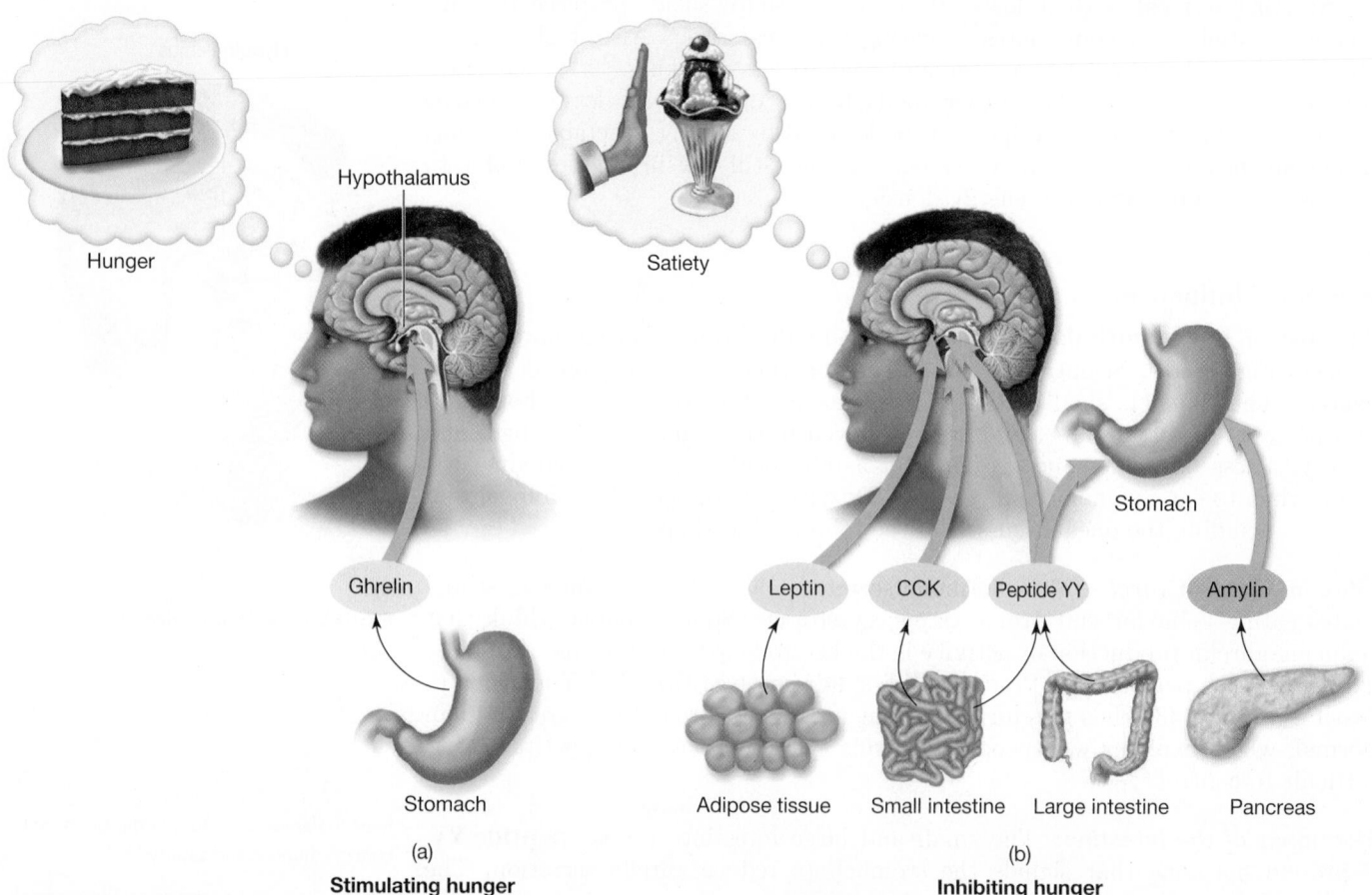

FIGURE 13.19 Hormones that influence hunger. Appetite regulation involves complex factors, including the secretion of proteins by the digestive tract and fat tissue that stimulate or inhibit a region of the hypothalamus. *(a)* Ghrelin stimulates hunger sensations. *(b)* Peptide YY, CCK, amylin, and leptin inhibit hunger sensations.

blood levels of adiponectin are associated with a lower risk of obesity and type 2 diabetes.[48] The hormone also inhibits the body's responses to inflammation, which may reduce the risk of cardiovascular disease. When fat cells accumulate too much triglyceride (fat), they lose their normal sensitivity to insulin, allow blood triglyceride levels to increase, and decrease their production of adiponectin.[48]

Other Influences

Other factors, including a person's environment, physical activity level, and psychological state, can modify the expression of genes that regulate body weight. Environmental influences play a major role in the development of obesity. Consider a family's eating behaviors during a typical holiday dinner that includes a variety of attractive, tasty foods. After eating the large meal, everyone's hunger should be satisfied, but as soon as pie or cake is placed on the table, family members "find room" in their stomach for dessert. When someone eats when he or she is not hungry, the environment is likely influencing the person's appetite. The senses of sight, smell, taste, and hearing contribute to one's appetite, even when the person is not hungry.

Food advertising is an aspect of the environment that has a powerful influence on people's food choices. Food ads typically appeal to consumers' senses, emphasizing the appearance and taste of food. In many instances, such ads do not mention the hefty caloric contents of the products. Recently, a television ad for a fast-food chain promoted a hamburger that had three beef patties, three slices of cheese, and six bacon slices topped with mayonnaise. According to information at the fast-food company's website, this burger provided 800 kcal. The site, however, did not explain that 800 kcal is more than one-third of a day's calorie needs for an average person!

Calorie Intake Overall, Americans consume significantly more food energy than they consumed in the early 1970s. Between 1971 and 1975, average intake for Americans who were 20 to 74 years of age was 1955 kcal/day, and by 2003–2004, this rose to 2269 kcal/day. After three decades of increasing calorie intake, however, recent reports indicate that the average calorie intake for adult Americans has *decreased* significantly (Fig. 13.20).[49] In 2009–2010, the average energy intake for American adults dropped to 2195 kcal/day.[49] The reasons for this decline are unclear. Perhaps consumers' greater awareness of the many serious health problems that are related to obesity is influencing the population's energy consumption.

Physical Inactivity The environment not only affects how much people eat, but also whether they choose to be sedentary (inactive) or physically active. At home, Americans rely on a variety of "energy-saving" devices such as dishwashing

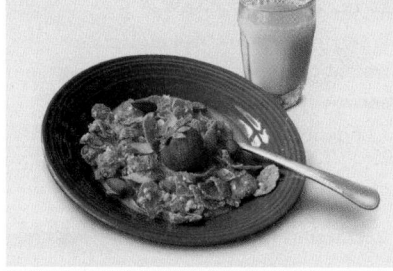

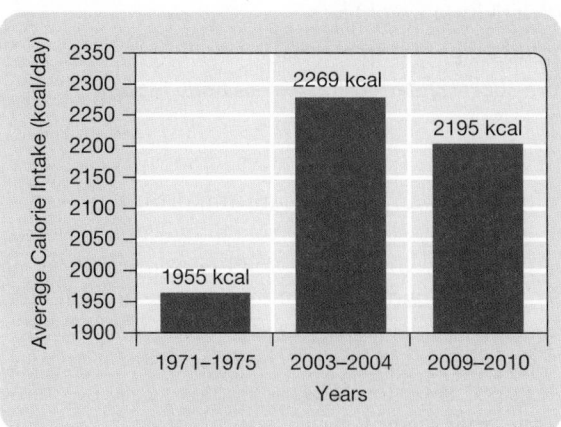

FIGURE 13.20 How much Americans eat, past and present. This graph shows average calorie intakes for Americans who were between 20 and 74 years of age during specific periods (1971–1975 to 2009–2010).

Source of data: Ford ES, Dietz WH: Trends in energy intake among adults in the United States: Findings from NHANES. *American Journal of Clinical Nutrition* 97(4):848, 2013.

Have you heard of the "freshman 15"? This is the idea that college students gain 15 pounds between high school graduation and the end of their freshman year. Recent research suggests that more than 70% of freshmen gain weight, usually in the first semester of college. However, they do not gain as much as 15 pounds; the average weight gain for a college freshman is 7.7 pounds.[53]

machines, TV remote controls, and garage door openers to work for them. Outside the home, people use cars, elevators, escalators, and other motorized devices, instead of their feet, to move them from place to place. With the help of machines, Americans' lives are considerably easier; however, the population consumes more calories than in the past while moving less.

By becoming more physically active, people can increase their energy output. Many Americans, however, have desk jobs that require little muscular movement. When people have leisure time, it is often spent performing tasks that involve sitting: watching television, texting friends, playing computer games, or chatting with people on the Internet. In a national survey conducted in 2010, approximately 25% of American adults reported that they did not engage in physical activity when they had leisure time during the month before the survey.[51]

According to experts with the American College of Sports Medicine, adults should perform 150 to 250 minutes per week of moderate−intensity physical activity to prevent weight gain.[52] An example of the minimal level of activity is 30 minutes of brisk walking on 5 days of the week. Overfat adults, however, may need to engage in more than 250 minutes of moderate−intensity activity per week to achieve clinically significant weight loss and to maintain the new lower body weight.[52] MyPlate.gov has information about physical activity, including tips for becoming more active (http://www.choosemyplate.gov/physical−activity).

Psychological Factors A person's mood and self−esteem, can also influence his or her eating behaviors. Many people eat not because they are hungry but because they are bored, anxious, angry, or depressed. Researchers, however, cannot easily determine whether being obese causes depression or being depressed contributes to obesity.

ASSESS YOUR PROGRESS

18 *What is the set-point theory?*
19 *Distinguish between hunger and appetite.*
20 *Identify at least three hormones that influence eating behaviors, and describe each hormone's particular effects.*
21 *Describe how the environment can influence a person's food intake and physical activity.*

13.8 Voluntary Weight Loss

LEARNING OUTCOMES

1 *Explain the importance of physical activity in weight loss.*
2 *Describe features of safe and reliable weight loss methods.*
3 *Identify practices of people who are successful at losing excess body fat and maintaining the reduced weight.*

Before embarking on an effort to lose (or gain) weight, an important first step is determining whether it is even necessary. The need to change one's weight should be based on overall health and family history of weight−related diseases. To determine goals for weight loss or weight gain, the following questions should be considered: *What is the person's BMI? Does the person's weight influence his or her physical health? If his or her BMI is within the healthy range, why is a change in weight necessary?* If a patient's BMI is above 24.9 or below 18.5, setting a reasonable and realistic goal weight is a useful next step.

It is important to note that an overfat person does not have to shed a lot of weight to reduce risk factors associated with CVD, stroke, and type 2 diabetes. Losing as little as 5 to 10% of excess body fat can increase beneficial high–density lipoprotein levels (HDL cholesterol), reduce elevated blood pressure and triglyceride levels, and improve glucose tolerance.[13]

The Importance of Physical Activity

Achieving a state of negative energy balance is the most important factor in weight loss and is usually the first recommendation for obesity treatment. It is difficult to burn much energy without being physically active. By being more physically active, people who are trying to lose weight do not need to limit their food intake as much as they would by relying on calorie reduction alone.

A person does not need to jog for 10 miles to reap the benefits of engaging in regular physical activity. Moderate–intensity activities are recommended for people who want to lose weight. Physical activity is also crucial in helping individuals maintain a healthy body weight and prevent weight gain. Chapter 15 discusses the healthful benefits of a physically active lifestyle.

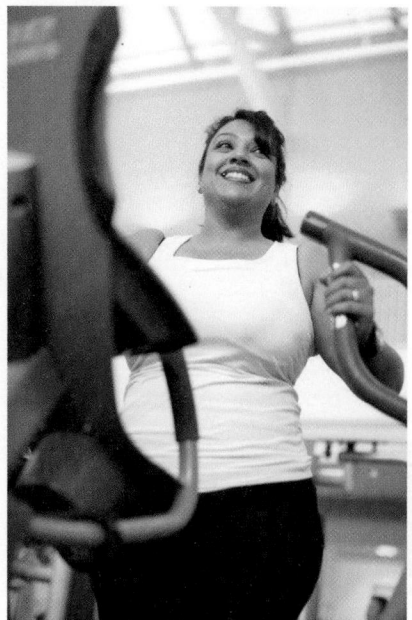

Behavioral Change

Controlling calorie intake and increasing physical activity are easier to accomplish when overfat persons analyze their unhealthy behaviors and identify their eating *cues* (signals) and "problem" behaviors. Once the cues and behaviors are identified, these individuals can develop ways to control the cues and change their responses.

Unhealthy eating cues are usually environmental factors that stimulate inappropriate eating behavior, such as smelling baked goods when walking past a bakery and then entering the store to buy a dozen brownies. Identifying such cues can enable people to recognize effects of the signals and avoid inappropriate ones, whenever possible. By analyzing their food–related behaviors, overfat individuals can often determine the circumstances in which they tend to overeat and learn strategies to help them resist the cues.

Although the process may seem slow, people are more likely to change ingrained food–related habits by focusing on changing one behavior at a time. For example, many people snack on energy–dense foods and drinks while watching television. To change this habit, a person could decide to eat only at the kitchen table and avoid all food and beverage consumption while sitting in front of a TV.

For individuals who want to lose (or gain) weight, keeping records (journals or diaries) of food intake and physical activities can be helpful for estimating daily calorie input and output. However, overfat persons often underestimate their calorie intake and overestimate their energy output.[54] Therefore, people need to record information about food choices and physical activity habits accurately. Many tools are available, including computer programs, mobile apps, and websites, for tracking caloric intake and expenditures during exercise.

Characteristics of Recommended Weight-Loss Methods

People often use a variety of methods to lose excess body fat. Some of these methods are safer than others and more likely to result in weight loss that is maintained over long periods.

The following is a list of characteristics of safe and effective weight–loss methods:

- Uses portion control at meals and snacks to help reduce calorie intake;

- Incorporates 3 to 4 servings of low–fat dairy foods;

- Emphasizes a variety of fresh fruits and vegetables;

- Spreads total calorie intake through the day by eating 4 to 5 meals or snacks, including breakfast;

- Involves a routine of self—monitoring, such as keeping a food diary or journal; and

- Suggests ways to reduce intake of energy—dense foods and monitor portion sizes when eating meals away from home.[55,56]

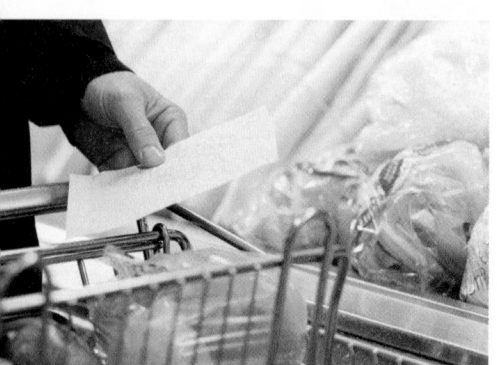

FRESH TIPS

The following tips can help you manage your weight:

Planning menus and grocery shopping

1. Plan meals and snacks to cover 3 or more days, then use the plan to prepare grocery lists.

2. Avoid labeling certain foods as "off limits." Depriving oneself of such items can result in bingeing on the "forbidden" food. Individuals can learn to analyze why they have difficulty controlling their intake of these foods and develop strategies to learn how to reduce their intake of them.

3. To reduce the likelihood of making impulsive food choices, shop from a grocery list and *after* eating.

4. Read food labels to compare calorie contents per serving.

Food preparation

1. Reduce the use of solid fat and added sugars in cooking; bake, broil, or roast meats instead of frying them.

2. Trim solid fat away from meat before cooking.

Eating behavior

1. Keep nutrient-dense, low-calorie snack foods, such as fresh fruits and vegetables, on hand.

2. Eat meals and snacks at scheduled times; do not skip meals, especially breakfast.

3. Never eat directly from a package containing several servings; instead remove a healthy portion of food from the container and serve it on a plate.[57]

4. Eat all food in a "dining" area, and avoid eating while engaged in other activities, such as reading a book or watching television.

5. Slow down the pace of meals by putting eating utensils down between mouthfuls and eating more slowly.

6. Beforehand, think about what you will eat and drink while attending the event. Practice polite ways to decline food.

7. Consider limiting food intake before the special occasion to avoid consuming too many calories for the day.

8. Eat a low-calorie snack about an hour before the occasion to help yourself feel full when tempting foods are available.

Restaurants

1. Avoid energy-dense food and monitor portion sizes.

2. Request salad dressing "on the side" to control the amount consumed.

3. Order an entrée and share it with another person. If choosing a dessert item, share it with another person.

4. When at fast-food outlets, make substitutions, such as ordering a salad instead of a fried fish sandwich, a regular hamburger instead of a specialty burger, or a roasted chicken sandwich instead of a breaded and fried chicken sandwich. Order an unsweetened ice tea or plain water instead of a soft drink. If possible, order a baked potato instead of fries.

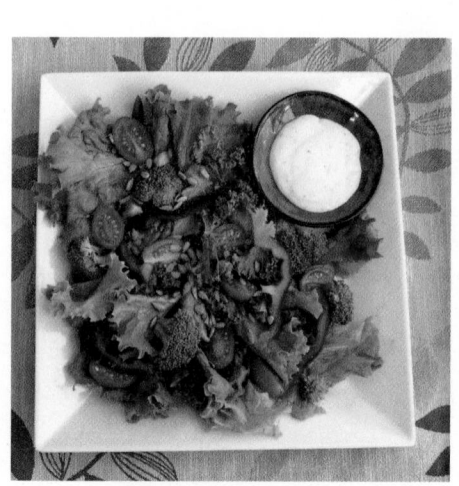

Salad with the dressing "on the side."

Self-monitoring

1. Keep a special notebook, computer log, or app to use as a food and exercise diary. If using a notebook, keep it in an obvious place, such as near the kitchen table, refrigerator, or pantry, for example. Note the time and place of eating, the type and amount of food eaten, and one's mood when the foods were eaten.

2. Use the diary to identify food-related problem areas, such as eating when bored or depressed.

3. In the exercise section of the diary, record the form of moderate-intensity exercise performed and the number of minutes spent each day. Try to achieve at least 150 minutes of moderate-intensity activities each week.

4. Weigh and measure your waistline at least once a week, preferably at the same time. However, do not rely on weight as the only indication of progress, because regular exercise can increase muscle mass and lead to failure in weight loss.

Lessons Learned from Successful Weight-Loss Experiences

Results of a national survey indicated that about half of American adults had tried to lose or maintain their weight at some point during the previous year.[58] However, the likelihood that obese people can achieve and maintain healthy weights without surgery is low. According to limited data, less than 20% of over-weight and obese people who intentionally lose weight can avoid regaining the weight for at least a year.[59]

Regular self-monitoring can be an important part of long-term weight-loss maintenance. In comparison to people who regain lost weight, those who are successful at maintaining a significant weight loss weigh themselves regularly.[60] Keeping daily records of body weight, physical activity, fruit and vegetable consumption, and water intake can aid in maintaining weight loss.[61] Weight regain is associated with waning motivation, which may be avoided through daily self-monitoring.[60]

The National Weight Control Registry

The National Weight Control Registry tracks a group of over 10,000 adult Americans, mostly women, who have lost at least 30 pounds and maintained the weight loss for at least 1 year.[62] Information about members' nutrition- and exercise-related practices provides insight into lifestyle habits that foster losing excess weight and maintaining the lower weight. Registry members tend to:

- Eat low-calorie, low-fat diets.

- Eat breakfast every day.

- Check body weight at least once a week.

- Exercise, on average, for 1 hour daily.

- Watch less than 10 hours of TV per week.[62]

Community-Based Weight-Loss Programs

Many communities offer a variety of weight-loss programs. Registered dietitians often conduct weight-loss classes at hospitals or universities. If a physician pre-scribes dietary counseling by a registered dietitian, the patient's health insurance may cover the cost of such treatment.

Some commercial weight-loss programs, such as *Weight Watchers*®, have diet plans that have been developed by dietitians. Members who have lost weight

REAL People, REAL Stories

Jan Haapala

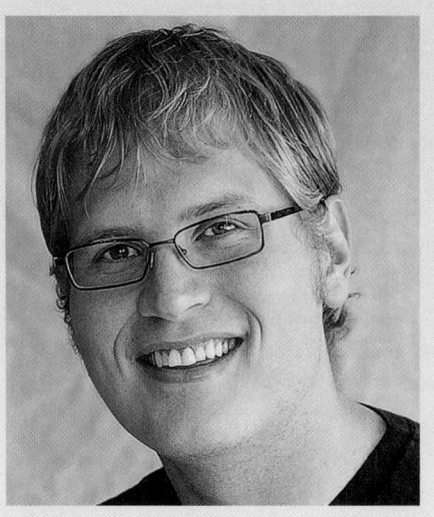

Early in 2005, 24-year-old Jan Haapala did not feel well. He slept poorly at night, and during the day, extreme fatigue seemed to be his constant companion. Frequent indigestion added to his general discomfort. During a physical exam, Jan was shocked to learn he had hypertension. The physician prescribed medication to reduce Jan's dangerously elevated blood pressure and told the young man to lose weight.

At the time of his doctor's appointment, Jan weighed 335 pounds and his BMI was over 45, which is in the "extremely obese" range. Taking medication can reduce elevated blood pressure and keep it under control, but losing excess fat often cures hypertension, making the medication unnecessary.

Jan was aware that his lifestyle contributed to his extreme obesity. He typically ate two doughnuts and a 20-ounce serving of a sugar-sweetened soft drink for breakfast. Lunches and dinners were "big" meals, often comprised of fast foods, especially double cheeseburgers and large portions of French fries and soft drinks. Candy bars were among his favorite snacks. "I knew those foods were unhealthy, but that didn't change what I ate once I sat down to eat," Jan says. In addition to his poor food choices, Jan was physically inactive.

To lose weight sensibly, Jan joined Weight Watchers. The personalized diet and exercise plan gave him the information and motivation he needed to change his lifestyle to a healthier one. In addition to choosing less fatty and sugary foods, he started a walking regimen that eventually became a jogging regimen. The pounds seemed to melt away from his body, and not long after he began to lose weight, he was able to discontinue taking the medication for hypertension. Although it took 3 years, Jan lost 125 pounds! The gradual but steady weight loss was an indication that he was making the kinds of behavioral and lifestyle changes that would be permanent.

Today, Jan is running 5K distance races and feeling great. When he was obese, he was embarrassed about exercising in public, but his self-confidence and high self-esteem helped him overcome his reluctance to work out while other people were around. His advice to overfat people who are worried about what strangers will think while they exercise: "Don't be embarrassed about doing something in public that's good for you. People won't judge you negatively for trying to become healthier." Clearly, Jan is a role model and inspiration for anyone who is overweight or obese and wants to get his or her weight (and life) under control.

while following the plan often conduct local meetings. Before joining any weight–loss program, consumers should obtain answers to the following questions:

- How much does the program cost? Do I pay when I attend meetings? Do I need to sign a contract? If so, for what length of time?

- Do I have to buy special foods or dietary supplements?

- Is nutrition counseling provided? Do the persons providing nutrition counseling and information have degrees in nutrition and dietetics from accredited colleges or universities? How much contact will I have with a counselor?

- Were the diet plans developed by dietitians? Do the plans emphasize the importance of making lifestyle changes, including ways to increase physical activity?
- Does the program's advertising include questionable weight—loss claims and deceptive testimonials?

ASSESS YOUR PROGRESS

22 *List at least six tips for modifying behavior to achieve weight loss.*

23 *List at least three practices of people who are successful at maintaining weight loss.*

13.9 Nonrecommended Methods of Weight Loss

LEARNING OUTCOMES

1 *Describe the typical features of fad diets.*

2 *Explain the pros and cons of following a low-carbohydrate diet.*

3 *Identify popular dietary supplements promoted for weight loss.*

Many overfat people seek "quick fixes" to lose weight, such as *fad diets* and dietary supplements promoted to "burn" or "melt" fat quickly. These plans rarely help people succeed in achieving their long—term weight—loss goals. This section pres— ents a number of popular weight—loss approaches that often lack formal scientific testing to document their safety and effectiveness.

fad diet trendy practice that has widespread appeal for a period, then becomes no longer fashionable

Fad Diets

A **fad diet** is a trendy weight—loss practice that has widespread appeal among a population. After a period, however, people lose interest in the practice, and it becomes no longer fashionable. Fad diets generally promote rapid weight loss without the need to "count" calories and exercise more. A fad diet often relies on a *gimmick*, a novel feature such as a device worn around the waist that "shrinks fat fast." A gimmick makes the diet seem to be unique and more likely to work than other diets. Some fad diets use gimmicks of emphasizing one food ("grapefruit diet") or consuming an exotic product or dietary supplement, such as açai juice or raspberry ketones. Weight loss occurs on these diets because the diet is low in calories, not because açai berries, raspberry ketones, cabbage soup, grapefruit, or another "special food" contains compounds that cause rapid weight loss. Following diets that emphasize eating a particular food for a few days often results in bore— dom and monotony. Eventually, dieters abandon such restrictive menu plans because they just cannot face another cup of cabbage soup or bowl of grapefruit.

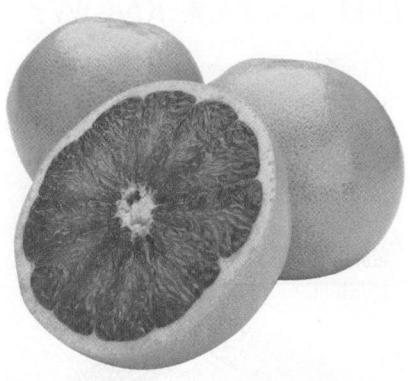

Although people often lose weight while following fad diets, they usually regain much of the weight that was lost while on the diet when they resume their prior eating and other lifestyle habits. Achieving a healthy body weight and maintaining that weight requires making lifestyle changes that a person adopts for the rest of his or her life.

Low-Carbohydrate Approaches

A weight—reduction diet is low carbohydrate if it eliminates or severely restricts the intake of carbohydrate—rich foods such as breads, cereals, fruits, vegetables, and sweets. Diets that limit carbohydrate intakes are high in protein and can be high in saturated fat. The lack of variety often leads to boredom with the selection of foods, and as a result, people lose weight because they tend to eat less. On the other hand, people who follow low–carbohydrate/high–protein diets tend to like the diet plan more and have less difficulty adhering to the diets than people who are on low–fat diets.[63]

Reduced–calorie, low–carbohydrate diets, such as the Atkins diet, usually produce rapid weight loss initially, primarily because the body loses water. When a person's carbohydrate intake is low, his or her body produces less glycogen and uses much of its stored glycogen to supply glucose for energy. Tissues maintain about 3 g of water with each gram of glycogen, so when the body's glycogen content decreases, the water that was stored with it needs to be eliminated in urine. Furthermore, a very–low–carbohydrate intake causes the liver to produce glucose, mostly from certain amino acids supplied by the body's tissue proteins. Protein tissue also contains a lot of water. When protein–rich tissues are dismantled and their amino acids used for energy, the water that was stored with the proteins also ends up in urine.

Low–carbohydrate diets that provide less than 35% of total kcal from carbohydrate may help overfat persons achieve greater weight loss than traditional reduced–calorie diets during the first 6 months of a diet plan. An analysis of 13 studies indicated that after 6 months, people on low–carbohydrate/high–protein diet plans lost an average of about 9 pounds more than people on low–fat/high–carbohydrate diets.[63] After 12 months, however, the people who were following the carbohydrate–restricted diets weighed only about 2 pounds less than people following the low–fat diets. Nevertheless, low–carbohydrate diets resulted in more favorable high–density lipoprotein ("good cholesterol") and triglyceride levels. Thus, low–carbohydrate diets may be as effective as or even more effective than low–fat diets for reducing weight and risk of CVD, but the benefits persist only for up to 1 year.[63] More studies, however, are needed to determine whether low–carbohydrate diets are safe and reduce the risk of CVD for longer periods.

Very-Low-Fat Approaches

Very–low–fat diets are very–high–carbohydrate diets. These diets supply approximately 5 to 10% of calories from fat and generally result in rapid weight loss when followed consistently. The most notable are the Pritikin Diet and Dr. Dean Ornish's "Eat More, Weigh Less" diet plans.

Very–low–fat diets that contain adequate amounts of essential fatty acids are not harmful for healthy adults, but they are difficult to follow for the long term. Fat contributes to the flavor and texture of foods. Thus, extremely low–fat diets are not tasty, and they eliminate many foods that are usually high on peoples' favorite foods' lists, such as ice cream and meat. Although grains, fruits, and vegetables are nutrient–dense foods, eating them repeatedly and without fat can cause "diet boredom" and waning interest in continuing the diet.

The Paleo Diet

The Paleo Diet™ is high in protein from meat and fish, low in fat, and moderate in carbohydrate (35 to 45% of calories). In addition to consuming high amounts of meat and fish, people who follow the diet eat low–glycemic–index (see Chapter 5) and unrefined foods, including nonstarchy fruits and vegetables. The Paleo Diet lacks grains and dairy items, as well as foods with added salt, sugar, and fat. Low–fat/high–meat diets may be helpful in lowering the risk of type 2 diabetes and CVD.[64] More research, however, is needed to support recommending such diets for weight loss.

Dietary Supplements for Weight Loss

Many people are attracted to dietary supplements for weight loss because they believe promoters' claims that their products are "magic bullets" for shedding

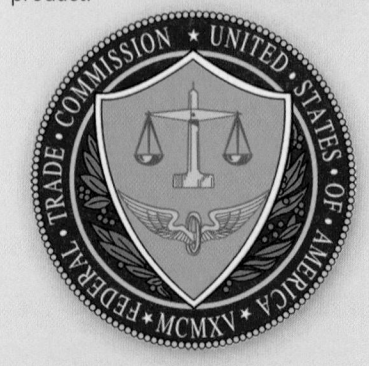

unwanted weight quickly and effortlessly.[65] Although several different types of weight–loss supplements are available, these products generally have not been scientifically tested in humans for safety and effectiveness.

Advertisements often claim that weight–loss products can help someone "Lose 30 pounds in just 30 days," or "Eat anything you want and still lose weight." In general, advertising claims that promise quick and easy weight loss are too good to be true. According to a survey conducted by the Federal Trade Commission (FTC) in 2011, more consumers were victims of fraudulent weight–loss than any other type of fraud that was included in the survey. According to FTC estimates, approximately 2% of American adults bought and used bogus weight–loss products in 2011.[66] See Chapter 2 for a discussion about ways to analyze information in weight–loss advertisements.

In 2004, the U.S. Food and Drug Administration (FDA) banned the sale of most dietary supplements that contained the natural stimulant ephedra ($eh-feh'-dra$) or ephedra–related compounds after the agency received reports of serious side effects and even deaths resulting from use of these products. The death in 2003 of Steve Bechler, Baltimore Orioles baseball player, was linked to ephedra. Table 13.9

TABLE 13.9 Summary of Selected Weight-Loss Supplements

Supplement	Usefulness	Side Effects/Safety Concerns (Usual Doses)
Açai berry	Not effective	Potentially dangerous; may be contaminated with an FDA-unapproved drug
Beta-hydroxy-beta-methylbutyrate	May decrease adipose tissue and increase lean body mass, but more research is needed.	None reported
Chia seed	No scientific support	None reported
Chinese diet pills	Not determined	Linked to illness and deaths in Japan May contain the active drug fenfluramine
Chitosan	A few studies show some usefulness, but more research is needed.	May cause gastrointestinal discomfort including nausea, constipation, and intestinal gas.
Chromium picolinate	May enhance weight loss to a small extent	None reported, but may damage DNA
Conjugated linoleic acid	Has minimal effect on reducing body weight	Appears to be safe, but can cause gastrointestinal upset
Green tea or extracts	May enhance weight loss to a small extent	Concentrated extracts linked to severe liver damage
Ephedrine (ma huang, ephedra, *Ephedra sinica, Sida cordifolia*, pinellia, and ephedrine with caffeine)	Ephedrine-containing products promote short-term weight loss but also increase risk of serious side effects. Ephedra-containing dietary supplements are banned in the United States.	May cause rapid heart rate, elevated blood pressure, dizziness, sweating, headache, and sleep disturbances. Linked to heart attacks, strokes, and deaths
Garcinia cambogia (hydroxycitric acid, HCA)	Overall evidence does not suggest usefulness.	May cause headache and gastrointestinal discomfort
Glucomannan	May be effective, but more research is needed	None reported
Guar gum	Not effective	May cause diarrhea and intestinal gas
Hoodia	Not effective	Vomiting, increased blood pressure and heart rate, signs of liver damage
Human chorionic gonadotropin (hCG)	Not effective	Unknown
Pyruvate	May be beneficial; more research is needed	None reported, but long-term safety is unknown
Spirulina (blue-green algae)	Not effective	Unknown

Sources: Food and Drug Administration: Public notification: "Acai Berry Soft Gel ABC" contains undeclared drug ingredient. October 18, 2011; Egras AM and others: An evidence-based review of fat modifying supplemental weight loss products. *Journal of Obesity 2011*, Article ID 297315, DOI: 10.1155/2011/297315; Nieman DC and others: Chia seed supplementation and disease risk factors in overweight women: A metabolomics investigation. *Journal of Alternative and Complementary Medicine* 18(7):700, 2012. Pittler MH, Ernst E: Dietary supplements for body-weight reduction: A systematic review. *American Journal of Clinical Nutrition* 79:529, 2004; Saper RB and others: Common dietary supplements for weight loss. *American Family Physician* 70:1731, 2004; Hursel R and others: The effects of green tea on weight loss and weight management: A meta-analysis. *International Journal of Obesity* advance online publication, 14 July 2009; DOI:10.1038/ijo.2009.135; Sarma DN and others: Safety of green tea extracts: A systematic review by the US Pharmacopeia. *Drug Safety* 31(6):469, 2008.

presents science—based findings about some popular weight—loss supplements, including their potential usefulness and safety concerns. At this point, medical experts do not recommend any dietary supplement for weight loss.[65]

ASSESS YOUR PROGRESS

24 Identify at least three typical features of fad diets.

25 What are the potential benefits and risks of following a low-carbohydrate diet for weight loss?

26 Discuss the major drawback of following a very-low-fat diet for weight loss.

27 Identify at least four popular weight-loss supplements, and indicate whether each supplement is safe and effective.

13.10 Medical Treatment of Obesity

LEARNING OUTCOMES

1 Identify medications that can aid in weight loss or weight management.

2 Discuss the three major types of bariatric surgery.

3 Describe some potential physical and psychological complications of bariatric surgery.

Obese patients often do not lose enough weight to improve their health by fol—lowing fad or recommended weight—loss diets. The frustration of repeated diet—ing leads some obese persons to turn to physicians for prescription medication and surgical procedures for managing their weight.

Weight-Loss Medications

At this time, Xenical®, Qsymia®, Belviq®, and Contrave® have been approved by the FDA for weight loss or weight management. These medications should be used with a weight—loss program that includes calorie restriction and physical activity.

Lipases secreted into the intestinal tract participate in the digestion of fat. When taken along with a meal, Xenical (*orlistat*) acts as a lipase inhibitor. As a result, orlistat reduces fat digestion by about 30%. The undigested fat is elim—inated in the stools and can cause an oily, unpleasant discharge. The fat carries fat—soluble vitamins along with it, so these micronutrients are eliminated in stools as well. Therefore, patients using orlistat often need to take a multiple vitamin supplement.

The typical patient who uses orlistat in addition to a weight—loss diet for up to 2 years loses only about 7 more pounds than he or she would have by dieting alone.[67] The medication's effects are too modest for obese people who need to lose substantial amounts of body fat. Nevertheless, the FDA has approved sales of the nonprescription form of orlistat ("Alli®") as a weight—loss aid for adults (Fig. 13.21).

In 2012, the FDA approved *Qsymia* (*kyoo—sim—ee'—uh*) for use with a reduced—calorie diet and physical activity to help with long—term weight man—agement.[68] Qsymia is a combination of *phentermine*, which suppresses appe—tite, and *topiramate*, which is used to treat certain types of seizures or prevent migraine headaches. Treatment with Qsymia along with a sensible weight—loss plan helped patients lose 6 to 9% more weight than patients in the placebo group.[68] This drug, however, is not safe for women who are pregnant or may become pregnant while taking the medication.

Lorcaserin (Belviq) alters the activity of the neurotransmitter *serotonin* in the brain, influencing satiety and reducing food intake as a result.[69] However, people who used lorcaserin for 1 year lost only 3 to 4% more weight than people in the placebo group who followed the same weight—loss plan but did not take the medication. Critics have raised concerns that this drug may increase risk of breast tumors or cause damage to heart valves.[69]

Contrave contains two active ingredients: *naltrexone*, which is often pre—scribed to treat alcoholism, and bupropion, an antidepressant. More research is needed to determine Contrave's long—term effectiveness as a weight—loss medication.

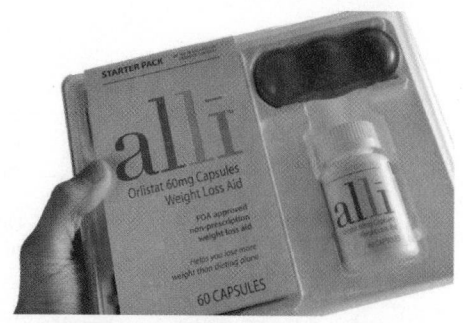

FIGURE 13.21 Alli. This weight-loss medication has the FDA's approval to be sold without the need for a prescription.

Bariatric Surgical Procedures

Bariatric (*ber—ee—a'—trik*) **medicine** is the medical specialty that focuses on the treatment of obesity. Bariatric surgery is an effective method of treating extreme obesity.[70] Such surgical procedures drastically reduce the size of an obese person's stomach, markedly limiting his or her food intake. As a result, obese patients may lose 50% or more of their excess weight during the first 2 years after the procedure.[71] Nevertheless, bariatric surgery is not a cure for obesity. Obese people who undergo one of the procedures still have to follow a nutritionally balanced, calorie—reduced diet and exercise regularly. However, the surgery often makes it easier for patients to eat less.

Aside from helping obese people lose considerable amounts of weight and maintain the loss, bariatric surgery can produce dramatic health benefits. Patients often achieve normal blood pressure, glucose levels, and triglyceride levels after surgery. Furthermore, overall death rates are lower for extremely obese people who lose weight after undergoing bariatric surgery. Such surgeries are relatively safe; fewer than 1% of patients die as a result of having a bariatric surgical procedure.[72]

bariatric medicine medical specialty that focuses on the treatment of obesity

Types of Bariatric Surgery

In the United States, two common surgical approaches to treating obesity are the **Roux—en—Y** (*ru—en—wi'*) **gastric bypass** and **gastric banding** procedures.[72] Bariatric surgeries often can be performed *laparoscopically*, that is, by using several small incisions that allow surgeons to insert instruments and a video camera into the abdomen. Laparoscopic bariatric surgical procedures reduce recovery time and the risk of infections.

During the Roux—en—Y operation, staples are placed surgically across the upper part of the stomach to create a small pouch. This procedure reduces the obese patient's stomach capacity to about 1 ounce, which is smaller than the volume of one egg. (Normally, the stomach's capacity is about 32 ounces.) Additionally, the small intestine is cut and attached to the lower end of the newly formed stomach pouch (Fig. 13.22a). Food no longer passes through the "bypassed" section of the intestine, so digestion and absorption are reduced as a result of the surgery.

Sleeve gastrectomy is another form of bariatric surgery that reduces the stomach's size. During this procedure, the stomach is stapled to form a banana—shaped pouch that holds about 2 to 5 ounces of food. The surgery does not involve bypassing a section of the small intestine, so nutrient absorption is not reduced (Fig. 13.22b). People who have undergone sleeve gastrectomy can eat only small portions of solid foods, which contributes to rapid weight loss. Sleeve gastrectomy surgery is irreversible, because the unused portion of the stomach is removed.

Roux-en-Y gastric bypass surgical approach to treating obesity

gastric banding surgical approach to treating obesity

sleeve gastrectomy surgical approach to treating obesity

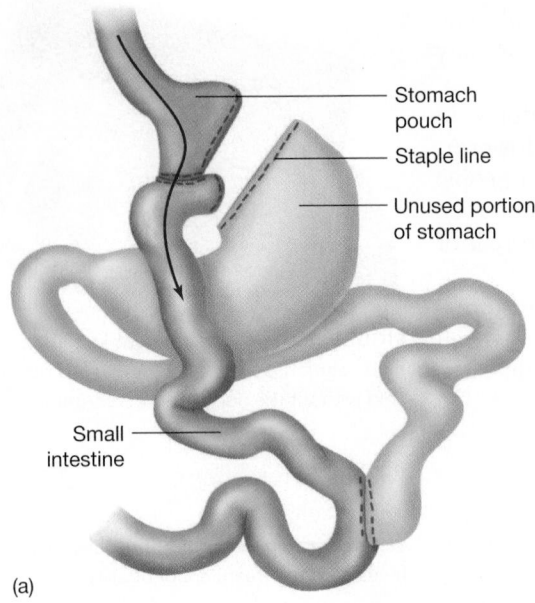

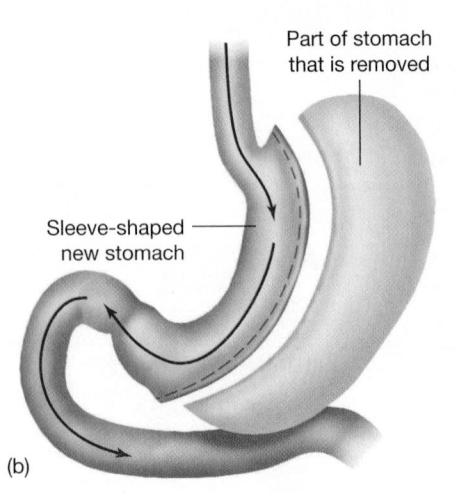

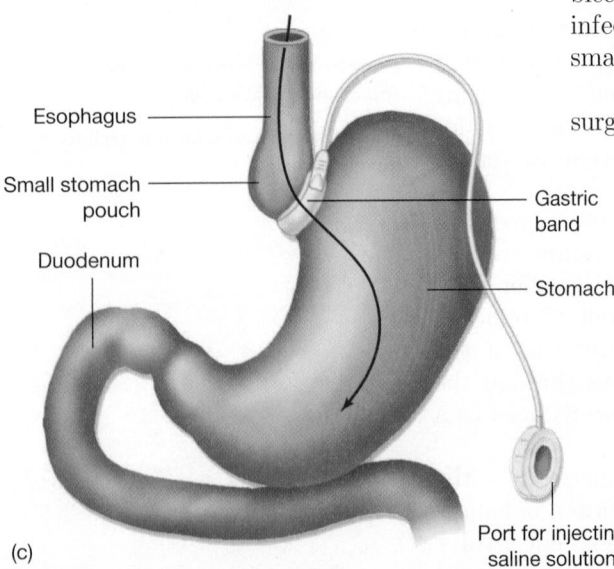

FIGURE 13.22 Bariatric surgeries. (a) The Roux-en-Y gastric bypass procedure, (b) sleeve gastrectomy, and (c) adjustable gastric banding procedure (also called the "lap band" procedure).

By performing the **adjustable gastric banding** procedure (also called the "lap band"), the bariatric surgeon creates the small stomach pouch with an adjustable band instead of fixed surgical staples (Fig. 13.22c). The surgeon determines the rate at which food leaves the pouch by altering the tightness of the band. The band is connected by a tube to a port placed directly under the skin. Saline can be added or removed via the port to increase or decrease the tightness of the band. The laparoscopic gastric banding procedure is easier to perform and safer than the other types of bariatric surgery.[70] The procedure is also relatively easy to reverse.

Outcomes of Bariatric Surgery

After bariatric surgery, patients lose an average of about 48 to 62% of their excess body weight.[8] However, up to 20% of Roux-en-Y gastric bypass patients struggle to maintain their initial weight loss 2 to 3 years after the surgery.[73] Researchers suggest this may be due to changes in hormones secreted from the gastrointestinal tract and a failure to adhere to strict portion sizes. Obese people who have gastric banding lose weight more slowly and lose less weight than those who undergo gastric bypass or sleeve gastrectomy procedures.

Bariatric surgeries result in weight loss partly because the stomach pouch fills quickly with food, so patients experience satiety sooner than they did prior to surgery. Moreover, overeating causes discomfort or vomiting. Thus, people who undergo such surgical procedures must make major lifestyle changes, such as learning to plan and consume frequent, small meals.

Patients, however, can be more successful at losing excess body fat and maintaining the lost weight if they learn how to plan nutritious meals, control food portions, change inappropriate food-related behaviors, and increase physical activity.[74]

Complications Following Bariatric Surgery Complications often associated with gastric bypass surgery include intestinal blockage and bleeding, leaks along the staple site, blood clot formation, and wound infections. The overall risk of death from bariatric surgery is very small (0.3%).[75]

"Dumping syndrome" is a common side effect of gastric bypass surgery that often occurs early in the recovery stage of the Roux-en-Y procedure.[76] This condition causes intestinal bloating, nausea, and diarrhea following consumption of simple carbohydrates. Treatment generally includes a diet that limits the consumption of simple carbohydrates.

After surgery, gastric bypass patients can develop micronutrient deficiencies due to malabsorption, diarrhea, and vomiting. Common deficiencies include fat-soluble vitamins, vitamin B-12, folate, iron, and calcium.[76] Calcium deficiency and rapid weight loss contribute to decreases in bone mineral density for bariatric surgery patients. However, patients can reduce their risk of nutrient deficiencies through counseling with a dietitian, regular monitoring, and lifelong use of vitamin and mineral supplements.

Psychological Concerns Following Bariatric Surgery Extremely obese people who want to undergo bariatric surgery are more likely to have experienced psychological stress than other obese persons.[8] After having the surgery, patients generally report improvements in their quality of life, sense of self—esteem, symptoms of depression and anxiety, and body image. Nevertheless, some bariatric patients do not maintain such positive feelings about their psychological well—being.

Candidates for bariatric surgery may think that undergoing the procedure and losing their excess weight will be the answer to all their problems. If, however, they had high expectations concerning how their lives will improve, they are likely to be disappointed when they fail to achieve goals that are not related to the weight loss that occurs after surgery.[8] Such goals may include enjoying more satisfying relationships and an improved body image.

People who were extremely obese and lose significant amounts of body fat after surgery experience sagging skin. Coping with the excess skin can lead to dissatisfaction with body image. The unneeded skin can be removed by having additional surgery ("cosmetic surgery"), which is costly and adds to patients' risk of complications.

Members of the health care team should assess each surgical candidate to identify patients who are likely to experience negative psychological outcomes after the bariatric procedure. Such patients may benefit from long—term and thorough postsurgical care to help them adjust psychologically to their weight loss.

adjustable gastric banding surgical approach to treating obesity, also called "lap band"

Liposuction

Liposuction is a surgical method of reducing the size of local subcutaneous fat deposits. Liposuction is not intended to treat obesity, but as a cosmetic surgery, the procedure can help a person improve the contours of his or her body. This procedure involves inserting a pencil—thin tube into an incision in the skin and suctioning the excess subcutaneous fat out of the body (Fig. 13.23).

Complications of liposuction are common and can be as minor as permanent dimpling of the skin at the suction site and as serious as death. Infection, blood clots, uncontrollable bleeding, fat droplets that enter the bloodstream (*fat emboli*), and punctures of internal organs are potentially lethal conditions that can occur as a result of liposuction.[77]

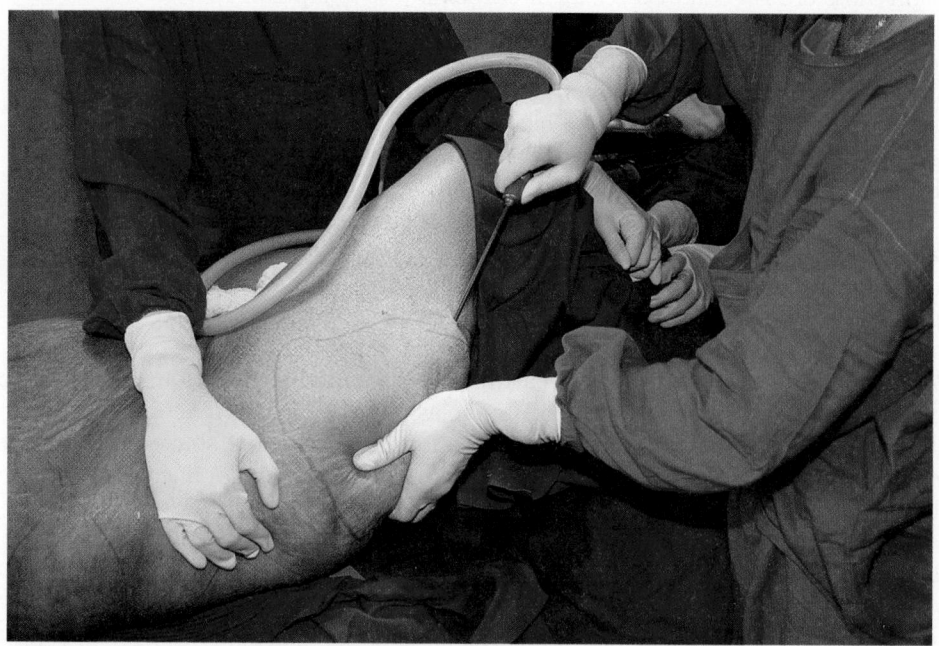

FIGURE 13.23 Liposuction. Liposuction is a surgical procedure that involves inserting a pencil-thin tube into an incision in the skin and suctioning subcutaneous fat out of the body.

ASSESS YOUR PROGRESS

28 *Discuss the effectiveness of prescribed weight-loss medications.*

29 *Describe the two most common types of bariatric surgery in the United States.*

30 *Why can bariatric surgery be an effective method of weight loss?*

31 *Identify at least two health-related concerns following bariatric surgery.*

13.11 Underweight

LEARNING OUTCOMES

1 *Explain the health consequences associated with being underweight.*

2 *Identify healthy ways to gain weight.*

underweight individual who has a BMI that is less than 18.5

An **underweight** individual has a BMI that is less than 18.5. In 2011–2012, 2.5% of Americans who were 20 to 39 years of age were underweight, and more women were likely to be underweight than men.[78] The percent of underweight Americans has decreased steadily since 1960–1962.

Multiple factors, including genetics, lifestyle, chronic diseases, and psycho-logical disturbances, often contribute to having a lower–than–average body weight. Individuals who inherit higher resting metabolic rates, tall body frames, or both, may find it difficult to gain weight. Excessive physical activity can result in low body weight. Compared to those of sedentary adults, the bodies of rapidly growing, physically active children and adolescents have higher energy needs. If these children do not consume enough energy, they can lose weight.

Having a BMI under 18.5 is associated with increased risk for early mortality, even in healthy, nonsmoking adults. People who are underweight are more likely to have a weakened immune system and have greater risk for illness or infection as a result. Underweight also increases the risk of osteoporosis.

Weight loss that occurs in people who are not intentionally trying to lose weight can be a sign of serious illness, such as a form of cancer that has spread in the body. **Cachexia** ($ka-kek'-see-ah$) is the medical term for a condition that is characterized by severe weight loss ("wasting"). When excessive, voluntary weight–loss efforts can also result in cachexia (see Chapter 14).

cachexia severe weight loss ("wasting")

If a person's BMI was within the healthy range before excessive weight loss occurred, an evaluation by a physician may be necessary to determine the cause or causes of the loss, especially when the underweight person has not tried to shed pounds. A thorough medical examination can rule out possible reasons for unintentional weight loss, such as hormonal imbalances, depression, cancer, and infectious or digestive tract diseases.

For an underweight person, gaining weight can be just as challenging as losing weight is for an overfat person. To gain weight, underweight adults can gradually increase their consumption of nutrient– and calorie–dense foods, especially those high in healthy fats. See the "Fresh Tips" on page 453 for examples of healthy snacks. Incorporation of energy–dense foods should focus on high–calorie nutri-tious food choices that are low in saturated–fat content. Additionally, under-weight people can replace beverages such as soft drinks with more nutritious calorie sources, such as 100% fruit juices, smoothies, and milk shakes made with peanut butter and fat–reduced ice cream. Following a regular meal and snack schedule also aids in weight gain and maintenance.

Many underweight individuals want to gain weight, especially muscle mass. Underweight persons can add muscle mass through a resistance–training (weight–lifting) program, but they must increase their calorie intake to support the additional exercise. Otherwise, gaining muscle tissue is not likely to occur.

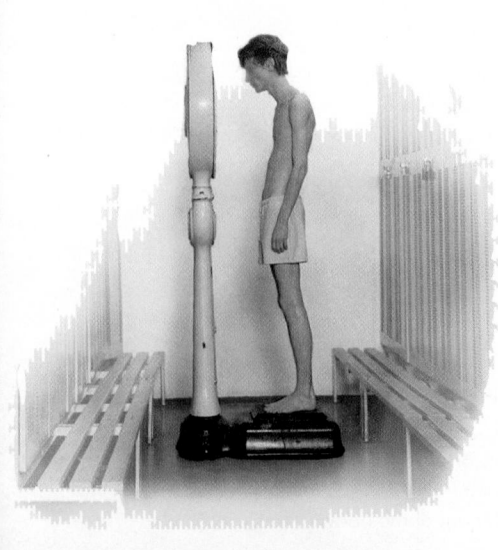

FRESH TIPS

Eating the following healthy foods may aid weight gain efforts:

- Fatty fish, such as salmon
- Olives, avocados, seeds, nuts, and butters made from seeds and nuts
- Granola with dried fruit
- Low-fat cheeses such as part-skim mozzarella sticks
- Smoothies made with milk, Greek yogurt, and peanut butter
- Dry or cooked cereals, such as raisin bran or oatmeal
- Bran muffins or breads made from bananas, zucchini, or carrots
- Oatmeal raisin cookies and/or fig bars

ASSESS YOUR PROGRESS

32 *Identify at least three health conditions associated with underweight.*

33 *Describe physical activities and dietary changes that can be used to gain weight in a healthy manner.*

SUMMARY

SECTION 13.1 Overweight and Obesity

- In the United States, overweight and obesity are widespread nutritional problems that have reached epidemic proportions. An overweight person has extra body weight that is contributed by bone, muscle, body fat, and/or body water. Obesity is characterized by excessive and unhealthy amounts of body fat.

SECTION 13.2 Body Mass Index

- Body mass index (BMI) is a numerical value based on the relationship between body weight and height.

SECTION 13.3 Body Composition and Fat Distribution

- Determining body composition involves measuring the components that make up the body's tissues. Methods of estimating body composition include underwater weighing, air displacement, dual-energy x-ray absorptiometry, bioelectrical impedance, and skinfold thickness.
- Distribution of excess body fat is important for assessing risk of health conditions associated with obesity.

SECTION 13.4 Energy Intake and Expenditures

- Total energy expenditure is made up of basal and resting metabolism, physical activity, thermic effect of food, and nonexercise activity thermogenesis.
- Many factors influence a person's metabolic rate. Basal metabolic rate can be estimated by using specific calculations.

SECTION 13.5 Measuring Energy Expenditure

- Energy expenditure can be measured through direct and indirect calorimetry. Methods of estimating energy expenditure include using heart rate monitors, accelerometry, and physical activity questionnaires.

SECTION 13.6 **The Body's Energy States**

- The concept of energy balance is critical to understanding why most people gain, lose, or maintain body weight. Positive energy balance contributes to weight gain; negative energy balance for an extended period of time contributes to weight loss.

SECTION 13.7 **Factors That Influence Body Weight**

- Genetic environmental, and psychological factors play major roles in the development of obesity.
- Physical activity level influences energy output and can alter body weight.

SECTION 13.8 **Voluntary Weight Loss**

- Safe and effective weight-loss methods involve achieving negative energy balance and regular physical activity. Regular self-monitoring is important for long-term weight-loss success.

SECTION 13.9 **Nonrecommended Methods of Weight Loss**

- Fad diets often contribute to short-term weight loss followed by regaining the lost weight. More research is needed to determine the safety and effectiveness of dietary supplements.

SECTION 13.10 **Medical Treatment of Obesity**

- Currently, four prescribed medications have been approved by the FDA for weight loss or management. Bariatric surgery is an effective method of treating extreme obesity.

SECTION 13.11 **Underweight**

- Being underweight is associated with increased risk for early mortality. To gain weight, underweight adults can gradually increase their consumption of calorie- and nutrient-dense foods.

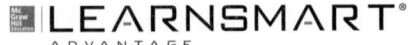 Get the most out of your study of nutrition with McGraw-Hill's innovative suite of adaptive learning products including McGraw-Hill LearnSmart®, SmartBook®, McGraw-Hill LearnSmart Achieve®, and McGraw-Hill LearnSmart Prep®. Visit www.learnsmartadvantage.com.

CASE STUDY RESPONSE

WEIGHT LOSS

TONY HAS A BMI OF 33.2, WHICH PLACES him in the "obese class I" category. Therefore, he has an elevated risk for chronic disease and early death. Tony's 42-inch waist circumference indicates he may have android obesity, which increases his risk of type 2 diabetes, hypertension, CVD, and metabolic syndrome. Tony's environment contributes to his excess body weight. The vending machine that is next to his office appeals to his senses. The presence, sight, and ease of access to empty-calorie food make it difficult for him to select a more healthful diet. Also, his desk job contributes to his sedentary lifestyle.

Tony can achieve a state of negative energy balance by reducing his calorie intake and increasing his physical activity. He can wake up 30 minutes earlier than usual and take the time to eat a simple breakfast, such as a bowl of whole-grain cereal with nonfat milk. He can also consume more low-calorie, nutrient-dense foods, such as fresh fruits and vegetables, and eat fewer energy-dense foods, including those in the break room vending machine. Tony can choose to switch from drinking sugar-sweetened soft drinks to drinking water or unsweetened iced tea. Perhaps at noon, he could eat a bag lunch that he has prepared at home and reserve some time to take a 30-minute walk.

TEST KITCHEN
Modifying Recipes for Healthy Living

Andre's BMI is 32.4. He would like some suggestions to reduce the amount of unhealthy fat and added sugar in one of his favorite recipes: a pumpkin pie that is made with melted vanilla ice cream. He's willing to try a pumpkin custard or soufflé recipe.

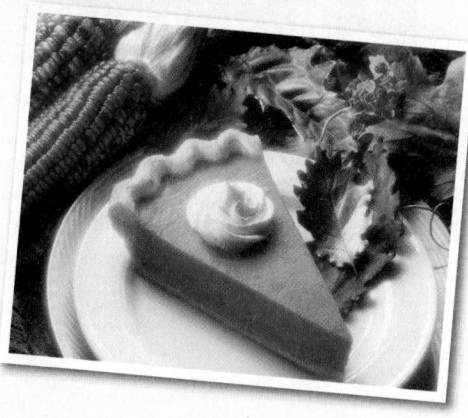

ANDRE'S PUMPKIN PIE

PREPARATION STEPS

1. Preheat the oven to 350°F.
2. Mix the first nine ingredients together until they are well blended.
3. Pour the mixture into the pie shell. Bake for about an hour or until a knife that is inserted into the pie filling is clean when it is removed.
4. Refrigerate. Serves eight.

STEP 1 Brainstorm

Use diet analysis software to analyze the calorie content of a one-eighth serving of Andre's pumpkin pie recipe.

STEP 2 Develop a modified recipe

Develop a modified version of his recipe that is lower in calories per serving.

STEP 3 Evaluate the modified dessert

Use diet analysis software to analyze the total calories, carbohydrates, fat, and protein in a serving of the dessert. Explain how the two versions of the pumpkin-based dessert differ nutritionally.

OPTIONAL ACTIVITIES

STEP 4 Test your new recipe

Keep notes on any changes you make to ingredient amounts as you prepare the modified dessert.

STEP 5 Reflect on your new recipe

Reflect on the sensory qualities (e.g., taste, texture) of the new dessert.

STEP 6 Add the recipe to your collection or repeat steps to improve the product

INGREDIENTS

1 can (15-oz) pumpkin puree

1 ½ cups melted vanilla ice cream

1 cup brown sugar

2 large eggs, lightly beaten

1 Tbsp all-purpose flour

½ tsp ground cinnamon

¼ tsp ground nutmeg

¼ tsp ground ginger

⅛ tsp ground cloves

1 unbaked 9" pie shell
(in an aluminum pan)

Critical Thinking

1. Explain why a person cannot claim to have 0% body fat.

2. An advertisement for a weight-loss supplement claims that the mixture of herbs in the product increases the metabolic rate by 150%. Explain why you would or would not recommend this product to someone who wants to lose weight.

3. Develop a table that lists the risks and benefits of bariatric surgery for obese adults.

4. Calculate your BMI. Which body weight classification is your BMI? Is it in the healthy range? If not, what is the healthy range, based on your height?

5. Discuss steps you can take to achieve and/or maintain a healthy body weight as you grow older.

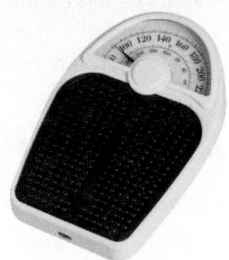

Practice Test

Select the best answer.

1. Body mass index (BMI) is
   a. a standard used to calculate a person's body fat percentage.
   b. based on a relationship between a person's weight and height.
   c. gradually being replaced by more reliable height/weight tables.
   d. used to estimate direct calorimetry.

2. Visceral fat is in the
   a. membranes of cells.
   b. skin.
   c. abdominal region.
   d. brain.

3. Andy's hip circumference is greater than his waist circumference. Based on this information, Andy has _____ obesity.
   a. visceral
   b. gynoid
   c. hormonal
   d. android

4. _____ relies on the principle that lean tissue is denser than water.
   a. Bioelectrical impedance
   b. Underwater weighing
   c. Dual-energy x-ray absorptiometry
   d. Direct calorimetry

5. A healthy percentage of body fat for women is _____ %.
   a. 10   b. 25   c. 38   d. 45

6. Eric rates his activity level as "average." Based on this information, basal metabolism accounts for _____ of his body's total energy use.
   a. 10–20%
   b. 21–49%
   c. 60–75%
   d. over 75%

7. Basal metabolism includes energy needs for
   a. breathing and circulating blood.
   b. performing physical activity.
   c. digesting food.
   d. absorbing nutrients.

8. Which of the following statements is true?
   a. Women generally have higher metabolic rates than men.
   b. Thyroid hormone influences BMR.
   c. A person who has more muscle mass will have a lower BMR than someone with less muscle tissue.
   d. When a person has a fever, his or her BMR drops below normal.

9. Negative energy balance occurs when
   a. the thermic effect of food equals NEAT.
   b. fat storage in the body increases.
   c. energy intake is higher than energy output.
   d. the body needs more calories than the diet supplies.

10. _____ is a hormone produced by fat tissue that reduces hunger.
    a. Pepsin
    b. Leptin
    c. Ghrelin
    d. Cholecystokinin

11. Members of the National Weight Control Registry tend to
    a. eat meals regularly, including breakfast.
    b. follow low-carbohydrate/high-protein diets.
    c. exercise 2 to 3 times per week.
    d. spend about 3 hours/day watching television.

12. Fat cells secrete
    a. adiponectin.
    b. insulin.
    c. cholecystokinin.
    d. ghrelin.

13. Peptide YY signals the
    a. kidneys to decrease fatty acid synthesis.
    b. thyroid gland to increase the metabolic rate.
    c. brain to increase glucose catabolism.
    d. stomach to reduce ghrelin secretion.

14. Leona's BMI is 18.2. According to this information, Leona's body weight is in the _____ range.
    a. underweight
    b. overweight
    c. healthy
    d. obese

15. Which of the following statements is true?

    a. At the present time, there is no direct way to measure a person's metabolic rate.

    b. A person's total daily energy output is the sum of calories used for metabolism and physical activity in a 24-hour period.

    c. A calorimetric chamber is used to measure a person's metabolic rate.

    d. Most people use more energy for NEAT than for resting metabolism.

ANSWERS TO PRACTICE TEST
1-b; 2-c; 3-b; 4-b; 5-b; 6-c; 7-a; 8-b; 9-d; 10-b; 11-a; 12-a; 13-d; 14-a; 15-c

---

ANSWERS TO CHAPTER 13 QUIZ Yourself

1. People can determine whether they have an unhealthy amount of body fat by measuring their waistline. **True** (p. 426)
2. The best way to lose weight and keep it off is to follow a low-carbohydrate, high-fat diet, such as the Atkins diet. **False** (p. 446)
3. Dietary supplements that contain ephedra can safely help a person lose 30 pounds in 30 days. **False** (p. 447)
4. When a person consumes more carbohydrates than needed, the excess may be converted to fat and stored in fat cells. **True** (p. 433)
5. Liposuction is an easy and safe way to eliminate excess body fat. **False** (p. 451)

References

1. National Institutes of Health, National Heart Lung and Blood Institute: *Aim for a healthy weight: What is overweight and obesity?* ND. http://www.nhlbi.nih.gov/health/public/heart/obesity/lose_wt/index.htm Accessed: February 15, 2014.

2. Ogden CL and others: Prevalence of childhood and adult obesity in the United States, 2011–2012. *Journal of the American Medical Association* 311(8):806,2014.

3. Centers for Disease Control and Prevention: *Overweight and obesity: Adult obesity facts.* Last updated September 2014. http://www.cdc.gov/obesity/data/adult.html Accessed: October 12, 2014.

4. Centers for Disease Control and Prevention: *Overweight and obesity: Childhood obesity facts.* Last updated September 2014. http://www.cdc.gov/obesity/data/childhood.html Accessed: October 12, 2014.

5. Ogden CL and others: Prevalence of obesity and trends in body mass index among US children and adolescents, 1999–2010. *Journal of the American Medical Association* 307(5):483, 2012.

6. World Health Organization: *Obesity and overweight.* Updated March 2013. http://www.who.int/mediacentre/factsheets/fs311/en/ Accessed: February 15, 2014.

7. Sikorski C and others: The stigma of obesity in the general public and its implications for public health—a systematic review. *BMC Public Health* 11:661, 2011. E-pub: August 23, 2011. DOI: 10.1186/1471-2458-11-661 PMCID: PMC3175190

8. Kubik JF and others: The impact of bariatric surgery on psychological health. *Journal of Obesity* 2013;2013:837989. DOI: 10.1155/2013/837989. Epub 2013 March 28.

9. Ter Maat S: Most health plans still resist covering weight-loss treatment. *American Medical News.* Posted: August 19, 2013. http://www.amednews.com/article/20130819/business/130819965/6/?utm_source=rss&utm_medium=&utm_campaign=20131104 Accessed: February 15, 2014.

10. Withrow D, Alter DA: The economic cost of obesity worldwide: A systematic review of the direct costs of obesity. *Obesity Reviews* 12:131, 2011.

11. Wang YC: Health and economic burden of the projected obesity trends in the USA and the UK. *Lancet* 378:815, 2011.

12. Centers for Disease Control and Prevention: *Overweight and obesity: Economic consequences: National estimated cost of obesity.* Updated April 2012. http://www.cdc.gov/obesity/causes/economics.html Accessed: February 15, 2014.

13. National Institutes of Health, National Heart Lung and Blood Institute: *Assessing your weight and health risk.* ND. http://www.nhlbi.nih.gov/health/public/heart/obesity/lose_wt/risk.htm Accessed: August 18, 2013.

14. Liebman B: Weighing the options? Do extra pounds mean extra years? *Nutrition Action Health Letter* 40(2):3, 2013.

15. Carpenter CL and others: Body fat and body-mass index among a multiethnic sample of college-age men and women. *Journal of Obesity.* E-pub: April 8, 2013. Article ID 790654; PMCID: PMC3649342. Accessed: November 13, 2013.

16. Romero-Corral A and others: Normal weight obesity: A risk factor for cardiometabolic dysregulation and cardiovascular mortality. *European Heart Journal* 31:737, 2010.

17. Marques-Vidal P and others: Prevalence of normal weight obesity in Switzerland: Effect of various definitions. *European Journal of Nutrition* 47(5):251, 2008.

18. Marques-Vidal P and others: Normal weight obesity: Relationship with lipids, glycaemic status, liver enzymes and inflammation. *Nutrition, Metabolism & Cardiovascular Diseases* 20:669e, 2010.

19. Saladin KS: *Anatomy & Physiology.* 7th ed. Boston: McGraw-Hill Publishing Company, 2015.

20. Avram MM: Cellulite: A review of its physiology and treatment. *Journal of Cosmetic and Laser Therapy* 6:181, 2004.

21. Bosy-Westphal A and others: Accuracy of bioelectrical impedance consumer devices for measurement of body composition in comparison to whole body magnetic resonance imaging and dual x-ray absorptiometry. *Obesity Facts* 1:319, 2008.

22. Dehghan M, Merchant AT: Is bioelectrical impedance accurate for use in large epidemiological studies? *Nutrition Journal* 7:26, 2008.

23. Peterson J and others: Accuracy of consumer grade bioelectrical impedance analysis devices compared to air displacement plethysmography. *International Journal of Exercise Science* 4(3):176, 2011.

24. American College of Sports Medicine: *ACSM's guidelines for exercise testing and prescription.* Baltimore, MD: Wolters Kluwer Lippincott Williams & Wilkins, 2010.

25. Food and Nutrition Board, National Institute of Health: *Dietary reference intakes for energy, carbohydrate, fiber, fat, fatty acids, cholesterol, protein, and amino acids (macronutrients).* Washington, DC: National Academies Press, 2005.

26. World Health Organization International Obesity Task Force: *Redefining obesity and its treatment.* 2000. http://www.who.int/nutrition/publications/obesity/09577082_1_1/en/index.html Accessed: February 15, 2014.

27. Barnett AH: The importance of treating cardiometabolic risk factors in patients with type 2 diabetes. *Diabetes & Vascular Disease Research* 5(1):9, 2008.

28. Klein S: The case of visceral fat: Argument for the defense. *Journal of Clinical Investigation* 113:1530, 2004.

29. Bray GA, Champagne CM: Dietary patterns may modify central adiposity. *Journal of the American Dietetic Association* 109:1354, 2009.

30. National Institutes of Health, National Heart Lung and Blood Institute: *Classification of overweight and obesity by BMI, waist circumference, and associated disease risks.* ND. http://www.nhlbi.nih.gov/health/public/heart/obesity/lose_wt/bmi_dis.htm Accessed: February 15, 2014.

31. Williams MH: *Nutrition for health, fitness, and sport.* 10th ed. New York: McGraw-Hill Publishing Company, 2012.

32. Roberts SB, Dallal GE: Energy requirements and aging. *Public Health Nutrition* 8(7A):1028, 2005.

33. Harris AM and others: Nonexercise movement in elderly compared with young people. *American Journal of Physiology. Endocrinology and Metabolism* 292: E1207, 2007; DOI:10.1152/ajpendo.00509.2006.

34. Hall KD and others: Energy balance and its components: Implications for body weight regulation. *American Journal of Clinical Nutrition* 95(4):989, 2012. DOI: 10.3945/ajcn.112.036350 PMCID: PMC3302369

35. Esposito L and others: Developmental perspectives on nutrition and obesity from gestation to adolescence. *Preventing Chronic Disease* 6(3), 2009. http://www.cdc.gov/pcd/issues/2009/jul/09_0014.htm Accessed: February 17, 2014.

36. Andres A and others: Body fat mass of exclusively breastfed infants born to overweight mothers. *Journal of the Academy of Nutrition and Dietetics* 112(7):991, 2012.

37. Ello-Martin JA and others: The influence of food portion size and energy density on energy intake: Implications for weight management. *American Journal of Clinical Nutrition* 82:236S, 2005.

38. Jequier E: Pathways to obesity. *International Journal of Obesity and Related Metabolic Disorders* 26:S12, 2002.

39. Rolls B. Don't be dense: Trim calories per bite to trim pounds. *Nutrition Action Health Letter* 39(2):7, 2012.

40. Perez-Escamilla R and others: Dietary energy density and body weight in adults and children: A systematic review. *Journal of the Academy of Nutrition and Dietetics* 112(5):671, 2012.

41. Raynor H and others: The effects of an energy density prescription on diet quality and weight loss: A pilot randomized controlled trial. *Journal of the Academy of Nutrition and Dietetics* 112(9):1397, 2012.

42. Douglas SM and others: Low, moderate, or high protein yogurt snacks on appetite control and subsequent eating in healthy women. *Appetite* 60:117, 2013.

43. Leidy HJ and others: Beneficial effects of a higher-protein breakfast on the appetitive, hormonal, and neural signals controlling energy intake regulation in overweight/obese, "breakfast-skipping," late-adolescent girls. *American Journal of Clinical Nutrition* 97(4):677, 2013.

44. Goldstone AP and others: Elevated fasting plasma ghrelin in Prader-Willi syndrome adults is not solely explained by their reduced visceral adiposity and insulin resistance. *Journal of Clinical Endocrinology and Metabolism* 89(4):1718, 2004.

45. Woods S: Gastrointestinal satiety signals I. An overview of gastrointestinal signals that influence food intake. *American Journal of Physiology Gastrointestinal and Liver Physiology* 286(1):G7, 2004.

46. Wasan KM, Looije NA: Emerging pharmacological approaches to the treatment of obesity. *Journal of Pharmacy and Pharmaceutical Sciences* 8:259, 2005.

47. Jequier E: Leptin signaling, adiposity, and energy balance. *Annals of the New York Academy of Sciences* 967:379, 2002.

48. Hivert M-F and others: Higher adiponectin levels predict greater weight gain in healthy women in the Nurses' Health Study. *Obesity* 19(2):409, 2011. DOI:10.1038/oby.2010.189

49. Ford ES, Dietz WH: Trends in energy intake among adults in the United States: Findings from NHANES. *American Journal of Clinical Nutrition* 97(4):848, 2013.

50. Ledikwe JH and others: Portion sizes and the obesity epidemic. *Journal of Nutrition* 135:905, 2005.

51. Moore L and others: Trends in no leisure-time physical activity—United States, 1988–2000. *Research Quarterly for Exercise and Sport* 83(4):587, 2012.

52. Donnelly JE and others: American College of Sports Medicine Position Stand: Appropriate physical activity intervention strategies for weight loss and prevention of weight regain for adults. *Medicine and Science in Sports and Exercise* 41(2):459, 2009.

53. Lloyd-Richardson EE and others: A prospective study of weight gain during the college freshman and sophomore years. *Preventive Medicine* 48:256, 2009.

54. Irwin ML and others: Estimation of energy expenditure from physical activity measures: Determinants of accuracy. *Obesity Research* 9:517, 2001.

55. Kong A and others: Self-monitoring and eating-related behaviors are associated with 12-month weight loss in postmenopausal overweight-to-obese women. *Journal of the Academy of Nutrition and Dietetics* 112(9):1328, 2012.

56. Seagle H and others: Position of the American Dietetic Association: Weight management. *Journal of the American Dietetic Association* 109(2):330, 2009.

57. Wansink B: Environmental factors that increase the food intake and consumption volume of unknowing consumers. *Annual Review of Nutrition* 24:455, 2004.

58. Weiss EC and others: Weight-control practices among U.S. adults, 2001–2002. *American Journal of Preventive Medicine* 31:18, 2006.

59. Wing RR, Phelan S: Long-term weight loss maintenance. *American Journal of Clinical Nutrition* 82:222S, 2005.

60. Reyes NR and others: Similarities and differences between weight loss maintainers and regainers: A qualitative analysis. *Journal of the Academy of Nutrition and Dietetics* 112(4):499, 2012.

61. Akers J and others: Daily self-monitoring of body weight, step count, fruit/vegetable intake, and water consumption: A feasible and effective long-term weight loss maintenance approach. *Journal of the Academy of Nutrition and Dietetics* 112(5):685, 2012.

62. National Weight Control Registry: *The National Weight Control Registry.* ND. http://www.nwcr.ws/ Accessed: April 25, 2014.

63. Hession M and others: Systematic review of randomized controlled trials of low-carbohydrate vs. low-fat/low-calorie diets in the management of obesity and its comorbidities. *Obesity Reviews* 10:36, 2009.

64. Wheeler ML and others: Macronutrients, food groups, and eating patterns in the management of diabetes: A systematic review of the literature. 2010. *Diabetes Care* 35(2):434, 2012. DOI: 10.2337/dc11-2216

65. Saper RB and others: Common dietary supplements for weight loss. *American Family Physician* 70:1731, 2004.

66. Federal Trade Commission: *Consumer Fraud in the United States, 2011: The Third FTC Survey.* http://www.ftc.gov/sites/default/files/documents/reports/consumer-fraud-united-states-2011-third-ftc-survey/130419fraudsurvey_0.pdf Accessed October 10, 2014.

67. Hollywood A, Ogden J: Taking Orlistat: Predicting weight loss over 6 months. *Journal of Obesity* 2011. DOI:10.1155/2011/806896.

68. Food and Drug Administration: *FDA approves weight-management drug Qsymia.* July 2012. http://www.fda.gov/NewsEvents/Newsroom/PressAnnouncements/ucm312468.htm Accessed: February 17, 2014.

69. Miller L: Lorcaserin for weight loss: Insights into US food and drug administration approval. *Journal of the Academy of Nutrition and Dietetics* 113(1):25, 2013.

70. O'Brien PE and others: Obesity, weight loss, and bariatric surgery. *Medical Journal of Australia* 183:310, 2005.

71. National Institutes of Health: *Medical encyclopedia: Gastric bypass surgery.* 2012. http://www.nlm.nih.gov/medlineplus/ency/article/007199.htm Accessed: February 17, 2014.

72. Guller U and others: Safety and effectiveness of bariatric surgery: Roux-en-Y gastric bypass is superior to gastric banding in the management of morbidly obese patients. *Patient Safety in Surgery* 3(10), 2009. DOI:10.1186/1754-9493-3-10

73. Meguid MM: Weight regain after Roux-en-Y: A significant 20% complication related to PYY. *Nutrition* 24(9):832, 2008.

74. Nijamkin M and others: Comprehensive nutrition and lifestyle education improves weight loss and physical activity in Hispanic Americans following gastric bypass surgery: A randomized controlled trial. *Journal of the Academy of Nutrition and Dietetics* 112(3):382, 2012.

75. Neff KJ, le Roux CW: Bariatric surgery: The challenges with candidate selection, individualizing treatment and clinical outcomes. *BioMed Central* 11:8, 2013. http://www.biomedcentral.com/1741-7015/11/8

76. Cello JP, Rogers SJ: Morbid obesity—the new pandemic: Medical and surgical management, and implications for the practicing gastroenterologist. *Clinical and Translational Gastroenterology* 4:335, 2013. DOI:10.1038/ctg.2013.6

77. Venkataram J: Tumescent liposuction: A review. *Journal of Cutaneous and Aesthetic Surgery* 1(2):49, 2008.

78. Fryar CD, Ogden CL: *Prevalence of underweight among adults 20 years and over: United States, 1960-1962 through 2011-2012.* Last updated September 19, 2014. http://www.cdc.gov/nchs/data/hestat/underweight_adult_11_12/underweight_adult_11_12.htm Accessed October 10, 2014.

14 Eating Disorders and Disordered Eating

Anorexia nervosa

BRANDY IS A 19-YEAR-OLD WOMAN WHO recently completed her first year of college. Before starting school, she was excited about moving away from home and her overprotective parents, but college life and her classes proved to be more stressful and difficult than she expected. After 9 weeks of school, she felt depressed about her grades and the sudden death of her beloved grandmother. When she moved into an all-girls dormitory, she became overly concerned about her body weight and shape, even though her body mass index (BMI) was 20.5.

To prevent putting on additional weight during her first year of college, Brandy avoided eating anything she thought would make her gain weight. She also recorded everything she ate and how many calories each item supplied in a notebook that she always carried with her. She did not like her "flabby legs," so within a few weeks of starting college, she was working out for 2 hours a day while eating no more than 800 kcal daily.

Brandy lost 20 pounds during her first year of college. Her BMI dropped to 16.1 by the end of that school year. Not long after she came home for the summer, her parents took her to see a physician who diagnosed the young woman as having an eating disorder.

- Based on the information about Brandy, which eating disorder does she likely have?
- What are some of the factors that may have contributed to Brandy's development of the eating disorder?
- Explain the kinds of treatment Brandy is likely to receive for the eating disorder.

The suggested Case Study Response can be found on page 476.

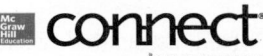

Check out the Connect site at www.mcgrawhillconnect.com to further explore this case study.

QUIZ Yourself

What is the difference between anorexia nervosa and bulimia nervosa? What factors contribute to the development of an eating disorder? What are typical signs of eating disorders? Test your knowledge of eating disorders by taking the following quiz. The answers are found on page 478.

1. Disordered eating behaviors can lead to development of an eating disorder. ___T ___F

2. Young men are more likely to develop eating disorders than young women. ___T ___F

3. Someone who is obese or overweight can have an eating disorder. ___T ___F

4. Anorexia and bulimia are the only types of eating disorders. ___T ___F

5. People with anorexia nervosa can die as a result of the condition. ___T ___F

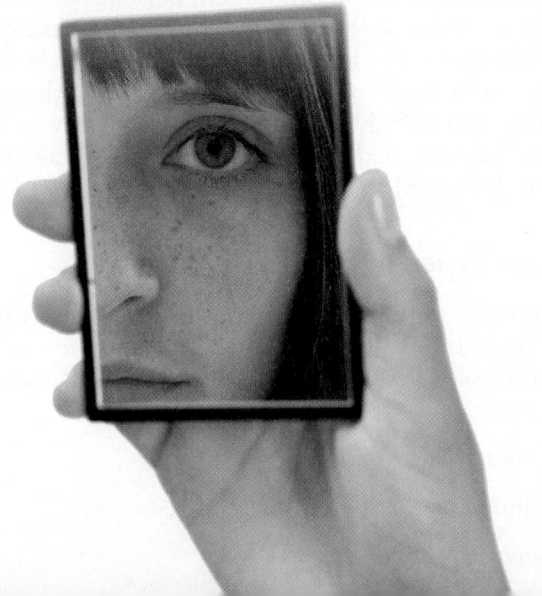

14.1 Introduction to Eating Disorders and Disordered Eating

LEARNING OUTCOMES

1 *Explain the difference between having an eating disorder and practicing disordered eating.*

2 *Identify factors that can contribute to the development of an eating disorder.*

Before the twentieth century in America, a "full–figured" woman such as the one shown in Figure 14.1a had an idealized body shape. At that time, she would have been considered desirable by many men because her shape was a sign that she was healthy, fertile, and prosperous. By the 1960s, the idealized female shape for most Americans had slimmed down considerably (Fig. 14.1b). As a result of this sociocultural shift, many American adolescents and young adults, especially females, are dissatisfied with their body shape and weight.

The media constantly bombards consumers with images of the "ideal" body shape, for both men and women. Television shows and movies often portray thin women or muscular men as happy, intelligent, and successful. As a result of such societal pressures, many young females are inspired to idealize an unhealthy, too–thin body build, and some young men feel the need to lift weights excessively to enlarge their muscle mass. In their efforts to pursue such unrealistic body shapes, young people often adopt unhealthy and potentially life–threatening eating practices. This chapter focuses on eating disorders and disordered eating behaviors.

Eating disorders are psychological disturbances that lead to abnormal food–related behaviors that can have dangerous physiological complications. An eating disorder is not the same as disordered eating. **Disordered eating** is chaotic and abnormal food–related practices, such as skipping meals, limiting food choices, following fad diets, and occasionally eating excessive amounts of food at one time. Disordered eating behaviors are temporary, and they often occur when a person is under a lot of stress or wants to lose weight quickly. When a person adopts disordered eating behaviors as a lifestyle, the practices can become harm–ful and lead to serious eating disorders.

Continuum of Eating Behaviors

The development of unhealthy food–related behaviors is often associated with concerns over body image. As illustrated by the staircase in Figure 14.2, such practices occur on a continuum that has normal and healthy eating behaviors and body image at the top and serious eating disorders and very negative or distorted body image at the bottom. With each step taken down the stairway, the person's eating patterns become more disordered and thoughts about his or her body image become increasingly negative. Not everyone who has disordered eating goes down to the last step and develops an eating disorder. However, the more steps that are taken downward, the greater the person's risk of long–term, harmful consequences.

Major Types of Eating Disorders

According to guidelines published by the American Psychiatric Association (APA) in the fifth edition of the *Diagnostic and Statistical Manual of Mental Disorders* (*DSM–5*), physicians can diagnose three main types of eating disorders:[1]

- Anorexia nervosa (AN);
- Bulimia nervosa (BN); and
- Binge–eating disorder (BED).

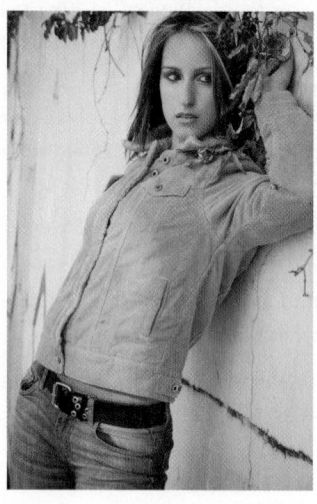

FIGURE 14.1 Idealized female shapes.
(*a*) French artist Edgar Degas made this drawing of a young woman in 1885. (*b*) By the late 1960s, the "ideal" body shape of a young woman had lost much of its curves.

eating disorders psychological disturbances that lead to certain physiological changes and serious health complications

disordered eating chaotic and abnormal food-related practices such as skipping meals, limiting food choices, following fad diets, and bingeing

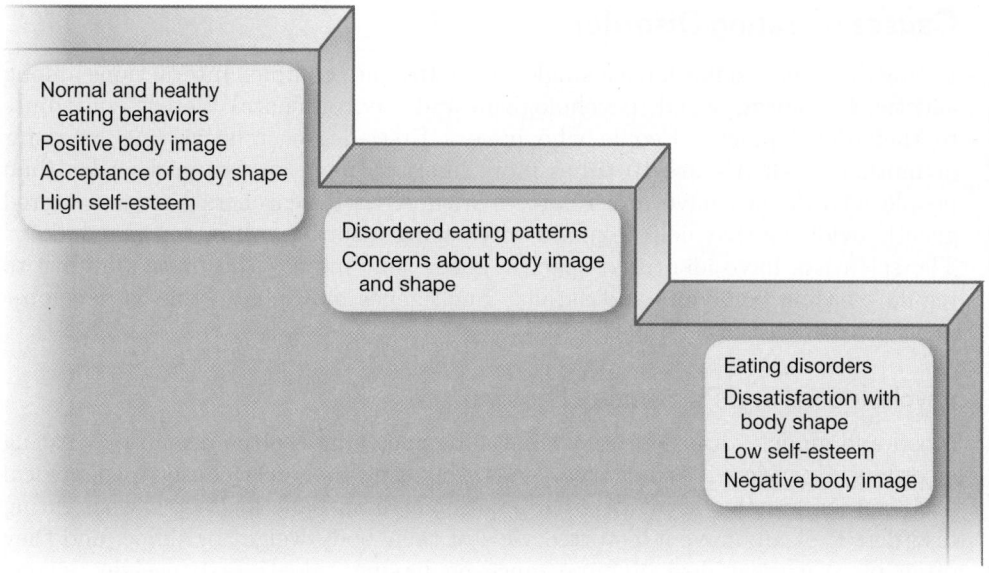

Normal and healthy
  eating behaviors
Positive body image
Acceptance of body shape
High self-esteem

Disordered eating patterns
Concerns about body image
  and shape

Eating disorders
Dissatisfaction with
  body shape
Low self-esteem
Negative body image

**FIGURE 14.2 Eating behaviors and
body image continuum.**

The *DSM−5* also describes "other specified" feeding and eating disorders, which include less severe versions of the three main eating disorders, as well as a condition called *night eating syndrome*. Physicians use the specific criteria reported in the *DSM−5* to diagnose individuals whom they suspect have eating disorders.

Eating Disorders: Risk Factors

As in cases of chronic diseases such as heart disease and cancer, eating disor−ders have risk factors that increase a person's likelihood of developing an eating disorder. These factors include being an adolescent female, having a history of frequent dieting, and having low self−esteem. Table 14.1 lists these and several other risk factors for eating disorders.[1,2]

A person's age is a major factor in predicting his or her risk of a particular eating disorder. Binge−eating disorder is more likely to occur in adults, while AN and BN tend to begin during adolescence.[2] Results of studies of adolescent girls conducted over a long period of time indicated that 13% developed an eating disorder.[3] In general, three factors contribute to an adolescent's vulnerability to develop AN or BN:

- Drastic changes in body weight and shape that normally occur during this life stage;

- Increased reliance on peers for support and approval; and

- Greater independence from parental control over food choices.

TABLE 14.1 Risk Factors for Eating Disorders

Being female
Being an adolescent (AN and BN)
Having a history of frequent dieting
Having a first-degree relative with an eating disorder
Placing a high degree of importance on having an "ideal" body shape
Being dissatisfied with one's body shape
Having a poor self-image and low self-esteem
Having a perfectionist personality
Being from a dysfunctional family
Being in an occupation or sport that emphasizes a lean body build

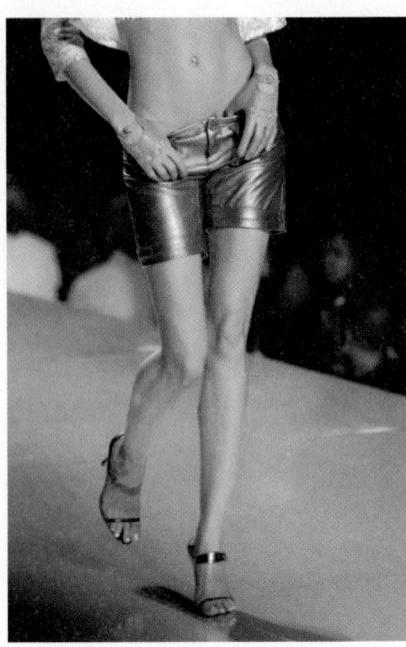

Modeling is an occupation that emphasizes extremely thin body builds.

Causes of Eating Disorders

Eating disorders do not have a single cause. Instead, complex interactions among genetic, biological, social, psychological, and environmental factors contribute to their development. People who have a first—degree relative (e.g., a sister or mother) with AN are 10 times more likely to have an eating disorder than people who do not have any relatives with AN.[4] Researchers have uncovered genetic evidence that helps explain why eating disorders often run in families.[1] The scientists have identified specific genes that modify the brain's ability to regulate eating behaviors and satiety. Such genes may play a role in develop—ment of eating disorders, particularly AN.[4]

Psychological and Personality Factors

Mood and anxiety disorders, as well as substance abuse, often accompany eating disorders. However, it is not clear whether eating disorders cause psychological problems or are the result of such emotional disturbances. People with eating disorders typically have a distorted view of their body weight or shape, and they often place a great deal of importance on having "ideal" body weight, shape, or specific body parts. Being dissatisfied with one's body shape, because it does not match the person's concept of an ideal shape, contributes to having a poor self—image, both of which are risk factors for developing an eating disorder.

People with eating disorders tend to have similar personalities. For exam—ple, people who are diagnosed with AN or BN typically are perfectionists, have obsessive tendencies, and are often fearful and anxious.[5,6]

Persons with binge—eating disorder (BED) or night eating syndrome tend to have a different set of personality traits than persons with AN or BN. People with BED or night eating syndrome often exhibit or express:

- Impulsive decision making;
- Excessive worrying;
- A negative outlook on life;
- Shyness; and
- A poor ability to adapt to different situations.[7]

Other Factors

National origin, income level, occupation, and lifestyle choices contribute to the development of eating disorders in people who are vulnerable to develop them. Eating disorders are most prevalent in industrialized, high—income countries such as the United States, Australia, Canada, Japan, and many European nations.[1] Individuals who participate in activities or occupations that encourage thinness such as ballet, acting, and fashion modeling have an increased risk for developing an eating disorder, especially AN and BN. Athletes, especially those participating in swimming, endurance running, and gymnastics, are at risk (Fig. 14.3).[2] Additionally, athletes who have to "make weight," such as wres—tlers and jockeys, have a higher incidence of eating disorders than athletes in other sports.

Sociocultural and ethnic backgrounds are not helpful in predicting a person's risk of an eating disorder. In the United States, a report indicated that rates of AN, BN, and BED were similar for non—Hispanic white persons, Hispanic Americans, Asians, and African—Americans.[8] In the United States, however, members of ethnic minorities who have an eating disorder are less likely to seek mental health services than are non—Hispanic whites.[8] Therefore, cases of eating disorders among minorities may be underreported and treated less frequently as a result.

FIGURE 14.3 Risky sport. Young people who train for and compete in sports, such as gymnastics, that emphasize small, lean body builds are at risk of certain eating disorders.

Stressful Life Events and Family Dynamics

Adolescents who are at risk of an eating disorder, such as AN, may develop the condition in response to a stressful life event (a "trigger"). For example, moving away from home to attend college is a stressful life event that can trigger an eating disorder.[9] Additionally, the stress of coping with a dysfunctional family can tip a vulnerable adolescent member of that family over the brink and into an eating disorder. Teenagers with eating disorders perceive their parents to be more controlling and less affectionate than the parents of healthy youths.[10] In particular, adolescents with AN report having overprotective and controlling parents, whereas young persons with BN report being a member of a family that is emotionally disengaged ("distant"). In general, individuals with eating disorders describe having a poor emotional connection to their family.

Parents can influence whether their children develop an eating disorder. Adolescents may model unhealthy behaviors of their parents, especially when the teens' mothers are overly focused on their own weight.[11] Furthermore, parents who tease their children about their body weight may foster the youths' development of disordered eating behaviors.[11,12] On a positive note, parents and other caregivers can play an important role in preventing eating disorders among their children by modeling healthy eating behaviors and expressing a positive attitude toward their own bodies.

The following sections provide more specific information about anorexia nervosa, bulimia nervosa, and binge-eating disorder. We also discuss other conditions that are characterized by unhealthy eating and exercise patterns, and we describe measures to prevent and treat these conditions.

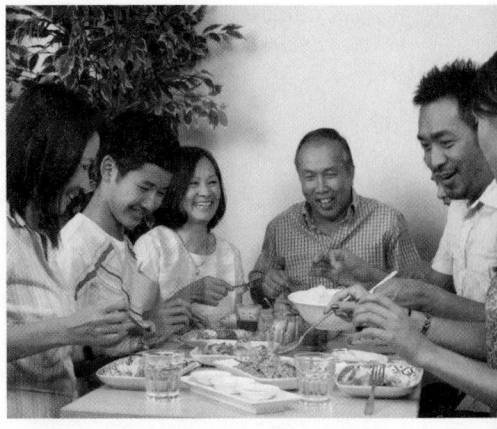

Adult caregivers can play an important role in preventing eating disorders among their children by displaying healthy eating behaviors.

DID YOU *KNOW?*

Sexual or physical abuse during childhood increases the abused child's risk of developing bulimia nervosa.[1]

ASSESS YOUR PROGRESS

1. *Describe the differences between an eating disorder, such as anorexia nervosa, and disordered eating practices.*

2. *How may an individual's personality, lifestyle choices, and family background influence his or her likelihood of developing an eating disorder?*

14.2 Anorexia Nervosa

LEARNING OUTCOMES

1 *Discuss anorexia nervosa, and describe the condition's primary signs and symptoms.*

2 *Identify major health consequences of anorexia nervosa.*

It is not unusual for *anorexia,* loss of appetite, to occur when a person is ill. The anorexia generally resolves as the individual recovers. **Anorexia nervosa (AN)** is a severe psychological disturbance characterized by self-imposed starvation that results in malnutrition and very low body weight **(emaciation)**.

According to estimates, about 0.5% of adolescent American females have AN.[13] Results of an 8-year prospective study of almost 500 American girls indicated that 1 in 120, developed anorexia nervosa by the age of 20.[3] Although males also develop AN, females comprise three times more cases than males.[14]

anorexia nervosa (AN) severe psychological disturbance characterized by self-imposed starvation

emaciation very low body weight

Signs and Symptoms

People with AN have distorted body images and severely restrict their food intake, which leads to rapid weight loss and maintenance of an unhealthy low body weight. Even when they are emaciated, the patients deny they are too thin, and

purging activities that limit calorie intake or increase calorie output

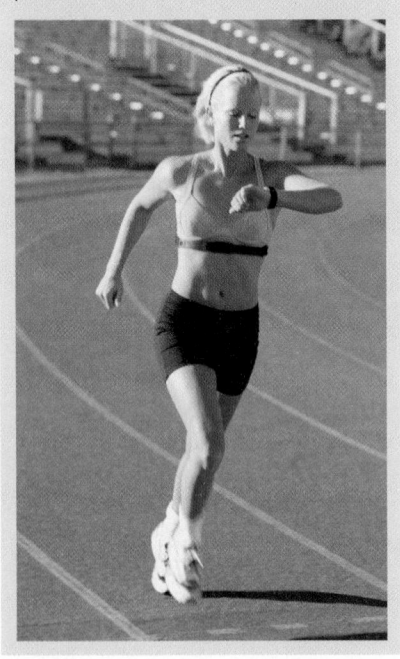

they are overly concerned about becoming fat. An intense fear of weight gain or "becoming fat" compels people with AN to act in ways that hinder weight gain. These behaviors can include frequent dieting, fasting, or exercising excessively.

Some forms of AN involve bingeing and purging behaviors. **Purging** includes activities that remove food (calories) from the body (e.g., self−induced vomiting) or increase calorie output by performing more physical activity than is necessary for optimal health. Although AN does not typically involve purging behaviors, when fasting or food restriction becomes difficult to maintain, someone with AN may try to compensate for eating by self−induced vomiting, misuse of laxatives or diuretics, or excessive exercise.[1]

Because people with AN are so thin, they lack adequate amounts of subcutaneous fat to insulate their bodies and have trouble maintaining their body heat as a result. Therefore, individuals with the disorder often wear layers of clothing to keep warm and hide their emaciated appearance.

People who have AN often display signs and symptoms of other psychological illnesses, particularly depression. Additionally, bipolar, anxiety, and obsessive compulsive disorders can occur with AN. It is not unusual for a person with AN to be preoccupied with thoughts of food and spend hours collecting recipes, hoarding food, or preparing food for others but not eating it.

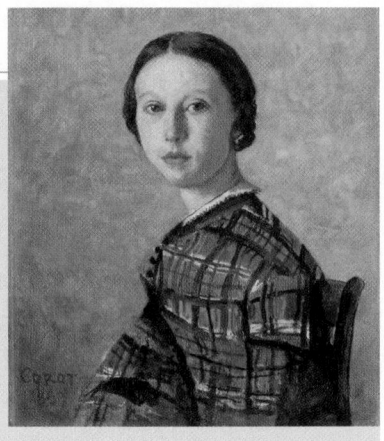

Young woman, mid-nineteenth century.

Diagnosis

To diagnose AN, a physician needs to determine whether the patient's weight is less than "minimally normal." A BMI of 18.5 kg/m^2 is the lowest limit of what is generally considered a normal or healthy body weight for adults.[17]

For children and adolescents, defining a less−than−normal body weight is more difficult. The Centers for Disease Control and Prevention (CDC) recommends using the percentile rank of *BMI−for−age* to assess children's body weight and defines *underweight* as weight that is below the 5th percentile.[1] AN, however, may be diagnosed in any child or adolescent, regardless of his or her weight, when the child meets diagnostic criteria and fails to maintain expected milestones of physical development. To access BMI−for−age charts, visit the CDC's website: http://www.cdc.gov/growthcharts/clinical_charts.htm.

Physiological Consequences

In cases of AN, the severe dietary restriction negatively affects most major organ systems. Table 14.2 lists some common physical consequences of AN. Several of the physiological abnormalities listed in Table 14.2 are reversible during recovery, but many former AN patients do not regain bone tissue that was lost as a result of the malnutrition.

AN has the highest mortality rate of any psychological disorder.[18] Almost 6% of people with AN eventually die as a result of the condition.[19] Primary causes of death include starvation, electrolyte imbalances, and suicide.[18]

Estrogen Insufficiency

If a girl develops AN during her teenage years, the lack of calories and nutritious food slows normal growth and alters normal physical maturation. **Menarche** (*men'—ark'—ee*) is the onset of the first menstrual cycle for female adolescents. A girl will not experience menarche until she has about 17% body fat.[20] **Amenorrhea** (*a—men'—or—ree'—ah*) occurs when regular menstrual cycles (menstruation) do not happen for 3 months or longer in a female who has previously experienced normal cycles. Many adolescent females with AN experience delayed menarche or amenorrhea, because they have lower—than—normal estrogen levels.

ASSESS YOUR PROGRESS

3 *List five signs or symptoms of anorexia nervosa.*

4 *Explain three health risks associated with anorexia nervosa.*

14.3 Bulimia Nervosa

LEARNING OUTCOMES

1 *Discuss bulimia nervosa, and describe the condition's major signs and symptoms.*

2 *Identify health consequences of bulimia nervosa.*

3 *Compare bulimia nervosa and anorexia nervosa.*

Bulimia nervosa (BN) is a severe psychological condition characterized by repeated episodes of *binge eating* followed by purging behaviors to prevent weight gain. **Binge eating** involves eating an amount of food that is much larger than what a normal person would eat in a brief period of time, such as 2 hours. Bingeing typically involves eating "forbidden" foods such as cakes, cookies, ice cream, and other high—fat, high—carbohydrate foods during binges.

People with BN feel they have no control over their eating behavior during binge episodes. After a binge, people with BN feel guilty and depressed. To prevent gaining weight, they purge by self—induced vomiting, abuse of laxatives and/or diuretics, fasting, or excessive exercise. As with AN, a major underlying personal characteristic of BN is having a distorted body image. Some people show behavioral characteristics of both anorexia nervosa and bulimia nervosa, because the illnesses can overlap. About half of the women originally diagnosed as having anorexia nervosa eventually develop signs or symptoms of bulimia.

An estimated 1.0 to 2.9% of Americans have bulimia nervosa.[3] BN usually begins in adolescence or young adulthood.[1] Results of an 8—year prospective study of almost 500 American girls indicated that almost 3% developed BN by the age of 20.[3] Females are 10 times more likely to have BN than males.[1]

Signs and Symptoms

Unlike people who have anorexia nervosa, individuals with bulimia nervosa are often difficult to identify by their appearances, because they tend to have BMIs in the normal or overweight range (between 18.5 and 30). However, people with

TABLE 14.2 Common Physiological Consequences of Anorexia Nervosa

Weakened immune system
Dehydration
Slow heart rate
Hypotension (low blood pressure)
Low bone mineral density
Muscle wasting and weakness
Lanugo (*la-new'-go*)—widespread, white, delicate, and dense hair
Cold intolerance
Low thyroid hormone
Decreased metabolic rate

Source: American Psychiatric Association. Feeding and eating disorders. In: *Diagnostic and Statistical Manual of Mental Disorders.* 5th ed. DOI: 10.1176/appi .books.9780890425596.323864, 2013.

lanugo widespread, white, delicate, and dense hair

menarche onset of the first menstrual cycle

amenorrhea cessation of menstruation for 3 months or longer

bulimia nervosa (BN) severe psychological condition characterized by repeated episodes of binge eating followed by unhealthy behaviors to prevent weight gain

binge eating eating an amount of food that is much larger than what a normal person would eat in a brief period of time

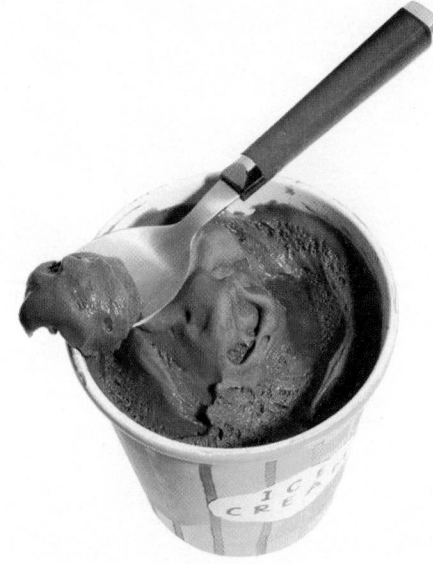

Excessive amounts of ice cream may be consumed during a food binge.

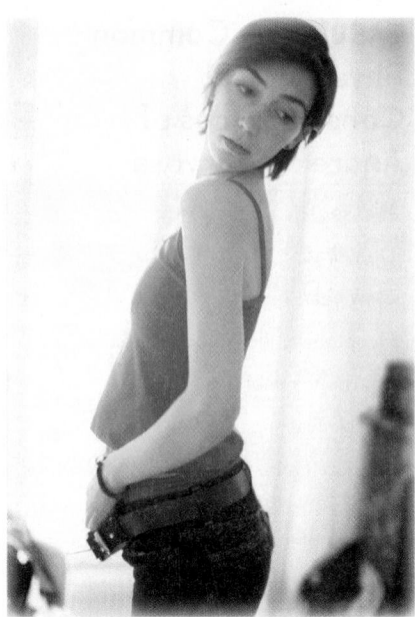

FIGURE 14.4 Binge trigger. Negative feelings about body shape can trigger binges in vulnerable persons.

BN are often ashamed of their food-related behaviors and attempt to conceal their binge-purge practices from others.

People with BN frequently induce vomiting by thrusting fingers deep into their mouths and, as a result, scrape their knuckles. Thus, characteristic signs of bulimia nervosa are bite marks and scars on the knuckles. Dentists often identify people who practice bulimia because the acid in vomit erodes the enamel on the surfaces of teeth, especially the backs of teeth. Eroded teeth develop many dental caries (cavities) and may become chipped and ragged in appearance.

Different triggers may bring on a binge, including social stress, excessive restraint over eating, and negative feelings about body weight and shape (Fig. 14.4). The bingeing activities can help the person with BN feel better in the short term; but guilt, emotional distress, and depression persist in the long term and worsen the disorder. The compelling need to binge and purge eventually becomes a preoccupation for people with BN, and as a result, they become less involved in social activities and more isolated.

Health Risks

The rapid loss of electrolytes and fluid due to self-induced vomiting and diuretic abuse can cause hypokalemia, low blood levels of potassium. Hypokalemia is the

REAL People, REAL Stories

Sarah Marie

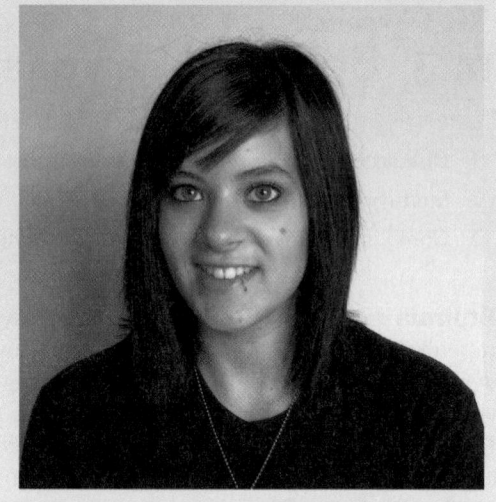

Twenty-year-old Sarah Marie loves animals. She loves them so much, she would like a career that involves animals, but she hasn't made up her mind yet. Underneath her seemingly happy and relaxed surface, Sarah suffers from a serious health condition that has no easy cure. Sarah has bulimia nervosa.

"When I was 12, I weighed 164 pounds and I was 5 feet, 1 inch tall," Sarah says. "My mom and I went on a diet, because she needed to lose weight, too. I just remember the first 10 days of the diet; all you ate was fruit. I don't recall much about the diet after that, but I followed it for 5 months and lost 45 pounds. Losing the weight made me so happy! After that, I got my first boyfriend, but the relationship didn't last and I didn't stay on the diet. I regained about 25 pounds. I tried to control the weight by 'on-and-off dieting'—yo-yo dieting—but it didn't work.

"When I was 16, I tried to do 'negative' calories. I'd walk for 2 hours every single day, and I still didn't think it was enough exercise. I also really limited my food. Some days, I would eat only 800 calories, and for me, that was a big accomplishment. I would eat all my calories within 2 hours early in the day, then I wouldn't eat anything for the rest of the day. I felt a lot of anxiety. . . . I worried about breaking the fast and eating, but I started losing weight again, and that made me feel good. When I looked at the scale, I thought when I reached a certain point, I would be happy. I kept losing weight, but I never felt happy. Soon my weight was 103 pounds. My dad told me that I looked like I walked out of a prison camp, and I took it as a compliment. If I hadn't started bingeing, I would've lost more weight.

"I feel relieved when I binge, but when I feel sick to my stomach, I realize what I've done, and I feel disgusting. I'm fearful that I'm going to gain weight, so I exercise after the binge.

"I've been to a few therapists, but I still have the disorder. I want fast results, but of course, that's not going to happen. I remember a time when I could eat and not worry about it. I wish I could go back then. If you have bulimia, you need to seek help," Sarah advises. "Don't keep it a secret. There's a lot of help out there."

main cause of serious cardiac *arrhythmias* (abnormal heartbeat rhythms), and the condition can cause skeletal muscle damage. Arrhythmias increase the risk of sudden death. Due to repeated vomiting, the salivary glands can become swollen, irritated, and infected. Frequent vomiting also causes tears, ruptures, or bleeding of the esophagus and stomach. Almost 4% of people with BN die as a result of the disorder.[21] One in four of these deaths are due to suicide.[18]

Several psychological disorders are associated with BN. Sometimes these disorders become evident at the same time as BN develops, but other times, the mental health conditions precede the eating disorder. Compared to people who do not have an eating disorder, people with BN are more likely to have low self—esteem, and bipolar, depressive, and personality disorders. Furthermore, some people with BN also abuse alcohol or other mind—altering drugs. Even after recovery, up to 30% of former BN patients continue to struggle with alcohol or drug abuse.[1]

ASSESS YOUR PROGRESS

⑤ Describe *five signs or symptoms of bulimia nervosa.*

⑥ What are *three health risks associated with bulimia nervosa?*

⑦ List *three similarities and three differences between anorexia nervosa and bulimia nervosa.*

14.4 Binge-Eating Disorder

LEARNING OUTCOMES

1 *Discuss binge-eating disorder, and describe the condition's signs and symptoms.*

2 *Compare binge-eating disorder with bulimia nervosa.*

3 *Identify major health consequences of binge-eating disorder.*

Binge—eating disorder (BED) is an eating disorder that features recurrent episodes of overeating that are not followed by purging behaviors.[1] It is common to overeat on holidays or special occasions; however, binge eating involves con—suming a much larger amount of food than most people would eat under similar circumstances in a brief period of time, such as within 2 hours. As observed in cases of BN, people with BED lack control over their eating behavior during a binging episode. People with BED can be normal weight, overweight, or obese. Table 14.3 lists the characteristics that physicians use to diagnose binge—eating disorder.

binge-eating disorder (BED) eating disorder featuring recurrent episodes of binge eating that are not followed by purging behaviors

TABLE 14.3 Common Signs and Symptoms of Binge-Eating Disorder

- Is extremely distressed over the binge-eating behavior
- Eats large amounts of food when not hungry
- Eats more rapidly than normal and until uncomfortably full
- Eats alone because of feeling embarrassed by how much is consumed
- Exhibits **food concocting** (i.e., making and eating strange food mixtures)
- Feels depressed, guilty, or disgusted with him- or herself after the binge
- Binge eats, on average, at least once a week for 3 months

food concocting making and eating strange food combinations

Source: American Psychiatric Association. Feeding and eating disorders. In: *Diagnostic and statistical manual of mental disorders.* 5th ed. DOI: 10.1176/appi.books.9780890425596.323864, 2013.

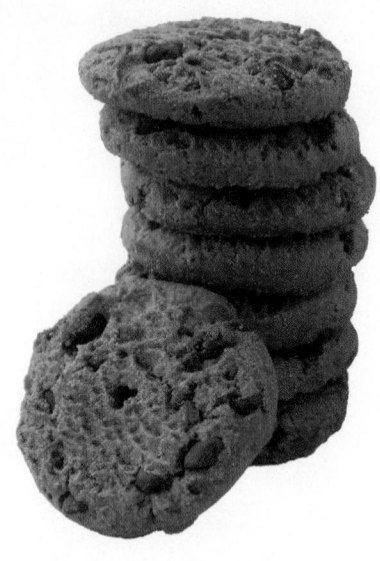

As in cases of the other eating disorders, BED usually begins during adolescence and young adulthood. However, people seeking treatment for BED are usually older than those seeking treatment for AN and BN.[1] People with BED often have other psychological illnesses, such as bipolar, depressive, anxiety, and substance use disorders. Stressful events and feelings of loneliness, anxiety, depression, anger, isolation, and frustration can trigger a food binge. During binges, a person with BED typically isolates him- or herself and consumes large quantities of calorie-dense foods, such as ice cream, cookies, and potato chips. While bingeing, the person may feel better, but after the episode of overeating, this individual usually feels depressed, ashamed, guilty, and disgusted with his or her abnormal eating behavior.

Prevalence and Health Risks

The prevalence of BED is difficult to estimate, but it may be more common than AN and BN.[2] According to one report, 3.5% of adult American women and 2% of adult American men have been diagnosed with binge-eating disorder.[14] An estimated 2.8% of Americans have BED at some point in their lives.

Because people with BED do not use compensatory mechanisms to purge calories, they are at high risk for obesity. Thus, people with BED are more likely to develop diabetes and hypertension than persons who are not obese.

ASSESS YOUR PROGRESS

8 *Describe the characteristics of people with binge-eating disorder.*
9 *What are some health consequences of binge-eating disorder?*
10 *How does binge-eating disorder differ from bulimia nervosa?*

14.5 Night Eating Syndrome and Other Feeding or Eating Disorders

LEARNING OUTCOMES

1 *Describe typical food-related behaviors associated with night eating syndrome.*
2 *Describe signs and symptoms of diabulimia, orthorexia nervosa, and muscle dysmorphia.*

"other specified" feeding or eating disorders disordered eating behavior that does not meet the full criteria for AN, BN, or BED

The *DSM-5* includes a section describing disordered eating behaviors **("other specified" feeding or eating disorders)** that do not meet the full diagnostic criteria for AN, BN, or BED.[1] Table 14.4 describes the "other specified" feeding or eating disorders that can be diagnosed by a physician. Some disordered eating behaviors, such as "diabulimia," are publicized in the media, but these unusual food-related practices are not recognized as eating disorders by the APA. The following sections describe night eating syndrome and some popularized unhealthy eating practices.

Night Eating Syndrome

night eating syndrome (NES) episodic food binges that are not followed by purging; binges take place after the evening meal and when the person wakens from sleep during the night

People with **night eating syndrome (NES)** experience episodic food binges that are not followed by purging. These binges take place after the evening meal and when the person wakens from sleep during the night. A person with NES may regularly consume 50% of his or her 24-hour calorie intake after the evening meal.[22] The condition is characterized by sleep disturbances, waking up during the night

TABLE 14.4 "Other Specified" Feeding or Eating Disorders

Other Specified Disorder	Description
Night eating syndrome	Repeated bouts of eating after awakening from sleep or excessive food intake after the evening meal
Atypical anorexia nervosa	Meets all of the criteria for AN except the affected person's weight is normal
Bulimia nervosa of low frequency and/or limited duration	Meets all of the criteria for BN except the disordered behaviors do not happen frequently enough or have been practiced for less than 3 months
Binge-eating disorder of low frequency and/or limited duration	Meets all of the criteria for BED except bingeing occurs, on average, less than once per week or the affected person has been bingeing for less than 3 months
Purging disorder	Recurrent purging behavior in attempt to lose weight or alter body shape without binge eating

Source: American Psychological Association: *Diagnostic and statistical manual of mental health disorders.* 5th ed. DOI: 10.1176/appi.books.9780890425596.323864, 2013.

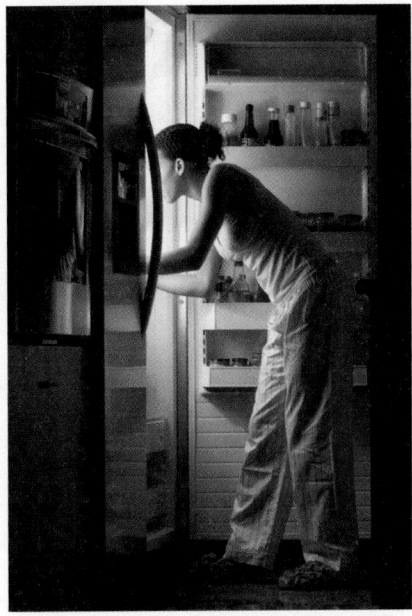

People who have night eating syndrome experience repeated bouts of eating after awakening from sleep or eating excessive food after the evening meal.

to binge eat, and the belief that one can only fall asleep after eating a large meal.[22] NES should not be confused with sleep walking, because people with NES are aware of their actions and can recall their overnight eating practices the next day.

Approximately 1 to 2% of the general population may have NES.[23,24] A major difference between BED and NES is that people with NES believe that they can only fall asleep by having a full stomach. Someone with NES will have no appetite in the morning and a depressed mood that worsens as the day progresses. It is common for people with NES to have erratic and unscheduled mealtimes during the day, which may contribute to their extreme eating behaviors at night.[22]

Anyone, regardless of his or her body weight, can have NES; however, the disorder is more likely to develop as body weight increases. Between 6 and 16% of the people seeking weight−loss treatment may have NES.[23] People with NES who are normal weight may compensate for night bingeing by eating less during the day or by burning more calories through increased physical activity.

Diabulimia, Orthorexia, and Muscle Dysmorphia

Some other disordered eating patterns, such as *diabulimia, orthorexia,* and *muscle dysmorphia,* are publicized in the media but are not recognized by the American Psychiatric Association to be included in the *DSM−5.* Although physicians do not have the criteria to diagnose these unhealthy behavioral patterns, it is important for health professionals, and dietitians in particular, to be aware of them.

It is not uncommon for a people with type 1 diabetes to forget to take their insulin, especially when they first begin treatment. However, some people with the chronic disease discover they can manipulate their body weight by skipping insulin injections or using less insulin than prescribed (Fig. 14.5). This abusive practice is often referred to as "**diabulimia**." An estimated 11 to 42% of young women with type 1 diabetes reduce or skip insulin to avoid weight gain or induce weight loss.[25] Table 14.5 lists signs and symptoms of diabulimia, some of which are signs of poorly controlled type 1 diabetes.

Complications of long−term diabulimia include blindness, kidney failure, hypertension, heart attack, permanent heart damage, stroke, and nerve damage.[26] When extensive, the nerve damage may require amputation of toes, fingers, and other extremities. Women with type 1 diabetes who use less insulin than pre−scribed have higher rates of disease complications and three times greater risk of death than women with type 1 diabetes who use insulin appropriately.[26]

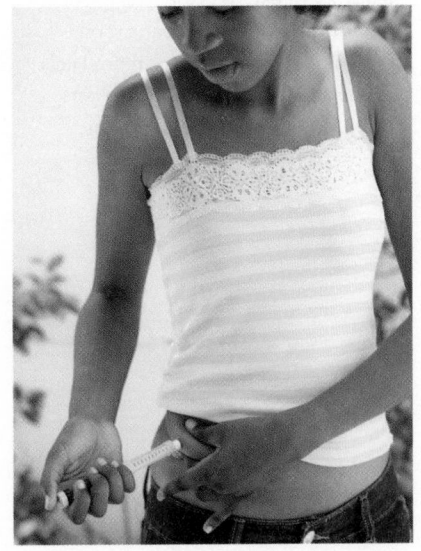

FIGURE 14.5 Diabulimia. Some people with type 1 diabetes manipulate their body weight by using less insulin than prescribed.

diabulimia term used to describe people with type 1 diabetes who manipulate their body weight by skipping insulin injections or using less insulin than prescribed

TABLE 14.5 Signs and Symptoms of Diabulimia

- High blood glucose levels
- Rapid change in body weight
- Obsession with food, weight, and/or body image
- Irregular eating patterns
- Hiding food and eating in secret
- Low energy levels
- Breath that smells "fruity"
- Frequent urination
- Repeated episodes of diabetic ketoacidosis (see Chapter 5)

orthorexia nervosa (ON) condition characterized by an extreme obsession with eating healthy foods

muscle dysmorphia unhealthy preoccupation with the body being too small or not muscular enough

DID YOU KNOW?

Students who choose to major in nutrition and/or dietetics may have a history of eating disorders. Results of studies suggest that registered dietitians/nutritionists are more likely to have disordered eating patterns than people in other professions.[30]

Insulin treatment for someone who is recently diagnosed with type 1 diabetes often leads to weight gain, and this situation can be difficult for someone with a poor body image. It is important for health care professionals to help adolescents with type 1 diabetes find safe ways to manage their weight.

"Orthorexia" (orthorexia nervosa or ON) is an extreme obsession with eating healthy foods, but the condition lacks official diagnostic criteria. Unlike other eating disorders in which the person's usual goal is weight loss, an individual with ON strives for the "perfect" and "pure" diet.

Orthorexia nervosa generally begins when a person makes an effort to select healthy foods. The behavior then evolves into a pattern of classifying foods as "good" or "clean," "bad" and "forbidden." The affected person avoids all foods that he or she believes are unhealthy or "impure." This behavior can lead to a diet that is nutritionally unbalanced and lacks moderation, and it can progress into a starvation diet. People who are at risk of developing ON include dietitians, medical students, dancers, and competitive athletes.[27,28]

Muscle dysmorphia is an unhealthy preoccupation with the body being too small or not muscular enough.[1] This condition occurs almost exclusively in men, and it is common among body builders. More than 50% of men with muscle dysmorphia have used anabolic steroids to help gain weight and increase muscle size.[29]

People with muscle dysmorphia exercise obsessively and may lift weights for hours every day. They can become so obsessed with exercise that they continue to train despite injury, and they allow exercise to take priority over work, school, and friends.

Like people who have AN, individuals with muscle dysmorphia tend to follow rigid diets, be preoccupied with their weight, have distorted body image, and abuse diet pills. However, people with muscle dysmorphia have an irrational pursuit of weight gain, rather than weight loss, as in cases of AN. People with muscle dysmorphia are more likely to drop out of school, and they have a high risk of suicide.[1]

DID YOU KNOW?

Researchers have identified a relationship between alcohol consumption, disordered eating, and physical activity among college students. Highly physically active college students are more likely to binge drink than their less active peers.[31] Individuals who binge drink may use exercise or fasting as a way to compensate for the extra calories consumed during a night of heavy drinking. This disordered behavior has been called "drunkorexia," but this is not a medically accepted term.

ASSESS YOUR PROGRESS

11 *What is night eating syndrome, and how does it differ from binge-eating disorder?*

12 *What are the consequences of diabulimia?*

13 *How is muscle dysmorphia similar to AN?*

14.6 Female Athlete Triad

LEARNING OUTCOMES

1 *Identify the components of the female athlete triad.*

2 *List the most serious health consequences of the female athlete triad.*

Adolescent girls and young women need to have the energy available from their diet to support reproductive and bone health. Women and girls participating in competitive sports or sports and activities that benefit from a low body mass, such as gymnastics, dance, and distance running, are at risk of developing one or more components of the **female athlete triad** (Fig. 14.6). This condition is characterized by three interrelated components:

- **Low energy availability** (negative energy balance);

- Menstrual disturbances that often include amenorrhea; and

- Reduced bone mineral density.

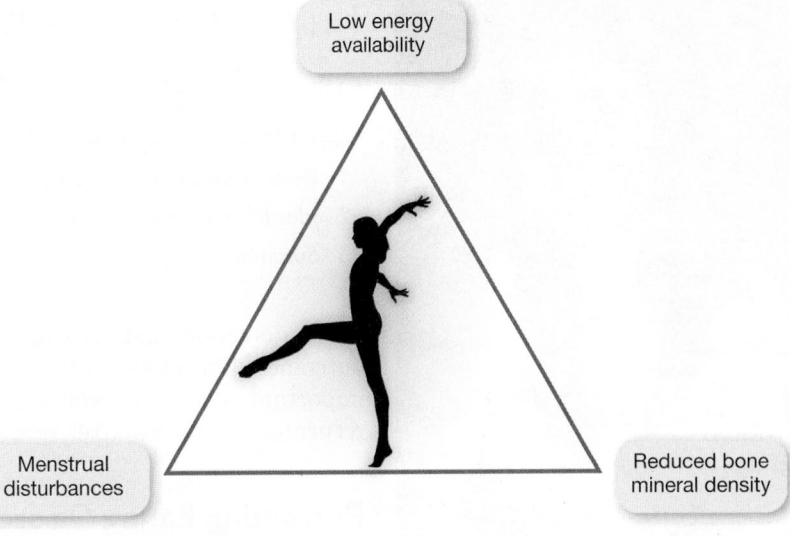

As many as 16% of female athletes have all three components of the triad.[32] Females participating in a sport that emphasizes a lean physique are more likely to have all three triad components than females who participate in sports that do not place much emphasis on leanness. It is also common for female athletes to exhibit one or two of the components, rather than all three. The most serious health outcomes of the triad are eating disorders, amenorrhea, and osteoporosis.

FIGURE 14.6 Female athlete triad.

female athlete triad condition that occurs as a result of the interrelationships among energy availability, menstrual function, and bone mineral density in female athletes

low energy availability state of negative energy balance

Health Consequences of the Female Athlete Triad

Female athletes have a higher risk of disordered eating practices and eating disorders than males and females who do not participate in sports.[33] The young women may intentionally restrict their calorie intake to improve athletic performance, lose weight, or maintain a lean physique. However, the low energy availability component of the triad may occur in the absence of an eating disorder. This situation can occur when female athletes lack the appetite, nutrition knowledge, or time to consume enough energy to meet their high needs and maintain a healthy BMI, especially during periods of intense physical training.

Females of childbearing age need adequate amounts of energy to maintain normal menstrual cycles. Low energy availability is associated with estrogen deficiency.[33] The lack of estrogen causes menstrual disturbances, such as longer−than−normal intervals between menstrual periods and amenorrhea.

Weight−bearing exercise normally contributes to high bone mineral density. However, female athletes who have low energy availability and amenorrhea can have low bone mineral density and an increased risk for fracture, especially stress fractures.

Estrogen is needed to build and maintain bone mineral mass. Thus, young women with low estrogen levels may not build bone mass normally, and their bones may lose bone mass. Almost 50% of an adult's bone mass is developed during adolescence. When the lack of estrogen occurs during such a critical time for bone growth, the female athlete's bone mineral density may not improve even after recovery from the triad.[34] Girls and young women who have low bone mineral density may experience serious and long−term consequences, including premature osteoporosis.

ASSESS YOUR PROGRESS

14 *What are the three components of the female athlete triad?*

15 *What are some of the long-term health consequences of the female athlete triad?*

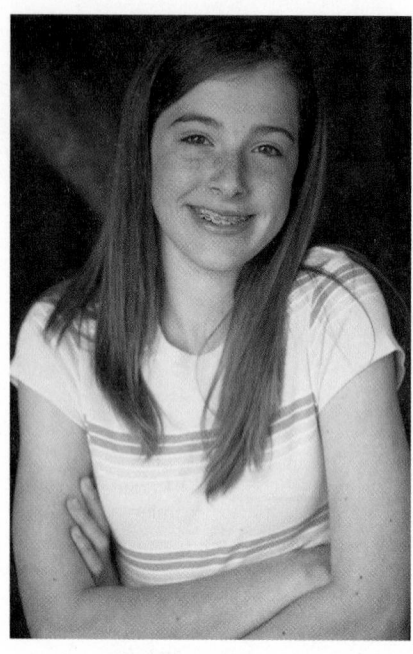

The best time to deliver education programs to help prevent eating disorders is when children are in early adolescence.

14.7 Prevention and Treatment of Eating Disorders

LEARNING OUTCOMES

1 *Discuss methods that may be used to prevent eating disorders.*
2 *Identify treatment goals for the three major eating disorders.*
3 *Summarize approaches to treatment of eating disorders.*

Early detection and treatment of eating disorders are important for the best outcomes. For adolescents with an eating disorder, parents and siblings can play important roles in prevention, recovery, and avoidance of *relapse*, which is the return of symptoms after recovery.[11]

Preventing Eating Disorders

According to the Academy of Nutrition and Dietetics, prevention may be one of the most cost—effective ways to approach eating disorders.[2] Early identification of people with risk factors, such as disordered eating patterns and distorted body images, can help prevent the development of eating disorders. Once someone has been identified as at risk for an eating disorder, prevention efforts should focus on fostering the individual's body acceptance, improving his or her self—confidence, and encouraging the person to challenge the idea that being thin is ideal.

Education programs designed to improve body image can help to prevent children from developing eating disorders.[35] The best time to deliver such programming is when adolescents are between 12 and 14 years of age. The positive benefits of the education remain for at least 6 months after the intervention.[35] More research is needed to determine whether eating disorder prevention programs are effective for longer terms.

The best approach to preventing the female athlete triad is to provide information about the disorder to parents and the people in sports who associate with the young women, including coaches and trainers.[34,36] Thus, a preparticipation screening of athletes could be required to assess the person's risk for the triad. An athlete who has one component of the triad, such as menstrual disturbances, should be screened for the other components.[34]

DID **YOU** KNOW?

Girls on the Run® is a nonprofit organization that provides girls in grades three through eight with tools to recognize their personal strengths and handle life's experiences effectively and confidently. The educational program also encourages the development of positive self-esteem, healthy food-related attitudes and behaviors, and body size satisfaction. Running is a core component of the girls' education. At the end of each 24-lesson program, members participate in a 5K noncompetitive running event that fosters a sense of accomplishment among the girls. For more information about the program, visit https://www.girlsontherun.org/.

Treating Eating Disorders

Treatment of eating disorders requires professional help from those with expertise in helping people with these conditions. If you or someone you know has an

FRESH TIPS

When you suspect someone has an eating disorder, it may be difficult to talk with that person about your concerns. Consider following these recommendations when approaching the individual to discuss his or her food-related behaviors:

1. Meet with the person privately and without distractions.

2. Share your feelings and concerns in a compassionate and supportive manner.

3. Describe occasions when you observed behaviors that were signs of an eating disorder and may indicate the person needs professional care.

4. Avoid using harsh or accusatory language and instead focus on explaining how you feel. For example, instead of stating, "You've lost too much weight. You look like you're starving!" say, "I feel very worried about how much weight you've lost."

5. Do not suggest simple solutions, such as: "If you'd just start eating meals with the family again, I know you'll eat and feel better!"

6. Suggest that the person discuss your concerns with an expert who is involved in the treatment of eating disorders, such as a psychotherapist, dietitian, physician, or nurse. Offer to help find such an expert, make an appointment, or accompany the individual on the first visit.

7. Avoid creating conflict. If the person denies that he or she has an eating disorder, repeat your concerns and indicate that you will be available to help in the future.

8. At the end of the conversation, share your desire to be supportive. For example, remind the person that you want him or her to be happy and healthy.[37]

eating disorder, it is important to seek medical care for the condition as soon as possible to avoid serious health consequences. In academic environments, professional help is often available at student health centers and student guidance or counseling facilities on campus.

A multidisciplinary group of experts in nutrition, mental health, and medicine is necessary for optimal treatment of eating disorders.[2] Treatment should include psychotherapy while also addressing critical nutritional needs and other existing medical conditions. Registered dietitians play a critical role in the assessment and treatment of eating disorders. Dietitians can answer patients' questions about foods and nutrition, and can provide information about healthy eating patterns. As members of the multidisciplinary treatment team, registered dietitians can improve patients' nutrient status by providing appropriate medical nutrition therapy. Furthermore, dietitians can play an important role in helping patients avoid relapse while their recovery is underway.[2]

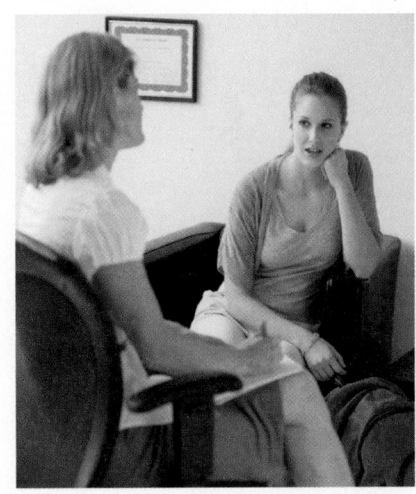

Professional counseling is often necessary for the treatment of eating disorders.

Treatment Settings and Approaches

Treatment for eating disorders can occur in several settings.[38] Inpatient hospitalization or residential care in a facility that specializes in the treatment of the disorders may be required when the patient's weight loss has been so extreme that the resulting medical complications become life threatening. However, eating disorder treatment generally occurs in outpatient care settings, which may involve group or family counseling. Supportive activities such as yoga, art, massage, and movement therapy may also be used during treatment. In addition, having patients participate in eating disorder support groups may help prevent relapse.

Medications Treatment of eating disorders may involve prescription medications. Only one prescription medication has been approved by the U.S. Food and

Drug Administration specifically for treatment of eating disorders.[38] Fluoxetine (Prozac®) has been shown to reduce binge episodes and aid in recovery of BN. Other medications may be prescribed to treat conditions that frequently occur with eating disorders, such as depressive, bipolar, anxiety, and obsessive–compulsive disorders. Medications that increase feelings of satiety may be prescribed to help prevent binges in patients with BN or BED.

cognitive behavioral therapy (CBT) psychological treatment approaches that address unhealthy behavior by challenging current beliefs and replacing them with more realistic thoughts

Behavioral Therapies **Cognitive behavioral therapy (CBT)** is a major treatment approach for BN and BED.[2] CBT is a general term used to describe therapy approaches that address unhealthy emotions and behavior. The therapy follows a goal–oriented, systematic process that challenges the patient's current beliefs and attempts to replace them with realistic thoughts. The most effective CBT approach for treating eating disorders involves three overlapping phases.[38] The first phase educates the patient about the dangers of the eating disorder in an effort to decrease his or her unhealthy behaviors. The second phase reduces the patient's use of dietary restraint and improves regular eating patterns. During this phase, consulting with a dietitian can help the patient with food planning. The last phase focuses on relapse prevention strategies. Successful behavioral therapy teaches people healthy coping strategies to use when under stress instead of fasting, bingeing, purging, or exercising excessively.[38]

dialectical behavioral therapy (DBT) form of psychotherapy that strives to improve skills used to manage stress, anxiety, or feelings of inadequacy

Treatment of eating disorders may include **dialectical behavioral therapy (DBT)**.[2] DBT is a form of psychotherapy that strives to improve skills used to manage stress, anxiety, or feelings of inadequacy. With this treatment, people with eating disorders attempt to replace high–risk behaviors such as bingeing and starvation with healthy eating habits that encourage dietary moderation. DBT is shown to be effective in treating BED and BN.[2] CBT and DBT can help patients learn to change unhealthy beliefs about themselves, accept themselves, and use alternative methods to cope with stressful situations.

Although family dysfunction contributes to the development of eating disorders, it is not a primary cause. However, family–based therapy can be an important part of the treatment plan, especially for adolescents with eating disorders.[2]

phototherapy exposure to certain wavelengths of light by use of a specific lamp for prescribed amounts of time

Treating "Other Specified" Feeding and Eating Disorders In addition to the therapies described above, phototherapy may be an important part of treating night eating syndrome (NES).[22] **Phototherapy** involves exposure to certain wavelengths of light through use of a specific lamp for prescribed amounts of time. The light exposure may regulate the sleep–wake cycle and improve sleep patterns. Also, use of progressive muscular relaxation to reduce stress may be helpful for treating NES.[22]

For someone with diabulimia, the treatment team should include health care professionals who have expertise in diabetes mellitus and insulin use, such as an endocrinologist and diabetes educator.[39] It is important to teach people with type 1 diabetes about the dangers of reducing insulin.

Treatment of the female athlete triad strives to create a state of energy balance by increasing calorie intake, decreasing energy expenditure, or a combination of both. Athletes should be advised to eat on a regular schedule and increase their caloric intake when their training intensifies.[34] Incorporating a weight–training or high–impact activity, such as jumping, into the patient's exercise regimen may help increase bone mineral density during treatment. Additionally, female athletes can learn ways to increase their calcium and vitamin D intakes.

Challenges to Recovery

A person with AN or BN may deny that there is a problem and resist treatment. Thus, treatment of eating disorders is most effective when the patient is ready to make changes to his or her harmful behaviors.

Although nearly half of patients fully recover from AN, the illness becomes chronic in about 20% of cases. Young patients who do not binge eat or purge and who have good relationships with their parents are more likely to recover. However, patients who begin treatment for AN at a later age or who abuse alcohol are more likely to have poor long—term outcomes than patients who obtain help at a younger age and do not abuse alcohol.[19] As mentioned earlier, AN has the highest mortality rate of any psychological disorder.[18]

Approximately 60% of persons with bulimia nervosa improve with treatment.[40] People with BN who struggle with relapse often suffer from more severe depression than those who respond well to treatment. Treatment of BED is successful when it reduces or stops binge episodes; however, weight loss does not always accompany recovery.[40]

ASSESS YOUR PROGRESS

16 *List the professionals who should be involved with the treatment of eating disorders.*

17 *What is cognitive behavioral therapy, and how is it used to treat eating disorders?*

18 *What are some of the challenges for patients recovering from eating disorders?*

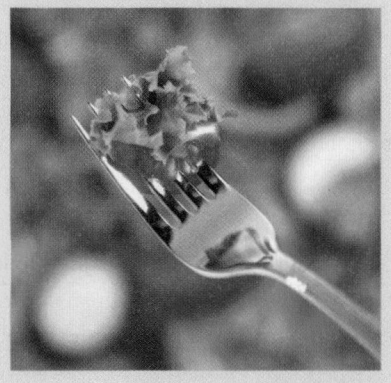

SUMMARY

SECTION 14.1 Introduction to Eating Disorders and Disordered Eating

- Eating disorders are psychological disturbances that cause abnormal physiological changes that have dangerous health consequences. The three types of eating disorders are anorexia nervosa, bulimia nervosa, and binge-eating disorder.

- Disordered eating is chaotic and abnormal food-related practices. Disordered eating behaviors are temporary.

- Risk factors for eating disorders include being a female, dieting frequently, and having low self-esteem. People who are diagnosed with the same eating disorder may share certain personality traits.

SECTION 14.2 Anorexia Nervosa

- Anorexia nervosa is a severe psychological disturbance characterized by self-imposed starvation that results in malnutrition and low body weight.

- A major underlying feature of anorexia nervosa is a distorted body image. Many people with the condition also display signs and symptoms of depression.

- People suffering from anorexia nervosa have a high risk of dying from starvation, electrolyte imbalances, or suicide.

SECTION 14.3 Bulimia Nervosa

- Bulimia nervosa is a severe psychological condition characterized by repeated episodes of binge eating followed by unhealthy compensatory behaviors in order to prevent weight gain.

- Persons with bulimia nervosa often have low self-esteem and feel guilty or depressed after a binge. The fluid and electrolyte imbalances caused by purging activities of bulimia nervosa can be life threatening.

SECTION 14.4 **Binge-Eating Disorder**

- Binge-eating disorder is an eating disorder featuring recurrent episodes of binge eating that are not followed by purging behaviors. BED increases risk of obesity, diabetes, and hypertension.

SECTION 14.5 **Night Eating Syndrome and Other Feeding or Eating Disorders**

- People with night eating syndrome experience episodic food binges (without purging) that take place after awakening from sleep or after the evening meal.
- Diabulimia, orthorexia nervosa, and muscle dysmorphia are not recognized as eating disorders by the American Psychiatric Association.

SECTION 14.6 **Female Athlete Triad**

- The female athlete triad is a condition characterized by low energy availability, abnormal menstrual function, and reduced bone mineral density in female athletes.

SECTION 14.7 **Prevention and Treatment of Eating Disorders**

- Early identification of people with disordered eating patterns and distorted body image is an important part of preventing eating disorders.
- Education programs designed to improve body image among adolescents may help prevent the development of eating disorders.
- Treatment of eating disorders requires a multidisciplinary approach. Cognitive behavioral therapy (CBT) is a major treatment approach for bulimia nervosa and binge-eating disorder.

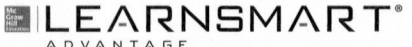 Get the most out of your study of nutrition with McGraw-Hill's innovative suite of adaptive learning products including McGraw-Hill LearnSmart®, SmartBook®, McGraw-Hill LearnSmart Achieve®, and McGraw-Hill LearnSmart Prep®. Visit www.learnsmartadvantage.com.

CASE STUDY RESPONSE

ANOREXIA NERVOSA

BASED ON THE INFORMATION PROVIDED, Brandy probably has anorexia nervosa (AN). Many factors may contribute to the development of Brandy's eating disorder. For example, she is female and, at 19 years old, is an age at which eating disorders are most likely to occur. Additionally, Brandy has controlling parents and recently experienced stressful changes in her life, including the often stressful transition from high school to college, death of a grandmother, and living away from her childhood home.

Brandy's treatment is likely to be a multidisciplinary approach that involves experts in nutrition, psychology, and medicine. Her treatment may be outpatient and will probably include psychotherapy, nutritional counseling, and possibly medication to help manage her depressive symptoms.

Critical Thinking

1. Sabrina's BMI is 23.2. You and her other friends are amazed because she eats lots of food without gaining weight and she is not physically active. After meals, she goes to the bathroom with her toothbrush, and when you use the bathroom after she has been in it, you notice the room has an unusual, unpleasant odor. Explain why you suspect Sabrina has an eating disorder.

2. A doll manufacturer wants to design male and female dolls with adult body shapes that would promote healthier and more realistic body images among the children who will play with them.

Describe how you would design the shapes of the new male and female dolls to meet the manufacturer's health-related concept for the toys.

3. Explain why eating disorders such as anorexia nervosa and binge-eating disorder are more common in developed countries than in poorer nations, such as Afghanistan, Bangladesh, and much of Africa.

4. Regardless of weather conditions, Karina spends at least 2 hours each day jogging on her high school's track. She only eats salads, apples, and plain canned tuna. She is 5-feet, 6-inches tall, and she weighs 110 pounds. Based on this information, which eating disorder do you suspect Karina has? Explain why you chose this particular disorder.

5. Your roommate is a dance major who you suspect has an eating disorder. She is very thin, spends several hours each day practicing ballet in the dance studio, and has some odd eating practices. Discuss how you approach your roommate to express your concerns about her health and well-being. Include resources that are available at your college or in your community to help persons with eating disorders.

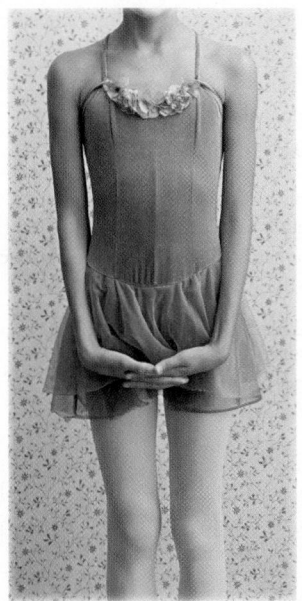

Practice Test

Select the best answer.

1. Joseph's BMI is 23. When he is under a lot of stress, he eats a large amount of empty-calorie foods. Soon after eating these foods, he goes to a bathroom and makes himself vomit. Based on this information, Joseph probably has
   a. diabulimia.
   b. anorexia nervosa.
   c. binge-eating disorder.
   d. bulimia nervosa.

2. Which of the following conditions is not an eating disorder that physicians can diagnose using criteria that are in the *DSM-5*?
   a. diabulimia
   b. anorexia nervosa
   c. binge-eating disorder
   d. bulimia nervosa

3. People who have anorexia nervosa typically
   a. have a distorted body image.
   b. consume most of their calories during the overnight hours.
   c. have BMIs between 18.5 and 20.0.
   d. consume foods that they think are healthy.

4. Which of the following behaviors is an example of a purging activity that is often used by people with bulimia nervosa to avoid weight gain?
   a. avoiding "white" foods, such as white sugar and flour
   b. abusing laxatives
   c. eating only organic foods
   d. sleeping for fewer than 6 hours per night

5. Having _____ is a sign of anorexia nervosa.
   a. a BMI of 19.4
   b. hypertension
   c. lanugo
   d. an increased metabolic rate

6. A person with _____ is more likely to die from the condition than from any other psychological disturbance.
   a. orthorexia nervosa
   b. diabulimia
   c. obsessive compulsive disorder
   d. anorexia nervosa

7. A major approach for treating binge-eating disorder is
   a. antipsychotic medication.
   b. electroshock treatment.
   c. cognitive behavioral therapy.
   d. bariatric surgery.

8. Phototherapy may be used to treat
   a. female athlete triad.
   b. muscle dysmorphia.
   c. anorexia nervosa.
   d. night eating syndrome.

9. Which of the following medications has been approved by the Food and Drug Administration to treat eating disorders?
   a. fluoxetine
   b. paroxetine
   c. citalopram
   d. bupropion

10. Which of the following conditions primarily affects men?

    a. night eating syndrome
    b. bulimia nervosa
    c. muscle dysmorphia
    d. binge-eating disorder

11. Fiona is very health conscious. She limits her diet to foods that she describes are "clean" or "pure." She will not eat red meat, sugar, flour, and milk because she believes they are not clean. Based on this information, Fiona probably has

    a. binge-eating disorder.
    b. orthorexia nervosa.
    c. muscle dysmorphia.
    d. anorexia nervosa.

12. Although Jemma's BMI is in the healthy range, she thinks her hips and thighs are too fat. She does not binge eat, but she often uses self-induced vomiting after eating to maintain her weight. Based on this information, Jemma probably has

    a. anorexia nervosa.
    b. diabulimia.
    c. orthorexia nervosa.
    d. purging disorder.

13. Jason lifts weights for at least 3 hours every other day. His shoulder and upper arm muscles are so large, he has difficulty raising his arms to comb his hair. Despite his muscular body build, Jason thinks he needs to increase the size of his muscles even more. Based on this information, Jason probably has

    a. bulimia nervosa.
    b. orthorexia nervosa.
    c. muscle dysmorphia.
    d. binge-eating disorder.

14. Which of the following characteristics is a sign of night eating syndrome?

    a. hyperactivity in the early evening
    b. lack of appetite in the morning
    c. purging immediately after bingeing
    d. inability to digest simple carbohydrates after midnight

15. Kayla has type 1 diabetes, but she frequently skips giving herself insulin because she does not want to gain weight. Based on this information, Kayla probably has

    a. anorexia nervosa.
    b. diabulimia.
    c. hyperinsulinemia.
    d. muscle dysmorphia.

1-d; 2-a; 3-a; 4-b; 5-c; 6-d; 7-c; 8-d; 9-a; 10-c; 11-b; 12-d; 13-c; 14-b; 15-b

ANSWERS TO PRACTICE TEST

ANSWERS TO CHAPTER 14 QUIZ Yourself

1. Disordered eating behaviors can lead to development of an eating disorder. **True** (p. 460)
2. Young men are more likely to develop eating disorders than young women. **False** (p. 461)
3. Someone who is obese or overweight can have an eating disorder. **True** (pp. 465, 467)
4. Anorexia and bulimia are the only types of eating disorders. **False** (p. 460)
5. People with anorexia nervosa can die as a result of the condition. **True** (p. 465)

References

1. American Psychiatric Association. Feeding and eating disorders. In: *Diagnostic and statistical manual of mental disorders.* 5th ed. DOI: 10.1176/appi. books.9780890425596.323864, 2013.

2. Ozier AD, Henry BW: Position of the American Dietetic Association: Nutrition intervention in the treatment of eating disorders. *Journal of the American Dietetic Association* 111(8):1236, 2011.

3. Stice E and others: Prevalence, incidence, impairment, and course of the proposed DSM-5 eating disorder diagnoses in an 8-year prospective community study of young women. *Journal of Abnormal Psychology* 122(2):455, 2013.

4. Pinheiro AP and others: The genetics of anorexia nervosa: Current findings and future perspectives. *International Journal of Child and Adolescent Health* 2(2):153, 2009.

5. Keel PK, Forney JK: Psychosocial risk factors for eating disorders. *International Journal of Eating Disorders* 46(5):433, 2013.

6. Kaye WH and others: Does a shared neurobiology for foods and drugs of abuse contribute to extremes of food ingestion in anorexia and bulimia nervosa? *Biological Psychiatry* 73:836, 2013.

7. Dalle Grave R and others: Personality features of obese women in relation to binge eating and night eating. *Psychiatry Research* 207:86, 2013.

8. Marques L and others: Comparative prevalence, correlates of impairment, and service utilization for eating disorders across US ethnic groups: Implications for reducing ethnic disparities in health care access for eating disorders. *International Journal of Eating Disorders* 44(5):412, 2011.

9. Attia E, Walsh BT: Anorexia nervosa. *American Journal of Psychiatry* 164(12):1805, 2007.

10. Dimitropoulos G and others: Inpatients with severe anorexia nervosa and their siblings: Non-shared experiences and family functioning. *European Eating Disorders Review* 21:284, 2013.

11. Quiles-Marcos Y and others: Peer and family influence in eating disorders: A meta-analysis. *European Psychiatry* 28:199, 2013.

12. Helfert S, Warschburger P: The face of appearance-related social pressure: Gender, age and body mass variations in peer and parental pressure during adolescence. *Child and Adolescent Psychiatry and Mental Health* 7(16):1, 2013.

13. Rosen DS and others: Clinical report—identification and management of eating disorders in children and adolescents. *Pediatrics* 126(6):1240, 2010.

14. Hudson JI and others: The prevalence and correlates of eating disorders in the national comorbidity survey replication. *Biological Psychiatry* 61:348, 2007.

15. Klein DA and others: Physical activity and cortisol in anorexia nervosa. *Psychoneuroendocrinology* 35(5):539, 2007.

16. Brumberg JJ: *Fasting girls: The history of anorexia nervosa.* New York: Vintage Books, 2000.

17. Centers for Disease Control and Prevention: *Healthy diet—it's not a diet, it's a lifestyle: About BMI for adults.* 2011. http://www.cdc.gov/healthyweight/ assessing/bmi/adult_bmi/index.html Accessed: January 26, 2014.

18. Smink FR and others: Epidemiology of eating disorders: Incidence, prevalence, and mortality rates. *Current Psychiatry Reports* 14:406, 2012.

19. Arcelus J and others: Mortality rates in patients with anorexia nervosa and other eating disorders: A meta-analysis of 36 studies. *Archives of General Psychiatry* 68(7):724, 2011.

20. Saladin KS: *Anatomy & Physiology.* 7th ed. Boston: McGraw-Hill Publishing Company, 2015.

21. Crow SJ and others: Increased mortality in bulimia nervosa and other eating disorders. *American Journal of Psychiatry* 66(12):1342, 2009. DOI: 10.1176/appi.ajp.2009.09020247. E-pub: October 15, 2009.

22. Berner LA, Allison KC: Behavioral management of night eating syndrome. *Psychology Research and Behavior Management* 6:1, 2013.

23. Fischer S and others: Night eating syndrome in young adults: Delineation from other eating disorders and clinical significance. *Psychiatry Research* 200:494, 2012.

24. Allison KC and others: An open-label efficacy trial of escitalopram for night eating syndrome. *Eating Behaviors* 14:199, 2013.

25. Gagnon C and others: Comorbid diabetes and eating disorders in adult patients: Assessment and considerations for treatment. *Diabetes Educator* 35:537, 2012.

26. Matheiu J: What is diabulimia? *Journal of the American Dietetic Association* 108(5):769, 2008.

27. Segura-Garcia C and others: Orthorexia nervosa: A frequent eating disordered behavior in athletes. *Eating and Weight Disorders* 17(4):e226, 2012 DOI: 10.3275/8272. E-pub: February 21, 2012.

28. Varga M and others: Evidence and gaps in the literature on orthorexia nervosa. *Eating and Weight Disorders* 18(2):103, 2013 DOI: 10.1007/s40519-013-0026-y. E-pub: April 12, 2013.

29. Murray SB and others: Muscle dysmorphia and the DSM-V conundrum: Where does it belong? A review paper. *International Journal of Eating Disorders* 43:483, 2010.

30. Houston CA and others: Eating disorders among dietetics students: An educator's dilemma. *Journal of the American Dietetic Association* 108(4):722, 2008.

31. Barry AE, Piazza-Gardener AK: Drunkorexia: Understanding the co-occurrence of alcohol consumption and eating/exercise weight management behaviors. *Journal of American College Health* 60(3):236, 2012.

32. Gibbs JC and others: Prevalence of individual and combined components of the female athlete triad. *Medicine and Science in Sports and Exercise* 45(5):985, 2013.

33. Nazem TH, Ackerman KE: The female athlete triad. *Sports Health* 4(4):302, 2012.

34. Thein-Nissenbaum J: Long term consequences of the female athlete triad. *Maturitas* 75:107, 2013.

35. Yager Z and others: What works in secondary schools? A systematic review of classroom-based body image programs. *Body Image* 10:271, 2013.

36. Nattiv A and others: American College of Sports Medicine position stand. The female athlete triad. *Medicine and Science in Sports and Exercise* 39(10):1867, 2007.

37. National Eating Disorder Association: *What should I say?* http://www.nationaleatingdisorders.org/what-should-i-say Accessed: June 28, 2013.

38. National Eating Disorder Association: Parent toolkit. http://www.nationaleatingdisorders.org/ Accessed: January 26, 2014.

39. Larranaga A and others: Disordered eating behaviors in type 1 diabetic patients. *World Journal of Diabetes* 15(2):89, 2011.

40. Berkman ND and others: Management of eating disorders. *Evidence Report/Technology Assessment* 135, 2006.

41. Bardone-Cone AM and others: The inter-relationships between vegetarianism and eating disorders among females. *Journal of the Academy of Nutrition and Dietetics* 112(8):1247, 2012.

15 Nutrition for Fitness and Sport

CASE STUDY

Training for a half-marathon

KYLIE IS A FORMER COLLEGIATE LACROSSE PLAYER who is now training for her first half-marathon (13.1 miles). She currently exercises for 60 minutes daily, 5 or 6 days a week, but she only recently started focusing on long-distance running. Over the next 16 weeks, Kylie will be following an online half-marathon training plan. Kylie has questions about fueling and hydrating her body to maximize her performance in her first half-marathon.

- Describe the energy system that will be most active in Kylie's body during the running of a half-marathon.
- Explain to Kylie the importance of following a diet that supplies plenty of carbohydrates during training and running of the half-marathon.
- Provide Kylie with a list of snacks to consume before a long training run.
- Describe the importance of hydration during the running of a half-marathon and how fluid needs can be met during the race.

The suggested Case Study Response can be found on page 520.

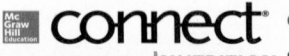
Check out the Connect site at www.mcgrawhillconnect.com to further explore this case study.

QUIZ Yourself

Are there certain foods you should eat before exercising to increase your endurance? Are there dietary supplements that can safely and effectively improve muscle strength and endurance? To test your nutrition and fitness knowledge, take the following quiz. The answers are found on page 522.

1. To meet physical activity recommendations, healthy adults should perform moderate-intensity physical activity for at least 150 minutes a week. __T __F

2. Low-fat chocolate milk is a good postexercise recovery beverage. __T __F

3. Protein is the body's preferred fuel during exercise. __T __F

4. Carbohydrate loading delays fatigue in athletes participating in events that last between 15 and 30 minutes. __T __F

5. Heatstroke is a serious illness that requires immediate professional medical treatment. __T __F

15.1 Physical Activity and Health

LEARNING OUTCOMES

1 *Explain the health benefits of performing regular physical activity.*

2 *Describe typical physical activity habits of Americans.*

Bicycling through quaint villages and over steep mountains in France; swimming for miles in the chilly English Channel while being buffeted by waves; lifting metal disks that weigh more than the weight lifter—the extent to which some people push their bodies is truly amazing. Superior athletes seem to thrive on performing grueling physical feats that require extraordinary stamina, strength, and energy. Millions of Americans admire competitive athletes for their physical accomplishments and enjoy watching them perform. Many Americans, however, lead sedentary lives; that is, their daily activities do not require much muscular exertion. In 2012, about half of all adults in the United States did not obtain recommended amounts of moderate or vigorous physical activity.[1] Moderate activities are those that cause small increases in the person's breathing or heart rate when performed for at least 150 minutes per week. Vigorous activities result in an even greater rise in breathing or heart rate and include activities such as jogging or swimming at a rapid pace.

What Is Physical Activity?

The human body is designed for **physical activity**, movement that results from skeletal muscle contraction. Most of the physical activities performed each day are unstructured; for example, shopping for groceries, walking to class, or doing household tasks. **Exercise** refers to physical activities that are usually planned and structured for a particular purpose, such as having fun or increasing muscle mass. Both forms of movement can benefit health.

Physical fitness is the ability to perform moderate— to vigorous—intensity activities without becoming excessively fatigued. A physically fit person has the strength, endurance, flexibility, and balance to meet the physical demands of daily living, exercise, and sports.

physical activity movement resulting from contraction of skeletal muscle

exercise physical activities that are usually planned and structured for a purpose

physical fitness ability to perform moderate- to vigorous-intensity activities without becoming excessively fatigued

Health Benefits of Regular Physical Activity

Regular physical activity has numerous health benefits, including weight control, improved body composition, and prevention of chronic disease.[2] Those who engage in regular physical activity have a reduced risk for many types of cancer, type 2 diabetes, hypertension, and cardiovascular disease (CVD).[3-6] In addition, regular physical activity helps people manage symptoms of depression and improve their sleep.[7,8] Adults who engage in higher levels of physical activity obtain even greater health benefits, particularly quality of life, which is a measure of both physical and mental well—being.[9] Youth who meet national physical activity guidelines are more likely to achieve age—appropriate physical fitness goals and have a healthier body mass index (BMI).[10]

Figure 15.1 illustrates physical as well as psychological benefits of regular moderate—intensity physical activity. Greater health benefits may be achieved by increasing the duration, frequency, and intensity (physical effort) of an exercise routine.

Physical Activity Habits of Americans

Despite recognized health benefits, fewer than half of all American adults meet the minimum physical activity recommendation of obtaining at least 2.5 hours a week of physical activity.[1] Various environmental factors contribute to whether or not an individual meets physical activity recommendations, including the

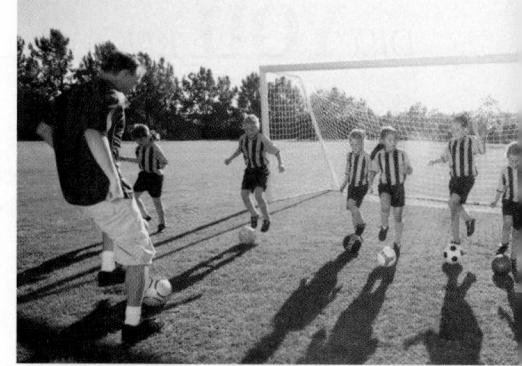

Youth who meet national physical activity guidelines are more likely to have a healthier body mass index.

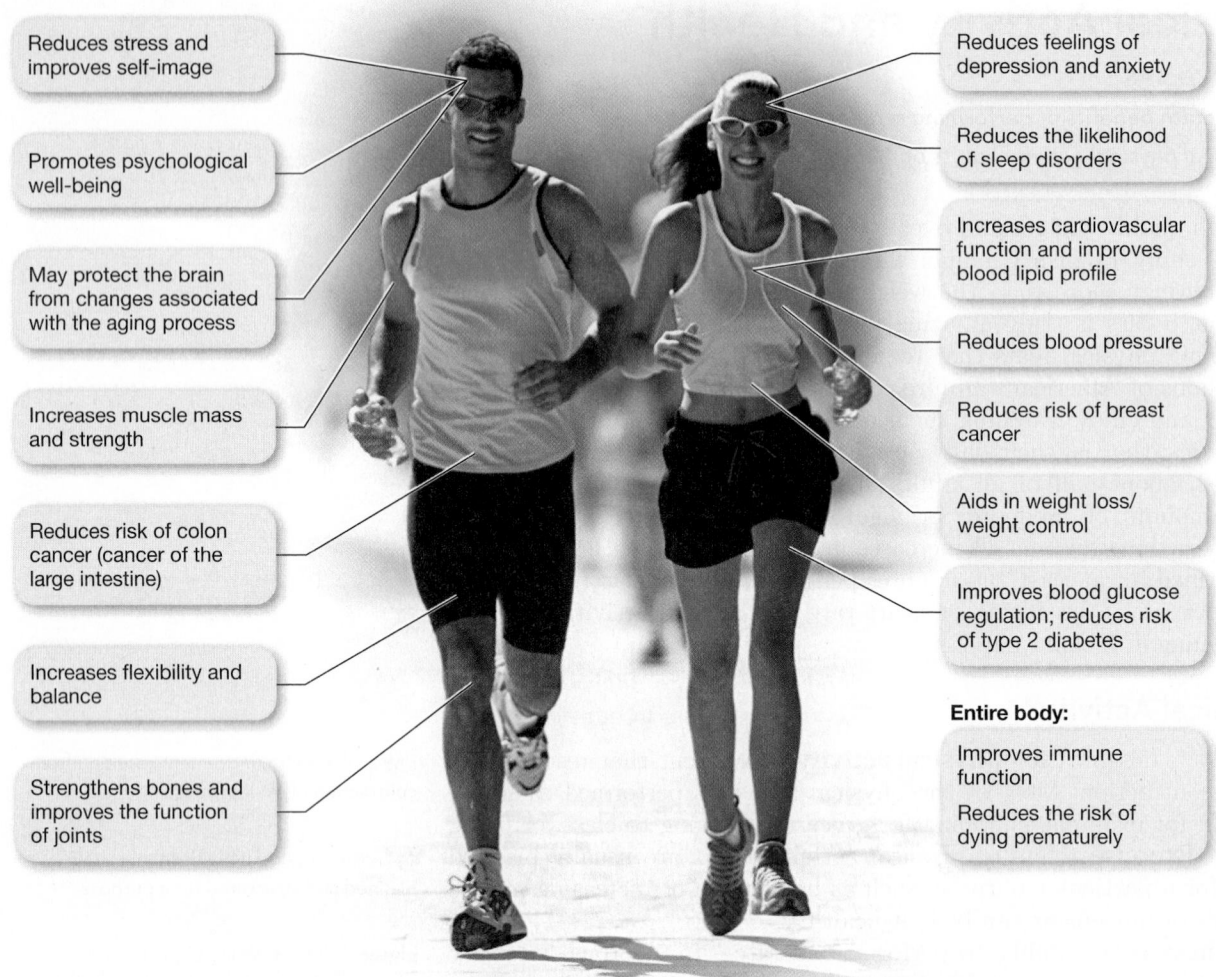

Reduces stress and improves self-image

Promotes psychological well-being

May protect the brain from changes associated with the aging process

Increases muscle mass and strength

Reduces risk of colon cancer (cancer of the large intestine)

Increases flexibility and balance

Strengthens bones and improves the function of joints

Reduces feelings of depression and anxiety

Reduces the likelihood of sleep disorders

Increases cardiovascular function and improves blood lipid profile

Reduces blood pressure

Reduces risk of breast cancer

Aids in weight loss/ weight control

Improves blood glucose regulation; reduces risk of type 2 diabetes

Entire body:

Improves immune function

Reduces the risk of dying prematurely

FIGURE 15.1 Benefits of physical activity. Regular physical activity improves health in several ways.

built environment human-made resources, including buildings, roads, parks, supermarkets, and restaurants, within a community

DID **YOU** KNOW?

Community fitness trails support physical activity for people who are currently active and promote physical activity among people who are sedentary.[14] One-third of Americans who engage in regular physical activity report frequent use of trails.[15]

location of a person's home (urban or suburban), safety of the neighborhood, ability to walk to destinations within the community, and availability of local parks, trails, and fitness centers.

The **built environment** refers to human-made resources, including buildings, roads, parks, supermarkets, and restaurants, within a community. A community's built environment often encourages more physical activity by both children and adults.[11,12] Safe streets and sidewalks, bikeable paths and street shoulders, and access to fitness facilities are all examples of built environment features that enable people to do more walking, cycling, rollerblading, and other forms of activity.[13] Having a built environment that supports walking is important because Americans who walk on a regular basis are most likely to meet physical activity guidelines. According to the Centers for Disease Control and Prevention (CDC), 56% of Americans reported walking on a regular basis in 2005; in 2010, that number increased to 62%.[1] Access to safe indoor and outdoor places to walk, including fitness facilities, churches, shopping malls, trails, and safe sidewalks, promotes physically active lifestyles.

Physical Activity Pyramid

Figure 15.2 shows a physical activity pyramid to help people add more physical activity into their daily routines. This pyramid presents various activities that need to be performed regularly and provides practical suggestions for increasing the intensity of various routine activities. For example, more physical effort will

FIGURE 15.2 Physical activity pyramid.

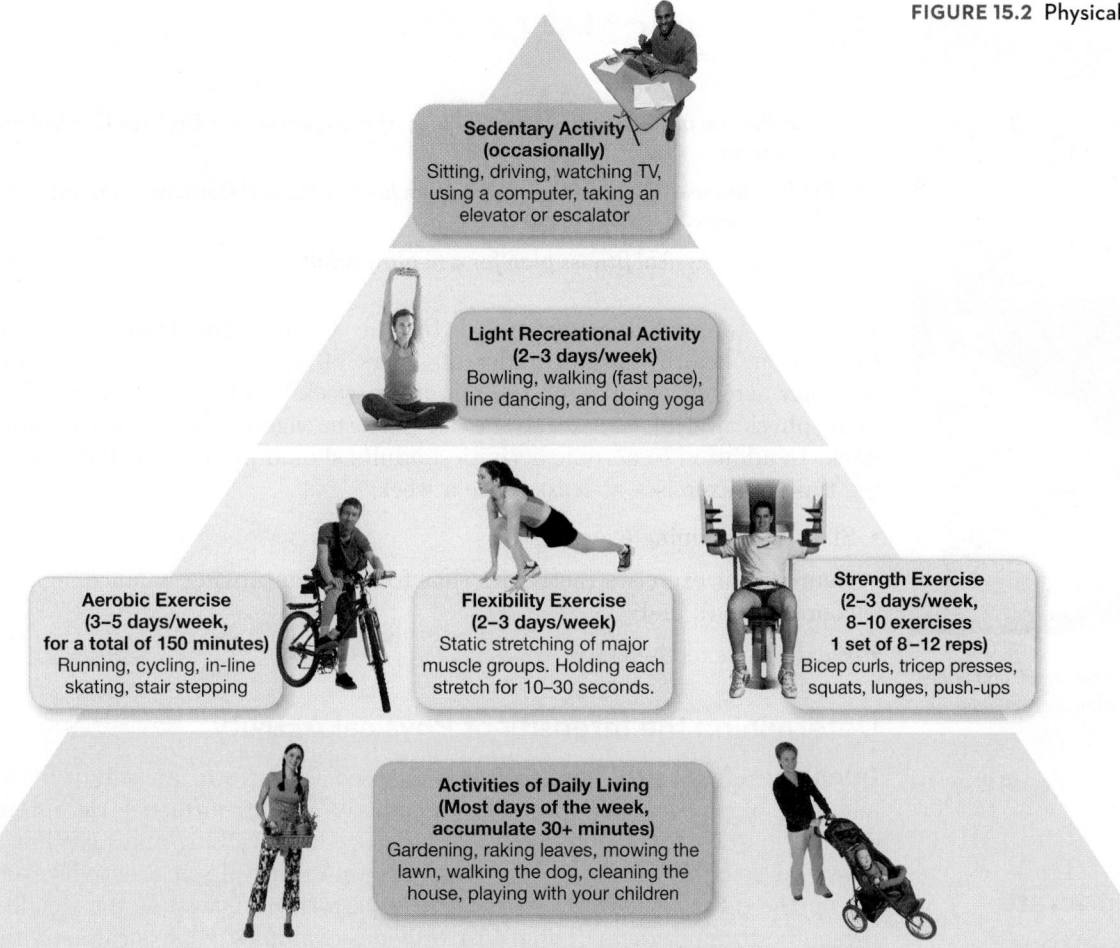

**Sedentary Activity
(occasionally)**
Sitting, driving, watching TV,
using a computer, taking an
elevator or escalator

**Light Recreational Activity
(2–3 days/week)**
Bowling, walking (fast pace),
line dancing, and doing yoga

**Aerobic Exercise
(3–5 days/week,
for a total of 150 minutes)**
Running, cycling, in-line
skating, stair stepping

**Flexibility Exercise
(2–3 days/week)**
Static stretching of major
muscle groups. Holding each
stretch for 10–30 seconds.

**Strength Exercise
(2–3 days/week,
8–10 exercises
1 set of 8–12 reps)**
Bicep curls, tricep presses,
squats, lunges, push-ups

**Activities of Daily Living
(Most days of the week,
accumulate 30+ minutes)**
Gardening, raking leaves, mowing the
lawn, walking the dog, cleaning the
house, playing with your children

be exerted and more energy expended when an individual uses stairs instead of elevators or jogs with instead of walking with the dog.

Low—intensity, unstructured physical activities that involve usual daily living activities, such as routine household chores, form the foundation of the physical activity pyramid. The next level of the activity pyramid recommends adding aer—obic exercise to foundation activities at least three times a week. **Aerobic exercise** involves sustained, rhythmic contractions of large muscle groups in the legs and arms. Such activities raise heart rate, giving the heart a more effective workout. Running, jogging, rapid walking, and swimming are aerobic activities. Additionally, the second level of the pyramid recommends performing resistance and stretching exercises at least two times a week to increase muscle mass, strength, and flexi—bility. **Resistance exercises**, such as weight lifting, can also increase bone density. The third level of the pyramid encourages regularly performing recreational activ—ities that are physical, such as yoga and dancing. The top of the pyramid depicts activities that expend little energy, such as watching television or using a personal computer. The pyramid recommends spending little time being sedentary.

aerobic exercise physical activities that involve sustained, rhythmic contractions of large muscle groups

resistance exercises physical activities, such as pull-ups and push-ups, that develop muscle strength and muscle endurance

ASSESS YOUR PROGRESS

1 *What is the difference between physical activity and exercise?*

2 *List at least five health benefits of performing moderate-intensity exercise regularly.*

3 *Identify components of the built environment that may help people in a community be more physically active.*

4 *Describe the main principles of the physical activity pyramid (Fig. 15.2).*

15.2 Physical Activity Guidelines

LEARNING OUTCOMES

1 *Describe the physical activity guidelines of the Centers for Disease Control and Prevention.*

2 *Explain the use of age-related maximum heart rate in determining the intensity of physical activity.*

3 *Develop a physical fitness plan for a healthy adult.*

According to guidelines promoted by the Centers for Disease Control and Prevention, healthy adults under 65 years of age should perform moderate—intensity aerobic activity for 150 minutes a week.[16] Adults who would like to do more physically intense workouts can perform vigorous activities 75 minutes a week. In addition to aerobic activities, adults should perform each of the following types of exercises at least twice a week:

- Strength—training exercises;

- Neuromotor exercises (activities that focus on improving balance, agility, and coordination); and

- Flexibility exercises.

Determining the Intensity of Physical Activity

Intensity refers to the level of exertion used to perform an activity. Duration and type of physical activity, as well as body weight, influence the intensity of skeletal muscle movement. Thus, activities such as walking and bicycling can be classified as either moderate— or vigorous—intensity physical activity, depending on the rate at which the activities are performed as well as the weight of the person performing them. Table 15.1 provides examples of physical activities that are generally classified as of moderate or vigorous intensity.

There are a few ways to determine the intensity of exercise. One way is to judge the level of exertion based on physical signs, such as breathing rate and sweat production. While exercising at the moderate—intensity level, individuals will be aware of their muscular effort, but they should also be able to chat with an exercise partner comfortably.

A popular method of estimating the intensity of exercise is to use a percentage of an individual's **age—related maximum heart rate**. To calculate age—related maximum heart rate, subtract a person's age from 220. The **target heart rate zone** is the range of heart rate that reflects the intensity of exertion during physical activity. For moderate—intensity physical activity, the target heart rate zone should be 50 to 70% of an individual's age—related maximum heart rate.[17] To determine the moderate—intensity "zone," take a person's age—related maximum heart rate and multiply this figure by 0.50 and 0.70. For example, the age—related maximum heart rate of a 20—year—old person is 200 beats per minute (220 minus 20). Multiply 200 beats per minute (bpm) by 0.50 to calculate the 50% value, and multiply 200 bpm by 0.70 to obtain the 70% level. This person's target heart rate zone for moderate—intensity activities is 100 to 140 bpm.

Moderate—intensity physical activities expend 3.5 to 7.0 kcal/min.[18] To "burn" (oxidize or metabolize) more energy and give the heart a more vigorous workout, an individual should engage in physical activities that expend more than 7 kcal/min.[18] Such physical activities usually require considerable muscular effort and result in significant increases in breathing rate and perspiration. Examples of vigorous physical activities include jogging, running, aerobic dancing, swimming laps, and bicycling uphill.

To exercise vigorously, the target heart rate should be 70 to 85% of an individual's age—related maximum heart rate.[17] To calculate this range, people can

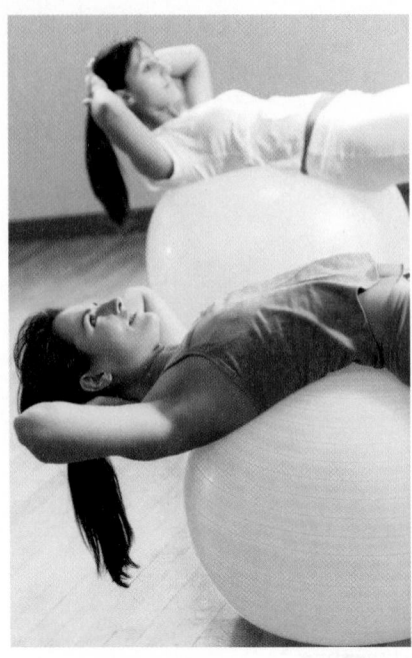

Exercise balls engage abdominal and upper leg muscles through balancing activities on the balls.

intensity level of exertion used to perform an activity

TABLE 15.1 Moderate- and Vigorous-Intensity Physical Activities

Moderate Intensity
Ballroom dancing
Bicycling (slower than 10 mph)
Gardening
Tennis (doubles)
Walking briskly (3 mph or faster)
Water aerobics

Vigorous Physical Activity
Aerobic dancing
Bicycling (faster than 10 mph)
Heavy gardening (e.g., digging)
Hiking uphill or with a backpack
Jumping rope
Speed walking, jogging, or running
Swimming laps
Tennis (singles)

Source: Centers for Disease Control and Prevention: *Measuring physical activity intensity.* Updated December 2011. http://www.cdc.gov/physicalactivity/everyone/measuring/index.html Accessed: March 8, 2014.

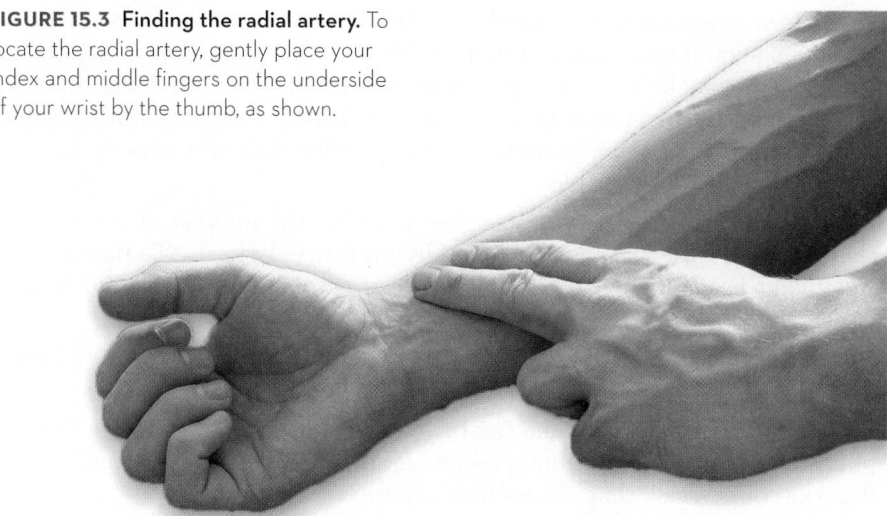

FIGURE 15.3 Finding the radial artery. To locate the radial artery, gently place your index and middle fingers on the underside of your wrist by the thumb, as shown.

follow the same formula that is used to determine the range for moderate–intensity activity, except they need to change "0.50 and 0.70" to "0.70 and 0.85." Those with serious health conditions should consult with a physician to determine a target zone for physical activity.

Measuring Heart Rate

Heart rate (pulse) can be measured using the radial artery in the wrist. The radial artery can be found by gently placing the index and middle fingers (not the thumb, because it has a pulse of its own) on the underside of the wrist by the thumb, as shown in Figure 15.3. Count the pulse for 10 seconds, and then multiply that number by 6 to determine heart rate for 1 minute. It is helpful for people to practice taking their pulse while resting. Because heart rate begins to decline as soon as an individual stops exercising, people should measure their heart rate while they are actively working out. Measuring heart rate while exercising at a vigorous intensity can be challenging, so some athletes use heart rate monitors, such as those that can be worn, to automatically measure and record heart rate.

age-related maximum heart rate normal maximum heart rate of an individual of a given age during exercise

target heart rate zone heart rate range that reflects intensity of physical exertion

Aerobic Training

An effective aerobic workout program should include the following components:

1. ***Warm–up:*** Warming up muscles can increase joints' range of motion (flexibility) and may decrease risk of injury. Stretching for 5 to 10 minutes is a good way to warm up. The person can start with smaller muscle groups such as the arms and progressively work toward stretching larger muscle groups in the legs and abdomen. It is important to hold the stretch for 15 seconds and not bounce. If stretching causes pain, the person should stop immediately. "No pain, no gain" is not true; pain is an indication of injury. Another way for a person to warm up is to perform 5 to 10 minutes of the anticipated activity, but at a low intensity. For example, if an individual is going to run for fitness, he or she can warm up by walking slowly for 5 minutes.

2. ***Aerobic workout:*** A comprehensive aerobic workout emphasizes the type, duration, frequency, intensity, and progression of exercise.

   • ***Type:*** The kind of exercise a person chooses should increase heart and breathing rates and involve rhythmic movements of large muscle groups in the legs. Examples include brisk walking, running, swimming, and cycling.

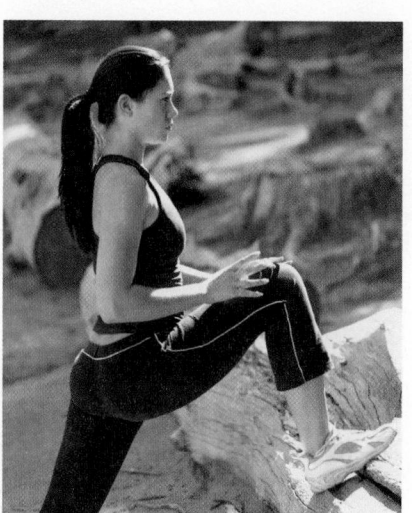

Stretching both before and after exercise can prevent injury and reduce muscle soreness following activity.

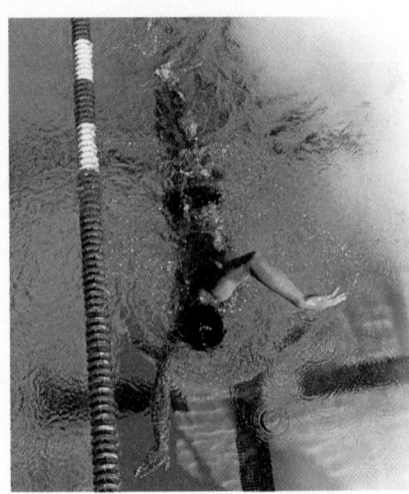

Aerobic exercise involves sustained rhythmic contractions of large muscle groups in the legs and arms.

- *Duration:* Duration is the amount of time spent in an exercise session. A session should generally last at least 20 to 30 minutes, depending on intensity, not including time spent warming up and cooling down. Ideally, the exercise session should be continuous (without stopping), but multiple 10—minute bouts of moderate to intense activity with rest periods in between are also acceptable.
- *Frequency:* The frequency of exercise describes the number of times that the activity is performed, generally on a weekly basis. To derive significant health benefits, the frequency of aerobic exercise should be at least 5 times per week.
- *Intensity:* Health benefits can occur when an individual achieves at least a moderate level of intensity during exercise.
- *Progression:* Progression, the final component of a comprehensive fitness plan, refers to the gradual increase in the frequency, intensity, and duration of exercise that occurs over a period of time.

3. *Cool—down:* To cool down, a person can repeat the same stretches performed during warming up for 5 to 10 minutes. Cooling down may prevent injury and reduce muscle soreness.

Strength Training

Strength training, such as weight lifting, is an important part of a compre—hensive physical fitness plan. Strength training should be performed at least 2 days per week. To start, the person should warm up by stretching for 5 to 10 minutes. After warming up, the individual performs a group of 8 to 10 exer—cises that strengthen major muscle groups of the upper body and lower body. After completing the strengthening exercises, the person should cool down for 5 to 10 minutes.

Fitness centers usually have different machines that provide resistance for various muscle groups. For resistance training outside of fitness facilities, simple elastic exercise cords designed to increase muscular strength can be used (Fig. 15.4). For increasing upper arm strength, a set of inexpensive handheld weights can be kept in a convenient location for performing resistance exercise regularly. The weight should be chosen so that it allows an individual to perform at least one set of 8 to 15 repetitions (the same actions). When 15 repetitions can be performed with relative ease, the weight can be increased slightly.

Developing a Physical Fitness Plan

Most healthy people can gradually increase their level of physical activity. Sedentary men who are 40 years of age or older, physically inactive women who are 50 years of age or older, and people who have exist—ing health problems may want to discuss their fitness goals with their physicians before beginning a fitness program. Health problems that require a preliminary medical evaluation include obesity, CVD (or family his—tory of CVD), hypertension, type 2 diabetes (or family history of the disease), shortness of breath after mild exertion, and arthritis. Additionally, pregnant women should consult with their physicians before starting an exercise regimen.

When developing a personalized physical fitness plan, health care practitioners should first consider the individual's fitness goals. For example, if weight loss is the primary goal, how much weight does the individual

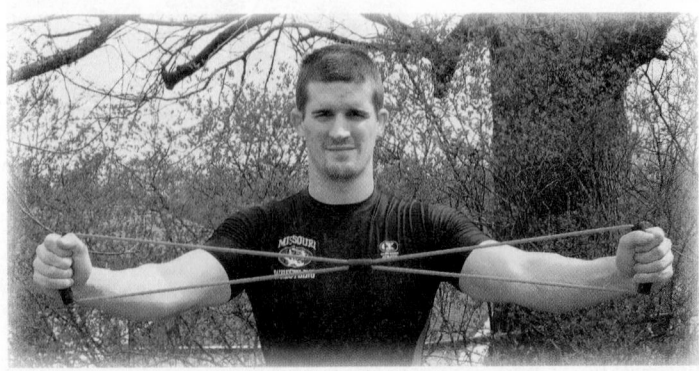

FIGURE 15.4 Increasing muscle strength. This individual is using a simple rubber exercise cord to increase muscular strength.

want to lose and how many weeks will it take to lose that amount? Does the individual want to focus more on resistance activities to strengthen muscles or exercises to improve aerobic capacity? Then, determine when the person can work out and whether he or she needs to join a fitness facility or purchase special equipment, such as handheld weights. For a comprehensive fitness program, make sure to include aerobic, resistance, and stretching activities in the client's weekly exercise regimen. The following fitness plan has three stages: initial, improvement, and maintenance phases.

Initiation

The first 3 to 6 weeks of an individual's new exercise program is the initiation stage. The person can start by incorporating short periods of physical activity into the daily routine. For example, walking more often, taking the stairs instead of the elevator, and doing more housework, gardening, or other activities that cause a person to "huff and puff" but not extensively.

The initial fitness goal is to accumulate a total of 150 minutes of moderate-intensity types of activity a week. If necessary, the time spent engaging in the activity each day can occur in three short intervals lasting at least 10 minutes. If the person does not have 30 minutes at a time to spend on exercising, he or she can increase the intensity of the activities that are performed during shorter bouts of exercise to obtain some health benefits.

Improvement

The next 5 or 6 months of the program is the improvement stage, in which the intensity and duration of exercises are increased. When beginning the improvement phase, an individual should strive to exercise at an intensity that is near the lower end of his or her target heart rate zone. As physical fitness improves, the person can increase the exercise intensity level by working out at a higher heart rate.

Maintenance

By the end of the improvement stage, the individual may notice that he or she has reached his or her goals, and no further gains in fitness are being achieved. This "plateau" marks the beginning of the maintenance stage. At this point, the fitness plan should be reevaluated and, if desired, new goals developed. A person who is satisfied with his or her current fitness level should continue with the existing program. Discontinuing the exercise program results in **detraining**, which is a gradual decline in physical fitness.

detraining declining physical fitness

Components of an Enduring Fitness Plan

Enduring fitness plans are those that include variety in the types of activities performed. For example, jogging one day might be followed by swimming the next day and playing basketball with friends the next day. Adding variety to a program not only prevents boredom with workouts, but also strengthens different muscle groups in the body and reduces risk of injury. Additionally, having a friend or family member as an exercise partner may provide additional motivation and encouragement to exercise regularly.

The following websites provide more information about the health benefits of physical fitness and developing a personalized fitness program:

www.choosemyplate.gov

www.shapeup.org

www.fitness.gov

www.presidentschallenge.org

FRESH TIPS

Some people who are overweight do not experience significant weight loss while following an exercise regimen. However, they still benefit from regular physical activity. Initially, exercise programs for some obese people, especially those who are morbidly obese, should emphasize non-weight-bearing activities, such as swimming, water aerobics, and bicycling. As obese people lose weight and become more fit, they can add weight-bearing activities to their fitness plan.

DID *YOU* KNOW?

Pedometers have become widely available and utilized as a tool to monitor and promote physical activity. Results of a review of 26 studies found that pedometer use is associated with significant increases in physical activity and significant decreases in body mass index and blood pressure.[19] People who wear a pedometer or use a smartphone-based tool to track their steps should aim for at least 5000 steps per day, which is about 2 ½ miles.

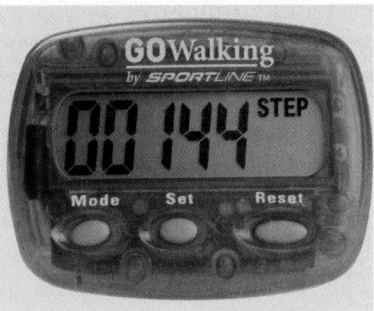

ASSESS YOUR PROGRESS

5 *Calculate the target heart rate range for a 24-year-old man performing moderate-intensity physical activity.*

6 *Identify two factors to consider when developing a physical fitness plan for an adult client.*

7 *Explain recommendations for the type, duration, frequency, intensity, and progression of aerobic physical activity.*

8 *Provide recommendations for initiating a strength-training exercise program.*

15.3 Energy Systems for Exercising Muscles

LEARNING OUTCOMES

1 *Describe how muscles obtain energy from the PCr-ATP, lactic acid, and oxygen systems.*

2 *Contrast the body's use of fat and carbohydrate during physical activities of different intensities.*

To move, skeletal muscles must contract, and to contract, the muscles must have a source of energy. Under normal conditions, most cells, including muscle cells, metabolize a mixture of biological fuels, especially glucose and fatty acids. Muscle cells also metabolize a small amount of amino acids from proteins to obtain energy.[18]

Energy Metabolism During Exercise

Recall from Chapter 8 that cells obtain energy through a complex series of chemical reactions that progressively catabolize macronutrients to release energy that is stored within them. Much of the energy is captured in the high-energy compound adenosine triphosphate (ATP). ATP forms when an inorganic phosphate group (P_i) bonds with adenosine diphosphate (ADP), trapping energy in the process (Fig. 15.5a). When a cell needs some energy to drive a chemical reaction, it uses an enzyme to break the bond between the last two phosphate groups of ATP (Fig. 15.5b). This process releases energy and reforms ADP and P_i. Thus,

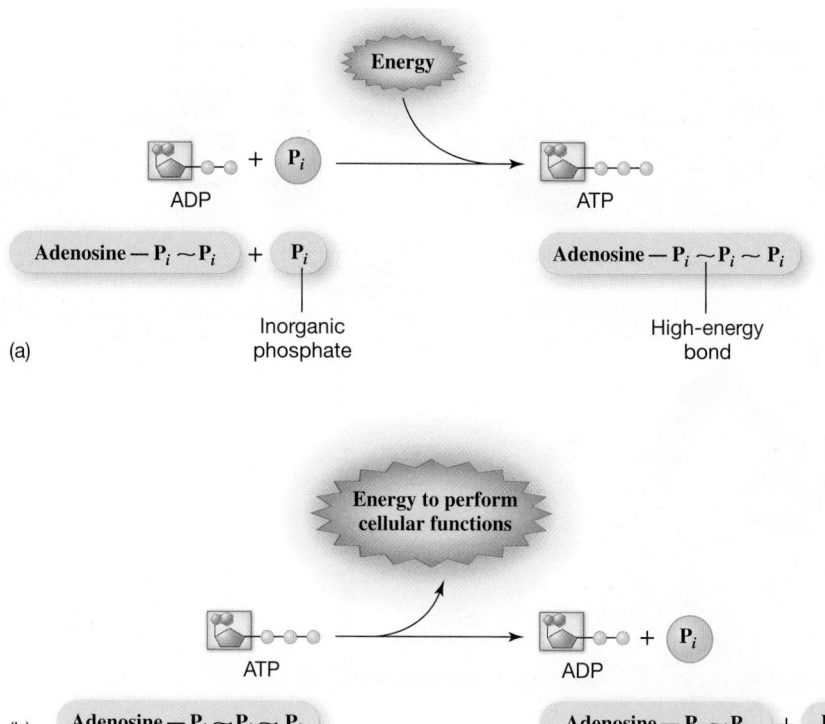

(a)

(b)

FIGURE 15.5 ATP. (*a*) Cells capture and store energy by forming ATP from ADP and inorganic phosphate (P_i). (*b*) When a cell needs energy to drive a chemical reaction, it uses an enzyme to break the bond between the last two phosphate groups of ATP, releasing energy and reforming ADP and P_i.

cells can recycle their supplies of ADP and P_i. Cells do not store much ATP, so they must constantly replace their supply of the high−energy compound by recycling ADP and P_i.

Glucose, triglycerides, and amino acids are all potential sources of ATP during exercise. Figure 15.6 summarizes the pathways that dietary carbohydrate, fat, and protein follow during energy metabolism. Chapter 8 provides a detailed explanation of the metabolism of each of these macronutrients.

Gram for gram, fat supplies more energy than carbohydrate or protein. Fatty acids, however, are not a very useful fuel for intense, brief exercise, such as a 100−meter sprint. Why? A fatty acid molecule has fewer oxygen atoms in relation to carbon atoms than a glucose molecule. Thus, cells need more oxygen to metabolize a fatty acid molecule than to burn a glucose molecule. During a brief bout of intense exercise, the heart and lungs do not have enough time to deliver much oxygen to muscles. Under these conditions, glucose is a major source of energy. For physical activities that last longer and are less intense, muscles can use more fat for energy, because the lungs are able to supply them with enough oxygen.

Muscle cells rely on three major systems to obtain energy: the *PCr−ATP*, *lactic acid*, and *oxygen systems*. The PCr−ATP and lactic acid systems do not need oxygen to produce ATP. Thus, these systems metabolize glucose under anaerobic conditions, such as may happen when a person holds his or her breath while sprinting or lifting a heavy load. As the duration of the activity increases, muscle cells need to form considerably more ATP. To meet this demand, muscle cells depend heavily on the oxygen system to metabolize glucose and fat, and protein, if necessary.

The three energy−releasing systems do not function independently of each other during intense physical exertion; each contributes ATP energy to power intense muscular activity. The following sections provide more information about these major energy systems.

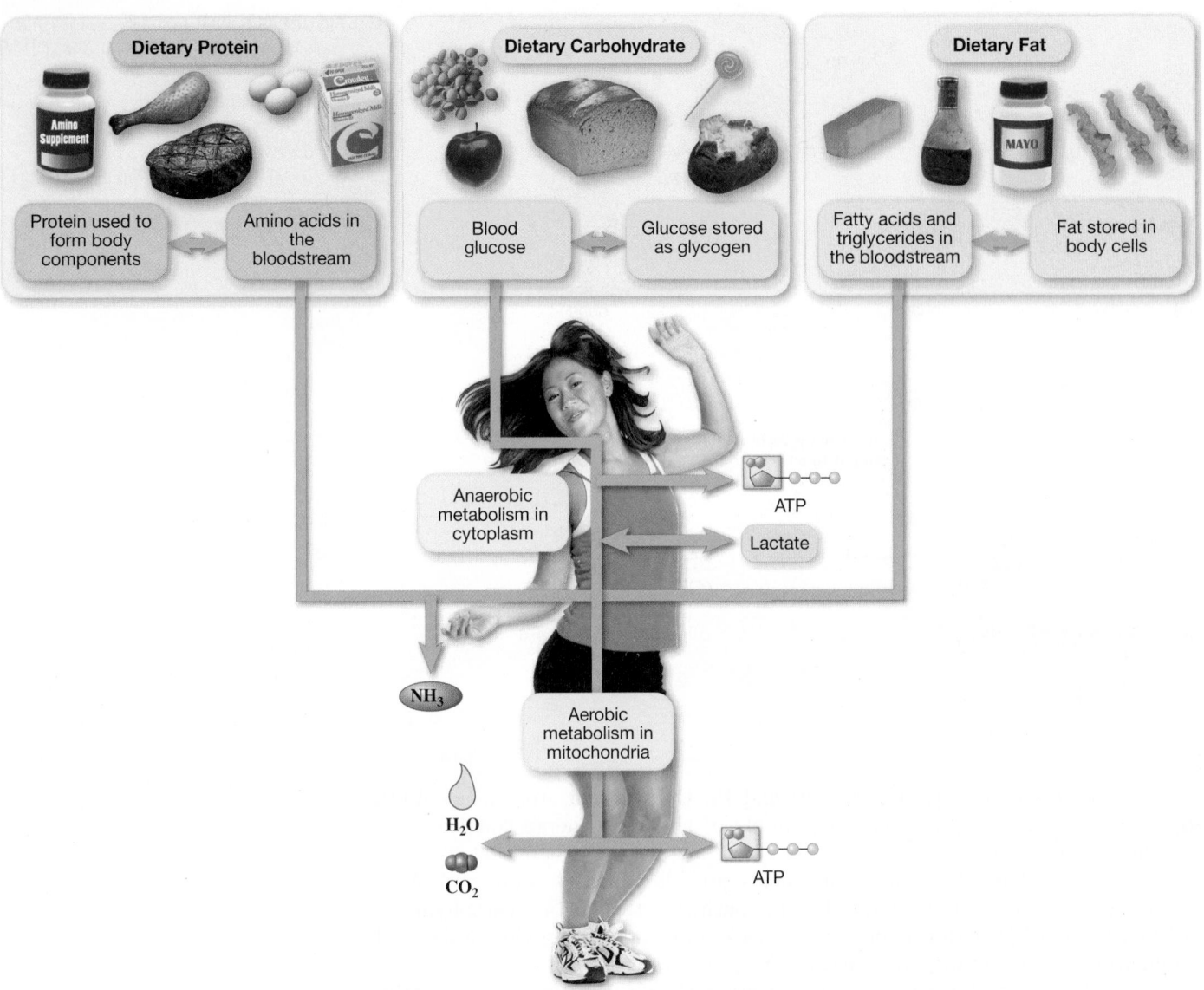

FIGURE 15.6 Summary of ATP formation. Protein, carbohydrate, and fat can be metabolized for ATP production. Amino acids from proteins may be channeled into aerobic energy pathways to generate ATP. Glucose (carbohydrate) can be broken down anaerobically, but the biological fuel generates relatively little ATP as a result. However, aerobic breakdown of pyruvate (a by-product of anaerobic glucose metabolism) in mitochondria generates more ATP. Products of fat breakdown can enter aerobic metabolic pathways as well.

phosphocreatine (PCr) high-energy compound used to reform ATP under anaerobic conditions; provides energy for short bouts of high-intensity activity

PCr-ATP Energy System

A resting muscle cell contains only a small amount of ATP that can be used immediately. Muscle cells have another type of high–energy compound—**phosphocreatine (PCr)**—that enables the cells to produce more ATP quickly under *anaerobic conditions*. To make the ATP, cells break down PCr into creatine and P_i, releasing energy to form ATP from ADP and P_i (Fig. 15.7). Cells do not use PCr directly to power their activities; the compound provides the energy to resupply ATP.

By breaking down PCr to form ATP, muscle cells can obtain enough energy to function during intense events, generally lasting only a few seconds.[18] However, the PCr–ATP system can be activated instantly, replenishing ATP fast enough to meet the energy demands of the swiftest and most powerful muscle move—ments, such as those involved in jumping, lifting, throwing, and sprinting. When the intense activity stops and there is no need to maintain high lev—els of ATP, an inorganic phosphate group bonds with creatine to recycle PCr (Fig. 15.7b). Muscle cells, however, do not make or store much PCr.

Lactic Acid Energy System

When physical activity lasts longer than a few seconds, the PCr–ATP energy system cannot keep up with the demand for energy, and muscle cells must metabolize glucose to generate more ATP. The immediate source of glucose for working muscles is glycogen that is stored in muscles.[18] The liver also helps sup—ply glucose for muscles by degrading glycogen and releasing glucose molecules into the bloodstream.

In anaerobic conditions, muscle cells metabolize glucose to pyruvate and then convert pyruvate to lactic acid (see Fig. 8.11). The degradation of glucose to lactic acid produces a small amount of ATP—only enough to sustain vigorous physical exertion for 30 to 40 seconds.[18] Lactic acid accumulates in muscles and converts to a related substance, lactate. Although certain muscle cells can use lactate as a fuel, some of the compound enters the bloodstream. Through the *Cori cycle*, the liver removes lactate from blood and can convert the compound into glucose. The liver may then release the glucose into the bloodstream to help meet muscles' demand for fuel or use the simple sugar to make glycogen.

Hydrogen ions (H^+) form as a result of the conversion of lactic acid to lac—tate. The accumulation of H^+ in muscle tissue contributes to muscle acidity, a condition that can lead to muscle fatigue and declining physical performance.

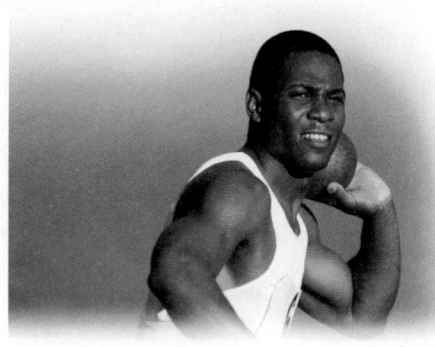

During a brief bout of intense anaerobic exercise, glucose is a major source of energy for working muscles.

FIGURE 15.7 PCr. Muscle cells break down PCr into creatine and inorganic phosphate, releasing energy to form ATP from ADP and P_i (a). When the intense activity stops and there is no need to maintain high levels of ATP, an inorganic phosphate group bonds with creatine to recycle PCr (b).

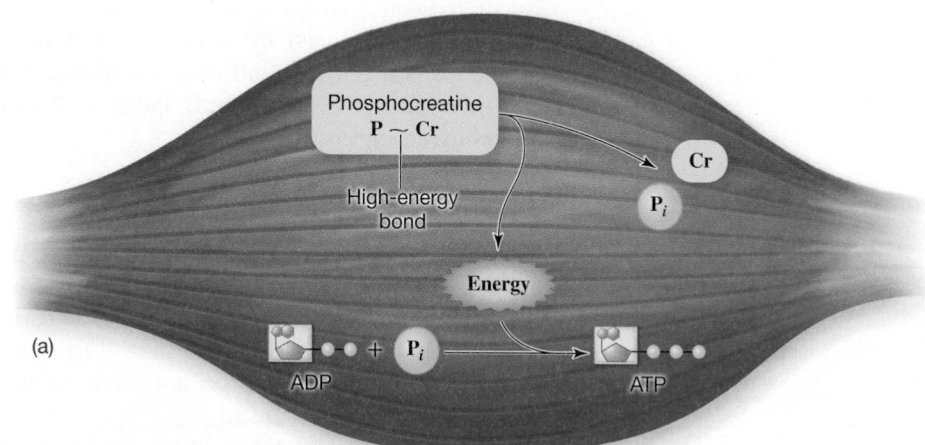

Actively Contracting Muscle

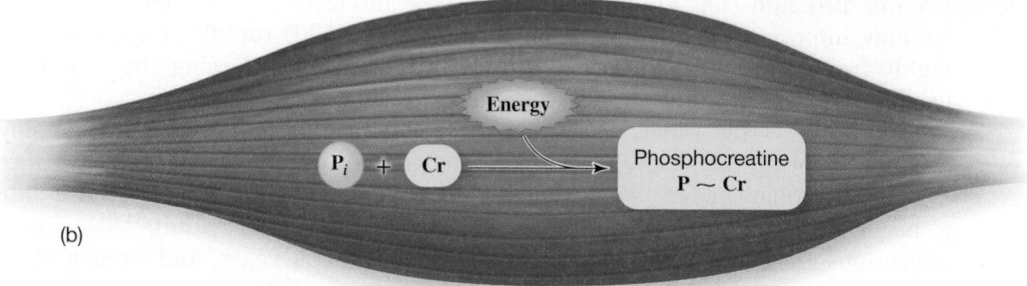

Relaxed Muscle

TABLE 15.2 Energy Sources for Muscles

Source/System*	When in Use	Examples of Activities
ATP	At all times	All types
Phosphocreatine (PCr)	All exercise initially; short bursts of exercise thereafter	Shot put, high jump, bench press
Carbohydrate		
Anaerobic	High-intensity exercise, especially lasting 30 seconds to 2 minutes	200-yard sprint
Aerobic	Exercise lasting 2 minutes to 3 hours or more; the higher the intensity of exercise, the greater the use	Basketball, swimming, jogging
Fat	At rest	Sitting
	Exercise lasting more than a few minutes; low- to moderate-intensity physical activities	30-minute brisk walk
Protein	Low amounts during all exercise, slightly more during endurance exercise, especially when carbohydrate fuel is lacking	Long-distance running

* Note that at any given time, more than one energy system is operating. Adapted from: Wardlaw GM, Smith AM: *Contemporary Nutrition*. 7th ed. New York: McGraw-Hill, 2009.

Oxygen Energy System

Activities such as walking at a fast pace, swimming laps, playing a game of soccer or basketball, or other continuous types of physical activity would not be possible if skeletal muscles depended only on the anaerobic energy systems. When muscle cells have plenty of oxygen, such as during low– to moderate–intensity exercise, they can metabolize glucose completely to CO_2 and H_2O. In fact, the availability of oxygen enables cells to produce about 18 times more ATP energy than the amount produced by anaerobic systems. The ability to obtain this amount of energy is useful for endurance athletes, because it allows their muscle cells to contract repeatedly for hours. Table 15.2 summarizes energy sources for resting and contracting muscles.

Aerobic Capacity

aerobic capacity (VO₂ max) maximal oxygen uptake; a measure of the amount of the maximal amount of oxygen consumed during physical activity

The ability of the cardiorespiratory system (the heart and lungs) to deliver oxygen to muscles determines capacity for intense aerobic physical activity. Scientists can use special equipment to estimate **aerobic capacity** (also called **VO₂ max**), maximal oxygen intake during vigorous physical exertion. A simple way to determine if a person is exercising near his or her aerobic capacity is for the individual to engage in vigorous exercise and note when the breathing rate increases to the point when he or she cannot carry on a conversation.

Aerobic exercise capacity can be increased by engaging in an endurance training program that gradually increases the intensity level of activities. Such training improves muscle cells' ability to generate ATP rapidly. However, even highly trained athletes experience muscle fatigue after increasing the time they usually spend performing intense muscular exertion.

As people grow older, their aerobic capacities decline with each passing decade. By being physically active, however, older adults can maintain a higher degree of aerobic capacity than their sedentary counterparts. It is never too late to begin a training program to improve physical fitness. Older adults with existing serious chronic health problems, men older than 40 years, and women older

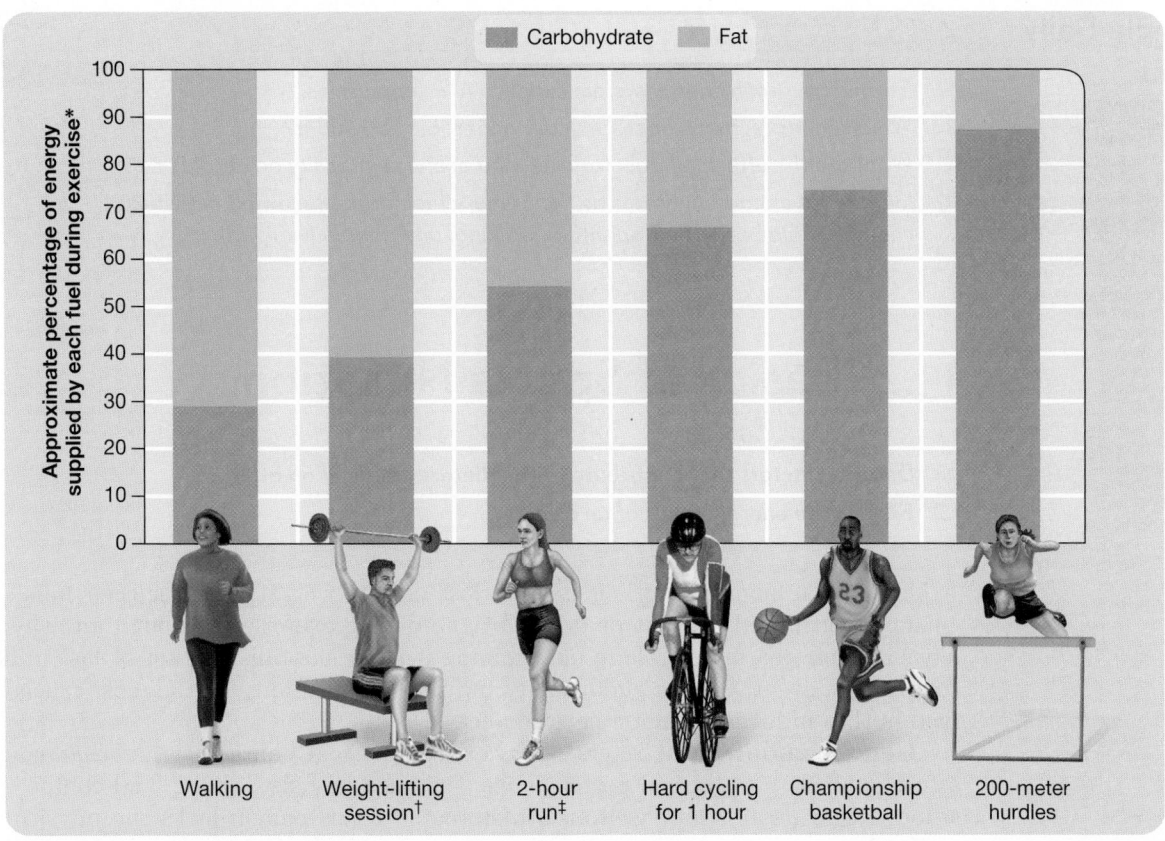

FIGURE 15.8 Rough estimates of energy usage during exercise. The intensity of an exercise largely influences the relative amounts of carbohydrate and fat that muscles metabolize for energy.

*Protein supplies a minor percentage of energy.
†Fat use generally is higher because much of the time spent weight lifting is for rest periods.
‡The values shown are for a runner consuming carbohydrate during the run; more fat and less carbohydrate would be used if carbohydrates were not consumed.

than 50 years should have a complete medical checkup and obtain a physician's okay before beginning a moderate—intensity fitness program.

Fat or Carbohydrate for Fueling Exercise?

The intensity of a physical activity largely influences the relative amounts of fatty acids and glucose that muscles metabolize for energy. Glucose supplies only about 40% of the energy needed to sustain a person who is resting or engaged in very light to light activities, such as watching TV, typing, and walking. Fat is the primary fuel muscles use while resting or engaged in low— to moderate—intensity physical activities.[20] During high—intensity exercise, the rate of fat oxidation decreases, while that of glucose oxidation increases. The chart in Figure 15.8 illustrates rough estimates of protein, carbohydrate, and fat metabolism during six forms of exercise. You'll notice that all six activities rely on all three sources of energy, just in different amounts.

An individual's level of training influences the ratio of glucose to fatty acids used by muscles during exercise. Trained endurance athletes tend to oxidize more fat when exercising at the same intensity than untrained persons.[21] As a result, muscle cells of trained athletes "spare" glycogen; that is, they conserve their supply of glucose. By sparing their glycogen supplies, athletes can exercise longer.

TABLE 15.3 Sample Daily 5000-kcal Menu

5000 kcal 66% carbohydrate 21% fat 13% protein
Breakfast
Fat-free milk, 1 cup
Cheerios, 2 cups
Bran muffins, 2
Orange, 1
Snack
Low-fat plain yogurt, 1 cup
Chopped dates, 1 cup
Lunch
Chicken enchilada, 1
Romaine lettuce, 1 cup
Garbanzo beans, 1 cup
Shredded carrots, ¾ cup
Chopped celery, ½ cup
Seasoned croutons, 1 oz
French dressing, 2 Tbsp
Whole-wheat bread, 2 slices
Butter or soft margarine, 1 Tbsp
Snack
Banana, 1
Bagel, 1
Cream cheese, 1 Tbsp
Dinner
Lean broiled beef, sirloin, 5 oz
Mashed potatoes, 2 cups
Butter or soft margarine, 2 tsp
Spinach egg noodles, cooked, 1 ½ cups
Grated parmesan cheese, 2 Tbsp
Green beans, 1 cup
Oatmeal-raisin cookies, 3
Snack
Air-popped popcorn, 2 cups
Raisins, ⅓ cup
Cranberry juice, 2 cups

ASSESS YOUR PROGRESS

9 *Explain how each energy system supplies ATP for muscles.*

10 *Which energy systems operate under anaerobic conditions?*

11 *What are the effects of age, training, and exercise intensity on aerobic capacity?*

12 *Identify fat or carbohydrates as the primary fuel for the following activities: championship basketball, sprinting, walking, and golfing (walking).*

15.4 Basics of Sports Nutrition

LEARNING OUTCOMES

1 *Describe factors that contribute to the dietary needs of an athlete.*

2 *Explain the energy needs of an athlete.*

Athletes often manipulate their diets to lose or gain weight, increase their muscular strength, and prevent or delay fatigue during exercise. Although an athlete's diet plays a major role in determining if he or she finishes first or last in a competitive event, genetic endowment and physical training are the most crucial factors that influence athletic performance.[18]

Genetic endowment refers to inherited physical characteristics that can affect an athlete's physical performance, such as body size, shape, and composition. Regardless of how well an athlete eats, if this person lacks the physical traits that are necessary for success in his or her chosen sport, the athlete will find it difficult to compete effectively. Athletes must also be highly motivated to compete and engage in a well–designed intensive training program to maximize their physical capabilities. Nevertheless, optimizing an athlete's diet may provide a competitive advantage, especially for sporting events in which hundredths of a second can mean the difference between finishing first and finishing second.

When determining the dietary needs of an athlete, multiple factors should be considered. These include age, gender, height, weight, body composition, type of training, frequency of training, environmental conditions (e.g., temperature and humidity), and current dietary habits. For example, the nutritional needs of a soccer player over the course of a 90–minute game on a hot and humid day are significantly different from those of a 50–yard dash sprinter who competes in a climate–controlled indoor arena.

Proper nutrition is essential for optimal physical fitness and sports performance. **Sports nutrition** focuses on applying nutrition principles and research findings to improving athletic performance and recovery following a training session. This section of Chapter 15 provides specific dietary recommendations that are appropriate for athletes and other physically active people.

Energy Needs

Compared to nonathletes, athletes generally need more energy to support their physically active lifestyles. Athletes who do not consume enough food energy can lose muscle mass and bone density, experience fatigue and menstrual irregularities (females), and be at risk of injury.[22] Thus, low energy intakes can hinder an athlete's chances of performing well.

Male athletes who train or compete aerobically for more than 90 minutes daily need at least 50 kcal/kg/day; their female counterparts need 45 to 50 kcal/kg/day.[23] Thus, athletes may require 3000 kcal/day or more to support their energy needs and maintain their weight. Table 15.3 presents a sample daily menu that is nutritionally adequate, supplies approximately 5000 kcal/day, and pro‐vides ample amounts of carbohydrate.

How can athletes tell if they are consuming enough energy? One way is to have them keep accurate food records and use the information to estimate their daily calorie intakes. Athletes can also monitor their body weight and have their body composition measured regularly. If their weight and body compo‐sition are within healthy ranges before training and they start to lose weight or muscle during training, the individuals should consume more food until they regain their pretraining weight and muscle. Consuming an additional 500 to 700 kcal/day, especially by eating calorie‐ and nutrient‐dense foods such as nuts and dried fruit, is a healthy way for anyone to boost his or her calorie intake. Athletes who gain too much body fat can increase their energy output by spending more time in training. Athletes who have excessive levels of body fat can also reduce their food intake by about 200 to 500 kcal/day, until they are in the healthy BMI range. In general, a good way to reduce energy intake is to limit portions of fatty foods. Chapter 3 provides general information to help people plan nutritious menus.

ASSESS YOUR PROGRESS

13 *List three factors that contribute to the dietary needs of an athlete.*

14 *What are some practical ways to assess whether an athlete's energy intake is adequate?*

15 *Describe the energy needs of male and female athletes engaged in 90 minutes or more of daily aerobic physical activity.*

15.5 Carbohydrate Needs of Athletes

LEARNING OUTCOMES

1 *Explain the importance of carbohydrates before, during, and after prolonged physical activity.*

2 *Identify carbohydrate recommendations for athletes.*

3 *Describe carbohydrate loading, and identify athletes who may benefit from this technique.*

Recommended diets for athletes should supply adequate amounts of energy from carbohydrates and fats. Although carbohydrates and fats are important energy sources for all athletes, carbohydrates are the primary fuel for high‐intensity anaerobic events lasting less than 60 seconds as well as high‐intensity aerobic events lasting more than 60 minutes. Thus, in addition to total caloric intake, many athletes should pay particular attention to their carbohydrate needs and intake.

Carbohydrate Needs

To maintain adequate muscle glycogen, athletes should consume 6 to 10 g of carbohydrate per kilogram of body weight daily.[22] Glycogen depletion is a major cause of fatigue during endurance exercise. By consuming several servings of grains, dairy foods, starchy vegetables, and fruits daily, an athlete can obtain enough carbohydrate to maintain adequate liver and muscle glycogen stores.

genetic endowment inherited physical characteristics that can affect athletic performance

sports nutrition practice of applying nutrition principles and research findings to improving athletic performance and recovery following a training session

DID YOU KNOW?

Olympic gold medalist swimmer Michael Phelps consumed nearly 12,000 per day when training for the Olympic Games. His typical daily diet included three fried egg sandwiches, a five-egg omelet, an entire cheese pizza, a ham and cheese sandwich, and 1000-Calorie drinks. The 12,000 provided the Olympian with the energy necessary for training 6 days a week—an intense regimen that totaled over 50 miles of swimming.

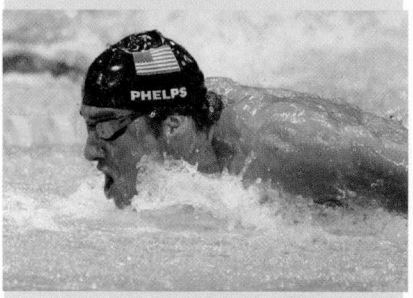

DID YOU KNOW?

A recent study of National Collegiate Athletic Association (NCAA) Division I female student-athletes found that only 9% of the students met their energy needs and 25% consumed the minimal recommendation for carbohydrates. Most of the young women skipped breakfast; about one-third consumed fewer than five meals per day; and only 16% monitored their fluid intake and hydration status during and after workouts. These findings reinforce the importance of nutrition education for collegiate athletes, especially female athletes.[24]

To calculate an individual's recommended range of carbohydrate intake, multiply his or her weight in kilograms by 6 and then by 10. For example, a 145−pound (66 kg) female athlete should consume between 396 and 660 g of carbohydrate each day. If she requires 3000 kcal/day to maintain her weight and physical activity level and she consumes 60% of her energy from carbohy−drates, she will obtain about 450 g of carbohydrate, which is within the recom−mended range.

It is important to keep in mind that there is no "one size fits all" diet plan that specifies amounts of carbohydrate−rich foods for pre−event, event, or post−event meals and snacks. Diets for athletes should be individualized and based on factors such as the athlete's gender, body composition and weight, sport and training level, and exposure to environmental conditions, as well as personal experiences and food preferences. Furthermore, athletes should test any dietary strategies during practices or trials several days or weeks before a competitive event to determine how they react to such changes to their rou−tine diet.

Pre-Event Meals and Snacks

About 3 to 4 hours before competing, athletes should consider eating a meal that supplies 200 to 300 g of carbohydrate, as such meals can improve performance.[22] Table 15.4 provides some menu ideas for high−carbohydrate, low−fat pre−event meals that supply approximately 200 g of carbohydrate. Eating fatty foods such as sausage, bacon, sauces, and gravies is not recommended because they take longer to digest than low−fat foods.[18] Although some nutritionists advise ath−letes to exclude high−fiber foods from pre−event meals, there is a lack of sci−entific evidence to support this recommendation. Nevertheless, athletes can have different responses to eating high−fiber diets prior to events; individuals who react negatively (e.g., excessive intestinal cramping and gas) may find it neces−sary to avoid eating high−fiber foods until after competing.

High−carbohydrate, low−fat food choices for pre−event meals or snacks include cereal with fat−free milk, bagels, dried fruit, pretzels and a sports drink, cooked oatmeal with fruit, pasta, baked potato topped with yogurt, and toasted bread with jelly. Table 15.5 presents commonly eaten foods that are high in carbohydrate and relatively low in fat. Blended or liquid foods pro−mote more rapid stomach emptying than solid foods. Examples of such foods are low−fat smoothies or liquid meal−replacement formulas, such as "instant breakfast" products. There are some athletes who perform optimally on a more empty stomach.[18]

The longer the period before the start of an event, the larger the meal can be, because there will be more time for the stomach to empty and some diges−tion to occur prior to the activity. Many athletes, however, are anxious before competing and may experience nausea and vomiting if they eat at this time. Other athletes feel comfortable consuming a high−carbohydrate, low−fat meal or snack prior to an event. Individual athletes should use trial and error to determine the timing and composition of snacks and meals that optimize their physical performance.

Carbohydrate Loading

A healthy person stores about 6 g of glycogen per kilogram of body weight. Therefore, an individual who weighs 165 pounds (75 kg) stores about 450 g of glycogen. This amount of glycogen supplies 1800 kcal, which is enough energy

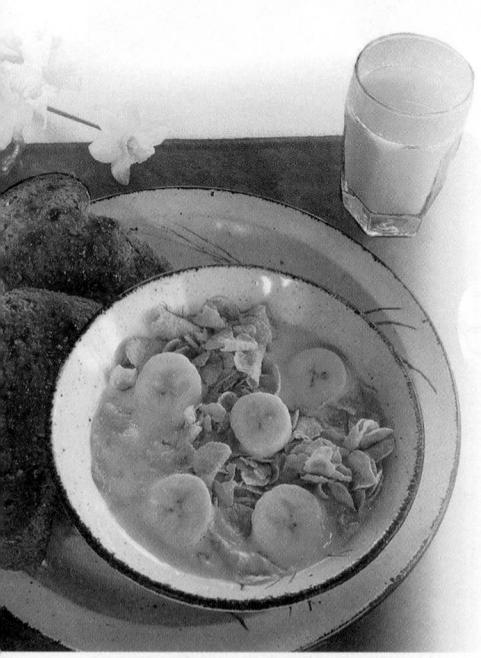

About 3 to 4 hours before performing vigorous exercise, athletes can eat a high-carbohydrate, low-fat meal that supplies 200 to 300 g of carbohydrate.

TABLE 15.4 High-Carbohydrate, Low-Fat Pre-Event Meals

Each menu supplies approximately 200 g of carbohydrate.		
Meal A	**Meal B**	**Meal C**
Instant oatmeal, cinnamon-flavored, 2 packets Fat-free milk, 8 oz	Pasta salad, 1½ cups French bread, 4 slices Soft margarine, 1 Tbsp	Corn Flakes®, ready-to-eat cereal, 1½ cups Fat-free milk, 8 oz Banana, medium
Canned peaches, light syrup, slices, 1 cup	Apple juice, 8 oz	Orange juice, 8 oz
Orange juice, 8 oz Raisin bran bread, toasted 2 slices Soft margarine, 1 Tbsp Jelly, 2 Tbsp	Frozen yogurt, 1 cup	English muffin, toasted Soft margarine, 1 Tbsp Jelly, 2 Tbsp Granola bar

TABLE 15.5 Energy and Macronutrient Contents of Selected Foods

Food and Amount	kcal	Carbohydrate (g)	Protein (g)	Fat (g)
Macaroni, plain, cooked, 1 cup	221	43.20	8.12	1.30
Spaghetti, cooked, 1 cup	220	42.83	8.12	1.30
Rice, instant, white, cooked, 1 cup	194	41.16	4.60	0.58
Egg noodles, cooked, 1 cup	221	40.26	7.26	3.31
Baked potato, ½ large	139	31.62	3.74	0.19
Corn, canned, drained, 1 cup	133	30.49	4.30	1.64
Bagel, ½, 4″ diam.	144	28.04	5.51	0.84
Grapes, 1 cup	104	27.33	1.09	0.24
Banana, 1 med. (approx. 7″ long)	105	26.95	1.29	0.39
Baked beans, ½ cup	119	26.85	6.03	0.47
Crackers, 6 rectangular saltines	154	25.53	3.32	4.09
Orange juice, unsweetened, 1 cup	110	25.05	1.99	0.69
Corn Flakes, 1 cup	101	24.28	1.88	0.03
Pretzels, 1 oz	108	22.61	2.93	0.75
Cooked oatmeal, plain, 1 cup	129	22.44	5.43	2.13
Apple, 1 med. (approx. 3″ diam.)	72	19.06	0.36	0.23
Yogurt, low-fat, plain, 1 cup	154	17.25	12.86	3.80
English muffin, ½	67	13.11	2.53	0.51
Bread, white, 1 slice	66	12.65	2.19	0.82
Fat-free milk, 1 cup	83	12.15	8.26	0.20
Tortilla, corn, ready-to-cook, 1 (6″ diam.)	58	12.12	1.48	0.65
Soy milk, 1 cup	127	12.08	10.98	4.70

Source: USDA: *USDA national nutrient database for standard reference*, release 19. 2006. www.nal.usda.gov/fnic/foodcomp/search/

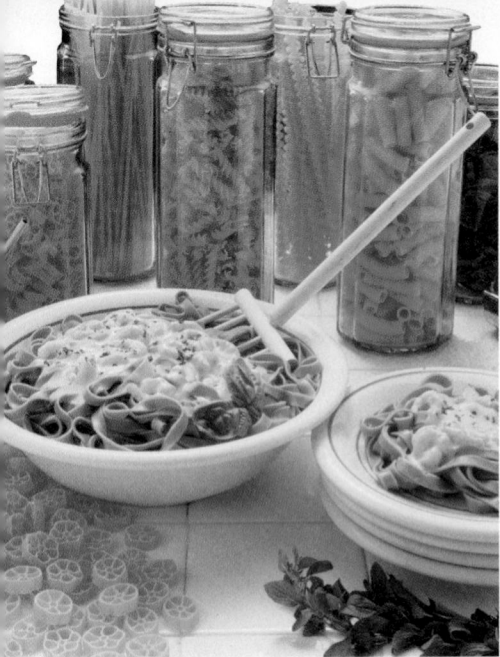

Pasta, rice, bread, potatoes, and cereal are examples of starchy foods that can boost an athlete's carbohydrate consumption.

carbohydrate loading practice of manipulating physical activity and dietary intake of carbohydrates to increase muscle glycogen stores

to enable the person to bicycle at 13 mph for about 4 hours and 15 minutes. Endurance athletes who have more muscle glycogen at the start of an event may be able to exercise longer than those who do not have as much muscle glycogen. **Carbohydrate loading** involves manipulating dietary and physical activity patterns 3 to 7 days before an event to increase muscle glycogen stores well above the normal range. The practice helps delay fatigue in athletes participating in events lasting more than 90 minutes.[25]

The original carbohydrate loading technique called for starting 7 days before an event. An athlete trained intensely during the first day to deplete his or her muscle glycogen stores. Over the next 3 days, the person gradually reduced the duration of his or her daily aerobic workouts (tapering), and during this period, the athlete ate a mixed diet that contained moderate amounts of carbohydrate (about 300 g/day). During the next 3 days, the athlete exercised lightly or rested. The athlete switched from a moderate-carbohydrate to a high-carbohydrate diet during these final 3 days of loading: one that supplied 400 to 800 g of carbohydrate/day. In recent years, a modified version of carbohydrate loading has been recommended. Unlike the original technique, the modified technique (1) does not require depletion exercise and (2) recommends a mixed diet on days 2 to 4, instead of the traditional low-carbohydrate diet during those days. With the modified technique, athletes start tapering their workouts starting 7 days before an event. This tapering continues with the transition from a moderate- to high-carbohydrate diet in the days leading up to the activity. Table 15.6 provides recommendations for both the original and modified carbohydrate loading techniques.

About 3 g of water are incorporated into muscle tissue along with each gram of glycogen. Thus, carbohydrate loading adds water to muscles. Although this fluid aids in maintaining proper hydration status, some individuals experience muscle stiffness and unwanted weight gain as a result of carbohydrate loading. Athletes who would like to determine whether a carbohydrate-loading regimen helps their performance should try the regimens during training to experience their effects and to determine which technique (original or modified) works

TABLE 15.6 Carbohydrate Loading Techniques

	Modified Technique	Original Technique
Day 1	Exercise: tapering	Exercise: depletion
Day 2	Exercise: tapering Diet: moderate-carbohydrate	Exercise: tapering Diet: low-carbohydrate
Day 3	Exercise: tapering Diet: moderate-carbohydrate	Exercise: tapering Diet: low-carbohydrate
Day 4	Exercise: tapering Diet: moderate-carbohydrate	Exercise: tapering Diet: low-carbohydrate
Day 5	Exercise: tapering Diet: high-carbohydrate	Exercise: tapering Diet: high-carbohydrate
Day 6	Exercise: tapering or rest Diet: high-carbohydrate	Exercise: tapering or rest Diet: high-carbohydrate
Day 7	Exercise: tapering or rest Diet: high-carbohydrate	Exercise: tapering or rest Diet: high-carbohydrate
Day 8	Competition	Competition

Source: Adapted from Williams MH and others: *Nutrition for health, fitness, and sport.* 10th ed. New York: McGraw-Hill, 2013.

best for them. Rather than promote carbohydrate loading, many nutrition and human performance experts simply recommend that athletes routinely follow a high–carbohydrate diet and consume certain forms of carbohydrate during pro–longed exercise.

Consuming Carbohydrate During Events

When athletes exercise vigorously for longer than 60 minutes, their glycogen supplies become depleted, resulting in hypoglycemia. At this point, athletes report they have "hit the wall"; that is, they feel exhausted and unable to main–tain a competitive pace. While performing prolonged physical activity, athletes can delay reaching "the wall" by consuming 30 to 60 g of carbohydrate per hour of activity.[22]

Sports drinks are a convenient way to obtain a source of glucose during lengthy and vigorous physical activities. Commercially available sports drinks are usually sweetened with nutritive sweeteners such as sucrose, glucose, fructose, or maltodextrin. Such beverages typically provide 15 to 27 g of carbohydrate per 12–ounce serving. Foods or drinks that are concentrated sources of fructose are not recommended, because large amounts of this particular simple sugar may cause gastrointestinal upset. In addition to supplying carbohydrate, sports drinks contain water and electrolytes, such as sodium, that can benefit athletes during prolonged physical effort. **Sports gels** are also good sources of simple carbohy–drates, but they generally supply very little fluid. Therefore, it is important for athletes who consume these products to drink enough water to maintain proper hydration during endurance events.

Consuming Carbohydrates During Exercise Recovery

After completing exhaustive physical activity, trained athletes can replenish nearly all of their glycogen stores within a few days, provided they rest and eat a high–carbohydrate diet. During a post–event meal, starchy foods such as whole–grain bread, mashed potatoes, rice, and pasta can be served to boost ath–letes' carbohydrate consumption.

Athletes who train intensely each day need to consume 8 to 10 g of carbo–hydrate/kg of body weight to replenish their muscle glycogen stores.[18] To restore their supply of muscle glycogen quickly after an event, athletes can consume sports drinks, candy, sugar–sweetened soft drinks, and fruit or fruit juices.

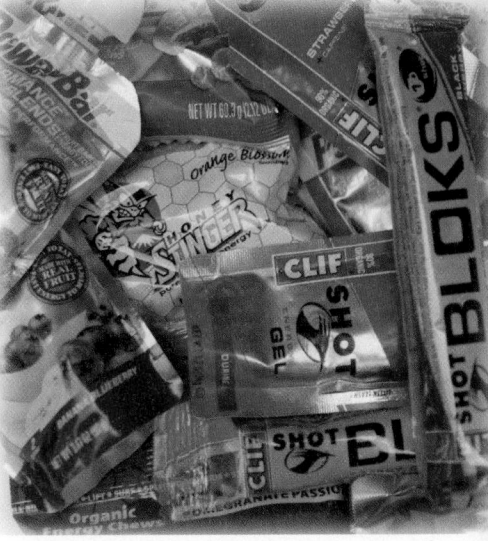

Sports or energy gels provide a concentrated source of carbohydrates and energy. Endurance athletes can easily carry the lightweight sports gels. Prior to competition, an athlete should try the sports gel on several training runs to ensure that the gel does not lead to nausea, which is the case for some individuals.

sports gels carbohydrate-rich gels developed for athletes, particularly those engaged in endurance training and competition

ASSESS YOUR PROGRESS

16 *Why should athletes be concerned about their carbohydrate intakes before, during, and after prolonged intense physical activity?*

17 *Identify at least five high-carbohydrate, low-fat foods.*

18 *Calculate the total daily carbohydrate needs of a 125-pound female athlete.*

19 *Describe the potential benefits of carbohydrate loading.*

20 *Explain carbohydrate needs before exercise, during exercise, and during exercise recovery.*

15.6 Fat Needs of Athletes

LEARNING OUTCOMES

1 *Explain how fats stored in muscle tissue and adipose tissue are used as energy sources during exercise.*

2 *Describe dietary fat recommendations for athletes.*

Along with carbohydrates, fats are a primary source of energy during exercise. As described in section 15.3, the amount of fat versus carbohydrate used as a fuel during exercise is dependent on a variety of factors, including intensity and duration of the activity.

Fats Utilization During Exercise

To fuel activity, muscle cells can use fatty acids from a variety of sources, including plasma free fatty acids (FFAs), intramuscular triglycerides, and plasma triglycerides transported as part of chylomicrons and very–low–density lipo–protein (VLDL). The chylomicrons and VLDL supply less than 10 percent of the fat energy during exercise.[18] Thus, plasma FFAs and intramuscular triglycerides are the primary sources of fat to fuel physical activity.

The amount of plasma FFAs available at any one time is very low. Therefore, plasma FFAs must be constantly replenished by using triglycerides stored in adipose tissue. Recall that, on average, humans store approximately 100,000 kcal of potential energy in adipose tissue. To use FFAs from the adipose tissue to fuel activity, the triglycerides in adipose cells must first be catabolized. Hormone–sensitive lipase (HSL), an enzyme found in adipose cells, facilitates the break–down of adipose cell triglycerides into glycerol and FFAs. The FFAs are then released into the plasma, where they are transported bound to the plasma pro–tein albumin. The plasma FFAs travel to the muscle tissue, where they can be absorbed and then metabolized for energy. Compared to the intramuscular triglycerides, which are an immediate source of energy for the muscles, it takes time for adipose cell triglycerides to be broken down, transported to the mus–cle tissues, and then utilized for energy. Because of this, use of plasma FFAs is greatest in low– to moderate–intensity physical activity. As exercise becomes more strenuous, the muscles rely more heavily on intramuscular triglycerides and carbohydrates as fuel sources.

Fat Needs

For most physically active people, fat should supply 20 to 35% of energy, which is within the range recommended for the general population.[26] Athletes should follow general dietary guidelines in terms of fat intake and focus on consuming health–promoting fats, including monounsaturated fatty acids and omega–3 fatty acids. As with those who are not physically active, sat–urated fat and cholesterol should be limited in the diet of an athlete. Nuts and seeds, hummus, peanut butter, and avocado are examples of foods rich in healthy fats that can be incorporated into snacks and meals for those who are physically active.

Fat Loading

Trained endurance athletes may adapt to long–term, very–high–fat diets (65% or more of total energy) without harming their performance.[27] Nevertheless, the bulk of scientific evidence does not support the use of high–fat diets for ath–letes.[18] Furthermore, very–low–fat diets (<20% of total energy from fat) are not beneficial for athletic performance.[18]

ASSESS YOUR PROGRESS

21 Compare the use of intramuscular triglycerides and free fatty acids during exercise.

22 As a general guideline, how much total fat should an athlete who consumes 2000 kcal/day consume daily?

15.7 Protein Needs of Athletes

LEARNING OUTCOMES

1 Explain the importance of proteins before, during, and after physical activity.

2 Identify protein recommendations for athletes.

3 Summarize the effects of protein supplements, including branched-chain amino acids and whey protein, in resistance and endurance athletes.

One of the most controversial topics in nutrition is the amount of protein needed to support athletic performance. Many athletes are convinced that consuming ample amounts of protein from animal foods and taking protein or amino acid supplements are necessary to improve their physical performance and body build.

Protein Intake of Athletes

The adult Recommended Daily Allowance (RDA) for protein is 0.8 g/kg of body weight.[26] A review of the nutritional practices of elite athletes indicated that individuals training for aerobic sports consumed 1.1 to 3.0 g of protein/kg of body weight per day (g/kg/day), whereas athletes training for anaerobic sports, such as weight lifting, consumed 1.1 to 3.2 g/kg/day.[23] Collegiate male athletes often do not know how much protein they should be consuming, and most of them consume approximately 2.0 g/kg/day.[28] Are such high protein intakes recommended or even necessary?

Importance of Protein for Physical Activity

Under normal conditions, carbohydrate and fat are the primary fuels for cellular activity, and protein provides no more than 10 to 15% of the body's energy needs. Thus, protein is not a major biological fuel. During prolonged physical activity, muscles lose some protein because they metabolize certain amino acids for energy.[18] To spare protein so the nutrient can be used for muscle tissue growth and repair instead of for energy, it is very important for physically active people to consume adequate amounts of carbohydrate and fat.

During moderate and intense physical activity, protein breakdown occurs in the muscles being exercised. After strenuous exercise, muscle cells repair themselves by using available amino acids to synthesize new proteins. Thus, having adequate amounts of amino acids in muscle tissue promotes positive nitrogen balance after exercise.[29] After engaging in intense physical activity, athletes may be able to enhance protein synthesis in their muscles by eating protein-rich foods.[18] Compared to nonathletes, however, the typical athlete consumes more food to meet his or her increased energy needs and, as a result, obtains plenty of dietary protein.[22] Therefore, healthy active Americans who eat varied diets that supply adequate energy do not need to take protein or amino acid supplements.[22] If people consume excess protein from foods or supplements and they do not need the energy, the amino acids in these proteins will not be used for building or repairing muscles. Instead, the body converts the extra amino acids into fat for storage in adipose tissue.

FIGURE 15.9 Branched-chain amino acids (BCAAs). Leucine, isoleucine, and valine are all BCAAs. Notice the similar "branch" points on each of the three structures.

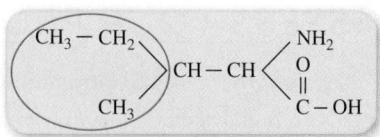

Valine   Leucine   Isoleucine

branched-chain amino acids (BCAAs) amino acids with a unique branched side chain; preferentially utilized by muscle cells for energy

Branched-Chain Amino Acids

The **branched—chain amino acids (BCAAs)** leucine, isoleucine, and valine are found in a wide variety of protein—rich foods (Fig. 15.9). Branched—chain amino acids may enhance exercise performance by delaying fatigue, sparing muscle glycogen, and decreasing protein degradation.[30,31] BCAAs are metabolized differently than other amino acids and may have a greater bioavailability for use during and after exercise. More research, however, is needed to determine the amount of BCAAs that provide optimal effects and the types of exercise in which they may be most effective.

Delayed Onset of Muscle Soreness

delayed onset of muscle soreness (DOMS) muscle soreness occurring in the 1 to 2 days following intense exercises

One to 2 days after performing intense exercise, such as sprinting downhill or lifting weights rapidly, many athletes experience muscle soreness. This **delayed onset of muscle soreness (DOMS)** is a result of microtears to muscle fibers. The microtears interfere with protein synthesis in the muscles, which results in the inability for muscles to repair themselves. By training properly, DOMS can be minimized. Treatment of DOMS often includes consuming a specialized diet or supplementing with certain nutrients, including BCAAs.[32–34]

Protein Recommendations for Athletes

Despite conventional wisdom that athletes have higher protein requirements than nonathletes, there are no specific protein RDAs for endurance or resistance athletes. Members of the National Academy of Sciences review scientific research and establish RDAs. According to experts with the academy, "No additional dietary protein is suggested for *healthy adults* undertaking resistance or endurance exercise."[26] Nevertheless, the RDA for protein (0.8 g of protein/kg of body weight/day) may not apply to athletes involved in training or competition. According to joint recommendations issued by the Academy of Nutrition and Dietetics, Dietitians of Canada, and the American College of Sports Medicine, endurance and resistance athletes should consume 1.2 to 1.4 g of protein/kg of body weight/day and 1.2 to 1.7 g of protein/kg of body weight/day, respectively.[22] Table 15.7 summarizes the protein recommendations based on activity type. Although these amounts of protein are considerably higher than the RDAs for nonathletes, they do not appear to be harmful for healthy, physically active people.

TABLE 15.7 Protein Recommendations for Athletes Engaging in Physical Training

Physical Activity Classification	Grams of Protein/kg of Body Weight/Day*
Adult RDA (nonathletes)	0.8
Endurance-trained athlete	1.2–1.4
Resistance-trained athlete, maintenance phase	1.2–1.4
High-intensity interval training	1.4–1.7
Resistance-trained athlete, building muscle phase	1.6–1.7

* Teenagers should increase their protein intake by up to 10% of the recommended amount.
Source: Williams MH and others: *Nutrition for health, fitness, and sport.* 10th ed. New York: McGraw-Hill, 2013.

Protein Intake Before Exercise

Consuming protein with carbohydrates before exercise appears to provide optimal support during activity. The protein and carbohydrate makeup of a preexercise meal or snack are highly dependent on the type, length, and frequency of activity, as well as an individual's fitness level. In general, athletes should consume 0.15 to 0.25 g of protein/kg of body weight 3 to 4 hours before a strenuous training session or competition.[35]

Protein Intake After Exercise

Consuming protein 1 to 3 hours after exercise can promote protein synthesis and maintain a net positive nitrogen balance.[29] However, sports experts do not agree on recommendations concerning optimal amounts and types of protein that should be consumed after exercise.[36] Research in young men engaged in resistance training indicated that consuming up to 20 g of high−quality protein after exercise optimally supports muscle protein synthesis.[37]

Low−fat chocolate milk has become a popular postexercise recovery drink for athletes, particularly those participating in endurance sports such as running, swimming, and soccer.[38] The carbohydrate−to−protein ratio in low−fat chocolate milk (approximately 32 g of carbohydrate and 8 g of protein in an 8−ounce serving) promotes energy and muscle recovery, and protein balance after exercise.[38] To achieve optimal benefits, low−fat chocolate milk should be consumed both immediately after exercise as well as 2 hours later.[39]

One cup of low-fat chocolate milk provides approximately 178 kcal, 32 g of total carbohydrate, 25 g of sugar, 2.5 g of fat, and 8 g of protein. The nutrient-dense beverage can promote recovery and replenish glycogen stores because of the unique balance of energy, carbohydrates, and protein.

Protein Supplements for Athletes

"Lasting energy," "fast fuel," "optimal energy": Such claims are used to promote so−called "energy" bars, gels, and drinks. Energy or sports bars are essentially cookies made from soy and milk proteins that are fortified with vitamins, minerals, and fiber. Sugary syrups hold these ingredients together. High−protein energy bars may appeal to athletes who think proteins are a source of energy and enhance muscular development. However, proteins are not a major biological fuel, and they are not "quick energy" sources, because the liver must process amino acids before they can be used for energy. Moreover, eating more protein than the body needs does not build muscle tissue. People need to follow a resistance training program to enlarge their skeletal muscles safely.

Yogurt, nuts, granola bars, and fresh or dried fruits are less expensive and more natural sources of energy and protein than energy or sports bars. Those consuming commercial energy bars should check the products' Nutrition Facts panels to determine amounts of carbohydrates and other nutrients that are in a serving. By eating several energy bars daily, a person may ingest high amounts of protein and micronutrients. Therefore, energy bars should be considered as

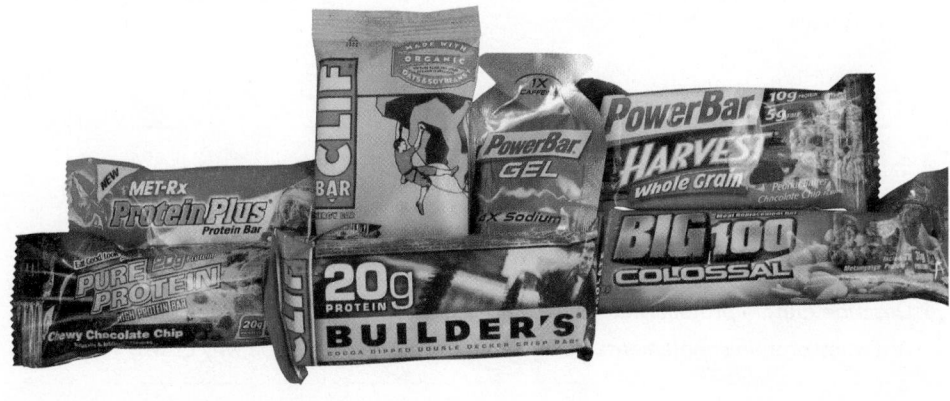

High-protein energy bars may appeal to athletes who think proteins are a source of energy and enhance muscular development. Many of these bars supply 20 to 30 g of protein per serving.

TABLE 15.8 Popular Energy Bars and Gels: Energy and Macronutrient Contents/100 g

Product	Energy (kcal/100 g)	Carbohydrates (g/100 g)	Protein (g/100 g)	Fat (g/100 g)
PowerBar® Performance (cookies & cream)	370	66.2	12.3	4.6
PowerBar ProteinPlus® (cookies & cream)	385	48.7	29.5	7.7
PowerBar PowerGel® (vanilla)	268	65.9	0	0
Luna Bar® (peanut butter cookies)	375	47.9	28.8	12.5
Clif Bar® (chocolate chip)	368	66.2	28.8	7.4
Clif Shot® (vanilla gel)	312	78.1	0	0
Balance Bar® (chocolate)	400	44.0	28.0	12.0
Balance CarbWell (chocolate peanut butter)	400	44.0	28.0	16.0

Sources: Clif Bar & Company, www.clifbar.com/; Luna Bar, www.lunabar.com/index_main.cfm; Balance Bar Food Company, www.balance.com/; Power Bar, www.powerbar.com/

occasional snacks and not as meal replacements. Table 15.8 presents approx—imate energy and macronutrient contents per 100 g of various popular energy bars and gels.

Whey Protein

whey protein nutrient-dense type of protein found in milk.

Milk contains two kinds of protein: casein and whey. Approximately 20% of the protein in cow's milk is whey.[40] **Whey proteins** can be isolated (separated) from the liquid that forms during cheese production. Most whey supplements are powders containing *whey protein isolates*. The powder can be used in many ways, including mixed with water, milk, or juice to form a drink; sprinkled on cereal; or incorporated into a smoothie.

Whey protein is nutrient dense, providing a rich mix of essential amino acids, vitamins, and minerals. Whey protein is also water soluble, can be mixed easily with watery fluids, and is quickly and readily digested.[41] For young adults engaged in heavy resistance training, whey protein supplementation has led to enhanced exercise recovery and increased muscle protein synthesis.[42,43] The effects of whey protein supplementation in endurance athletes are not as well researched as the effects for resistance training. However, coupling whey protein with a source of carbohydrate appears to provide beneficial results for endurance athletes as well.[44] Researchers continue to evaluate the specific effects of whey protein on performance and recovery in resistance and endur—ance activities.

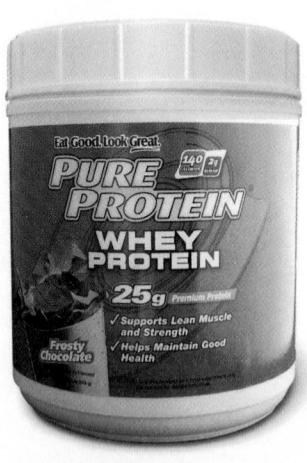

Whey protein supplements are usually found in powder forms containing whey protein isolates. The supplement provides a concentrated balance of essential amino acids.

ASSESS YOUR PROGRESS

23 *Explain the role of protein during and after physical activity.*

24 *Why are branched-chain amino acids important to those who exercise regularly?*

25 *How much daily protein should the following 150-pound athletes consume: endurance trained and resistance trained (maintenance phase)?*

26 *Describe dietary protein recommendations before and following exercise.*

27 *Are whey protein supplements beneficial for athletes? Describe why or why not.*

15.8 Micronutrient Needs of Athletes

LEARNING OUTCOMES

1 *Explain the importance of antioxidant vitamins in physical activity.*

2 *Describe the incidence of iron deficiency anemia and recommendations for prevention in athletes.*

3 *Summarize the roles of vitamin D and calcium in bone health of athletes and exercise performance.*

Vitamins and minerals play essential roles in hemoglobin formation, immune function, and bone health as well as serving as cofactors involved in energy metabolism, but they are not a source of energy themselves. Antioxidant vitamins are also important for protecting the body against oxidative stress and damage. Physical activity may increase the need for certain vitamins and minerals because of (1) increased energy metabolism to support the activity, (2) enhanced turn-over and loss from the body, and (3) consumption of low–calorie diets by some athletes.

Athletes consuming nutritionally inadequate and unbalanced diets may benefit from vitamin and mineral supplementation to meet micronutrient needs. However, vitamin and mineral supplements do not improve performance in athletes consuming nutritionally balanced diets.[22] This section will review the role of antioxidant vitamins, vitamin D, and the minerals iron and calcium in physically active adolescents and adults, and discuss recommendations for intake and supplementation of these micronutrients.

Antioxidant Vitamins

During aerobic physical activities, skeletal muscles use more oxygen and generate more free radicals than resting muscle tissue.[45] Exercise can produce a temporary imbalance between free radical generation and the ability of antioxidants to counteract them. Scientific evidence suggests that such oxidative stress may contribute to muscle fatigue and damage. Nevertheless, results of studies that examined whether antioxidant vitamin supplements enhanced athletic performance generally concluded that performance was not improved, unless there was a preexisting deficiency of those particular vitamins.

Findings of some scientific studies indicate that free radicals generated during intense exercise may stimulate the body's natural antioxidant defense system. Thus, the oxidative stress produced during exercise might have benefits, and blocking this process by taking antioxidant vitamin supplements may not be desirable.[22]

Currently, antioxidant vitamin supplements are not recommended for athletes.[22] Athletes should be cautious about taking such supplements based on anecdotes or advertising claims, because there is not enough scientific evidence concerning the long–term effects of using these products. Results of a meta–analysis on vitamin E supplementation found that vitamin E supplementation increased the risk of stroke by 10 to 20% in healthy adults.[46] Rather than experiment on themselves with antioxidant supplements, athletes should follow diets that contain foods naturally rich in antioxidants, such as fruits, vegetables, whole–grain breads and cereals, and vegetable oils.

Vitamins C and E and Exercise Performance

In addition to their antioxidant properties, vitamins C and E may increase aerobic endurance capacity by enhancing oxygen delivery to muscles and promoting integrity of red blood cells. While some studies have shown a beneficial effect of vitamin supplementation, recent evidence does not support vitamin E in enhancing aerobic performance.[47] Despite the lack of evidence, many athletes still

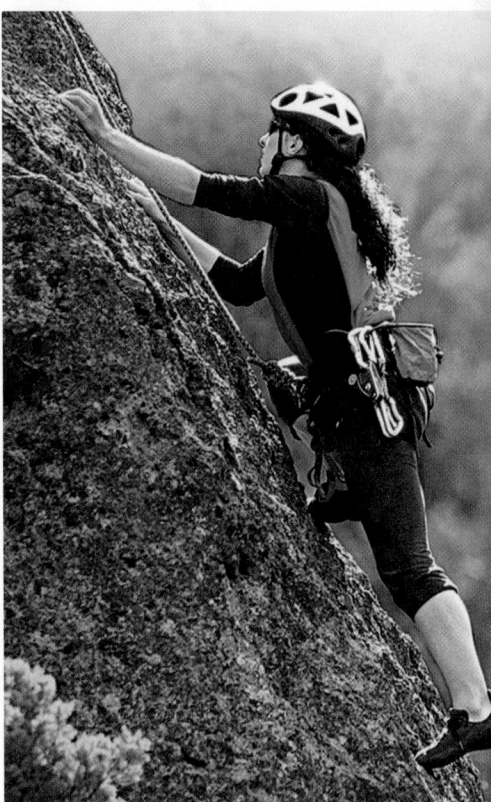

Intense exercise may stimulate the body's natural antioxidant defense system.

supplement their diets with vitamins C and E. Among ultraendurance athletes, over 60% reported using vitamin supplements, with 98% of those taking vitamin C and 78% vitamin E.[48]

Iron

The body needs iron to produce red blood cells, synthesize the oxygen–carrying proteins hemoglobin and myoglobin, and form enzymes involved in energy production.[22] Thus, iron deficiency can negatively affect athletic performance. A study of adolescent female athletes found that 52% were deficient in iron and 9% had iron deficiency anemia.[49] In adult female athletes, approximately 50 to 80% have low iron status, as measured by blood levels of ferritin.[18] Gymnasts and endurance runners have the highest rate of low iron status. However, other elite athletes, including female soccer and basketball players, have iron deficiency.[50] A study of FIFA Women's World Cup soccer players reported that 57% had iron deficiency and 29% had iron deficiency anemia.[51]

As with nonathletes, young female athletes are more likely to develop iron deficiency than male athletes because of their menstrual blood losses: bleeding is a cause of iron deficiency. Athletes who follow low–calorie or vegetarian (especially vegan) diets are also at risk of iron deficiency, because their food choices may be low in iron. Additionally, distance runners may develop low iron status, because intense prolonged workouts can lead to gastrointestinal bleeding.

In the early phase of their training, endurance athletes often develop **sports anemia**, a temporary condition that results from an increase in the liquid portion of blood (plasma), rather than from iron deficiency.[18] The effects of sports anemia on physical performance are unknown. Nevertheless, it can be difficult to differentiate between sports anemia and true iron deficiency anemia. It is a good idea for athletes, especially females, to have their iron status checked at the beginning of a training season and at least once during midseason. If an athlete is iron deficient, a physician needs to determine the cause and prescribe treatment. Taking an iron supplement without the recommendation and monitoring of a physician can result in iron overload, a potentially very serious condition that can result in liver failure. Therefore, health professionals recommend iron supplements should only be given following very careful evaluation and prescription by a licensed health care provider.[18]

Calcium and Vitamin D

Athletes, especially those who are total vegetarians or restrict their consumption of dairy products because of lactose intolerance or to lose weight, can have marginal or low vitamin D and calcium intakes. This practice may result in weak bones that fracture easily, as well as in osteoporosis later in life. In a study of junior elite female soccer players, 67% did not meet the Dietary Reference Intake for calcium, and 100% did not meet recommendations for vitamin D. Half of the young athletes also had depleted blood levels of vitamin D.[52]

Dietary consumption of calcium and vitamin D are essential for maintaining optimal bone health, particularly in cases of estrogen deficiencies. As discussed in Chapter 9, vitamin D enhances the absorption of calcium from the gastrointestinal tract and works with calcium and phosphorus in promoting optimal bone strength. In the United States, only 25% of healthy female adults consume the Adequate Intake (AI) for calcium and 23% for vitamin D.[18,53]

Vitamin D deficiency is most common in athletes who train primarily indoors throughout the course of the year. In addition, athletes training at northern latitudes tend to have the lowest vitamin D status.[22] Even for athletes training closer to the equator, the amount of time spent outdoors during peak daylight hours is the most important determinant of vitamin D status.[53] Poor vitamin D status, in conjunction with inadequate calcium intake, contributes to reduced bone density.

sports anemia temporary condition that develops during the early stages of training in endurance athletes; a result of an increase in the liquid portion of blood (plasma) that results in low hemoglobin levels

DID **YOU** KNOW?

The number of cheerleading-related injuries is on the rise.[54] Approximately 60% of cheerleading injuries in the United States occur during stunts.[55] Fractures, muscle strains, and concussions are the most common cheerleading injuries. The sites most likely to be reinjured while training and performing are the ankle, lower back, and wrist. Low bone density may contribute to bone injury and reinjury in cheerleaders. Therefore, it is important for cheerleaders to meet daily needs for calcium and vitamin D.

Vitamin D and Athletic Performance

The relationship between vitamin D status and athletic performance has been investigated for many years.[56] Early research explored the relationship between sun exposure, fatigue, and athletic performance in athletes. We now know that sun exposure, specifically ultraviolet (UV) light, promotes vitamin D synthesis. UV exposure significantly improves aerobic fitness, muscle strength, and optimal performance in timed sprints.[56]

In recent years, scientists have begun to study the relationship between vitamin D status and athletic performance. In older adults, low blood levels of vitamin D have been associated with reduced reaction time, poor balance, and an increased risk of falling.[57] Based on this and similar findings of other studies, researchers are now exploring the effects of vitamin D on athletic performance in healthy adult athletes. Supplementation with vitamin D appears to improve performance, but further research is needed to examine the magnitude of the effect and the amount of vitamin D necessary to obtain optimal physical fitness.[58] At this time, athletes should meet recommendations for vitamin D intake to ensure optimal athletic performance. Athletes who train predominately indoors should consider taking a vitamin D supplement under the guidance of their health care provider.[53]

The Female Athlete Triad

As described in Chapter 14, the female athlete triad is characterized by disordered eating and low energy intake resulting in abnormal menstrual cycles and low bone mass. Female athletes who have irregular or no menstrual cycles may be deficient in the hormone estrogen. Estrogen is necessary for maintaining healthy bones; therefore, a deficiency contributes to low bone mass. Female athletes who develop menstrual cycle abnormalities should consult a physician to determine the cause. Decreasing the amount of training or increasing the amount of energy consumed may restore a regular menstrual pattern and help protect against stress fractures and bone loss.

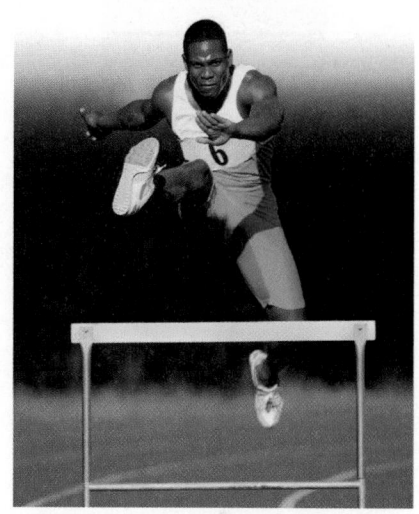

Athletes who train and compete outdoors generally have higher blood levels of vitamin D because of exposure to UV light. Athletes who train exclusively indoors or who train only early in the morning and late at night are at a greater risk for a vitamin D deficiency.

ASSESS YOUR PROGRESS

28 *Explain why you would or would not recommend that an athlete take antioxidant supplements.*

29 *Explain how iron deficiency can impair an athlete's physical performance.*

30 *Identify athletes at the greatest risk for iron deficiency anemia.*

31 *For young female athletes, what is the significance of having irregular or no menstrual cycles for bone health?*

32 *Describe characteristics of athletes at the greatest risk for calcium and vitamin D deficiency.*

15.9 Fluid and Electrolyte Needs of Athletes

LEARNING OUTCOMES

1 *Describe the fluid recommendation for athletes.*

2 *Compare heat cramps, heat exhaustion, and heat stroke.*

3 *Explain the composition of sports drinks and recommendations for consumption by athletes.*

Proper hydration is essential for athletes to optimize athletic performance, delay fatigue, and prevent some forms of heat illness. A deficiency of water and associated electrolytes can result in dehydration and possible death. This section will

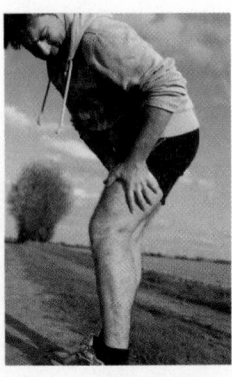

Dehydration can contribute to muscle cramping. Adequate fluid is necessary to prevent and treat this type of cramping.

heat cramps heat-related illness characterized by painful muscle contractions

heat exhaustion heat-related illness that can occur after intense exercise and is characterized by weakness or dizziness

heatstroke most dangerous form of heat-related illness; potentially fatal condition characterized by body temperatures of greater than 104°F

TABLE 15.9 Heat-Related Illnesses: Signs and Symptoms

Heat Cramps
Painful muscle spasms

Heat Exhaustion
Muscle ("heat") cramps
Low-grade fever
Heavy sweating
Weakness
Light-headedness or dizziness
Headache
Nausea

Heatstroke
Severe weakness
High fever (over 104°F)
Lack of sweating
Rapid, shallow breathing
Irritability and confusion
Coma

review fluid recommendations for athletes, as well as causes and treatment of heat–related illnesses.

Fluid Recommendations

The AI for total water intake is approximately 11 cups (2.7 L) and 15.5 cups (3.7 L) for young women and men, respectively. Athletes generally require more water than nonathletes to keep their bodies cool during muscular activity. Many factors, however, influence a person's hydration status. Among athletes in particular, dif–ferences in sports, fitness levels, and environmental conditions affect fluid needs. For example, sweating can cause runners to lose 3 to 8 cups (750 to 2000 mL) of water per hour.[59] Even a small degree of dehydration can lead to declines in an athlete's endurance, strength, and overall performance. Dehydration can result in a fluid and electrolyte imbalance, which contributes to muscle cramping.[60] Moreover, body temperature rises when dehydration occurs, increasing the risk of heat–related illness.

Heat-Related Illness

As the environmental temperature and humidity increase, the evaporation of sweat from skin slows, and the body has difficulty cooling itself by perspiring. Ineffective sweating contributes to fatigue, makes the heart work harder, and raises the risk of heat–related illness. Table 15.9 presents three major types of heat–related illness and their common signs and symptoms.

Heat Cramps

Many athletes have experienced **heat cramps**. These painful muscle spasms (involuntary contractions) can affect any muscle, but they usually occur in the back, abdominal, or calf muscles. The cause of heat cramps is unclear, but the spasms may result from the loss of electrolytes in sweat.[18] Treatment for heat cramps includes resting, drinking juice or a sports drink, and gently stretching and massaging the affected muscles.

Heat Exhaustion

Heat exhaustion can occur after heavy exercise in warm conditions, especially when fluid intake has been inadequate. A person suffering from heat exhaustion experiences heat cramps, sweats excessively, and has an elevated body tempera–ture with a rectal temperature of up to 104°F.[61] Other signs of the illness include cool, moist, gray–colored skin and rapid, weak pulse. To treat heat exhaustion, move the victim to a cool or shady place and have the person lie on his or her back, with legs slightly elevated above chest level. Furthermore, cool the person by fanning, spraying with cool water, or giving a cool sponge bath. It is also very important to have the victim drink cool water or a sports drink. People with heat exhaustion should be monitored closely, because the condition can rapidly develop into heatstroke.

Heatstroke

Heatstroke is the most dangerous form of heat–related illness. Signs of heat–stroke include elevated body temperature (more than 104°F); lack of sweating; rapid, shallow breathing; irritable and confused behavior; and loss of conscious–ness (coma).[61] Heatstroke is a medical emergency that needs to be treated by trained medical staff. If a person appears to have heatstroke, emergency medical assistance needs to be summoned immediately (dial 911) and the victim should be moved to a cool environment. While waiting for professional medical care to arrive, the patient can be given cool water to drink (if he or she is conscious) and sprayed or sponged with cool water.

DID **YOU** KNOW?

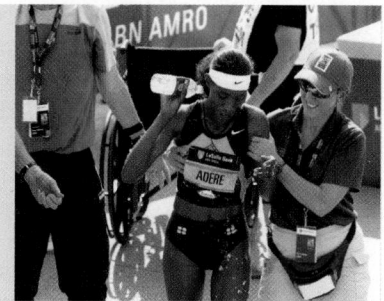

In October 2007, thousands of runners gathered for the annual Chicago marathon. The race began at 8 A.M., and by 10 A.M., the temperature had risen well into the 80s, which was much higher than normal for a fall morning in Chicago. Runners quickly began to experience signs of heat illness and seek medical help at the 15 emergency aid stations along the race route. A 35-year-old man collapsed and died at the eighteenth mile of the race, and more than 300 people were transported by ambulance to hospitals with symptoms of nausea, heart palpitations, and dizziness. Because of the heat, number of ill runners, and chaos on the marathon course, race organizers stopped the event at 11:30 A.M.

Replenishing Fluids

To reduce the risk of dehydration and heat illnesses, athletes and other physi-cally active people should avoid exercising under extremely hot, humid conditions and should replace fluid losses that occur during prolonged exertion. Table 15.10 summarizes recommendations from the American College of Sports Medicine's Position Stand on Exercise and Fluid Replacement. These recommendations

TABLE 15.10 Fluid Needs Before, During, and After Physical Activity

During the Days Leading Up to Training and/or Competition	• Drink adequate amounts of fluid to stay well hydrated. • Avoid alcoholic beverages that may contribute to dehydration.
At Least 4 Hours Before Exercise	• Drink about 5–7 mL/kg of body weight of water or a sports drink. • If no urine is produced or the urine is dark, drink another 3–5 mL/kg of body weight about 2 hours before exercise. • Urine should be a clear yellow color prior to training or competition.
During Exercise	• Drink about 0.4–0.8 L of fluids per hour of physical activity. This is approximately 14 to 28 ounces of fluid during the hour or between 3 and 7 ounces every 15 minutes. Fluid needs will depend on body size and sweat loss. • Fluid needs can be met with cold water in many athletes exercising less than 60 minutes. • For activities lasting longer than 1 hour, beverages containing 6–8% carbohydrate and small amounts of electrolytes are recommended.
After Exercise	• Consume fluids to achieve optimal hydration. • Drink 16–24 ounces of fluid for every pound of body weight lost during exercise. • Consume sports drinks or other rehydration beverages (e.g., low-fat chocolate milk) to replace fluid, carbohydrate, and electrolyte losses.

DID **YOU** KNOW?

Sweat losses during professional tennis matches can be significant with rates of 0.5 to over 5 L per hour in elite male and female tennis players. To avoid dehydration, tennis players should consume 200 mL of fluid containing electrolytes every changeover (the time when players switch sides of the court) when playing in mild to moderate temperatures. When the temperature is greater than 80°F, 400 mL or more fluid should be consumed at each changeover. Fluids containing carbohydrates and electrolytes are often recommended.[63]

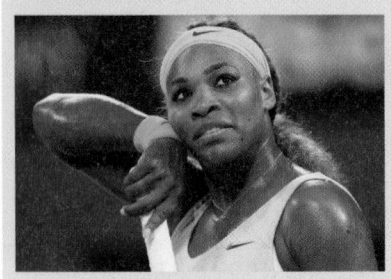

provide guidance for fluid intake before, during, and after exercise.[62] The full position statement can be accessed at www.journals.lww.com/acsm−msse.

Measuring Fluid Needs Through Changes in Body Weight

Athletes should monitor change in body weight and avoid losing more than 2% of their body weight during exercise.[22] To estimate the amount of fluids needed to replace water loss during exercise (rehydration), athletes can weigh themselves prior to exercising and then calculate 2% of their body weight (0.02 × weight). After working out, athletes should weigh themselves again. If the difference between preexercise and postexercise body weights is more than 2%, fluid replacement is necessary during such activities. For example, if an athlete weighs 150 pounds, 2% of that weight is 3 pounds (0.02 × 150). Therefore, the individual should drink enough fluids to avoid losing 3 or more pounds when he or she trains or competes. In general, drinking 2 to 3 cups (16 to 24 fluid ounces) of fluid can replace each pound lost during exercise.[22] If an athlete's usual weight is 150 pounds and he or she weighs 149 pounds immediately after exercising, this person has lost 1 pound of body fluids during the activity. The next time the person exercises under sim−ilar conditions, he or she can consume 2 to 3 cups of water during the activity to maintain body water balance.

Why does a person need to drink 50% more fluids than the amount lost in sweat? After exercise, rehydration may stimulate the kidneys to produce more urine than normal; thus, extra fluids may be necessary to achieve proper hydra−tion.[22] As noted in Chapter 11, alcoholic beverages have a diuretic effect on the body and are not recommended for rehydration.

Sports Drinks

Sports drinks provide some nutritional benefits beyond those of plain water. These beverages usually contain three main ingredients: water, carbohydrates, and electrolytes, particularly sodium and potassium. Simple carbohydrates in sports drinks provide a rapidly absorbed source of energy that can enhance per−formance during endurance activities. Sucrose, glucose, fructose, high−fructose corn syrup, and maltodextrin (a glucose polymer composed of a long chain of glucose molecules) are the most common sources of carbohydrate in sports drinks.

The type of simple carbohydrate in a sports drink does not significantly influence exercise performance.[18] However, a mix of simple carbohydrates pro−vides optimal energy during physical activity.[64] Athletes should carefully read the ingredients list on sports drink labels and consider trying different sports drinks before exercising to determine which one promotes the best performance.

Table 15.11 compares the carbohydrate sources of several popular commer−cially available sports drinks. Recommended products contain about 21 g of car−bohydrate per 12−ounce serving, or about 6% carbohydrate by weight. Drinks with sugar contents above 10%, such as soft drinks or fruit juices, are not recom−mended because they may cause intestinal discomfort. Sodium and other elec−trolytes in sports beverages help maintain blood volume, enhance the absorption of water and carbohydrate from the intestinal tract, and stimulate thirst.

Water

Water is the recommended source of fluid for most athletes exercising at a low to moderate intensity for less than 30 to 60 minutes. Although electrolytes are lost in sweat, the quantities lost in shorter periods can be easily replaced by consuming foods and beverages, such as water or fruit juice, after the event. For events lasting longer than 30 to 60 minutes, high−intensity activities, and when exercising in excessive heat and humidity, sports drinks are often warranted.

Sports drinks are generally not necessary for children participating in youth sports. The sugar content of sports drinks can be excessive for children who do not exercise long enough or at a high enough intensity to necessitate carbohydrate

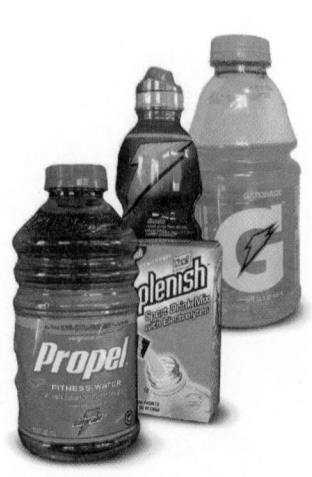

Sports drinks provide some nutritional benefits beyond those of plain water.

TABLE 15.11 Composition of Popular Sports Drinks (per 8-oz Serving)

Sports Drink	Carbohydrate Source	Carbohydrate (% of Concentration by Weight)	Carbohydrate (g)	Sodium (mg)	Potassium (mg)	Energy (kcal)
Accelerade™	Sucrose, trehalose (disaccharide), fructose	6	14	127	43	80
CarbBoom™	Maltodextrin, sucrose, glucose, fructose	7	17	160	50	70
Cytomax®	Amylopectin, maltodextrin, fructose, dextrose	5	11	60	7	45
Gatorade®	Sucrose, glucose, fructose	6	14	110	30	50
Gatorade Endurance Formula™	Sucrose, glucose, fructose	6	14	200	90	50
Powerade®	High-fructose corn syrup	6	14	100	25	56
Powerade Endurance Formula®	Maltodextrin, fructose, dextrose	3	7	76	4	28
Ultima®	Maltodextrin	1.5	3	37	75	10

Source: Adapted from Williams MH and others: *Nutrition for health, fitness, and sport.* 10th ed. New York: McGraw-Hill, 2013.

consumption. Nevertheless, results of a large study of over 1400 children found that 1% of the youngsters regularly consumed sports drinks.[65]

Hyponatremia

It is possible to drink too much water and develop water intoxication (see Chapter 11). Under trained endurance athletes who exercise at relatively low intensities for prolonged periods do not sweat as much as better—trained athletes who exercise at higher intensities. Therefore, those exercising at the lower intensity do not need to replace as much water as those exercising at higher intensities. Regardless of their training level, athletes who drink too much water can dilute the level of sodium in their blood and develop low blood sodium, **hyponatremia** (*high—poe—nay—tree'—mee—ah*). Hyponatremia results in serious and even deadly side effects. Headaches, confusion, vomiting, bloating, and seizures are symptoms of hyponatremia. Immediate treatment is necessary to prevent death.

Although sports drinks generally contain sodium, these beverages are mostly water; therefore, consuming excessive amounts of sports drinks can contribute to fluid overload. To avoid water intoxication and hyponatremia, athletes should drink water according to their fluid losses, primarily through sweat. If an athlete gains weight while exercising, he or she may be retaining too much fluid. Some athletes prevent hyponatremia by eating pretzels during the second part of an endurance event, such as an ultramarathon or triathlon. In addition, vulnerable athletes should be sure they are consuming adequate amounts of sodium in the days leading up to an event.

ASSESS YOUR PROGRESS

33 *Identify at least three reasons athletes generally require more water than nonathletes.*

34 *What are major signs and symptoms of heat cramps, heat exhaustion, and heatstroke?*

35 *Summarize the fluid needs of an athlete before, during, and immediately after exercise.*

36 *When is consuming a sports drink a better choice than plain water for rehydration?*

37 *Explain the causes and treatment of hyponatremia.*

DID YOU KNOW?

The formula for Gatorade was developed in 1960 by Dr. Robert Cade at the University of Florida. Dr. Cade developed the glucose-electrolyte solution, which was the first of its kind, to restore nutrients lost through sweat. The name *Gatorade* came from the "Gators," the nickname for collegiate athletes on the University of Florida's teams.

hyponatremia low blood sodium

15.10 Ergogenic Aids

LEARNING OUTCOMES

1 *Summarize trends in the use of ergogenic aids by athletes.*

2 *Identify commonly used ergogenic aids.*

3 *Describe the ergogenic effects of creatine, energy drinks, and caffeine.*

4 *Explain the safety of ergogenic aids and how supplements are categorized based on safety.*

erogenic aids foods, devices, dietary supplements, or drugs used to try to improve physical performance

anabolic steroid drug that mimics the action of the male sex hormone testosterone

Athletes and coaches often believe misinformation concerning the value of dietary supplements, certain foods, and fad diets for optimizing physical health and performance. Such beliefs can lead to diet—related practices that are use—less and a waste of money. In some cases, these practices are harmful or even deadly.

According to results of a study of college students, 86% had used energy drinks, dietary supplements, or prescription medications within the past year to enhance athletic performance. Energy drinks were the most frequently used (80%), followed by dietary supplements (64%) and prescription medications (53%). Intercollegiate student athletes had the highest use, but club and intramural ath—letes also reported high use of these potentially performance—enhancing aids.[66] Many college athletes use ergogenic aids, but do they work?

What Is an Ergogenic Aid?

Ergogenic aids are foods, dietary supplements, devices, and even drugs ("dop—ing") used by athletes to try to improve physical performance. Creatine, sodium bicarbonate, caffeine, protein supplements, amino acid supplements, energy drinks, and DHEA (*dehydroepiandrosterone*) are all examples of products claiming to be ergogenic agents. **Anabolic steroids** are drugs that are designed to mimic the action of the male sex hormone testosterone to stimulate the devel—opment of muscle tissue. Anabolic steroids pose serious health risks, and are regulated by the Food and Drug Administration (FDA) and Drug Enforcement Administration under the Controlled Substances Act.[67]

Ergogenic aid use is common in athletes of all ages and at all levels of competition. Use of such aids is highest in males, individuals who participate in individual sports, and elite athletes (90% of this class of athletes).[18,68,69] The following sections focus on the use of creatine and caffeine among athletes. Table 15.12 summarizes science—based findings regarding these and some other dietary supplements and ergogenic aids that are popular among athletes.

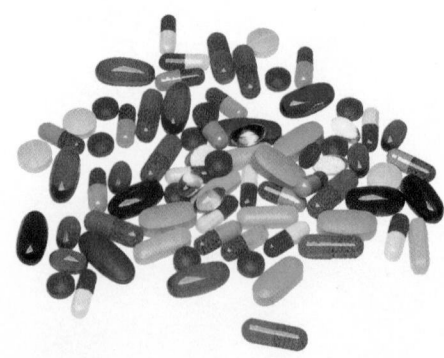

Ergogenic aids include dietary supplements such as caffeine pills and antioxidant vitamin supplements.

TABLE 15.12 Evaluation of Some Popular Ergogenic Aids

Substance	Claim	Current Evidence-Based Findings Concerning Claims	Side Effects
Anabolic steroids	Increase muscle mass and strength	Increase protein synthesis In the United States, legal use requires physician's prescription.	Side effects include blood liver cysts; increased risk of CVD, hypertension, and reproductive problems; mood swings and aggressive behavior ("roid rage"); sleep disturbances Banned by many sports organizations
Bee pollen	Shortens muscle recovery time Increases muscular strength and endurance	No benefit	May cause allergic reactions in sensitive persons
Beta-hydroxy-beta-methylbutyrate (HMB)	Decreases protein metabolism, increasing muscle mass	May increase muscle mass, but evidence is weak	None reported, but results of long-term use are unknown
Branched-chain amino acids	Provide energy for muscles	May enhance muscle recovery after intense physical activity	None reported
Caffeine	Enhances fat metabolism Delays depletion of muscle glycogen Increases alertness	Consuming 3 to 6 mg of caffeine/kg of body weight about 1 hour before exercise can benefit certain athletes.	High doses can cause nervousness, shakiness, and sleep disturbances. Intakes of more than 600 mg (6 to 8 cups of coffee) can produce levels of caffeine in urine that are banned by NCAA.
Chromium	Increases lean mass	No benefit	Toxicity effects unknown
Creatine	Enhances muscular endurance and strength Increases lean muscle mass	May enhance performance of sprinters and weight lifters	High doses may cause kidney damage, especially in persons with kidney disease.
DHEA and androstenedione ("andro")	Increases the body's steroid production Increases testosterone and estrogen levels	No benefit	May be dangerous Banned by International Olympic Committee
Energy drinks	Increases alertness and focus Enhances anaerobic and endurance performance Increases fat metabolism	Results vary based on the composition of the energy drink Some energy drinks may enhance performance of athletes and promote a small amount of fat loss.	See "Caffeine." Elevated heart rate and blood pressure Increased likelihood of engaging in risky behaviors
Gamma hydroxybutyric acid (GHB)	Increases muscle mass by acting like an anabolic steroid	Illegal: FDA has not approved GHB for production or sale in the United States.	Vomiting, dizziness, shakiness, and seizures May cause death
Ginseng	Combats fatigue and improves stamina	May have mild stimulant effects	Adverse effects on the immune system Headache, nausea, and sleep disturbances
Glucosamine	Aids in repairing damaged joints	Mixed results, but generally no beneficial results	None reported
Human growth hormone	Increases muscle mass and fat metabolism	Most studies indicate no benefit.	May increase height in children and adolescents as well as size of the heart and other internal organs at any stage of the life cycle Very dangerous, can be deadly
Sodium bicarbonate (baking soda)	Reduces lactic accumulation	May enhance performance, particularly in exercises that rely primarily on the lactic energy system (e.g., 400-meter sprint)	May cause nausea, vomiting, and diarrhea

Sources: American Dietetic Association: Position of the American Dietetic Association, Dietitians of Canada, and the American College of Sports Medicine—Nutrition and athletic performance. *Journal of the American Dietetic Association* 109:509, 2009; Campbell B and others: International Society of Sports Nutrition position stand: Energy drinks. *Journal of the International Society of Sports Nutrition* 10:1, 2013; Higgins JP and others: Energy beverages: Content and safety. *Mayo Clinic Proceedings* 85:1033, 2010; Williams MH and others: *Nutrition for health, fitness, and sport.* 10th ed. New York: McGraw-Hill, 2013.

creatine nitrogen-containing substance found in muscles; can combine with phosphate to form phosphocreatine

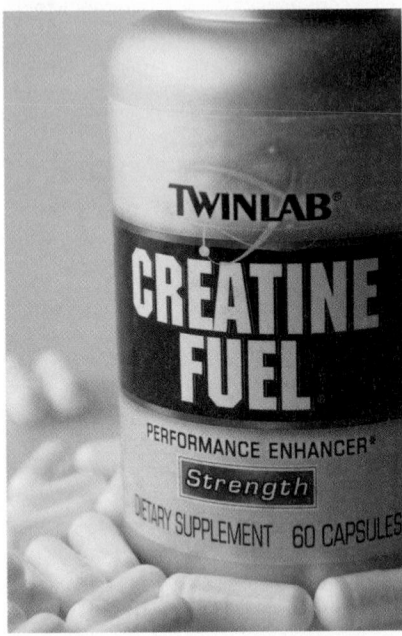

Athletes who use creatine supplements should read the product label carefully for dosing recommendations.

Creatine

Creatine $(kree'-ah-tin)$ is the ergogenic aid used most frequently by athletes who want to build muscle and promote muscle recovery after exercise.[18] Creatine itself does not directly increase muscle mass. Athletes use creatine to increase the amount of the high−energy compound creatine phosphate (CP) in muscles. CP works to replenish ATP in muscles, thus providing the muscles with a quick source of energy (see Fig. 15.7). Creatine is most effective for athletes engaging in activities that rely heavily on the PCr−ATP energy system, such as sprinting and weight lifting. There is no benefit of creatine supplementation for endurance activities, because the PCr−ATP system only provides energy for the first few seconds of an activity. Thus, athletes who perform high−intensity, short−duration activities can benefit from creatine supplementation.[22]

The safety of creatine supplementation has been questioned, because of reports that the compound may damage kidneys and cause diarrhea and nausea. However, results of studies indicate that creatine supplementation is associated with few serious adverse effects.[70,71] Creatine use among young athletes has increased significantly over the past 10 years. Such widespread supplementation has raised concerns about the effects of creatine on growth and development of children and adolescents.[72] The American Academy of Pediatrics opposes use of ergogenic agents, including creatine, in children and adolescents under the age of 18 years.[73]

Caffeine

Worldwide, **caffeine** is the most widely used ergogenic aid. Caffeine is a component of energy drinks and energy shots, as well as natural food and beverage sources, such as coffee, tea, sodas, and chocolate. Some athletes also take pills that contain caffeine.

Caffeine raises the level of fatty acids in the blood, and as a result, exercising muscles can use more fat for energy. By using more fat as an energy source, muscles are able to maintain higher levels of glycogen, which is called glycogen sparing. Caffeine also enhances the ability of skeletal and heart muscles to contract and increases mental alertness. Consumption of caffeine by athletes can dampen pain perception and perceived exertion during exercise.[74]

Although consuming even small amounts of caffeine may help endurance athletes, the National Collegiate Athletic Association limits the amount of caffeine that athletes can have in their bodies during competition. Athletes who have more than 15 micrograms of caffeine per milliliter (µg/mL) in their urine can be banned. Nevertheless, the World Anti−Doping Agency (WADA) removed caffeine from the restricted list in 2004 and does not prohibit the use of caffeine. The WADA continues to monitor caffeine use in athletes as part of its "Monitoring Program" for substances that are not prohibited in sport but have the potential for misuse.[75]

People who are not regular caffeine consumers may experience shakiness, rapid heart rate, sleep disturbances, diarrhea, and frequent urination after ingesting relatively high amounts of the stimulant drug. Caffeine is addictive; discontinuing its use results in withdrawal and temporary unpleasant side effects, especially headache.

caffeine drug found in many beverages and food products, including coffee, tea, and cola drinks, that stimulates the central nervous system and may enhance physical activity

Table 15.13 compares the caffeine and calorie contents of popular beverages, including energy drinks. Note that the amount of caffeine in brewed coffee can vary widely, depending on preparation methods. "Stay awake" pills and chewing gums are concentrated sources of caffeine that can be purchased without a prescription.

TABLE 15.13 Caffeine Content of Selected Beverages

Beverage and Amount	Energy (kcal)	Caffeine (mg)
Chocolate drink, 8 oz	120	2
Coffee, Starbucks® Coffee Grande, 16 oz*	5	330
Coffee, brewed from grounds, unsweetened, 8 oz	2	95
Coffee, instant plain, prepared, 8 oz	5	62
Cola with caffeine, 12-oz can	136–151	29–99
5-Hour ENERGY SHOT®, original, 2-oz bottle[†]	4	215
5-Hour ENERGY SHOT, extra-strength, 2-oz bottle[†]	4	242
5-Hour ENERGY SHOT, decaf, 2-oz bottle[†]	4	6
Monster Energy Drink®, 8-oz can[†]	100	92
Mountain Dew®, 12-oz can[‡]	170	54
Red Bull®, 8.3-oz can	115	76
Rockstar® energy shot, 2.5-oz bottle[‡]	10	229
Tea, brewed, unsweetened, 8 oz	2	47
Tea, ready-to-drink, 12-oz can	89	11

*Starbucks Beverages: Nutrition information www.starbucks.com Accessed: October 31, 2013.
[†]The buzz on energy drink caffeine. *Consumer Reports* December 2012. http://www.consumerreports.org/cro/magazine/2012/12/the-buzz-on-energy-drink-caffeine/index.htm Accessed: October 31, 2013.
[‡]Brands: Pepsi-Cola™ www.pepsicobeveragefacts.com Accessed: October 31, 2013.
Source: U.S. Department of Agriculture: *USDA national nutrient database for standard reference*, release 26. 2011. www.nal.usda.gov/fnic/foodcomp/search

Energy Drinks

Energy drinks are now the second most popular dietary supplement, behind only multivitamins, among adolescents and young adults in the United States.[76] In recent years, use of energy shots in these same populations has also increased significantly.[77] Energy drinks are different from sports drinks in that they contain higher amounts of carbohydrate as well as other ingredients, such as caffeine, vitamin B–6, vitamin B–12, niacin, and *taurine* (an amino acid), that have the potential to improve perceptions of attention and increase alertness.[78] Energy shots are similar to energy drinks, but the "shots" provide a concentrated source of caffeine and certain micronutrients in 2– to 4–ounce servings. Compared to other persons, individuals who are 11 to 35 years of age are most likely to consume energy drinks and energy shots.[79]

The International Society of Sports Nutrition (ISSN) recently published a position paper concerning the use of energy drinks among athletes.[78] According to the ISSN, energy drinks that are consumed 10 to 60 minutes before exercise may improve mental focus, alertness, and sports performance in some athletes. The potential positive effects of energy drinks in athletes may result primarily from the caffeine in the beverages and not from the other added "energy" ingredients. The ISSN urges caution in the use of energy drinks and shots because of the potential for negative effects on physical and mental health. Reported side effects from the use of energy drinks include elevated heart rate and blood pressure, anxiety, increased likelihood of engaging in risky behaviors, and even death.[80]

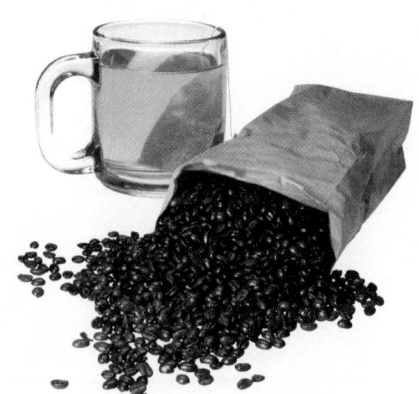

Coffee and tea are natural sources of caffeine.

energy drinks highly caffeinated beverages containing a variety of product-specific "energy blends"

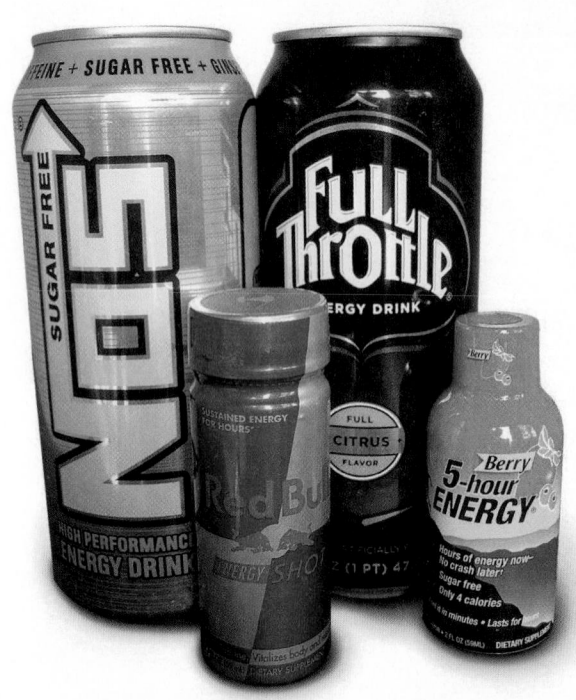

Energy drinks and energy shots are readily available in the United States. The beverages are often conveniently located at the checkout lines.

Powdered Pure Caffeine

In 2014, the FDA warned Americans about the dangers of using powdered pure caffeine. Such products are often marketing through Internet outlets. According to the FDA, consuming a teaspoon of pure caffeine is roughly comparable to drinking 25 cups of caffeinated coffee. People who ingest very small amounts of pure caffeine can experience accidental overdose. Signs and symptoms of caffeine toxicity generally include vomiting, diarrhea, and disorientation; excess caffeine consumption may also cause rapid or dangerously erratic heartbeat, seizures, and death. As of July 2014, FDA was aware of one fatality that was attributed to the use of the powdered caffeine.

Safety and Effectiveness of Ergogenic Aids

Consumers should use caution when evaluating the claims for the effectiveness of ergogenic aids. Many kinds of ergogenic agents are dietary supplements that enter the marketplace without being tested for effectiveness and safety. Other ergogenic aids are produced and obtained illegally. Table 15.12 lists the primary health concerns associated with use of popular ergogenic agents. In addition to such known safety concerns with particular ergogenic agents, there is also concern over contamination with illegal and unlabeled substances in many supplements. In some instances, ergogenic supplements contain high levels of anabolic steroids.[81] Unlabeled ingredients, including anabolic steroids, pose a health risk to the athlete as well as the potential for testing positive on a drug test.

A study of male college athletes found that those using performance—enhancing substances were more likely to use tobacco products, marijuana, cocaine, and prescription drugs without a prescription for the medications. In addition, these young men were more likely to engage in sensation—seeking activities (e.g., driving a car excessively fast) and to consume alcohol and marijuana as coping techniques during stressful times.[82]

Classifying Ergogenic Aids

The American College of Sports Medicine, the Academy of Nutrition and Dietetics (formerly the American Dietetic Association), and the Dietitians of Canada have classified ergogenic agents into one of four safety categories.[22] According to these organizations, an ergogenic aid may be classified as:

1. Effective, safe, and permissible. Although scientific research supports the product's effectiveness, not all athletes may respond positively to its use, because there is individual variability in effectiveness.

2. Possibly effective, safe, and permissible, but there is insufficient scientific evidence to support a more definitive recommendation. Additional research is needed to classify these agents as effective, safe, and permissible.

3. Not effective and the aid's activity does not support claims.

4. Dangerous, banned, or illegal and, therefore, should not be used.

Table 15.14 identifies several ergogenic agents and their classification into one of these four effectiveness and safety categories.

TABLE 15.14 Categorizing Ergogenic Aids Based on Effectiveness and Safety

Ergogenic aids that are effective, safe, and permissible*	Ergogenic aids that may be effective, are safe, and are permissible but for which there is insufficient evidence to support recommendation	Ergogenic aids that are not effective and do not improve performance as claimed	Ergogenic aids that are dangerous, banned, or illegal and, therefore, should not be used
Caffeine	Aspartate salts	Antioxidant vitamins	Anabolic steroids
Creatine	Beta-arginine	Arginine	Androstenediol
Sports drinks, gels, and bars	Colostrum	B vitamin complex	Androstenedione
Sodium bicarbonate	Glycerol	Bee pollen	DHEA
Water	Phosphate salts	Boron	Ephedra
	Protein and essential amino acid supplements	Calcium	Human growth hormone
	Pseudoephedrine	Choline	Synephrine
	Whey protein	Conjugated linoleic acid	Yohimbine
		Coenzyme Q10	
		Ginseng	
		Glucosamine	
		Glycine	
		Niacin	
		Ornithine	
		Pyruvate	
		Ribose	
		Selenium	
		Tryptophan	
		Vitamins A, C, D, E	
		Wheat germ oil	
		Zinc	

*Upper limits have been established for some of these substances.
Sources: American Dietetic Association: Position of the American Dietetic Association, Dietitians of Canada, and the American College of Sports Medicine—Nutrition and athletic performance. *Journal of the American Dietetic Association* 109:509, 2009; Williams MH and others: *Nutrition for health, fitness, and sport.* 10th ed. New York: McGraw-Hill, 2013.

Banned Substances and Testing of Athletes

The World Anti–Doping Agency provides information on dietary supplements that have been banned or are being monitored. Visit www.wada–ama.org for a list of prohibited ergogenic aids (click on "Prohibited List"). The National Collegiate Athletic Association monitors use of ergogenic aids through random urine testing of student athletes. The NCAA posts a list of banned substances and limits on the use of certain ergogenic aids. For more information about the NCAA's list of banned substances, visit www.ncaa.org.

ASSESS YOUR PROGRESS

38 Describe current trends in ergogenic aid use among adolescent and adult athletes.

39 Why do so many athletes use ergogenic aids?

40 Develop a chart summarizing the usage characteristics, efficacy, and safety of creatine, energy drinks, and caffeine.

41 List the four categories used to categorize the effectiveness and safety of ergogenic aids. Identify at least two substances in each category.

42 Identify at least three ergogenic aids that have been banned by at least one athletic association.

SUMMARY

SECTION 15.1 Physical Activity and Health

- Physical fitness refers to the ability of an individual to perform moderate- to vigorous-intensity physical activity without becoming excessively fatigued. Regular physical activity has numerous health benefits, including weight control and prevention of heart disease.
- Aerobic exercises raise heart rate, and resistance exercises build muscle mass, muscle strength, and bone density.

SECTION 15.2 Physical Activity Guidelines

- Adults under 65 years of age should perform moderate-intensity aerobic activity for at least 150 minutes per week. For moderate-intensity physical activity, an individual should exercise at 50 to 70% of their age-related maximum heart rate.
- At least 2 days per week, adults should engage in strength-training exercises, neuromotor exercises, and flexibility exercises.
- Physical fitness plans should be individualized and include three stages: initiation, improvement, and maintenance.

SECTION 15.3 Energy Systems for Exercising Muscles

- The PCr-ATP energy system does not require oxygen and provides energy for quick bursts of physical activity. The lactic acid energy system does not require oxygen. The degradation of glucose to lactic acid provides energy during high-intensity physical activity that lasts up to 30 to 40 seconds.
- The oxygen energy system is the primary source of energy for most exercising muscles. The aerobic system enables cells to produce significantly more ATP energy than the PCr-ATP or lactic acid energy systems.
- The rate of intensity and duration of physical activity determine the fuel source for that activity. Muscle cells rely on a balance of carbohydrate and fat for fuel.

SECTION 15.4 Basics of Sports Nutrition

- Compared to nonathletes, athletes generally need more energy to support their physically active lifestyles. Many athletes require an additional 500 to 700 kcal/day, but caloric needs depend on the individual athlete, type of training, and amount of training.
- Athletes should chose nutrient-dense foods to boost daily energy intake.

SECTION 15.5 Carbohydrate Needs of Athletes

- Carbohydrates are necessary for optimal muscle glycogen in athletes.
- Athletes should consume 6 to 10 g of carbohydrate per kilogram of body weight daily. About 3 to 4 hours before competing, athletes should consume a meal containing 200 to 300 g of carbohydrates.
- Carbohydrate loading may delay fatigue in athletes participating in certain endurance activities. Athletes exercising vigorously or for a prolonged period of time can optimize performance by consuming 30 to 60 g of carbohydrate per hour of physical activity.
- Glycogen stores should be replenished following physical activity.

SECTION 15.6 Fat Needs of Athletes

- Intramuscular triglycerides and plasma free fatty acids are used to fuel exercise. Plasma free acids must be constantly replenished, predominately by breaking down triglycerides stored in adipose tissue.
- Like nonathletes, athletes should consume a diet with 20 to 35% of total calories being supplied by fat.

SECTION 15.7 **Protein Needs of Athletes**

- Protein is not a major energy source during exercise. Protein is important for muscle tissue growth and repair.
- There are no specific protein RDAs for athletes. According to recommendations, endurance athletes should consume 1.2 to 1.4 g of protein/kg of body weight/day. Resistance athletes should consume 1.2 to 1.7 g of protein/kg of body weight/day.
- Consuming protein with carbohydrates before and after exercise provides support for the physical activity and the body's recovery.
- Protein supplements are unnecessary. By eating their usual diet, most athletes meet their protein needs.

SECTION 15.8 **Micronutrient Needs of Athletes**

- Antioxidant vitamin supplements are not recommended for athletes.
- Young female athletes are at the greatest risk for iron deficiency. Athletes who follow low-calorie or vegan diets are also at risk of iron deficiency. Sports anemia is a temporary condition that develops in the early phases of endurance training as a result of an increase in the liquid portion of blood.
- Vitamin D or calcium deficiency in athletes results in low bone mass, increasing the risk of injury during physical activity.
- Athletes who consistently train indoors are at the greatest risk for a vitamin D deficiency. These athletes should consume adequate amounts of vitamin D-rich foods and consider supplementation, if dietary intake is inadequate.

SECTION 15.9 **Fluid and Electrolyte Needs of Athletes**

- Proper hydration is essential for athletes to optimize athletic performance, delay fatigue, and prevent some forms of heat illness. Heat-related illnesses can impair physical performance and cause serious health concerns. Exercising in extremely hot and humid conditions increases the risk for heat-related illness.
- Fluid intake before, during, and after exercise is important in preventing dehydration. An athlete's fluid needs during and following exercise can be determined by measuring changes in body weight. Athletes should avoid losing more than 2% of their body weight during exercise.
- Sports drinks may be beneficial for some athletes. The source of carbohydrate varies based on the variety of sports drink.
- Hyponatremia can result when athletes drink too much water and dilute the level of sodium in their blood.

SECTION 15.10 **Ergogenic Aids**

- Ergogenic aids are used by athletes to try to improve physical performance.
- Scientific evidence does not support the use of most potentially ergogenic agents, and the long-term safety of such products has not been determined. Certain ergogenic aids are restricted or banned by various athletic organizations.

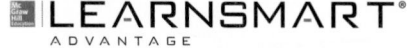

CASE STUDY RESPONSE

TRAINING FOR A HALF-MARATHON

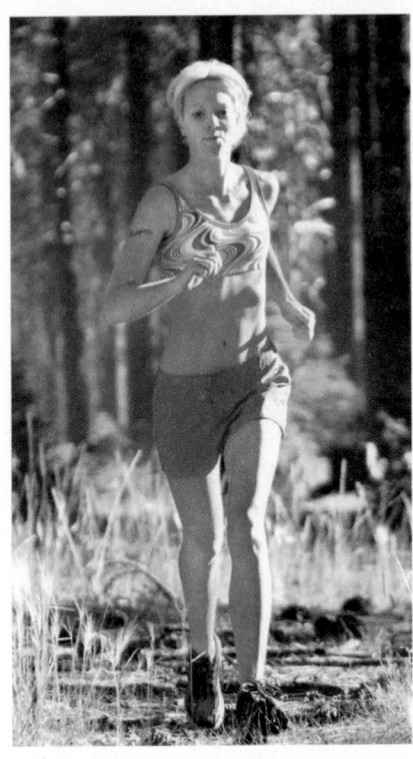

KYLIE'S SKELETAL MUSCLES WILL rely predominately on the oxygen energy system during the running of the half-marathon. A half-marathon is considered a low- to moderate-intensity endurance activity.

Carbohydrates are the primary source of energy during aerobic activities lasting more than 60 minutes. Consuming adequate amounts of carbohydrates (6 to 10 g of carbohydrate per kg of body weight) will enhance her muscle glycogen levels and help provide a sustained source of energy for the endurance activity.

Pretraining and pre-event snacks for endurance activities should be rich in complex carbohydrates and lean protein. Kylie should consume snacks such as a bagel with peanut butter, dried fruit, Greek yogurt with fresh fruit or nuts, pretzels mixed with nuts, or an energy bar.

It is important for Kylie to consume adequate amounts of fluid every day. Approximately 4 hours before a long training run or the half-marathon, she should drink about 5 to 7 mL/kg of body weight of water or a sports drink. While running, Kylie should continue to consume small amounts of water or sports drink, approximately 3 to 7 ounces every 15 minutes. How much fluid Kylie should consume will depend on several factors, including the air temperature, humidity, and length of the run. When exercising under extremely hot and humid conditions, Kylie will sweat more and, therefore, have a greater need for fluids. Following her run, Kylie should consume fluids to achieve optimal hydration. She should drink 16 to 24 ounces of fluid for every pound of body weight lost during exercise. Sports drinks are important for endurance athletes to replenish both fluids and electrolytes as well as to provide a source of energy.

The following 10-week plan provides guidance for an individual training for his or her first half-marathon. Before engaging in any form of strenuous exercise, including training for an endurance event, it is important to have a physical examination. In this plan, the mileage for each run is provided.

	Sunday	Monday (miles/day)	Tuesday	Wednesday (miles/day)	Thursday (miles/day)	Friday	Saturday (miles/day)
Week 1	Rest	3	Rest	3	3	Rest	4
Week 2	Rest	3	Rest	4	3	Rest	5
Week 3	Rest	3	Rest	4	3	Rest	6
Week 4	Rest	3	Rest	5	3	Rest	8
Week 5	Rest	3	Rest	5	3	Rest	10
Week 6	Rest	4	Rest	5	4	Rest	11
Week 7	Rest	4	Rest	6	4	Rest	12
Week 8	Rest	4	Rest	5	4	Rest	9
Week 9	Rest	3	Rest	4	3	Rest	8
Week 10	Rest	3	Rest	3	Walk 2	Rest	RACE DAY!

Critical Thinking

1. Using the recommendations provided in this chapter, analyze your weekly physical activity habits. Does your participation in various activities meet the minimum recommendations? If not, which physical activities are you willing to include in your weekly routine to improve your fitness level?

2. Why is protein not a major source of energy for the body during physical activity?

3. Describe how taking a creatine supplement may improve performance in activities requiring short bursts of intense energy.

4. Develop a chart summarizing the fluid needs of a 170-pound male endurance runner before, during, and after a 3-hour race. Assume the runner lost 2 pounds of body weight during the race.

5. Explain why low-fat chocolate milk is considered a good recovery drink for athletes.

TEST KITCHEN
Modifying Recipes for Healthy Living

Miguel is a 19-year-old college student who exercises at the student fitness facility 6 days per week for 60 to 90 minutes. He rotates his workout a little every day. For example, one day he takes a spinning class, another day he lifts weights and does sprints, and another day he runs for 45 minutes and then takes a 30-minute core workout group class. Miguel generally works out in the late afternoon after his classes have ended for the day. Lately, Miguel has been feeling sluggish during his workouts. Using Miguel's typical lunch sub sandwich meal as a guide, develop a modified version of the meal to provide Miguel with optimal energy during his workout.

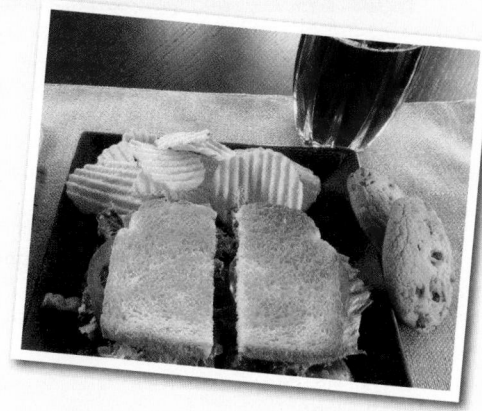

STEP 1 Brainstorm

Use diet analysis software to analyze the nutrient and calorie content of Miguel's lunch. List the total calories, carbohydrates, fat, and protein in the meal. How do you rate the overall quality of the meal?

STEP 2 Develop a modified version of this meal

Provide a detailed modified version of Miguel's lunch to promote optimal energy during his workout later in the afternoon.

STEP 3 Evaluate the modified meal

Use diet analysis software to analyze the total calories, carbohydrates, fat, and protein in the meal. Explain how the two versions of the meal differ nutritionally.

OPTIONAL ACTIVITIES

STEP 4 Shop for the ingredients for the modified lunch

Were the ingredients readily available?

STEP 5 Test your new recipe

Keep notes on any changes you make to ingredient amounts as you prepare the modified lunch.

STEP 6 Reflect on the modified lunch

TYPICAL LUNCH (EATEN 3 TO 4 HOURS BEFORE WORKING OUT)

Homemade BLT sandwich made with 4 slices bacon, 1 lettuce leaf, and 2 slices tomato on white bread with regular mayonnaise (3 Tbsp)

1 small bag potato chips

2 chocolate chip cookies

1 large (20-oz) bottle sweet tea

Practice Test

Select the best answer.

1. Miranda is physically fit. She has
   a. an increased risk of osteoporosis.
   b. the strength, endurance, and flexibility to meet the demands of daily living.
   c. a greater need for vitamins and minerals than other women.
   d. the endurance to run an ultramarathon.

2. A _____ physical activity generally requires a high degree of exertion.
   a. vigorous
   b. basic
   c. moderate
   d. precise

3. Which of the following statements is true?
   a. Resistance exercises do not help build bone mass.
   b. Sedentary activities do not require much energy to perform.
   c. Anaerobic energy systems need large quantities of oxygen to produce ATP.
   d. Contracting muscles rely primarily on protein for energy.

4. What is the target heart rate zone for a 40-year-old male who wants to engage in moderate-intensity physical activity?
   a. 72 to 104 bpm
   b. 88 to 116 bpm
   c. 90 to 126 bpm
   d. 104 to 134 bpm

5. Tom is on his college's track team. While he competes in the 200-meter hurdles, his muscles use primarily _____ for energy.
   a. fat
   b. carbohydrates
   c. protein
   d. vitamins

6. The energy system most active in high-intensity activities lasting for a few seconds is the _____ energy system.
   a. PCr-ATP
   b. oxygen
   c. lactic acid
   d. gluconeogenesis

7. Carbohydrate loading
   a. provides a competitive edge for award-winning sprinters, body builders, and weight lifters.
   b. involves manipulating dietary patterns and physical activities prior to an endurance event.
   c. often results in short-term weight loss and positive energy balance.
   d. is generally recommended for long-term weight control for athletes.

8. A pre-event meal should be consumed _____ before competing.
   a. 5 to 6 hours
   b. 3 to 4 hours
   c. 1 to 2 hours
   d. 30 minutes

9. Which of the following foods is high carbohydrate and low fat?
   a. whole milk
   b. dried apricots
   c. avocados
   d. cream cheese on a bagel

10. According to recommendations, a healthy adult who participates in regular high-intensity interval training should consume _____ of body weight of protein per day.
    a. 0.8 g/kg
    b. 1.2 to 1.4 g/kg
    c. 1.4 to 1.7 g/kg
    d. 1.6 to 2.0 g/kg

11. Drinking at least 6 L of water daily
    a. is recommended by the National Academies of Sciences.
    b. is necessary for healthy persons, even if they are not thirsty.
    c. can result in water intoxication.
    d. improves athletic performance.

12. Sports drinks
    a. are the best source of fluid for most athletes.
    b. contain a mix of complex carbohydrates.
    c. provide carbohydrates and electrolytes in addition to water.
    d. are calorie-free.

13. Iron deficiency is most common in which of the following athletes?
    a. male gymnasts
    b. female gymnasts
    c. male short-distance runners
    d. female short-distance runners

14. Which of the following beverages does not contain caffeine?
    a. Red Bull
    b. tea
    c. chocolate milk
    d. fruit juice

15. Ergogenic aids
    a. have been evaluated for safety and effectiveness by the Food and Drug Administration.
    b. are banned by most sports organizations.
    c. are natural substances produced in the body.
    d. include caffeine and certain amino acids.

ANSWERS TO CHAPTER 15 QUIZ Yourself

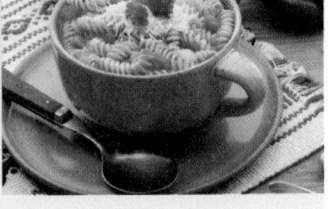

1. To meet physical activity recommendations, healthy adults should perform moderate-intensity physical activity for at least 150 minutes a week. **True** (p. 481)

2. Low-fat chocolate milk is a good postexercise recovery beverage. **True** (p. 503)

3. Protein is the body's preferred fuel during exercise. **False** (p. 488)

4. Carbohydrate loading delays fatigue in athletes participating in events that last between 15 and 30 minutes. **False** (p. 498)

5. Heatstroke is a serious illness that requires immediate professional medical treatment. **True** (p. 508)

References

1. Centers for Disease Control and Prevention: *U.S. physical activity statistics,* 2012. http://www.cdc.gov/physicalactivity/data/ Accessed: March 10, 2014.

2. Clark JE: An overview of the contribution of fatness and fitness factors, and the role of exercise, in the formation of health status for individuals who are overweight. *Journal of Diabetes and Metabolic Disorders* 11:19, 2012.

3. Ballard-Barbash R and others: Physical activity, biomarkers, and disease outcomes in cancer survivors: A systemic review. *Journal of the National Cancer Institute* 104:815, 2012.

4. Sanz C and others: Physical exercise for the prevention and treatment of type 2 diabetes. *Diabetes and Metabolism* 36:346, 2010.

5. Whelton SP and others: Effect of aerobic exercise on blood pressure: A meta-analysis of randomized, controlled trials. *Annals of Internal Medicine* 136:493, 2002.

6. Centers for Disease Control and Prevention: *Strategies to prevent obesity and other chronic diseases: The CDC guide to strategies to increase physical activity in the community.* Atlanta: U.S. Department of Health and Human Services, 2011.

7. Blumenthal JA and others: Is exercise a viable treatment for depression? *American College of Sports Medicine Health & Fitness Journal* 16:14, 2012.

8. Lira FS and others: Exercise training improves sleep pattern and metabolic profile in elderly people in a time-dependent manner. *Lipids in Health and Disease* 10:113, 2011.

9. Anokye NK and others: Physical activity and health related quality of life. *BMC Public Health* 12:624, 2012.

10. Morrow JR and others: Meeting physical activity guidelines and health-related fitness in youth. *American Journal of Preventative Medicine* 44:439, 2013.

11. McCromack GR, Shiell A: In search of causality: A systemic review of the relationship between the built environment and physical activity among adults. *International Journal of Behavioral Nutrition and Physical Activity* 8:125, 2011.

12. Ding D and others: Neighborhood environment and physical activity among youth: A review. *American Journal of Preventative Medicine* 41:442, 2011.

13. Saelens BE and others: Environmental correlates of walking and cycling: Findings from the transportation, urban design, and planning literatures. *Annals of Behavioral Medicine* 25:80, 2003.

14. Starnes HA and others: Trails and physical activity: A review. *Journal of Physical Activity and Health* 8:1160, 2011.

15. Librett JJ and others: Characteristics of physical activity levels among trail users in a U.S. national sample. *American Journal of Preventative Medicine* 31:399, 2006.

16. Centers for Disease Control and Prevention: Physical activity: *How much physical activity do adults need?* Last updated March 2014. http://www.cdc.gov/physicalactivity/everyone/guidelines/index.html Accessed: September 7, 2014.

17. Centers for Disease Control and Prevention: Target heart rate and estimated maximum heart rate. Updated March 2011. http://www.cdc.gov/physicalactivity/everyone/measuring/heartrate.html Accessed: March 10, 2014.

18. Williams MH and others: *Nutrition for health, fitness, and sport.* 10th ed. New York: McGraw-Hill, 2013.

19. Bravata DM and others: Using pedometers to increase physical activity and improve health: A systemic review. *Journal of the American Medical Association* 298:2296, 2007.

20. Jeppesen J, Kiens B: Regulation and limitations to fatty acid oxidation during exercise. *Journal of Physiology* 590:1059, 2012.

21. Yeo WK and others: Fat adaptation in well-trained athletes: Effects on cell metabolism. *Applied Physiology, Nutrition, and Metabolism* 36:12, 2011.

22. American Dietetic Association: Position of the American Dietetic Association, Dietitians of Canada, and the American College of Sports Medicine—Nutrition and athletic performance. *Journal of the American Dietetic Association* 109:509, 2009.

23. Economos CD and others: Nutritional practices of elite athletes: Practical recommendations. *Sports Medicine* 16:381, 1993.

24. Shriver LH and others: Dietary intakes and eating habits of college athletes: Are female college athletes following the current sports nutrition standards? *Journal of the American College of Health* 61:10, 2013.

25. Wismann J, Willoughby D: Gender differences in carbohydrate metabolism and carbohydrate loading. *Journal of the International Society of Sports Nutrition* 3(1):28, 2006.

26. Otten JJ and others (eds.): Institute of Medicine of the National Academies: *Dietary reference intakes: The essential guide to nutrient requirements.* Washington, DC: National Academies Press, 2006.

27. Lambert EV and others: High-fat diet versus habitual diet prior to carbohydrate loading: Effects of exercise metabolism and cycling performance. *International Journal of Sports Nutrition and Exercise Metabolism* 11:209, 2011.

28. Fox EA and others: Perceived protein needs and measured protein intake in collegiate male athletes: An observational study. *Journal of the International Society of Sports Nutrition* 8:9, 2011.

29. Poole C and others: The role of post-exercise nutrient administration on muscle protein synthesis and glycogen synthesis. *Journal of Sports Science and Medicine* 9:354, 2010.

30. Howatson G and others: Exercise-induced muscle damage is reduced in resistance-trained males by branched-chain amino acids: A randomized, double-blind, placebo controlled study. *Journal of the International Society of Sports Nutrition* 9:20, 2012.

31. Blomstrand E and others: A role for branched-chain amino acids in reducing central fatigue. *Journal of Nutrition* 136:544S, 2006.

32. Nelson N: Delayed onset of muscle soreness: Is massage effective? *Journal of Bodywork and Movement Therapy* 17:475, 2013.

33. Torres R and others: Effect of single bout versus repeated bouts of stretching on muscle recovery following eccentric exercise. *Journal of Science and Medicine in Sports* 16:583, 2013.

34. Jackman SR and others: Branch-chained amino acid ingestion can ameliorate soreness from eccentric exercise. *Medicine and Science in Sports and Exercise* 42:962, 2010.

35. Kerksick L and others: The effects of protein and amino acid supplementation on performance and training adaptations during ten weeks of resistance training. *Journal of Strength and Conditioning Research* 20;643, 2006.

36. Aragon A, Schoenfeld B: Nutrient timing revisited: Is there a post-exercise anabolic window? *Journal of the International Society of Sports Nutrition* 10:5, 2013.

37. Moore D and others: Ingested protein dose response of muscle and albumin protein synthesis after resistance exercise in young men. *American Journal of Clinical Nutrition* 89:161, 2009.

38. Lunn WR and others: Chocolate milk and endurance exercise recovery: Protein balance, glycogen, and performance. *Medicine and Science in Sports and Exercise* 44:682, 2012.

39. Pritchett K, Pritchett R: Chocolate milk: A post-exercise recovery beverage for endurance sports. *Medicine and Sport Science* 59:127, 2012.

40. Krissansen GW: Emerging health properties of whey proteins and their clinical implications. *Journal of the American College of Nutrition* 26:713S, 2007.

41. Wilson J, Wilson GJ: Contemporary issues in protein requirements and consumption for resistance trained athletes. *Journal of the International Society of Sports Nutrition* 3:7, 2006.

42. Hulmi JJ and others: Effect of protein/essential amino acids and resistance training on skeletal muscle hypertrophy: A case for whey protein. *Nutrition and Metabolism* 7:51, 2010.

43. Joy JM and others: The effects of 8 weeks of whey or rice protein supplementation on body composition and exercise performance. *Nutrition Journal* 12:86, 2013.

44. Hill KM and others: Co-ingestion of carbohydrate and whey protein isolates enhance PGC-1α mRNA expression: A randomized, single blind, cross over study. *Journal of the International Society of Sports Nutrition* 10:8, 2013.

45. Powers SK and others: Dietary antioxidants and exercise. *Journal of Sports Sciences* 22:81, 2004.

46. Schurks M and others: Effects of vitamin E on stroke subtypes: Meta-analysis of randomized controlled trials. *British Medical Journal* 341:c5702, 2010.

47. Taghiyar M and others: The effect of vitamins C and E supplementation on muscle damage, performance, and body composition in athlete women: A clinical trial. *International Journal of Preventative Medicine* 4:S24, 2013.

48. Knez WL, Peake JM: The prevalence of vitamin supplementation in ultraendurance triathletes. *International Journal of Sport Nutrition and Exercise Metabolism* 20:507, 2010.

49. Sandstrom G and others: Iron deficiency in adolescent female athletes—is iron status affected by regular sporting activity? *Clinical Journal of Sports Medicine* 22:495, 2012.

50. Dubnov G, Constantini NW: Prevalence of iron depletion and anemia in top-level basketball players. *International Journal of Sport Nutrition and Exercise Metabolism* 14:30, 2004.

51. Landahl G and others: Iron deficiency and anemia: A common problem in female elite soccer players. *International Journal of Sport Nutrition and Exercise Metabolism* 15:689, 2005.

52. Gibson JC and others: Nutrition status of junior elite Canadian female soccer athletes. *International Journal of Sport Nutrition and Exercise Metabolism* 21:507, 2011.

53. Ogan D, Pritchett K. Vitamin D and the athlete: Risks, recommendations, and benefits. *Nutrients* 5:1856, 2013.

54. Bagnulo A: Cheerleading injuries: A narrative review of the literature. *Journal of the Canadian Chiropractic Association* 56:292, 2012.

55. Shields BJ and others: Epidemiology of cheerleading stunt-related injuries in the United States. *Journal of Athletic Training* 44:586, 2009.

56. Cannell JJ and others: Athletic performance and vitamin D. *Medicine and Science in Sports and Exercise* 41:1102, 2009.

57. Campbell PMF, Allain TJ: Muscle strength and vitamin D in older people. *Gerontology* 52:335, 2006.

58. Close GL and others: Assessment of vitamin D concentration in non-supplemented professional athletes and healthy adults during the winter months in the UK: Implications for skeletal muscle function. *Journal of Sports Science* 31:344, 2013.

59. Coyle EF: Fluid and fuel intake during exercise. *Journal of Sports Science* 22:39, 2004.

60. Miller KC and others: Exercise-associated muscle cramps: Causes, treatment, and prevention. *Sports Health* 2:279, 2010.

61. American College of Sports Medicine and others: American College of Sports Medicine position stand: Exertional heat illness during training and competition. *Medicine and Science in Sports and Exercise* 39:556, 2007.

62. Sawaka MN and others: American College of Sports Medicine position stand: Exercise and fluid replacement. *Medicine and Science in Sports and Exercise* 39:377, 2007.

63. Ranchordas MK and others: Nutrition for tennis: Practical recommendations. *Journal of Sports Science and Medicine* 12:211, 2013.

64. Garth AK, Burke LM: What do athletes drink during competitive sporting activities? *Sports Medicine* 43:539, 2013.

65. Tomlin DL and others: Sport drink consumption and diet of children involved in organized sport. *Journal of the International Society of Sports Nutrition* 10:38, 2013.

66. Hoyte CO and others: The use of energy drinks, dietary supplements, and prescription medications by United States college students to enhance athletic performance. *Journal of Community Health* 38:575, 2013.

67. U.S. Food and Drug Administration: *Controlled substances act.* Updated June 2009. http://www.fda.gov/regulatoryinformation/legislation/ucm148726.htm Accessed: March 12, 2014.

68. Maughan RJ and others: Dietary supplements for athletes: Emerging trends and recurring themes. *Journal of Sports Science* 29 Suppl 1:S57, 2011.

69. Giannopoulou I and others: Performance level affects the dietary supplement intake of both individual and team sports athletes. *Journal of Sports Science and Medicine* 12:190, 2013.

70. Groeneveld GJ and others: Few adverse effects of long-term creatine supplementation in placebo-controlled trial. *International Journal of Sports Medicine* 26:307, 2005.

71. Lugaresi R and others: Does long-term creatine supplementation impair kidney function in resistance-trained individuals consuming a high-protein diet? *Journal of the International Society of Sports Nutrition* 10:26, 2013.

72. McDowall JA: Supplement use by young athletes. *Journal of Sports Science and Medicine* 6:337, 2007.

73. Gomez J: Use of performance-enhancing substances. Position statement of the American Academy of Pediatrics Committee on Sports Medicine and Fitness. *Pediatrics* 115:1103, 2005.

74. Davis JK, Green JM: Caffeine and anaerobic performance: Ergogenic value and mechanisms of action. *Sports Medicine* 39:813, 2009.

75. World Anti-Doping Agency: *Questions and answers on 2014 prohibited list,* 2014. http://www.wada-ama.org/en/Resources/Q-and-A/2014-Prohibited-List/ Accessed: March 10, 2014.

76. Hoffman JR: Caffeine and energy drinks. *Strength and Conditioning Journal* 32:15, 2010.

77. Wolf BJ and others: Toxicity of energy drinks. *Current Opinions in Pediatrics* 24:243, 2012.

78. Campbell B and others: International Society of Sports Nutrition position stand: Energy drinks. *Journal of the International Society of Sports Nutrition* 10:1, 2013.

79. Ballard SL and others: Effects of commercial energy drink consumption on athletic performance and body composition. *Physiology and Sports Medicine* 38:107, 2010.

80. Higgins JP and others: Energy beverages: Content and safety. *Mayo Clinic Proceedings* 85:1033, 2010.

81. Braume N and others: Research of stimulants and anabolic steroids in dietary supplements. *Scandinavian Journal of Medicine and Science in Sports* 16:41, 2006.

82. Buckman JF and others: Risk profile of male college athletes who use performance-enhancing substances. *Journal of Studies on Alcohol and Drugs* 70:919, 2009.

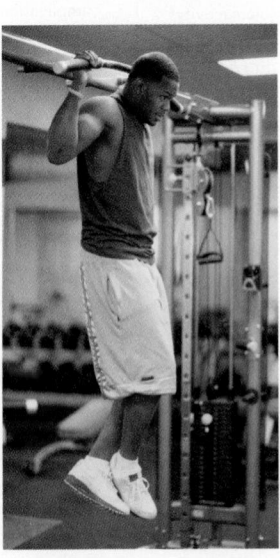

16 Pregnancy and Lactation

Diet during pregnancy

JIA IS EXPECTING HER FIRST BABY. Her prepregnancy BMI was 27; she is currently in her twenty-eighth week of pregnancy and has gained 20 pounds. She takes the daily multivitamin/mineral supplement that was prescribed by her physician. When she discovered that she was pregnant, she stopped drinking alcohol and smoking cigarettes.

Jia's typical breakfast is a chocolate iced coffee drink with a large muffin from a coffee shop. For lunch, she visits a fast-food outlet near her home and has a hamburger, French fries, and a soft drink. At night, she prepares dinner at home and spends the evening watching television.

- If Jia had come to you for preconception counseling, what recommendations would you have given her?

- Assess Jia's weight gain compared to the recommended weight gain for a pregnant woman with a BMI of 27. At this point in her pregnancy, is her weight gain appropriate?

- Provide Jia with an example of an easy-to-prepare, nutrient-dense breakfast and lunch menu that she can make at home.

The suggested Case Study Response can be found on page 548.

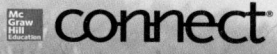 Check out the Connect site at www.mcgrawhillconnect.com to further explore this case study.

QUIZ Yourself

How much weight should a woman gain during pregnancy? Should a pregnant woman "eat for two"? Is breast milk the perfect food for infants? Check your knowledge of pregnancy and breastfeeding by taking the following quiz. The answers are found on page 551.

1. A woman's dietary choices before she becomes pregnant have no effect on the health of her developing offspring. ___T ___F

2. Physicians recommend that women gain at least 25 pounds during pregnancy. ___T ___F

3. Breast milk may not contain enough vitamin D to meet an infant's needs. ___T ___F

4. Babies who consume infant formula have fewer intestinal and respiratory infections than breastfed babies. ___T ___F

5. A 40-year-old pregnant woman has a higher risk of giving birth to a baby with Down syndrome than a 20-year-old pregnant woman. ___T ___F

16.1 Preparing for Pregnancy: Nutrition Concerns

LEARNING OUTCOMES

1 *Define the preconception period, and explain why proper nutrition is important during this period.*

2 *Identify the two groups of females who have a higher risk of complications from pregnancy and the potential causes of the complications.*

gestation pregnancy

conception point at which a woman's egg is fertilized by a sperm; fertilization

preconception period time before pregnancy

fertility ability to conceive

prenatal time from conception until birth

If you are a female, there is an 85% chance that you will have a baby by the time you reach age 40. Thirty years ago, most women began having children in their 20s; today, many women are delaying pregnancy (**gestation**) until they are 30 to 40 years of age and beyond.[1]

A woman who enters pregnancy in the best physical condition and with adequate nutrient stores in her body is likely to achieve two major positive outcomes: a healthy newborn and healthy new mother. Positive lifestyle choices are also important for the father-to-be, as healthy choices may affect the quality of his sperm. When planning a pregnancy, both women and men should consider adopting healthy lifestyles that include:

- Consuming a nutritionally optimal diet;
- Having a healthy BMI;
- Avoiding harmful drugs, including alcohol and nicotine; and
- Exercising regularly.

The Preconception Period

Conception (*fertilization*) is the point at which a woman's egg (ovum) is fertilized by a sperm and pregnancy occurs. The time before pregnancy is the **preconception period**. It is important for both partners to be in good health for conception to occur and for the woman to maintain the pregnancy. According to the Centers for Disease Control and Prevention (CDC), couples should seek preconception health counseling before they begin efforts to conceive.[2] During counseling, the physician or other health care provider discusses aspects of health that have been shown to increase **fertility**, the ability to conceive. Women who have chronic medical conditions such as diabetes and hypertension may need to learn ways to stabilize or improve their health prior to and during pregnancy. Men may be counseled to avoid anabolic steroids and exposure to a variety of environmental toxins, because both can damage sperm's genetic material.[3,4]

Despite the importance of preconception counseling, about one-half of couples experience unplanned pregnancies in the United States.[5] Girls and women should schedule an appointment with a health professional as soon as pregnancy is confirmed. During the initial appointment, the health care provider begins routine **prenatal** (before birth) care, including monitoring the pregnant woman's weight and her blood pressure level.

Mother's Age and the Outcome of Pregnancy

The mother's age when she conceives can significantly influence the outcome of the pregnancy. Teenage (adolescent) girls and women over age 35 years tend to have more health complications during pregnancy than women in their 20s or early 30s.[6]

In the United States, the teenage pregnancy rate is the highest of all developed countries. In 2010, 3.4% of all 15- to 19-year-old girls became pregnant.[6]

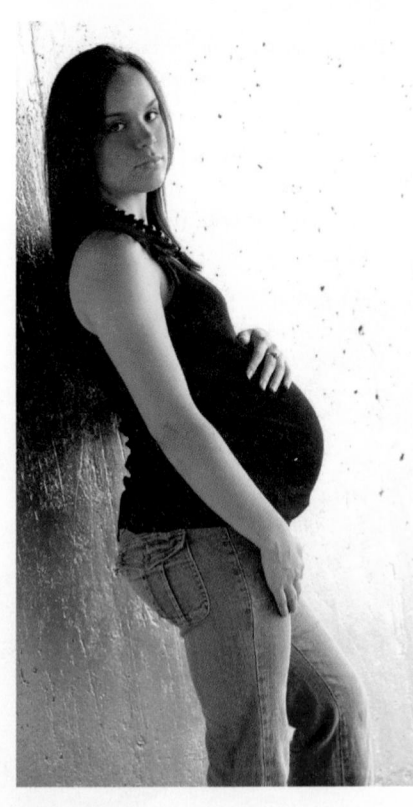

A girl who becomes pregnant within 2 years after she begins menstruating has a higher risk of having complications during pregnancy than older girls and young adult women.

Because her body is still growing, a girl who becomes pregnant within 2 years after she begins menstruating has a higher risk of complications during pregnancy than older girls and young adult women.

The pregnant adolescent needs enough nutrients to support both her fetus's and her own growth. If the teenager's nutritional needs are not met, her baby is likely to have a lower than desirable birth weight or be born before the thirty-seventh week of pregnancy **(preterm)**. Low birth weights and preterm births place newborns' lives in danger. Pregnant teenagers are more likely to have preterm deliveries than pregnant women who are 20 to 30 years of age.[6]

About 20% of American women have their first child after they are 35 years of age.[6] Older women can have healthy pregnancies and normal babies, but the risk of giving birth to a child with birth defects, especially *Down syndrome*, increases as a woman nears the end of her childbearing years. Down syndrome results when a person has 47 chromosomes instead of the normal 46 chromosomes. A baby with Down syndrome has various abnormalities, including characteristic facial features, delayed physical development, and impaired intellectual abilities (Fig. 16.1). A 20-year-old woman has only one chance in 1200 of giving birth to a baby with Down syndrome. By age 40, a woman's risk of having an infant with Down syndrome is one in 100; at age 49 and older, one in 10 women give birth to a child with Down syndrome.[7]

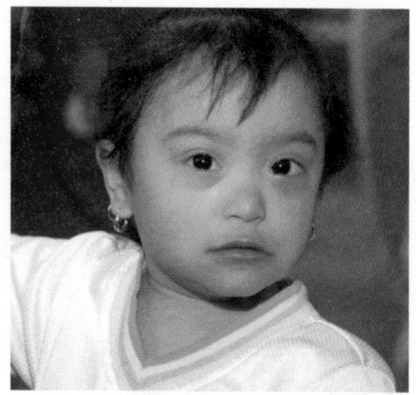

FIGURE 16.1 Child with Down syndrome.

ASSESS YOUR PROGRESS

1. *Why is it important for a woman to eat a nutritious diet prior to pregnancy?*
2. *What are two undesirable outcomes of pregnancy that occurs in adolescence?*
3. *What is Down syndrome?*

preterm describes an infant born before the thirty-seventh week of gestation

full term describes an infant born between 38 and 40 weeks of gestation

trimester three-month period of pregnancy

ovulation release of an ovum (egg) from an ovary

zygote egg that has been fertilized by a sperm

16.2 The Prenatal Period

LEARNING OUTCOMES

1. *Summarize the major physiological milestones that occur during each of the three trimesters of pregnancy.*
2. *Discuss how the placenta develops and the major functions of this organ.*

The prenatal period is the time from conception until birth. The length of most pregnancies is 38 to 40 weeks **(fullterm)**, depending on the method used to calculate the duration of pregnancy. The prenatal period is often divided into three **trimesters**, and each trimester lasts about 13 weeks.

The First Trimester

Pregnancy begins with **ovulation**, the release of an egg cell from an ovary (Fig. 16.2). If sperm are present in the fallopian tube, one of them is likely to fertilize the egg, resulting in a **zygote**. During the first few days after conception, the zygote divides repeatedly in the fallopian tube and eventually forms

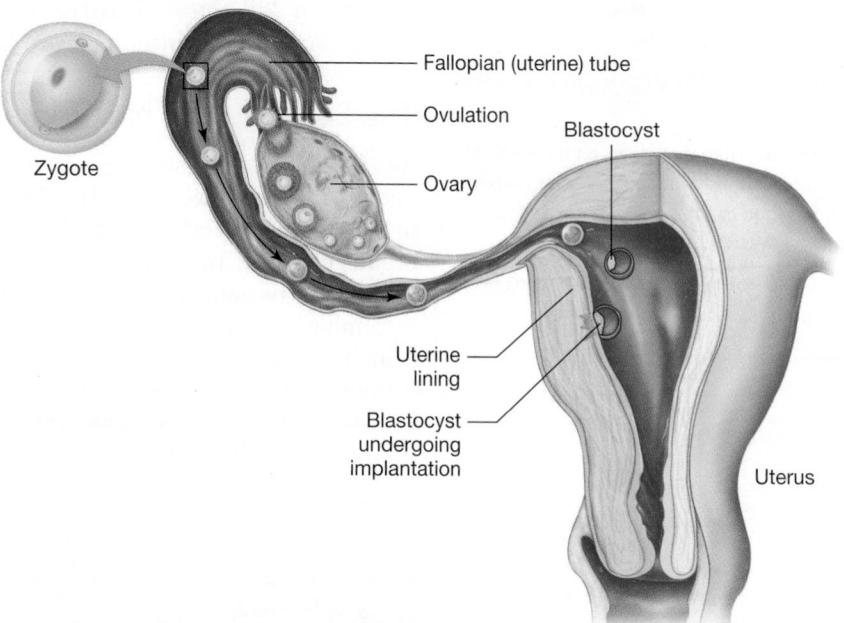

FIGURE 16.2 Conception and implantation.

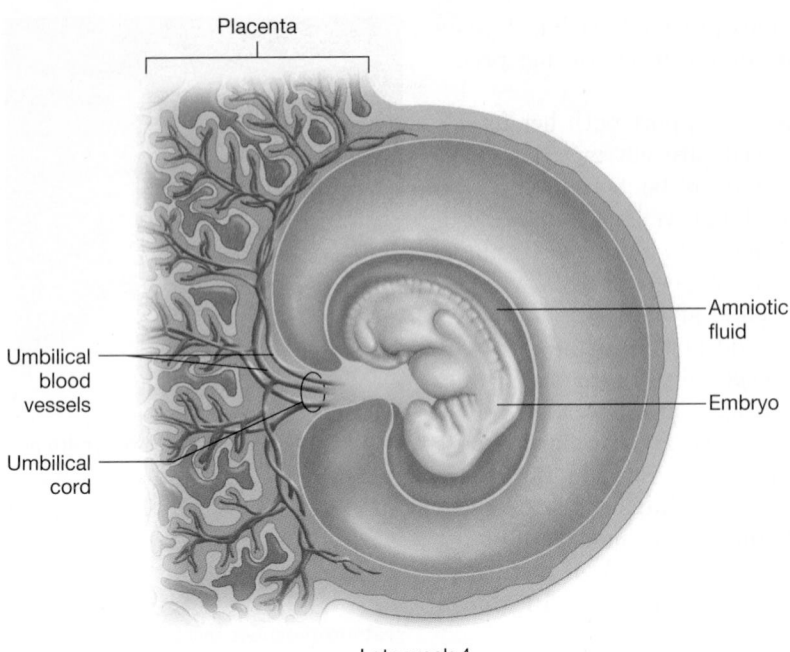

Placenta

Amniotic fluid

Embryo

Umbilical blood vessels

Umbilical cord

Late week 4

FIGURE 16.3 Placenta and umbilical cord. By the end of the fourth week of development, the placenta forms on the lining of the mother's uterus.

a mass of cells (**blastocyst**), which enters the cavity of the **uterus**, the female reproductive organ that protects the developing organism. In the process of *implantation*, the blastocyst imbeds itself in the uterine lining (see Fig. 16.2). The developing blastocyst receives nourishment from nutrients that are stored in the lining of the uterus. Thus, the nutritional status of the mother before conception is very important. The zygote and blastocyst form during the *pre−embryonic* stage of development. From 2 to 8 weeks after conception, the developing offspring is called an **embryo**. After 8 weeks and until birth, the off−spring is a **fetus**.

The Placenta

During the early weeks of pregnancy, the **placenta** forms on the lining of the mother's uterus. The embryo depends on this structure for survival (Fig. 16.3). The **umbilical cord** that extends from the embryo/fetus to the pla−centa contains blood vessels that enter and leave the developing offspring (Fig. 16.3).

The placenta enables oxygen and nutrients to pass from the mother's bloodstream to the embryo/fetus and allows carbon dioxide and other waste products from the embryo/fetus's bloodstream to be eliminated by the mother's body. The transport of nutrients and respiratory gases (oxygen and carbon dioxide) between **maternal** (the mother's) blood and blood of the embryo/fetus occurs by diffusion. Although all nutrients are necessary for a healthy pregnancy outcome, those involved in cell production, such as folate, are extremely important during the first trimester. This stage of embryonic/fetal development is a critical period, because organs are forming.

The placenta acts as a barrier by preventing potentially harmful substances that are in the maternal bloodstream from entering the embryo/fetus. The pla−centa, however, does not prevent transfer of various *teratogens* to the embryo/fetus. Teratogens are environmental substances that cause abnormalities (birth defects) or kill the embryo/fetus. Many drugs, including alcohol and nicotine; viruses; and excess vitamin A are teratogens.

The Second and Third Trimesters

As the second trimester begins, the fetus is very tiny—about 3 ½ inches in length and 1½ ounces in weight.[8] By 5 months of gestation, the fetus is about 7 ½ inches in length and weighs about 1 pound. During the second trimester, the fetus's organs continue to grow and mature in their ability to function.

The fetus gains the most of its birth weight during the third trimester. At the beginning of the last trimester, the fetus weighs less than 2 pounds and is about 9 inches long (from crown to rump). The rate of weight gain increases to about ½ ounce per day during the seventh month of pregnancy. During the last 2 months of gestation, the fetus gains about 1 ounce per day. At birth, healthy full−term infants generally weigh between 7 and 8 pounds and are about 20 inches in length.

blastocyst mass of cells that develops after fertilization and implants in the uterine lining

uterus female reproductive organ that houses the embryo/fetus before birth

embryo refers to the offspring from 2 to 8 weeks after conception

fetus refers to the offspring from 8 weeks until birth

placenta organ that forms on the lining of the uterus and functions to deliver nutrients and oxygen to the embryo/fetus and remove wastes

umbilical cord structure that extends from the embryo/fetus to the placenta

maternal referring to a mother

ASSESS YOUR PROGRESS

4. *Distinguish between the trimesters of pregnancy in terms of embryonic and fetal development.*

5. *Why is a healthy placenta important during pregnancy?*

16.3 Pregnancy: Maternal Physiological Adjustments

LEARNING OUTCOMES

1 *Identify the major changes that occur in a woman's body during pregnancy.*
2 *Describe recommendations for weight gain during pregnancy.*

During pregnancy, it is normal for a woman's body to experience many physio—logical changes, including those listed in Table 16.1. Most of these adjustments are necessary to ensure that the developing offspring receives all the nutrients it needs to thrive. This section discusses major signs of pregnancy, as well as developmental and physiological changes that occur in a healthy pregnant woman's body.

Common Signs and Symptoms of Pregnancy

In the first trimester, most women experience signs and symptoms of pregnancy such as mild nausea and extreme tiredness. Experiencing these conditions can be unpleasant, but they usually do not create serious complications or harm the mother or fetus. Some of the common signs and symptoms of pregnancy include:

- *Breast changes:* An early sign of pregnancy is tender and enlarged breasts. Breasts continue to grow throughout pregnancy as estrogen levels increase, but breast tissue does not produce milk, because high levels of the hormone *progesterone* inhibit milk production.[9]

- *Nausea:* Perhaps the most well—known early symptom of pregnancy is **morning sickness**, which is nausea that is sometimes accompanied by vomiting. The name "morning sickness" is misleading because the queasy feeling can occur at any time of the day. Most pregnant women experience some degree of nausea, which usually begins between the fourth and seventh week of pregnancy and typically ends by the twentieth week of pregnancy. The cause of morning sickness is unclear, but it may result from the adaptation of a pregnant woman's body to high levels of certain hormones. The "Fresh Tips" on page 530 has dietary steps that may prevent morning sickness. Some pregnant women experience severe nausea and vomiting, which we will discuss in section 16.6.

- *Fatigue and sleepiness:* Many women complain of being tired and needing frequent naps during the first trimester. Many pregnant women report having more energy during the second trimester, but fatigue often returns in the third trimester.

morning sickness nausea and/or vomiting during pregnancy

TABLE 16.1 Physiological Adjustments of Pregnancy

Physiological Change	Maternal Effects
Increased synthesis and secretion of hormones *estrogen* and *progesterone*	Facilitates uterine and breast enlargement and suppresses ovulation Slows gastrointestinal tract movements, which enhances nutrient digestion and absorption but can lead to constipation (progesterone)
Synthesis and secretion of the hormone *human placental lactogen*	Increases metabolic rate
Increased synthesis and secretion of the hormone *prolactin*	Stimulates cells in the breast to prepare for milk production
Increased blood levels of the hormone *aldosterone*	Increases blood volume, which may increase blood pressure during the first trimester (after the first trimester, blood pressure normally drops) Lowers concentration of red blood cells in bloodstream (*hematocrit*) Increases likelihood of edema late in pregnancy

Both ginger and vitamin B-6 have been used to reduce nausea in pregnant women;[10] however, some medical experts are concerned about the safety of consuming excessive amounts of ginger during pregnancy.[11] In 2013, the Food and Drug Administration (FDA) approved the use of the medication Diclegis®, which contains a form of vitamin B-6, to treat morning sickness.

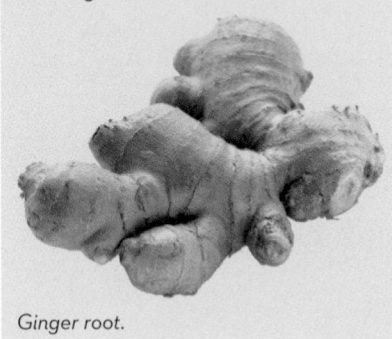

Ginger root.

food craving sudden urge for a particular food or an unusual combination of foods

food aversion intense dislike of a food that was previously enjoyed

pregravid before pregnancy

- *Frequent urination:* Beginning in the early weeks of gestation, many women experience frequent urination, which may last for the duration of pregnancy. By the end of pregnancy, the size of the enlarging uterus presses on the bladder, which reduces the amount of urine the organ can hold (Fig. 16.4). As a result, the pregnant woman makes frequent trips to the bathroom to urinate.

- *Food cravings and aversions:* A **food craving** is characterized by a sudden urge for a particular food or an unusual combination of foods. A **food aversion** is an intense dislike of a food that was previously enjoyed. It is common for pregnant women to experience food cravings as well as food aversions. The causes of cravings and aversions are unclear.

FRESH TIPS

Dietary strategies that are often recommended to control morning sickness include:

- Eating small, frequent meals every 2 to 3 hours. Keeping some food in the stomach may decrease nausea;

- Avoiding fried or spicy foods;

- Choosing carbohydrates that are easy to digest, such as white rice, dry toast, plain baked potato, and plain pasta; and

- Keeping crackers by the bed and eating 1 or 2 before getting up.

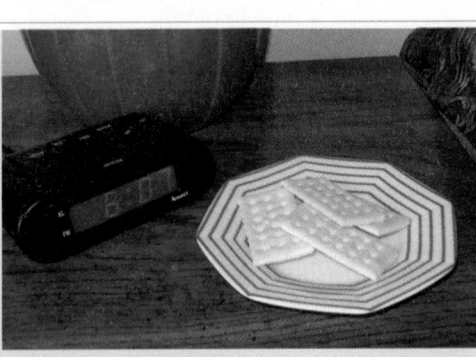

Maternal Weight Gain During Pregnancy

For most pregnant females, the most obvious physical change that occurs during this stage of life is weight gain. Gaining an appropriate amount of weight is very important during pregnancy. Inadequate or excessive maternal weight gain results in the risk of complications and poor pregnancy outcomes.

The total amount of weight gained by the end of pregnancy depends on the woman's prepregnancy **(pregravid)** weight. Experts with the American College of Obstetricians and Gynecologists (ACOG) and the Institute of Medicine rec—ommend that women whose pregravid weight was in the normal range should gain between 25 and 35 pounds, while those who were underweight prior to pregnancy should gain at least 28 pounds.[12] The recommended weight gain for women who

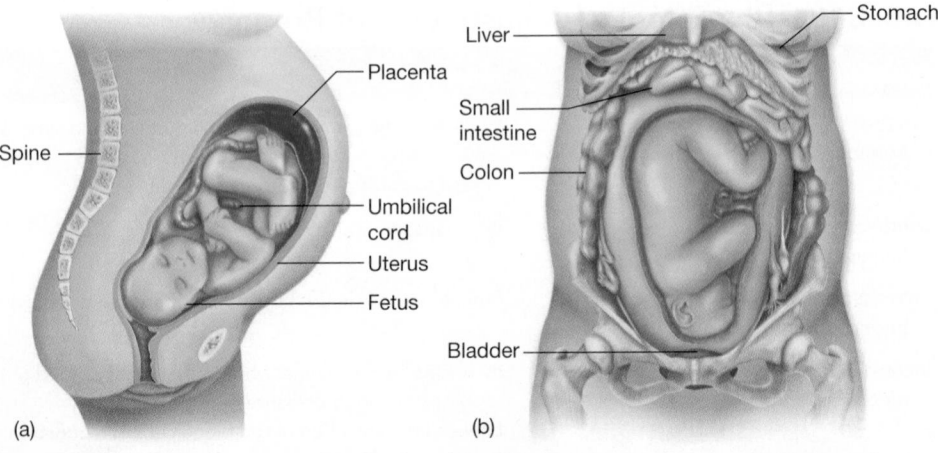

FIGURE 16.4 Position of full-term fetus. (*a*) Cross section showing the normal position of fetus before birth. (*b*) Frontal view showing the extent to which the fetus compresses its mother's bladder and displaces her abdominal organs.

Spine — Placenta — Umbilical cord — Uterus — Fetus

Liver — Stomach — Small intestine — Colon — Bladder

(a) (b)

TABLE 16.2 Weight Gain Recommendations

	Recommended Weight Gains	
Pregravid Weight Status	For Single Birth	For Twin Birth
Underweight (BMI <18.5)	28–40 pounds	*Not established*
Normal weight (BMI 18.5–24.9)	25–35 pounds	37–54 pounds
Overweight (BMI 25–29.9)	15–25 pounds	31–50 pounds
Obese (BMI > 30)	11–20 pounds	25–42 pounds

Source: National Research Council: *Weight gain during pregnancy: Reexamining the guidelines.* Washington, DC: National Academies Press, 2009.

were overweight before pregnancy is 15 to 25 pounds, and the recommendation for women who were obese before pregnancy is to limit their weight gain to no more than 20 pounds. A woman who is pregnant with more than one fetus needs to gain more weight, depending on the number of fetuses. Table 16.2 includes ranges of recommended weight gain based on pregravid weight status, as well as for single or twin pregnancies.

According to the CDC, less than 30% of pregnant women in the United States gain an amount of weight that is within their recommended range.[13] Women who gain too much weight during pregnancy often have difficulty losing the weight after delivery and have a greater chance of developing complications, which are discussed in section 16.6. Additionally, they are more likely to give birth to a **high birth weight (HBW)** infant. At birth, HBW babies weigh more than 4000 g (approximately 8.8 pounds). A large baby is difficult to deliver vag–inally. Such deliveries often require birth by **caesarian section**, which involves surgical removal of the fetus from the mother's uterus.

In contrast, women who do not gain the recommended minimum weight during pregnancy have a greater chance of delivering a **low birth weight (LBW)** infant. A LBW newborn's weight is less than 2500 g (5.5 pounds). LBW infants are more likely to have respiratory distress, heart problems, visual impairment, bleeding in the brain, and intestinal problems than those born with weights in the recommended range.[14] Women who experience inadequate weight gain, particu–larly during early pregnancy, may have a small or poorly developed placenta. A smaller–than–normal placenta means that fewer nutrients can reach the fetus, which can result in delivery of a LBW baby.

Rate of Weight Gain

For a pregnant woman, the rate of weight gain is as important as the total amount she gains. During the first trimester, healthy women usually gain only 1 to 5 pounds. Recommendations for the rate of weight gain during the second and third trimesters are based on the woman's pregravid weight status, based on the BMI (see Chapter 13). Table 16.3 lists the recommended rates for women who are pregnant with a single fetus. Note that regardless of the pregnant wom–an's prepregnancy weight, she should gain about 1.0 to 4.5 pounds during the first trimester.[13] Table 16.4 indicates the components of healthy pregnancy that contribute to weight gain.

Physical Activity in Pregnancy

Being physically active during pregnancy reduces the likelihood that an expectant woman will gain an excessive amount of weight. According to the ACOG, certain activities are appropriate during pregnancy.[15] Most pregnant woman can walk, swim, cycle, and engage in low–impact aerobics safely. During the later stages of pregnancy, women should avoid activities that involve rapid, jerky movements

high birth weight (HBW) infant whose birth weight is greater than 4000 g (approximately 8.8 pounds)

caesarian section surgical removal of the fetus from its mother's uterus

low birth weight (LBW) infant whose birth weight is less than 2500 g (5.5 pounds)

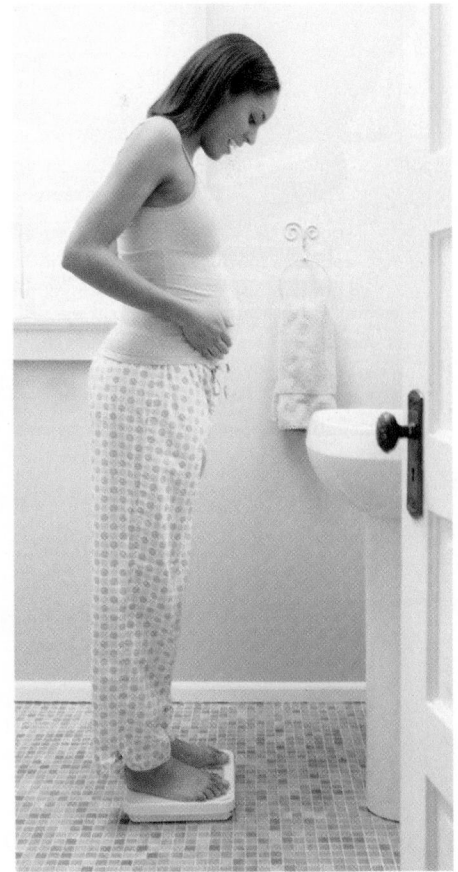

During pregnancy, the rate of weight gain is as important at the total amount of weight gained.

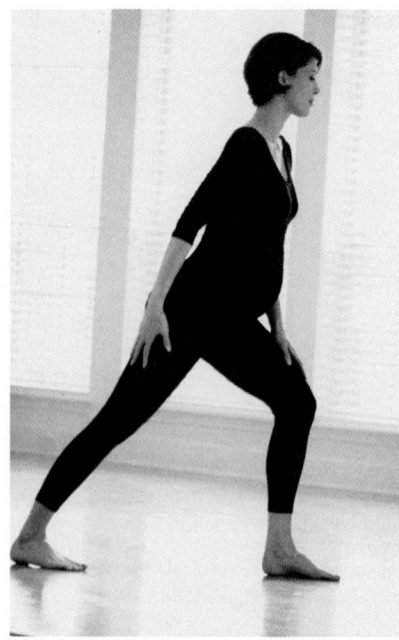

such as tennis and racquetball. Activities that have an increased risk of impact injuries to the abdomen ("contact" sports) or falling, such as gymnastics, downhill or water skiing, and horseback riding, should be avoided throughout pregnancy.[15]

TABLE 16.3 Recommendations for Weight Gain by Trimester of Pregnancy

Prepregnancy Weight Classification (Based on BMI)	Total Weight Gain (Pounds) First Trimester	Weight Gain (Pounds/Week) Second and Third Trimesters
Underweight	1.0–4.5	1
Healthy weight	1.0–4.5	1
Overweight	1.0–4.5	0.6
Obese	1.0–4.5	0.5

Source: National Research Council: *Weight gain during pregnancy: Reexamining the guidelines.* Washington, DC: National Academies Press, 2009.

TABLE 16.4 Distribution of Weight Gain During Pregnancy

Tissue or Component	Approximate Pounds
Maternal	
Blood	4
Breasts	2
Uterus	2
Fat	7
Retained fluid	4
Fetus	7.5
Placenta	1.5
Amniotic fluid (fluid surrounding embryo/fetus)	2.0
TOTAL	30.0

Source: National Research Council: *Weight gain during pregnancy: Reexamining the guidelines.* Washington, DC: National Academies Press, 2009.

ASSESS YOUR PROGRESS

6 List major changes and conditions that a woman is likely to experience during pregnancy.

7 What is the recommended weight gain for a woman whose pregravid BMI was 17?

8 List at least three physical activities that are not recommended for pregnant women.

16.4 Nutrition for a Healthy Pregnancy

LEARNING OUTCOMES

1 Discuss the importance of adequate energy and nutrient intake for pregnant women.

2 Explain why pregnant women should limit certain foods and beverages during pregnancy.

3 Describe the WIC program and its importance.

To meet her increased nutrient and energy needs, a pregnant woman does not need to double her food intake. Even though she may be "eating for two," her embryo/fetus needs a relatively small amount of energy and most nutrients. Women who have well-balanced diets before pregnancy need to make very few dietary changes during pregnancy. To help plan meals and snacks that are nutritionally adequate, pregnant as well as breastfeeding women can follow MyPlate recommendations that are available at http://www.choosemyplate.gov/moms-pregnancy-breastfeeding.

Energy, Protein, and Essential Fatty Acid Needs

During the first trimester, a pregnant woman's daily energy requirement is essentially the same as before pregnancy (Table 16.5). However, during the second and third trimesters, the pregnant woman requires additional energy to support the growth of her enlarging placenta, breasts, and fetus.

Vegetarians who include dairy and eggs in their diets appear to have ample protein intakes during pregnancy. However, it may be difficult for the pregnant *vegan* to consume at least 71 g protein/day, which is her RDA for protein. Vegans should be encouraged to include soy "burgers," meat analogs, and a variety of legumes and other protein-rich vegetables in their diets to ensure ample protein intake. For more information about vegetarianism, see Chapter 7.

For pregnant adults, the Dietary Reference Intake (DRI) for the omega-3 fatty acid alpha-linolenic acid (ALA) increases from 1.1 to 1.4 g/day, while the DRI for linoleic acid increases from 12 to 13 g/day (Table 16.5). During pregnancy, adequate intake of the omega-3 fatty acids eicosapentaenoic acid (EPA) and docosahexaenoic (DHA) is necessary for proper fetal brain and retina development.[16,17] (See Table 6.8 for food sources of DHA.)

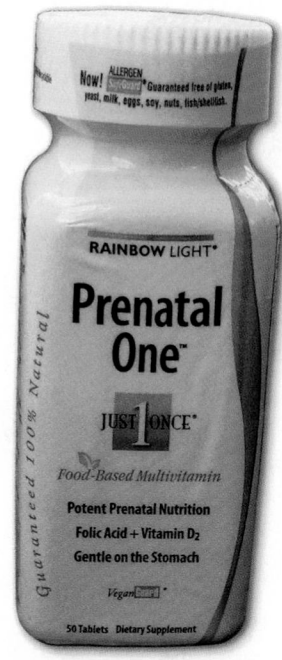

Taking a prenatal dietary supplement daily is often recommended for pregnant women.

Vitamin and Mineral Needs

According to the DRIs, pregnant women require additional amounts of several vitamins and minerals (Table 16.6). In many cases, eating a varied diet that follows MyPlate recommendations will provide the extra amounts. Obtaining enough folate, vitamin D, and iron from food sources can be difficult without taking a dietary supplement that contains these micronutrients.

Vitamin D

Vitamin D deficiency is widespread among women in the United States and throughout the world.[18] The Recommended Dietary Allowance (RDA) for vitamin D during pregnancy is 15 µg/day. According to some medical experts, pregnant

FRESH TIPS

Many ready-to-eat breakfast cereals are fortified with several micronutrients, including folic acid. For example, a single serving of many popular breakfast cereals can provide 600 µg folic acid. For a complete list of cereals that are fortified with folic acid, visit http://www.cdc.gov/ncbddd/folicacid/cereals.html.

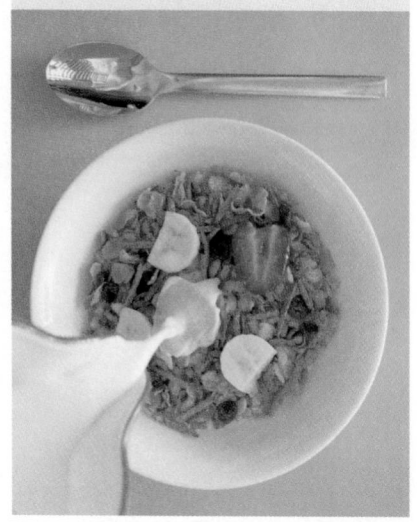

TABLE 16.5 Comparison of Selected Energy and Macronutrient Dietary Reference Intakes: 25-Year-Old Nonpregnant and Pregnant Women

Energy or Nutrient	Nonpregnant	Pregnant
Kilocalories	Estimated Energy Requirement (EER)	First Trimester EER + 0 kcal
		Second Trimester EER + 340 kcal
		Third Trimester EER + 452 kcal
Carbohydrate	103 g	175 g
Fiber	25 g	28 g
Linoleic acid	12 g	13 g
Alpha-linolenic acid	1.1 g	1.4 g
Protein	46 g	71 g

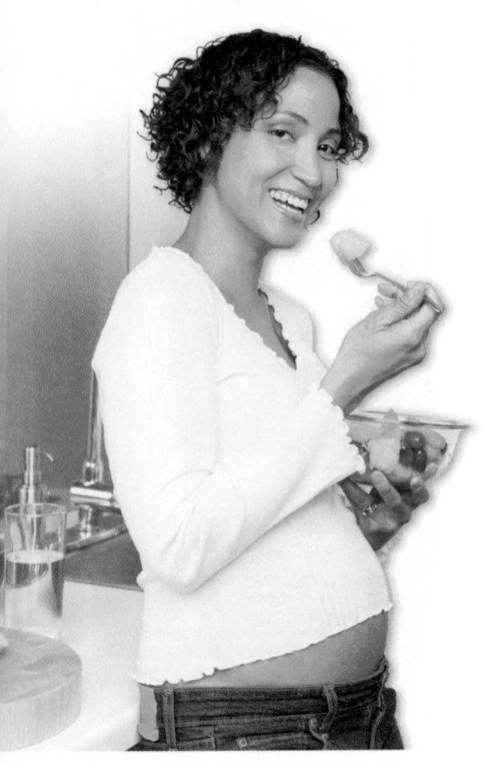

TABLE 16.6 Comparing Recommended Intakes and Upper Limits (ULs)* for Selected Vitamins and Minerals: 25-Year-Old Nonpregnant and Pregnant Woman

Nutrient	Nonpregnant RDA	Pregnant RDA	UL*
Vitamin A	700 µg	770 µg	3000 µg
Folate (DFE)	400 µg	600 µg	1000 µg
Vitamin B-12	2.4 µg	2.6 µg	No UL
Vitamin C	75 mg	85 mg	2000 mg
Vitamin D	15 µg (600 IU)	15 µg (600 IU)	100 µg (4000 IU)
Calcium	1000 mg	1000 mg	2500 mg
Iron	18 mg	27 mg	45 mg
Iodine	150 µg	220 µg	1100 µg

*ULs are the same for nonpregnant and pregnant women.

women can safely consume 100 µg/day, which is the Upper Limit (UL) for the micronutrient (see Table 9.3).[18] More research, however, is necessary to recommend this level of intake for pregnant women.

Vitamin A

Recall from Chapter 9 that vitamin A is required for normal reproduction and cell growth. The UL for vitamin A is 3000 µg/day. During pregnancy, high intake of vitamin A in the forms of retinol or retinoic acid has the potential to be toxic to both the mother and fetus. Excess vitamin A may act as a teratogen, and thus cause birth defects, when the micronutrient is taken by mouth or used topically in skin creams. Some skin treatments for acne, such as isotretinoin and Retin−A®, are derived from vitamin A, and pregnant women should consult their doctors before using these products.

Iron

The RDA for iron is much higher for pregnant women than for nonpregnant women. During pregnancy, the RDA for iron increases 50% from the 18 mg for nonpregnant women, to 27 mg. The additional iron is needed to support increased maternal hemoglobin synthesis that occurs when blood volume expands. Additionally, a pregnant woman's body transfers iron to her fetus, so the developing offspring can produce its own hemoglobin. Pregnant women who are iron deficient have a high risk of giving birth prematurely and having a LBW infant.[19] According to the Dietary Guidelines, iron is a "nutrient of public health concern" for pregnant women.

Pica Some people, especially pregnant women, crave and eat nonfood items such as dirt, clay, or laundry starch on a regular basis. This practice is called **pica** (*pie′−kah*). Some medical researchers think that eating clay or dirt is a *response* to being iron deficient, but it is unclear whether pica causes iron deficiency or is the result of the deficiency. The components of dirt, clay, or raw starch may include the toxic mineral lead that binds to trace minerals such as iron or may compete with mineral absorption.[20] Furthermore, certain bacterial infections or worm infestations may result from eating contaminated soil.[21]

pica eating nonfood substances

Iodine

The RDA for iodine increases from 150 µg for nonpregnant women to 220 µg for pregnant women. The body needs iodine to synthesize thyroid hormone, which is critical for normal fetal brain development. In Chapter 12, we discussed the risk of cretinism in children who are born to mothers who had severe iodine deficiency during pregnancy. Pregnant women who avoid using iodized salt should ask their physician about the need to take a prenatal supplement that contains the rec—ommended amount of iodine.

Calcium

The RDA for calcium does not increase during pregnancy, primarily because absorption of the mineral increases. Many American women, however, do not consume enough calcium—rich foods.[22] In the third trimester, fetal bone miner—alization occurs at a rapid rate, as about 150 mg calcium/day cross the placenta to meet the fetus's demand for the mineral.[23] Women who are in a calcium—depleted state when they become pregnant and consume low amounts of the mineral during pregnancy are likely to have difficulty replacing the calcium after their babies are born. Therefore, it is important for women to enter pregnancy with ample calcium reserves.

Special Supplemental Nutrition Assistance Program for Women, Infants, and Children

In the United States, the federal government manages the **Special Supplemental Nutrition Assistance Program for Women, Infants, and Children**, commonly known as **WIC**. WIC provides funds to state governments so they can help spe—cific populations obtain certain supplemental foods, basic health care services, and nutrition education. Such populations are low—income, nutritionally at—risk pregnant women; women who have recently given birth and are breastfeeding or formula—feeding their infants; and children under 5 years of age who are con—sidered at "nutritional risk." Nutritional risks may be medically based, such as having anemia, being underweight or obese, or having a history of pregnancy complications. Nutritional risks may also be diet—based, such as having food allergies, gastrointestinal disorders, or poor dietary practices.[24]

To obtain foods, beverages, and infant formulas that are allowed by the WIC program, participants receive vouchers or checks that are redeemable at partici—pating grocery stores. WIC—eligible foods are those that are rich in iron, calcium, vitamins A and C, and protein. Such foods include iron—fortified infant and adult cereals, eggs, milk, cheese, peanut butter, dried beans and peas, canned fish, and certain fruit and vegetable juices. Other eligible foods include soy beverages, tofu, baby foods, whole—wheat breads and grain options, and fresh fruits and vegetables.

In 2013, approximately 8.6 million women, infants, and children received WIC benefits each month.[24] Results of studies indicate that participation in the WIC program provides important public health benefits for infants and children, including:[25]

- Reduced incidence of fetal death, low birth weight, and infant mortality;

- Improved growth of nutritionally at—risk infants and children;

- Decreased incidence of iron deficiency anemia in young children; and

- Improved intellectual development.

Special Supplemental Nutrition Assistance Program for Women, Infants, and Children (WIC) federal program that provides funds to state governments so they can help specific populations obtain certain supplemental foods, basic health care services, and nutrition education

ASSESS YOUR PROGRESS

9 *Discuss the importance of adequate energy and nutrient intakes during pregnancy.*

10 *Explain why a woman's needs for folate, iron, and iodine increase by 50% during pregnancy.*

11 *What is WIC?*

16.5 Substances to Limit or Avoid During Pregnancy

LEARNING OUTCOMES

1 *Identify the recommendation concerning alcohol consumption during pregnancy.*
2 *Explain the possible effects of alcohol and caffeine consumption on an embryo/fetus.*
3 *Explain how a pregnant woman's exposure to lead or arsenic may affect her baby.*
4 *Summarize recommendations for avoiding mercury or methylmercury during pregnancy.*

A great deal of emphasis is placed on what pregnant women should consume to increase the likelihood of having a healthy baby. What substances should she avoid? Can she drink alcohol without harming her developing offspring? This section of the chapter focuses on substances that should be avoided or limited during pregnancy.

Alcohol

When a pregnant woman drinks a beverage that contains alcohol, her embryo/fetus also "drinks" the alcohol, because the drug passes freely from the mother's bloodstream, through the placenta, and into her offspring's bloodstream. Exposure to alcohol can damage neurons in the brain of the embryo/fetus, which can result in psychological, *cognitive* (thought processes), and behavioral problems. Alcohol exposure can also injure other tissues in the developing offspring and, in extreme cases, cause its death.[26] The toxic effects of alcohol are most devastating to an embryo, because this is the critical period when organs are forming. Unfortunately, many women are not aware that they are pregnant during this early stage of their offspring's development.

Fetal alcohol spectrum disorders (FASDs) is the umbrella term for conditions that can affect a child whose mother drank alcohol during pregnancy. The most devastating form of FASDs is **fetal alcohol syndrome (FAS)**, a condition characterized by severe birth defects that occur in infants whose mothers drank *excessively* during pregnancy. Babies who are born with FAS have distinct facial abnormalities (Fig. 16.5). They also have heart abnormalities as well as extensive, irreversible damage to their nervous system that causes intellectual impairment and behavioral problems. Children who have FAS also experience delayed physical development.

Medical experts do not know how much alcohol is safe to consume during pregnancy, and they do not know whether there is a particular period during gestation when it is safe to consume alcohol. Preventing FASDs involves completely avoiding alcohol during pregnancy or when conception is likely to occur. Thus, experts with the American College of Obstetricians and Gynecologists recommend that pregnant females as well as females who are planning a pregnancy should not consume alcohol.[27]

fetal alcohol spectrum disorders (FASDs) group of conditions that result in a child due to alcohol consumption by the mother during pregnancy

fetal alcohol syndrome (FAS) severe physical and intellectual deficits that develop in a fetus whose mother drank excessively during pregnancy

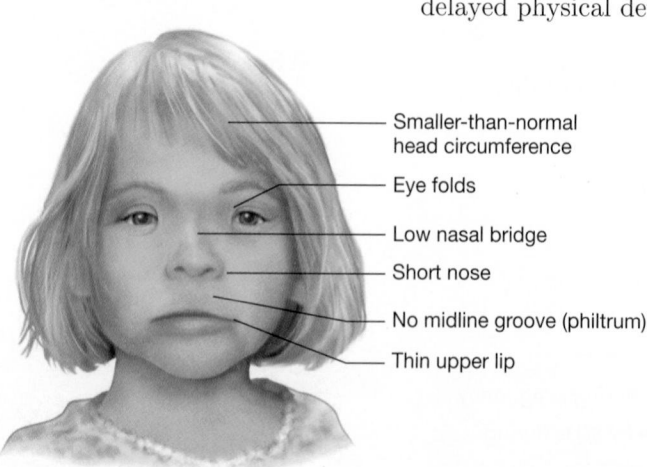

— Smaller-than-normal head circumference
— Eye folds
— Low nasal bridge
— Short nose
— No midline groove (philtrum)
— Thin upper lip

FIGURE 16.5 Child with FAS. This illustration shows typical signs of FAS.

Caffeine

Caffeine is a stimulant drug that can pass through the placenta and enter the embryo/fetus. The drug may depress the flow of blood in the placenta, which may be harmful to the developing offspring. At present, there is no conclusive scientific evidence that a pregnant woman's consumption of caffeinated beverages contributes to **miscarriage**. A miscarriage is the death of an embryo or fetus that occurs before the twentieth week of gestation. Nevertheless, pregnant women are advised to limit their caffeine consumption to 200 mg/day, which is approximately the amount found in 1.5 cups of regular brewed coffee.[28]

miscarriage death of an embryo or fetus that occurs before the twentieth week of gestation

Lead and Arsenic

A pregnant woman's past or present exposure to the nonnutrient mineral lead places her embryo/fetus at risk for lead toxicity.[29] Women who live in old houses are at risk of lead poisoning, especially if the home has lead–based paint that is peeling off the walls or lead pipes and fixtures. When a pregnant woman breathes in or swallows lead, the mineral enters her blood and eventually passes through the placenta and into her developing offspring.[30]

If a pregnant woman was exposed to lead before she became pregnant, her body may have stored the mineral in her bones. During pregnancy, the lead can be mobilized from her bones, enter her bloodstream, and eventually reach her embryo/fetus. Exposure to high levels of lead may cause miscarriage, preterm delivery, low birth weight, and developmental and cognitive delays in the offspring.[29–31]

Arsenic, a mineral that is in soil and some sources of drinking water, is a well–known toxin (see Chapter 12). A pregnant woman who is exposed to arsenic has a greater chance of developing hypertension and anemia than a pregnant woman who is not exposed to the mineral.[32] When arsenic passes through the placenta and into the fetus, the toxic mineral impairs fetal growth and increases the risk of fetal and infant *mortality* (death).[29,32]

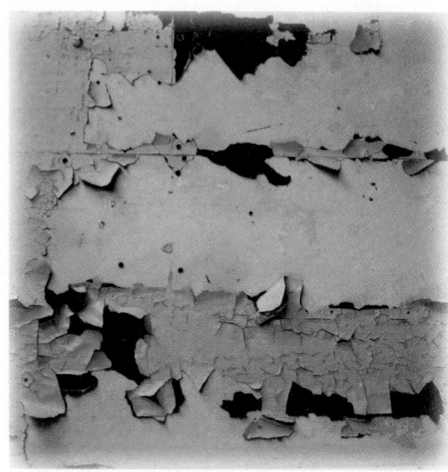

Pregnant women should avoid exposure to toxic lead-based paint in old homes.

DID **YOU** KNOW?

Toxoplasmosis is a condition caused by the microscopic protozoan *Toxoplasma gondii* (*T. gondii*), which may be present in undercooked meats, unwashed fruits and vegetables, water, garden soil, and dust. *T. gondii* can also be present in cat feces.[33] According to the FDA, toxoplasmosis infects between 400 and 4000 fetuses and is responsible for 80 infant deaths each year.[33] In the fetus, *T. gondii* can cause hearing loss, intellectual impairment, and visual problems. To avoid exposure to *T. gondii*, pregnant women should not clean cat litter boxes. If no one else is available to do the job, the mother-to-be should always wear protective gloves while cleaning the box and wash her hands thoroughly with soap and warm water afterward.

toxoplasmosis condition caused by infection with *Toxoplasma gondii*

Methylmercury

Although fish and shellfish are excellent sources of many minerals, omega–3 fatty acids, and high–quality protein, most contain very small amounts of the toxin **methylmercury**, an organic form of mercury. Methylmercury may form naturally from mercury that is in the environment, but the toxic compound can also be a pollutant that forms as a result of industrial activity. Methylmercury accumulates in the tissues of fish, and it is most concentrated in large fish that eat smaller fish. For this reason, experts at the FDA and Environmental Protection Agency advise pregnant women to avoid eating large fish, including swordfish, shark, king mackerel, and tilefish (see Chapter 3).[34] Methylmercury exposure during the prenatal period is associated with nervous system damage in the offspring, which may lead to learning disabilities.[35]

methylmercury organic form of mercury

12 *What are the risks of consuming alcohol during pregnancy?*

13 *What is the recommended limit for caffeine consumption during pregnancy?*

14 *List three environmental factors (excluding alcohol) that can harm the embryo/fetus.*

16.6 Pregnancy: Nutrition-Related Health Conditions

LEARNING OUTCOMES

1 *List recommendations for managing diabetes during pregnancy.*

2 *Describe dangers of hypertension in pregnant women, particularly preeclampsia.*

3 *Discuss maternal complications associated with anemia during pregnancy and strategies for treating the condition.*

4 *Explain the difference between morning sickness and hyperemesis gravidarum.*

5 *Identify factors that contribute to constipation and heartburn in a woman during pregnancy.*

In the United States, the majority of women have uncomplicated pregnancies and deliver healthy, full–term infants. However, many women enter pregnancy with existing obesity, diabetes, hypertension, or other chronic health conditions. Some women develop serious medical problems during pregnancy that can be life–threatening. Conditions and diseases that are associated with pregnancy and have nutritional significance are discussed in this section of the chapter.

Diabetes in Pregnancy

Advances in prenatal health care have greatly improved the outlook for women who have diabetes during this stage of life, especially when the pregnant women follow the advice of their professional health care providers. Recommendations to manage diabetes during pregnancy include monitoring blood glucose levels, eating healthy foods, and participating in regular exercise. Women who had dia–betes and were using insulin prior to becoming pregnant may need to increase their insulin dosages, especially in the third trimester.[36] Chapter 5 provides an in–depth discussion of diabetes, including diabetes that develops during preg–nancy (gestational diabetes).

Hypertensive Disorders of Pregnancy

During pregnancy, normal hormonal changes cause various tissues to retain fluid during pregnancy (edema). Swelling in the ankles and feet is the most notice–able sign of edema and results from the expanding uterus putting pressure on the veins that return blood from the lower limbs. Although some swelling of the lower limbs is common in pregnancy, severe edema can be a sign of a hyperten–sive disorder during pregnancy.

Hypertension affects 8 to 10% of pregnant woman.[37] Hypertension in preg–nancy is among the leading causes of maternal death, preterm labor, and com–plications that affect the newborn infant.[37] Elevated blood pressure damages the blood supply to the placenta, which can interfere with the fetus's weight gain.

Gestational hypertension occurs when a pregnant woman is diagnosed with elevated blood pressure for the first time after 20 weeks of gestation and her

gestational hypertension form of hypertension that occurs after 20 weeks of gestation and returns to normal by 12 weeks after the baby is delivered

blood pressure returns to normal by 12 weeks after the baby is delivered (*post–partum*). This condition was formerly known as "pregnancy–induced hypertension." If the new mother's blood pressure remains elevated after 12 weeks postpartum, she has chronic hypertension.

Preeclampsia and Eclampsia

Gestational hypertension that is accompanied by sudden weight gain, **proteinuria** (protein in the urine), and edema is known as **preeclampsia** (*pre–ih–clamp'–see–ah*), a condition that is often associated with maternal kidney and liver damage (Fig. 16.6). Preeclampsia occurs in 5 to 8% of pregnancies, and the cause of the condition is unknown.[38,39] Several risk factors for preeclampsia are listed in Table 16.7.

A pregnant woman who is diagnosed with preeclampsia needs close medical supervision, and she may receive instructions to stay in bed as much as possible. In severe cases, a woman with preeclampsia may develop seizures **(eclampsia)**, which is life–threatening for the pregnant woman and her fetus. Women with eclampsia may need to undergo medically induced labor. Once the fetus is delivered, the majority of women experience the return of their blood pressure to normal levels and recovery from edema and proteinuria.

Anemia of Pregnancy

Maternal anemia occurs when a pregnant woman has a hemoglobin level that is less than 11 g/dL or a hematocrit that is less than 33%.[40] Recall from Chapter 12 that hemoglobin is the iron–containing protein in red blood cells; **hematocrit** is the ratio of red blood cells to total blood volume. Even though a deficiency of iron, folate, or vitamin B–12 may cause anemia, iron deficiency is the most common cause of the disorder. Based on CDC data, 7% of American women are anemic in the first trimester, 12% in the second trimester, and 34% in the last trimester.[41]

proteinuria protein in the urine

preeclampsia condition that occurs during pregnancy; characterized by proteinuria and edema

eclampsia severe stage of preeclampsia that results in seizures

hematocrit ratio of red blood cells to total blood volume

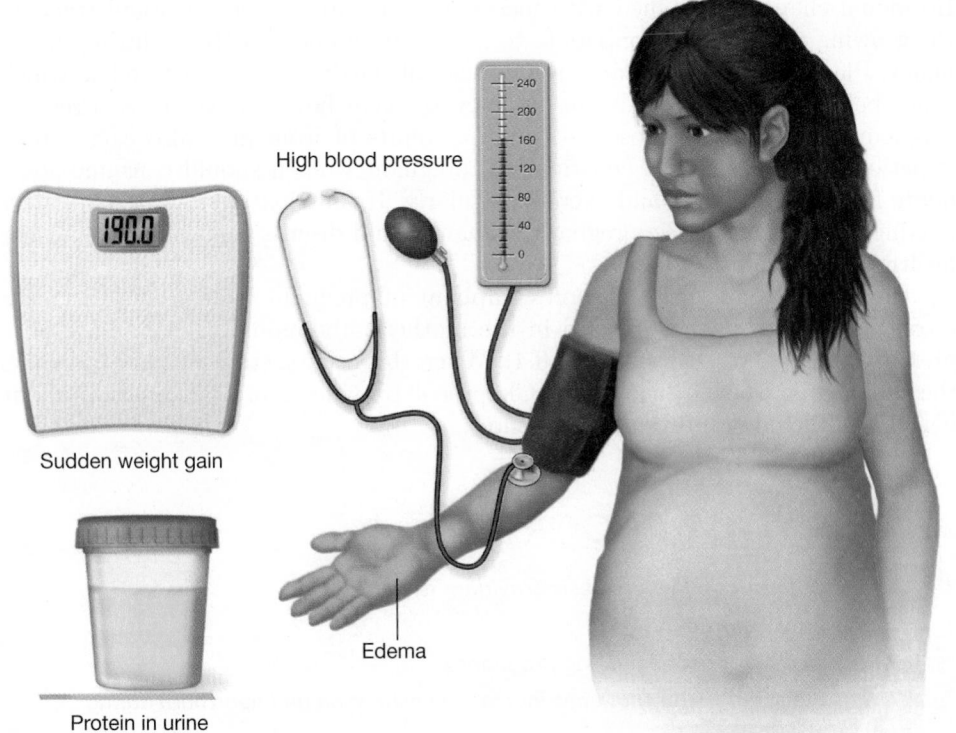

Sudden weight gain

High blood pressure

Edema

Protein in urine

FIGURE 16.6 Signs of preeclampsia.

TABLE 16.7 Risk Factors for Preeclampsia

- First pregnancy
- History of preeclampsia in a previous pregnancy
- Chronic hypertension
- Younger than 18 years of age or older than 40 years of age
- Carrying twins, triplets, or other multiples
- Diabetes or kidney disease
- Obesity
- Very low calcium and/or vitamin D intake
- African-American or American Indian ancestry

Adapted from: Preeclampsia Foundation: *FAQs.* (ND). http://www.preeclampsia.org/health-information/faq#five Accessed: March 20, 2014.

There are two main causes of anemia during pregnancy. The first results from expansion of the mother's blood volume to approximately 150% of the nonpregnancy level, which is a normal physiological adjustment. The number of red blood cells, however, increases only 20 to 30%. As a result, the hemoglobin level of the pregnant woman's blood also decreases.

The second major cause of anemia is poor dietary intake of iron. It is a challenge for most nonpregnant women to consume the recommended 18 mg iron/day, so it is even more difficult for a pregnant woman to consume the 27 mg/day that are recommended during this stage of life. Inadequate iron results in reduced hemoglobin production and, subsequently, iron–deficiency anemia.

During prenatal visits, health care providers routinely check the mother's blood hemoglobin or hematocrit levels to determine whether she has anemia. Women who are diagnosed with mild anemia are given dietary supplements that supply 30 to 60 mg/day. Parenteral (by injection) iron may be necessary to treat cases of severe iron–deficiency anemia.

Gastrointestinal Problems

As mentioned in section 16.3, many women experience morning sickness early in pregnancy. The following sections discuss some gastrointestinal conditions that are associated with pregnancy.

Hyperemesis Gravidarum

About 10% of women with morning sickness continue to be somewhat affected by the condition during the entire 40 weeks of pregnancy.[42] **Hyperemesis gravidarum** (*hy′–per–em′–e–sis grav–ih–dah′–rum*) is a severe form of nausea and vomiting that affects one in 200 pregnant women.[43] The condition is characterized by persistent vomiting, dehydration, ketosis, electrolyte disturbances, and weight loss. Treatment of hyperemesis gravidarum often includes hospitalization and the administration of intravenous fluids that contain glucose, electrolytes, and vitamins.

Constipation and Heartburn

Hormonal changes combined with increasing pressure on the intestinal tract by the growing uterus often contribute to constipation and heartburn during pregnancy. Placental hormones cause the muscles of the digestive tract to relax, which slows peristalsis and reduces the urgency to have bowel movements. Prenatal supplements, especially those with high amounts of iron, may also cause constipation. To help prevent constipation, pregnant women should consume adequate fiber, drink fluids, and exercise regularly. If constipation still persists after making these changes, the pregnant woman should discuss this concern with her health care provider.

Heartburn is another common complaint of pregnant women. As the fetus grows, the uterus pushes upward in the mother's abdominal cavity and applies pressure on her stomach (see Fig. 16.4). When this occurs, stomach acid can enter the esophagus, causing heartburn. Chapter 4 provides more information about heartburn, including preventive measures.

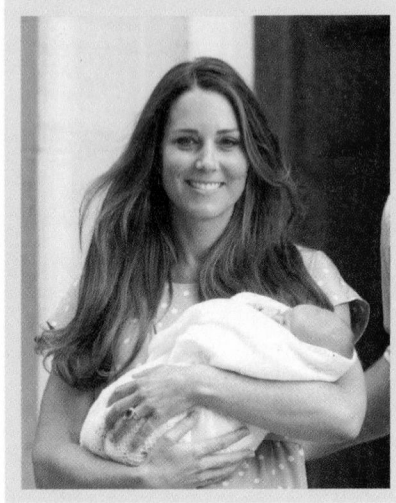
hyperemesis gravidarum severe form of nausea and vomiting that occurs during pregnancy

ASSESS YOUR PROGRESS

15 *List characteristics of hyperemesis gravidarum.*

16 *What is preeclampsia?*

17 *Identify a cause of anemia during pregnancy.*

18 *What is the major factor that contributes to constipation and heartburn during pregnancy?*

16.7 Physiology of Lactation and Breastfeeding

LEARNING OUTCOMES

1 *Describe the physiology of the human breast and the hormones that are involved in milk production.*

2 *Compare the three stages of breast milk production.*

3 *Discuss recommendations for the duration of breastfeeding and circumstances under which a mother should not breastfeed.*

As her delivery date approaches, a pregnant woman needs to decide how to feed her newborn infant. Should she allow the newborn to **suckle** (draw milk) from her breasts or feed the baby from a bottle filled with **infant formula**, a synthetic food that simulates human milk?

Trends in Breastfeeding

Two hundred years ago, a new mother who could not breastfeed likely faced the death of her infant—unless a *wet nurse* (a woman who was producing breast milk) could be located to suckle the infant. In the late 1940s, the practice of feeding infants formula in a bottle became popular, and the practice of breast—feeding rapidly declined among new mothers. By 1972, only 22% of infants in the United States were breastfed, and most of those babies were born to women who could not afford infant formula.[46] Over the following decades, breastfeeding increased in popularity as information about the benefits of the practice emerged. In 2013, 76.5% of babies born in the United States had been breastfed at some point.[47]

Physiology of Lactation and Breastfeeding

The human breast contains adipose tissue and special—ized structures that form milk after the baby is born (Fig. 16.7a). **Lactation** is the production of milk by cells that line the *mammary alveoli* (mammary glands) in breast tissue (Fig. 16.7b). Mammary gland cells synthesize lactose, proteins, and some fatty acids that will be incorporated into the milk. The cells also remove vitamins and minerals from the mother's bloodstream and add them to milk. Therefore, the mother's nutritional status influences the quality of milk she produces.

After delivery, progesterone and estrogen levels in the mother's body decrease. This decrease triggers the release of **prolactin**, the hormone that stimulates milk produc—tion within a woman's breasts. A second hormone that aids in lactation is **oxytocin**, which is secreted by the pituitary gland in the brain. Oxytocin signals tiny muscles around the mammary alveoli to contract and release milk into a system of ducts that eventually drains to an area near the nipple (Fig. 16.7b). The milk is released through the *nipple pores*, tiny holes in the end of the nipple. The release of milk from the breast is known as **let—down reflex**. Shortly before milk begins to flow, a lactating woman may feel a tingling sen—sation in her breasts and nipples, a signal that let—down is occurring. Figure 16.8 illustrates the roles of oxytocin and prolactin in the let—down process.

suckle to draw milk

infant formula synthetic food that simulates human milk

lactation production of milk by mammary glands

DID YOU KNOW?

In China, employment of wet nurses increased dramatically after the 2008 infant formula scandal in which contaminated infant formula poisoned thousands of babies and a few infants died after consuming it.[44] The formula was contaminated with melamine, a nitrogen-containing substance that is used to make hard plastics. The formula manufacturer added melamine to elevate the nitrogen content of the formula, which gave the false impression that the product had a higher protein content.[45]

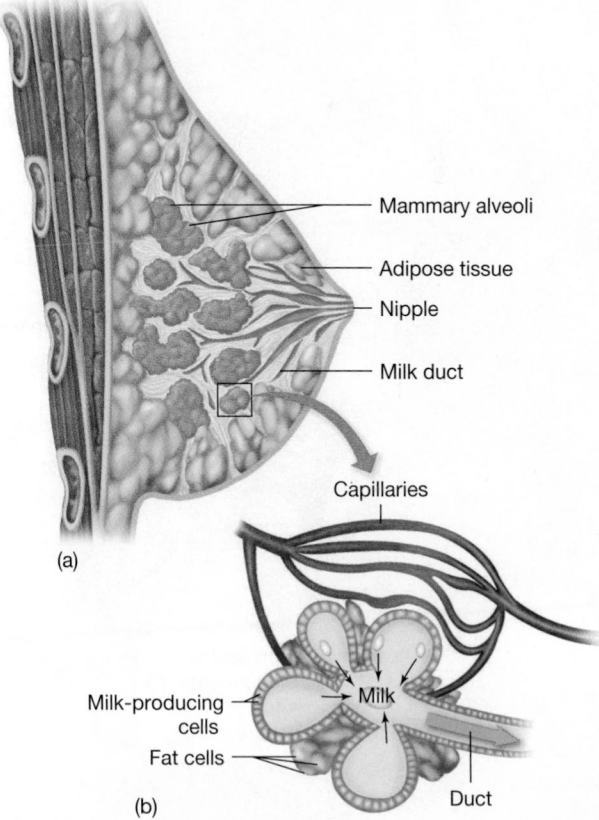

FIGURE 16.7 Human breast during lactation (side view). (*a*) Cross section of human breast during lactation that shows milk-producing glands and related structures. (*b*) Cross section of a mammary alveolus that shows milk-producing cells and the duct for conveying milk to the nipple area.

prolactin hormone that stimulates milk production

oxytocin hormone that stimulates the release of milk from the breast

let-down reflex reflex that enables milk to be released from breasts

let-down failure condition that occurs when the let-down reflex is blocked

colostrum form of milk that is secreted from a woman's breast during the first few days after birth

Embarrassment, emotional stress and tension, pain, and fatigue can easily block the let–down reflex, a condition known as **let–down failure**. If let–down failure occurs, the hungry baby becomes frustrated and angry, and the mother may respond by becoming even more tense and upset, setting up a vicious cycle. At this point, new mothers often give up breastfeeding, reporting that they tried to nurse (breastfeed) their babies but were unable to "produce" milk.

In contrast, when lactation and breastfeeding are well established, the let–down reflex often occurs without the need for the infant's suckling. For example, the let–down reflex may be triggered just by thinking about *nursing* (breast–feeding the baby) or hearing a baby cry. This could lead to a little milk leaking through the mother's clothing. Wearing special pads over the nipples and inside a nursing bra that is designed for breastfeeding women can help absorb the milk.

Stages of Breast Milk

During the first 3 to 4 days after giving birth, a woman's breasts secrete **colostrum** (*co–loss'–trum*), a yellow substance that does not resemble cow's milk. If a woman is unaware that colostrum is secreted by breasts soon after birth, she may think something is wrong with her ability to produce milk or that her milk

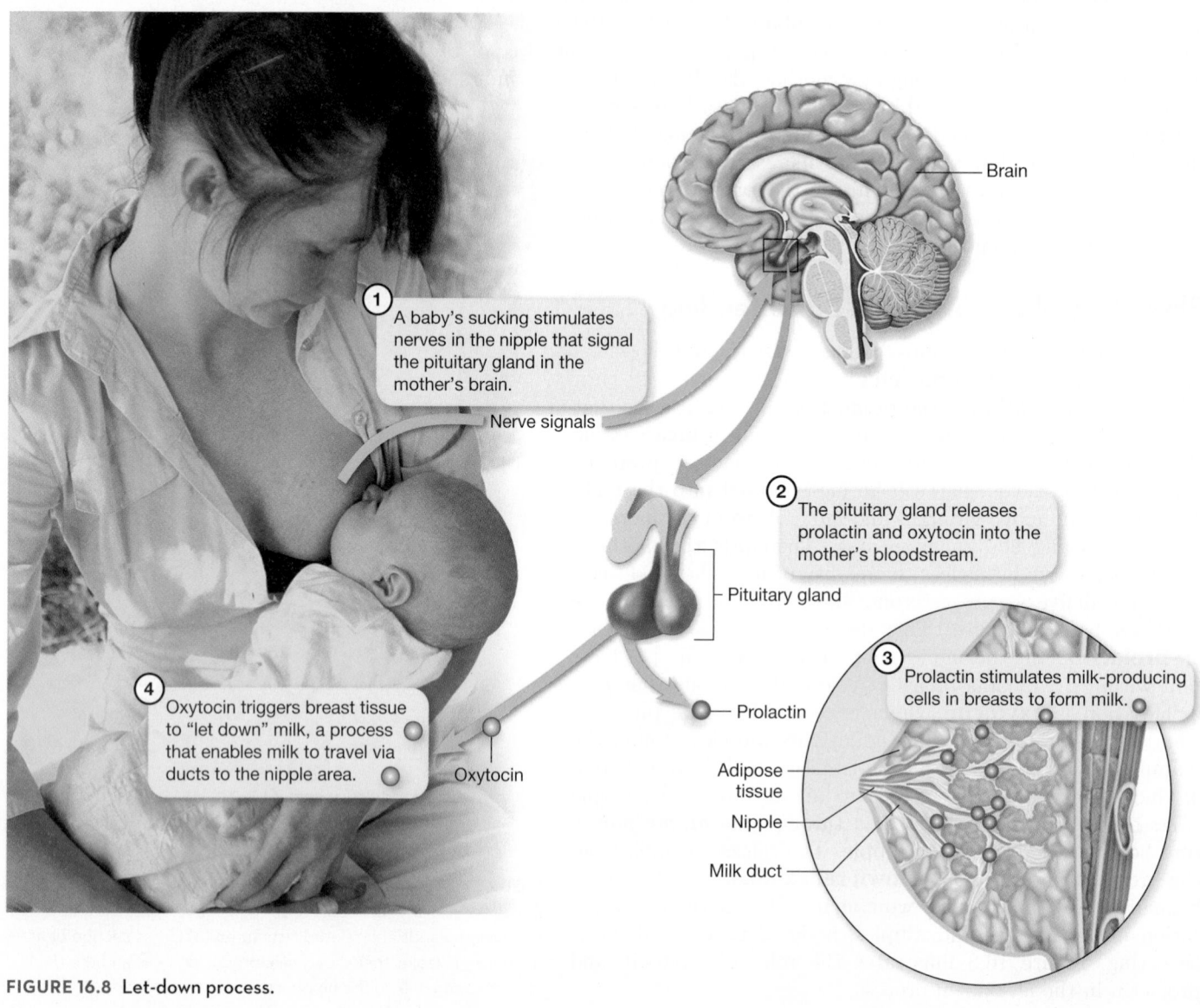

① A baby's sucking stimulates nerves in the nipple that signal the pituitary gland in the mother's brain.

Nerve signals

Brain

② The pituitary gland releases prolactin and oxytocin into the mother's bloodstream.

Pituitary gland

③ Prolactin stimulates milk-producing cells in breasts to form milk.

Prolactin

④ Oxytocin triggers breast tissue to "let down" milk, a process that enables milk to travel via ducts to the nipple area.

Oxytocin

Adipose tissue

Nipple

Milk duct

FIGURE 16.8 Let-down process.

is contaminated. However, colostrum is a very important first food for babies, because it is rich in protein and other nutrients needed to support early growth and development.

By the end of the first week, lactating breasts produce **transitional milk**, which is a combination of colostrum and **mature milk**. After about 2 weeks, all of the milk that is synthesized by the breasts is mature and higher in fat, carbo—hydrates, minerals, and vitamins. The appearance of mature human milk differs from that of cow's milk; breast milk is more watery than cow's milk and may have a slightly bluish tint.

Supply and Demand

Typically, a lactating woman produces over 3 cups of milk per day.[9] It is import—ant to recognize that milk production relies on supply and demand. The more the infant suckles (demand), the more milk his or her mother's breasts produce (supply). However, if milk is not fully removed from the breasts, milk production soon ceases. This is likely to occur when infants are not hungry because they have been given formula or solid foods to supplement breast milk feedings.

Recommendation for the Duration of Breastfeeding

In the United States, organizations representing maternal and child health pro-fessionals, including the American Academy of Nutrition and Dietetics, American Academy of Pediatrics, and American College of Obstetricians and Gynecologists, recommend that new mothers breastfeed their babies exclusively for 6 months.[48] Even though more than 76% of women breastfeed their newborn infants soon after giving birth, only a few of them follow the recommendation to breastfeed exclusively for 6 months. Of the infants born in 2011 who were breastfed, about 11% were exclusively breastfed through the first 3 months, while only 6% were exclusively breastfed for at least 6 months.[49]

ASSESS YOUR PROGRESS

19 *What are the three stages of human milk?*

20 *Why it colostrum a valuable first food for breastfed babies?*

21 *How does supply and demand regulate the amount of milk that a lactating woman's breasts produce?*

22 *In the United States, what is the recommended duration for exclusively breastfeeding an infant?*

16.8 Breastfeeding

LEARNING OUTCOMES

1 *Describe the nutritional content of breast milk.*

2 *List some factors present in breast milk that help protect an infant from some common infectious diseases.*

3 *Summarize the advantages and disadvantages of breastfeeding for new mothers.*

4 *Explain the benefits and potential disadvantages of consuming human milk for the breastfed infant.*

5 *Summarize the nutritional recommendations for breastfeeding women.*

Human milk is uniquely formulated to provide infants with most nutrients—in the correct amounts—required for optimal health and growth. Breastfeeding also

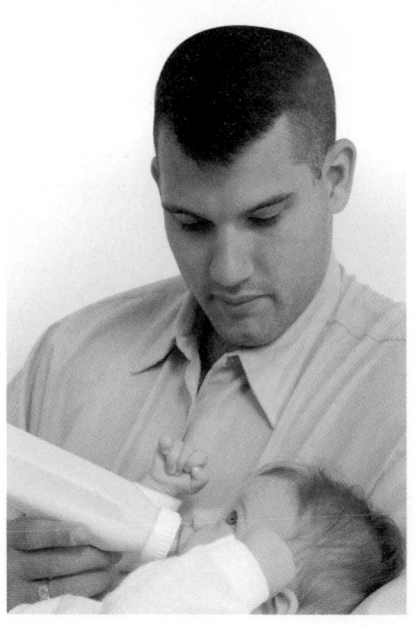

Breast milk can be placed in a bottle so the father and other caregivers can feed the baby.

transitional milk combination of colostrum and mature milk

mature milk form of milk that is secreted by the breast about 2 weeks after delivery

provides many advantages for the lactating mother and her infant, but there are some possible disadvantages, too. This section of the chapter focuses on the nutrient composition of human milk, pros and cons of breastfeeding, and the nutritional needs of breastfeeding women.

Nutritional Qualities of Human Milk

The nutrient composition of breast milk changes during the weeks and months that the mother nurses her baby. The changes that breast milk undergoes are adaptations that reflect the changing nutritional needs of the growing infant.

Carbohydrates

The main carbohydrate in human milk is lactose. Breastfeeding promotes growth of certain bacteria, such as *Lactobacillus bifidus*, in an infant's digestive tract. Such bacteria are beneficial because they aid lactose digestion and help control the growth of potential harmful bacteria in the baby's gastrointestinal tract. Human milk also contains oligosaccharides, which are comprised mainly of glucose and galactose (see Chapter 5). The oligosaccharides in human milk act as natural prebiotics by promoting the growth of beneficial bacteria in the large intestine, which plays an important protective role in reducing intestinal infections during infancy.[50,51]

Fats and Cholesterol

The fat content of human milk varies greatly among mothers. A study of 71 mothers found that fat content ranged from 22 g/L to 41 g/L.[52] The type of fat in human milk reflects the type of fats that the mother consumes. A mother whose diet is high in the DHA will produce milk higher in that fat, which may support brain development in the young child.[16]

On average, more than 55% of the calories in mature human milk are from fat. An interesting feature of human milk is that its fat content changes during each feeding. In the beginning of the session, the mother's milk, known as *foremilk*, is low in fat, but as her infant continues to nurse, the fat content of her milk gradually increases. The higher fat content of the *hindmilk* may make the baby feel satisfied and, as a result, discontinue feeding. Mothers should make sure the baby drains one breast before moving to the second. Babies who do not suckle long enough to receive the hindmilk may become hungry soon after the feeding.

Breast milk has four times more cholesterol than infant formula. As a result, breastfed infants have higher total and LDL blood cholesterol levels during infancy. However, when these infants become adults, their blood cholesterol levels are lower, indicating that breastfeeding may have a long-term protective effect against the development of abnormal lipid levels.[53]

Protein

Even though the protein content in human milk is lower than the protein in infant formulas, human milk provides the amount needed to support normal infant growth. About 80% of protein in colostrum is the easily digested **whey**, while the remaining 20% is the curd-forming casein. The whey-to-casein ratio makes human milk ideal for the immature digestive tracts of young infants. In contrast, casein is the main protein in cow's milk, which makes it more difficult for infants to digest.

whey water-soluble protein in milk

Vitamins and Minerals

Generally, the vitamin content of human milk reflects maternal intake.[54] A well-nourished mother produces milk that contains ample amounts of most vitamins and minerals. However, most health care practitioners advise new mothers to continue taking prenatal supplements during lactation. The two vitamins that may be low in human milk are vitamins B–12 and D. A vegan mother who does not take B–12 supplements should give her breastfed infant a B–12 supplement as advised by her physician. Because vitamin D content of human milk is reflective of the mother's sun exposure and dietary intake, amounts of the micronutrient in breast milk can vary widely. Therefore, breastfed infants should be given 10 µg (400 IU) of vitamin D each day.[55]

Immunological Qualities of Human Milk

Colostrum is very high in antibodies and other immunological proteins that can be absorbed by the infant's immature digestive tract and help defend against infectious illnesses. Mothers who plan to bottle–feed should be encouraged to nurse their newborns for the first few days, so the infants will receive immunological benefits of colostrum. Breast milk contains other substances, including *lysozymes*, *lactoferrin*, and *bifidus factor*, that help protect the nursing infant from infections. As a result of consuming these immunological factors, breastfed infants, especially those who are exclusively breastfed, have lower risks of gastrointestinal, respiratory, and ear infections and pneumonia than formula–fed infants.[55] Furthermore, breastfed babies are less likely to develop childhood asthma, allergies, leukemia, obesity, sudden infant death syndrome (SIDS), and type 1 diabetes than infants who are not breastfed.[55,56]

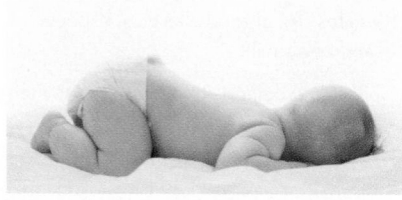

Breastfed babies are less likely to die of sudden infant death syndrome than babies who are not breastfed.

Dietary Planning for Lactating Women

Milk production requires approximately 800 kcal every day. However, the lactating woman's daily energy needs can be met by adding only about 300 to 400 kcal to her prepregnancy EER. The difference between the energy needed for milk production and the recommended energy intake can enable the new mother to lose the extra body fat she accumulated during pregnancy. This loss is more likely to occur if she continues breastfeeding her baby for 6 months or more and increases her physical activity level. To help plan meals and snacks that are nutritionally adequate, she can follow MyPlate recommendations at www .choosemyplate.gov.

No special foods are necessary to sustain milk production. However, a lactating woman should drink fluids every time her infant suckles to help her maintain adequate milk volume and keep her body properly hydrated. For as long as she breastfeeds her baby, the lactating mother should limit her intake of alcohol– and caffeine–containing beverages because her body secretes these drugs into her milk. A woman who breastfeeds her baby should also check with her physician before using any medications, even over–the–counter and herbal products, because such substances may also end up in her breast milk.

Benefits for the Mother

Breastfeeding can provide many benefits for the mother. The oxytocin that is secreted by the mother's body as she nurses helps shrink her uterus to its pre–pregnancy size. Mothers who breastfeed their babies have lower risks of breast and ovarian cancers,[48] as well as type 2 diabetes—if they did not have gestational diabetes.[55] The physical contact between the mother and infant during nursing increases the pair's bonding[57] and may reduce the mother's risk of postpartum depression.[58]

Many women find that breastfeeding is more convenient and economical than feeding infant formula. Human milk is readily available; there is no need to

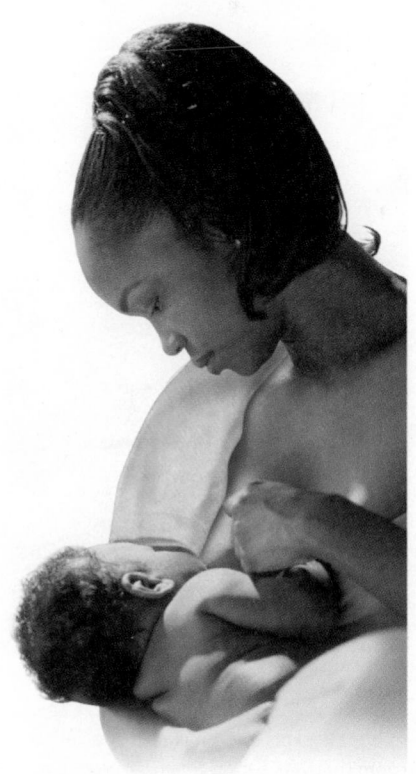

Breastfeeding may enhance a new mother's emotional bonding to her baby.

TABLE 16.8 Pros and Cons of Breastfeeding

Advantages for Infants	Disadvantages for Infants
Human milk:	**Human milk:**
Is nutritionally adequate for most full-term infants. Is free of bacteria as it leaves the breast.	May be low in vitamins D and B-12.
Supplies antibodies and immune cells.	May contain undesirable flavors, odors, and or food components that contribute to intestinal gas.
Is easily digested.	May contain food allergens from the mother.
Reduces risk of food allergies, especially to proteins in infant formulas and cow's milk.	
Changes in composition over time to meet the changing needs of a growing infant.	
Contains zinc, iron, and other minerals in highly absorbable forms.	
Decreases risks of ear, intestinal, and respiratory infections.	
May reduce the risk of asthma, obesity, and type 1 diabetes in childhood.	
Advantages for New Mothers	**Disadvantages for New Mothers**
Breastfeeding:	**Breastfeeding:**
Reduces uterine bleeding after delivery.	May make it difficult to return to work or school.
Promotes shrinkage of the uterus to its prepregnancy size.	May make it difficult for others to feed the baby.
May decrease the risk of breast cancer (before menopause) and ovarian cancer.	Requires avoiding or limiting alcohol and caffeine consumption.
May promote maternal weight loss.	May require the mother to stop taking certain medications.
May enhance bonding with the infant.	
Is less expensive and more convenient than feeding infant formula.	

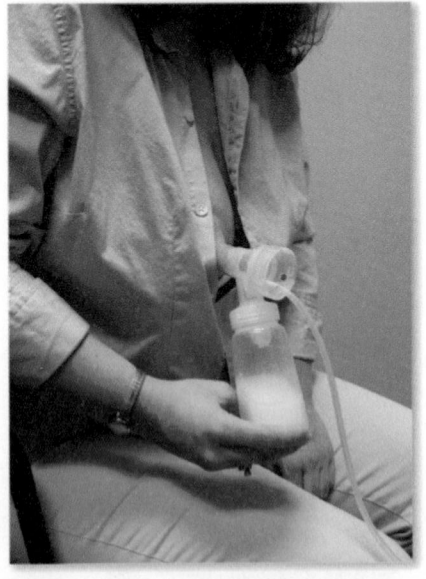

FIGURE 16.9 Expressing milk. This new mother is expressing milk in a special room that was set up for this purpose at her workplace. She will refrigerate the milk and take it home for later bottle feeding.

purchase cans of formula and go to the trouble of preparing and washing bottles or finding a refrigerator to store the formula–filled bottles. As milk leaves the breast, it is always fresh, free of bacteria, and ready to feed without mixing or warming.

Table 16.8 summarizes the major advantages and disadvantages of breast–feeding. Note that some of the disadvantages may be resolved by having a con–sultation with a medical professional or lactation consultant.

Choosing Not to Breastfeed

Breastfeeding is not always the best choice for some new mothers. Many drugs can leave the mother's bloodstream and enter her breast milk. Therefore, most women who drink excessive amounts of alcohol or take certain prescription medicines, including some mood stabilizers and migraine medicines, should not breastfeed. Women with serious chronic infectious diseases, particularly HIV or active tuber–culosis, both of which may be transmitted to the infant through breast milk, also should not breastfeed.

Many women choose not to breastfeed because they think it will interfere with returning to school or work. Such responsibilities can present a challenge for many new mothers who want to continue breastfeeding. Some progressive employers, especially those that employ a large number of females, allow breaks and provide a secluded room so women can express milk from their breasts and store it for later use (Fig. 16.9).

DID **YOU** KNOW?

Some hospitals have a certified lactation consultant, a credentialed health care professional, on staff, whereas others have women experienced in breastfeeding to teach new mothers the skill. Many breastfeeding support groups are also available, such as the La Leche League (http://www .llli.org). Such resources are very helpful for women who are inexperienced with breastfeeding and have questions concerning how to manage problems relating to feedings.

ASSESS YOUR PROGRESS

23 *Discuss the energy and nutrient composition of breast milk.*

24 *List at least three benefits that infants derive from consuming breast milk.*

25 *List three advantages of breastfeeding for the lactating woman and three possible disadvantages.*

26 *Compare the energy needs of a breastfeeding woman to her needs before pregnancy.*

SUMMARY

SECTION 16.1 **Preparing for Pregnancy: Nutrition Concerns**

- The nutritional status of both a woman and a man affects their fertility. A teenage girl who becomes pregnant needs enough nutrients to support both the fetus's and her own growth. Adolescents and women over 40 years of age are at risk for complications during pregnancy.

SECTION 16.2 **The Prenatal Period**

- After an egg is fertilized by a sperm, it divides into a blastocyst that is composed of many cells. Between the second and eighth weeks of pregnancy, all organs of the embryo have formed; the organs grow and develop during the fetal period.

- The placenta connects the mother and embryo/fetus via the umbilical cord. Nutrients and oxygen are delivered to the embryo/fetus, and waste products from the embryo/fetus are removed by this connection.

SECTION 16.3 **Pregnancy: Maternal Physiological Adjustments**

- Many of the changes that occur in a woman's body during pregnancy help her developing offspring receive the nutrients it needs to survive. Common signs and symptoms of pregnancy include morning sickness, breast soreness, frequent urination, and fatigue.

SECTION 16.4 **Nutrition for a Healthy Pregnancy**

- A pregnant woman should focus on eating nutrient-dense foods to support growth of the fetus and expansion of tissues in her body. An additional 340 kcal/day and 452 kcal/day are needed in the second and third trimesters, respectively.

SECTION 16.5 **Substances to Limit or Avoid During Pregnancy**

- Women should not drink alcoholic beverages, should limit caffeine consumption, and should avoid foods that contain lead, arsenic, and methylmercury.

SECTION 16.6 **Pregnancy: Nutrition-Related Health Conditions**

- During pregnancy, 1 in 200 women develop hyperemesis gravidarum that may require hospitalization. Gestational hypertension may result in maternal death, preterm labor, and complications affecting the newborn, and may lead to preeclampsia or eclampsia.

- About 34% of pregnant women are diagnosed with iron-deficiency anemia in the last trimester.
- Constipation and indigestion are common gastrointestinal complaints during the later weeks of pregnancy.

SECTION 16.7 Physiology of Lactation and Breastfeeding

- Hormonal changes result in milk production. Prolactin stimulates the breasts to produce milk, whereas oxytocin triggers the let-down reflex.
- Colostrum is the first substance secreted from a woman's breast after delivery. Colostrum is rich in protein, other nutrients, and anti-infective substances needed to support early growth, development, and immunity.

SECTION 16.8 Breastfeeding

- Human milk is uniquely formulated with most nutrients an infant requires for optimal health and growth. Colostrum contains high amounts of antibodies and other immunological proteins.
- A lactating mother should consume 300 to 400 more kilocalories than she did before pregnancy. Breastfeeding provides emotional, physical, and economic advantages to the lactating mother.

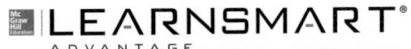

Get the most out of your study of nutrition with McGraw-Hill's innovative suite of adaptive learning products including McGraw-Hill LearnSmart®, SmartBook®, McGraw-Hill LearnSmart Achieve®, and McGraw-Hill LearnSmart Prep®. Visit www.learnsmartadvantage.com.

CASE STUDY RESPONSE

DIET DURING PREGNANCY

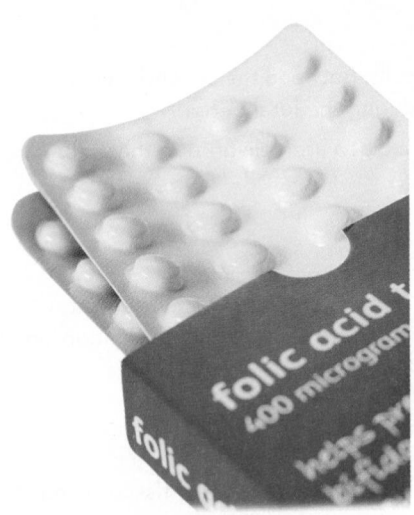

IF JIA HAD OBTAINED PRECONCEPTION COUNSELING, she would have been advised to stop drinking alcohol and smoking cigarettes, and begin taking a supplement of folic acid during the preconception period. Other recommendations would include losing enough weight to reduce her BMI to within the healthy weight range. Weight loss could be achieved by modifying her diet to meet MyPlate food group recommendations and limiting the calories she consumes from solid fat and added sugars. Additionally, Jia may have been advised to begin a moderate exercise program that includes 30 to 60 minutes of physical activity each day.

Based on her BMI, Jia was overweight before pregnancy, and her weight gain since conception has been excessive. A woman who is overweight when she enters pregnancy should gain 1 to 4.5 pounds during the first trimester (13 weeks) and 0.6 pounds per week during the last two trimesters. Therefore, Jia's weight gain should be between 9 and 13.5 pounds, instead of 20 pounds at 28 weeks of pregnancy.

Examples of simple, nutrient-dense breakfast and lunch menus that Jia can prepare at home are:

Breakfast
100% whole-wheat, fortified ready-to-eat cereal
Banana
Fat-free milk
Lunch
Grilled chicken strips
Pasta salad
Fresh blueberries with reduced-fat plain yogurt
Low-fat or nonfat milk

TEST KITCHEN
Modifying Recipes for Healthy Living

You are working with a client who is in her twentieth week of pregnancy. Her prepregnancy BMI was 23, and at this point, she has gained 12 pounds since conception. She has recently been diagnosed with iron-deficiency anemia. She has a recipe for bean burritos that she would like to modify to make the burrito provide more iron per serving. Indicate how to modify the recipe so it is a better source of iron than the original recipe.

BEAN BURRITO

PREPARATION STEPS

1. In a small saucepan, heat the cooked rice with beans and 2 tablespoons of salsa until warm. If necessary, add a tablespoon of water to keep the mixture from sticking to the pan.
2. Place the tortilla on a large plate, and add the rice-bean-salsa mixture to the bottom third of the tortilla. Sprinkle 1 tablespoon of shredded cheese over the mixture.
3. Roll the filling end of the tortilla over the rice mixture once, then fold the sides of the tortilla toward the center, before rolling up the burrito completely.
4. Top the burrito with the remaining salsa and the shredded cheese.
5. Heat in a microwave oven for about 45 seconds (high) or until the cheese is melted and bubbly. Recipe makes 1 burrito.

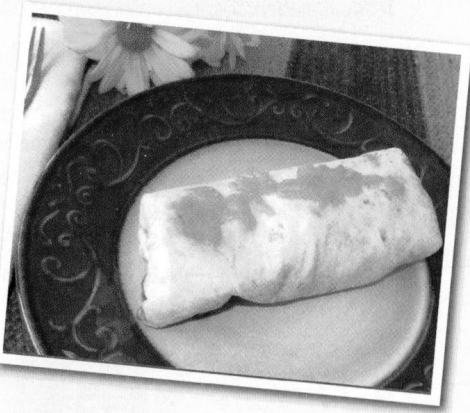

INGREDIENTS

¼ cup cooked white rice

2 Tbsp canned black beans

3 Tbsp mild salsa (commercially prepared)

2 Tbsp shredded Colby cheese

1 8" flour tortilla

STEP 1 Brainstorm

Examine the recipe. What ingredients can you add to the recipe to make it a better source of iron and provide an acceptable texture and flavor?

STEP 2 Develop a modified version of this recipe

List ingredients and amounts needed.

List the preparation steps.

STEP 3 Analyze nutrient contents of the original and modified recipes by using a computer software program or Internet website

Develop a table that compares the number of kcal and amounts of iron in the original and modified recipes.

How did your modifications change the nutrient composition of the burrito?

OPTIONAL ACTIVITIES

STEP 4 Test your new recipe

Keep notes on any changes you make to ingredient amounts as you prepare the burrito.

STEP 5 Reflect on your findings

Rate the burrito's appearance and taste.

STEP 6 Add the recipe to your collection or repeat steps to improve the product

Critical Thinking

1. One of your friends just found out that she is pregnant. Although her BMI is in the healthy range, she is concerned about gaining too much weight during pregnancy. What advice would you give your friend about the need to gain some weight during pregnancy?

2. When Danielle began to breastfeed her newborn baby, she was alarmed because her breast milk did not look like cow's milk. What would you tell Danielle about lactation that would calm her concerns?

3. Heather is pregnant and was recently diagnosed with iron deficiency. What kinds of information does a health care practitioner need to know about Heather to make appropriate dietary recommendations?

4. Thirty-year-old Karena did not exercise much before becoming pregnant. What would you tell her concerning the benefits of exercise during pregnancy, and which forms of physical activity would you recommend as being safe for an expectant woman?

5. Tamara is a 16-year-old high school junior who is expecting her first baby in 3 months. Discuss factors that are likely to influence her decision on whether she will breastfeed her baby.

Practice Test

Select the best answer.

1. Theresa is in the thirtieth week of a normal pregnancy. Based on this information, Theresa is
   a. reporting mild edema in her feet and urinating frequently.
   b. experiencing a decline in her estrogen level.
   c. having morning sickness and proteinuria.
   d. gaining weight at the rate of 3 pounds/week.

2. Holly is planning to become pregnant. To have a healthy pregnancy and baby, when should she be the most concerned about her nutritional status and the nutritional quality of her diet?
   a. during preconception
   b. between the eighth and thirteenth weeks of pregnancy
   c. during the second trimester of pregnancy
   d. between the twenty-sixth and thirty-fourth weeks of pregnancy

3. According to current recommendations, a woman who is pregnant with one fetus and whose pregravid BMI was 31 should gain _____ pounds during pregnancy.
   a. 3 to 10
   b. 11 to 20
   c. 25 to 35
   d. 30 to 40

4. To reduce the risk of toxoplasmosis, pregnant women should
   a. avoid cleaning a cat's litter box.
   b. eat fatty fish at least once a week.
   c. gain between 25 and 35 pounds.
   d. take a daily prenatal dietary supplement.

5. Which of the following statements is true?
   a. An infant whose birth weight is 7 ½ pounds is more likely to have visual impairments than an infant whose birth weight is 5 ½ pounds.
   b. An infant who weighs 7 pounds 10 ounces at birth is considered to be a high birth weight infant.
   c. A pregnant woman who is over 45 years of age has a higher risk of having a baby with Down syndrome than a pregnant woman who is 25 years of age.
   d. A woman who takes a daily folic acid supplement during the preconception period is more likely to give birth to a baby with heart defects than a woman who did not take the vitamin supplement daily during the preconception period.

6. To have a healthy baby and pregnancy, a woman whose pregravid BMI was 23 should gain _____ pounds during pregnancy.
   a. 10 to 15
   b. 15 to 25
   c. 25 to 35
   d. 35 to 45

7. A woman whose pregravid BMI was 21 should consume an additional _____ kcal/day during the second trimester and _____ kcal/day during the third trimester.
   a. 215; 305
   b. 340; 452
   c. 425; 475
   d. 495; 585

8. Pregnant women
   a. who consume lead have a high risk of giving birth to a baby with cretinism.
   b. should restrict their weight gain to prevent edema.
   c. generally need twice as many calories and three times as much protein as nonpregnant women.
   d. should avoid dietary supplements that have high amounts of vitamin A.

9. Which of the following statements is true?
   a. The consumption of nonfood substances is called pica.
   b. Sodium and vitamin C deficiencies are known causes of pica.
   c. Anemia causes pica.
   d. Pica is a safe way to obtain mineral nutrients.

10. Which of the following conditions is a cause of maternal deaths in the United States?
    a. pica
    b. hyperemesis gravidarum
    c. gestational hypertension
    d. protein malnutrition

11. Pregnant women who have _____ experience persistent vomiting, dehydration, electrolyte disturbances, and weight loss.
    a. hyperemesis gravidarum
    b. pica
    c. morning sickness
    d. iron deficiency anemia

12. Emily is breastfeeding her 2-week-old baby. What is the main type of protein in the milk Emily is producing?

    a. casein
    b. albumin
    c. oligosaccharide
    d. whey

13. A day after giving birth, Chelsea complained that she could not produce milk. Based on this information, Chelsea had experienced

    a. pica.
    b. let-down failure.
    c. oxytocin.
    d. hyperemesis gravidarum.

14. Often, the level of vitamin ____ in human milk is inadequate for an infant.

    a. B-6
    b. C
    c. A
    d. D

15. According to results of studies, infants and children who receive WIC benefits are ____ than infants and children who do not receive WIC benefits.

    a. less likely to have food allergies
    b. more likely to develop type 2 diabetes later in life
    c. less likely to develop iron deficiency anemia
    d. more likely to have developmental problems

ANSWERS TO CHAPTER 16 QUIZ Yourself

1. A woman's dietary choices before she becomes pregnant have no effect on the health of her developing offspring. **False** (p. 526)
2. Physicians recommend that women should gain at least 25 pounds during pregnancy. **False** (p. 532)
3. Breast milk may not contain enough vitamin D to meet an infant's needs. **True** (p. 545)
4. Babies who consume infant formula have fewer intestinal and respiratory infections than breastfed babies. **False** (p. 545)
5. A 40-year-old pregnant woman has a higher risk of giving birth to a baby with Down syndrome than a 20-year-old pregnant woman. **True** (p. 527)

ANSWERS TO PRACTICE TEST
1-a; 2-a; 3-b; 4-a; 5-c; 6-c; 7-b; 8-d; 9-a; 10-c; 11-a; 12-d; 13-b; 14-d; 15-c

---

References

1. Ventura S and others: Estimated pregnancy rates and rates of pregnancy outcomes for the United States, 1990–2008. *National Vital Statistics Reports* 60:7, 2012. http://www.cdc.gov/nchs/data/nvsr/nvsr60/nvsr60_07.pdf Accessed: March 4, 2014.

2. Centers for Disease Control and Prevention: *Preconception health and health care: Information for health professionals.* Last updated July 2013. http://www.cdc.gov/preconception/hcp/ Accessed: March 4, 2014.

3. de Souza G, Hallak J: Anabolic steroids and male infertility: A comprehensive review. *British Journal of Urology International* 108(11):1860, 2011.

4. Mortimer D and others: What should it take to describe a substance or product as "sperm-safe"? *Human Reproductive Update* Suppl 1:i1, 2013. DOI: 10.1093/humupd/dmt008

5. Centers for Disease Control and Prevention: *Preconception health and health care: Reproductive life plan tool for health professionals.* Last updated July 2013. http://www.cdc.gov/preconception/rlptool.html Accessed: March 4, 2014.

6. Martinez G and others: Fertility of men and women aged 15–44 years in the United States: National Survey of Family Growth, 2006–2010. *National Health Statistics Reports*, no. 51. Hyattsville, MD: National Center for Health Statistics, 2012. http://www.cdc.gov/nchs/data/nhsr/nhsr051.pdf Accessed: March 4, 2014.

7. National Down Syndrome Society: *What is Down syndrome?* ND. http://www.ndss.org/Down-Syndrome/What-Is-Down-Syndrome/ Accessed: March 4, 2014.

8. Saladin KS: *Anatomy & physiology.* 7th ed. Boston: McGraw-Hill Publishing Company, 2015.

9. Neville MC, McManaman JL: Milk secretion and composition. In Thuree P, Hay W (eds): *Neonatal nutrition and metabolism.* 2nd ed. New York: Cambridge University Press, 2006.

10. Ensiyeh J, Sakineh MA: Comparing ginger and vitamin B6 for the treatment of nausea and vomiting in pregnancy: A randomised controlled trial. *Midwifery* 25(6):649, 2009.

11. Tiran D: Ginger to reduce nausea and vomiting during pregnancy: Evidence of effectiveness is not the same as proof of safety. *Complementary and Therapeutic Clinical Practice* 18(1):22, 2012. DOI: 10.1016/j.ctcp.2011.08.007

12. American College of Obstetricians and Gynecologists, Committee on Obstetric Practice: Committee Opinion No. 548: Weight gain during pregnancy. *Obstetrics and Gynecology* 121(1):210, 2013. DOI: 10.1097/01.AOG.0000425668.87506.4c

13. National Research Council: *Weight gain during pregnancy: Reexamining the guidelines.* Washington, DC: National Academies Press, 2009.

14. March of Dimes: *Your premature baby.* Last reviewed September 2012. http://www.marchofdimes.com/baby/low-birthweight.aspx Accessed: March 4, 2014.

15. American Congress of Obstetricians and Gynecologists: *Exercise during pregnancy.* 2011. www.acog.org Accessed: March 4, 2014.

16. Hadders-Algra M: Effect of long-chain polyunsaturated fatty acid supplementation on neurodevelopmental outcome in full-term infants. *Nutrients* 2(8):790, 2010. DOI: 10.3390/nu2080790

17. Morse NL: Benefits of docosahexaenoic acid, folic acid, vitamin D and iodine on foetal and infant brain development and function following maternal supplementation during pregnancy and lactation. *Nutrients* 4(7):799, 2012. DOI: 10.3390/nu4070799

18. Dawodu A, Akinbi H: Vitamin D nutrition in pregnancy: Current opinion. *International Journal of Women's Health* 5:333, 2013. E-pub: June 24, 2013. DOI: 10.2147/IJWH.S34032

19. Bánhidy F and others: Iron deficiency anemia: Pregnancy outcomes with or without iron supplementation. *Nutrition* 27(1):65, 2011. E-pub: April 8, 2010. DOI: 10.1016/j.nut.2009.12.005

20. Young, S: Pica in pregnancy: New ideas about an old condition. *Annual Review of Nutrition* 30:403, 2010.

21. Khan Y, Tisman G: Pica in iron deficiency: A case series. *Journal of Medical Case Reports* 4:86, 2010. DOI: 10.1186/1752-1947-4-86

22. United States Department of Agriculture, Agricultural Research Service: What we eat in America 2011-2012. Last modified October 2014. http://www.ars.usda.gov/Services/docs.htm?docid=18349 Accessed: November 11, 2014.

23. Kovacs C. Vitamin D in pregnancy and lactation: Maternal, fetal, and neonatal outcomes from human and animal studies. *American Journal of Clinical Nutrition* 88(2):520S, 2008.

24. U.S. Department of Agriculture: *Women, Infants and Children (WIC): Frequently asked questions about WIC.* Updated April 2104. http://www.fns.usda.gov/wic/frequently-asked-questions-about-wic Accessed: October 12, 2014.

25. U.S. Department of Agriculture: *Women, Infants and Children (WIC): About WIC—How WIC helps.* ND. http://www.fns.usda.gov/wic/about-wic-how-wic-helps Accessed: February 6, 2014.

26. Centers for Disease Control and Prevention: *Fetal alcohol spectrum disorders.* Last updated January 2014. http://www.cdc.gov/ncbddd/fasd/ Accessed: March 4, 2014.

27. American College of Obstetricians and Gynecologists: Women and alcohol. 2011. *Frequently asked questions: FAQ 068: Women's health.* http://www.acog.org/Search?Keyword=Alcohol%20and%20women Accessed: March 2, 2014.

28. March of Dimes: *Eating and nutrition: Caffeine in pregnancy.* 2012. http://www.marchofdimes.com/pregnancy/caffeine-in-pregnancy.aspx Accessed: March 4, 2014.

29. Bellinger D: Prenatal exposures to environmental chemicals and children's neurodevelopment: An update. *Safety and Health at Work* 4(1):1, 2013. E-pub: March 11, 2013. DOI: 10.5491/SHAW.2013.4.1.1

30. Centers for Disease Control and Prevention, Work Group on Lead and Pregnancy; National Center for Environmental Health (U.S.), Division of Emergency and Environmental Health Services: *Guidelines for the identification and management of lead exposure in pregnant and lactating women.* 2010. http://www.cdc.gov/nceh/lead/publications/leadandpregnancy2010.pdf Accessed: March 4, 2014.

31. Lin C and others: In utero exposure to environmental lead and manganese and neurodevelopment at 2 years of age. *Environmental Research* 123:52, 2013. E-pub: April 8, 2013. DOI: 10.1016/j.envres.2013.03.003

32. Vahter M: Effects of arsenic on maternal and fetal health. *Annual Review of Nutrition* 29:381, 2009. DOI: 10.1146/annurev-nutr-080508-141102

33. Food and Drug Administration: *Food safety for moms-to-be: Before you're pregnant—Toxoplasma.* Last updated October 2013. http://www.fda.gov/food/foodborneillnesscontaminants/peopleatrisk/ucm082328.htm Accessed: March 4, 2014.

34. Food and Drug Administration: *What you need to know about mercury in fish and shellfish.* Updated June 2013. http://www.fda.gov/food/resourcesforyou/consumers/ucm110591.htm Accessed: March 4, 2014.

35. Environmental Protection Agency: *Mercury.* Updated July 2013. http://www.epa.gov/mercury/effects.htm Accessed: March 4, 2014.

36. American Diabetes Association: *Prenatal care.* Last edited November 2013. http://www.diabetes.org/living-with-diabetes/complications/pregnancy/prenatal-care.html Accessed: March 4, 2014.

37. Mustafa R and others: A comprehensive review of hypertension in pregnancy. *Journal of Pregnancy* 2012. Article ID 105918 http://www.hindawi.com/journals/jp/2012/105918/

38. Preeclampsia Foundation: *What is HELLP syndrome?* (ND). http://www.preeclampsia.org/health-information/hellp-syndrome Accessed: March 4, 2014.

39. Backes CH and others: Maternal preeclampsia and neonatal outcomes. *Journal of Pregnancy* 2011; 2011:214365. E-pub: April 4, 2011. DOI: 10.1155/2011/214365

40. Lee I, Okam M: Anemia in pregnancy. *Hematology/Oncology Clinics of North America* 25(2): 241, 2011.

41. Centers for Disease Control and Prevention: *Pediatric and pregnancy nutrition surveillance system: Pregnancy data tables by health indicators.* http://www.cdc.gov/pednss/pnss_tables/pdf/national_table2.pdf Accessed: March 4, 2014.

42. Niebyl J: Nausea and vomiting in pregnancy *New England Journal of Medicine* 363(16):1544, 2010. DOI: 10.1056/NEJMcp1003896

43. Ayyavoo A and others: Hyperemesis gravidarum and long-term health of the offspring. *American Journal of Obstetrics and Gynecology* November 23, 2013. PII: S0002-9378(13)02149-2. DOI: 10.1016/j.ajog.2013.11.035 [E-pub ahead of print]

44. Fowler G, Ye J: Got Milk? Chinese crisis creates a market for human alternatives. *Wall Street Journal* September 24, 2008.

45. Hau AK: Melamine toxicity and the kidney. *Journal of the American Society of Nephrology* 20(2):245, 2009.

46. Wright A, Schanler R: The resurgence of breastfeeding at the end of the second millennium. *Journal of Nutrition* 131(2):421S, 2001.

47. Centers for Disease Control and Prevention: *Breastfeeding report card—United States, 2013.* http://www.cdc.gov/breastfeeding/pdf/2013BreastfeedingReportCard.pdf Accessed: March 4, 2014.

48. Department of Health and Human Services: *The Surgeon General's call to action to support breastfeeding.* 2011. http://www.cdc.gov/breastfeeding/promotion/calltoaction.htm Accessed: March 2, 2014.

49. Centers for Disease Control and Prevention: *2011 pediatric nutrition surveillance: National summary of breastfeeding indicators: Children aged less than five years.* http://www.cdc.gov/pednss/pednss_tables/html/pednss_national_table3.htm Accessed: March 4, 2014.

50. Jantscher-Krenn E, Bode L: Human milk oligosaccharides and their potential benefits for the breast-fed neonate. *Minerva Pediatrica* 64(1):83, 2012.

51. Peterson R and others: Glycoconjugates in human milk: Protecting infants from disease. *Glycobiology* 2013. DOI: 10.1093/glycob/cwt072

52. Kent JC and others: Volume and frequency of breastfeedings and fat content of breast milk throughout the day. *Pediatrics* 117:e387, 2006.

53. Owen C and others: Does initial breastfeeding lead to lower blood cholesterol in adult life? A quantitative review of the evidence. *American Journal of Clinical Nutrition* 88 (2):305, 2008.

54. Chapman D, Normsen-Rivers L: Impact of maternal nutritional status on human milk quality and infant outcomes: An update on key nutrients. *Advances in Nutrition* 3:351, 2012. DOI: 10.3945/an.111.001123

55. American Academy of Pediatrics: Policy Statement: Breastfeeding and the use of human milk. *Pediatrics* 129; e827, 2012; originally published online February 27, 2012; http://pediatrics.aappublications.org/content/129/3/e827.full.html

56. Hauck F and others: Breastfeeding and reduced risk of sudden infant death syndrome: A meta-analysis. *Pediatrics* 128:103, 2011.

57. Svensson K and others: Effects of mother-infant skin-to-skin contact on severe latch-on problems in older infants: A randomized trial. *International Breastfeeding Journal* 8:1; 2013. DOI: 10.1186/1746-4358-8-1

58. Watkins S and others: Early breastfeeding experiences and postpartum depression. *Obstetrics and Gynecology* 118(2 Pt 1):214, 2011. DOI: 10.1097/AOG.0b013e3182260a2d

17 Infants, Children, and Adolescents

CASE STUDY

School lunches from home

SIX-YEAR-OLD GEORGIA IS ABOUT to enter first grade in an elementary school that became "nut free" at the beginning of the new school year. Georgia's mother, Robin, wants to prepare nutritionally well-balanced lunches that do not contain nuts or nut products for her daughter to take to school. Georgia is not a picky eater, so she will consume a wide variety of foods. Also, Robin has a small insulated container to keep foods cold until lunchtime. Georgia can purchase low-fat milk at school, and she has access to water in the school's cafeteria.

- Using MyPlate as a guide, list some "child-friendly" and easy-to-prepare menu items under each food group that would be appropriate for Georgia's lunches.
- Suggest at least two nutrient-dense lunches that Robin can prepare for her daughter to take to school.

The suggested Case Study Response can be found on page 577.

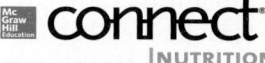 Check out the Connect site at www.mcgrawhillconnect.com to further explore this case study.

QUIZ Yourself

How much weight should a healthy infant gain during its first year of life? What environmental factors contribute to the development of obesity during childhood? Before reading Chapter 17, test your knowledge of infant, child, and adolescent nutrition by taking the following quiz. The answers are found on page 578.

1. A healthy infant doubles his or her birth weight by 4 to 6 months of age and triples his or her birth weight by 1 year of age. __T __F

2. Experts with the American Academy of Pediatrics recommend that babies should be fed fruit juice within the first month of life. __T __F

3. Breast milk provides enough high-quality protein to meet a 4-month-old infant's needs. __T __F

4. The percentage of American children and adolescents who are obese is at an all-time low. __T __F

5. In the United States, the average adolescent girl consumes more calcium than the RDA. __T __F

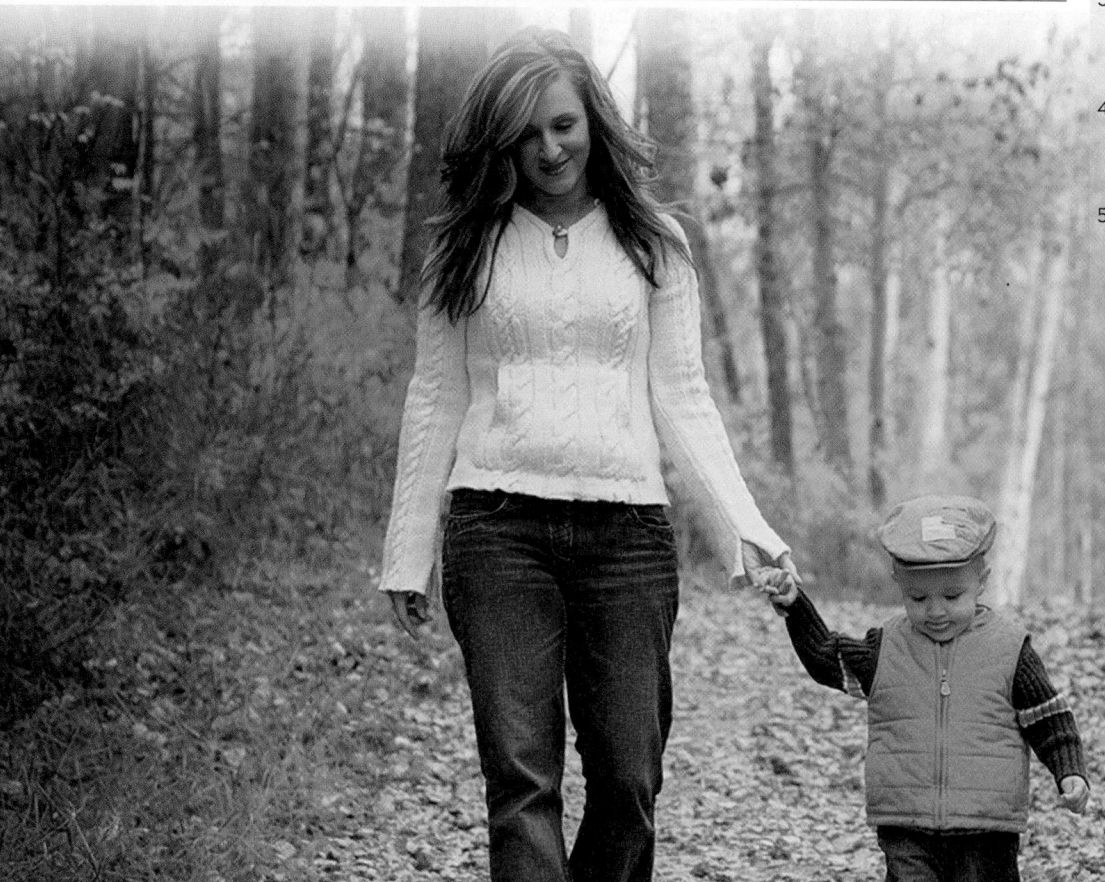

17.1 Infancy: Birth to 12 Months

LEARNING OUTCOMES

1 *Describe three nutrition-related reflexes that healthy infants have at birth.*
2 *Compare the nutrient compositions of human milk and iron-fortified infant formula.*
3 *Discuss the nutrient needs of healthy infants.*
4 *Identify physiological milestones that indicate an infant is ready to eat solid foods.*
5 *Discuss nutrition-related problems that are common among infants.*
6 *Identify foods that should not be given to infants, and explain why the items are inappropriate.*

infancy period from birth to 12 months of age

meconium first feces passed by a newborn shortly after birth

Proper nutrition is critical to support the rapid growth and development that occur during **infancy**, the period from birth to 12 months of age. The term *new-born* is used to describe an infant during its first 4 weeks of life.

At birth, a newborn's weight, length, and head circumference are measured and recorded. During the first few days after birth, the newborn typically loses about 5% of his or her birth weight; breastfed infants tend to lose more of their weight than bottle-fed ones.[1] The early weight loss is normal and attributed to some fluid loss and to the passage of **meconium** (*meh–ko'–ne–um*). Meconium is the first feces eliminated by a newborn shortly after birth; it is black and composed mainly of intestinal epithelial cells, mucus, and bile. The weight that a healthy newborn loses is usually regained within the first 7 to 10 days of life.

On average, a healthy infant doubles his or her birth weight by about 4 to 6 months of age and triples his or her birth weight by his or her first birthday (Fig. 17.1). Additionally, an infant's length increases by 50% during the first year of life. In general, exclusively breastfed infants gain weight more rapidly during the first 2 to 3 months of life than formula-fed infants. From 6 to 12 months of age, weight gain is slower for breastfed infants than for formula-fed babies.[1]

Brain growth occurs at a remarkably rapid rate during infancy. Health care providers can estimate the infant's brain growth by monitoring the expansion of an infant's head circumference (see Fig. F.6). If undernutrition occurs during

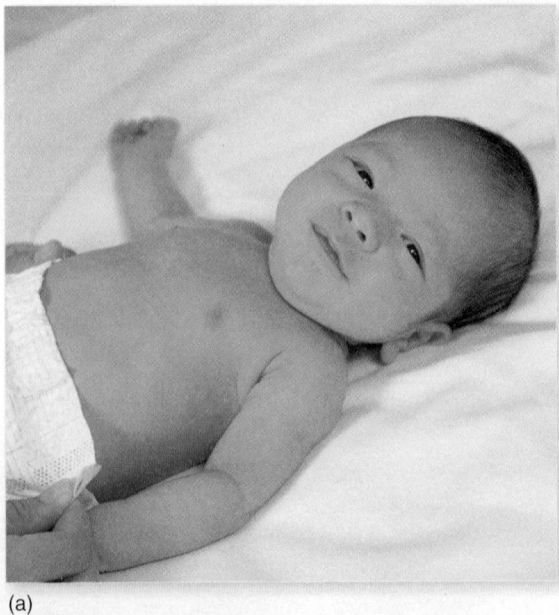
(a)

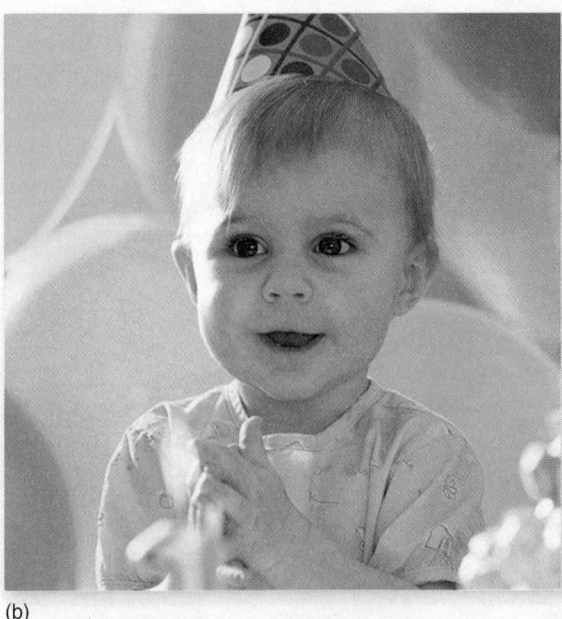
(b)

FIGURE 17.1 From birth to first birthday. A healthy newborn baby (a) grows rapidly during its first year. By 1 year of age (b), the infant's birth weight has tripled and its length has increased by 50%.

infancy, affected children may have a brain that is smaller than average, which can result in impaired *cognitive* (intellectual skills) development and behavioral problems.[2,3] Growth charts used to assess an infant's growth and development are available at http://www.cdc.gov/growthcharts/.

Reflexes

The muscular movements of a newborn occur primarily as uncoordinated **reflexes**. A reflex is an involuntary muscular reaction that occurs in response to a stimulus, such as a loud sound or caregiver's touch. Healthy newborns typically exhibit three nutrition–related reflexes:

- The **suck reflex** enables an infant to draw milk and swallow when a nipple is put into its mouth.

- The **rooting reflex** causes an infant to turn its head and open its mouth as the baby's cheek is stroked. Rooting is a survival mechanism that helps a newborn find the nipple of a breast or bottle to begin sucking.

- The **extrusion reflex** causes a baby's tongue to thrust forward when a solid or semisolid object is placed in his or her mouth. This reflex helps prevent young infants from eating foods before they are able to digest them. The extrusion reflex also enables young infants to reject solid foods that may cause choking.

The suck, rooting, and extrusion reflexes help infants obtain and consume liquid food (breast milk). These reflexes disappear by the age of 4 to 6 months, which is around the age when an infant is physiologically ready to consume solid foods.

Developmental Milestones

Developmental maturation is generally measured against *milestones*, skills or characteristics that a healthy infant is expected to acquire within a specific time frame. Milestones generally have age ranges that represent what is normal. Physical milestones occur in a sequential fashion, which means that a child will need to develop a particular ability involving skeletal muscles (*motor skills*) before he or she can progress to more advanced ones (Table 17.1). For example, most infants can hold up their heads without support for the first time at about

reflexes involuntary muscular reactions that occur in response to a stimulus

suck reflex involuntary response that enables an infant to draw milk and swallow when a nipple is put into his or her mouth

rooting reflex involuntary response in infants in which the child turns and opens his or her mouth as the child's cheek is stroked

extrusion reflex involuntary response in which the young infant's tongue thrusts forward to remove solid or semisolid objects placed in the mouth

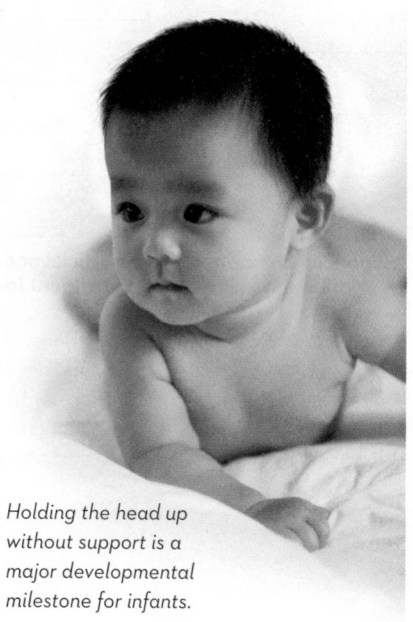

Holding the head up without support is a major developmental milestone for infants.

TABLE 17.1 Major Nutrition-Related Developmental Milestones from Birth to 12 Months

Approximate Age in Months When Skills Are Often Acquired	Milestones
1–2	Briefly follows objects with eyes Holds head up without support
3–4	Grasps a toy or bottle with palms of hands Begins to lose extrusion and rooting reflexes
5–6	Sits with back support
7–8	Has the strength and coordination to self-feed with a bottle Sits without support Has first teeth emerge Moves tongue from side to side and closes lips over spoon
8–10	Self-feeds finger foods Begins to drink from cup
11–12	Uses spoon to feed him- or herself; drinks liquids from a cup Has several teeth and good control over chewing ability

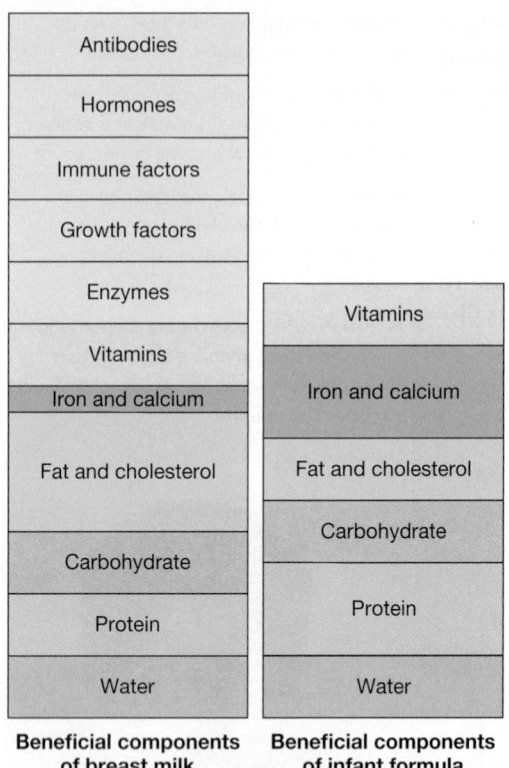

Beneficial components of breast milk

- Antibodies
- Hormones
- Immune factors
- Growth factors
- Enzymes
- Vitamins
- Iron and calcium
- Fat and cholesterol
- Carbohydrate
- Protein
- Water

Beneficial components of infant formula

- Vitamins
- Iron and calcium
- Fat and cholesterol
- Carbohydrate
- Protein
- Water

FIGURE 17.2 Comparing compositions. The nutrient contents of human milk and commercially prepared infant formulas are similar, but breast milk has several beneficial components that are not duplicated in formulas (light blue components).

4 months of age, and they can sit up with back support at 6 months. Infants must acquire these two muscular skills before they are ready to be fed solid foods.

Infant Formula

In Chapter 16, we discussed human lactation and the benefits of breast‐feeding for new mothers and breast milk for their infants. In the United States, however, about 21% of parents choose to feed infant formula to their newborns.[4] Of the new mothers who initiate breastfeeding while in the hospital, the majority do not exclusively breastfeed their infants by the time the babies are 3 months old. The mothers either supplement breastfeedings with infant formula or discontinue breastfeeding entirely.

Feeding fresh fluid cow's milk to infants is not recommended during the first year of life.[5] Cow's milk does not supply enough iron, vitamins E and C, and essential fatty acids for babies, and the beverage contains more protein, sodium, potassium, and chloride than an infant's imma‐ture kidneys can process. Additionally, an infant's digestive system does not break down the protein and fat in cow's milk as easily as the protein and fat in breast milk.

Popular infant formulas are based on cow's milk. Formula manu‐facturers modify the milk so infant formulas have a nutrient composition similar to that of human milk. Table 17.2 compares the approximate energy and selected nutrient contents of human milk, cow's milk, and cow's milk–based, iron–fortified infant formulas (per ounce).

Although the energy and nutrient compositions of commer‐cially prepared infant formulas are similar to human milk, formu‐las do not have the numerous beneficial biological substances that enter breast milk when it is being made by human milk–producing cells (Fig. 17.2).[6] According to the American Academy of Pediatrics (AAP), "… all substitute feeding preparations differ markedly from it [breast milk], making human milk uniquely superior for infant feeding."[7]

TABLE 17.2 Comparing Approximate Compositions of Human Milk, Cow's Milk, and Iron-Fortified Infant Formulas (Per Ounce)

Milk or Iron-Fortified Formula	Energy (kcal/oz)	Protein (g/oz)	Carbohydrate (g/oz)	Fat (g/oz)	Cholesterol (mg/oz)	Iron (mg/oz)	Calcium (mg/oz)
Human milk	22.0	0.32	2.12	1.35	4.00	0.01	10.0
Cow's milk, whole	19.0	0.96	1.46	0.99	3.00	0.01	34.0
Cow's milk, fat-free	10.0	1.03	1.52	0.02	1.00	0.01	37.0
Cow's milk protein-based formulas							
Similac® with iron	20.0	0.41	2.10	1.08	1.00	0.36	16.0
Enfamil® with iron	19.0	0.42	2.19	1.07	0.00	0.36	16.0
Soy protein-based formulas							
ProSobee® with iron	19	0.50	1.86	1.07	0.00	0.36	21.0
Similac Isomil® with iron	20	0.49	2.04	1.09	0.00	0.36	21.0

Source of data: U.S. Department of Agriculture, Agricultural Research Service. *What's in the foods you eat search tool*, 5.0. http://www.ars.usda.gov/services/docs.htm?docid=17032 Accessed: February 20, 2014.

DID YOU KNOW?

In the early 1900s, many infants were bottle fed home-prepared formulas made with canned evaporated cow's milk, corn syrup, and water. To prevent scurvy and rickets, babies were also given orange juice and cod liver oil to supply vitamins C and D. In the 1940s, commercially prepared infant formulas that were made from cow's milk and had micronutrients added to them became more widely used in the United States.

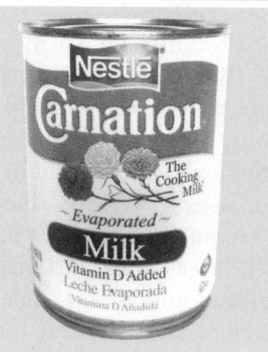

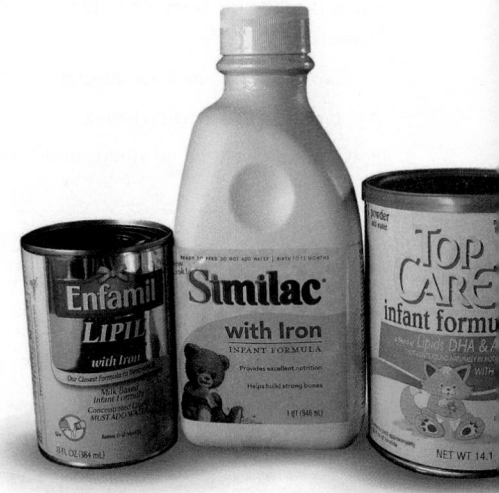

Commercially prepared infant formulas are available in ready-to-use, liquid concentrate, and powdered forms.

Forms of Infant Formula

Three basic forms of commercial infant formulas are available:

- *Ready-to-feed* formulas are poured directly from the container into a baby bottle. Such formulas are more expensive than the other types of formula, but they are convenient to use. The container must be refrigerated after opening to avoid spoiling.

- *Concentrated formulas* are packaged in 13-ounce cans and require the addition of an equal amount of water. Although concentrated formulas are less expensive than ready-to-feed infant formulas, the concentrate requires a sterile source of water, and the product must be refrigerated after opening. Thirteen ounces of bottled water may be used to reconstitute a can of concentrated formula. If tap water is used instead of bottled water, the water should be boiled for 2 minutes, then cooled to room temperature to ensure the water is sterile.[8]

- *Powdered formula* is useful for breastfeeding mothers who occasionally supplement with formula.[9] Powdered formula is less expensive than other forms of infant formulas, and the powder requires no refrigeration. Like concentrated formula, powdered formula requires a sterile source of water for reconstitution. Care must be taken to add the proper amount of water to the powder to ensure it has the necessary concentration of nutrients for infants.

Specialized Infant Formulas. In the United States, 2 to 3% of infants are allergic to proteins in cow's milk.[10] **Eczema** (a type of skin rash) is the major sign of cow's milk allergy. Other signs of cow's milk allergy may include diarrhea, refusal to eat, frequent respiratory infections, and **colic** (*excessive crying infant syndrome*), a condition in which a young infant cries excessively for no apparent reason. Many children outgrow milk allergy by the time they are 3 years of age.[10]

Infants who cannot tolerate cow's milk–based formulas are given a specialized formula. Formulas that are based on soy protein can be used by families who are strict vegans. Babies who are allergic to the proteins in cow's milk or soy–protein formulas are often given protein **hydrolysate formulas** (e.g., Nutramigen® or Pregestimil®). Hydrolysate formulas contain proteins that have been hydrolyzed (broken down) into polypeptides or free amino acids. Switching to a hydrolysate formula may reduce the symptoms of colic.[11] However, the hypothesis that exposure to cow's milk or soy proteins can cause colic in infants is controversial.[10]

Energy and Nutrient Needs

Most of an infant's energy intake is used for growth. During its first 6 months, a healthy infant generally needs about 49 kcal/lb/day (108 kcal/kg), which is

DID YOU KNOW?

Some parents try to save money by adding extra water to infant formula. Adding too much water to formula results in an undernourished baby, because the formula's energy and nutrient contents are inadequate to support growth. Overdilution can also result in water intoxication and hyponatremia, which can be life threatening for infants (see Chapter 11).

eczema type of skin rash

colic condition in which a young infant cries excessively for no apparent reason

hydrolysate formulas infant formulas that contain protein that has been hydrolyzed to polypeptides or free amino acids

FRESH TIPS

The following signs indicate that an infant is ready for complementary foods. The child:

- Can sit with some back support;
- Has lost the extrusion reflex;
- Can hold its head up steady and straight;
- Shows interest in consuming foods that adult caregivers and older children eat; and
- Opens his or her mouth when he or she sees food.

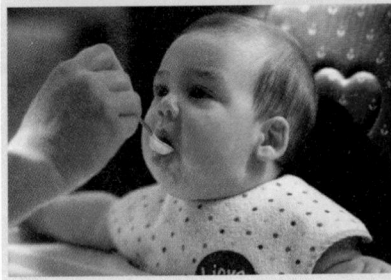

higher than the number of calories required during any other time in life.[12] If a 150−pound adult consumed 49 kcal/lb/day, he or she would be obtaining 7350 kcal/day!

Protein is a critical nutrient for the infant's growth and development. During the first 6 months, an infant's Adequate Intake (AI) for protein is 1.52 g/kg body weight. Breast milk and infant formula provide enough high−quality protein to meet the young infant's needs. After 6 months of age, an infant's growth rate slows, and the baby's Recommended Dietary Allowance (RDA) for protein decreases to 1.2 g/kg body weight.[12]

Even though there are no recommendations for total lipid intake for infants, both breast milk and infant formula provide about 55% of calories from fat. The high amount of fat ensures a concentrated source of energy for the infant and provides the essential fatty acids, linoleic acid and alpha−linolenic acid. Breast milk naturally provides arachidonic acid and docosahexaenoic acid, whereas these two fatty acids are added to most commercially prepared infant formulas.

The main carbohydrate in a young infant's diet is lactose, either from breast milk or from cow's milk–based infant formulas. Cereals or other starchy foods are not appropriate for infants who are under 4 months of age, because the babies do not have adequate amounts of the enzyme amylase that is required for efficient starch digestion.[13]

Micronutrients

Table 17.3 lists the Dietary Reference Intakes (DRIs) for selected micronutrients. An infant who consumes a commercially prepared, iron−fortified infant formula obtains adequate amounts of most vitamins and minerals.

Healthy full−term infants are born with a supply of iron (as ferritin) that lasts until they double their birth weight, which is normally around 4 to 6 months of age. At this age, the addition of iron−containing foods is recommended. Formula−fed infants usually receive much more than the AI for iron (0.27 mg iron/day), because most infants are given iron−fortified infant formula that provides 12 mg/L of iron.[9] Because cow's milk is a poor source of iron, infants who drink cow's milk have a high risk of iron deficiency anemia.[14] To reduce the risk of iron deficiency, most infants who are not consuming an iron−fortified infant formula should receive a supplemental dose of 8 to 10 mg of iron per day.[14] Breastfed babies do not need to be given as much iron, because the iron in breast milk is well absorbed.

Preterm or low−birth−weight infants as well as babies born to mothers who were iron deficient during pregnancy have lower iron stores at birth than infants born to women with adequate iron status during pregnancy. Thus, preterm and low−birth−weight infants deplete their iron stores earlier than other infants. Experts with the AAP recommend that such infants be given an iron supplement daily, regardless of whether they are breastfed or formula−fed.[15]

Iron needs increase dramatically to 11 mg/day for infants who are 6 to 12 months of age. Bottle−fed infants receive the recommended amount of the mineral from their daily consumption of iron−fortified formula. Breastfed infants, however, should be given iron−containing foods such as meats and iron−fortified cereals.

The recommended intake of fluoride for infants who are 6 to 12 months of age is 0.5 mg/day. Recall from Chapter 12 that fluoride reduces the risk of

TABLE 17.3 Dietary Reference Intakes for Selected Micronutrients During Infancy

Age in Months	Iron (mg)	Fluoride (mg)	Calcium (mg)	Vitamin A (µg)	Vitamin C (mg)	Vitamin D (µg) (IU)
Birth–6	0.27	0.01	200	400	40	10 (400)
6–12	11	0.5	260	500	50	10 (400)

decayed teeth (dental caries); however, ingesting too much fluoride may result in dental fluorosis, a condition that causes discoloration of the teeth before they erupt through the gums. The level of fluoride added to municipal water supplies twice the level of the mineral that infants need. Therefore, adding fluoridated water to powdered or concentrated infant formula may cause bottle—fed babies to have excessive intake of fluoride.[16] To reduce the risk of dental fluorosis, care—givers can use purified, distilled, or fluoride—free bottled water to reconstitute the formula.

The placenta does not efficiently transfer vitamin D to the fetus, so newborns may have inadequate amounts of vitamin D stored in their bodies. Furthermore, vitamin D deficiency is common in women during pregnancy and lactation.[17] To reduce the likelihood of vitamin D deficiency occurring in infants, exclusively breastfed infants should receive 10 μg (400 IU) of vitamin D each day within the first few days after birth and throughout their first year of life.[18] Commercial infant formulas contain vitamin D.

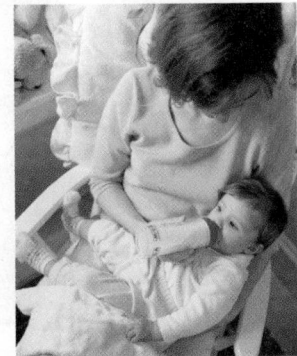

Keeping a baby upright for 30 minutes after a bottle or breastfeeding can reduce the likelihood of the infant vomiting some food.

Water

Human milk and infant formula provide all the water infants need, unless an infant sweats excessively during hot weather or loses fluid by vomiting or hav—ing diarrhea. In these cases, a supplemental bottle of 2 to 4 ounces of water may be necessary, but the volume of water depends on the volume of fluids that was lost. Dehydration can occur rapidly in infants, especially in extreme heat or severe illnesses. To treat dehydration, the infant's physician may recommend **oral rehydration therapy (ORT)**, the administration of products that contain electrolytes (primarily sodium and chloride), water, and glucose.

oral rehydration therapy (ORT) treatment for dehydration that contains electrolytes, water, and glucose

DID **YOU** KNOW?

"Infant reflux" occurs when stomach contents flow back into the esophagus after a feeding, and the baby often vomits a small amount of food ("spits up") as a result. About 50% of babies experience infant reflux several times a day during their first 3 months of life.[19] To reduce the likelihood of "spitting up," both bottle-fed and breastfed infants should be kept upright for 30 minutes after eating. It is also helpful to interrupt each feeding session a few times to "burp" the baby by sitting the child upright and gently rubbing or patting its back. Most babies do not require treatment for infant reflux, because the condition often resolves by itself.

If a baby forcibly vomits ("projectile vomiting") or fails to gain weight, caregivers should contact the child's physician. Treatment depends on the cause of the vomiting, but in severe cases, medication or surgery may be necessary.[19]

DID **YOU** KNOW?

Many caregivers think adding complementary foods to infants' diets before they are 4 months of age helps babies sleep through the night, but there is no scientific evidence to support the practice. As an infant's nervous system matures, the baby stays awake more often during the day and sleeps for longer periods at night. Thus, staying asleep between midnight and 5 A.M. is a developmental milestone that the majority of healthy babies reach when they are 3 months of age, regardless of what they are eating.[21]

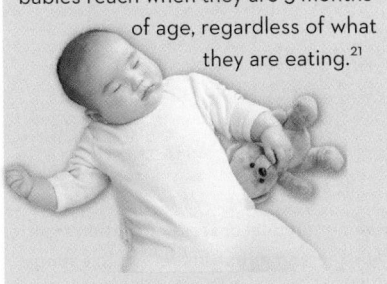

Complementary Foods

Complementary baby foods are solid, pureed (ground up, moistened, and blended), or mashed foods as well as beverages other than breast milk or for—mula.[8] Caregivers should introduce complementary foods when the infant is 4 to 6 months of age.[20] Caregivers, however, should also wait to do so until they observe the signs listed in the "Fresh Tips" box on the previous page that indi—cate the infant is ready to eat solid foods.

Until recently, health care practitioners recommended that caregivers avoid introducing certain foods (e.g., eggs, fish, and peanuts) to infants because of the risk of food allergy. According to experts with the Academy of Nutrition and Dietetics, there is a lack of science—based evidence to support the practice of withholding such foods *after* the infant is 4 to 6 months of age.[20]

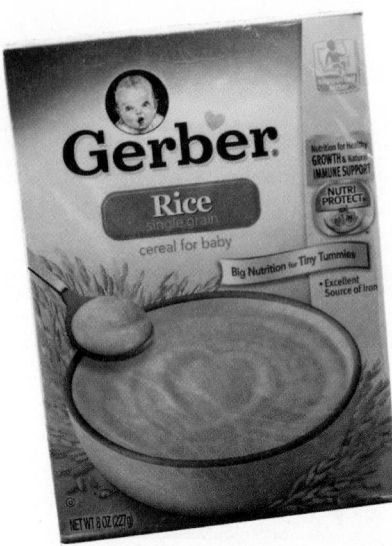

FIGURE 17.3 Infant cereal. For many American infants, rice cereal is their first solid food.

Infant Cereal

Most pediatricians recommend iron–fortified rice cereal, especially for breastfed infants, as the first complementary food (Fig. 17.3). Infant cereals made with rice are easily digested and less likely to cause allergies than other foods.[8] To intro–duce infant cereal to an infant, the caregiver can combine about 1 tablespoon of cereal with 4 to 5 tablespoons of breast milk or formula. This semisolid mixture is then spoonfed to the baby. After the infant becomes accustomed to eating the cereal, the amount of fluid added to it can be gradually decreased until the food has the consistency of cooked oatmeal.

Introducing Other Complementary Foods

Experts with the American Academy of Allergy, Asthma & Immunology recom–mend the gradual introduction of new foods to babies.[22] Adding a new food to feedings for a period of time (4 or 5 days) can help caregivers determine if the baby has adverse responses that may indicate allergies, such as wheezing, vom–iting, or itchy skin, to the particular food.

To complement cereal feedings, babies are usually given single vegetables or fruits before meats are introduced. Fruits and vegetables, however, are not sources of heme iron. Therefore, infants who either have or are at risk of iron deficiency can benefit from consuming meat before being offered fruits and veg–etables, because meat contains heme, the easily absorbed form of iron.

After caregivers determine that an infant can consume individual foods without having an allergic reaction, those items may be served as combinations, such as peas with carrots or carrots with turkey. Commercially prepared baby foods are available in different stages, based on an infant's age and chewing ability. However, caregivers can make their own baby foods from items that they eat. Many babies can be fed soft, finely cut up, or mashed versions of foods that are served to older family members.

Caregivers should prepare or purchase products that are plain with no added sugar, salt, starch, or fat. Although "baby desserts" may be appealing to adults, such foods are not necessary for infants.

DID **YOU** KNOW?

Caregivers can make their own baby food by taking plain, unseasoned cooked foods and pureeing them in a blender. If a large amount of an item is blended, the puree can be poured into an ice-cube tray that is then sealed in a plastic bag and placed in the freezer. When it is feeding time, an ice-cube-sized portion of baby food can be popped out of the tray and warmed.

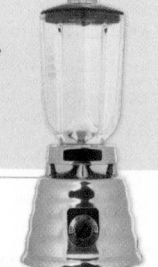

Physiological Readiness for Weaning

After a healthy infant is 6 months of age, he or she is physiologically ready for **weaning**, the gradual process of shifting from breastfeeding or bottle feeding to eating solid foods and drinking from a cup. Infants must reach certain phys–iological milestones before weaning. A significant and noticeable nutrition–related milestone is the emergence of the first primary tooth, which generally occurs at about 6 to 8 months of age. Usually, the first teeth to erupt are the two bottom front teeth. Most children have all 20 primary teeth by age 2 ½ to 3 years.

weaning gradual process of shifting from breastfeeding or bottle feeding to eating solid foods and drinking from a cup

Gross motors skills are abilities to control large muscles of the arms, legs, and back. A healthy 6−month−old baby has acquired enough control over his or her gross muscles to sit up alone without assistance, such as sitting in a high chair. **Fine motor skills** involve abilities to control the movement of smaller muscles, such as those found in the fingers. Mastery of fine motor skills enables babies to move their fingers in a coordinated, purposeful manner.

By the eighth or ninth month of life, the infant has developed the **pincer grasp**, which enables the baby to pick up objects with its thumbs and forefingers. The baby uses its pincer grasp to feed itself finger foods, small pieces of food such as ripe bananas, cooked string beans, or cooked chicken (Fig. 17.4). Finger feeding is usually a messy process, and the baby can appear to be "playing with food" to some adults (Fig. 17.5). Babies, however, need to practice the skills needed to feed themselves. As the infant's fine motor skills mature, he or she is able to use a spoon and hold a cup.

As infants' muscular coordination improves, beverages such as water or infant formula can be offered from a cup at meal times. Sugar−sweetened, caffeinated, carbonated, or artificially sweetened beverages are not appropriate for babies. Added sugars promote dental caries; caffeine interferes with sleep; and long−term consequences for infants who consume carbonated beverages and artificial sweeteners are unknown.

According to recommendations of the American Academy of Pediatrics, babies should not be given fruit juice before they are 6 months of age.[23] Fruit juice lacks the fiber content of whole, mashed, or pureed fruit, and children may consume the beverages in place of more nutritious foods. Pear, apple, or prune juices contain high amounts of the sugars sorbitol and fructose that may cause infants to experience diarrhea, gas, or abdominal pain. Intake of fruit juice should limited to 4 to 6 ounces/day for children who are 6 months to 6 years of age.[23]

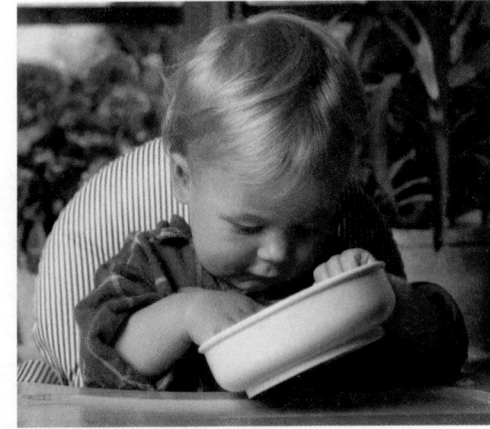

FIGURE 17.4 Pincer grasp. Older infants use their pincer grasp to pick up foods and feed themselves.

gross motors skills control of the large muscles

fine motor skills control of the small muscles, particularly thumb and fingers

pincer grasp use of the thumb and forefinger to pick up small objects

nursing bottle caries form of dental decay that occurs in young children who suck on a bottle that contains any sugar-containing substance for several hours at a time

DID **YOU** KNOW?

Nursing bottle caries is a form of dental decay that occurs in young children who suck on a bottle that contains any sugar-containing substance (including formula or juice) for several hours at a time. As a result of this practice, the child's teeth are bathed in a sugary solution that oral bacteria can metabolize for energy. The bacteria produce lactic acid, which damages tooth enamel. To prevent caries, nighttime bottles should contain only water, and bottles of formula or juice should be offered only during regular feedings.

What Not to Feed Infants

By the end of the first year, babies should be eating a variety of foods. However, the following foods and beverages are not recommended for infants:

- *Honey* may contain spores of *Clostridium botulinum* that can produce a potentially fatal toxin in children under 1 year old (see Chapter 5).

- *Peanut butter or other nut butters* have a sticky consistency that makes them difficult for a young child to swallow safely.

- *Regular, low−fat, or skim cow's or goat's milks* contain more protein and minerals than the infant's immature kidneys can excrete and are low in iron, folate, and vitamin C.

- *Unpasteurized (raw) milk* may be contaminated with bacteria or viruses.

- *Cookies, candy, chips, pastries, or anything with added sugar, solid fat, or salt* provide too many calories and sodium in relation to an infant's

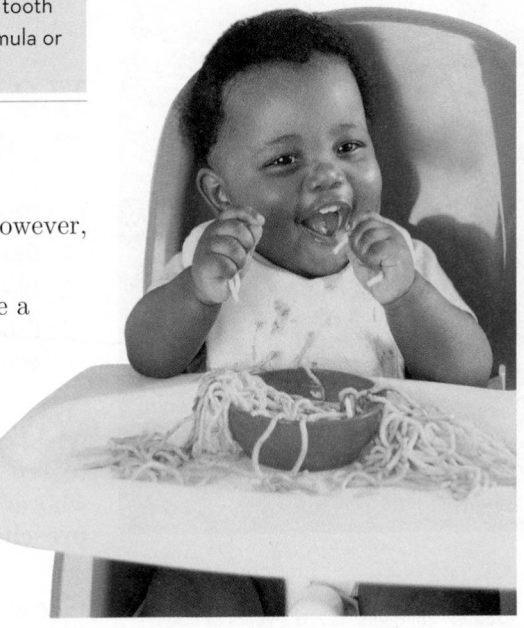

FIGURE 17.5 Self-feeding. Learning to feed one's self is often a messy process!

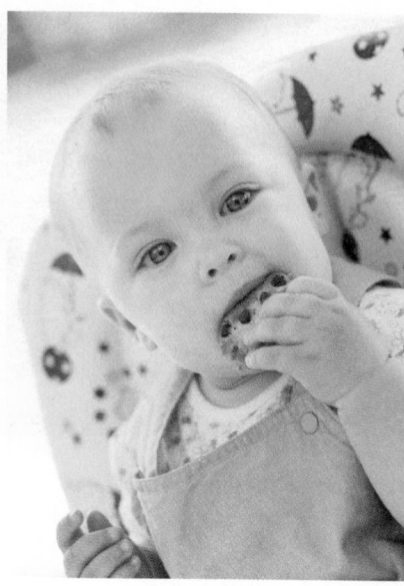

Cookies are not recommended for babies because they contain too many calories and may displace more nutrient-dense foods from the child's diet.

energy and sodium needs. Furthermore, such empty–calorie foods are likely to displace more nutrient–dense items from the child's diet.

- *Small pieces of hard or coarse foods that do not dissolve quickly,* such as whole nuts, grapes, large chunks of cooked meat, raw carrots, popcorn, peanut butter, and hot dogs, can cause choking. Caregivers should supervise meals to keep infants or young children from stuffing too much food into their mouths at one time and administer first aid in case choking occurs.
- *Rare poultry, beef, or pork* might be contaminated with bacteria that are common causes of food–borne illness.

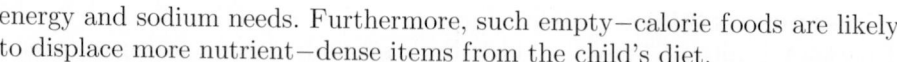

DID **YOU** KNOW?

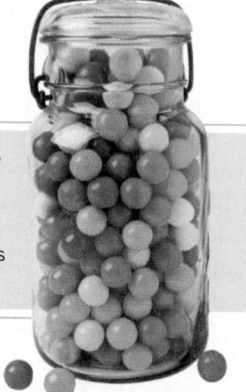

Most cases of choking that involve young children occur while they are eating food. Hard candy and chewing gum are responsible for 19% of choking cases. Common nonfood causes of choking among children include coins, toy parts, and balloons.[24] Chapter 4 provides instructions for administering first aid to a choking infant.

ASSESS YOUR PROGRESS

1 *List the three reflexes that are present at birth and the role of each as related to infant feeding.*
2 *Identify at least two developmental milestones that an infant needs to reach before being weaned.*
3 *James is a healthy newborn who weighs 6.5 pounds and is 18 inches in length. What weight and length would his caregivers expect him to be when he is 12 months of age?*
4 *List three forms of infant formula and some pros and cons of using each form.*
5 *What can caregivers do to reduce the likelihood of infant reflux?*
6 *List at least three finger foods that are appropriate for a 10-month-old infant.*

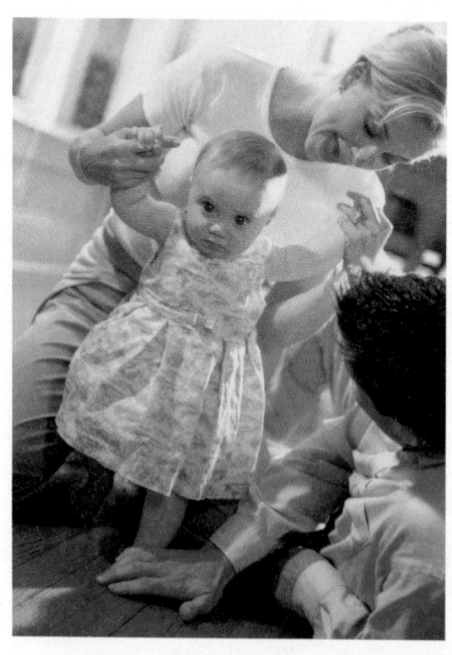

17.2 Toddlers and Preschool-Age Children

LEARNING OUTCOMES

1 *Describe normal growth patterns of children who are between 1 and 5 years of age.*
2 *Discuss the energy and nutrient needs of young children.*
3 *Explain diet-related problems that are common among young children and how adults should handle them.*

At 12 months of age, an infant matures into a toddler. The term **toddler** refers to the stiff, unsteady walking gait (toddle) that is characteristic of children who are between 1 and 3 years of age and have recently learned to walk. A **preschool–age** child is between 3 and 5 years of age.

Growth and Development

toddler child who is 1 to 3 years of age

preschool-age child who is 3 to 5 years of age

The rapid growth rate that characterizes the first 12 months tapers off quickly during the toddler and preschool years. From ages 1 to 2 years, a healthy child gains about 6 pounds. During the preschool years, the child gains 4 to 5 pounds/year. Increases in body length average about 2 ½ to 3 inches/year. A child's weight and height continue to be monitored during routine medical checkups as important indicators the youngster's health status.

The toddler period is a time of transition—physically, emotionally, cognitively, and nutritionally. Most 2–year–old children have a full set of teeth, which makes chewing easier. By the age of 3 years, most healthy children can eat with a fork or spoon, but they need assistance cutting up food. Toddlers are beginning to develop **autonomy**, which refers to independence from caregivers and the ability to make decisions.

Adult caregivers have a major influence on young children's food choices. If toddlers observe their caregivers enjoying broccoli and carrots, the children may be willing to sample these foods. If caregivers regularly indulge in chips, candy, cookies, and soft drinks, children are likely to prefer these foods over more nutritious items.

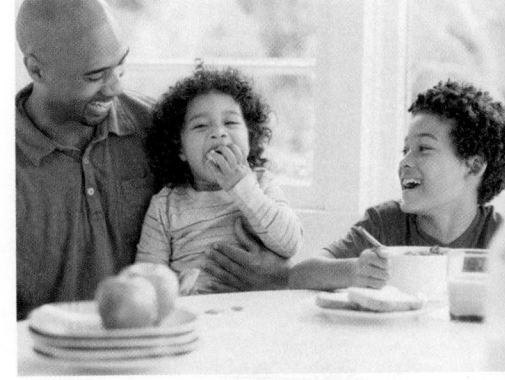

Adult caregivers have a major influence on young childrens' food choices.

Energy and Nutrient Needs

Between the ages of 2 and 10 years, a healthy child grows at a steady pace.[25] As the child's bones, muscles, and blood volume enlarge, his or her energy and nutrient intakes must be adequate enough to support this growth.

autonomy independence and the ability to make decisions

Energy

The number of calories a child needs varies by body size, gender, and physical activity level. The Institute of Medicine created the following formula to calculate the Estimated Energy Requirement (EER) for toddlers.[12]

$$EER = ([89 \, kcal/kg/day] \times [weight \; in \; kg]) - 80$$

Therefore, a child who weighs 28 pounds (12.7 kg) needs 1050 kcal/day based on the calculations below:

$$(89 \; kcal/kg/day \times 12.7 kg = 1130.3) - 80 = 1050 \; kcal/day$$

For information about converting a child's energy needs into servings of foods from MyPlate food groups, visit https://www.supertracker.usda.gov/myplan.aspx.

Macronutrients

A toddler's RDA for protein is 13 g/day, and a preschool–age child's RDA for protein is 19 g/day. Most healthy children can easily meet their RDA for protein by consuming a varied, nutrient–dense diet. For example, a toddler who drinks 2 cups of milk (16 g protein) and eats 2 ounces of chicken (14 g protein), 2 slices of whole–wheat bread (14 g protein), and 1 tablespoon of peanut butter (7 g protein) during a day obtains 51 g of protein just from those foods.

According to results of the National Health and Nutrition Examination Survey, 2005–2008, preschool children ate a considerable amount of their total carbohydrate in the form of added sugars. Preschool–age girls and boys consumed 13.1 and 13.5%, respectively, of their total calories from added sugars.[26]

Caregivers can help children obtain adequate amounts of fiber by serving unprocessed vegetables, whole fruits, and whole grains. Preschool–age children typically do not eat recommended amounts of fruits and vegetables.[27] According to one report, American children between 2 and 5 years of age consume, on average, only about 12 g of fiber daily.[28] For children who are 1 to 3 years of age, the AI for fiber is 19 g/day. For children who are 4 to 8 years of age, the AI for fiber is 25 g/day.[12]

Some fat, especially sources of essential fatty acids, is needed for normal growth and brain development. Toddlers should consume between 30 to 40% of total kcal from fat, whereas older children should limit their fat intake to 25 to

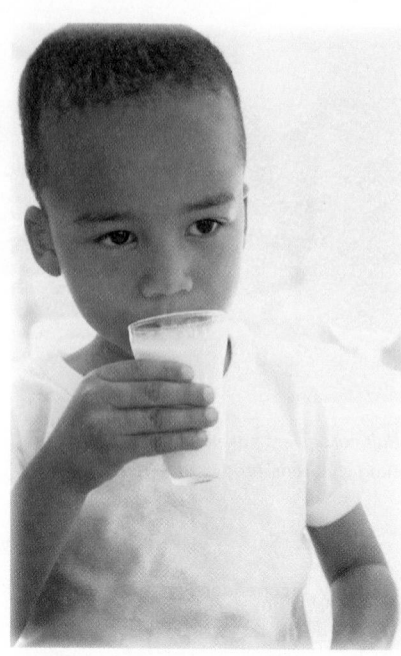

To reduce the risk of developing cardiovascular disease later in life, children who are over 2 years of age should consume low-fat or fat-free dairy products.

FRESH TIPS

Adults can use the following tips to reduce children's intake of sweet treats:

- Serve small portions of sweets and do not serve them regularly.

- Avoid buying or serving sugary soft drinks. At restaurants, order water, juice, or low-fat or fat-free milk, if appropriate.

- Use a checkout lane at the supermarket that does not display candy, if possible.

- Do not offer sweets as rewards.

- Serve fruit, especially fresh fruit, for dessert.

Adapted from: U.S. Department of Agriculture, Choose MyPlate.gov: DG tip sheet no. 13: *Cut back on your kid's sweet treats; 10 tips to decrease added sugars.* Revised January 2016. http://www.cnpp.usda.gov/sites/default/files/dietary_guidelines_for_americans/DGTipsheet13CutBackonSweetTreats.pdf Accessed: January 28, 2016.

food jags periods in which a young child refuses to eat a food that he or she liked in the past or wants to eat only a particular food

35% of total kcal.[29] Many toddlers and preschoolers eat more than the recommended amount of unhealthy saturated fats.[27] Because arterial plaque formation (precursor of atherosclerosis) begins early in life, it is advisable for caregivers to encourage young children to eat foods that supply "healthy fats," such as seeds, nuts, and avocadoes (see Chapter 6).

Milk and some other dairy products are rich sources of protein, calcium, magnesium, and vitamin D (if fortified). Whole milk, however, is major source of saturated fat in young children's diets. According to the American Academy of Pediatrics, reduced–fat forms of milk can be given to children who are between 1 and 2 years of age, but only as part of a diet that supplies 30% of total calories from fat.[30] To reduce the risk of developing cardiovascular disease later in life, children over age 2 years should consume low–fat or fat–free dairy products.[30]

Vitamins and Minerals

Consuming adequate amounts of vitamin D, calcium, and iron may be a challenge for some toddlers and preschool–age children. Most ready–to–eat cereals are fortified with many vitamins and minerals. If a child drinks 2 cups of vitamin D–fortified milk or soy milk each day, his or her vitamin D and calcium intakes are likely to be adequate. As mentioned earlier, cow's milk is a poor source of iron. A recent report shows that young children who drink more than 2 cups of milk each day are at increased risk of iron deficiency.[31]

Almost 16% of toddlers ages 1 to 2 years are iron deficient.[4] Iron deficiency can lead to decreased physical stamina, compromised learning ability, and lowered resistance to infection. To reduce the likelihood of iron deficiency, caregivers can limit milk consumption to 2 cups/day and include foods that are good sources of iron, such as lean meat and enriched breads and cereals, in meals and snacks. Chapter 12 provides more information about foods that are high in iron.

Diet-Related Concerns

Diets of toddlers and preschoolers typically provide too much sodium and less than recommended amounts of potassium.[27,28] Recall from Chapter 11 that sodium and potassium are involved in fluid balance. Excessive intakes of sodium and inadequate intakes of potassium are associated with increased risk of hypertension.

The incidence of caries is increasing among toddlers and preschoolers. According to the National Institutes of Health, about 28% of children 2 to 5 years of age have dental caries affecting their primary teeth.[32] Added sugar consumption contributes to tooth decay. Children who consume an excess of calories, including too many empty–calorie foods that contain added sugars, may also develop obesity.

The "Fresh Tips" box on this page lists suggestions from MyPlate that can help caregivers reduce children's intake of added sugars. The MyPlate website (www.choosemyplate.gov) provides suggestions for developing healthy eating habits among preschool–age children, including ways to increase intakes of vegetables, whole fruit, and whole grains (Fig. 17.6).

Food Jags

Food jags are periods in which a young child refuses to eat a food that he or she liked in the past or wants to eat only a particular item, such as peanut butter and jelly sandwiches or cereal and milk. These behaviors usually begin in the toddler years and may continue throughout the preschool period. During a food jag, adults should continue to offer a variety of nutrient–dense foods to the child,

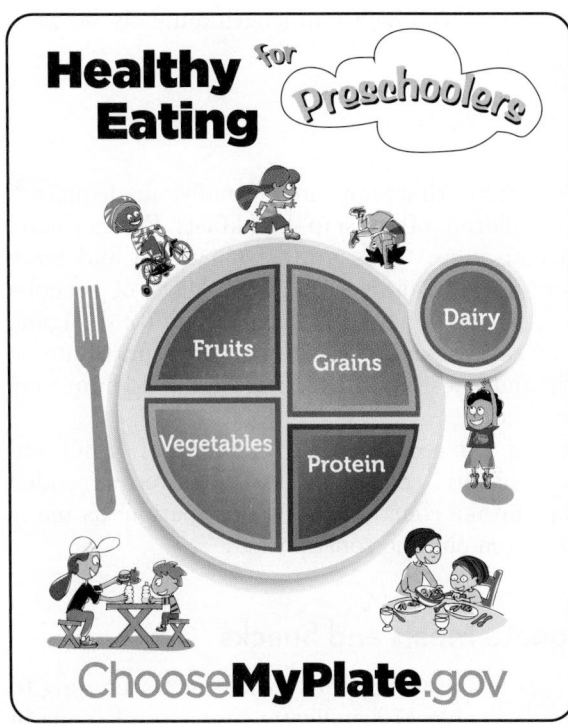

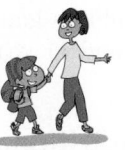

Get your child on the path to healthy eating.

Focus on the meal and each other.
Your child learns by watching you. Children are likely to copy your table manners, your likes and dislikes, and your willingness to try new foods.

Offer a variety of healthy foods.
Let your child choose how much to eat. Children are more likely to enjoy a food when eating it is their own choice.

Be patient with your child.
Sometimes new foods take time. Give children a taste at first and be patient with them. Offer new foods many times.

Let your children serve themselves.
Teach your children to take small amounts at first. Let them know they can get more if they are still hungry.

Cook together.
Eat together.
Talk together.
Make meal time family time.

FNS-451
October 2012
USDA is an equal opportunity provider and employer.

FIGURE 17.6 MyPlate for preschool-age children.

DID **YOU** KNOW?

Many preschoolers, especially physically active ones, can benefit from eating between-meal snacks. An appropriate snack for children should be nutrient dense and provide about 50 to 75 kcal. Caregivers can consider offering a snack that includes a fruit, vegetable, or whole grain, such as a short stick of celery stuffed with a teaspoon of peanut butter or ⅓ cup plain, fat-free yogurt mixed with pieces of fresh fruit and topped with some granola.

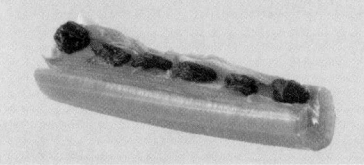

such as whole fruits, whole–grain breads and cereals, and nut butters. After a while, the youngster is likely to become bored with eating the same food repeat–edly and be more willing to add some variety to his or her diet.

ASSESS YOUR PROGRESS

7 *Provide an example of a food jag.*

8 *What steps can adults take to reduce the risk of dental caries among young children?*

9 *List three nutrient-dense snacks that would be appropriate for toddlers.*

school-age child who is 6 to 11 years of age

17.3 School-Age Children

LEARNING OUTCOMES

1 *Discuss major diet-related concerns of school-age children.*

2 *Discuss the nutrients that tend to be excessive and those that are inadequate in school-age children's diets.*

3 *Describe factors that influence the food choices of school-age children , including school lunches.*

Food–related behaviors continue to develop during the **school–age** years (middle childhood), which are defined in this chapter as ages 6 to 11 years. During this stage, a healthy child has a steady but slow growth rate.[25] On average, healthy

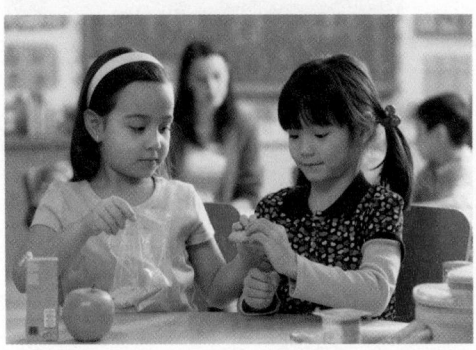

Food-related behaviors continue to develop during the school-age years.

children gain about 5 pounds and grow 2 to 3 inches in length annually between 6 and 11 years of age.

Nutritional Concerns

Many school–age children adopt diets that are nutritionally inadequate.[33] Compared to preschoolers, older children often skip breakfast. Furthermore, school–age children tend to consume more foods away from home and more fried items and sweetened beverages than younger children. Diets of school–age children tend to provide excessive amounts of saturated fat, total sugars, and sodium.[28] Excessive intakes of saturated fat and sugar may contribute to the development of atherosclerosis and obesity, and high intake of sodium may contribute to hypertension among children.

School–age children often do not eat recommended amounts of fruits and vegetables, and the youngsters typically consume less–than–recommended amounts of dietary fiber. Low fiber intake contributes to constipation; as many as 10% of American children suffer from chronic constipation.[34]

Planning Nutritionally Adequate Meals and Snacks

As with younger children, school–age children's appetites fluctuate according to their growth rates and activity levels. Table 17.4 indicates amounts of foods in MyPlate food groups that are recommended for school–age children who need 1200 to 2000 kcal/day. Such information can help caregivers plan nutritious and balanced meals and snacks for the youngsters.

Factors That Influence Children's Food Choices

Factors that affect a school–age child's diet can be positive, such as having health–conscious parents who serve whole–grain products and fresh fruit with meals and snacks. Other factors, however, are negative influences, such as viewing television advertisements for sugary fruit drinks and carbonated beverages. Adults can help offset negative influences on youngsters' food choices by making healthy foods available for them to eat. Parents, for example, can plan nutrient–dense, well–balanced meals that are prepared and eaten at home. Parents and other caregivers can also set limits on children's consumption of empty–calorie foods.

School Lunches

After the end of World War II, the U.S. Congress passed the *National School Lunch Act of 1946* to help improve the nutritional status of American school–age children. The National School Lunch Act established the **National School Lunch Program**, a federally assisted school meal program. School breakfasts

National School Lunch Program federally assisted school meal program

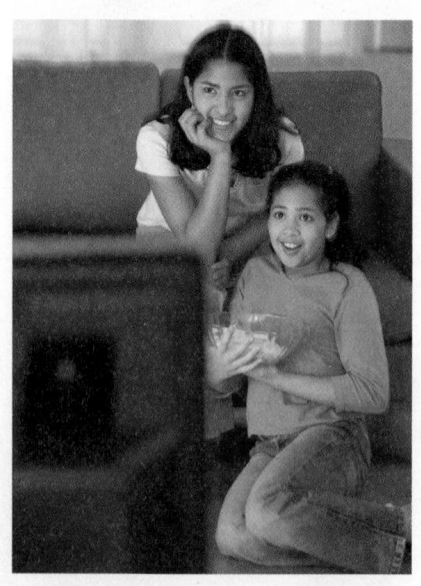

Caregivers can help reduce the risk of obesity among children by limiting their "screen time" to fewer than 2 hours per day.

TABLE 17.4 School-Age Children: Daily Food Plans (MyPlate)

Food Group	1200 kcal	1400 kcal	1600 kcal	1800 kcal	2000 kcal
Grains	4 oz	4 oz	5 oz	6 oz	6 oz
Vegetables	1.5 cups	1.5 cups	2 cups	2.5 cups	2.5 cups
Fruits	1 cup	1.5 cups	1.5 cups	1.5 cups	2 cups
Dairy	2 cups	2 cups	2 cups	3 cups	3 cups
Protein foods	3 oz	4 oz	4 oz	5 oz	5 ½ oz

were added to the program in 1966.[35] Today, many American children eat lunch as well as breakfast and a snack at school.

In the United States, public and nonprofit private schools and residential child care institutions can participate in the National School Lunch Program. The program provides nutritionally balanced, low−cost or free lunches to chil−dren each school day. School lunches must meet meal pattern and nutrition standards that are based on the Dietary Guidelines for Americans. The cur−rent meal pattern has more fruit, vegetables, and whole grains in the school menu than previous menus. Additionally, schools with a high percentage of low−income children are required to serve breakfast. For more information about the National School Lunch Program, visit http://www.fns.usda.gov/nslp/national−school−lunch−program−nslp .

Healthy, Hunger-Free Kids

The U.S. Congress passed the *Healthy, Hunger−Free Kids Act of 2010* to improve the nutrient content of school lunches and other foods sold in public schools. As a result of this act, school food service operations must provide more servings of fruits, vegetables, and whole grains, and reduce amounts of solid fats and sodium in school meals.[35] Additionally, schools must only serve low−fat or fat−free milk at meals. The federal government, however, does not regulate "bag lunch" foods that children bring to school or items served during classroom parties. For more information about the Healthy, Hunger−Free Kids Act, visit: http://www.fns.usda.gov/cnd/Governance/Legislation/CNR_2010.htm.

MyPlate for Children

The MyPlate website (www.chooseMyPlate.gov) is a valuable resource to help caregivers, school educators, and children learn about nutritious foods and healthy eating practices. The website includes *MyPlate Kids' Place*, which is designed for children ages 6 to 11 years (Fig. 17.7). The site has games and other activities to help children learn basic dietary and physical activity concepts of MyPlate. To access this site, visit http://www.choosemyplate.gov/kids/index.html.

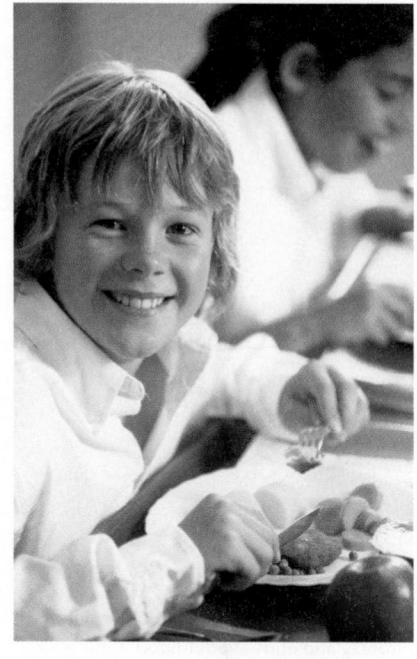

As a result of the National School Lunch Program, millions of American children consume nutritionally balanced, low-cost or free lunches each school day.

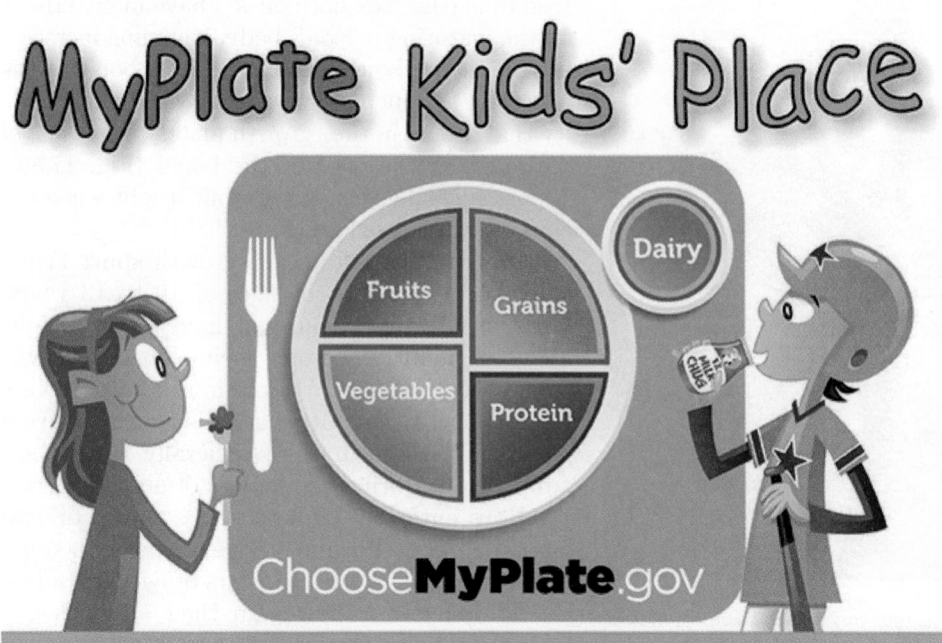

FIGURE 17.7 MyPlate Kids' Place. The MyPlate website provides information about foods and nutrition for caregivers, educators, and children who are 6 to 11 years of age.

ASSESS YOUR PROGRESS

10 *How does a child's diet often change when he or she reaches school age?*

11 *Which nutrients are often consumed in excessive amounts by American school-age children?*

12 *What factors influence a school-age child's food choices?*

13 *Describe the National School Lunch Program.*

14 *What is a major objective of the Healthy, Hunger-Free Kids Act?*

17.4 Adolescence

LEARNING OUTCOMES

1 *Describe physiological changes that normally occur during the adolescent growth spurt.*

2 *Compare the typical growth pattern of girls to that of boys during adolescence.*

3 *Identify nutrients that tend to be low in diets of adolescents.*

adolescence period of life that begins at puberty and ends at adulthood

puberty time at which a child matures physically and sexually into an adult

Adolescence is the life stage that begins at **puberty**, the period in which a child undergoes numerous physiological changes that eventually enable the young person to be capable of reproduction. The timing of puberty varies but usually occurs between ages 9 and 15 years.[25] By the end of adolescence, the individual has reached *adulthood*—physical and reproductive maturity, which generally occurs around 18 to 21 years of age. In this chapter, we refer to children who are 12 to 19 years of age as adolescents.

Growth and Development

growth spurt period characterized by a rapid increase in growth

Adolescence is the second most rapid period of physiological growth that occurs after birth. (An infant grows at a faster rate than an adolescent.) During adolescence, nearly every organ in the body increases in size as healthy children gain weight and become taller. The final period of rapid growth, which may be referred to as "the adolescent **growth spurt**," is associated with puberty.

During the adolescent growth spurt, a female's ovaries secrete high levels of estrogen, and a male's testes secrete high levels of testosterone. Estrogen and testosterone (the "sex hormones") have many effects on the maturing person's body, including increasing the rate of bone growth. The long bones in the arms and legs increase in length by cellular activity that occurs in the "growth plates" (*epiphyseal plates*) near the ends of the bones (Fig. 17.8a). A person reaches his or her adult height when the epiphyseal plates close (Fig. 17.8b).

In girls, the adolescent growth spurt typically begins around the ages of 10 to 13 years. Girls usually experience an increase in weight about 6 months before their stature growth spurt occurs. Skeletal growth is almost complete about 2 years after a girl's first menstrual period. Thus healthy girls generally reach their adult height during the middle of adolescence.

Boys enter the growth spurt a year or two later than girls. For most boys, the growth spurt begins between 12 and 15 years of age, but adolescent males usually attain their adult height later than girls.

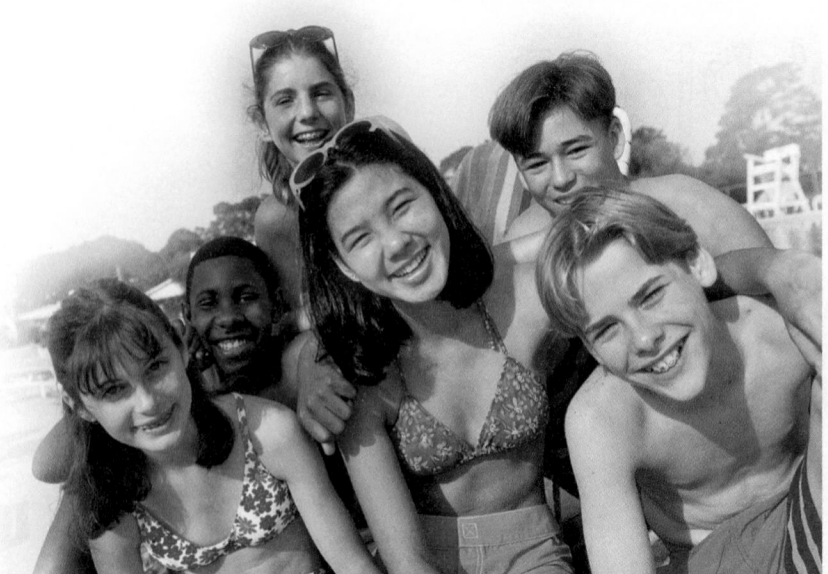

Although these adolescents are about the same age, they vary in their levels of physical maturity.

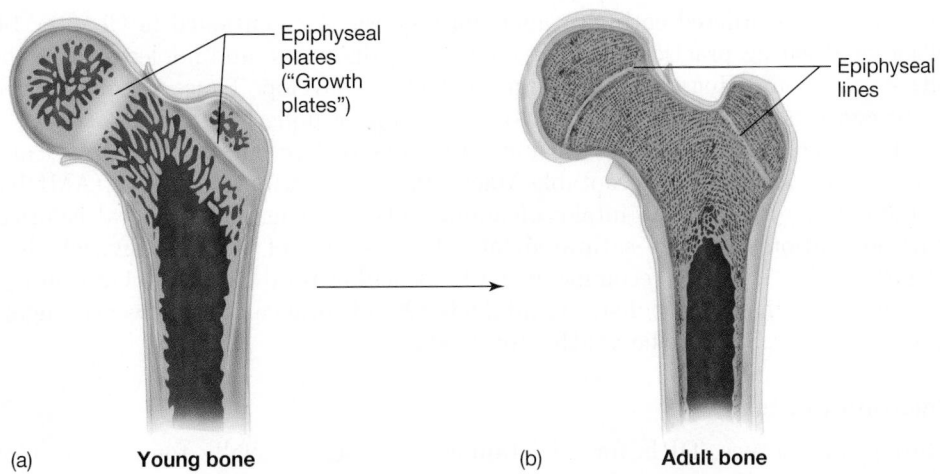

(a) **Young bone**   (b) **Adult bone**

FIGURE 17.8 Growth of long bones. (*a*) The long bones in the arms and legs increase in length by cellular activity that occurs in the "growth plates" near the ends of the bones. (*b*) A person reaches his or her adult height when the epiphyseal plates close. The epiphyseal lines are where the growth plates had been.

The timing of puberty and growth spurts can vary widely among adolescents, primarily as a result of interactions among genetic, environmental, and nutritional factors. Obese girls, for example, typically enter puberty earlier than their nonobese peers.[36] If a girl experiences puberty earlier than the norm, she is likely to be shorter as an adult than a girl who enters puberty later.[37] The shorter stature results from the earlier–than–normal closure of her epiphyseal plates.

Nutrient Recommendations and Status

The amount of energy and nutrients required during adolescence reflects the individual's stage of growth and level of physical activity. Early in adolescence, when a girl is at the peak of her growth spurt, she consumes more calories than a boy of the same age, especially if she is involved in sports. By age 13 or 14 years, girls' growth rate slows and boys' growth spurts begin. As a result, adolescent boys' food intake typically surpasses that of adolescent girls.

Energy and Macronutrients

Energy needs for adolescents range from less than 1400 kcal/day for an inactive girl who has not entered the growth spurt to more than 3200 kcal/day for an active boy who is still in his growth spurt (Table 17.5). Many teens consume more calories than needed for their physical activity level, which results in a high prevalence of obesity in teenagers. Youths whose energy intake is balanced by the energy they expend tend to choose foods that are low in many essential nutrients.[38]

Inadequate energy intake results in underweight, which is defined as having a body mass index (BMI) that is less than 18.5. Underweight in adolescence may

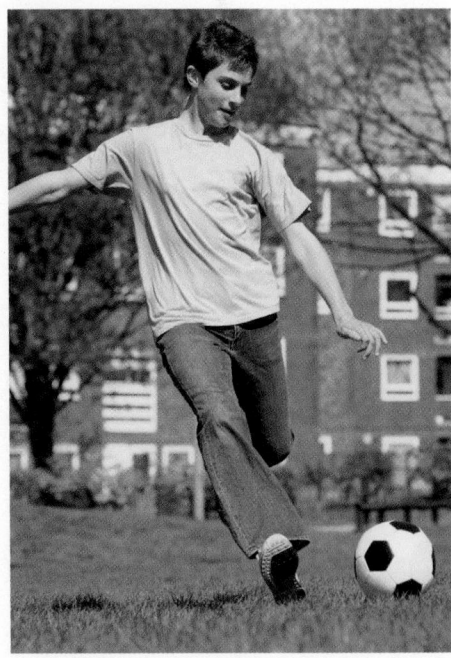

A physically active adolescent male who is in his growth spurt may need at least 3200 kcal per day.

TABLE 17.5 Estimated Energy (kcal) Needs per Day Based on Age, Sex and Activity Level

Age (Years)	Boys			Girls		
	Sedentary	Moderately Active	Active	Sedentary	Moderately Active	Active
12–13	1800–2000	2200	2400–2600	1600	2000	2200
14–18	2000–2400	2400–2800	2800–3200	1800	2000	2400
19–20	2600	2800	3000	2000	2200	2400

Source: U.S. Department of Agriculture, U.S. Department of Health and Human Services: *2015–2020 Dietary Guidelines for Americans* 2015. http://health.gov/dietaryguidelines/2015/guidelines/appendix-2/ Accessed: January 28, 2016.

be a sign of disordered eating or anorexia nervosa. As mentioned in Chapter 14, disordered eating practices may become eating disorders, and adolescence is the life stage when eating disorders are most likely to develop. Thus, caregivers need to be concerned about the health and well−being of underweight adolescents.

On average, adolescents consume amounts of protein, carbohydrate, and fat than are within the Acceptable Macronutrient Distribution Range (AMDR). Although the average fat intake of adolescents is about 33% of total calories, this population's average saturated fat intake is 11% of total energy, which is slightly higher than the recommended 10% or less of total calories.[28] On average, an adolescent male's carbohydrate intake is 52% of total calories; however, sugars comprise about 25% of the youth's total calories.[28]

Micronutrients

During adolescence, DRIs for all vitamins increase, especially for the vitamins that are involved in new cell synthesis (folate and vitamin B−12), collagen for− mation (vitamin C), protein metabolism (vitamin B−6), and bone development (vitamins A, D, and K). Adolescents' average intakes of vitamins A, D, K, and folate (girls) are lower or marginal than the DRIs for these micronutrients.[28]

For adolescents, RDAs for most minerals, including calcium, are higher than for school−age children. On average, males between 12 and 19 years of age con− sume more than the RDA for calcium (1300 mg/day), but the average calcium intake of girls in this age range is less than 75% of the RDA for micronutrient.[28] Both men and women generally achieve their peak bone mass before they are 25 years of age. Low calcium intakes during adolescence places youths, especially teenage girls, at increased risk of developing osteoporosis later in life.[39]

The RDA for iron increases to 15 mg/day for girls who are 14 to 18 years of age. The higher RDA is necessary to make up for increased losses of iron that occur during menstrual bleeding. According to findings of the National Health and Nutrition Examination Survey 2011−2012, females between 12 and 19 years of age consume, on average, 12 mg/iron/day.[28] About 9% of teenage girls expe− rience iron deficiency.[4]

Nutrition-Related Concerns of Adolescents

The national Youth Risk Behavior Surveillance System (YRBSS) monitors key health−related behaviors of American high schools students. Some diet−related findings of the 2011 YRBSS survey are shown in Table 17.6. According to the results of the survey, most high school students did not eat enough fruits, veg− etables, and dairy, and students drank too many sugar−sweetened soft drinks.[38]

TABLE 17.6 Youth Risk Behavior Surveillance System: Key Nutrition-Related Findings, 2011

Diet- and Health-Related Behaviors	Girls (Approx. Percentage)	Boys (Approx. Percentage)
Ate fruit or drank 100% fruit juice 3 or more times/day (during the 7 days before the survey)	20	25
Drank a can, bottle, or glass of a sugar-containing soft drink 1 or more times/day (during the 7 days before the survey)	24	31.4
Ate vegetables (other than French fries, fried potatoes, and potato chips) less than 3 times/day (during the 7 days before the survey)	86	83.4
Described themselves as overweight	35	24
Did not participate in 60 minutes of physical activity (on any day during the 7 days before the survey)	18	10

High school–age girls were almost twice as likely as high school–age boys to be physically inactive.

Adolescent girls who have poor eating habits and nutritionally inadequate diets are a concern of public health experts. Teenage girls may become pregnant, and their bodies' lack of adequate nutrient stores could lead to serious complications during pregnancy and poor pregnancy outcomes. Furthermore, girls who have poor eating habits as adolescents may continue to make unhealthy food choices after they reach adulthood. As discussed in Chapter 16, a woman who does not have adequate nutrient stores in her body when she becomes pregnant is also at risk of having complications and poor pregnancy outcomes.

ASSESS YOUR PROGRESS

15 *Compare the typical growth pattern of a healthy adolescent girl to the growth pattern of a healthy boy who is the same age.*

16 *Which vitamins and minerals are often low in teenagers' diets?*

17.5 Overweight and Obesity in Children

LEARNING OUTCOMES

1 *Provide definitions for overweight, obesity, and extreme obesity in childhood.*

2 *Discuss the prevalence of and factors that contribute to childhood obesity.*

3 *Identify health problems associated with obesity in childhood.*

4 *List strategies for preventing and treating childhood obesity.*

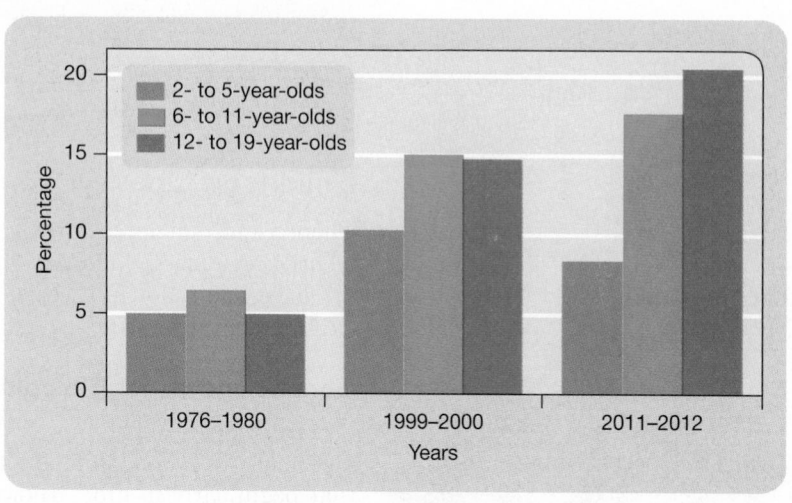

FIGURE 17.9 Prevalence of childhood obesity from 1976–1980 to 2011–2012 (United States).[41]

Over the past few decades, U.S. public health officials became concerned about the increasing prevalence of obesity among children and adolescents ("childhood obesity"). Approximately 17% of American children who are between the ages of 2 and 19 years are obese.[41] Since 1980, obesity prevalence among American children has increased dramatically (Fig. 17.9). There is some good news: Obesity rates among low–income preschoolers are declining.[42] Nevertheless, more obese American children are classified as having "extreme" obesity than in the past.[43]

Defining Obesity in Children

Health care professionals use *BMI–for–age charts* that are available from the Centers of Disease Control and Prevention (CDC) to determine children's and adolescents' weight status. The BMI for children is calculated in the same way as for adults, but BMIs for children are plotted on sex–specific growth charts that define BMI–to–age percentiles for each weight classification. To access these charts, visit the CDC website (http://www.cdc.gov/growthcharts/). Table 17.7 lists weight classifications for children and adolescents.

TABLE 17.7 Weight Status Classifications: Children and Adolescents (Ages 2 to 19)

Classification	BMI-to-Age Percentile
Desirable weight	> 5th to < 85th
Overweight	≥ 85th to < 95th
Obese	≥ 95th
Extreme obesity*	≥ 97th

*No official definition for children and adolescents

Health Problems Associated with Childhood Obesity

Compared to children who have healthy body weights, obese children and adolescents are more likely to have elevated blood pressure, cholesterol, and glucose levels.[42] These chronic conditions are risk factors for cardiovascular disease (CVD). According to results of one study, 70% of obese children had at least one risk factor for CVD, and 39% of obese children had two or more risk factors.[44] Table 17.8 lists chronic health problems that obese children are more likely to have than children with healthy body weights.

Many obese children and adolescents do not "grow out" of their excess body fat (Fig. 17.10). Overweight or obese preschool–age children are five times as likely as preschool children who have healthy weights to be overweight or obese as adults.[42] Furthermore, overweight or obese children are more likely to be *extremely* obese when they are adults.[44]

TABLE 17.8 Chronic Health Problems Associated with Childhood Obesity

- Impaired glucose tolerance, insulin resistance, and type 2 diabetes
- Breathing problems, including sleep apnea and asthma
- Musculoskeletal problems, including joint discomfort
- Fatty liver disease, gallstones, and gastroesophageal reflux (heartburn)
- Social and psychological problems, such as discrimination and poor self-esteem

Source: Centers for Disease Control and Prevention: *Overweight and obesity: Basics about childhood obesity.* Updated April 2012. http://www.cdc.gov/obesity/childhood/basics.html Accessed: January 23, 2014.

Childhood Obesity: Contributing Factors

There is no single cause of excess body fat in children, but researchers have identified multiple factors that are associated with the development of the condition.[45] The following sections examine the role of some genetic, biological, and environmental factors that contribute to childhood obesity.

Genetic and Other Biological Factors

Scientific evidence supports the role of inherited (genetic) and other biological factors in the development of childhood obesity, especially in cases of obesity that begin early in life.[46] Biological factors that contribute to obesity include:

- **Having overfat parents**. If both parents are obese, the child has 10 times the risk of obesity as a child who has only one obese parent.

- **Having a mother who was overfat during pregnancy**. When compared to children whose mothers have healthy body weight during pregnancy, babies born to overweight mothers are nearly three times as likely to be overweight. Furthermore, obese women are more likely than healthy women to have large babies, and such infants have a high risk of childhood obesity.

- **Gaining too much weight and/or having diabetes during pregnancy**. Women who gain too much weight during pregnancy or have diabetes are more likely to give birth to high–birth–weight (HBW) babies. Such children are at risk of developing excess body fat in childhood.

- **Smoking during pregnancy**. Although the reasons are unclear, women who smoke during pregnancy set the stage for the future development of overweight and obesity in their babies.

- **Being undernourished during prenatal development**. Undernutrition during pregnancy contributes to delivery of a low–birth–weight (LBW)

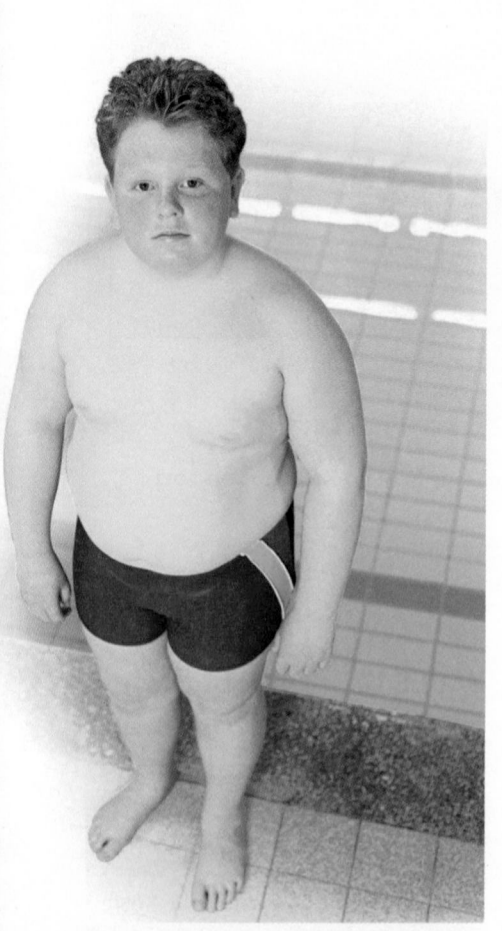

FIGURE 17.10 Childhood obesity. Obese school-age children have a high risk of maturing into obese adolescents and adults.

infant. LBW infants are more likely to develop hypertension, CVD, and type 2 diabetes later in life, which are chronic diseases associated with obesity. At this point, scientists have been unable to explain why prenatal undernutrition contributes to hypertension, CVD, and type 2 diabetes in adulthood.

Biological factors, however, are not entirely responsible for the current obesity epidemic. In many cases, it is difficult to determine whether genes play a more important role than environmental factors in the development of childhood obesity. Is a child obese because the youngster inherited genes from his or her parents that "program" for obesity? Or is a child obese because his or her caregivers provide the child with an excess of empty-calorie, energy-dense foods and do not encourage the child to be physically active?

Impact of the Child's Environment

In the United States, many children are exposed to an environment that encourages overeating and consumption of empty-calorie foods. Additionally, the environment often does not provide children with opportunities to participate in enough physical activity. Table 17.9 lists these and other environmental factors that contribute to childhood obesity.

Preventing Childhood Obesity

The Institute of Medicine developed a set of policy recommendations that may reduce the likelihood of obesity among preschool-age children.[47] Some of the institute's major recommendations focused on specific physical activity and dietary behaviors:

- New mothers should breastfeed their babies exclusively for the first 6 months of life and continue breastfeeding along with introducing appropriate foods after 6 months.

- Communities and child care providers should provide opportunities for children to be physically active throughout the day.

- Children's exposure to TV and forms of digital media ("screen time") should be limited to less than 2 hours per day

Specific dietary steps that caregivers can take to help children achieve and maintain a body weight are listed in the "Fresh Tips" box on this page.

To be healthy, children need opportunities to be physically active daily.

TABLE 17.9 Environmental Factors That Contribute to Childhood Obesity

- Easy access to empty-calorie foods and drinks at or near schools
- Limited access to healthy and affordable foods, particularly in areas with many convenience stores and fast-food restaurants
- Advertising of empty-calorie foods that targets youth
- Lack of established periods for daily physical activity in schools and safe places to be active in many communities
- Large portion sizes of foods sold from vending machines and in restaurants and grocery stores
- Excess exposure to television and other media
  - TV viewing and use of other digital media contribute to childhood obesity because the sedentary activities can reduce the time children spend being physically active.

Source: Centers for Disease Control and Prevention: *Overweight and obesity: A growing problem: What causes childhood obesity?* Last updated April 2013. http://www.cdc.gov/obesity/childhood/problem.html Accessed: March 8, 2014

FRESH TIPS

To help children achieve and maintain a healthy weight, caregivers can:

- Provide plenty of vegetables, fruits, and whole-grain products;

- Include low-fat or nonfat dairy products;

- Serve lean meats, poultry, fish, lentils, and beans for protein;

- Serve "child-size" portions;

- Encourage children to drink water; and

- Limit sources of saturated fat and added sugar.

Adapted from: Centers for Disease Control and Prevention: *Healthy weight—it's not a diet, it's a lifestyle! Tips for parents—ideas to help children maintain a healthy weight.* 2011. http://www.cdc.gov/healthyweight/children/index.html #prevention Accessed: May 15, 2014.

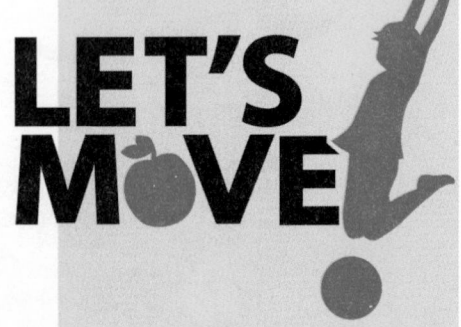

Treating Childhood Obesity

The treatment goal for managing overweight and obese young children and adolescents is to slow the rate of weight gain without interfering with normal growth and physical development. This goal can be accomplished by balancing the calories children consume with the calories they use for physical activity and need for normal growth. Caregivers should not place a child or youth on a weight reduction diet without consulting the child's physician.[48] For severely obese adolescents, treatment approaches that go beyond dietary changes and increased physical activity are often necessary. Such interventions may include prescription medication and weight–loss surgery (see Chapter 13).

Bariatric Surgery for Youth

Bariatric (weight–loss) surgery can improve the health of adolescents with extreme obesity.[50] According to a review of bariatric surgery outcomes in the United States, the surgeries are safe for adolescents. At this time, however, the adjustable gastric banding procedure has not been approved for use with patients who are under 18 years of age.

To qualify for bariatric surgery, an adolescent should have:

- Extreme obesity (BMI >40);

- Failed to lose weight after 6 months of trying to reduce his or her weight;

- Attained his or her adult height (skeletal maturity), which is generally at 13 years of age for girls and 15 years of age for boys; and

- Serious chronic conditions that are associated with obesity, such as type 2 diabetes or sleep apnea, which may improve after surgery.[50]

Regardless of one's age, bariatric surgery is a drastic measure to lose excess body weight and involves some risks. Thus, caregivers and health care providers should carefully assess adolescents who are potential candidates for bariatric surgery to determine whether they are emotionally ready to handle the surgery and make the necessary lifestyle changes to achieve good health and well–being after the procedure.

ASSESS YOUR PROGRESS

17 *Define* overweight, obese, *and* extremely obese *for children as defined by the Centers for Disease Control and Prevention.*

18 *List at least three factors that contribute to cases of childhood and adolescent obesity.*

19 *List at least three practical steps caregivers can take to help children to have healthy weights.*

SUMMARY

SECTION 17.1 Infancy: Birth to 12 Months

- Infants have a rapid growth rate. Sucking, rooting, and extrusion reflexes are observed in newborns.

- Most infant formulas are made from modified cow's milk that has been formulated to be nutritionally similar to breast milk. Some infants cannot tolerate cow's milk–based formulas, so alternative formulas, such as soy-based products, may be used.

- Caregivers should introduce complementary foods when an infant doubles his or her birth weight, which is generally around 4 to 6 months of age. At this age, healthy babies have reached certain physiological milestones that allow for eating solid foods. The first complementary foods for babies are usually an iron-fortified rice cereal followed by single-ingredient foods with no added sugar, salt, or fat.

- Physical growth slows when an infant is 6 to 12 months of age. Primary teeth begin to emerge through the infant's gums, motor skills improve, and children are physiologically ready for chewing solid foods and feeding themselves.

SECTION 17.2 Toddlers and Preschool-Age Children

- The growth rate of toddlers and preschoolers is slower than the growth rate of infants. Energy and nutrient intake must be adequate to support the child's growth and his or her activity level.

SECTION 17.3 School-Age Children

- Many school-age children adopt diets that are nutritionally inadequate. Compared to preschoolers, older children often skip breakfast, consume more foods away from home, eat larger portions of foods, and consume more fried items and sweetened beverages. Many school-age children do not consume recommended amounts of fruits and vegetables.

SECTION 17.4 Adolescence

- After the first year of life, adolescence is the second most rapid period of growth in the life cycle. The adolescent growth spurt typically begins in a girl around the ages of 10 to 13 years and between 12 and 15 years of age in boys.

- The amount of energy and nutrients required during adolescence reflects the stage of growth and types of activity in which the teen is engaged.

SECTION 17.5 Overweight and Obesity in Children

- Since 1980, obesity prevalence among American children who are between 6 and 19 years of age has increased dramatically. Obese children and adolescents are more likely to have elevated blood cholesterol, high blood pressure, and type 2 diabetes than children with healthy body weights.

- Overweight or obese preschool-age children are five times as likely as preschool-age children with healthy weights to be overweight or obese as adults.

- Many factors contribute to the development of childhood obesity. In many cases, it is difficult to determine whether genes play a more important role than environmental factors in the development of childhood obesity.

- Treating childhood obesity involves increasing physical activity, reducing intake of empty-calorie foods, and, in some cases, prescribing medication and having surgery.

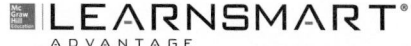

Modifying Recipes for Healthy Living

Stephen is the father of three physically active children, ages 3, 8, and 12 years. He is concerned about his children's health because they experience frequent constipation. The favorite family "treat" is homemade oatmeal cookies. Stephen would like to make the cookies higher in fiber and lower in sugar and solid fat than the original recipe. How can Stephen modify the following recipe to increase its fiber content and reduce its solid fat and added sugars content?

GRANDMA'S OATMEAL COOKIES

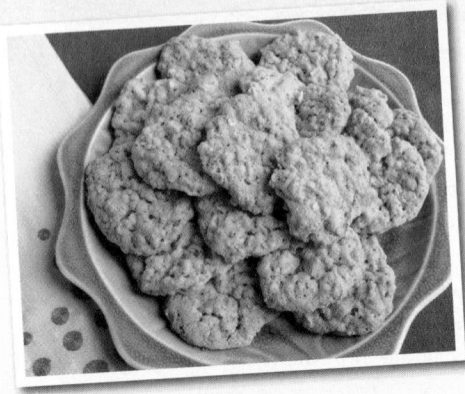

INGREDIENTS

1 cup butter, softened

1 cup white granulated sugar

1 cup brown sugar, packed

2 eggs

1 tsp vanilla extract

2 cups all-purpose flour

1 tsp baking soda

1 tsp salt

2 tsp ground cinnamon

3 cups quick-cooking oats

PREPARATION STEPS

1. Mix together butter, white sugar, and brown sugar. Beat in eggs one at a time. Add vanilla and stir to distribute the vanilla through the mixture.

2. Combine flour, baking soda, salt, and cinnamon; stir these dry ingredients into the butter, sugar, and egg mixture. Mixture will be stiff.

3. Stir in oats; cover, and chill the dough for at least 1 hour.

4. Preheat the oven to 375 °F (190 °C). Roll the dough into 1-inch balls about the size of a walnut, and place 2 inches apart on a greased cookie sheets. Bake for 8 to 10 minutes.

5. Allow cookies to cool on baking sheet for 5 minutes before transferring to a plate.

STEP 1 Brainstorm

Examine the recipe. What ingredients can you use in place of some or all of the butter that would increase the fiber and decrease the fat contents? (Refer to Table 1.7 for substitutions.) What ingredients can be used in place of the all-purpose flour to increase the fiber?

STEP 2 Develop a modified version of this recipe

List ingredients and amounts needed.

List the preparation steps.

STEP 3 Analyze nutrient contents of the original and modified recipes by using a computer software program

Develop a table that compares the number of kcal and amounts of fat and calories in the two recipes.

How did your modifications change the nutrient composition of the cookies?

OPTIONAL ACTIVITIES

STEP 4 Test your new recipe

Keep notes on any changes you make to ingredient amounts as you prepare, bake, and taste the cookies.

STEP 5 Reflect on your findings

How did the cookies look and taste?

STEP 6 Add the recipe to your collection or repeat steps to improve the product

CASE STUDY RESPONSE

SCHOOL LUNCHES FROM HOME

ROBIN CAN VISIT THE MYPLATE WEBSITE for ideas to help her plan nutritious lunches that incorporate items from each food group that her daughter will eat, are acceptable to take to school, and can be stored safely in an insulated school lunch container until lunchtime. For example, Robin can pack:

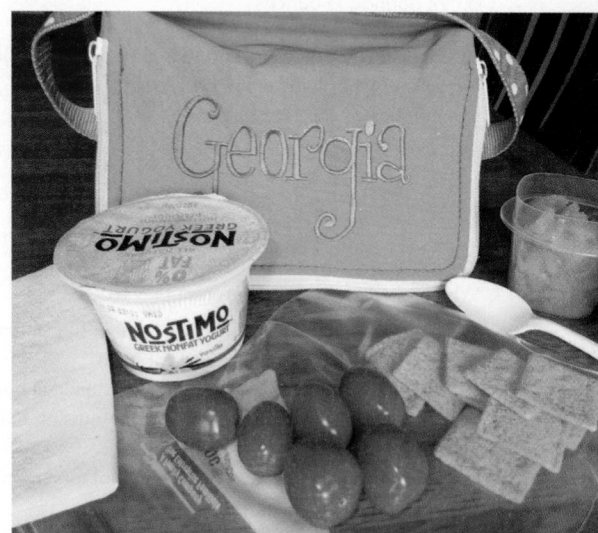

Dairy
Yogurt
Reduced-fat cheese
Reduced-fat milk

Grains
Whole-grain crackers, bagels, and breads
Ready-to-eat cereal

Vegetables
Cherry tomatoes
Celery and carrot sticks
Bell pepper slices

Fruits
Raisins, dried cranberries, and other dried fruit
Fresh apple, orange, clementine, and banana
Unsweetened applesauce

Protein
Sliced turkey or chicken breast
Hummus
Hard-cooked egg
Unsalted sunflower and pumpkin seeds

Two examples of "child-friendly," easy-to-prepare, nutrient-dense lunches are:

Lunch 1: A 6-ounce container of Greek yogurt, 6 cherry tomatoes, ½ cup unsweetened applesauce, 10 whole-wheat crackers, and water

Lunch 2: A 1-ounce serving of sliced turkey on 1 slice of whole wheat bread, 4 to 6 red pepper slices to dip in 2 Tbsp hummus, a clementine, and an 8-ounce carton of low-fat milk

Critical Thinking

1. You are working for an international relief organization in southern Europe. A physician with the organization has asked you to help Amira, a refugee from Syria. The doctor is concerned because Amira's 2-month-old daughter is not growing properly. What questions should you ask Amira to determine why her infant is not thriving?

2. A physician has referred a 28-year-old mother of two children to you for nutrition counseling concerning weight management. When you meet the family, you observe that the mother and her 4-year-old daughter and 19-month-old son are obese. What kinds of information do you need to obtain from the mother to make some practical lifestyle recommendations for this family?

3. Ben is worried about his 8-year-old son's nutritional status, because the child's appetite seems to fluctuate. The child's physician has indicated that the boy is healthy and his growth rate is normal. What information can you give to Ben to assure him that his child's development is normal?

4. Liang is the mother of an active 3-year-old daughter Janey. Liang is concerned because Janey refuses to eat the same foods that the rest of the family eats. The only foods she will consume are apples,

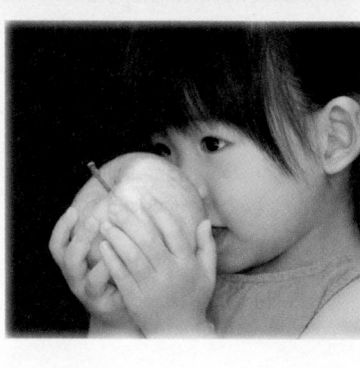

peanut butter with jelly on bread, and soy milk. Liang asks you for advice about her daughter's eating habits. What would you tell her?

5. Gerald is a 16-year-old high school student who is 5-feet, 9-inches tall and weighs 205 pounds. After obtaining his driver's license, Gerald got a part-time, after-school job at a fast-food restaurant. He is so busy, he often skips the breakfasts and dinners that his mother prepares for him and his brothers. Although he eats lunch at school, his dinner is usually a couple of double cheeseburgers, two large orders of French fries, and a milk shake at the fast-food restaurant where he works. Gerald's mother thinks her son is too heavy and he needs some suggestions for improving his diet. What would you tell her?

Practice Test

Select the best answer.

1. Jewel is a healthy newborn infant who weighs 6 pounds, 4 ounces. Based on this information, how much can she be expected to weigh by her first birthday?

   a. 12 pounds, 8 ounces
   b. 18 pounds, 12 ounces
   c. 20 pounds, 8 ounces
   d. 24 pounds, 12 ounces

2. At birth, Jewel is healthy and 18 inches in length. Based on this information, her length can be expected to be _____ inches when she celebrates her first birthday.

   a. 25
   b. 26
   c. 27
   d. 28

3. Which of the following statements is true?

   a. The majority of babies who are born in the United States are fed an iron-fortified infant formula at birth.
   b. Newborns have adequate stores of vitamin D because the placenta transfers the vitamin to the fetus efficiently during the last trimester.
   c. Under normal conditions, breastfed infants need to consume at least 4 ounces of water daily.
   d. Healthy full-term infants who do not consume an iron-fortified formula need a source of iron by the time they are 4 to 6 months of age.

4. The _____ reflex enables newborn baby Jackson to locate his mother's nipple when she brushes it against his cheek.

   a. rooting
   b. nursing
   c. extrusion
   d. grasp

5. Healthy infants are physically ready to start eating complementary solid foods when they are _____ months of age.

   a. 2 to 4
   b. 4 to 6
   c. 8 to 10
   d. 10 to 12

6. A healthy 9-month-old infant relies on the _____ to pick up solid foods, such as a cooked string bean.

   a. rooting reflex
   b. pincer grasp
   c. self-feeding response
   d. grab stimulus

7. Which of the following statements is true?

   a. The rapid growth rate that characterizes infancy continues during the toddler and preschool years.
   b. Infancy is the stage of life when a person develops autonomy.
   c. Food jags are common among preschool children.
   d. American preschool-age children typically eat recommended servings of fruit.

8. Which of the following foods is most likely to cause choking in an 18-month-old child?

   a. ready-to-eat cereal with milk
   b. French fries with no salt
   c. chewing gum
   d. ripe banana

9. Which of the following statements is true?

   a. The appetite of a school-age child increases when the youngster is experiencing a growth spurt.
   b. During early adolescence, the child's rate of physical growth normally decreases.
   c. Diets of school-age children tend to provide excessive amounts of potassium and vitamin C.
   d. Compared to older children, preschoolers typically do not eat breakfast.

10. Compared to preschoolers, school-age children are more likely to consume

   a. meals at home.
   b. breakfast.
   c. sweetened beverages.
   d. nutritionally adequate diets.

11. As a result of the _____, school food service operations must provide more servings of fruits, vegetables, and whole grains, and reduce amounts of solid fats and sodium in school meals.

   a. Affordable Care Act
   b. National School Lunch Program
   c. Women, Infants, and Children Program
   d. Healthy, Hunger-Free Kids Act

12. Which of the following standards are used to determine children's and adolescents' weight status?

   a. BMI estimates
   b. height/weight tables
   c. BMI-for-age charts
   d. waist-to-hip ratios

ANSWERS TO PRACTICE TEST
1-b; 2-c; 3-d; 4-a; 5-b; 6-b; 7-c; 8-c; 9-a; 10-c; 11-d; 12-c

ANSWERS TO CHAPTER 17 QUIZ Yourself

1. A healthy infant doubles his or her birth weight by 4 to 6 months of age and triples his or her birth weight by 1 year of age. **True** (p. 554)

2. Experts with the American Academy of Pediatrics recommend that babies should be fed fruit juice within the first month of life. **False** (p. 561)

3. Breast milk provides enough high-quality protein to meet a 4-month-old infant's needs. **True** (p. 558)

4. The percentage of American children and adolescents who are obese is at an all-time low. **False** (p. 571)

5. In the United States, the average adolescent girl consumes more calcium than the RDA. **False** (p. 570)

References

1. Grossman X and others: Neonatal weight loss at a U.S. baby-friendly hospital. *Journal of the Academy of Nutrition and Dietetics* 112(3):410, 2012. DOI: 10.1016/j.jada.2011.10.024

2. Galler JR and others: Socioeconomic outcomes in adults malnourished in the first year of life: A 40-year study. *Pediatrics* 130(1):e1-7, 2012. E-pub: June 25, 2012. DOI: 10.1542/peds.2012-0073

3. Galler JR and others: Infant malnutrition predicts conduct problems in adolescents. *Nutritional Neuroscience* 15(4):186, 2012. E-pub: April 3, 2012. DOI: 10.1179/1476830512Y.0000000012

4. Centers for Disease Control and Prevention: *Breastfeeding report card: United States 2014.* www.cdc.gov/breastfeeding/pdf/2014breastfeedingreportcard.pdf Accessed: November 12, 2014.

5. National Institutes of Health: Cow's milk—infants. Updated 2011. *Medline Plus* http://www.nlm.nih.gov/medlineplus/ency/article/002448.htm Accessed: March 7, 2014.

6. Ballard O, Morrow AL: Human milk composition: Nutrients and bioactive factors. *Pediatric Clinics of North America* 60(1):49, 2013.

7. U.S. Department of Health and Human Services: *The Surgeon General's call to action to support breastfeeding.* 2011. http://www.cdc.gov/breastfeeding/promotion/calltoaction.htm Accessed: March 2, 2014.

8. U.S. Department of Agriculture, WIC Works Resource System: *Infant feeding guide.* 2009. http://wicworks.nal.usda.gov/infants/infant-feeding-guide Accessed: March 6, 2014.

9. Oliveria V and others: *The infant formula market: Consequences of a change in the WIC contract brand,* ERR-124, U.S. Department of Agriculture, Economic Research Service. August 2011.

10. Kattan JD and others: Milk and soy allergy. *Pediatric Clinics of North America* 58(2): 407, 2011. DOI:10.1016/j.pcl.2011.02.005

11. Hall B and others: Infantile colic: A systematic review of medical and conventional therapies. *Journal of Paediatric and Child Health* 48(2):128, 2012. E-pub: April 7, 2011. DOI: 10.1111/j.1440-1754.2011.02061.x

12. Institute of Medicine: *Dietary reference intakes for energy, carbohydrate, fiber, fat, fatty acids, cholesterol, protein, and amino acids.* Washington, DC: National Academy Press, 2002.

13. Stephen A and others: The role and requirements of digestible dietary carbohydrates in infants and toddlers. *European Journal of Clinical Nutrition* 66(7):765, 2012.

14. MedlinePlus: *Iron deficiency anemia—children.* Updated 2012. http://www.nlm.nih.gov/medlineplus/ency/article/007134.htm Accessed: March 6, 2014.

15. Baker R and others: Diagnosis and prevention of iron deficiency and iron-deficiency anemia in infants and young children (0–3 years of age). *Pediatrics* 126:1040, 2010. DOI: 10.1542/peds.2010-2576

16. Berg J and others: Evidence-based clinical recommendations regarding fluoride intake from reconstituted infant formula and enamel fluorosis: A report of the American Dental Association Council on Scientific Affairs. *Journal of the American Dental Association* 142(1):79, 2011.

17. Dawodu A, Tsang RC: Maternal vitamin D status: Effect on milk vitamin D content and vitamin D status of breastfeeding infants. *Advances in Nutrition* 3(3): 353, 2012. E-pub: May 4, 2012. DOI: 10.3945/an.111.000950. PMCID: PMC3649470

18. Casey CF and others: Vitamin D supplementation in infants, children, and adolescents. *American Family Physician* 81(6):745, 2010.

19. National Digestive Diseases Information Clearinghouse: *Gastroesophageal reflux (GER) and gastroesophageal reflux disease (GERD) in infants.* Last updated September 2013. NIH Publication No. 13-5419. http://digestive.niddk.nih.gov/ddiseases/pubs/gerdinfant/ Accessed: March 6, 2014.

20. Academy of Nutrition and Dietetics: *Reducing the risk from food allergies.* Revised January 2014. http://www.eatright.org/Public/content.aspx?id=8052 Accessed: March 6, 2014.

21. Cook F and others: Baby business: A randomized controlled trial of a universal parenting program that aims to prevent early infant sleep and cry problems and associated parental depression. *BioMed Central Pediatrics* 12:13, 2012. http://www.biomedcentral.com/1471-2431/12/13

22. American Academy of Allergy Asthma & Immunology: *Prevention of allergies and asthma is children: Tips to remember.* 2013. http://www.aaaai.org/conditions-and-treatments/library/at-a-glance/prevention-of-allergies-and-asthma-in-children.aspx Accessed: March 6, 2014.

23. American Academy of Pediatrics, Committee on Nutrition: The use and misuse of juice in pediatrics. *Pediatrics* 107(5):1210, 2001. Reaffirmed August 2013. DOI: 10.1542/peds.107.5.1210

24. American Academy of Pediatrics, Committee on Injury, Violence, and Poison Prevention: Policy statement—prevention of choking among children. *Pediatrics* 125(3):601, 2010. DOI: 10.1542/peds.2009-2862

25. MedlinePlus: *Normal growth and development.* Last updated February 2014. http://www.nlm.nih.gov/medlineplus/ency/article/002456.htm Accessed: March 6, 2014.

26. Ervin RB and others: Consumption of added sugar among U.S. children and adolescents, 2005–2008. *NCHS Data Brief* 87, March 2012.

27. Briefel RR: New findings from the Feeding Infants and Toddlers Study: Data to inform action. *Journal of the American Dietetic Association* 110(12 Suppl):S5, 2010. DOI: 10.1016/j.jada.2010.10.016

28. United States Department of Agriculture, Agricultural Research Service: *What we eat in America 2011–2012.* Last modified October 2014. http://www.ars.usda.gov/Services/docs.htm?docid=18349 Accessed: November 12, 2014.

29. U.S. Department of Agriculture, U.S. Department of Health and Human Services: *2015–2020 Dietary Guidelines for Americans.* 2015. Appendix 7, Table A7-1. http://health.gov/dietaryguidelines/2015/guidelines/appendix-7/ Accessed: January 28, 2016.

30. American Academy of Pediatrics: Expert panel on integrated guidelines for cardiovascular health and risk reduction in children and adolescents: Summary report. *Pediatrics* 128(S5):S213, 2011. DOI: 10.1542/peds.2009-2107C

31. McGuire JL and others: The relationship between cow's milk and stores of vitamin D and iron in early childhood. *Pediatrics* 131(1):e141, 2013.

32. National Institutes of Health, National Institute of Dental and Craniofacial Research: *Dental caries (tooth decay) in children (age 2 to 11): Dental caries in primary teeth.* Last updated January 2014. http://www.nidcr.nih.gov/DataStatistics/FindDataByTopic/DentalCaries/DentalCariesChildren2to11 Accessed: March 6, 2014.

33. Reeding J, Krebs-Smith S: Dietary sources of energy, solid fats, and added sugars among children and adolescents in the United States. *Journal of the American Dietetic Association* 110(10):1477, 2010.

34. Kranz S: What do we know about dietary fiber intake in children and health? The effects of fiber intake on constipation, obesity, and diabetes in children. *Advances in Nutrition* 3(1):47, 2012.

35. Food and Nutrition Board, U.S. Department of Agriculture: *National school lunch program: Program fact sheet: National School Lunch Program.* 2012. http://origin.www.fns.usda.gov/cnd/Lunch/ Accessed: March 6, 2014.

36. Biro FM, Wien M: Childhood obesity and adult morbidities. *American Journal of Clinical Nutrition* 91(5):1499S, 2010. E-pub: March 24, 2010. DOI: 10.3945/ajcn.2010.28701B

37. Proos L, Gustafsson J: Is early puberty triggered by catch-up growth following undernutrition? *International Journal of Environmental Research and Public Health* 9(5):1791, 2012. E-pub: May 9, 2012. DOI: 10.3390/ijerph9051791

38. Centers for Disease Control and Prevention: Youth Risk Behavior Surveillance—United States, 2011. http://www.cdc.gov/healthyyouth/yrbs/index.htm Accessed: March 6, 2014.

39. National Institutes of Health, Osteoporosis and Related Bone Diseases National Resource Center: Osteoporosis handout on health. 2011. http://www.niams.nih.gov/Health_Info/Bone/Osteoporosis/osteoporosis_hoh.asp Accessed: March 6, 2014.

40. Eichenfield L and others: Evidence-based recommendations for the diagnosis and treatment of pediatric acne. *Pediatrics* 131(3):S163, 2013. DOI: 10.1542/peds.2013-0490B

41. Fryar CD and others: Prevalence of obesity among children and adolescents: United States, trends 1963–1965 through 2011–2012. *NCHS Health E-Stat.* Updated September 2014. http://www.cdc.gov/nchs/data/hestat/obesity_child_11_12/obesity_child_11_12.htm Accessed: October 14, 2014.

42. Centers for Disease Control and Prevention: Progress on childhood obesity. Updated August 2013. *CDC Vital Signs.* http://www.cdc.gov/VitalSigns/ChildhoodObesity/ Accessed: February 20, 2014.

43. Pan L and others: Trends in the prevalence of extreme obesity among US preschool-aged children living in low-income families, 1998–2010. *Journal of the American Medical Association* 308 (24): 2563, 2012.

44. Centers for Disease Control and Prevention: Overweight and obesity: *Basics about childhood obesity*. Updated April 2012. http://www.cdc.gov/obesity/childhood/basics.html Accessed: March 6, 2014.

45. Centers for Disease Control and Prevention: *Overweight and obesity: A growing problem: What causes childhood obesity?* Updated April 2013. http://www.cdc.gov/obesity/childhood/problem.html Accessed: February 20, 2014.

46. Dattilo AM and others: Need for early interventions in the prevention of pediatric overweight: A review and upcoming directions. *Journal of Obesity* 2012; 2012: 123023. E-pub: May 17, 2012. DOI: 10.1155/2012/123023. PMCID: PMC3362946

47. Institute of Medicine, Committee on Obesity Prevention Policies for Young Children: *Early childhood obesity prevention policies*. Washington, DC: National Academies Press, 2011. www.nap.edu Accessed: February 20, 2014.

48. Centers for Disease Control and Prevention: *Healthy weight—it's not a diet, it's a lifestyle! Tips for parents—ideas to help children maintain a healthy weight*. 2011. http://www.cdc.gov/healthyweight/children/index.html Accessed: February 20, 2014.

49. Let's Move! America's Move to Raise a Healthier Generation of Kids. (ND) http://www.letsmove.gov/ Accessed: February 20, 2014

49. National Institute of Diabetes and Digestive and Kidney Diseases, Weight Control Information Network: *Bariatric surgery for severe obesity: Bariatric surgery for youth*. Last modified January 2014. http://win.niddk.nih.gov/publications/gastric.htm Accessed: February 20, 2014.

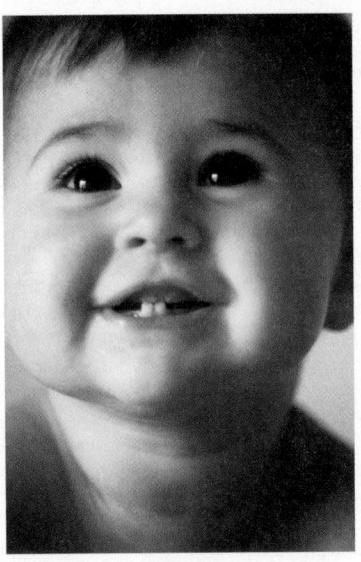

18 Nutrition for Older Adults

CASE STUDY

Urinary incontinence

DIEGO IS 72 YEARS OF AGE AND LIVES with his wife in an apartment complex for independent older adults. Like many people his age, Diego suffers from *urinary incontinence*, a condition in which urine leaks out of his bladder. To remain "dry" while he is away from home, he limits his fluid intake a few hours before leaving his house and avoids drinking fluids while he is away from home.

Two months ago, Diego noticed that his feet and ankles were swollen. When he showed his swollen lower extremities to his daughter, the young woman was alarmed and took her father to his doctor's office for a blood pressure check. According to the physician, Diego's blood pressure was 175/100 mm Hg. The physician told Diego that he had hypertension and explained that edema can be caused by high blood pressure. The physician prescribed a diuretic (*furosemide*) for him to take twice a day. Although Diego is pleased that the diuretic reduced his edema, he thinks the medication has made his incontinence worse. To avoid getting up several times during the night to urinate, he drinks no fluids after 5 P.M.

- What complications might occur if Diego limits his fluid intake while taking a diuretic?
- What steps can Diego take to control his blood pressure?

The suggested Case Study Response can be found on page 599.

Mc Graw Hill Education **connect** | NUTRITION Check out the Connect site at www.mcgrawhillconnect.com to further explore this case study.

The suggested Case Study Response can be found on page 599.

QUIZ Yourself

Are there any foods people can eat to reduce their risk of Alzheimer's disease? Can being overfat benefit an older adult? What is *sarcopenia*? Check your knowledge about nutrition for older adults by taking the following quiz. The answers are found on page 602.

1. People in the United States can expect to live for about 65 years. ___T ___F

2. Gout is the most common form of arthritis. ___T ___F

3. Compared to people living in other countries, Americans have the highest life expectancy. ___T ___F

4. Diets of older adults generally do not supply adequate amounts of calcium. ___T ___F

5. To prevent Alzheimer's disease, people should follow a gluten-free diet. ___T ___F

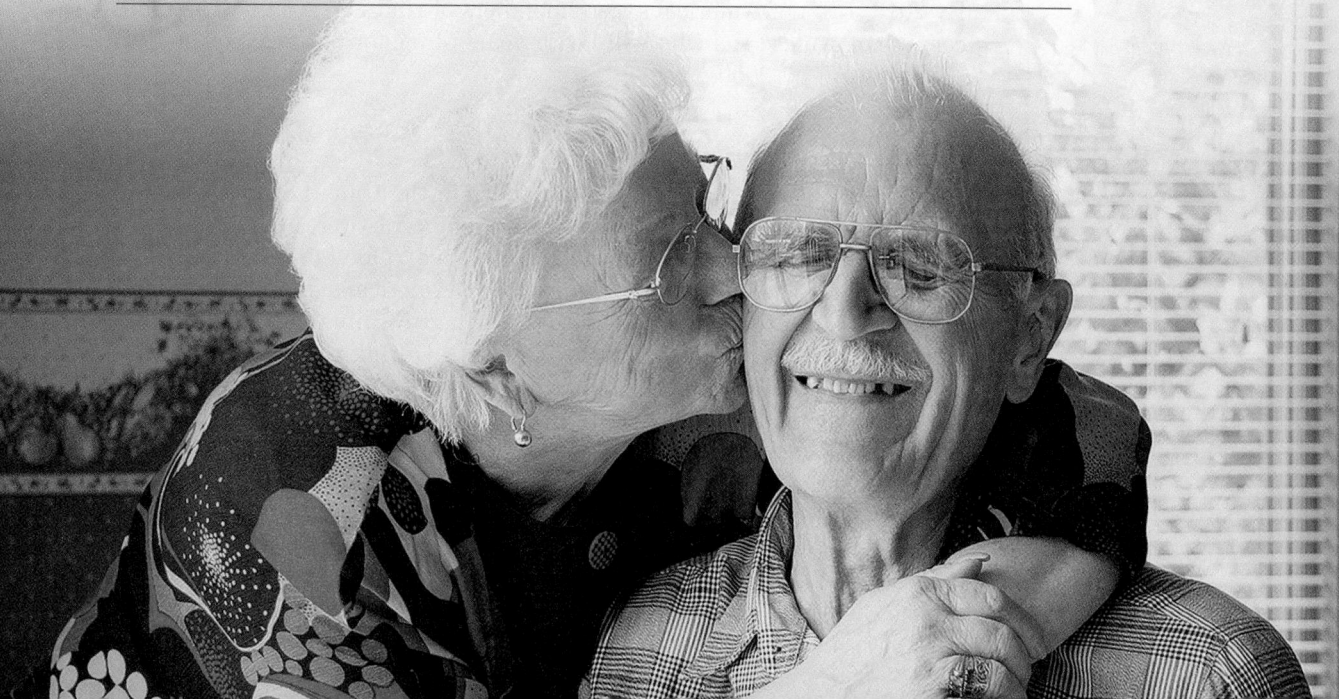

18.1 Older Adults

LEARNING OUTCOMES

1 *Distinguish between* life expectancy *and* life span.

2 *Summarize how life expectancy has changed since 1900, and give some reasons for the change.*

3 *Discuss at least one theory of aging.*

Regardless of one's age, many factors influence a person's health and well–being, including diet, physical activity, medications, income, and social support. As a person grows older, his or her body undergoes observable and measurable changes that are associated with the normal aging process. Many of these physiological changes can negatively affect the aging individual's nutritional status.

Senescence (*se–ness'–enz*) refers to declining organ functioning and increasing vulnerability to disease that occur with advanced age. **Geriatrics** is the medical specialty that focuses on health care needs and medical conditions that are associated with older adults. This chapter includes information about older adults in the United States and some of their medical concerns, especially diseases and conditions that often influence their nutritional state.

senescence declining organ functioning that occurs with advanced age

geriatrics specialty of health care that focuses on older adults

Defining *Older Adult*

The specific age used to define *older adults* varies greatly. Officials with the World Health Organization (WHO) consider people in certain underdeveloped counties to be "old" when they reach 50 years of age, but WHO officials use 60 years and older for people living in developed countries.[1] The Dietary Reference Intakes (DRIs) have a separate category for dietary standards for people who are 51 to 70 years of age and another category for persons who are older than 70 years. Sixty–five years is the minimum age used by the U.S. Census Bureau to classify the "older population."[2]

In 1900, only 3% of the U.S. population were 65 years of age or older. In 2012, 13.7% of the U.S. population were 65 years of age or older (Fig. 18.1).[2] By 2050, government experts estimate that about 21% of Americans will be in this age group.[3] Americans who are the "oldest old"—85 years of age or older—comprise one of the fastest–growing segments of the U.S. population. In 1900, only 0.1% of Americans were 85 years of age or older. By 2010, 1.8% of Americans were members of that age group.[4] The percentage of Americans who will be 85 years of age or older is expected to be about 5% by 2050.[4]

life expectancy average length of time a person born in a specific year can expect to live

What Is Life Expectancy?

In 1900, the life expectancy of a baby born in the United States was only 47 years. **Life expectancy** is the average length of time a person born in a specific year, such as 1900, can expect to live.[4] One hundred years ago, the top three leading causes of death for Americans were pneumonia, influenza, and other infectious diseases. By 2013, life expectancy in the United States had risen to almost 79 years.[5] During the twentieth century, several factors contributed to increased life expectancy, including improved diets, housing conditions, and public sanitation, as well as advances in medical care such as the development of antibiotics, vaccines, and reliable ways to diagnose diseases.

The United States ranks fifty–first out of 223 countries in life expectancy, even though Americans spend more on health care than people of any other country.[5] Poor diet, physical inactivity, and other typical lifestyle habits of Americans are largely responsible for our

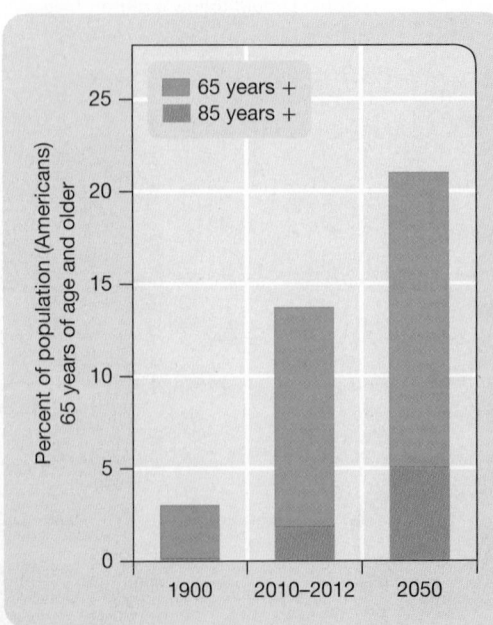

FIGURE 18.1 Older adult population of the United States: Then, now, and in the future.

nation's unimpressive world ranking for life expectancy. Unhealthy lifestyles increase the risk of chronic diseases, including heart disease, cancer, and stroke. Such diseases are the leading causes of death among older American adults (see Fig. 1.6).[6]

Healthy life expectancy is the number of years a person can expect to spend without being disabled or having serious diseases. Although more Americans are living longer than their ancestors, they are not necessarily living well. Many older adult Americans are in poor health, have limited mobility (ability to move around), and depend on others for their care.

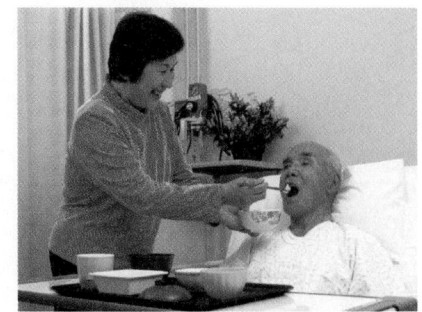

Many older American adults are in poor health and depend on others for their care.

Longevity

Growing old is a normal and natural process; however, some people show the signs of aging at an earlier age than others. Scientists have found a strong genetic component to human **longevity**, the capability of living a long life. A person who has ancestors who are very old or lived to be 95 years of age or older may have inherited genes that contribute to longevity. Such character-istics could be having an immune system that functions better than average or cells that can divide more times to replace themselves without becoming can-cerous. If a person's ancestors died of natural causes at a relatively young age, that person can still control the rate at which he or she ages to some extent. How? By making responsible healthy lifestyle decisions while he or she is still young, such as selecting a nutritious diet, exercising regularly, and avoiding tobacco. The focus should not be simply on living longer but rather on living longer *and* healthier.

healthy life expectancy number of years a person can expect to spend without being disabled or having serious diseases

longevity capability of living a long life

Who Are the Centenarians?

Life span refers to the maximum number of years an organism can live. To date, Frenchwoman Jeanne Calment (1875–1997) had the longest documented human life span (122 years). Very few people live to be 100, but the num-ber of **centenarians** (people who have reached the age of at least 100 years) is increasing in the United States. Based on 2010 census data, 53,364 centenarians were in the United States.[7] By 2050, it is estimated, the number will increase to 1 million.[4]

life span maximum number of years an organism can live

centenarian individual who has lived for 100 years or more

Compared to other regions in the world, Okinawa, Japan, may have the high-est concentration of centenarians within the population (five per 10,000 people).[8] Much of the longevity that occurs among Okinawans may be related to their traditional diet, which is low in calories yet nutrient dense. The traditional Okinawan diet is very high in carbohydrate (90% of total calories) and consists primarily of abundant vegetables and fruits that are rich sources of micronutrients and phytochem-icals.[9] Some scientists, however, predict that younger members of Okinawa's population will not live as long as their ancestors, because they have adopted a more Western lifestyle.[10]

Theories on Aging

The aging process begins at conception and is characterized by a number of predictable physical changes. What causes people to age is unclear, but medical researchers have proposed various theories to explain why aging occurs.[11] In this chapter, we will focus on two major categories of biological aging theories: programmed theories and damage or error theories.

Programmed Theories

Programmed theories imply that aging is genetically programmed and follows a biological sequence, similar to

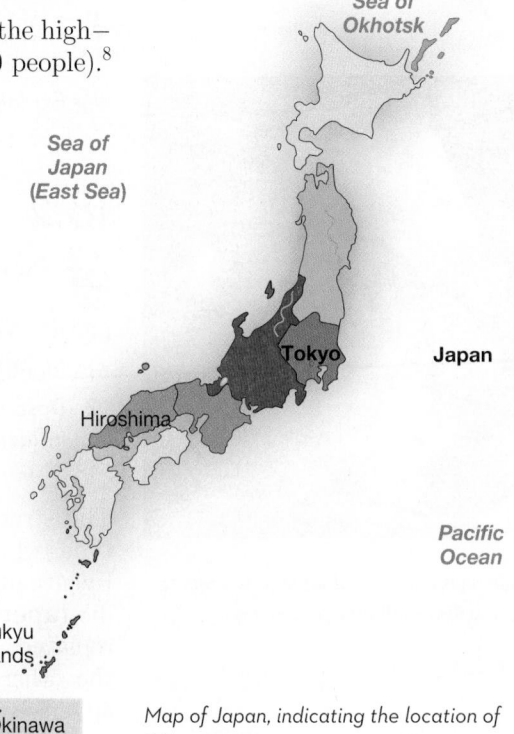

Map of Japan, indicating the location of Okinawa.

the milestones of a child's growth and development. Programmed theories may include the following notions:

• Over time, the activity of certain genes results in aging;

• Changes in hormones, particularly decreases in estrogen or growth hormone levels, act as biological "clocks" that contribute to aging; and

• The immune system is programmed to decline over time, which makes people more susceptible to diseases and ultimately results in their death.[11]

According to programmed theories, aging is inevitable and healthy dietary and lifestyle choices have little influence on the rate at which the aging process occurs.

Damage or Error Theories

Damage or error theories have the premise that organs simply wear out with use and abuse, largely from a combination of damage that results from lifestyle, which may include poor diet, smoking, and excessive alcohol consumption. One particular damage or error theory focuses on the effects of *free—radical injury* to cells. Such injury causes the accumulation of damaged material in cells that interferes with their ability to function normally, and eventually, organ failure occurs as a result. The nucleic acids, lipids, and proteins that are within cells are susceptible to free—radical attack and destruction. If this theory is correct, fol—lowing a diet that is high in antioxidants might delay the aging process.

Another damage or error theory proposes that an increase in the number of *cross—linked proteins* in cells causes damage to tissues and organs, slowing down bodily processes, which results in senescence. The *glycation theory* suggests that elevated levels of glucose or other sugars in the body bind to proteins, lipids, and nucleic acids **(glycation)**. **Advanced glycation end products (AGEs)** form in people who have poorly controlled diabetes. Eventually, AGEs cause inflammation and disrupt organ functioning.[12] Thus, maintaining healthy blood glucose levels through—out one's lifetime may reduce AGEs damage and extend one's life expectancy.

glycation condition that occurs when sugars bind to proteins, lipids, and nucleic acids in the body

advanced glycation end products (AGEs) substances formed by glycation that cause inflammation and organ damage

ASSESS YOUR PROGRESS

1 *Define life expectancy, life span, and longevity.*
2 *Provide one reason why an American's life expectancy was shorter in 1900 than in 2010.*
3 *Explain at least one theory of aging.*

18.2 Physiological Aspects of Normal Aging

LEARNING OUTCOMES

1 *Identify normal physiological changes that are associated with the aging process.*

2 *Describe how the physiological changes that normally occur with increasing age can influence an older adult's nutritional status.*

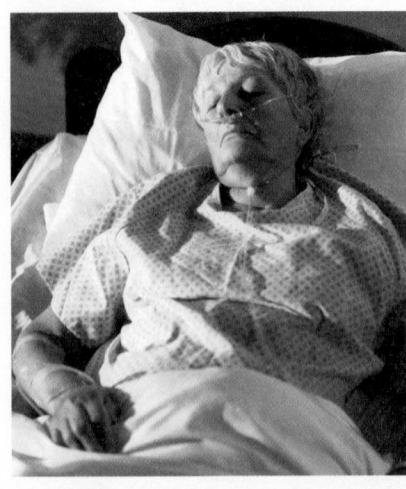

When an organ fails, other organs begin to fail, and eventually, the person dies.

The structure and function of cells in the body break down and decline with time, which results in many of the physiological changes shown in Table 18.1. Eventually, most cells lose their ability to regenerate their organelles, and they die **(apoptosis)**. As the number of dying cells in an organ increases and are not replaced, the organ begins to lose its functional capacity. When one organ fails, the other organs begin to fail, and eventually, the body's organ systems are adversely affected to the extent that the person dies.

Some of the physiological changes that are associated with the normal aging process can have adverse effects on the older adult's nutritional state. For

apoptosis cellular death

TABLE 18.1 Age-Related Physiological Changes

Body System	Changes
Digestive	Reduced saliva, gastric acid, and intrinsic factor secretion; increased likelihood of heartburn and constipation; reduced number of taste buds; and delayed swallowing rate
Integumentary (skin, hair, and nails)	Reduced skin elasticity, increased wrinkles and dryness; decreased efficiency in vitamin D synthesis from sun exposure; decreased hair thickness; reduced hair color (graying)
Musculoskeletal	Decreased activity of osteoblasts, resulting in bone loss that can lead to tooth loss and bones that fracture easily Decreased joint flexibility Decreased muscle mass, resulting in loss of strength and stamina
Nervous	Decreased brain weight; reduced production of neurotransmitters; delayed transmission of nerve impulses; loss of short-term memory; and reduced sensory abilities (e.g., vision, hearing, smell, and taste)
Lymphatic (immune)	Reduced functioning, resulting in increased vulnerability to cancer and infections
Circulatory	Reduced flexibility of arteries, reduced cardiac output, and increased risk of blood clots
Endocrine	Decreased production of growth and thyroid hormones
Respiratory	Reduced lung capacity and increased vulnerability to respiratory infections
Urinary	Increased loss of functional kidney cells, resulting in decreased blood filtration rate
Reproductive	**Men:** Decreased male hormone production and sperm count **Women:** Decreased female hormone production, resulting in cessation of menstrual cycles and loss of fertility

example, declines in digestive system functioning can interfere with the older person's ability to chew, swallow, and digest food. Other changes may negatively influence the older adult's appetite. To enjoy eating, for example, people must be able to taste the flavor and smell the aroma of foods.

With advancing age, a person's senses of smell and taste typically become less acute. By 60 years of age, approximately 25% of people lack the ability to smell (*anosmia*), and the prevalence of anosmia increases with advancing age.[13] The sense of taste, especially the ability to taste sweet and salty foods, also tends to decrease after 60 years of age.[14] The most common causes of taste disorders are the use of certain medications and zinc deficiency.[15] As a person's ability to enjoy the aroma and flavor foods declines, his or her caloric and nutrient intake usually declines as well. Adding spices to foods may help enhance their taste and stimulate an older adult's interest in eating.

ASSESS YOUR PROGRESS

4 *List at least five physiological changes that occur as a result of the normal aging process.*

5 *Explain how less acute senses of taste and smell can affect an older adult's nutritional status.*

18.3 Nutrient Needs of Healthy Older Adults

LEARNING OUTCOMES

1 *Identify nutrients that are often low in the diets of older Americans.*

2 *Describe how the aging process affects energy needs.*

3 *Discuss the effects of dehydration on older adults.*

Diets of older Americans, especially older women, often provide inadequate amounts of vitamins A, D, and B–12, and minerals, particularly calcium and

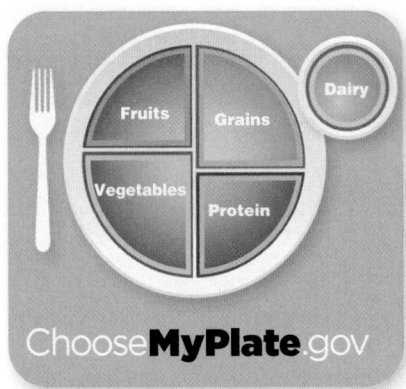

Older adults can use recommendations from MyPlate to plan nutritious menus.

TABLE 18.2 What Americans 71 Years of Age and Older Eat Compared to MyPlate Recommendations

	Food Group				
	Fruit (cups)	Vegetables (cups)	Grains (oz equivalents)	Dairy (cups)	Protein (oz equivalents)
MyPlate recommendations*					
Men	2	2.5	6	3	5.5
Women	1.5	2	5	3	5
Percentage of people who consumed recommended amount (estimated)					
Men†	23	12	55	7	46
Women†	34.5	13	53	3.6	40

*Amounts are for people who are 51 years of age and older, and obtain fewer than 30 minutes/day of moderate physical activity beyond their normal daily activities.
Adapted from Krebs-Smith SM and others: Americans do not meet federal dietary recommendations. *Journal of Nutrition* 140(10):1832, 2010.
† 71 years of age and older

potassium.[16] In the United States, fewer than half (41.8%) of older adults consume 2 or more servings of fruit each day, and fewer than a third (29.6%) of this population eats 3 or more servings of vegetables each day.[17] Furthermore, over 80% of people who are 71 years of age and older consume more empty calories than recommended.[18] Table 18.2 shows recommended amounts from U.S. Department of Agriculture MyPlate food groups and percentages of men and women ages 71 years and older who meet the recommendations.

The University of Florida Extension Service and Tufts University have each developed their own version of MyPlate for older adults. The Florida version (http://edis.ifas.ufl.edu/pdffiles/FY/FY126000.pdf) includes age–specific recommendations such as "Use fortified foods or supplements to meet your vitamin D and vitamin B–12 needs." The Tufts version (http://www.nutrition.tufts.edu/research/myplate–older–adults) emphasizes the need to consume more vegetables and 8 servings of fluids daily. The following sections provide more specific information about the nutrient intakes of older Americans.

Energy

As the human body ages, its need for energy decreases from a combination of physical inactivity and reduced metabolic rate.[19] The Estimated Average Requirement for energy is 2000 kcal for older men and 1600 kcal for older women. Average energy intakes of Americans who are 70 years of age or older are close to these values: approximately 2020 kcal for men and 1555 for women.[16]

Hypothyroidism, which contributes to a slower metabolic rate and weight gain, is common among older adults. According to findings of various studies, 1 to 10% of the older adult population has hypothyroidism; the condition is more likely to develop in women.[20] Signs and symptoms of hypothyroidism include fatigue, lack of concentration, depression, dry skin, puffy eyes (edema), cold sensitivity, constipation, and weight gain.[20] Because these signs and symptoms can be physiological aspects of the normal aging process, physicians may over–look the possibility that an older adult patient has hypothyroidism. Therefore, it is important for physicians to screen older adults for the condition and consider treating affected patients with oral medication, usually *L–thyroxine*, the synthetic form of thyroid hormone.[20]

Calorie-Restricted Diets and Longevity

In the 1930s, researcher Clive McKay proposed that the life span could be prolonged by following a calorie–restricted (CR) diet. In his studies of laboratory rats, the rodents that were given a CR diet (30% fewer kcal) lived longer and had fewer cases of age–related diseases than controls that ate a standard diet. Since McKay's work, results of other studies involving nonprimates indicate that CR diets prolong life, as long as the diet provides all essential nutrients.[21] Whether CR will extend lifespan in humans is not yet known, but it appears that moderate CR coupled with adequate micronutrient intake may protect against many of the chronic conditions associated with old age, such as hypertension, cancer, type 2 diabetes, and obesity.[21,22]

Macronutrients

Americans generally consume adequate amounts of carbohydrates, fats, and proteins.[16] Diets of most older Americans meet or exceed the Recommended Dietary Allowance (RDA) for protein (0.8 g/kg body weight) that is set by the Institute of Medicine. However, as much as 1.6 g protein/kg body weight may be required to maintain muscle mass in older adults.[23] Foods that provide high–quality protein, such as beef, chicken, and fish, are often more expensive and difficult to prepare than carbohydrate–rich foods. Older adults who are on limited incomes, live alone, or are physically unable to shop for and cook food are at risk of developing protein malnutrition.

Water

The body's water content decreases with advancing age: About 60% of the body weight of younger adults is water, whereas water comprises about 50% of the body weight of healthy older adults. With advancing age, thirst sensation declines, kidneys are less able to conserve fluids, and frail older persons may find it difficult to drink water regularly because they lack good mobility. Poor mobility can limit an older adult's ability to get to sources of water. Additionally, some medications, such as furosemide, which is taken to control high blood pressure, increase urination and/or depress thirst perception. Many older adults avoid drinking fluids simply because they want to avoid frequent trips to the bathroom or urinary incontinence. **Urinary incontinence** is a condition characterized by urine leaking out of the bladder.

urinary incontinence condition in which urine leaks out of the bladder

Dehydration is a common problem, especially among people who are 85 years of age and older (see Chapter 11). Signs of dehydration include weakness, constipation, and mental confusion. If untreated, dehydration can lead to coma and death. To avoid dehydration, older adults often need to be reminded to drink water and other fluids.

Vitamin D

Recall from Chapter 9 that vitamin D_3 must be hydroxylated in the liver and the kidneys to become the active calcitriol form of the vitamin. As one ages, the liver and kidneys become less able to activate the vitamin D_3 precursor. Furthermore, most older adults do not obtain sufficient exposure to sunlight, so they are unable to synthesize adequate amounts of vitamin D. Thus, the RDA for vitamin D increases from 15 to 20 μg (600 to 800 IU) for people who are over 70 years of age.

Table 9.6 lists foods that are good sources of vitamin D. On average, Americans over the age of 70 consume considerably less than the recommended amount of vitamin D from food sources.[16] Therefore, health experts often recommend

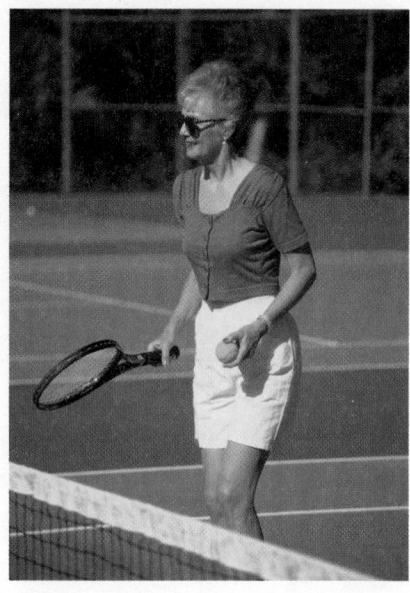

Even with exposure to sunlight, the body of an older adult does not synthesize as much vitamin D as it did when it was young.

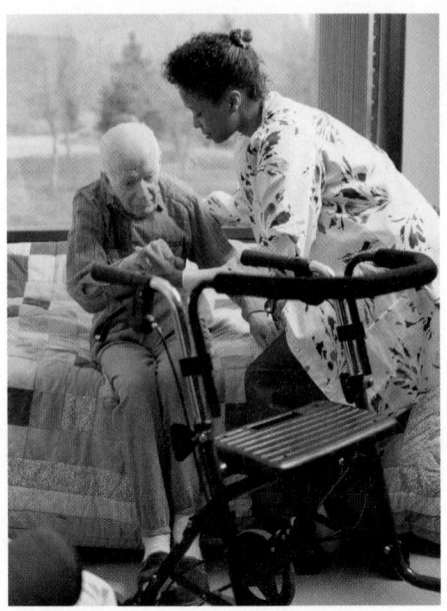

For frail older adults, recovery after a broken hip or spine may require months of rehabilitation, and many patients are unable to walk without assistance after recovering from the injury.

that older adults take a daily supplement that supplies 400 IU of vitamin D. Supplements that contain the calcitriol form of the vitamin are a good choice for older adults, because the vitamin is in the active form.

Vitamin B-12

The DRI for vitamin B–12 is 2.4 µg for all individuals who are over 14 years of age. On average, older Americans consume more than this amount of vitamin B–12 from food sources.[16] However, low vitamin B–12 status is common among the older adult population,[24] because absorption of vitamin B–12 is diminished in older persons (see section 18.4).

Recall from Chapter 10 that the natural form of vitamin B–12 is bound to protein, which renders it difficult to absorb unless the micronutrient is released from the protein by the steps described in Figure 10.12. Dietary supplements contain unbound ("free") vitamin B–12, which is easier to absorb than the natural form. Many adults ages 50 and older are encouraged to consume foods that have been fortified with free vitamin B–12, such as fortified grain products, or take vitamin B–12 supplements.[25] According to results of one national survey, about 36% of older Americans reported taking a dietary supplement that contained vitamin B–12 in the past month.[26]

Increasing the daily intake of vitamin B–12 to between 6 and 10 µg may be beneficial for older adults who have adequate absorption of the micronutrient. Higher doses of vitamin B–12 and even injections of the vitamin may be appropriate for people with impaired absorption.[27]

Calcium

The calcium RDA for adults ages 70 years and above is 1200 mg/day. Most adults do not meet their RDA for calcium by consuming foods.[28] Therefore, calcium supplementation among older Americans is common: 62% of people over age 70 take a daily calcium supplement.[29] Prevention of osteoporosis and related bone fractures is the main reason older adults should be concerned about their calcium intake (see Chapter 11). Recovery after any broken bone may require months of rehabilitation, especially for frail older adults. Many older persons are unable to walk without assistance after recovering from a broken hip or spine.

Sodium and Potassium

Older adults consume about twice as much sodium as recommended, but they obtain less than the recommended potassium (Fig. 18.2).[16,19] This mineral imbalance is of particular concern because almost 70% of adults over 60 years of age have hypertension.[30] The best dietary approach to treating hypertension is the DASH diet (see Chapter 11), which is low in sodium and recommends fruits and vegetables that are rich sources of potassium. Excessive dietary sodium is also associated with loss of calcium from bones; inadequate potassium intake increases the risk of osteoporosis, stroke, and kidney stones.

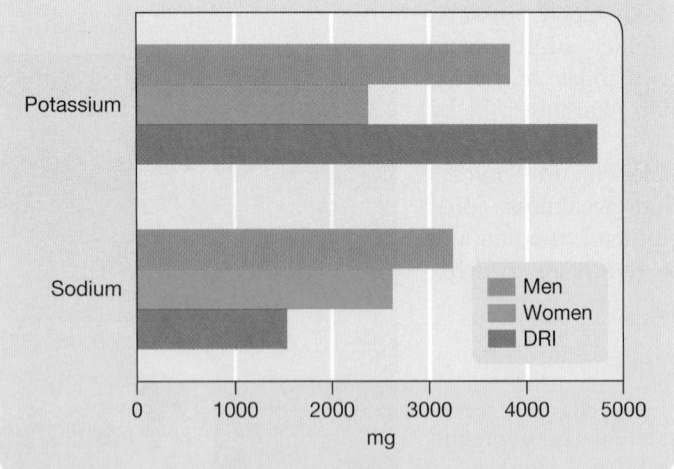

FIGURE 18.2 Sodium and potassium intakes: Older adults (U.S.).

ASSESS YOUR PROGRESS

6 *Describe energy intakes of older adults.*

7 *Why is dehydration a serious problem for older adults?*

8 *Older adults often have low intakes of which micronutrients?*

18.4 Common Health Concerns of Older Adults

LEARNING OUTCOMES

1 *Discuss common health concerns of older adults, including sarcopenia, vision problems, arthritis, heart failure, and depression.*

2 *Describe common diseases or conditions of the digestive system that can negatively affect the health of older adults.*

3 *Explain why polypharmacy is common among older adults, and discuss the nutritional implications of the condition.*

A variety of chronic diseases and age—related conditions affect the health and well—being of older adults. In many instances, the individual has more than one of the diseases or conditions. In this section, we discuss physiological health diseases or conditions that often affect older adults, including sarcopenia, cataracts, and arthritis.

Weight Loss

It is not unusual for people to lose some weight after they are 70 years of age. Several factors can contribute to weight loss among older adults. For example, older persons may eat less because they have lost the ability to taste and smell food. In addition, loss of teeth and difficulty swallowing can result in decreased food consumption. Table 18.3 lists factors that contribute to reduced food intake.

Sarcopenia

The weight loss that often occurs after the age 70 years is partially a result of the loss of muscle mass (sarcopenia).[31] In people with sarcopenia, some muscle cells shrink or die, and loss of muscular strength results. Among older adults, sarcopenia is a major cause of reduced mobility and independence.[32] The loss of muscular mass also increases the risk of falls and diminished ability to recover from serious illness.

Obesity

After a person reaches 50 years of age, his or her metabolic rate declines by approximately 4% per decade.[32] Most older adults are less physically active than when they were younger. Thus, older persons generally need fewer calories for basal metabolism and physical activity than when they were 25 years of age. If older individuals do not reduce their caloric intake to accommodate their reduced energy needs, they experience an increase in body fat.

The aging body tends to gain fat tissue in the intra—abdominal region and lose subcutaneous fat in other areas of the body, especially the legs and face. Increased abdominal fat results from hormonal changes, overeating, and lack

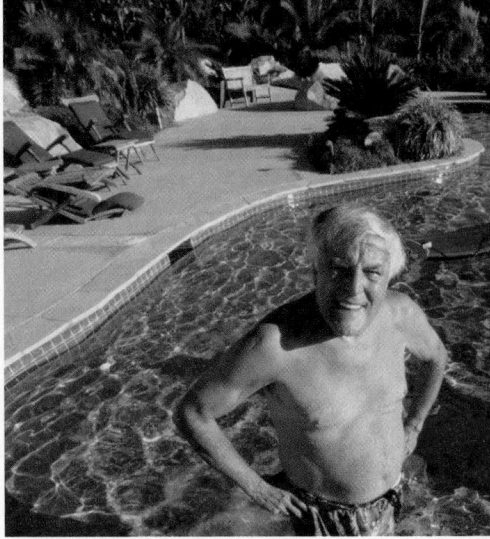

Having some sarcopenia is normal for an aging person.

TABLE 18.3 Factors That Contribute to Reduced Food Intake Among Older Adults

- Reduced ability to taste and smell food
- Difficulty swallowing (*dysphagia*)
- Loss of teeth
- Loss of normal cognitive function
- Low income
- Depression
- Reduced mobility and flexibility

of physical activity; but even athletic and lean people usually gain some central body fat after they are 50 years of age.

An estimated 24.3% of Americans who are 65 years of age and older are obese.[17] Being overweight or obese may be beneficial to the survival of older adults, especially older men.[33] In older adults, obesity reduces the likelihood of hip and spine fractures, but excess body fat increases the risk of ankle and upper arm fractures.[34]

Sarcopenic Obesity

sarcopenic obesity type of obesity that is characterized by the loss of skeletal muscle mass combined with excessive body fat

Older people may develop **sarcopenic obesity**: the loss of skeletal muscle mass and strength combined with an increase in body fat. A combination of lack of exercise and excessive caloric intake contributes to the development of sarcopenic obesity. People with sarcopenic obesity are more likely to experience mobility problems than people who do not have the condition.[35]

Healthy people are never too old to gain some benefits from aerobic and strength–training exercise. The "Real People, Real Stories" feature on this page is about Paul Appelbaum, an 88–year–old who works out almost every day. Before embarking on a program to increase physical fitness, however, sedentary older adults should consult their physicians concerning appropriate activities.

REAL People, **REAL** Stories

Paul Appelbaum

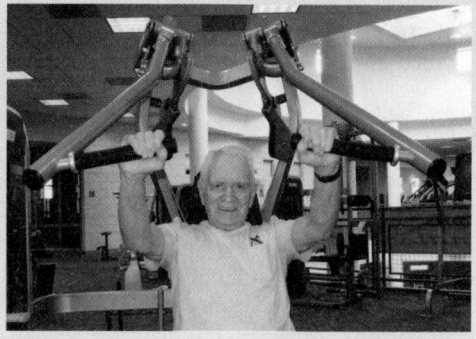

Paul Appelbaum is a healthy 88-year-old father of three children, grandfather of two children, and great-grandfather of one child. He's been married for 53 years. Several years ago, he retired from working as a businessman, but he hasn't retired from taking excellent care of himself.

Some clues to Paul's good health are in his lifestyle—past and present. "I grew up during the Great Depression," he says. "I paid no attention to my diet, but I never went hungry. I ate a lot of home-cooked foods . . . vegetables, fruits, dairy foods, meat, seafood, chicken. . . . I ate a balanced diet. I wasn't fond of sweets . . . I've never been overweight." Paul's height is 5-feet, 8-inches, and his weight is 160 pounds.

"I've always been physically active. When I was a boy, my friends and I didn't have sports teams. We just found empty spaces and played sandlot baseball and football," he recalls. "In high school, I was on the track team. I was a good runner.

"I never had a desk job," Paul says. "I was always on my feet, moving around. . . . That's partially what I owe my longevity and health to." Compared to the average person who is his age, Paul *is* very active. For the last 20 years, he has maintained an impressive workout regimen. Six days a week, he walks for an hour and a half at a nearby community gymnasium. When Paul doesn't walk, he rides a stationary bike for 20 minutes at an average speed of 12 miles per hour. In addition to his aerobic activity routine, he performs resistance exercises that focus on the muscles of his upper body three days a week. On three alternating days, he focuses on doing exercises that strengthen his lower body muscles. "I like working out! But I also like to keep my brain well-stimulated," Paul says. "I read books and play bridge [a complex card game]."

Paul reports he had no serious health problems until he was in his early 80s. "When I was 82," he says, "I had to have a triple bypass [surgery to restore blood flow to areas of the heart that were supplied by three blocked arteries]. My doctors are all very happy with me!" According to Paul, "Longevity is fine, but quality of life is more important. Keep physically fit and follow a healthy diet, and you'll have it all."

Diseases and Conditions That Affect Vision

To obtain food and prepare meals, a person must be able to drive (or walk) to the store, select groceries from the aisles, take the groceries home, and use the stove to cook the foods. Visual impairments negatively affect all aspects of meal preparation, from grocery shopping to cooking.

Figure 18.3 shows the major anatomical components of the eye. By the age of 40 years, the lens of the eye begins to harden and the muscle fibers around the lens lose their ability to control the shape of the lens. As a result of these normal changes, it becomes more difficult for the eyes to focus on objects that are close, such as print on the pages of a book. The loss of this focusing ability is called **presbyopia**. With advancing age, the likelihood of presbyopia increases, and eventually, everyone's eyes lose some ability to focus on close objects clearly.[36] Reading glasses or contact lenses often can correct presbyopia and enable older people to read food labels and recipes, and prepare meals.

Other more serious vision problems can lead to permanent blindness. A **cataract** develops when proteins in the lens of the eye are damaged, causing the lens to become translucent or opaque. About 25% of Americans who are 65 to 69 years of age have a cataract; the prevalence of cataract increases to almost 70% of the population who are 80 years of age or more.[37] Cataracts occur more frequently in smokers and people with diabetes. Exposure to sources of ultraviolet light, including sunlight, also contributes to cataract formation. A cataract can be treated by surgically removing the clouded lens and replacing it with an artificial lens. As a result of the surgery, vision is usually restored.

Age–related macular degeneration (AMD) is characterized by loss of vision in the center of the visual field (the *macula*) of the eye (Fig. 18.3). A healthy macula is necessary for sharp central vision. People with AMD cannot see a clear image when they look straight ahead. Only 3% of Americans who are 75 to 79 years of age have AMD, but the prevalence of the condition increases to almost 12% of the population who are 80 years of age or older.[38] AMD is more common in people who smoke, have a family history of the disease, and have elevated blood pressure or elevated blood cholesterol levels.[39]

Glaucoma occurs when the fluid pressure in the *anterior chamber* of the eye is higher than normal. The increased pressure damages the optic nerve (Fig. 18.3), which can result in blindness. About 10% of white Americans who are 80 years of age and older have glaucoma.[40]

Cataracts, glaucoma, and **diabetic retinopathy** are collectively referred to as *diabetic eye disease*, because these conditions are complications of poorly controlled diabetes. Diabetic retinopathy is the most common type of diabetic eye disease.[41] This condition is caused by elevated blood glucose and subsequent AGEs damage to the small blood vessels of the retina. In some cases, the tiny blood vessels in the retina swell and leak fluid into the *vitreous*, the gel–like substance that fills much of the inner eye. In other cases, the vessels become blocked, which signals the development of new blood vessels in the retina. The new vessels, however, are delicate and may leak blood, which interferes with vision.

In the early stages of diabetic retinopathy, people usually do not have any symptoms, but as the condition worsens, affected individuals report seeing floating "spots" or having blurry vision. Long–term good control of blood pressure, cholesterol, and glucose levels reduces the risk that diabetic retinopathy will progress to blindness.[41] Laser eye surgery is used to treat advanced cases of diabetic retinopathy.

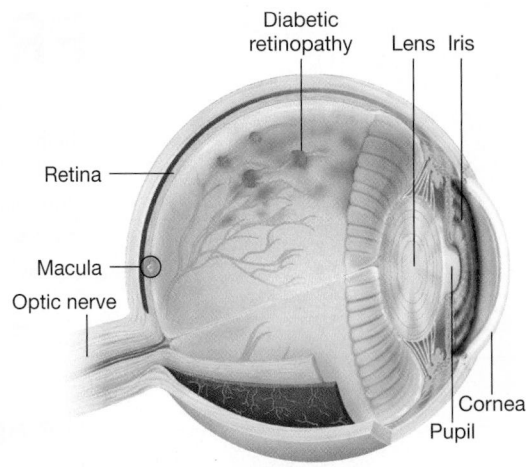

FIGURE 18.3 Human eye. Note the position of the macula.

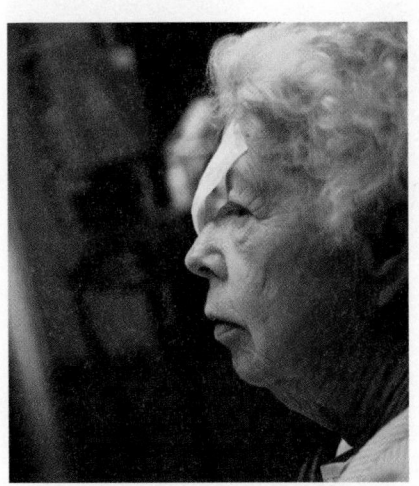

Laser eye surgery may be used to treat glaucoma and diabetic retinopathy.

presbyopia decline in near vision that occurs with aging

cataracts condition characterized by abnormal changes in the lens of the eye that can cause blindness

glaucoma condition characterized by increased pressure within the anterior chamber that damages the optic nerve

diabetic retinopathy damage to the retina caused by glycation

FRESH TIPS

According to experts with the American Optometric Association, a diet high in fruits and vegetables that contain the carotenoids lutein and zeaxanthin may protect against age-related vision problems, particularly age-related macular degeneration and cataracts. Some of the richest food sources of lutein and zeaxanthin are dark green, leafy vegetables, such as spinach, collards, and kale.[42]

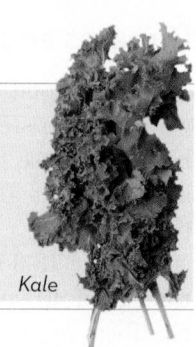

Kale

The Aging Digestive Tract

As a person ages, his or her gastrointestinal tract usually secretes less digestive juices, and the muscles of the digestive tract weaken. The result of such changes can be the development of gastrointestinal disorders and a reduced ability to digest food and absorb nutrients.

Teeth and Mouth

In the 1950s, surveys of Americans indicated that the majority of older adults had lost all their natural teeth. Since then, the percentage of older persons who retain all or most of their teeth has increased in the United States. On average, an older American has only 19 of his or her 32 natural teeth remaining. Moreover, 23% of Americans who are 65 years or older have lost all their natural teeth **(edentulism)**.[43]

Excessive tooth loss can lead to poor nutrition. People who lack teeth often avoid crisp or chewy foods, such as fresh fruits, vegetables, whole-grain cereals, and meat.[44] Although dentures that replace natural teeth can enable some people to chew normally, many older adults do not like to wear them because they can be uncomfortable. When a person has difficulty chewing food, serving soft foods such as ground meats, cooked vegetables, pureed fruits, and puddings can stimulate the individual's appetite. By following recommended dental hygiene practices, obtaining regular dental care, and avoiding tobacco use, people can greatly increase their chances of keeping most of their teeth as they age.

Xerostomia (*zeer-o-sto'-me-ah*), or "dry mouth," results from a lack of saliva secretion. A review of the medical literature shows that 17 to 29% of older adults have xerostomia; women are more likely than men to have the condition.[45] X-rays of the oral cavity, chemotherapy, and certain medications are common causes of dry mouth, although the condition may develop spontaneously, that is, without a clear cause. Recall from Chapter 4 that saliva makes food easier to swallow and increases the flavor and palatability of foods. Thus, xerostomia interferes with a person's ability to taste food, which generally results in reduced intake.

Esophagus, Stomach, and Intestines

Older adults are more likely to develop gastroesophageal reflux disease (GERD) than any other disorder of the upper gastrointestinal tract.[46] As an adult grows older, the lower esophageal sphincter may "wear out" and lose its ability to constrict, which enables acidic gastric juice to enter the esophagus. Dietary treatment of GERD is described in Chapter 4.

As a person ages, his or her stomach secretes less hydrochloric acid and intrinsic factor. These changes can contribute to poor absorption of vitamin B-12 and the development of vitamin B-12 deficiency and pernicious anemia. Many

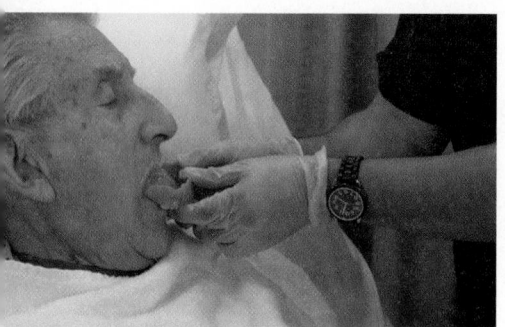

One-fourth of Americans who are 65 years of age or older have lost all of their teeth.

edentulism condition characterized by the loss of all teeth

xerostomia dry mouth

older adults are able to meet their vitamin B—12 needs by eating foods that have been fortified with the micronutrient or by taking vitamin B—12 supplements. Other persons with vitamin B—12 deficiency must take injections of the vitamin to prevent pernicious anemia (see Chapter 10).

Older persons are also at risk of iron deficiency, because reduced stomach acid production may hinder iron absorption. Furthermore, many older adults take aspirin regularly, and this practice can cause intestinal bleeding that can lead to iron deficiency anemia. Intestinal ulcers and cancer can also cause blood loss from the digestive tract. The discovery of blood in bowel movements needs to be reported to a physician—regardless of one's age.

Constipation is a major complaint of older adults. By increasing their intake of fiber—rich foods, such as whole—grain products and vegetables, older adults may be able to have more regular bowel movements (see the "Fiber" section of Chapter 5). Dehydration also contributes to constipation, so older persons should make sure their fluid intake is adequate.

Arthritis

Arthritis is inflammation of a joint that is usually accompanied by pain, swelling, and stiffness. In the United States, arthritis affects more than 50 million adults (one in five), making it the most common health problem in the nation. Arthritis can strike people of any age, but it is more common in older adults.[47] **Osteoarthritis**, the most common form of arthritis, affects 21 million Americans. The condition results from progressive degeneration of the bones and cartilage, particularly in the fingers, wrists, knees, hips, and spine. The pain of osteoarthritis can be so severe, it interferes with a person's ability to shop, prepare food, and eat.

The primary risk factor for osteoarthritis is obesity, but the condition also develops in people who have experienced trauma to a joint earlier in life. For example, after years of overuse and injury, joggers and retired professional football and soccer players often develop osteoarthritis in their knees.

Treatment of osteoarthritis includes controlling pain, improving joint function, and weight loss in individuals who are obese. Pain is treated by *NSAIDs* (*nonsteroidal anti—inflammatory drugs*), which increase the risk of gastrointestinal bleeding and subsequent anemia. Dietary supplements that contain *glucosamine sulfate* may be helpful in reducing the discomfort and slowing the joint damage that occur in osteoarthritis, but more research is needed to support the use of such products.[48]

Gout

Gout is a form of inflammatory arthritis that is caused by a buildup of crystals that contain uric acid in joints, particularly a joint in the big toe. **Uric acid** is derived from the breakdown of *purines*, which are nitrogen—containing compounds made in the body and found in animal foods. The condition affects about 3 to 5% of Americans and is most common in older adults.[49] People who are overweight or obese, have hypertension, consume alcohol, take diuretics, and/or consume high amounts of meat and seafood are more likely to develop gout than people who do not have these characteristics.

Although gout is a chronic disease, people with the condition tend to have times when they are free of symptoms (remission). An acute bout of the disease is called a "flare," which is characterized by joint pain and swelling of the affected joint. Treatment usually includes anti—inflammatory medication, such as NSAIDs and steroids. To prevent flares, gout patients may need to take medications (*allopurinol*, for example) that lower blood uric acid levels.

arthritis inflammation of a joint

osteoarthritis condition characterized by degeneration of the bones and cartilage

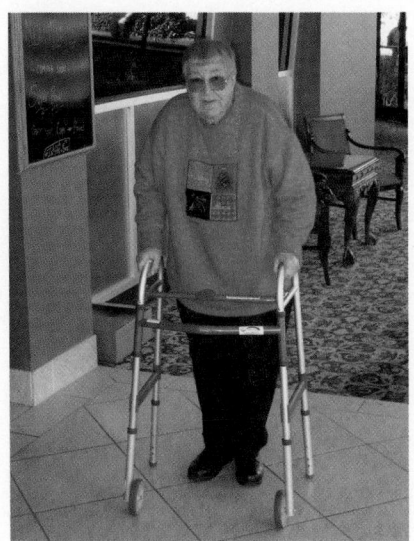

Obesity is the primary risk factor for osteoarthritis.

gout form of arthritis caused by the buildup of uric acid crystals in joints

uric acid derivative of purine metabolism

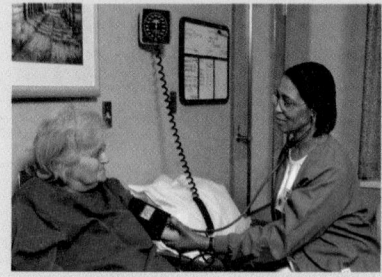

Depression

About 5% of community—dwelling older persons and as many as 15% of older persons living in long—term care facilities suffer from depression.[50] Situations that contribute to depression among the older adult population include chronic illness, loss of mobility, and isolation and loneliness as family members and friends die or move away. If the depressed person loses interest in cooking and eating, weight loss and nutrient deficiencies are likely to occur. In many instances, depression can be managed with medication, but social support and psychological counseling may be necessary as well. Without proper treatment, depressed persons are at risk of alcoholism and suicide. Suicide rates of older adult Americans, especially older white men, are higher than rates for members of other age groups.[51]

FRESH TIPS

The following suggestions can help improve nutrient intakes of older persons:

- Emphasize nutrient-dense foods when planning daily menus.
- Try new foods, seasonings, and ways of preparing foods.
- Serve meals in well-lit or sunny areas, and plan appealing meals by using foods with different flavors, colors, shapes, textures, and smells.
- Plan occasions for the older adult to share cooking responsibilities and eat meals with friends or relatives.
- Encourage the older person to eat at a senior center whenever possible.
- Investigate community resources for helping the older adult obtain groceries, cook, or manage other daily care needs.
- Encourage the older adult to be physically active.
- If biting and chewing are difficult for an older person, chop, grind, or blend tough or crisp foods.

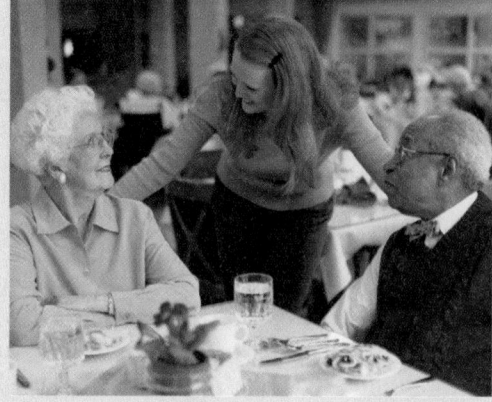

Eating meals at a senior center can help stimulate the appetite of a lonely older adult.

Heart Failure

By age 65 years, most Americans have some form of cardiovascular disease (CVD), which causes progressive damage to the heart. Heart disease, a form of CVD, is the number one cause of death of older adults.[17] As the heart becomes too weak to pump an adequate amount of blood throughout the body, **heart failure (HF)** develops. Signs and symptoms of HF include shortness of breath, fatigue, and edema, especially in the legs. The prevalence of heart failure increases with advancing age, and the majority of cases are diagnosed in people who are 75 years of age and older.

Treatment of heart failure consists of medications and dietary modifications. Medications such as beta—blockers and ACE inhibitors may improve heart func—tion. Diuretics such as furosemide are prescribed to increase urine output, and anticoagulants such as warfarin are given to reduce the likelihood of developing blood clots.[53] Patients with HF may need to consult with a registered dietitian for individualized medical nutrition therapy.

heart failure (HF) condition in which the heart cannot pump effectively

Polypharmacy and Food-Drug Interaction

People who are over 65 years of age make up only 13.7% of the American popu—lation, but they take one—third of all prescription and 40% of all nonprescription medications that are sold in the United States.[54] **Polypharmacy** (taking five or more medicines each day) is a common practice among older adults, especially in individuals who have multiple chronic diseases.[55] According to the CDC, about 37% of Americans aged 65 years or older use five or more prescription drugs per day.[56] An 88—year—old woman, for example, may take *hydrochlorothiazide* to lower her blood pressure, *lovastatin* to reduce her elevated cholesterol level, *citalopram* to combat depression, *metformin* to help control her diabetes, and *levothyroxine* to boost her level of thyroid hormone. Additionally, she takes over—the—counter products that contain vitamin D to treat her vitamin D defi—ciency and low—dose aspirin to reduce inflammation.

Cholesterol—lowering medications (statins) are the most frequently used class of drugs, followed by *beta—blockers* that help regulate heartbeat. The third most frequently used class of drugs are diuretics.[56] Although diuretics can help reduce blood pressure, these medications can cause serious side effects, including dizziness and dehydration.

Although medications can improve health and quality of life of older persons, some drugs interfere with the body's absorption and/or use of certain nutrients.[55] Prescription medications can have a variety of effects on a person's nutritional status, such as by:

- Altering taste (*dysgeusia*);
- Causing gastrointestinal bleeding or diarrhea;
- Causing anorexia or increased appetite; and
- Altering blood glucose levels.

Certain dietary supplements, including herbal products, can reduce or amplify the effects of prescribed medications. Therefore, older adults should notify their physicians about their use of all dietary supplements. A few foods also interfere with the metabolism of prescribed drugs. Grapefruit juice, for example, can alter the potency of certain statins that are used to lower blood cholesterol.

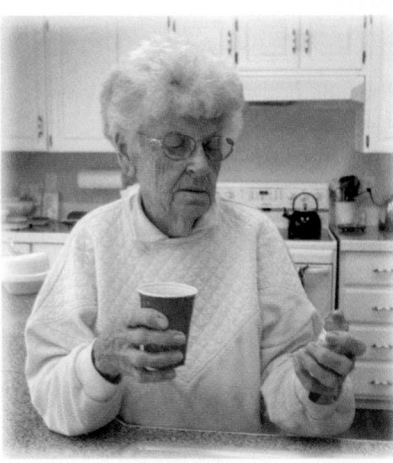

People who are over 65 years of age make up only 13.7% of the American population, but they take one-third of all prescription medications that are sold in the United States.

polypharmacy condition that occurs when a person takes five or more medications each day

ASSESS YOUR PROGRESS

9 *Identify at least five physiological changes associated with the normal aging process that can affect the nutritional status of an older adult.*

10 *Describe the three main diabetic eye diseases.*

11 *List at least three signs or symptoms of heart failure.*

12 *Identify factors that contribute to depression among older adults.*

13 *Define polypharmacy.*

18.5 Dementia

LEARNING OUTCOMES

1 *Explain what happens to the brain of an aging person that can negatively affect cognition.*

2 *Discuss the different forms of age-related dementia, including common causes of the conditions and how dementia can affect a person's nutritional status.*

The number of functioning neurons (nerve cells that transmit information) in the brain decreases with age. A reduction in the number of neurons in the brain

dementia decline in mental functioning that affects daily living

negatively affects mental functioning (cognition). Memory, language skills, and the abilities to reason, pay attention, and solve problems are cognitive functions. **Dementia** results from the decline in cognition. Some people with dementia also lose control over their emotions. Dementia can be so severe that it interferes with the person's ability to carry out tasks of daily living. Age–related dementia is associated with advancing age, but it is important to recognize that dementia is not a normal aspect of the aging process.[57]

Some forms of dementia are reversible and not related to advanced age. Reversible dementia might result from poor dietary practices, hormonal imbalances, or medications. For example, a deficiency of thiamin or vitamin B–12, or dehydration can cause reversible dementia. Treating reversible dementia may simply involve modifying the diet of the older adult to improve its thiamin content or giving the person a vitamin B–12 supplement. Most forms of age–related dementia, including vascular dementia and *Alzheimer's disease*, are irreversible. This section of the chapter focuses on common forms of age–related dementia.

Age-Related Dementia

Alzheimer's disease (AD) most common form of irreversible dementia that affects older adults

As the name implies, the risk of developing an age–related dementia increases with advancing age. **Alzheimer's disease (AD)** is the most common form of irreversible, degenerative, age–related dementia among older Americans.[58] AD affects about 5% of people who are 65 to 74 years of age, but the prevalence increases to between 25 and 50% of the population who are 85 years of age and older. AD is the fifth leading cause of death in persons age 65 years and older.[58] Although AD is more likely to occur in older adults, the condition can begin in persons who are younger than 60 years of age.[58]

During the early stages of AD, the degree of cognitive impairment is mild; affected individuals may have difficulty following directions or become lost while driving in an area that was formerly familiar to them. As the disease progresses, persons with AD may forget where they live and names of family members. Eventually, individuals with AD are unable to care for themselves and need 24–hour care. Death usually occurs 3 to 20 years after the disease is first suspected, depending on how quickly the disease worsens.[59] People with AD usually die as a result of complications from infection or organ failure.

Physicians often have difficulty diagnosing AD because many of the disease's signs and symptoms are the same as those of other forms of dementia. Medical practitioners need to rule out other causes of dementia, such as stroke or brain tumor. Currently, the only way to determine whether a person had AD is to microscopically examine a sample of his or her brain tissue after death to find specific signs of tissue degeneration.[59]

DID **YOU** *KNOW?*

In the past, theories about the causes of AD included exposure to lead, aluminum, and mercury that resulted in the accumulation of these toxic minerals in the body. According to scientific evidence, however, the presence of lead, aluminum, and mercury in the body is not related to the development of AD.[59]

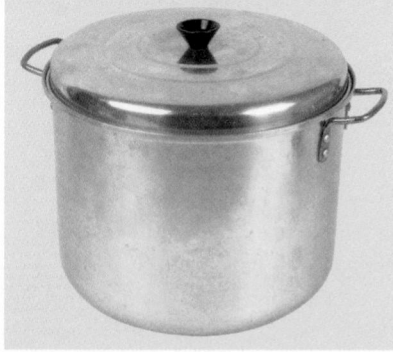

Vascular-Degenerative Dementia

Vascular dementia occurs when the blood supply to the brain is reduced, which damages brain tissue. This form of dementia usually occurs after a person has had several small strokes.[57] Vascular dementia is more common in people with hypertension or atherosclerosis; therefore, dietary strategies described in Chapters 6 and 11 to control these diseases may reduce a person's chances of developing this form of dementia.

The majority of people who were at least 80 years of age and had dementia when they died probably had "mixed dementia" (*mixed vascular–degenerative dementia*).[57] Results of some studies indicate that mixed vascular–degenerative dementia is the most common cause of severe cognitive decline in older adults.

Table 18.4 lists major risk factors for age–related dementia.[57] Note that several of the risk factors are modifiable. The Fresh Tips on page 597 provides ways to improve diets of people with dementia.

vascular dementia condition that occurs when the blood supply to the brain is reduced

TABLE 18.4 Age-Related Dementia: Risk Factors

- **Age.** The risk increases with advanced age.
- **Alcohol use.** Consuming large amounts of alcohol increases the risk of dementia, while drinking a moderate amount may be protective.
- **Atherosclerosis.** This inflammatory process leads to a thickening of the vessel walls, which can reduce the flow of blood that reaches the brain, leading to stroke or another brain injury. High levels of LDL cholesterol can raise the risk for vascular dementia and Alzheimer's disease.
- **Diabetes.** Poorly controlled diabetes is risk factor for stroke and cardiovascular disease-related events, which in turn increase the risk for vascular dementia.
- **Down syndrome.** Many people with Down syndrome develop early-onset AD by the time they reach middle age.
- **Genetics.** Some types of dementia are inherited.
- **Hypertension.** Chronic high blood pressure has been linked to cognitive decline, stroke, and types of dementia that affect the regions of the brain involved in cognition.
- **Smoking.** Smokers often develop circulatory problems that can interfere with normal blood flow to the brain.

Although there are a few medications that can be prescribed to slow the progression of Alzheimer's disease, there is no way to prevent or cure the disease. Some steps people can take that might reduce their risk of AD and, possibly, other forms of irreversible dementia include:[59]

- Eating cold–water fish (such as tuna, salmon, and mackerel) that are rich sources of omega–3 fatty acids at least two to three times per week;

- Reducing intake of linoleic acid, which is in margarine, butter, and dairy products;

- Choosing fruits and vegetables that contain carotenoids, vitamin E, and vitamin C (antioxidants);

- Maintaining normal blood pressure; and

- Keeping intellectually and socially active.

Parkinson's Disease

Another possible cause of dementia is **Parkinson's disease**, a disease that affects at least a half million people in the United States.[60] Parkinson's disease usually strikes people who are over 50 years of age.[61] The disease is a neurological disor–der that results from the loss of dopamine–producing cells in the brain. Without dopamine, the nerve cells of the brain cannot send messages properly, which leads to the loss of muscle function, shaking (tremors), stiffness, and impaired balance. As the disease progresses, the affected person eventually has difficulty swallowing, chewing, and speaking.

There is no cure for Parkinson's disease, but the medications *levodopa* and *carbidopa* often provide relief for some signs of the condition. Because levodopa is an amino acid, it competes with other amino acids for absorption. Therefore, foods high in protein should not be eaten close to the time that levodopa is taken. Also, high–fat diets should be avoided, because the presence of fat in the small intestine slows the absorption of levodopa.[62]

Parkinson's disease neurological disorder that results from a lack of dopamine

FRESH TIPS

Caregivers of people who have an irreversible form of dementia can consider the following tips when feeding the affected person:

- **Limit distractions.** Serve meals in a quiet area of the house.

- **Use plain plates and placemats to avoid visual confusion.**

- **Limit utensils.** Prepare easy-to-eat meals that require either a fork or a spoon.

- **Serve only one food at a time.** Offering too many food choices may overwhelm the individual.

- **Be patient during meals.** As the dementia progresses, the person may forget how to chew and swallow, so gently remind him or her to chew and swallow carefully.

- **Eat with the person who has dementia and provide directions on how to use utensils.**

Adapted from: Alzheimer's Association: *Food, eating and Alzheimer's.* http://www.alz.org/care/alzheimers-food-eating.asp#ixzz2fdmuhRTd

ASSESS YOUR PROGRESS

14 *Describe at least two physiological changes that can occur to the brain of an older adult that contribute to dementia.*

15 *Identify a type of dementia that is irreversible.*

16 *What causes vascular dementia?*

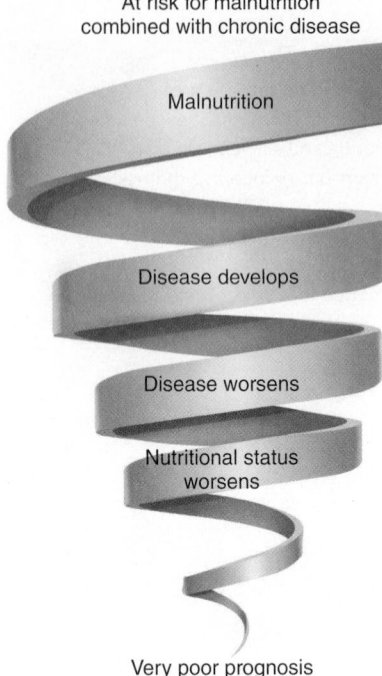

At risk for malnutrition combined with chronic disease

Malnutrition

Disease develops

Disease worsens

Nutritional status worsens

Very poor prognosis

FIGURE 18.4 Spiral of malnutrition and health in older adults. In older adults, undernutrition causes a downward spiraling effect on overall health and contributes to poor outcomes.

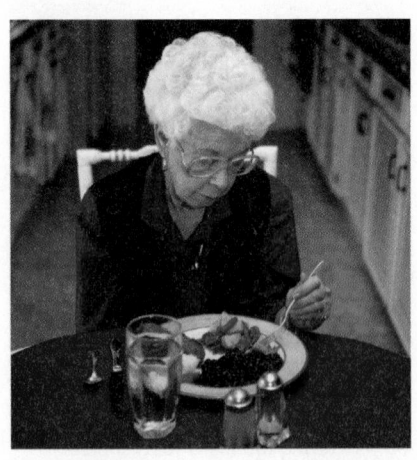

DID YOU KNOW?

Having multiple chronic diseases results in high health care expenditures; on average, more than 12% of older adults' total expenditures go to health care, which is higher than for any other age bracket.[52] Lower-income older adults must often decide between paying for food or paying for medications and other health-related expenditures.

18.6 Food Insecurity Among Older Adults

LEARNING OUTCOMES

1 *Describe factors that place older adults at risk for malnutrition.*
2 *Discuss the major goals of the Elderly Nutrition Program.*

In the United States, older adults are a diverse population. Some members of this population are healthy, have adequate incomes, and live independently, whereas others suffer from multiple chronic diseases, cannot care for themselves, and live in poverty. In 2011, about 9% of adults over 65 years of age were classified as poor, which the federal government defines as living below the poverty level; rates were higher among African–American and Hispanic older adults.[63] An impoverished person is at risk of *food insecurity*, the situation that occurs when the individual is concerned about running out of food or not having enough money to buy more food.

Food insecurity can result in poor nutritional status, because the food-insecure person does not have enough money to buy nutrient–dense foods. Consuming nutritionally inadequate diets often worsens existing chronic diseases and impairs physical and cognitive functioning. If, for example, an older adult's diet is low in protein, vitamin B–12, and iron, he or she is likely to experience sarcopenia and anemia, which limit the person's ability walk, shop, and prepare foods. As the older adult's nutritional status deteriorates, his or her immune system function becomes weakened. Lowered immunity makes a person susceptible to infections such as pneumonia, a leading cause of death among older Americans. As Figure 18.4 illustrates, undernutrition causes a downward spiraling effect on overall health and contributes to poor outcomes, especially for older adults who have multiple chronic diseases.

The Elderly Nutrition Program

To combat food insecurity and undernutrition among older Americans, the federal government provides funds for nutrition assistance programs. The Elderly Nutrition Program was established under Title III of the Older Americans Act of 1965. The Older Americans Act had three major goals:

• Reducing hunger and food insecurity;

• Promoting socialization; and

• Promoting good health and well–being of older individuals.[64]

To learn more about the government–sponsored nutrition–related programs for older adults, visit the following websites: National Institute on Aging, www.nia.nih.gov; American Geriatrics Society, www.americangeriatrics.org; and Administration on Aging, www.aoa.gov. Chapter 20 includes information concerning food insecurity and federal food assistance programs, including programs for older adults.

ASSESS YOUR PROGRESS

17 *In 2011, what percentage of older adult Americans were living in poverty?*
18 *Explain the role that poverty plays in malnutrition.*
19 *List major goals of the Elderly Nutrition Program.*

SUMMARY

SECTION 18.1 Older Adults

- Senescence refers to declining organ functioning and increasing vulnerability to disease that occur with advanced age. Scientists have found a strong genetic component to human longevity.
- Life expectancy is the number of years a person will live; life span refers to the maximum number of years an organism can live; and longevity refers to a long duration of life.
- Programmed theories and damage or error theories provide possible reasons for why people age.

SECTION 18.2 Physiological Aspects of Normal Aging

- As a person ages, every organ system in his or her body experiences physiological changes that are normal but can contribute to nutrient deficiencies.

SECTION 18.3 Nutrient Needs of Healthy Older Adults

- Many factors influence the nutrient needs and intake of older adults. Energy needs decrease about 4% for each decade over age 50. Following a calorie-restricted, nutrient-dense diet may increase longevity.
- Older adults generally do not eat enough fruits, vegetables, and dairy products, and they exceed recommendations for consumption of empty-calorie foods. Many older adults have diets that are deficient in vitamins B-12 and D, calcium, and potassium.

SECTION 18.4 Common Health Concerns of Older Adults

- Sarcopenia, problems affecting vision, osteoarthritis, constipation, and depression are common health concerns of older adults. Gout is a type of arthritis. Edentulism, xerostomia, and reduced production of stomach acid can negatively affect the nutritional status of older adults. Among many older adults, polypharmacy is common.

SECTION 18.5 Dementia

- The prevalence of dementia increases with advancing age. Risk factors for age-related dementia include advanced age, smoking, diabetes, and hypertension. Alzheimer's disease is the most common form of age-related dementia that affects older Americans. Other causes of age-related dementia include conditions that reduce the blood supply to the brain and Parkinson's disease.

SECTION 18.6 Food Insecurity and Older Adults

- In the United States, about 9% of adults over 65 years of age are poor. Food insecurity can result in poor nutritional status.
- The Elderly Nutrition Program aims to reduce hunger and food insecurity, as well as promote socialization, good health, and well-being of older individuals.

Get the most out of your study of nutrition with McGraw-Hill's innovative suite of adaptive learning products including McGraw-Hill LearnSmart®, SmartBook®, McGraw-Hill LearnSmart Achieve®, and McGraw-Hill LearnSmart Prep®. Visit www.learnsmartadvantage.com.

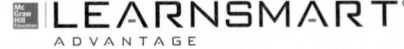

CASE STUDY RESPONSE

URINARY INCONTINENCE

DIEGO NEEDS TO UNDERSTAND THE IMPORTANCE of maintaining adequate fluid intake. He might develop dehydration if he restricts his fluid intake. Signs of dehydration include constipation, weakness, mental confusion, and coma. If untreated, dehydration can result in death.

To control his blood pressure, Diego should take his medication as prescribed, not limit his water intake, and follow the DASH diet, because it recommends fruits and vegetables that are rich sources of potassium. If necessary, he can lose excess body fat and exercise more.

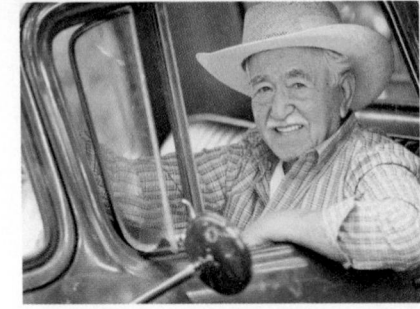

Modifying Recipes for Healthy Living

You are consulting with Sam concerning his diet. Sam is an 85-year-old widower who lives alone in a small apartment. He is relatively healthy for his age; his major health-related complaint is frequent constipation. His income is low but adequate enough to enable him to buy nutrient-dense food.

Since his wife's death, he consumes two slices of buttered toast and coffee for breakfast. He has a stove, but he likes to use his toaster and microwave oven. He relies heavily on single-serving, frozen microwavable foods for meals. His family has referred Sam to you for advice about ways to improve his diet and relieve his constipation. During the consultation, Sam tells you that he likes cooked oatmeal with brown sugar and cinnamon.

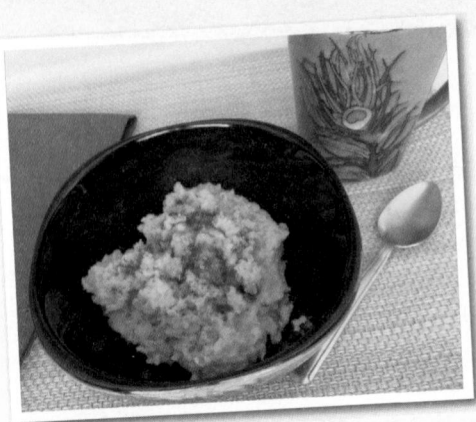

INGREDIENTS

½ cup of quick-cooking oats

1 cup water

1 tsp brown sugar

Dash of ground cinnamon

BASIC OATMEAL RECIPE

PREPARATION STEPS

1. Place oats in a bowl and add water to the oats. Place the bowl of cereal on a flat plate, which will collect any oatmeal that boils over the top of the bowl.

2. Cook in the microwave (on "high") for 1 ½ minutes. Sprinkle with brown sugar and cinnamon.

STEP 1 Brainstorm

What ingredients could be added to the recipe to increase the cereal's fiber, protein, micronutrient, and phytochemical contents?

STEP 2 Strategies for preparing the cooked oatmeal

Provide a detailed list of strategies that Sam can implement to obtain the additional foods to boost the nutrient content of the oatmeal. Include strategies for purchasing the ingredients at a reasonable cost.

OPTIONAL ACTIVITIES

STEP 3 Prepare the cooked oatmeal recipe

Did you follow all of the strategies listed in Step 2? Why or why not?

STEP 4 Reflect on the process

Based on information in this chapter, are there any other actions Sam's family can take within their community to obtain nutritious meals for Sam on a regular basis?

Critical Thinking

1. You are asked to present a 45-minute lesson on healthy eating to a group of women who are over 70 years of age and living independently. List three possible nutrition-related topics you would select to present to this population group, and explain why you chose the topics.

2. Are any of your parents, grandparents, or great grandparents still alive? If any of your ancestors died before they were 65 years of age, can you identify their causes of death and factors that contributed to their deaths? What lifestyle changes can you make now that can help you achieve a longer, healthier lifetime?

3. Use the MyPlate website (www.choosemyplate.gov) to design a day's menu for a 70-year-old woman whose height is 5-feet, 5-inches and weight is 140 pounds. Also, this woman performs 30 to 60 minutes of physical activity daily.

4. David is 79 years of age and was diagnosed with age-related dementia 7 years ago. His caregiver would like some suggestions for making meals easier for David to eat. Provide some food-related recommendations that would be practical for his caregiver to implement at mealtimes.

5. Use one of the assessment tools in Appendix F to evaluate the nutritional status of an older adult relative, such as a grandparent.

Practice Test

Select the best answer.

1. By the year 2050, government sources predict that _____ percent of the U.S. population will be 85 years of age or older.
   a. 3
   b. 5
   c. 10
   d. 14

2. The natural decline of organ functioning that occurs with advancing age is
   a. apoptosis.
   b. incontinence.
   c. presbyopia.
   d. senescence.

3. Which of the following is true?
   a. In 2010, the life expectancy of Americans was 85 years of age.
   b. As the American life expectancy increases, more Americans under 25 years of age are dying earlier than normal.
   c. Life expectancy in the United States is longer than for any other developed country in the world.
   d. People may inherit genes that code for longevity.

4. Which of the following conditions is not a normal physiological change that occurs with advancing age?
   a. Alzheimer's disease
   b. presbyopia
   c. thinning hair
   d. reduced saliva secretion

5. Advanced glycation end products are associated with
   a. reduced risk of osteoporosis and osteoarthritis.
   b. increased risk of urinary incontinence.
   c. long-term elevated blood glucose.
   d. high intakes of phytochemicals.

6. The term _____ refers to having no teeth.
   a. *caries*
   b. *edentulism*
   c. *fluorosis*
   d. *dementia*

7. The condition in which an older person loses skeletal muscle mass and gains excessive body fat is
   a. cystic fibrosis.
   b. geriatric malnutrition.
   c. sarcopenic obesity.
   d. Parkinson's disease.

8. In the United States, diets of older adults often supply inadequate amounts of
   a. potassium.
   b. thiamin.
   c. vitamin B-6.
   d. niacin.

9. A common type of irreversible age-related dementia in older adults is
   a. metabolic syndrome.
   b. age-related macular degeneration.
   c. advanced glycation.
   d. Alzheimer's disease.

10. Which of the following behaviors may reduce a person's risk of Alzheimer's disease?
    a. consuming a caffeine-free diet
    b. adding 50 g of oleic acid to the diet each day
    c. consuming fish that are rich sources of omega-3 fatty acids regularly
    d. avoiding products that contain gluten

11. Which of the following diseases or conditions is a common cause of blindness in older adults?
    a. presbyopia
    b. glaucoma
    c. gout
    d. dementia

12. According to results of scientific studies involving animals, a _____ diet can extend longevity.
    a. calorie-restricted
    b. gluten-free
    c. very-low-sodium
    d. high-linoleic

13. Eighty-year-old Maxine takes nine different medications each day to manage her chronic diseases. Maxine's son is concerned that she began to shows signs of dementia when she began taking the last prescription drug. Based on this information, Maxine probably has
    a. gout.
    b. presbyopia.
    c. polypharmacy.
    d. elevated uric acid.

14. Which of the following statements is true?

    a. A major goal of the Elderly Nutrition Program is to reduce the calorie intake of older adults to extend their life expectancy.

    b. The average older adult American spends 5% of his or her total expenditures on health care.

    c. An undernourished older adult is more susceptible to developing gout, which is a leading cause of death among older Americans.

    d. Older adults who consume nutritionally inadequate diets are likely to experience impaired cognitive functioning.

15. Which of the following conditions is the primary risk factor for osteoarthritis?

    a. gout

    b. obesity

    c. sarcopenia

    d. vitamin B-12 deficiency

ANSWERS TO PRACTICE TEST

1-b; 2-d; 3-d; 4-a; 5-c; 6-b; 7-c; 8-a; 9-d; 10-c; 11-b; 12-a; 13-c; 14-d; 15-b

ANSWERS TO CHAPTER 18 QUIZ Yourself

1. People in the United States can expect to live an average of 65 years. **False** (p. 582)
2. Gout is the most common form of arthritis. **False** (p. 593)
3. Compared to people living in other countries, Americans have the highest life expectancy. **False** (p. 582)
4. Diets of older adults generally do not supply adequate amounts of calcium. **True** (p. 588)
5. To prevent Alzheimer's disease, people should follow a gluten-free diet. **False** (p. 597)

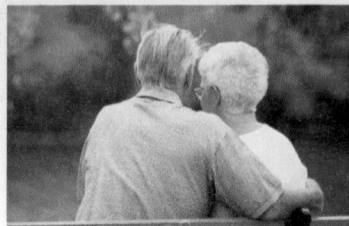

References

1. World Health Organization: *Definition of older or elderly person.* http://www.who.int/healthinfo/survey/ageingdefnolder/en/ Accessed: March 10, 2014.

2. U.S. Census Bureau: *Statistical Abstract of the United States: 2012.* http://www.census.gov/compendia/statab/. Accessed: March 10, 2014.

3. United Nations, Department of Economic and Social Affairs: *World population ageing: 1950–2050.* http://www.un.org/esa/population/publications/worldageing19502050/ Accessed: March 10, 2014.

4. Federal Interagency Forum on Aging-Related Statistics: *Older Americans 2012: Key indicators of well-being.* Washington, DC: U.S. Government Printing Office. July 2012. http://www.agingstats.gov/Main_Site/Data/2012_Documents/Population.aspx Accessed: March 10, 2014.

5. United Nations, Department of Economic and Social Affairs: *The world factbook 2013.* https://www.cia.gov/library/publications/the-world-factbook/rankorder/2102rank.html Accessed: March 10, 2014.

6. Hoyert D, Xu J: Deaths: Preliminary data 2011. *National Vital Statistics Reports* 61:6, 2012. http://www.cdc.gov/nchs/data/nvsr/nvsr61/nvsr61_06.pdf Accessed: March 10, 2014.

7. Meyer J: *Centenarians 2010. 2010 Census special reports.* 2012. http://www.census.gov/prod/cen2010/reports/c2010sr-03.pdf Accessed: March 10, 2014.

8. *Okinawa Centenarian Study.* http://www.okicent.org/cent.html Accessed: March 10, 2014.

9. Davinelli S and others: Extending healthy aging: Nutrient sensitive pathway and centenarian population. *Immunity & Ageing* 9(9), 2012. DOI:10.1186/1742-4933-9-9 http://www.immunityageing.com/content/9/1/9 Accessed: March 10, 2014.

10. Gavrilova NS, Gavrilov, LA: Comments on dietary restriction, Okinawa diet and longevity. *Gerontology* 58:221, 2012. DOI: 10.1159/000329894

11. Kunlin J: Modern biological theories of aging. *Aging and Disease* 1(2):72, 2010. http://www.ncbi.nlm.nih.gov/pmc/articles/PMC2995895/ Accessed: March 10, 2014.

12. Semba R and others: Does accumulation of advanced glycation end products contribute to the aging phenotype? *Journals of Gerontology: Series A, Biological Sciences and Medical Sciences.* 65(9):963, 2010. DOI: 10.1093/gerona/glq074. E-pub: May 17, 2010.

13. Karpa M and others: Prevalence and neurodegenerative or other associations with olfactory impairment in an older community. *Journal of Aging Health* 22(2):154, 2010. DOI: 10.1177/0898264309353066

14. Nation Library of Medicine, National Institutes of Health: Taste—impaired. *MedLinePlus,* 2013. http://www.nlm.nih.gov/medlineplus/ency/article/003050.htm Accessed: March 10, 2014.

15. Imoscopi A and others: Taste loss in the elderly: Epidemiology, causes and consequences. *Aging Clinical and Experimental Research* 24(6):570, 2012. DOI: 10.3275/8520

16. United States Department of Agriculture, Agricultural Research Service: *What we eat in America 2011–2012.* Last modified October 2014. http://www.ars.usda.gov/Services/docs.htm?docid=18349 Accessed: November 11, 2014.

17. Centers for Disease Control and Prevention, U.S. Department of Health and Human Services: *The state of aging and health in America 2013.* 2013. http://www.cdc.gov/aging/pdf/state-aging-health-in-america-2013.pdf Accessed: March 10, 2014.

18. Krebs-Smith SM and others: Americans do not meet federal dietary recommendations. *Journal of Nutrition* 140(10):1832, 2010.

19. Otten JJ and others: *Dietary Reference Intakes: The essential guide to nutrient requirements.* Institute of Medicine of the National Academies. Washington, DC: National Academies Press, 2006.

20. Bensenor IM and others: Hypothyroidism in the elderly: Diagnosis and management. *Clinical Interventions in Aging* 7:97, 2012. E-pub: April 3, 2012. DOI: 10.2147/CIA.S23966

21. McDonald R, Ramsey J: Honoring Clive McCay and 75 years of caloric restriction research. *Journal of Nutrition* 140(7):1205, 2010. DOI:10.3945/jn.110.122804

22. Cava E, Fontana L: Will calorie restriction work in humans? *Aging* 5(7):507, 2013.

23. Position of the Academy of Nutrition and Dietetics: Food and nutrition for older adults: Promoting health and wellness. *Journal of the Academy of Nutrition and Dietetics* 112(8):1255, 2012.

24. Hughes C and others: Vitamin B_{12} and ageing: Current issues and interaction with folate. *Annals of Clinical Biochemistry* 50(4):315, 2013.

25. National Institute on Aging: What's on your plate?: *Vitamins and minerals.* ND. https://www.nia.nih.gov/health/publication/whats-your-plate/vitamins-minerals Accessed: January 28, 2016.

26. Bailey RL and others: Dietary supplement use in the United States, 2003–2006. *Journal of Nutrition* 141(2):261, 2011.

27. Vogiatzoglou A and others: Dietary sources of vitamin B-12 and their association with plasma vitamin B-12 concentrations in the general population: The Hordaland Homocysteine Study. *American Journal of Clinical Nutrition* 89(4):1078, 2009.

28. Bailey RL and others: Dietary supplement use is associated with higher intakes of minerals from food sources. *American Journal of Clinical Nutrition* 94(5):1376, 2011.

29. Bailey RL: Estimation of total usual calcium and vitamin D intakes in the United States. *Journal of Nutrition* 140(4):817, 2010.

30. Roger V and others: Heart disease and stroke statistics—2012 update: A report from the American Heart Association. *Circulation* 125(1):e2, 2012.

31. Patel H and others: Prevalence of sarcopenia in community-dwelling older people in the UK using the European Working Group on Sarcopenia in Older People (EWGSOP) definition: Findings from the Hertfordshire Cohort Study (HCS). *Age and Ageing* 42(3):378. E-pub: February 5, 2013. DOI: 10.1093/ageing/afs197

32. Sakuma K, Yamaguchi A: Sarcopenic obesity and endocrinal adaptation with age. *International Journal of Endocrinology* Volume 2013, Article ID 204164. http://dx.doi.org/10.1155/2013/204164

33. Auyeung TW and others: Survival in older men may benefit from being slightly overweight and centrally obese—A 5-year follow-up study in 4,000 older adults using DXA. *Journals of Gerontology Series A: Biological Sciences and Medical Sciences* 65A(1):99, 2010.

34. Dimitria P and others: Obesity is a risk factor for fracture in children but is protective against fracture in adults: A paradox. *Bone* 50(2):457, 2012.

35. Li Z, Heber D: Sarcopenic obesity in the elderly and strategies for weight management. *Nutrition Review* 70(1):57, 2012. DOI: 10.1111/j.1753-4887.2011.00453.x

36. National Eye Institute: *Facts about presbyopia.* 2010. http://www.nei.nih.gov/health/errors/presbyopia.asp Accessed: March 10, 2014.

37. National Eye Institute: *2010 U.S. age-specific prevalence rates for cataracts by age, and race/ethnicity.* http://www.nei.nih.gov/eyedata/cataract.asp#1 Accessed: March 10, 2014.

38. National Eye Institute: *2010 U.S. age-specific prevalence rates for AMD by age, and race/ethnicity.* http://www.nei.nih.gov/eyedata/amd.asp#1 Accessed: March 10, 2014

39. National Eye Institute: *Facts about age-related macular degeneration.* 2013. http://www.nei.nih.gov/health/maculardegen/armd_facts.asp Accessed: March 10, 2014.

40. National Eye Institute: *2010 U.S. age-specific prevalence rates for glaucoma by age, and race/ethnicity.* http://www.nei.nih.gov/eyedata/glaucoma.asp#1 Accessed: March 10, 2014.

41. National Eye Institute: *Facts about diabetic retinopathy.* 2012. http://www.nei.nih.gov/health/diabetic/retinopathy.asp Accessed: March 10, 2014.

42. American Optometric Association: *Lutein and zeaxanthin.* http://www.aoa.org/patients-and-public/caring-for-your-vision/diet-and-nutrition/lutein Accessed: March 10, 2014.

43. Centers for Disease Control and Prevention: Edentulism. *Health Data Interactive.* http://205.207.175.93/HDI/TableViewer/tableView.aspx?ReportId=110 Accessed: March 10, 2014.

44. Mann T and others: The association between chewing and swallowing difficulties and nutritional status in older adults. *Australian Dental Journal* 58(2):200, 2013. DOI: 10.1111/adj.12064

45. Wiener RC and others: Hyposalivation and xerostomia in dentate older adults. *Journal of the American Dental Association* 141(3):279, 2010.

46. Chait MM: Gastroesophageal reflux disease: Important considerations for the older patients. *World Journal of Gastrointestinal Endoscopy* 2(12):388, 2010. ISSN 1948-5190 (online)

47. Centers for Disease Control and Prevention: *Arthritis: Meeting the challenge of living well: At a glance 2013.* http://www.cdc.gov/chronicdisease/resources/publications/aag/arthritis.htm Accessed: March 10, 2014.

48. Reginster J-Y and others: Review article: Role of glucosamine in the treatment of osteoarthritis. *Rheumatology International* 32(10):2959, 2012.

49. Centers for Disease Control and Prevention: Gout. 2011. http://www.cdc.gov/arthritis/basics/gout.htm Accessed: March 10, 2014.

50. Centers for Disease Control and Prevention: Depression is not a normal part of growing older. 2012. http://www.cdc.gov/aging/mentalhealth/depression.htm Accessed: March 10, 2014.

51. Conwell Y and others: Suicide in older adults. *Psychiatry Clinics of North America* 34(2):451, 2011. DOI: 10.1016/j.psc.2011.02.002

52. U.S. Department of Health and Human Services. Administration on Aging: *A profile of older Americans: 2012.* http://www.aoa.gov/Aging_Statistics/Profile/2012/14.aspx Accessed: March 10, 2014.

53. Dunaly S and others: Medication adherence among community-dwelling patients with heart failure. *Mayo Clinic Proceedings* 86(4):273, 2011. DOI: 10.4065/mcp.2010.0732

54. Riker G, Setter S: Polypharmacy in older adults at home: What it is and what to do about it—Implications for home healthcare and hospice. *Home Healthcare Nurse* 30(8):474, 2012. DOI: 10.1097/NHH.0b013e31826502dd

55. Crentsil V and others: A pharmacoepidemiologic study of community-dwelling, disabled older women: Factors associated with medication use. *American Journal of Geriatric Pharmacotherapy* 8(3):215, 2010. DOI: 10.1016/j.amjopharm.2010.06.003

56. Centers for Disease Control and Prevention. *Health, United States, 2012.* http://www.cdc.gov/nchs/data/hus/hus12.pdf#091 Accessed: March 10, 2014.

57. National Institutes of Health, National Institute of Neurological Disorders and Stroke: *Dementia: Hope through research.* Last updated January 2014. http://www.ninds.nih.gov/disorders/dementias/detail_dementia.htm Accessed: March 10, 2014.

58. Centers for Disease Control and Prevention: *Alzheimer's disease.* Updated 2011. http://www.cdc.gov/aging/aginginfo/alzheimers.htm Accessed: March 10, 2014.

59. Nation Library of Medicine, National Institutes of Health: *MedlinePlus: Alzheimer's disease.* 2011. http://www.nlm.nih.gov/medlineplus/ency/article/000760.htm Accessed: March 10, 2014.

60. National Institutes of Health, National Institute of Neurological Disorders and Stroke: *NINDS Parkinson's disease research web overview.* http://www.ninds.nih.gov/research/parkinsonsweb/index.htm Accessed: March 10, 2014.

61. National Institutes of Health, National Institute of Neurological Disorders and Stroke: *NINDS Parkinson's disease information page.* http://www.ninds.nih.gov/disorders/parkinsons_disease/parkinsons_disease.htm Accessed: March 10, 2014.

62. Cereda E and others: Controlled-protein dietary regimens for Parkinson's disease. *Nutritional Neuroscience* 13(1):29, 2010. DOI: 10.1179/147683010X12611460763760

63. U.S. Department of Health and Human Services. Administration on Aging: *A profile of older Americans: 2012: Poverty.* http://www.aoa.gov/AoARoot/Aging_Statistics/Profile/2012/10.aspx

64. U.S. Department of Health and Human Services. Administration on Aging: *Nutrition services (OAA Title IIIC).* http://www.aoa.gov/AoARoot/AoA_Programs/HCLTC/Nutrition_Services/index.aspx#purpose Accessed: March 10, 2014.

19 Food and Water Safety

Food-borne illness from raw milk

LAST SPRING, MARY PURCHASED RAW MILK at a local grocery store for her 7-year-old son, Chris. She had researched the Internet for information about potential health benefits of raw milk for young children, and she found a local dairy farm that marketed its milk as "tested for harmful bacteria." After a few weeks of drinking the raw milk, Chris developed fatigue and abdominal pain, and within 24 hours, his symptoms worsened and included frequent diarrhea. After Mary noticed blood in her son's stools, she took the child to the hospital.

A couple of days after Chris was hospitalized, his physicians reported that he had a bacterial infection that was destroying his red blood cells and damaging his kidneys. The physicians told Mary that her child was in acute renal failure.

Within days, public health investigators learned that three other young children were admitted to local hospitals around the same time who had signs and symptoms that were similar to Chris's. The investigators determined that all of the sickened children had consumed raw milk processed from the same dairy and that the milk had been contaminated with bacteria called *Escherichia coli* (*E. coli*) O157:H7.

After spending 3 weeks in the hospital, Chris was well enough to return home. Before leaving the hospital, a registered dietitian provided Mary with information about food-borne illnesses and how to protect her family against them in the future.

- What are food-borne illnesses, and what are their potential causes?
- Why were all of the victims young in this outbreak?
- Why is raw milk a potential source of harmful bacteria?
- What are some food safety practices that Mary could implement to prevent future food-borne illnesses?

The suggested Case Study Response can be found on page 637.

QUIZ Yourself

What is the safest way to store food after cooking? If the water supply is interrupted, what sources of drinkable water are available in the home? Take the following quiz to test your knowledge of food and water safety. The answers are found on page 638.

1. Pregnant women are more likely to experience food-borne illness than other healthy women of similar age. __T __F

2. Eggs and milk are examples of potentially hazardous foods. __T __F

3. Hot foods should sit out at room temperature for a few hours to cool before placing in the refrigerator. __T __F

4. A new food additive must be approved by the Food and Drug Administration before being added to foods. __T __F

5. Melted ice cubes, water drained from a water heater, and water from the tank of a toilet are safe sources of drinking water in case of an emergency. __T __F

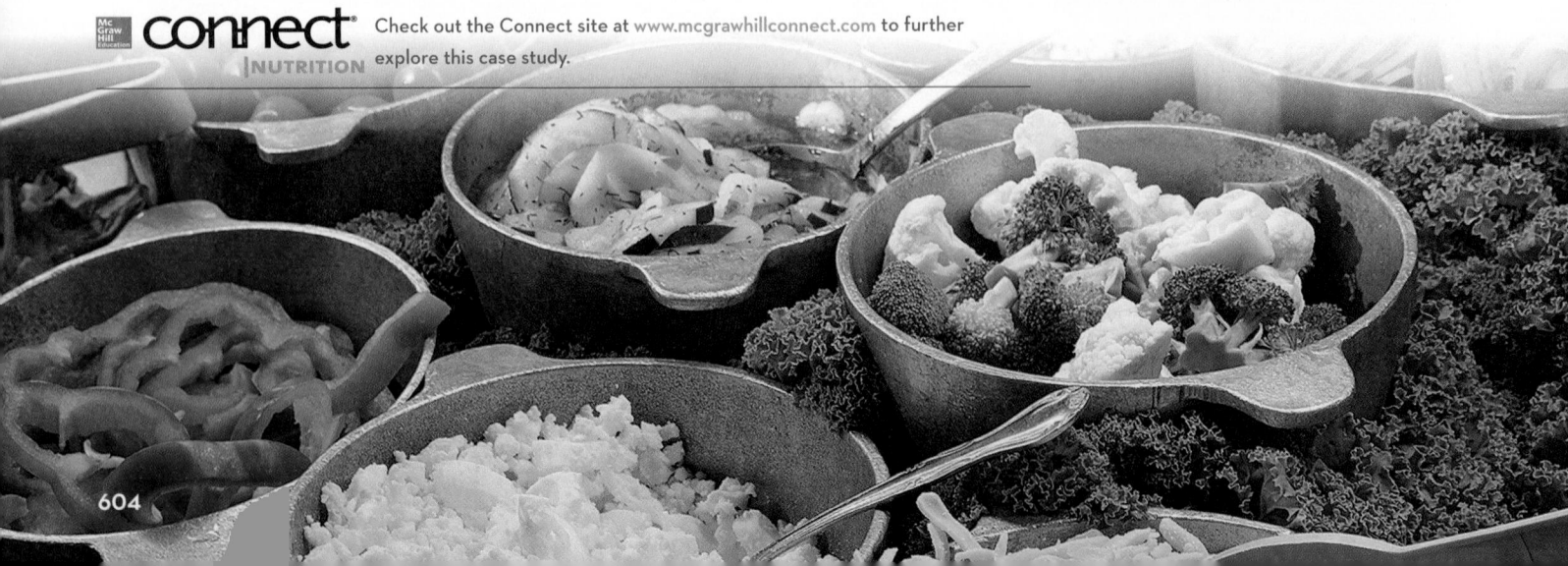

19.1 Protecting the Food Supply

LEARNING OUTCOMES

1 *Define food-borne illness.*

2 *List the federal agencies involved in food and water safety and the role each plays.*

3 *Explain how local health departments protect the public from food-borne illness.*

4 *Describe the Food Code and its use by state and local health departments.*

Food—borne illnesses can occur when microscopic agents (*microbes*) or their toxic by—products enter food or water and then are consumed. Infections spread through the ingestion of contaminated food or beverages are common, debilitating, and sometimes life—threatening diseases for millions of people around the world. Each year, an estimated 48 million Americans become sick from food-borne illnesses, and of those persons who contract such ailments, 128,000 require hospitalization and over 3000 die.[1]

Although these statistics seem to be high, the United States has one of the safest food and water supplies in the world, primarily the result of cooperating federal, state, and local agencies that regulate and monitor the production and distribution of food and sanitation of water. The Food and Drug Administration (FDA) of the U.S. Department of Health and Human Services and the U.S. Department of Agriculture (USDA) are the key federal agencies that protect consumers by regulating the country's food industry. Other team members include the Environmental Protection Agency (EPA), the Centers for Disease Control and Prevention (CDC), the Federal Trade Commission (FTC), and state and local governments.

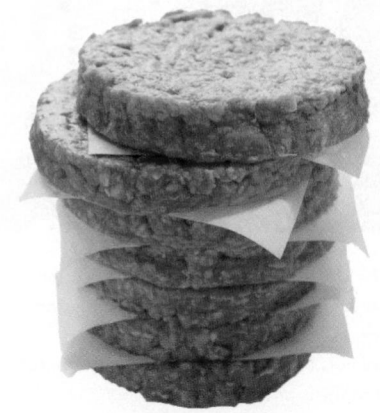

High-risk foods include raw or undercooked ground meat.

food-borne illness infection caused by microscopic disease-causing agents in food

History of Food Safety Legislation

Food safety legislation has been in place for over 100 years and is frequently modified as new information becomes available. In January 2011, Congress passed the Food Safety Modernization Act (FSMA), the most significant food—safety law enacted in over 70 years.[2] The FSMA improves the safety of the nation's food supply by strengthening the authority of federal regulating agencies and shifting focus from reaction to prevention of food—borne illnesses. Passage of this law made it possible for the FDA to require, rather than only request, food companies to recall potentially unsafe foods. FSMA also includes mandatory inspection of all imported foods and requires food manufacturers to develop better regulations concerning how food should be handled before being distributed to the public.

Key Federal Food Safety Agencies

To help protect the U.S. food supply, the FDA's Center for Food Safety and Applied Nutrition performs many important tasks, such as regulating nearly all domestic and imported food sold in interstate commerce and enforcing federal food safety laws. Additionally, the FDA establishes standards for safe food manufacturing practices, such as **Hazard Analysis and Critical Control Point (HACCP)** programs. HACCP is a science—based, systematic approach to preventing food—borne illness by predicting which hazards are most likely to occur in a food production facility. When a hazard is identified, food manufacturers can then take appropriate measures to eliminate the hazard. If necessary, FDA officials can take certain enforcement actions, such as detaining or recalling potentially unsafe foods before they reach consumers. Another important function of the FDA is educating the general public about safe food—handling practices.

Hazard Analysis and Critical Control Point (HACCP) science-based, systematic approach to preventing food-borne illness by predicting which hazards are most likely to occur in a food production facility

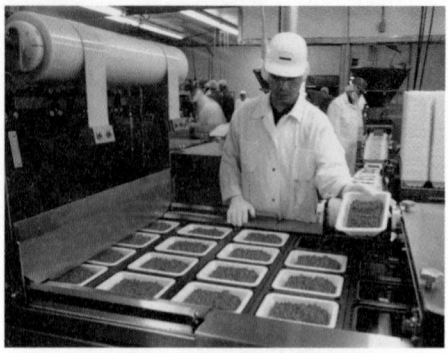

The USDA's Food Safety and Inspection Service is responsible for inspecting the nation's beef, poultry, and other food animals to ensure food safety and sanitation standards are met.

pathogen disease-causing microorganism

Although the FDA oversees the safety of most foods, the USDA's Food Safety and Inspection Service (FSIS) enforces food safety laws for domestic and imported meat and poultry products. FSIS staff inspect beef, poultry, and other food animals for diseases before and after slaughter, and the agency ensures that meat and poultry processing plants meet federal standards. Additionally, FSIS staff collect and analyze food samples to check for the presence of microbial and other unwanted and potentially harmful material in foods. If a food hazard is identified, FSIS officials can require meat and poultry processors to recall their unsafe products. Food safety experts with FSIS conduct programs and publish a magazine (*be FoodSafe*) to educate people about proper food-handling practices. For more information, visit the FSIS website at www.fsis.usda.gov/.

The EPA, FTC, and CDC are other team members of the federal government that provide support to the FDA and USDA in safeguarding the food and water supply. The EPA oversees the quality of our drinking water by establishing safe drinking water standards and assisting state officials in their efforts to monitor water quality. Furthermore, EPA staff regulate toxic substances and wastes to prevent their entry into foods and the environment. In an effort to prevent consumer fraud, the FTC collaborates with the FDA in regulating labels on food and dietary supplements. Finally, the CDC aims to control and prevent diseases, including food-borne illnesses, by investigating and monitoring **pathogens** (disease-causing microorganisms). The CDC uses multiple surveillance systems such as the Foodborne Disease Active Surveillance Network (FoodNet) to track food-borne diseases.

State and Local Health Departments

State and local officials work with FDA and other federal agency staff to implement national food safety standards for foods produced and sold within their state's borders. Local health departments, for example, are responsible for inspecting restaurants, grocery stores, dairy farms, and local food processing companies. In many communities, restaurants are required to post their sanitation rating where customers can easily see it (Fig. 19.1). Local health departments can close restaurants that do not receive high enough ratings and prevent them from reopening until food safety hazards have been corrected. The FDA publishes a guidance document called the *Food Code* every 4 years that assists state and local health officials in developing regulations. Visit the FDA's website at http://www.fda.gov/food/guidanceregulation/retailfoodprotection/foodcode/default.htm to access the latest version of the *Food Code*.

After consumers bring food into their home, it becomes their responsibility to reduce the risk of food-borne illness by handling the items properly. If consumers suspect that something they consumed made them or a family member sick, they should contact their physicians for treatment. Physicians may decide to report cases of food-borne illness to local public health officials so they can investigate and determine the source of the infection.

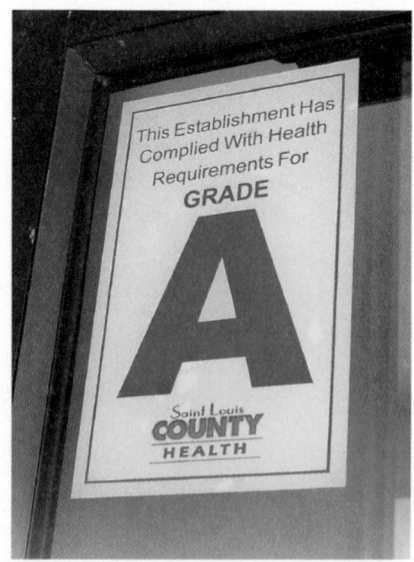

FIGURE 19.1 Sanitation scores. In many communities, restaurants must display their rating for sanitation where customers can easily see it. Local health departments can close restaurants that do not receive high enough ratings and not allow them to reopen until food safety hazards have been corrected.

ASSESS YOUR PROGRESS

1 *What causes food-borne illnesses?*

2 *Describe the roles of the FDA, USDA, EPA, FTC, and CDC in protecting the nation's food and water supply.*

3 *What is an HACCP plan?*

4 *Explain the importance of the* Food Code.

19.2 Pathogens in Food

LEARNING OUTCOMES

1 *Describe ways pathogens can contaminate food.*

2 *Identify potentially hazardous foods.*

3 *Explain characteristics of potentially hazardous foods.*

For thousands of years, people have used certain microbes to produce a variety of foods, including hard cheeses, yogurt, leavened breads, pickled foods, and alcoholic beverages. These foods are generally termed *cultured foods*. When microorganisms metabolize nutrients in food, they often secrete substances that alter the color, texture, taste, and other characteristics of the food in beneficial and desirable ways.

Other kinds of microbes grow and multiply in food, but their metabolic by–products spoil the food, making it unfit for human consumption. When pathogens are in food, they can make the item unsafe to eat.

A **contaminated food** (or beverage) is no longer wholesome, that is, pure or safe for human consumption. Contamination occurs when something enters food or beverages unintentionally. Such contaminants include pathogens, insect parts, residues of compounds used to kill insects that destroy food crops, and metal fragments from food–processing equipment. Contaminants may or may not be harmful, but pathogens are always harmful. The following section discusses how pathogens can contaminate our food.

Where Are Pathogens Found?

The microbes that cause food–borne illness can be found practically anywhere—in air, water, soil, and sewage, and on various surfaces. Human skin, nasal passages, and large intestine have vast colonies of many different kinds of microbes, some of which can be pathogenic. Animals, including cats, dogs, reptiles, cattle, and poultry, can also harbor harmful microbes on and in their bodies, especially in their intestinal tracts. In addition to microbes, viruses and parasitic worms can act as pathogens. A **parasite** is a life form that lives on or in another organism and takes advantage of its host.

Common routes for pathogenic contamination include transmission from *vermin*, improper personal hygiene practices, poor food–handling practices, and improper heating of foods. In this section, the emphasis is on how contamination occurs; sections 19.4 and 19.5 provide more detail about common pathogens and prevention of food–borne illnesses.

Vermin

One common route for transmitting harmful microbes involves **vermin**, animals that often live around sewage or garbage, such as flies, cockroaches, mice, and rats. When vermin land on or crawl across filth, they pick up pathogens on their feet. Then, if the vermin comes in contact with food, they can transfer the pathogens to humans. To reduce the risk of food–borne illness, keep flies, cockroaches, and other vermin away from food.

Personal Hygiene

Poor personal hygiene practices frequently transfer microbes to food. People can contaminate their hands with pathogens when they come in contact with feces, such as while using the toilet or changing a baby's soiled diaper. Furthermore, animals

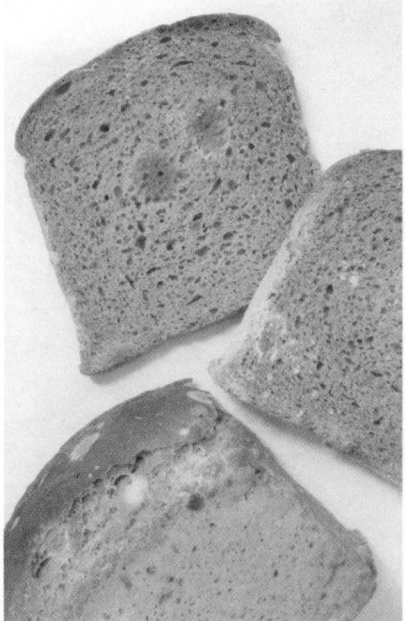

Mold growing on bread is an example of a contaminated food.

contaminated food item that is impure or unsafe for human consumption

parasite life form that lives on or in another organism and takes advantage of its host

vermin animals that often live around sewage or garbage, such as flies, cockroaches, mice, and rats

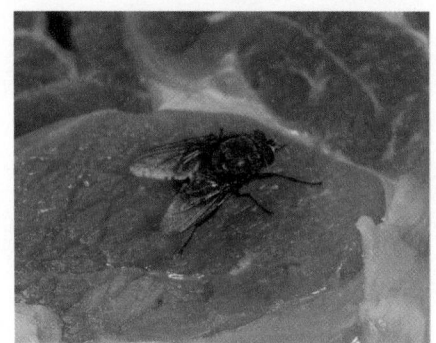

To reduce the risk of food-borne illness, keep flies, cockroaches, and other vermin away from food.

harbor pathogens in their feces as well as on their skin and fur. If children prepare or eat foods after touching animals at petting zoos or playing with pets, they can transmit these microbes to themselves or others. Thus, it is important for people to wash their hands before preparing or eating foods.

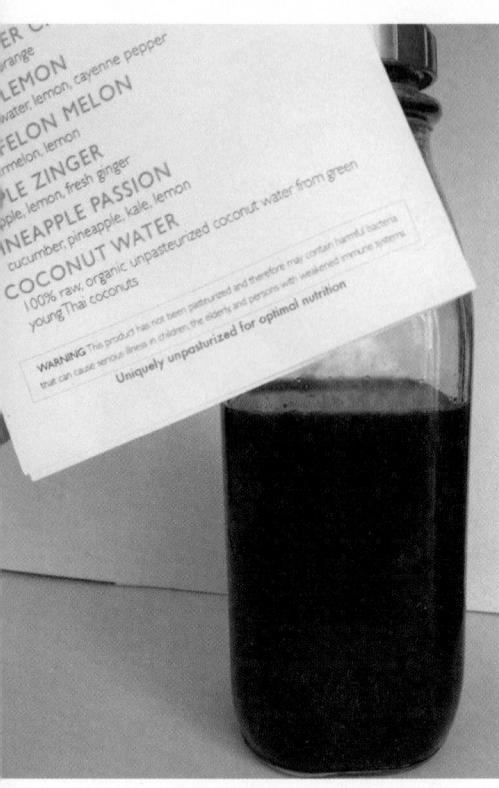

Raw milk and some juices may not be pasteurized and, therefore, should be consumed with caution. This cold-pressed juice is unpasteurized: The label and product information clearly indicates this and provides a warning for consumers.

cross-contamination transferring of pathogens from a contaminated food or surface to an uncontaminated food or surface

pasteurization process that kills the pathogens in foods and beverages as well as many microbes responsible for spoilage

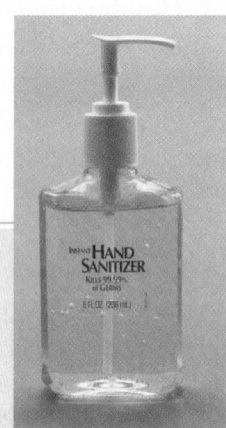

FRESH TIPS

If washing your hands with soap and very warm water is not an option, hand sanitizers are a good alternative. According to the CDC, effective alcohol-based sanitizers should contain at least 60% alcohol. Although sanitizers can quickly reduce the number of microorganisms on hands, they do not eliminate all pathogens.[3] They are also not as effective when hands are visibly dirty.

Food Handling

Improper food handling frequently results in food–borne illness. A common mis–take is failing to wash cutting boards and food preparation utensils after they come in contact with raw meat or poultry and then using the contaminated boards and utensils to prepare other foods, such as raw carrots for a salad. Pathogens from the raw meat or poultry can be transferred to the carrots and could produce food–borne illness. This transfer of pathogens is called **cross–contamination**.

Heating Food

Failing to cook foods properly can also increase the likelihood of food–borne ill–ness. **Pasteurization** is a special heating process used by many commercial food producers to kill pathogens. In the United States, for example, most juices and milk have been pasteurized before they are marketed. The nutrient composition of pasteurized foods may be slightly lower than that of unpasteurized foods, but the benefits of pasteurization far outweigh the loss of nutrients.

Potentially Hazardous Foods

Not all foods are likely to harbor pathogens. To survive and multiply, most microbes need warmth, moisture, and a source of nutrients, and some also require oxygen. In general, **potentially hazardous foods** are warm and moist, contain some protein, and they have a neutral or slightly acidic pH. Many of the foods Americans eat every day, such as meats, eggs, milk, and even some produce, fit this description. Table 19.1 presents some potentially hazardous foods and the common food–borne pathogens they may contain.

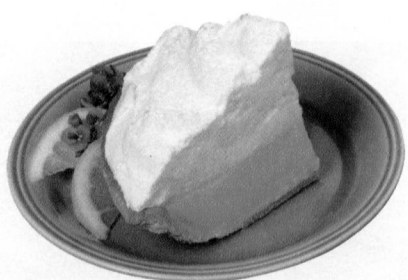

Meringue is made by whipping egg whites into foam. If homemade meringue is not baked long enough to kill pathogens, it is a potentially hazardous food. It is important to remember that all meringue pies should be kept chilled rather than left out at room temperature.

ASSESS YOUR PROGRESS

5 List common contaminants of food and beverages.

6 Identify at least two ways that pathogens can contaminate foods.

7 Discuss factors that contribute to a food's potential to harbor pathogens, and list at least five potentially hazardous foods.

TABLE 19.1 Summary of Potentially Hazardous Foods and Their Primary Pathogens

Food Source	Typical Menu Item	Common Pathogen
Beef	Undercooked ground beef; steak tartare	*E. coli* O157:H7
Poultry or eggs	Undercooked chicken or turkey; stuffing cooked inside the bird cavity; undercooked or raw eggs or products made with these, including Hollandaise sauce, homemade mayonnaise, homemade ice cream, meringue pies	*Salmonella* species
Fish	Sushi with raw fish; ceviche	*Anisakis*; *Vibrio vulnificus*
Shellfish	Raw oysters	*Vibrio vulnificus*; norovirus
Milk and dairy products	Unpasteurized milk or cheeses made with unpasteurized milk	*Salmonella*; *Campylobacter jejuni*; *Listeria monocytogenes*
Produce	Raw sprouts such as alfalfa sprouts; cut tomatoes or melon; leafy salad greens; prepared salads	*E. coli* O157:H7; *Salmonella*; *Shigella*; norovirus
Cooked plant food	Rice; beans; tofu; potatoes or baked potato	*Bacillus cereus*; *Clostridium botulinum*

Sources: National Restaurant Association: *ServeSafe Coursebook*. 5th ed. Chicago: National Restaurant Association Solutions, LLC, 2008; FDA: *Annex 3–hazard analysis for managing food safety: A manual for the voluntary use of HACCP principles for operators of food service and retail establishments*, updated 2011. http://www.fda.gov/Food/FoodSafety/RetailFoodProtection/ManagingFoodSafetyHACCPPrinciples/Operators/ucm078069.htm.

19.3 Food-Borne Illness

LEARNING OUTCOMES

1 *Identify the typical signs and symptoms of food-borne illness.*

2 *Explain the difference between food-borne illness and food intoxication.*

3 *Describe high-risk populations for food-borne illness.*

Signs and symptoms of food−borne (and water−borne) illnesses generally involve the digestive tract and include nausea, vomiting, diarrhea, and intestinal cramps. Most pathogens have an **incubation period**, a length of time in which they grow and multiply in food or the digestive tract before they can cause illness. Incubation periods can range from 1 hour to several days. Thus, if a person develops signs and symptoms of a food−borne illness, he or she might have difficulty identifying the source of the illness.

Causes of Food-Borne Illness

Bacteria, viruses, tiny worms, and even chemicals can result in food−borne illness. Many kinds of food−borne pathogens infect the digestive tract, inflaming the tissues and causing an "upset stomach" within a few hours after being ingested. A few types of food−borne pathogens multiply in the human intestinal tract, enter the bloodstream, and cause general illness when they invade other tissues. These are examples of food−borne illnesses related to infection from the pathogen.

Other pathogens do not sicken humans directly. Instead, these organisms contaminate food and secrete toxins. **Toxins** are poisonous substances. In many instances, toxins cannot be visually detected or identified through tasting or smelling of the food, nor can toxins be destroyed through usual cooking or freezing methods. When the contaminated food is eaten, the toxins irritate the intestinal tract and cause a type of food−borne illness called **food intoxication** (or *food poisoning*). In some cases, food intoxication can lead to death.

In most cases, otherwise healthy individuals who suffer from common types of food−borne illness or intoxication recover completely and without professional

potentially hazardous foods foods that promote pathogen growth; these foods typically have high moisture content, neutral pH or low acidity levels, and/or high protein amounts

incubation period length of time in which bacteria can grow and multiply in food or the digestive tract before they cause illness

toxins poisonous substances produced by living organisms

food intoxication type of food-borne illness caused by toxins in the food or beverage

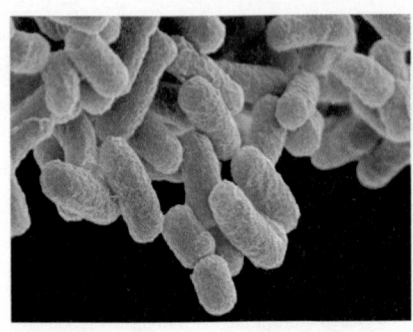

Escherichia coli *bacteria of the strain O157:H7, which is one of hundreds of strains of this bacterium. Although most strains are harmless and live in the intestines of healthy humans and animals, this strain produces a powerful toxin that can be deadly.*

medical care within a few days. However, vomiting, diarrhea, and other signs of illness can be so severe that the person requires hospitalization. A person should consult a physician when an intestinal disorder is accompanied by one or more of the following signs: fever (oral temperature above 101.5°F), bloody bowel movements, prolonged vomiting that reduces fluid intake, diarrhea that lasts more than 3 days, or dehydration.[4]

Differences Between Food-Borne Illness and "Stomach Flu"

Many people mistakenly report that they have the "stomach flu" when in reality they are suffering from a food– or water–borne illness. "Flu," or *influenza*, is an infectious disease caused by specific viruses that invade the respiratory tract. Influenza is characterized by coughing, fever, weakness, and body aches. In contrast, food–borne illness primarily affects the digestive system and not the respiratory system. Intestinal cramps, diarrhea, and vomiting are not typical signs and symptoms of influenza, especially in adults. Coughing is *not* a usual sign of a food–borne illness. Thus, it is inaccurate to call a bout of diarrhea and intestinal cramps the "stomach flu."

High-Risk Populations

A number of factors influence whether an individual becomes ill after consuming a food or beverage that has been contaminated with a pathogen or toxin. The number of pathogenic microbes in a food or the amount of toxin it contains can contribute to the risk and severity of a food–borne illness. Furthermore, individuals vary in their vulnerability to many food–borne pathogens, mainly due to differences in how their immune systems respond. In general, high–risk groups are pregnant women, very young children, older adults, and persons who suffer from serious chronic illnesses or weakened immune systems. Very young children typically have underdeveloped immune systems, increasing their susceptibility, whereas older adults can have decreased immune responses due to the aging process. In addition, older adults may produce less gastric acid, which can reduce their ability to kill any bacteria consumed in foods.[5]

listeriosis food-borne illness that results from ingesting *Listeria monocytogenes*

Listeria monocytogenes

The bacterial species *Listeria monocytogenes* is a pathogen that can be present in milk and dairy products that have not undergone proper pasteurization. The food–borne illness that results from ingesting *Listeria monocytogenes* is called **listeriosis**. Foods typically associated with listeriosis include raw milk; soft cheeses made from raw milk; raw, undercooked, and smoked seafood; and ready–to–eat processed meats, such as hot dogs, luncheon meats, or deli meats. A pregnant woman is 13 to 14 times more likely to contract listeriosis than is a nonpregnant woman.[6] According to CDC, about one in six of the individuals diagnosed with listeriosis are pregnant women.

Listeria bacteria can be passed from mother to her unborn offspring through the placenta and result in miscarriages, premature delivery, or serious health problems for the newborn.[7] Signs include fever and other nonspecific symptoms such as fatigue and aches. Because the bacterium is not destroyed by salt and other food preservatives, pregnant women should avoid eating foods that are not heated adequately.[7] Hot dogs and deli meats can be safely consumed as long as they have been heated until steaming, either in the oven or in a microwave oven.

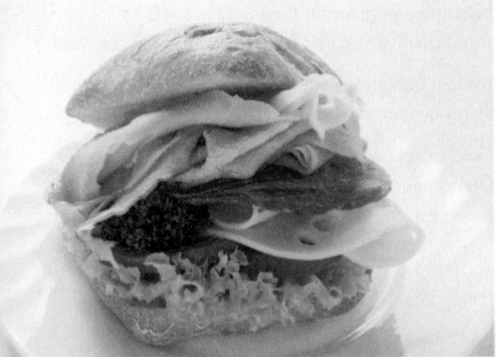

Pregnant women and other high-risk individuals should avoid eating deli meats unless they are thoroughly heated to the reduce risk of listeriosis.

DID YOU *KNOW?*

While a rare circumstance, commercial farmers and food producers can be held legally accountable for the safety of their foods. In 2013, two cantaloupe farmers were arrested and faced with criminal charges after the FDA and CDC found that their cantaloupes were not adequately cleaned before being sold to the public. The contaminated cantaloupes from a farm in Colorado were linked to a listeriosis outbreak in 2011 that sickened 147 people across 28 states and resulted in 33 deaths.[8]

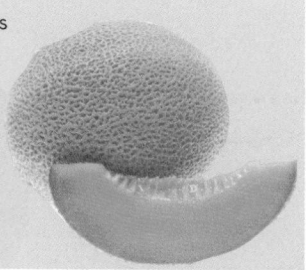

ASSESS YOUR PROGRESS

8 *Describe three typical signs and symptoms of food-borne illness.*

9 *Explain the difference between food-borne illness and food intoxication.*

10 *Explain why it is not appropriate to refer to diarrhea and intestinal cramps as the "stomach flu."*

11 *Identify four high-risk populations for food-borne illness.*

12 *Why do pregnant women need to be careful about consuming hot dogs and deli meats?*

19.4 Common Food-Borne Pathogens

LEARNING OUTCOMES

1 *Identify specific types of pathogens that cause food-borne illness.*

2 *Compare the effects of pathogenic bacteria, viruses, and protozoans when ingested as contaminants.*

3 *Describe characteristics of specific bacteria, viruses, and other pathogens that cause food-borne illness.*

bacteria single-cell microorganisms

The major kinds of food–borne pathogens are bacteria, viruses, and protozoa. Less common pathogens include toxins, produced by fungi or in seafood; tiny worms; and prions. In the United States, bacteria and viruses are responsible for most cases of food–borne illness (Fig. 19.2). The following sections provide information about some of the major pathogens that can cause food–borne illness.

Bacteria

Bacteria are single–cell microorganisms that do not have the complex array of organelles that plant and animal cells contain. While the majority of bacteria require foods with moist environments, warm temperatures, and a neutral pH to grow, some species of bacteria have more unusual needs. For example, certain pathogenic bacteria can live *anaerobically* (without oxygen), such as in canned or vacuum–packed foods (foods packaged by removing all the air from the container before sealing), whereas other types of bacteria grow well in the cold temperature of a refrigerator. There are even a few species of bacteria that can transform into inactive resistant forms called *spores* when their food environment is less than ideal. If the environment becomes more hospitable, the spores revert to the active bacterial state.

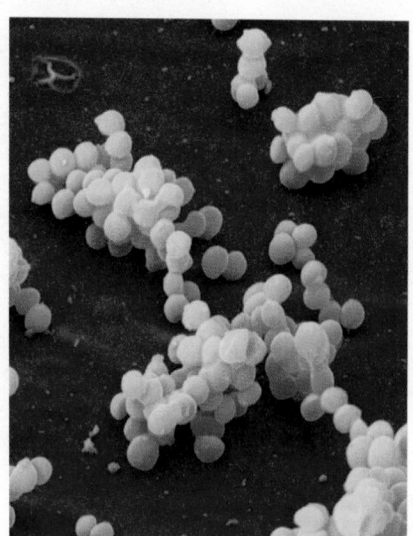

Improperly cooked or handled meat, poultry, eggs, and foods made with eggs are common sources of the bacterium Staphylococcus aureus.

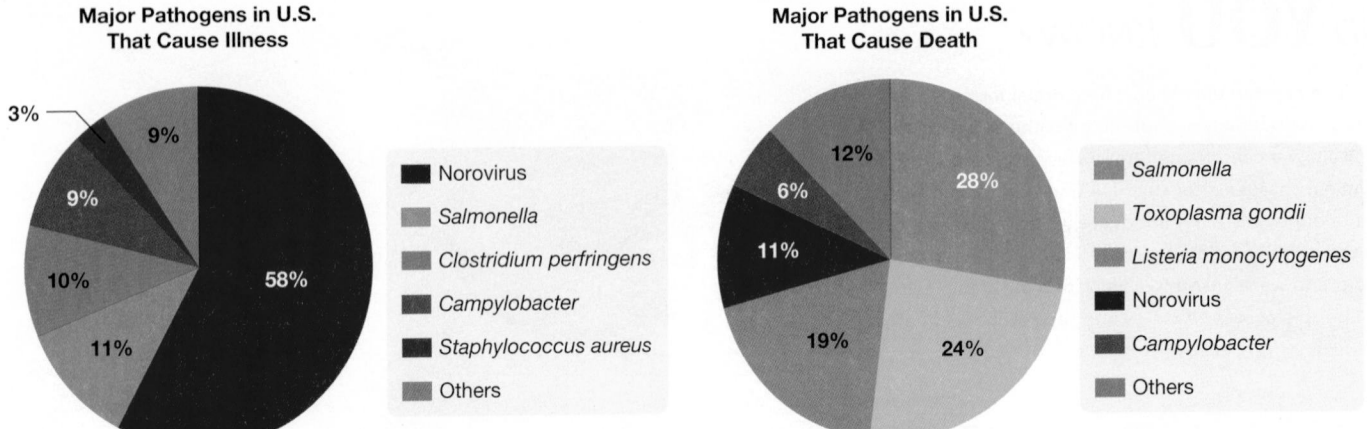

FIGURE 19.2 Major pathogens in the United States. These graphs illustrate the leading pathogens that cause food-borne illness and death in the United States.

Adapted from CDC: http://www.cdc.gov/foodborneburden/2011-foodborne-estimates.html

FRESH TIPS

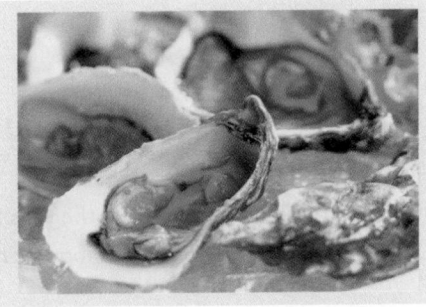

Have you ever heard the old saying that it's safe to eat raw oysters as long as there is an "R" in the month? *Vibrio vulnificus* bacteria thrive in warm coastal water, where they can contaminate oysters. However, 40% of cases of infection occur during the colder months, September through April, and the names of these months contain an "R."[9] Thus, raw oysters can be a source of food-borne illness throughout the year.

Once bacteria have contaminated a food source, they can grow and reproduce very quickly. Under the ideal conditions, bacterial concentrations in food can double every 20 minutes.[10] The majority of bacteria are killed when foods are heated properly, but toxins and even some spores can withstand the high temperatures of cooking.

Many kinds of bacteria are pathogens that cause food-borne illness, including forms of *Campylobacter*, *Clostridium*, *Escherichia*, *Listeria*, *Salmonella*, and *Staphylococcus* (*kam'−pih−low−bak'−ter, klo−strid'−e−um, esh'−ah−rik'−e−ah, lis−te'−re−ah, sal−mo−nell'−ah, staff'−il−lo−caw−kiss*). Table 19.2 summarizes some general information about common bacterial sources of food-borne illness in the United States.

virus microbe consisting of a piece of genetic material coated with protein

Viruses

Viruses are another common source of food-borne infection. A **virus** is simply a piece of genetic material coated with protein (Fig. 19.3). Viruses must invade a living cell to produce more viruses. Unlike certain bacteria, viruses do not secrete toxins, and therefore, they do not cause food intoxication. Contaminated food or water, however, can transmit viruses to humans and cause *food infection*. The most common virus-contaminated foods include shellfish, salads, and ready-to-eat foods. Table 19.3 summarizes the most common viruses found in foods.

Viruses are typically transmitted from person to person or person to food as a result of poor hygienic practices such as improper hand washing. Vaccines that

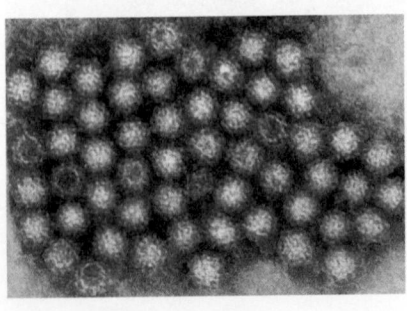

FIGURE 19.3 *Norovirus.*

protect against hepatitis A and rotaviral infections are available; however, one has not been developed yet for the norovirus, the leading cause of gastroenteritis in the United States.

TABLE 19.2 Common Food-Borne Pathogens: Bacteria

Bacterium	Potentially Hazardous Foods	Approximate Time of Onset	Typical Signs and Symptoms
Bacillus cereus (toxin)	Rice or other starchy foods; sauces, puddings, soups or casseroles; meats	30 minutes–15 hours	Watery diarrhea, abdominal cramps and pain, nausea, and vomiting
Campylobacter jejuni	Raw, undercooked poultry; unpasteurized milk or cheeses; contaminated water	2–5 days	Fever, diarrhea (often watery or bloody), abdominal cramps and pain, and vomiting
Clostridium botulinum (toxin)	Home-canned low-acid vegetables (corn, peppers, green beans, beets) and meats; vacuum-packed foods; garlic-in-oil mixtures; honey may contain spores that can infect infants	18–36 hours	Double or blurred vision, difficulty swallowing, and muscle weakness
Clostridium perfringens (toxin)	Improperly handled cooked meats or meat-containing foods	16 hours	Watery diarrhea and abdominal cramps
Escherichia coli O157:H7 (toxin)	Raw or undercooked beef and ground beef; unpasteurized milk and juices; bagged lettuces; alfalfa sprouts	1–9 days	Watery diarrhea with blood and severe abdominal cramps; may develop kidney failure
Listeria monocytogenes	Unpasteurized milk and cheeses; hot dogs and deli meats; raw and smoked fish; raw meats and poultry	3 hours–3 days Severe form: 3 days–3 months	Fever, muscle aches, nausea, and vomiting; severe form may impact nervous system
Salmonella species	Raw or undercooked meat, poultry, seafood, and eggs; raw produce (fruits and vegetables); unpasteurized juices	6–72 hours	Nausea, vomiting, abdominal cramps, diarrhea, fever, and headache
Shigella species	Contaminated water; raw produce and ready-to-eat foods; poor personal hygiene of food staff	8–50 hours	Diarrhea (often bloody), fever, and stomach cramps
Staphylococcus aureus (toxin)	Meats; poultry and eggs; prepared deli salads; cream-filled pastries	1–7 hours	Nausea, abdominal cramping, vomiting, and diarrhea
Vibrio vulnificus	Raw oysters and other seafood	12 hours	Fever, diarrhea, abdominal cramps, nausea, and vomiting; may result in septicemia (bacterial infection in blood)
Yersinia enterocolitica	Meats, especially undercooked pork; oysters, fish, and crabs; unpasteurized milk	1–11 days	Diarrhea, vomiting, fever, and abdominal pain

Source: U.S. Food and Drug Administration: *Bad bug book: Handbook of foodborne pathogenic microorganisms and natural toxins.* 2nd ed. 2012. http://www.fda.gov/Food/FoodborneIllnessContaminants/CausesOfIllnessBadBugBook/

TABLE 19.3 Common Food-Borne Pathogens: Viruses

Virus	Potentially Hazardous Foods	Approximate Time of Onset	Typical Signs and Symptoms
Norovirus	Salad ingredients or other ready-to-eat foods; fruits; oysters; contaminated swimming water	24–48 hours	Severe vomiting, watery diarrhea, abdominal cramps, and nausea
Rotavirus	Raw, undercooked poultry; unpasteurized milk or cheeses; contaminated water	48 hours	Diarrhea, vomiting, and fever
Hepatitis A virus (HAV)	Water; shellfish; salads; foods or water contaminated from feces	15–50 days	Fever, anorexia, nausea, vomiting, diarrhea, hepatitis, and sometimes jaundice

Source: U.S. Food and Drug Administration: *Bad bug book: Handbook of foodborne pathogenic microorganisms and natural toxins.* 2nd ed. 2012. http://www.fda.gov/Food/FoodborneIllnessContaminants/CausesOfIllnessBadBugBook/

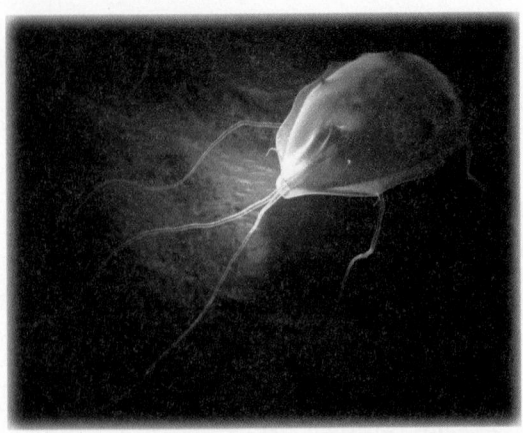

Giardia is a parasitic protozoan, a single-celled microorganism that has a more complex structure than bacteria.

Protozoa and Parasitic Worms

Protozoa are single-celled microorganisms with a complex cell structure. *Giardia (jee–ar'–de–ah)* and *Cryptosporidium (krip'–toe–spo–rid'–ee–um)* are examples of protozoa that are pathogenic to humans. Consumption of contaminated water and food, as well as contact with feces that contain protozoa, are the common routes of infection. Protozoa often live and reproduce in the tissues of their host, at times for an extended length of time before being detected. Diarrhea and other gastrointestinal symptoms are typical of infections from protozoa. For more information about common protozoa that infect food and water sources in the United States visit http://www.fda.gov/Food/FoodborneIllnessContaminants/CausesOfIllnessBadBugBook/.

The tiny parasitic worms that may contaminate food can cause muscle pain and malnutrition.[11] Most Americans who become infected with parasitic worms recover when they receive proper treatment. Nevertheless, some infected persons suffer long–term health problems and even die as a result of the illnesses. The FDA website has more information about parasitic worms that cause food–borne illness (http://www.fda.gov/Food/FoodborneIllnessContaminants/CausesOfIllnessBadBugBook).

FRESH TIPS

Travelers' diarrhea (TD) results from consuming contaminated food or water, typically when traveling in countries where sanitary water supplies are not always available. To reduce your risk of TD when traveling to high-risk areas, the CDC suggests:

- Carry alcohol-based hand sanitizer and thoroughly clean hands before eating;
- Avoid consuming food or beverages purchased from street vendors;
- Make sure meats are fully cooked before consuming;
- Avoid raw foods that have been washed in water before serving, such as fruits, vegetables, and salads;
- Avoid tap water, ice, and beverages made with ice;
- Consume beverages that are bottled and sealed, such as bottled water, bottled juices, and bottled alcoholic beverages; and
- Use bottled water to brush teeth, wash hands, and take medicine.

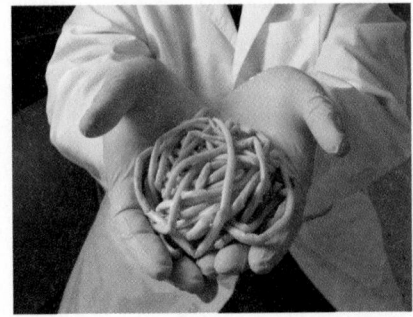

This mass of parasitic worms (Ascaris lumbricoldes) was in the feces of a child from Kenya, Africa. Initial infection typically occurs when people consume eggs in contaminated water or food. The worm then hatches and invades the mucosa of the human small intestine.

protozoa single-celled microorganisms that have complex cell structures

fungi simple organisms that live on dead or decaying organic matter

Toxins

As mentioned earlier, toxins are poisonous substances that can be produced naturally in foods by living organisms. Some pathogenic bacteria cause food intoxication by releasing toxins. In this section, we discuss other common sources of toxins in foods.

Fungal Toxins

Fungi, such as molds, yeast, and mushrooms, are simple life forms that live on dead or decaying organic matter. Certain fungi, including button mushrooms and the mold in blue cheese, are beneficial and edible. Other fungi are responsible for spoiling foods, such as bread molds, or causing respiratory problems or allergic reactions in sensitive people.[12]

A serious concern is the toxicity of several varieties of wild mushrooms. Cases of severe illness and even death have been reported as a result of people picking and eating toxic wild mushrooms after mistaking them for edible varieties (Fig. 19.4). Nevertheless, fungi are not a major source of food−borne intoxication in the United States.

Certain molds produce **aflatoxins**, substances that can cause severe illness, particularly liver damage, and even death when consumed. Tree nuts, peanuts, and corn that are stored under warm, humid conditions can become sources of aflatoxins. In some regions of the world, especially Africa and Southeast Asia, people often eat foods that are contaminated with aflatoxin−producing molds. Rates of liver cancer are high in these places. Thus, medical researchers think there is an association between ingestion of aflatoxins and development of liver cancer, presumably because the liver cannot excrete the toxins. No outbreaks of food−borne intoxication caused by aflatoxins have been reported in the U.S. population.[13]

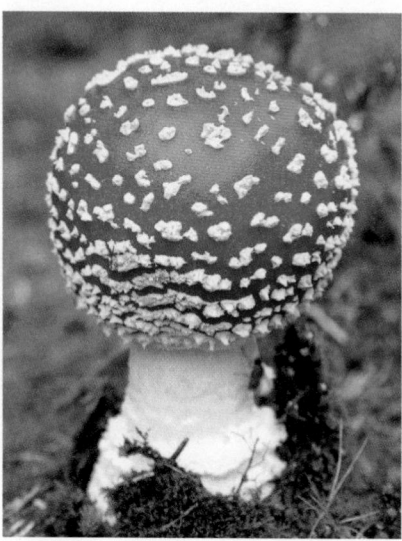

FIGURE 19.4 Deadly mushroom.
Poisonous fly agaric mushroom growing outdoors in autumn.

Seafood Toxins

Certain varieties of shellfish and fish, such as barracuda and grouper, are commonly associated with toxin−related food−borne illnesses. Some toxins are produced by specific types of marine algae (dinoflagellates) that accumulate in the flesh of fish or shellfish that consume the algae. **Scombrotoxin** results from the bacterial breakdown of fish tissue that has been improperly stored.[13] As bacteria begin to break down the protein in fish, *histamine* compounds are produced. When a person consumes the spoiled fish, the high levels of histamines from the fish tissue can cause an immune response that includes allergy−like symptoms such as headaches, diarrhea, itchy skin, and a rash.

Prions

Prions (*pree'−onz*) are similar to viruses in that they are not living organisms but rather infectious proteins that are folded improperly. Unlike typical food−borne pathogens that cause nausea, vomiting, and other gastrointestinal disorders, prions are responsible for *neurodegenerative* diseases (diseases that damage cells of the brain and spinal cord). Neurodegenerative diseases can occur in both animals and humans. The disease spreads when the abnormal, infectious proteins cause normal proteins to fold incorrectly.

The most notable prion disease is **bovine spongiform encephalopathy (BSE)**, otherwise known as "mad cow disease." When people consume certain tissues from infected cows, the humans may develop *variant Creutzfeldt−Jakob disease (vCJD)*. Fortunately, BSE is very rare in the United States due to strict food−safety regulations.[14]

aflatoxins substances produced from molds that can have toxic effects when consumed

scombrotoxin toxin that forms as a result of bacterial breakdown of fish tissue that has been improperly stored

prions infectious pathogens that are composed of misfolded proteins

bovine spongiform encephalopathy (BSE) neurodegenerative disease in cattle that is caused by prions; also referred to as "mad cow disease"

ASSESS YOUR PROGRESS

13 *List potentially hazardous foods at risk for carrying the following bacteria:* Clostridium botulinum, Listeria monocytogenes, *and* Vibrio vulnificus.

14 *Name at least two specific viruses that cause food-borne illness in the United States, along with potentially hazardous foods and major signs and symptoms of illness.*

15 *Identify two nonbacterial sources of toxins that may result in food-borne illness.*

16 *What do viruses and prions have in common? How are they different?*

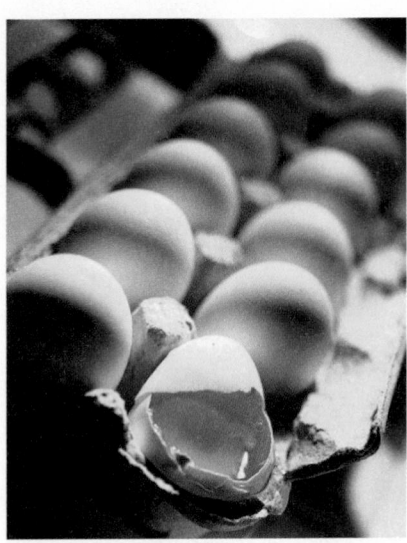

Before purchasing eggs, open the carton and inspect the eggs. Do not buy cartons that have any cracked eggs.

19.5 Preventing Food-Borne Illnesses

LEARNING OUTCOMES

1 *List strategies for proper food selection, including fresh produce, packaged foods, dairy, eggs, and meats and fish.*

2 *Explain why it is important to separate meat, fish, and poultry from other groceries.*

3 *Describe ways to avoid cross-contamination during food preparation.*

4 *Identify the temperature "danger zone" for potentially hazardous foods.*

5 *List strategies for proper food cooking, including of fresh produce and packaged foods, dairy, eggs, and meats and fish.*

In many instances, consumers cannot control the safety of foods that are prepared in restaurants or other places outside the home. However, consumers can greatly reduce the risk of food–borne illness by following some important rules at home, most of which require changing risky food selection, preparation, and storage practices.

Food Selection

Food selection guidelines emphasize selecting unexpired foods, purchasing fresh produce, and keeping cold or frozen foods at the proper temperature during transport home. To reduce the risk of food–borne illness:

Packaged and fresh perishable foods

- Check "best by" dates on packaged perishable foods. Choose meats and other animal products with the latest dates.

- Do not buy food in damaged containers; for example, avoid cans that leak, bulge, or are severely dented, or jars that are cracked or have loose or bulging lids.

Dairy and eggs

- Open egg cartons and examine eggs; do not buy cartons that have cracked eggs.

- Purchase only pasteurized milk and cheese, as well as fruit and vegetable juices (check the label).

- Store whole eggs in their cartons, even if the refrigerator has a place for storing eggs. Egg cartons are designed to keep eggs fresh longer than a refrigerator's egg compartment.

Meats, fish, and frozen foods

- When shopping in a supermarket, select frozen and cold foods last, especially potentially hazardous foods such as meats, poultry, dairy, or fish.

- Pack meat, fish, and poultry in separate plastic bags, so their drippings do not contaminate each other and other groceries.

- After shopping for food, take groceries home immediately. Refrigerate or freeze meat, fish, egg, and dairy products promptly.

Food Preparation

Even if individuals are careful when shopping, it is possible for foods to become contaminated during food preparation. The following sections describe

FRESH TIPS

Fruits that grow on the ground, such as cantaloupe and watermelon, can collect pathogens on their peels. Unlike many other fruits, however, cantaloupe is not very acidic. Thus, sliced cantaloupe is a good environment for bacteria to grow. To enjoy cantaloupe, be sure to purchase undamaged melons and scrub their peels with a clean, sturdy produce brush under running water before cutting. If purchasing precut cantaloupe, be sure it is refrigerated. Discard any cut cantaloupe if it has been left out at room temperature for longer than 2 hours.

several aspects of food preparation as they apply to the safety of packaged or canned foods, fresh produce, and animal foods, including the potential for cross—contamination.

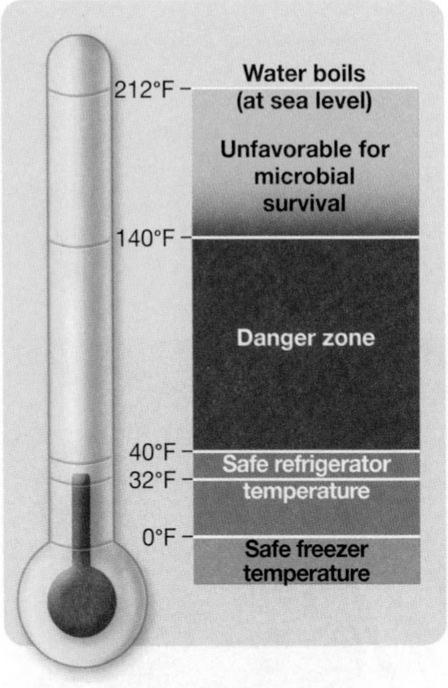

Canned Foods and Fresh Produce

It is often helpful for consumers to use common sense when evaluating the safety of canned foods and fresh produce. To reduce the risk of food—borne illness:

- Do not use foods from containers that have damaged safety seals, because the food they contain may have been contaminated.

- Do not taste or use food that spurts liquid or has a bad odor when the can or jar is opened.

- Before preparing fresh produce, carefully wash the foods under running water to remove dirt and bacteria clinging to the surface.

- Avoid eating moldy foods. Small amounts of mold on hard cheeses and on firm fruits and vegetables can be removed by cutting away the mold along with at least 1 inch of food that surrounds the moldy area.[12] If mold is too extensive, discard the entire food.

- When in doubt, throw the food out.

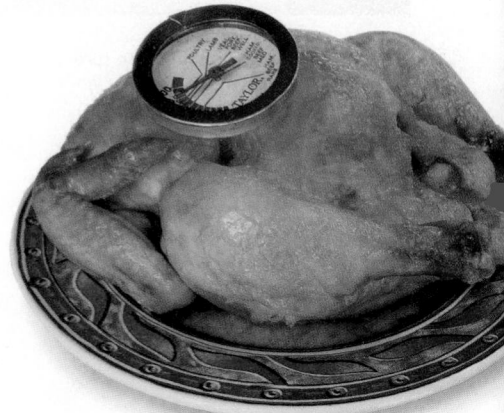

FIGURE 19.5 Temperature guide for food safety.

Maintaining Proper Temperature of Foods

Most microbes grow well when the temperature of a potentially hazardous food is between 40°F and 140°F—the "danger zone" (Fig. 19.5).[15] Cooking foods to the proper temperature destroys food—borne pathogens, such as norovirus and *E. coli* O157:H7. To be safe, a product must be cooked to an internal temperature that is high enough to destroy harmful pathogens and certain bacterial toxins. Using a meat thermometer is a reliable way to ensure that meat, poultry, thick pieces of fish, and egg—containing dishes have reached the proper internal temperature without overcooking.

When removing veal, beef, lamb, or pork from the oven or grill, allow it to "rest" for 3 minutes before carving. While the meat "rests," its temperature remains constant or rises slightly, helping to kill microorganisms. Table 19.4 indicates recommended minimum internal temperatures for cooking these foods. Check out the "Test Kitchen" recipe for a safe and healthy Broccoli and Cheddar Cheese Quiche at the end of this chapter.

Meat thermometers must be used properly to give accurate values. In general, the thermometer should be placed in the thickest part of the muscle tissue, away from bone, fat, or gristle (Fig. 19.6). If the thermometer is inserted incorrectly

FIGURE 19.6 Meat thermometer. Using a meat (or food) thermometer is a reliable way to ensure that the cooked item has reached the proper internal temperature.

TABLE 19.4 USDA Recommended Safe Minimum Internal Temperatures

Beef, pork, and lamb steaks or roasts	145°F
Ground beef, pork, or lamb	160°F
Poultry (whole or ground)	165°F
Eggs	160°F
Seafood	145°F
Casseroles, stuffing, or other mixed dishes	165°F

Source: U.S. Department of Agriculture: Fact Sheets: Safe food handling: Safe minimum internal temperature chart. Last modified: October 16, 2012. http://www.fsis.usda.gov/factsheets/Safe_Minimum_Internal_Temperature_Chart/index.asp

or placed in the wrong area, the reading may not accurately reflect the internal temperature of the product. The following information includes some guidelines for proper heating of foods. To reduce the risk of food−borne illness:

Packaged and fresh perishable foods

- Give picnic foods special attention, because outdoor temperatures may favor rapid bacterial growth. Keep cold salads and desserts on ice. Meats should be cooked completely at a picnic site. Do not partially cook foods in advance and plan to finish cooking them at the picnic.

Meat, fish, and eggs

- Cook beef, poultry, pork, thick pieces of fish, and egg−containing dishes thoroughly, using a meat thermometer to check for doneness.

- Cook eggs until the yolk and white have solidified and no runniness remains.

- Properly cooked seafood should not be shiny but be firm and flake easily when touched with a fork.

- Bake stuffing separately from poultry, or alternatively, wash the poultry cavity thoroughly and stuff the bird immediately before cooking. Do not stuff the bird ahead of time, because bacteria will have more chance to grow. Make sure the temperature of the stuffing reaches 165°F during cooking. After cooking, transfer the stuffing to a clean bowl for serving or storage.

- Serve meat, poultry, and fish on a clean plate.

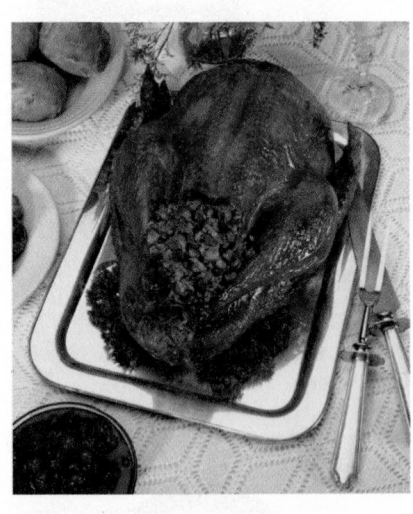

When cooking stuffed poultry, be sure the stuffing also reaches 165°F to kill any potential bacteria that might have transferred from the meat to the stuffing.

Microwave Cooking

Microwave cooking can result in uneven heating that does not destroy microbes in the cool spots. While cooking a food in a microwave oven, keep the dish cov−ered, and stop the oven occasionally to stir the food. Stirring the food reduces uneven heating. Cook the food until it reaches 165°F. Microwave cooking is not recommended for stuffed foods, because during cooking, the temperature of the stuffing may not be high enough to kill pathogens.[16]

Chilling Foods

Chilling food, when done appropriately, slows the growth of microbes in the items, but some bacteria can grow even at proper refrigeration temperatures. To chill correctly, foods should be divided into shallow containers and cooled rapidly to less than 40°F. Freezing does not kill bacteria or inactivate viruses in food; the process just halts the microbes' ability to multiply. As frozen food thaws, the bacteria and viruses resume their activities and can cause illness.

Keeping Hot Foods Hot and Cold Foods Cold

A major challenge for food handlers involves keeping large amounts of high−risk foods at safe temperatures when they are served from a single container. Food that is near the sides of the container may stay hotter or colder than food that is near or in the center of the container. As shown in Figure 19.7, chilled foods should be kept covered and served from a shallow container filled with ice. Hot foods should be kept covered and be served from shallow, heated pans.

The best simple advice to follow is, "Keep hot foods hot and cold foods cold." To reduce the risk of food−borne illness:

- Always thaw high−risk foods in the refrigerator, under cold running water, or in a microwave oven.

- Cook foods immediately after thawing.

- Marinate food in the refrigerator, and if marinating meat, fish, or poultry, discard the marinade.

- Do not remove cold foods from the refrigerator or hot foods from the stove until it is time to serve them.

Preventing Cross-Contamination

Cross—contamination is the passing of contaminants from one food to another. The most frequent cause of cross—contamination is failure to wash hands and kitchen tools during food preparation. To reduce the risk of food—borne illness:

Hands

- Wash hands thoroughly with very warm, soapy water for at least 20 seconds before and after touching food. If clean water for hand washing is not available, use sanitizing hand wipes.

- If you are preparing more than one type of food, such as cutting up chicken and dicing carrots, wash hands in between.

- Use a fresh paper towel or clean hand towel to dry hands. Reserve dish towels for drying pots, pans, and cooking utensils that are not washed and dried in a dishwasher.

Surfaces

- Before preparing food, clean food preparation surfaces, including kitchen counters, cutting boards, dishes, knives, and other food preparation equipment, with hot, soapy water.

- Sanitize food preparation surfaces and equipment that have come in contact with raw meat, fish, poultry, and eggs as soon as possible. *Sanitizing* is a process that uses heat or chemicals to destroy pathogens. Most pathogens on surfaces can be killed by using a sanitizing solution made by adding a tablespoon of bleach to 1 gallon of cool water.[17] However, avoid getting bleach solution on colored fabrics or surfaces that can be damaged by bleach (granite, for example).

Cutting boards

- The FDA recommends using cutting boards with unmarred surfaces made of easy—to—clean, nonporous materials, such as plastic, marble, or glass. If you prefer to use wooden cutting boards, make sure they are made of a nonabsorbent hardwood, such as oak or maple, and have no obvious seams or cracks.

- Replace cutting boards when they become streaked with cuts, because these grooves can be difficult to clean thoroughly and may harbor bacteria.

- If possible, have a cutting board reserved for meats, fish, and poultry; another cutting board for fruits and vegetables; and a third board for breads.

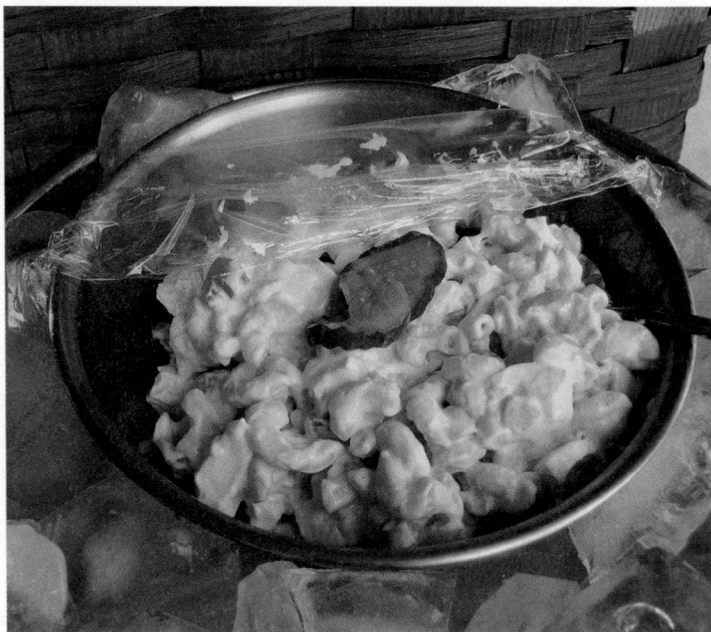

FIGURE 19.7 Keep cold foods cold. Chilled foods, especially picnic items, should be kept covered, in a shallow container, and placed in another container that is filled with ice.

DID **YOU** *KNOW?*

More is not always better, especially when it comes to using chlorine bleach as a sanitizer for items in contact with food. Chlorine is the ingredient in bleach that effectively eliminates pathogens, yet the chemical can also be very toxic and dangerous if used in excess of 1 tablespoon per gallon of cool water. Additionally, only *regular* bleach is safe to use for sanitizing equipment and surfaces in food service settings. Bleaches that contain fragrances, thickeners (i.e., "no-splash"), and other additives are not safe to use in the kitchen and should be limited to use in cleaning other areas of a house or food service operation.

FRESH TIPS

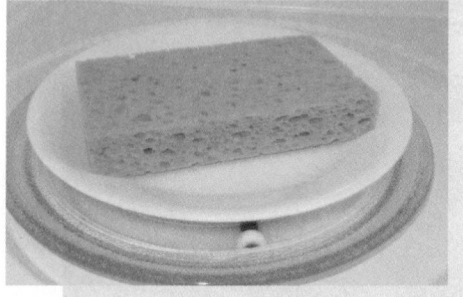

Utensils and other equipment

- Do not reuse cooking utensils such as tongs, knives, or spoons that have previously touched raw meat, fish, poultry, or eggs unless they have been sanitized first.

- Sanitize kitchen sponges and wash kitchen towels frequently.

Raw Fish

Eating raw fish, such as in sushi, can be safe for most healthy people if the fish is very fresh before being commercially frozen and then thawed. While frozen, the fish must maintain an internal temperature of −4°F or less for at least 7 days.[19] The freezing step is important because very cold temperatures can kill pathogenic worms that are often in fish tissues. If a person chooses to eat uncooked fish, it should be purchased from reputable establishments that have high standards for quality and sanitation. Nevertheless, it is a good idea to avoid eating any raw animal products, including fish.

Ground Meats, Poultry, and Cooked Fish

Ground meats, poultry, and fish are highly perishable and must be thoroughly cooked to avoid being a source of food−borne illness. The interior portion of an intact piece of raw animal flesh is normally free of bacteria, because the tissues are not exposed to air. However, ground meats, fish, and poultry products are often contaminated with microbes.

Prior to being ground up, the surface of a chunk of meat, fish, or poultry may contain relatively harmless concentrations of pathogens. The grinding process, however, mixes the pathogens throughout the meat. At the same time, grinding the meat greatly increases its surface area, exposing more of the protein−rich tissues to microbes in air. Furthermore, the meat grinder can be a source of pathogens and spread them to the food product, especially if the machine was not properly cleaned after its last use. The particles of food that remained in the grinder can provide food for pathogenic microorganisms. Therefore, surfaces that touch ground meats should be cleaned carefully.

Storing and Reheating Food

After food is cooked, careless food handling continues to set the stage for the growth of pathogens. Food−borne pathogens thrive at "room temperature," temperatures that are between 60°F and 110°F. Although it is common practice in many homes to leave food in serving dishes and on the table for several hours after meals, to be safe, cover leftovers and refrigerate or freeze them as soon as people have finished eating, or within 2 hours. If environmental temperatures are above 90°F, refrigerate the leftovers within 1 hour.[20]

Before storing, separate the food into as many shallow pans as needed to provide a large surface area for faster cooling. There is no need to let hot foods cool on a counter before chilling or freezing them. To reduce the risk of food−borne illness, follow these food storage tips:

- Check the refrigerator's temperature regularly to make sure it stays below 41°F. Keep the refrigerator as cold as possible without freezing milk and lettuce.

- Cook ground meats and poultry soon after purchasing. If this is not possible, freeze the ground items.

- Note that raw fish, shellfish, and poultry are highly perishable. It is best to cook these foods or freeze them the day they are purchased.

- Use refrigerated ground meat and patties within 1 to 2 days, and use frozen meat and patties within 3 to 4 months after purchasing them.

- Use refrigerated leftovers within 4 days.

- Reheat leftovers to 165°F; reheat gravy to a rolling boil to kill pathogenic bacteria that may be present.

Table 19.5 presents recommended time limits for refrigeration and freezer storage of foods. Foods that are stored in the freezer for longer periods often develop unappealing flavors. Note that ground meats are more perishable than intact cuts of meat.

Cross–contamination is a threat not only during food preparation, but also during food storage. Therefore, keep all foods, including leftovers, covered while they are in the refrigerator. This practice can prevent drippings from foods that are often contaminated, such as raw chicken, from tainting other foods. Furthermore, store raw meats, fish, poultry, and shellfish on lower shelves of the refrigerator, so they are separated from foods that are to be eaten raw. Examine Figure 19.8. Are there at least two examples of improperly stored refrigerated foods?

TABLE 19.5 Cold Storage Time Limits for Perishable Foods

Product	Storage Period in Refrigerator (40°F)	Storage Period in Freezer (0°F)
Fresh meat		
Ground meat	1–2 days	3–4 months
Steaks and roasts	3–5 days	4–12 months
Fresh pork		
Chops	3–5 days	4–12 months
Ground	1–2 days	3–4 months
Roasts	3–5 days	4–12 months
Cured meats		
Luncheon meat, open package	3–5 days	—
Unopened package	2 weeks	—
Sausage	1–2 days	1–2 months
Fresh fish	1–2 days	—
Fresh chicken or turkey (whole)	1–2 days	12 months
Parts	1–2 days	9 months
Giblets	1–2 days	3–4 months
Dairy products		
Cheese (swiss, brick, processed cheese)	3–4 weeks	(Not recommended)
Milk	5 days	—
Eggs		
Fresh, in shell	3–5 weeks	—
Hard-cooked	1 week	—

Source: USDA, FSIS: Kitchen companion. 2008. http://www.fsis.usda.gov/PDF/Kitchen_Companion.pdf; *Freezing and food safety.* 2013. http://www.fsis.usda.gov/wps/portal/fsis/topics/food-safety-education/get-answers/food-safety-fact-sheets/safe-food-handling/freezing-and-food-safety/ct_index Accessed: February 9, 2014

FIGURE 19.8 Storing risky foods in the refrigerator. In this photograph, are there at least two risky foods that are stored improperly? What could be done to store these foods safely?

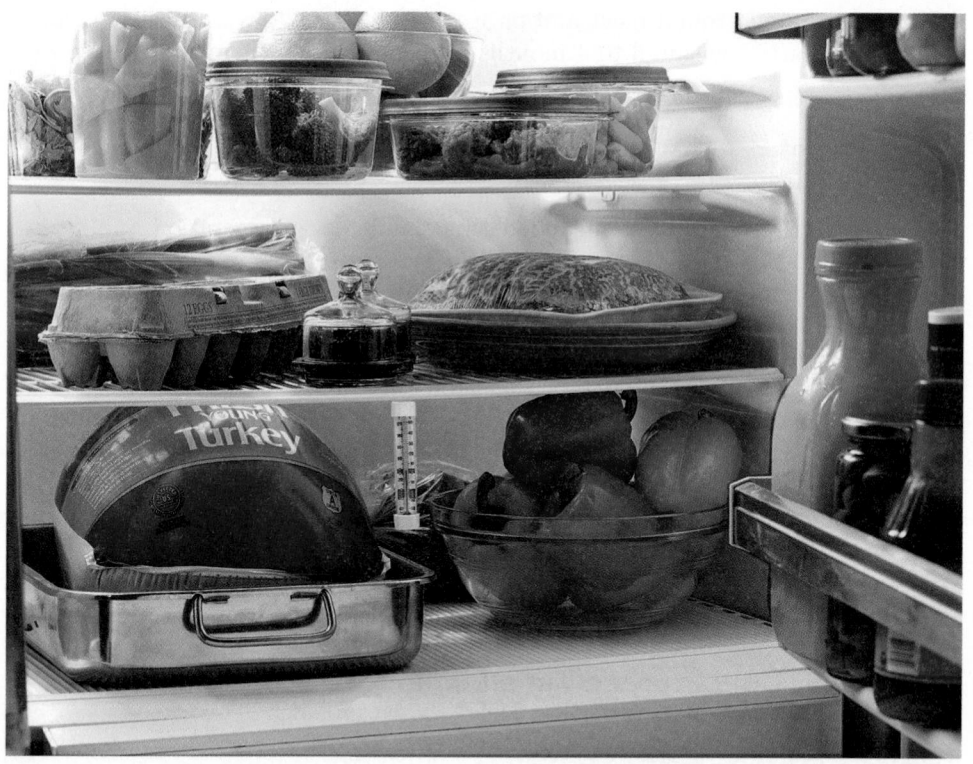

Check Your Steps Program

Food safety educators with the federal government condensed food safety rules into four simple actions for consumers to utilize as a part of their Check Your Steps program (see www.foodsafety.gov):

1. ***Clean:*** Wash hands and surfaces often.

2. ***Separate:*** Do not cross–contaminate.

3. ***Cook:*** Cook to proper temperatures.

4. ***Chill:*** Refrigerate promptly.

In addition to the Check Your Steps website, reliable information about food–borne illness is available at www.homefoodsafety.org. For general food safety questions, consumers can call the FDA's food safety hotline at 1–888–723–3366.

ASSESS YOUR PROGRESS

17. List at least three ways to reduce the risk of food-borne illness when selecting foods.

18. What are five ways to reduce food-borne illness caused by canned foods and fresh produce?

19. List at least three guidelines for the proper heating of foods, including fresh perishable foods, meat or fish, and eggs.

20. Identify the temperature range of the "danger zone," and explain why foods should not remain in this temperature for long.

21. Your friend says she uses only one cutting board for preparing a meal because it's easier to clean up afterward. What suggestions would you make to help her avoid food-borne illness?

19.6 Food Preservation

LEARNING OUTCOMES

1 *List methods of preserving food.*

2 *Describe canning and food irradiation as food-preservation techniques.*

3 *Identify the main bacterium of concern in home-canned foods.*

If nothing is done to preserve a fresh food, the item soon undergoes various chemical changes that eventually result in spoilage. Preserving food extends its shelf life. **Shelf life** refers to the period of time that a food can be stored before it spoils. Techniques to preserve food include heating, chilling or freezing, drying, and fermenting. This section of the chapter provides information about common food preservation methods.

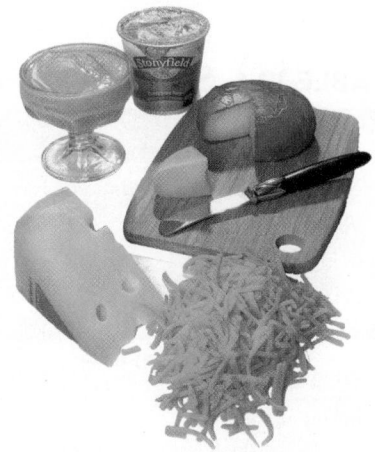

Fermentation is used to produce foods such as yogurt and cheese.

Food Preservation Techniques

Heating is one of the oldest ways to preserve foods. Heat can kill or deactivate pathogens, and the process also destroys naturally occurring enzymes in foods that can contribute to food spoilage. **Fermentation** is another ancient method of food preservation that is still used to produce a variety of foods, including yogurt, wine, cheese, and sauerkraut. The fermentation process involves adding certain bacteria or yeast to food. These microbes use sugars in the food to make acids and alcohol, chemicals that hinder the growth of other types of bacteria and yeast that can spoil food.

For centuries, people preserved meats, fruits, and other foods that had high water contents by adding salt or sugar to them. Adding sugar or salt to foods draws water out of cells, including cells of bacteria, fungi, protozoa, and worms. As a result, these pathogens are less likely to survive in sugary or salty foods. Drying of foods reduces their water content, making it difficult for pathogens to grow due to the absence of moisture. Dried fruits such as raisins, for example, have a longer shelf life than grapes, their natural counterparts.

Today, we can add pasteurization, refrigeration, freezing, canning, irradiation, additives, and *aseptic processing* to the list of food preservation techniques (Table 19.6). Aseptic processing involves sterilizing a food and its package separately, before the food enters the package. The **sterilization** process destroys all microorganisms and viruses, as compared to pasteurization, which is a less extensive heating process that kills most pathogens. After undergoing aseptic packaging, boxes of sterile foods and beverages, such as milk or juices (Fig. 19.9), can remain free of microbial growth for several years while sitting on supermarket or pantry shelves. However, once the containers of these products are opened, the foods or beverages have the same shelf life as their counterparts that have not undergone aseptic processing.

shelf life period of time that a food can be stored before it spoils

fermentation process used to preserve or produce a variety of foods

sterilization process that kills or destroys all microorganisms and viruses

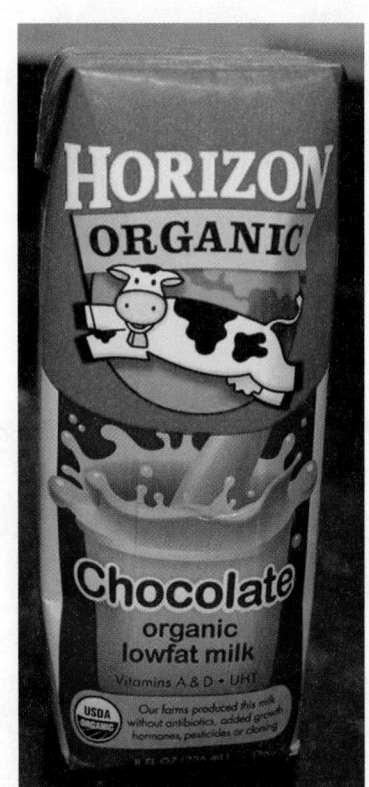

FIGURE 19.9 Aseptic packaging. Aseptically packaged milk, when stored at room temperature, can stay fresh for up to 7 months without needing refrigeration or preservatives due to the lack of bacteria in the milk.

Canned Foods

When food is canned, commercial food production methods require heating the food to certain temperatures for specified times. Thus, unless the can or jar has been damaged, properly processed canned foods should be free of pathogens. Certain home–canned foods, however, may contain the microorganism *Clostridium botulinum* (*C. botulinum*) that produces the botulism toxin. The home–canning process may kill *C. botulinum* bacteria in the food, but their spores or toxin may remain. That is why home–canned, *low–acid* foods such as beans and corn should be boiled for 10 minutes before eating to destroy any toxin. Foods made with vinegar, tomatoes, or citrus juices are usually high–acid foods, and as a result, such items are not likely to be sources of *C. botulinum*.

TABLE 19.6 Summary of Food Preservation Methods

Method	Means of Effectiveness	Examples of Foods
Heating (cooking, pasteurization, aseptic processing)	Kills or deactivates pathogens; destroys enzymes that result in food spoilage	Most foods, dairy products
Adding salt or sugar	Binds water, decreasing amount available for microbes	Ham, bacon, jellies or preserves, pickled foods
Smoking	Kills spoilage microbes; destroys enzymes that result in food spoilage	Meats, fish
Curing	Retards growth of *Clostridium botulinum* and stabilizes the flavor of the food	Luncheon meats, smoked fish
Chilling or freezing	Slows molecular movement, retarding microbial and enzymatic activity	Most foods
Drying (dehydration)	Removes much of the moisture in food that microbes need to survive	Fruits, herbs, meat jerkies, seeds
Fermenting	Produces acids and alcohol that interfere with the survival of unwanted microbes	Alcoholic beverages, yogurt, cheeses, soy sauce
Canning	Kills spoilage microbes; destroys enzymes in food that result in spoilage; removes oxygen that certain microbes need to survive	Meat, fish, poultry, fruits, vegetables, milk
Irradiating	Destroys most pathogens; delays sprouting (potatoes)	Spices, raw meat and poultry, fresh fruits and vegetables

Sources: Pacific Northwest Extension: *Smoking fish at home—safely.* PNW 238, 2009. extension.oregonstate.edu/ http://cru.cahe.wsu.edu/cepublications/pnw238/pnw238.pdf; National Center for Home Food Preservation: *USDA complete guide to home canning, 2009 revision.* http://www.uga.edu/nchfp/publications/publications_usda.html.

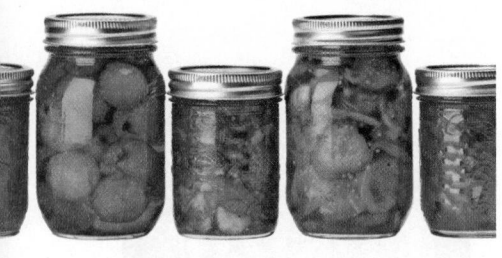

Certain home-canned foods can be a potential source of Clostridium botulinum.

Nevertheless, any home—canned food should be discarded if the lid has lost its seal or has "popped up."

The *C. botulinum* toxin is highly poisonous even in tiny amounts; never taste a home—canned, low—acid food before boiling it. For more information about proper home canning of foods, obtain a copy of the U.S. Department of Agriculture's *Complete Guide to Home Canning* (http://www.uga.edu/nchfp/publications/publications_usda.html) or contact a food and nutrition specialist at your community's university extension office.

Irradiation

The process of food irradiation preserves food by using a high amount of energy (ionizing radiation) to kill pathogens such as *Salmonella* and *E. coli* O157:H7 (Fig. 19.10). These methods do not make the items radioactive. The energy passes through the food, as in microwave cooking, and no radioactive material is left behind. The energy is strong enough to destroy the genetic material as well as cell membranes or cell walls of insects and microbes. As a result, irradiation is a highly effective way of killing insects, bacteria, protozoa, and worms that may be in foods. Irradiation, however, is not an effective way to destroy viruses or prions that may have contaminated food.[21] Furthermore, irradiated foods, especially meats, can still become contaminated once their packaging has been opened.

Irradiation extends the shelf life of spices, meats, poultry, certain shellfish, seeds, shell eggs, and fresh fruits and vegetables.[22] Except for dried season—ings, packages that contain irradiated foods must be labeled with the interna—tional food irradiation symbol, the Radura, and include a statement indicating the product has been treated by irradiation (Fig. 19.11).

Irradiation of food is not a new technology; in 1963, U.S. food manufactur—ers were given approval to irradiate wheat flour. Today, France, Canada, the Netherlands, and China are among the countries that use irradiation to pre—serve various foods.[23] Nevertheless, some consumer groups claim that irradiation diminishes the nutritional value of food and leads to the formation of harmful compounds, such as carcinogens, cancer—causing substances. According to med—ical experts with the World Health Organization, FDA, and CDC, irradiated

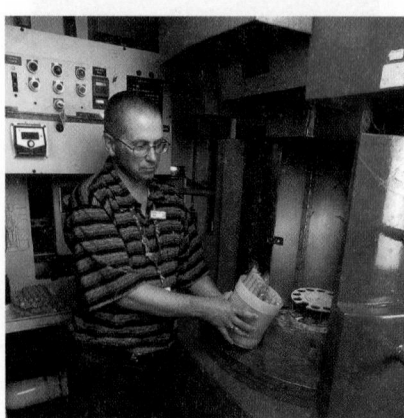

FIGURE 19.10 Irradiating food. U.S. Department of Agriculture microbiologist Glenn Boyd places a batch of hot dogs into the gamma radiation source to rid them of food-borne pathogens.

foods are safe to eat.[21] Furthermore, irradiation causes few or no nutritive losses because foods are not heated during the process. Despite such assurances, many Americans are skeptical about the safety of irradiated foods, and they avoid purchasing such products.

FIGURE 19.11 Radura symbol. The Radura symbol on a food package indicates that the food has been treated with irradiation.

ASSESS YOUR PROGRESS

22 *Identify four methods of food preservation, and explain how each method extends the shelf life of foods.*

23 *What specific bacterium is of concern in home-canned foods?*

24 *Explain how food irradiation preserves foods and extends shelf life.*

19.7 Food Additives

LEARNING OUTCOMES

1 *Differentiate between intentional and unintentional food additives, and give examples of each.*

2 *Explain the acronym GRAS.*

3 *Discuss the Delaney Clause and its impact on food additives.*

4 *Define accidental food contaminants and give examples.*

5 *Identify common categories of pesticides that can contaminate foods.*

food additive any substance that becomes incorporated into food during production, packaging, transport, or storage

intentional additive food additive added purposefully by a food manufacturer to enhance the food

color additives dyes, pigments, or other substances that provide color to food

indirect or **unintentional food additives** substances that are accidently in foods

A **food additive** is any substance that becomes incorporated into food during production, packaging, transport, or storage. Food manufacturers incorporate direct or **intentional additives** into their products for a variety of reasons, including making the food easier to process, more nutritious, able to stay fresh longer, or better tasting. Most additives are added to influence a food's sensory characteristics, including taste or color.

Intentional and Unintentional Food Additives

Many intentional food additives help maintain the safety of foods by limiting the growth of bacteria that cause food–borne illness. Other additives protect against the action of enzymes that can lead to undesirable changes in the food's color and taste. These unwanted chemical changes occur when enzymes that are naturally present in certain foods are exposed to the oxygen in air. Antioxidant additives, including vitamins E and C and a variety of sulfites, can prevent oxygen from reacting with these enzymes. **Color additives** include dyes, pigments, or other substances that provide color to foods, drugs, or cosmetics, such as beta–carotene in margarine and FD&C (Food, Drug, & Cosmetic) Red No. 40 in cherry–flavored cough syrup. Table 19.7 lists common types of direct food additives (including color additives), their uses, examples of products that contain the additives, and names of specific additives.

Indirect or **unintentional food additives**, such as compounds from a food's wrapper or container, can enter food as it is packaged, transported, or stored. Indirect additives, however, have no purpose. The FDA and certain international organizations regulate *all* food additives to ensure that processed foods and their packaging are safe.[24]

Food Safety Legislation: Food Additives

By the 1950s, hundreds of ingredients were being added to foods during process–ing. Many of these substances had long histories of being safe; others were deemed

DID YOU KNOW?

Some natural color additives come from interesting and unusual sources. Beets contain pigments that can be used to add pink or red color to foods. Annatto is a yellow or orange coloring made from the seeds of the achiote tree, a tropical plant. Cochineal extract and carmine are red dyes that are extracted from cochineal, an insect (*Dactylopius coccus*).

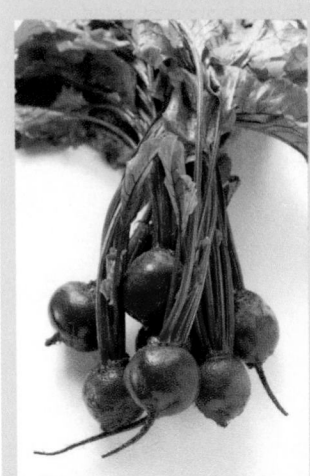

Beets

TABLE 19.7 Common Types of Direct Food Additives

Type of Additive	Functions	Typical Products	Examples of Specific Ingredients
Preservatives	Prevent food spoilage	Jellies, beverages, baked goods, cured meats, cereals, snack foods	Ascorbic acid, citric acid, sodium benzoate, calcium propionate, sodium erythorbate, BHA, BHT, EDTA, sulfites
Sweeteners	Add sweetness	Processed foods, beverages, baked goods, sugar substitutes	Sucrose, glucose, mannitol, corn syrup, aspartame, sucralose
Flavors and spices	Add specific flavors	Puddings, pie fillings, gelatins, cake mixes, candies, soft drinks	Natural flavorings, artificial flavorings, spices
Flavor enhancers	Enhance flavors already present	Snack foods	Monosodium glutamate (MSG), hydrolyzed soy protein
Nutrients	Replace nutrients lost during processing, boost levels of nutrients naturally in food	Flour, grains, cereals, margarine, juice, energy bars	Thiamine hydrochloride, riboflavin, niacin, niacinamide, folic acid, beta-carotene, ascorbic acid
Emulsifiers	Keep oily and watery ingredients from separating	Salad dressings, peanut butter, chocolate, frozen desserts	Soy lecithin, mono- and diglycerides, polysorbates
Leavening agents	Promote rising of certain baked goods	Baked goods	Baking soda, monocalcium phosphate, calcium carbonate
Stabilizers, thickeners, binders	Provide uniform texture and improve "mouth feel"	Frozen desserts, puddings, sauces	Gelatin, pectin, guar gum, carrageenan
Color additives	Enhance natural colors, provide color to colorless and "fun" foods as well as to medications and cosmetics	Processed foods, including candies, snack foods, margarine, cheese, soft drinks, gelatin, drug capsules, cough syrup, lipstick	FD&C Blue No. 1, FD&C Red No. 40, beta-carotene, caramel color

Source: International Food Information Council and U.S. Food and Drug Administration: *Food ingredients & colors.* 2010. http://www.foodinsight.org/Resources/Detail.aspx?topic=Food_Ingredients_Colors

Food Additives Amendment U.S. legislation that requires evidence that a new food additive is safe before it can be marketed for use

Generally Recognized as Safe (GRAS) ingredients thought to be safe

Delaney Clause component of the 1958 Food Additives Amendment that prevents manufacturers from adding carcinogenic compounds to foods

safe after undergoing scientific testing. In 1958, the U.S. Congress enacted the **Food Additives Amendment**. According to this amendment, an ingredient that had been in use prior to 1958 was **Generally Recognized as Safe (GRAS)** when qualified experts generally agreed that the substance was safe for its intended use. The Food Additives Amendment excluded GRAS substances from being defined as food additives.[25] Thus, modern food manufacturers can use substances on the GRAS list as ingredients without testing them for safety or getting prior approval from the FDA. Examples of GRAS substances include sucrose, acetic acid, caffeine, and guar gum.[26]

As a result of the 1958 Food Additives Amendment, the manufacturer of a *new* food additive (one developed after 1958) must provide evidence of the substance's safety to the FDA before the additive can be used.[27] When evaluating the safety of a newly developed food additive, FDA experts consider the chemical composition and characteristics of the substance, the amount of the substance that Americans would typically ingest, and the additive's effects on the body. If the additive is safe in amounts that people are likely to consume, FDA experts establish a level of the substance that can be added to foods.

According to the **Delaney Clause** of the Food Additives Amendment, food manufacturers cannot add a new compound that causes cancer at *any* level of intake. Thus, if an additive causes cancer, even though very high doses may be necessary to cause the disease, no amount of the additive is considered to be safe, and none is allowed in food. Evidence for cancer risk could come from either laboratory animal or human studies. The FDA allows very few exceptions to this clause.

The FDA cannot ban unintentional food additives—which include various industrial chemicals, pesticide residues, and mold toxins—from foods, even though some of these contaminants may be carcinogenic. The Food Quality Protection Act of 1996 established the safety standard of "a reasonable certainty of no harm" for pesticide residues in foods. As a result of this act, the "no risk" provision of the Delaney Clause does not apply to pesticide residues. However, the Delaney Clause remains in effect for food additives.[28] The following section discusses chemical contaminants and other unintentional food additives.

Accidental Food Contaminants

Many substances can accidentally enter food during processing. These *accidental food additives* include common biological and physical food contaminants such as insect parts, rodent feces or urine, dust and dirt, and bits of metal or glass from machinery used to process food. Although some of these substances may not be harmful to health, most people find it unappealing to have such unintentional ingredients in their foods.

According to the Federal Food, Drug, and Cosmetic Act, **adulterated food** contains objectionable and unsanitary material, and it cannot be distributed. However, the FDA permits very small amounts of unavoidable, naturally occurring substances such as dirt and insect parts in foods, because they are not harmful when consumed in tiny amounts. The FDA established guidelines ("action levels") concerning amounts of certain materials that are permitted in specific foods, such as mold and rodent hairs in paprika or insect eggs in canned orange juice. According to the FDA, "...it is economically impractical to grow, harvest, or process raw products that are totally free of nonhazardous, naturally occurring, unavoidable defects. Products harmful to consumers, however, are subject to regulatory action whether or not they exceed the action levels."[29]

Chemical contaminants also enter foods unintentionally. Toxic metals, such as lead, cadmium, and mercury, are naturally in our environment, and these elements may also be in our food. Poisonous human–made compounds such as benzene and polychlorinated biphenols (PCBs) are in the environment as well. Toxic metals or poisonous compounds resulting from manufacturing practices can pollute sources of water used by consumers (well water, for example). Americans who drink water from municipal supplies can be assured that the water is analyzed regularly to determine its concentrations of toxic substances. However, people who rely on privately owned wells should have the water tested routinely.

adulterated food food that has been intentionally or unintentionally altered and made impure

What Is Benzene?

Late in 2005, the FDA received reports that low levels of benzene had been detected in some soft drinks that contained ascorbic acid (vitamin C) and a group of food additives called benzoate (*ben'–zo–ate'*) salts. Benzene is a cancer–causing agent present in the environment from natural and manufactured sources. After receiving the reports, the FDA's Center for Food Safety and Applied Nutrition surveyed benzene levels in soft drinks. The survey's findings indicated that the vast majority of beverages sampled, including those containing both benzoate salts and ascorbic acid, contained either no detectable amounts of benzene or amounts that were very low and within the range allowed by the U.S. water standard.[30] Thus, FDA scientists concluded that the levels of benzene in soft drinks did not pose a safety concern. Nevertheless, agency officials determined it was necessary to contact beverage manufacturers to ensure that processing conditions avoid or minimize benzene formation.

What Is Acrylamide?

Acrylamide is a naturally occurring compound in foods that was not discovered until 2002. The compound forms when foods containing sugars and the amino acid asparagine are heated to high temperatures, such as when foods are roasted,

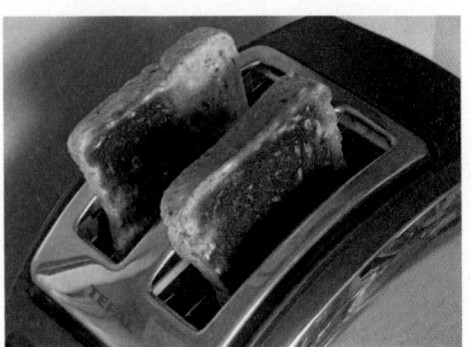

Burnt toast can be a source of acrylamide, a naturally occurring compound that may be carcinogenic.

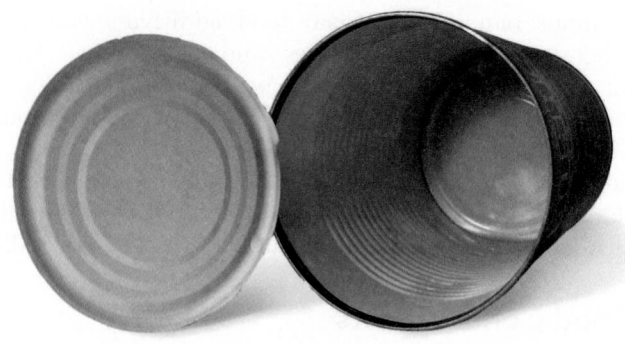

FIGURE 19.12 BPA and epoxy resins. The epoxy resin that is used to coat the inside of cans contains BPA.

fried, or baked. Acrylamide tends to form mostly in plant−based foods, especially grains, potatoes and products made with potatoes, and coffee beans. The FDA has been actively researching the safety of acrylamide; in November 2013, the FDA released guidance to the food industry on how to limit acrylamide in processed foods.[31] Consumers can avoid producing acrylamide during cooking by boiling, steaming, and microwaving potatoes and grains. Sources of acrylamide include overly browned potato− and grain−based foods, so it is wise to avoid eating burnt bread or French fries.

What Is BPA?

Bisphenol A (biss'−feenol), or *BPA*, has received quite a lot of attention lately, even though the synthetic chemical is not a common food contaminant. Since the 1960s, manufacturers have used BPA to make polycarbonate plastics and epoxy resin. The plastics and resin are used in the production of disposable and reusable beverage bottles. The layer of epoxy resin that lines the inside of some food cans prevents the can's metal from coming in contact with and being damaged by the food (Fig. 19.12).[32] Small amounts of BPA, however, can migrate into the foods or liquids held inside these containers.

Experts with the National Toxicology Program of the National Institute of Environmental Health Sciences have "some concern" about the effects of BPA on the brain, behavior, and prostate gland (male) of fetuses, infants, and children. Although the FDA does not feel the low levels are cause for concern in humans,[33] the agency supports efforts to find safer alternatives. Plastic containers that contain BPA are marked with the symbol shown in Figure 19.13. The "Fresh Tips" feature on this page lists steps consumers can take to reduce their exposure to BPA.

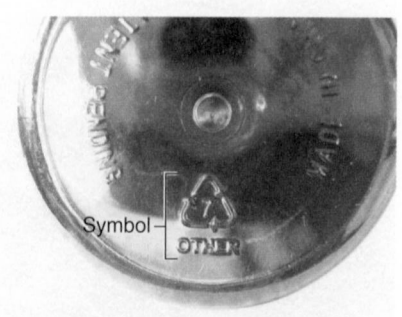

FIGURE 19.13 Where's the BPA? This symbol indicates that the plastic used to make this water bottle contains BPA.

FRESH TIPS

To reduce your exposure to BPA, consider taking these actions:

- Avoid heating foods in polycarbonate plastic containers.
- Avoid plastic containers that have the symbol shown in Figure 19.13.
- Do not wash polycarbonate containers in the dishwasher or with harsh detergents.
- Reduce your intake of canned foods.
- Cook or store foods and beverages in glass, porcelain, or stainless steel containers.
- Avoid serving foods (especially hot foods or liquids) on or in polycarbonate dishware, cups, or eating utensils.
- Avoid using older baby bottles and plastic chew toys that may have been made with BPA.

What Are Pesticides?

A **pesticide** is any substance that people use to control or kill unwanted insects, weeds, rodents, fungi, or other organisms. There are several different kinds of pesticides. **Insecticides** control or kill insects; **rodenticides** kill mice and rats; **herbicides** destroy weeds; and **fungicides** limit the spread of fungi, such as mold and mildew. Over 5 *billion* pounds of pesticides are used in the United States annually.[34] Herbicides are the most widely used type of pesticide in agriculture.[34]

Pesticide Residue Tolerances The use of pesticides in modern farming practices has helped increase crop yields, reduce food costs, and protect the quality of many agricultural products. However, many pesticides leave small amounts of pesticide residues in or on treated crops, including fruits, vegetables, and grains, even when they are applied correctly. Concentrations of pesticide residues often decrease as food crops are washed, stored, processed, and prepared. Nevertheless, some of these substances may remain in fresh produce, such as apples or peaches, as well as in processed foods derived from the produce, such as canned applesauce or peaches.

The EPA regulates the proper use of pesticides. The agency can limit the amount of a pesticide that is applied on crops, restrict the frequency or location of the pesticide's application, or require the substance be used only by specially trained, certified persons. The EPA also sets **pesticide tolerances**, maximum amounts of pesticide residues that can be in or on each treated food crop. A pesticide tolerance includes a margin of safety, so the maximum pesticide residue that is allowed to be in or on a food is much lower than amounts that can cause negative health effects.[34]

Nonchemical Methods of Pest Management Although the EPA focuses on chemical methods of managing pests, the agency also promotes nonchemical pest management techniques that may be safer for humans and the environment. Integrated pest management (IPM) involves using a variety of methods for controlling pests while limiting damage to the environment. IPM methods include growing pest−resistant crops, using predatory wasps to control crop−destroying insects, and trapping adult insect pests before they can reproduce. Biologically based pesticides are becoming increasingly popular among farmers (Fig. 19.14). Examples of these pesticides include sex hormones (*pheromones*) that attract pesky insects to predators or traps and viruses that infect harmful insects and weeds. Such methods are often safer for humans than traditional chemical pesticides.

It is important to note that IPM permits the use of chemical pesticides but only as needed to enhance the effects of nonchemical methods. Studies suggest

pesticide substance used to kill or control unwanted insects, weeds, or other organisms

insecticides substances used to control or kill insects

rodenticides substances used to kill mice and rats

herbicides substances used to destroy weeds

fungicides substances used to limit the spread of fungi

pesticide tolerances maximum amounts of pesticide residues that can be in or on each treated food crop

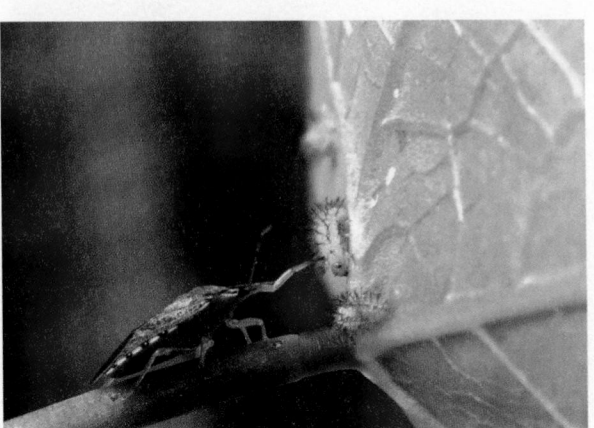

FIGURE 19.14 Helpful insects. The spined soldier bug (left) makes a meal of a Mexican bean beetle larva. Bean beetle larvae are devastating pests of snap beans and soybeans. The spined soldier bug's pheromone may help farmers control many insects that eat crops.

that IPM techniques generally increase crop yields and economic profits, while reducing the use of chemical pesticides.[34] As IPM programs become more widely adopted, conventional farmers will depend less on the use of chemical pesticides.

Fruits and vegetables grown without use of pesticides are available and may bear an "organic" label (see Chapter 3 for information about organic foods). These products generally are more expensive than those grown using pesticides, and they are not necessarily safer or more nutritious than conventionally produced foods.[35] However, organic products are generally more "environmentally friendly" than conventional produced foods.

How Safe Are Pesticides? Pesticides help protect the food supply and make food crops available at reasonable cost. Nevertheless, pesticides have the potential to harm humans, animals, or the environment because they are designed to kill or otherwise negatively affect organisms. If a pesticide is applied improperly to cropland, it may remain in the soil, be taken up by plant roots, decompose to other compounds, or enter groundwater and waterways. Winds may carry pesticides in air and dust to distant locations. In addition, pesticides remain in the soil, in some cases for many years, after application. Each path can be a route to the human food chain (Fig. 19.15).

The potential harmful effects of a pesticide in food depend on the particular chemical and how effectively the body can eliminate it, its concentration in the food, how much and how often it is eaten, and the consumer's vulnerability to the substance. Tolerable amounts of pesticide residues on or in foods are extremely small. However, it is possible that regular exposure to small amounts of these chemicals may enable the substances to accumulate in the body and produce toxicity or initiate cancer.[36] Health experts have studied rates of cancers among people who have close contact with pesticides, such as farmers and pesticide applicators. Among the people who applied pesticides, the likelihood of developing certain cancers, including breast, prostate, non–Hodgkin lymphoma, and leukemia, was increased.[37] Because of such concerns, environmental health experts continue to monitor the effects of pesticides on humans.

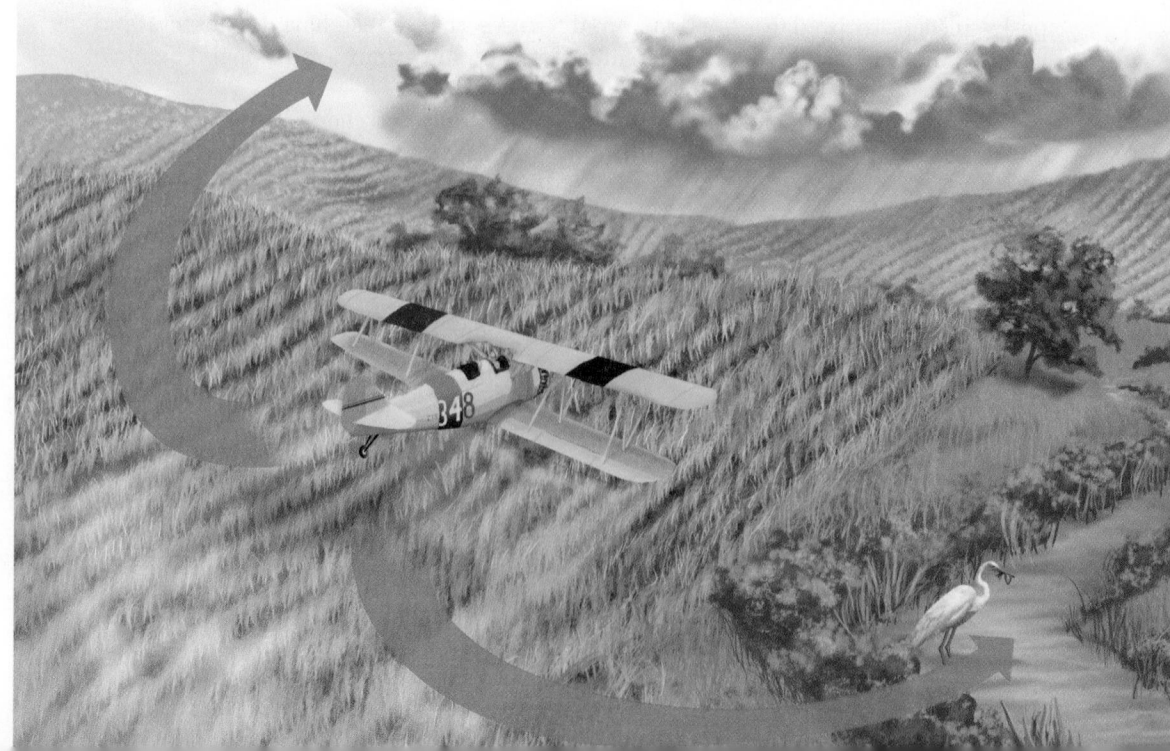

FIGURE 19.15 Pesticide pathways. If a pesticide is applied to cropland, it may remain in the soil, be taken up by plant roots, decompose to other compounds, or enter the groundwater and waterways. Winds may carry pesticides in the air and dust to distant locations. Each path can be a route to the human food chain.

ASSESS YOUR PROGRESS

25 Contrast intentional and unintentional food additives.

26 Explain the difference between GRAS substances and other intentional food additives.

27 Explain the role of the Delaney Clause in protecting the U.S. food supply.

28 Identify at least three examples of unintentional food additives.

29 Identify the federal agency that regulates the use of pesticides.

19.8 Public Water Supply and Safety

LEARNING OUTCOMES

1 **Identify the key federal agencies that regulate the safety of drinking water.**

2 **Compare tap water and bottled water.**

Today, preparing for a class often involves bringing into the classroom a notebook, something to write with, and a bottle of cold water. On average, Americans drink 3.9 cups of plain water each day, with 61% coming from a faucet ("tap water") and 39% from bottled water.[38]

The EPA regulates the sanitation of public water supplies in the United States. Most Americans can trust the safety of their tap water because the vast majority of municipal water systems in the United States are regulated by the Safe Drinking Water Act (SDWA). As a result of this law, most tap water undergoes a thorough purification process and is constantly tested for safety. Public availability of annual reports on water safety is required by the SDWA, and public notification of any violations is mandatory. If such testing indicates the water supply may pose a threat to public health, consumers are warned through media, and a "boil order"—requirement to boil water for 10 minutes to kill harmful microorganisms—may be issued.[39]

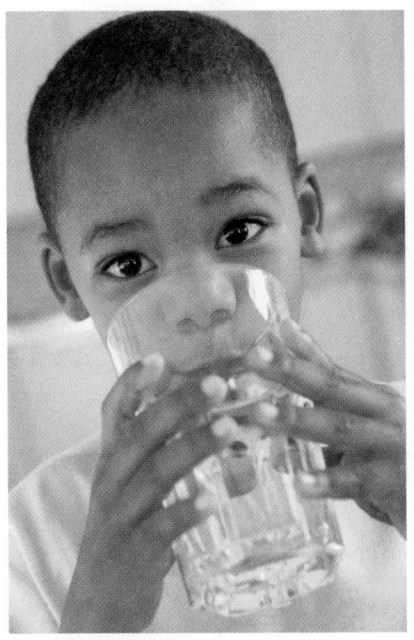

The U.S. Environmental Protection Agency is responsible for ensuring water intended for human consumption is safe.

Comparing Bottled and Tap Water

Millions of Americans have been turning away from the tap and choosing to drink bottled water instead. According to the Beverage Market Corporation and International Bottled Water Association, each American consumed 30.8 gallons of bottled water in 2012.[40] That amount of bottled water is over 50% more than the amount consumed in 2000. The U.S. population drinks more bottled water than milk, juice, or any other beverage, except carbonated soft drinks.

Why do so many Americans drink bottled water when tap water is much less costly? Among adults, taste, convenience, and health concerns were major reasons they chose bottled water over other beverages. For most Americans, however, bottled water is usually unnecessary and expensive, because it is often very similar to tap water. Consumers need to be aware that the water in some bottled water products comes from a municipal water supply. However, when public water supplies are disrupted by hurricanes, tornadoes, or earthquakes, drinking bottled water may be a consumer's only option (see section 19.9, "Preparing for Disasters").

Regulation of Bottled Water

While the EPA regulates tap water, the FDA is responsible for regulating bottled water products that are marketed for interstate commerce. The FDA defines bottled water as water intended for human consumption that is sealed in

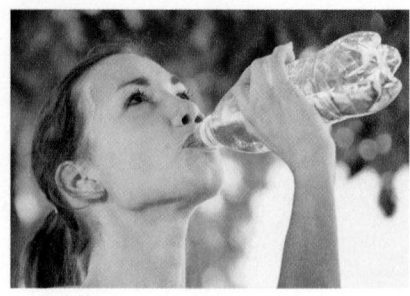

The FDA ensures that bottled water is safe to drink, while the EPA regulates the safety of the public water supply.

containers and has no added ingredients other than a substance that prevents the growth of microbes such as bacteria.[41] Bottled water may have fluoride added, but amounts must meet FDA guidelines. If bottled water manufacturers add flavorings or other ingredients to their products, the name of the product must indicate the added ingredients: "Bottled Water with Cherry Flavor," for example. These drinks are often called "flavored water beverages." Flavored waters may simply contain additives that make the beverage taste good, but a growing number of flavored waters also have added nutrients other than sugars, such as sodium, potassium, and amino acids. The beverage's label must identify the additives in the list of ingredients.

The FDA uses place of origin to classify some bottled waters. "Artesian well water," for example, must come from a well that taps an aquifer, a body of water found between porous layers of rock, sand, and earth. Common types of water used for bottling purposes and their FDA definitions are available at http://www.fda.gov/food/foodborneillnesscontaminants/buystoreservesafefood/ucm077079.htm.

Safety standards for bottled water are similar to those established by the EPA for tap water.[41] According to FDA guidelines, bottled water manufacturers are responsible for producing safe products. Production procedures for bottled water must follow manufacturing regulations established and enforced by the FDA. For example, the FDA has regulations concerning maximum levels of contaminants permitted in bottled water. Such contaminants include microbes, chemicals, and minerals. Prior to being bottled, the water must be sampled, analyzed, and found to be safe and clean. Additionally, the FDA inspects water bottling facilities regularly.

Because of FDA regulations and oversight, consumers can be assured that their supply of bottled water is safe to drink. Although the beverage is safe, the plastic bottle used to contain it may have toxic effects on health or the environment. As noted in section 19.7 "Food Additives," water bottles may contain BPA, which can leach from the polycarbonate plastic containers and enter the water that is stored inside of them.

ASSESS YOUR PROGRESS

30 *Compare the agencies responsible for regulating the safety of tap water versus bottled water.*

31 *Identify two pros and two cons for drinking both tap water and bottled water.*

32 *Is bottled water safer than tap water? Explain.*

19.9 Preparing for Disasters

LEARNING OUTCOMES

1 *Identify at least five foods that are appropriate for an emergency food supply.*

2 *Describe safe and unsafe sources of drinking water for situations in which public water supplies are disrupted.*

In late October 2012, Hurricane Sandy devastated the East Coast of the United States, as well as other countries on the Atlantic seaboard. The storm took the lives of 285 individuals and caused more than $50 billion in damages to homes and workplaces in the United States. Widespread power outages lasted for days in many areas and impacted millions of people. In this section, we consider steps a person can take to have enough water and food available to survive hurricanes, earthquakes, or other serious emergency situations.

Emergency Water Supply

A supply of clean water and wholesome food is necessary for surviving disasters such as hurricanes and earthquakes. People can be more prepared for natural disasters by storing at least 1 gallon of water per person per day. Ideally, keep at least a 3– to 5–day supply of drinking water, or at least 5 gallons of water for each person in a household. Children and breastfeeding women may need more than 1 gallon of water per day. Also, more water may be necessary for people living in warm climates.

To maintain a safe emergency supply of drinking water, consumers should:

- Maintain the water in a cool place and in sturdy plastic bottles with tight–fitting lids.

- Avoid storing water in areas where toxic substances, such as gasoline and pesticides, are stored. Over time, toxic vapors from these products may penetrate the plastic and contaminate the water.

- Change stored water every 6 months.

- Drink only bottled, boiled, or treated water until certain the public water supply is safe.

When there is time to prepare, people can fill a bathtub with water to use if necessary. The water, however, will need to be sanitized before being consumed. If the emergency water supply becomes inadequate or contaminated, a person can consume melted ice cubes from the freezer, canned fruit juices, and water drained from an undamaged water heater. Water stored in the tank of the toilet (not the bowl) is also fit to drink. Pets can drink toilet bowl water that has not been treated with a toilet bowl sanitizer. Water in swimming pools and spas can be used for personal hygiene needs but not for drinking. Never drink water from car radiators, home heating systems, or water beds. Alcoholic beverages contribute to dehydration and therefore should be avoided.

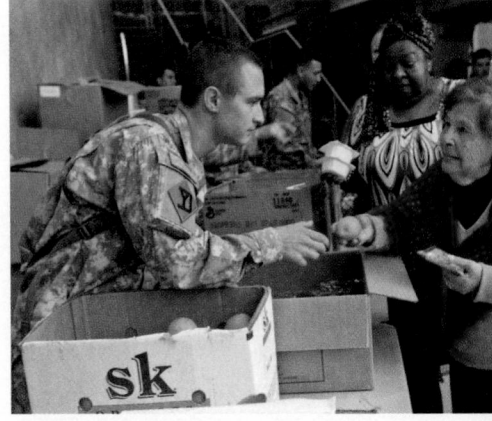

Specialist Anthony Monte along with soldiers from the 50th Infantry Brigade Combat Team, New Jersey National Guard, mobilized for Hurricane Sandy to provide assistance and food to displaced residents at an emergency shelter.

FRESH TIPS

If clean water is not available, water can be safely sanitized by:[43]

- Boiling for 1 minute, covered, and allowing it to cool. If at altitudes greater than 6562 feet, boil water for 3 minutes.

- Adding tablets that contain chemicals, such as chlorine or iodine. These tablets can be purchased at outdoor and camping stores and should be used only according to package instructions, because adding chemicals to water can be unsafe when not done in the appropriate ratios.

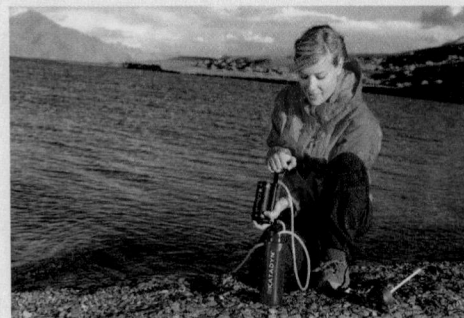

Water filters can remove bacteria and protozoa from drinking water.

- Using water filters. Such filters can remove bacteria and protozoa, but they may not remove viruses. A guide for purchasing water filters can be found at http://www.cdc.gov/parasites/crypto/gen_info/filters.html.

- Using portable units that produce ultraviolet light, which can effectively sanitize small amounts of clear water. These units are often sold at camping stores.

Emergency Food Supply

A natural disaster can easily disrupt one's access to safe food; therefore, a person should store at least a 3–day supply of food for emergency use. Choose foods that have a long storage life, require no refrigeration, and can be eaten without cooking, such as canned meats, fruits, and vegetables. (If pets are in the household, people should also keep a supply of pet foods.) Also store bat—teries, flashlights, matches, a radio, a manual can opener, paper plates, and eating utensils.

If stored under proper conditions, the majority of unopened canned or boxed foods will remain fresh for about 2 years beyond the date stamped on the pack—age. Before storing food, use a permanent marking pen to write the date on the package. Use and replace foods before they lose their freshness or reach their expiration dates. An ideal food storage location is a cool, dry, dark place. Protect foods from rodents and insects by storing them in airtight containers or plastic storage bins.

If there is no electricity, people should consume perishable food that is in the refrigerator or freezer before using the emergency food supply. However, discard cooked foods after they have been at room temperature for 2 hours. Do not eat food that appears or smells spoiled or is from cans that are leaking or bulging. To prepare meals safely after a disaster, store the following items:

- A camp stove or charcoal grill and matches.

- Fuel for cooking, such as charcoal. Never cook food on a camp stove or charcoal grill indoors. The fumes contain carbon monoxide, a deadly odorless gas.

- Cooking and eating utensils, paper plates, cups, and towels.

For more information about emergency preparedness, visit the Centers for Disease Control and Prevention's website: www.bt.cdc.gov/disasters/.

ASSESS YOUR PROGRESS

33 *How much water should a person store in the home to be prepared for an emergency?*

34 *In case public water supplies are disrupted, identify at least three safe sources of drinking water in the home.*

35 *Identify at least five foods people could store in their homes as part of an emergency food supply.*

SUMMARY

SECTION 19.1 **Protecting the Food Supply**

- The United States has one of the safest food supplies in the world with FDA and the USDA being the key federal agencies that protect consumers by regulating the country's food industry.

- Other regulatory agencies include the EPA, the CDC, the FTC, and state and local governments.

- Food regulations can help protect individuals from food-borne illness.

SECTION 19.2 **Pathogens in Food**

- Pathogens are disease-causing microorganisms that can be found in foods, making them unsafe to eat. Common ways pathogens contaminate foods include contact by vermin, poor personal hygiene practices, and improper food handling.

SECTION 19.3 **Food-Borne Illness**

- Signs and symptoms of food-borne illness include nausea, vomiting, diarrhea, and intestinal cramps. In most cases of food-borne illness or intoxication, healthy individuals recover completely and without professional medical care within a few days; however, severe vomiting, diarrhea, and other signs of illness may require hospitalization.

- In general, high-risk groups are pregnant women, very young children, older adults, and persons who suffer from serious chronic illnesses or weakened immune systems.

SECTION 19.4 **Common Food-Borne Pathogens**

- Pathogens causing food-borne illness include bacteria, viruses, protozoa, tiny parasitic worms, and prions. In the United States, bacteria and viruses are responsible for most cases of food-borne illness.

SECTION 19.5 **Preventing Food-Borne Illnesses**

- One can greatly reduce the risk of food-borne illness by following some important safety guidelines in selecting, preparing, and storing food. Maintaining appropriate temperatures is important because most microbes grow well when temperatures of potentially hazardous foods are between 40°F and 140°F.

SECTION 19.6 **Food Preservation**

- Food preservation is important to extend a food's shelf life. Methods of preservation include heating, fermentation, chemical preservatives, smoking, curing, chilling or freezing, drying, canning, and irradiation.

- Boiling home-canned, low-acid foods for 10 minutes before eating can reduce one's risk for food-borne illness from *Clostridium botulinum*.

SECTION 19.7 **Food Additives**

- Food additives are any substances that become incorporated into food during production, packaging, transport, or storage. Intentional food additives are used to make food easier to process, more nutritious, able to stay fresh longer, or better tasting or looking.

- Unintentional food additives have no purpose for being in the food and can accidently enter food as it is packaged, transported, or stored; unintentional food additives include biological, physical, and chemical contaminants.

- The FDA and other agencies regulate all food additives to ensure that processed foods and their packaging are safe.

- The Delaney Clause of the Food Additives Amendment ensures that new direct food additives that cause cancer at any level of intake are prohibited for use in foods.

SECTION 19.8 **Public Water Supply and Safety**

- The EPA regulates the sanitation of public water supplies in the United States under the Safe Drinking Water Act; however, bottled water is regulated by the FDA.

- Although bottled water is safe to drink, the plastic bottle may have toxic effects on health or the environment.

SECTION 19.9 **Preparing for Disasters**

- Having a 3- to 5-day supply of at least 1 gallon of bottled water per person in a household is ideal. Store at least a 3-day supply of foods that have a long storage life, require no refrigeration, and can be eaten without cooking.

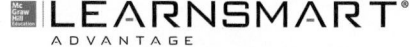

Modifying Recipes for Healthy Living

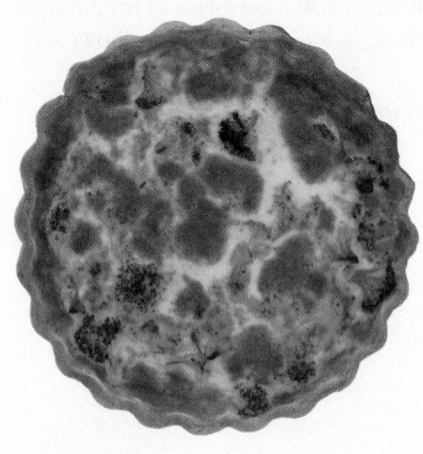

Last week, Shantal made a broccoli and cheddar cheese quiche for a potluck lunch with four of her coworkers. She prepared the quiche the night before the luncheon. When she opened the egg carton that she purchased 6 weeks earlier, she noticed that almost all of the eggs had small cracks in their shells. The egg carton had been stored in the refrigerator, under the heavy milk jug. Shantal did not have time to shop for fresh eggs, so she used the cracked eggs. The recipe called for baking the quiche for 40 minutes. However, Shantal thought the quiche looked done and took it out of the oven after 25 minutes. A few days after the potluck meal, Shantal and her four coworkers were unable to work because they were sick with nausea, vomiting, and diarrhea. After questioning Shantal, her coworkers suspected the quiche was the source of the food-borne illness.

This weekend, Shantal is planning on making the quiche again for a brunch with friends. She definitely does not want to make anyone sick! Using the recipe below and information you know about preventing food-borne illness, provide Shantal with advice on how to prepare the quiche safely.

BROCCOLI AND CHEDDAR CHEESE QUICHE

INGREDIENTS

1 9-inch piecrust, prebaked according to package instructions

1 cup broccoli florets, rinsed

¾ cup of 2% shredded cheddar cheese

1 cup sliced or diced cherry tomatoes

6 large eggs

½ cup 1% milk

⅓ cup light sour cream

½ tsp salt

¼ tsp black pepper

PREPARATION STEPS

1. Preheat oven to 375°F.
2. Bring a medium pot of water to a boil and blanch the broccoli florets by boiling for 1 minute. Strain florets from the water and transfer to a bowl of ice cold water to stop the cooking process. Once cooled, drain the broccoli well.
3. Sprinkle one half of the shredded cheese evenly in bottom of the pie shell and top evenly with broccoli florets and tomatoes.
4. In a medium bowl, beat eggs, milk, sour cream, salt, and pepper with a fork or whisk until blended. Carefully pour into pie shell.
5. Transfer quiche to the center of the oven and bake about 40 minutes, or until a knife inserted into the center of the quiche comes out clean when removed. Check final temperature of dish; the dish should be at or above 160°F.
6. Let quiche sit for 5 minutes before cutting into six wedges and serving.

STEP 1 Brainstorm

What ingredients in the quiche are most likely to cause food-borne illness? How did Shantal's food storage and preparation practices likely contribute to the food-borne illness?

STEP 2 Strategies for preparing a safe recipe

Provide a detailed list of strategies that Shantal can implement to reduce the risk of food-borne illness. Include strategies for purchasing, storing, and cooking (minimum internal temperature) eggs.

OPTIONAL ACTIVITIES

STEP 3 Prepare the Broccoli and Cheddar Cheese Quiche recipe

Did you follow all of the strategies listed in Step 2? Why or why not?

STEP 4 Reflect on the process

Do you regularly follow the strategies listed in this chapter to prevent food-borne illness? Which strategies are you most likely to follow, and which are you least likely to follow?

CASE STUDY RESPONSE

FOOD-BORNE ILLNESS FROM RAW MILK

SOME CONSUMERS CHOOSE RAW MILK because they consider it a "living food" that provides beneficial bacteria and natural food enzymes that *may* be lost through traditional pasteurization. Mary's son, Chris, became very ill after consuming raw milk from a local dairy farm. The cause of his illness was traced to *E. coli* O157:H7 that had contaminated the milk.

Young children are more vulnerable to food-borne illnesses because their immune systems are immature and still developing. Other high-risk groups include pregnant women, infants, older adults, and persons who suffer from serious chronic illnesses or weakened immune systems.

Raw milk has not undergone pasteurization, a heat treatment used by many commercial food processors to kill the majority of pathogens that may be present in foods and beverages. Because of its high water and protein content and neutral pH, milk is a potentially hazardous food that may harbor pathogens such as *Listeria monocytogenes*, *Salmonella*, and *E. coli* O157:H7. Raw milk and cheeses are more likely to cause outbreaks of food-borne illness than pasteurized milk and dairy products.

To reduce her family's risk of future food-borne illnesses, Mary can:

- Purchase only pasteurized milk, cheeses, and fruit and vegetable juices.
- Cook foods to proper temperatures.
- Wash hands and cooking surfaces frequently.
- Refrigerate foods and leftovers quickly.
- Avoid cross-contamination.

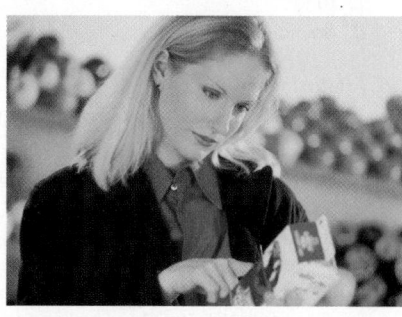

Inspecting the package and reading the ingredient label can help ensure that certain foods have been pasteurized.

Critical Thinking

1. Prepare a food safety checklist that can be used in your household.

2. Consider your usual food selection, preparation, and storage practices. After having read Chapter 19, list any of these practices you have that are unsafe.

3. For lunch on Monday, you visited a restaurant and ordered a hamburger, French fries, baked beans, and a container of orange juice. Two days later, you developed nausea, vomiting, fever, chills, headache, abdominal cramps, and diarrhea. You suspect Monday's lunch made you sick. Considering the foods that you ate for

lunch on Monday, which one was the most likely source of your infection? Why? In the future, what steps can you take to reduce the likelihood that the food will make you sick again?

4. Develop a pamphlet to educate consumers about food-borne illness.

5. A friend refuses to drink tap water because she thinks it is contaminated. She drinks only bottled water or well water. If she asked you to explain why you drink tap water, what would you tell her?

Practice Test

Select the best answer.

1. _____ are disease-causing microbes.
   a. Pathogens
   b. Toxins
   c. Teratogens
   d. Oxidants

2. The _____ is the primary government agency that oversees the safety of most foods in the United States.
   a. Food and Drug Administration (FDA)
   b. Federal Trade Commission (FTC)
   c. Centers for Disease Control and Prevention (CDC)
   d. Environmental Protection Agency (EPA)

3. Which of the following foods is considered a potentially hazardous food?
   a. overripe bananas
   b. raisins
   c. raw ground meat
   d. commercially canned tomato soup

4. Food-borne illnesses are usually characterized by
   a. flulike signs and symptoms.
   b. coughing, sneezing, and respiratory inflammation.
   c. megaloblastic anemia and nervous system defects.
   d. abdominal cramps, diarrhea, and vomiting.

5. In the United States, common sources of food-borne illness include all of the following, except

    a. norovirus.
    b. *Staphylococcus aureus.*
    c. fungi.
    d. *Salmonella.*

6. Aflatoxins are

    a. responsible for 30% of food-borne illnesses in the United States.
    b. harmful compounds produced by certain molds.
    c. a type of parasitic worm.
    d. medications that are effective against viral toxins.

7. Which of the following practices increases the growth of food-borne pathogens?

    a. washing hands before preparing food
    b. keeping cold foods cold and hot foods hot
    c. cooking foods to proper internal temperatures
    d. using the same cutting board to prepare all parts of a meal

8. Which of the following substances are not direct food additives?

    a. color additives
    b. sweeteners
    c. pesticide residues
    d. flavor enhancers

9. Irradiation of food is

    a. an untested technology.
    b. not recommended, because the process increases nutrient losses.
    c. widely used in Spain, Russia, and Mexico.
    d. a common method of food preservation in the United States.

10. To reduce the risk of food-borne illness, raw poultry should be cooked to an internal temperature of at least

    a. 125°F.
    b. 145°F.
    c. 165°F.
    d. 185°F.

11. _____ is the commercial heating process that destroys pathogens in milk and fruit juices.

    a. Fermentation
    b. Homogenization
    c. Detoxification
    d. Pasteurization

12. Which of the following practices is not a safe food preparation practice?

    a. washing hands thoroughly with soap and warm water for at least 20 seconds before handling foods
    b. cutting away mold on block cheeses as long as you can cut away about 1 inch from the mold
    c. selecting wooden cutting boards for raw meats, rather than nonporous materials such as plastic or marble
    d. heating alfalfa sprouts until they are steaming to reduce potential pathogens

13. Stephanie developed a food-borne illness after eating ice cream made with raw eggs. The pathogen that was most likely contaminating her food was

    a. *Salmonella.*
    b. *Vibrio vulnificus.*
    c. *Giardia.*
    d. *Toxoplasma gondii.*

14. _____ is the most reliable method of making water that contains pathogens safe to drink.

    a. Detoxification
    b. Straining
    c. Boiling
    d. Carbonation

15. Food additives that are thought to be safe without extensive research are called

    a. GRAS.
    b. direct food additives.
    c. indirect food additives.
    d. color additives.

ANSWERS TO PRACTICE TEST
1-a; 2-a; 3-c; 4-d; 5-b; 6-b; 7-d; 8-c; 9-d; 10-c; 11-d; 12-c; 13-a; 14-c; 15-a

---

ANSWERS TO CHAPTER 19 QUIZ Yourself

1. Pregnant women are more likely to get food-borne illness compared to other healthy women of similar age. **True** (p. 610)
2. Eggs and milk are examples of potentially hazardous foods. **True** (p. 609)
3. Hot foods should sit out at room temperature for a few hours to cool before placing in the refrigerator. **False** (p. 620)
4. A new food additive must be approved by the Food and Drug Administration before being added to foods. **True** (p. 626)
5. Melted ice cubes, water drained from a water heater, and water from the tank of a toilet are all safe sources of drinking water in case of an emergency. **True** (p. 633)

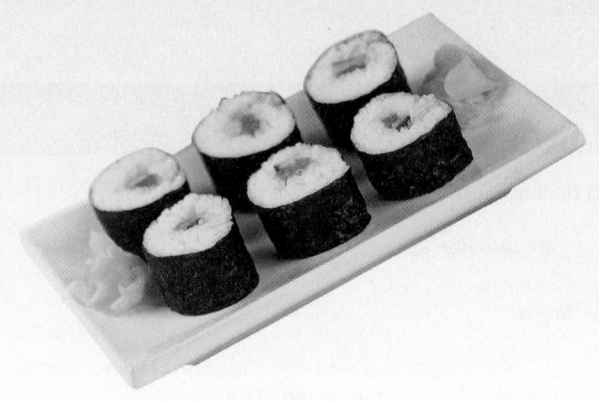

References

1. Centers for Disease Control and Prevention: *Estimates of foodborne illness in the United States.* 2011. http://www.cdc.gov/foodborneburden/ Accessed: March 15, 2014.

2. U.S. Food and Drug Administration: The New FDA Food Safety Modernization Act (FSMA). Updated March 2014. http://www.fda.gov/food/guidanceregulation/fsma/default.htm Accessed: March 15, 2014.

3. Centers for Disease Control and Prevention: *Handwashing: Clean hands save lives.* Updated December 2013. http://www.cdc.gov/handwashing/ Accessed: March 15, 2014.

4. Centers for Disease Control and Prevention: *Foodborne safety: General questions: When should I consult my doctor about a diarrheal disease?* Updated September 2012. http://www.cdc.gov/foodsafety/facts.html Accessed: March 15, 2014.

5. Kirk MD and others: Gastroenteritis and food-borne disease in elderly people living in long-term care. *Clinical Infectious Diseases* 50(3):397, 2010.

6. Dean J, Kendall P: *Food Safety During Pregnancy.* Updated January 2014. http://www.ext.colostate.edu/pubs/foodnut/09372.html Accessed: March 15, 2014.

7. Centers for Disease Control and Prevention: *Listeriosis (Listeria) and pregnancy.* Updated December 2011. http://www.cdc.gov/pregnancy/infections-listeria.html Accessed March 15, 2014.

8. Centers for Disease Control and Prevention: *Multistate outbreak of listeriosis linked to whole cantaloupes from Jensen Farms, Colorado.* Updated September 2012. http://www.cdc.gov/listeria/outbreaks/cantaloupes-jensen-farms/index .html Accessed: March 15, 2014.

9. U.S. Food and Drug Administration: Food: *Raw oyster myths: Vibrio vulnificus health education kit.* Updated March 2013. http://www.fda.gov/food/resourcesforyou/healtheducators/ucm085385.htm Accessed: March 15, 2014.

10. National Restaurant Association: *ServeSafe coursebook.* 5th ed. Chicago: National Restaurant Association Solutions, LLC, 2008.

11. Centers for Disease Control and Prevention: Parasites: *Food.* Updated March 2014. http://www.cdc.gov/parasites/food.html Accessed: March 15, 2014.

12. USDA Food Safety and Inspection Service: Safe food handling: *Molds on food: Are they dangerous?* Updated August 2013. http://www.fsis.usda.gov/wps/portal/fsis/topics/food-safety-education/get-answers/food-safety-fact-sheets/safe-food-handling/molds-on-food-are-they-dangerous_/ Accessed: March 15, 2014.

13. U.S. Food and Drug Administration: *Bad bug book: Handbook of foodborne pathogenic microorganisms and natural toxins.* 2nd ed. 2012. http://www.fda .gov/Food/FoodborneIllnessContaminants/CausesOfIllnessBadBugBook/ Accessed: March 15, 2014.

14. Centers for Disease Control and Prevention: *About prion diseases.* Updated December 2012. http://www.cdc.gov/ncidod/dvrd/prions Accessed: March 15, 2014.

15. U.S. Department of Health and Human Services: *Keep foods safe: Cook.* ND. http://www.foodsafety.gov/keep/basics/cook Accessed: March 15, 2014.

16. U.S. Department of Agriculture, Food Safety and Inspection Service: Appliances and thermometers: *Microwave ovens and food safety.* Updated August 2013. http://www.fsis.usda.gov/wps/portal/fsis/topics/food-safety-education/get-answers/food-safety-fact-sheets/appliances-and-thermometers/microwave-ovens-and-food-safety/ct_index Accessed: March 15, 2014.

17. Food and Agricultural Products Research and Technology Center: *Guidelines for the use of chlorine bleach as a sanitizer in food processing operations.* http://ucfoodsafety.ucdavis.edu/files/26437.pdf Accessed: March 15, 2014.

18. Home Food Safety: *Do's and don'ts of kitchen sponge safety.* http://homefoodsafety.org/safety-tips/wash/dos-and-donts-of-kitchen-sponge-safety Accessed: March 15, 2014.

19. U.S. Food and Drug Administration: *Food Code 2009: Chapter 3—Food.* http://www.fda.gov/Food/GuidanceRegulation/RetailFoodProtection/FoodCode/ucm186451.htm Accessed: March 15, 2014.

20. U.S. Department of Agriculture, Food Safety and Inspection Service: *Food safety information: Basics for handling food safely.* Updated August 2013. http://www.fsis.usda.gov/wps/portal/fsis/topics/food-safety-education/get-answers/food-safety-fact-sheets/safe-food-handling/basics-for-handling-food-safely/ct_index Accessed: March 15, 2014.

21. Centers for Disease Control and Prevention, National Center for Emerging and Zoonotic Infectious Diseases: *Irradiation of food.* Updated November 2009. http://www.cdc.gov/nczved/divisions/dfbmd/diseases/irradiation_food/ Accessed: March 15, 2014.

22. Food irradiation: What you need to know. *FoodFacts: From the U.S. Food and Drug Administration,* p. 2, June 2011. http://www.fda.gov/downloads/Food/IngredientsPackagingLabeling/UCM262295.pdf Accessed: March 15, 2014.

23. International Consultative Group on Food Irradiation. *Facts about food irradiation.* 1999. http://www.iaea.org/Publications/Booklets/foodirradiation.pdf Accessed: March 15, 2014.

24. International Food Information Council and U.S. Food and Drug Administration: *Food ingredients and colors.* Revised April 2010. http://www.fda.gov/downloads/Food/IngredientsPackagingLabeling/ucm094249.pdf Accessed: March 15, 2014.

25. Center for Food Safety and Applied Nutrition, U.S. Food and Drug Administration: *Frequently asked questions about GRAS.* 2004. Updated February 2014. http://www.fda.gov/Food/GuidanceRegulation/GuidanceDocumentsRegulatoryInformation/IngredientsAdditivesGRASPackaging/ucm061846.htm Accessed: March 15, 2014.

26. U.S. Food and Drug Administration: Food: *Alphabetical list of SCOGS substances.* Updated June 2013. http://www.fda.gov/Food/IngredientsPackagingLabeling/GRAS/SCOGS/ucm084104.htm Accessed: March 15, 2014.

27. U.S. Food and Drug Administration: Food: Ingredients, packaging and labeling: Food additives and ingredients: *Determining the regulatory status of a food ingredient.* Updated March 2013. http://www.fda.gov/Food/IngredientsPackagingLabeling/FoodAdditivesIngredients/ucm228269.htm Accessed: March 15, 2014.

28. Congressional Research Service Report for Congress, Pesticide legislation: *Food Quality Protection Act of 1996 (P.L. 104-170) II 96-759 ENR.* http://www .ncseonline.org/programs/science-policy/crs-reports Accessed: March 15, 2014.

29. U.S. Food and Drug Administration: *Defect levels handbook: The food defect action levels: Levels of natural or unavoidable defects in foods that present no health hazards for humans.* May 1998. Updated March 2014. http://www.fda .gov/Food/GuidanceRegulation/GuidanceDocumentsRegulatoryInformation/SanitationTransportation/ucm056174.htm#CHPT3 Accessed: March 15, 2014.

30. U.S. Food and Drug Administration: *Data on benzene in soft drinks and other beverages.* 2007. Updated March 2013. http://www.fda.gov/Food/FoodborneIllnessContaminants/ChemicalContaminants/ucm055815.htm Accessed: March 15, 2014.

31. U.S. Food and Drug Administration: *Draft guidance for industry: Acrylamide in foods.* Updated November 2013. http://www.fda.gov/Food/GuidanceRegulation/GuidanceDocumentsRegulatoryInformation/ChemicalContaminantsMetalsNaturalToxinsPesticides/ucm374524.htm Accessed: March 15, 2014.

32. U.S. Food and Drug Administration: *FDA continues to study BPA.* March 2012. Updated August 2013. http://www.fda.gov/ForConsumers/ConsumerUpdates/ucm297954.htm Accessed: March 15, 2014.

33. U.S. Department of Health and Human Services: *Bisphenol A (BPA) information for parents.* ND. http://www.hhs.gov/safety/bpa/ Accessed: March 15, 2014.

34. Environmental Protection Agency: Pesticides: Fact sheets: *The EPA and food security.* Updated May 2012. http://www.epa.gov/pesticides/factsheets/securty .htm Accessed: March 15, 2014.

35. Forman J, Silverstein J: Organic foods: Health and environmental advantages and disadvantages. *Pediatrics* 130(5):1406, 2012.

36. Centers for Disease Control and Prevention: *Fourth national report on human exposure to environmental chemicals.* Updated September, 2013. May 2012. http://www.cdc.gov/exposurereport/ Accessed: March 15, 2014.

37. Alavanja M and others: Increased cancer burden among pesticide applicators and others due to pesticide exposure. *CA* 63(2):120-142, 2013.

38. Sebastian RS and others: Drinking water intake in the U.S. *What we eat in America: NHANES 2005-2008,* 2011. http://www.ars.usda.gov/SP2UserFiles/Place/12355000/pdf/DBrief/7_water_intakes_0508.pdf Accessed: March 15, 2014.

39. U.S. Environmental Protection Agency: *Water on tap: What you need to know.* 2009. http://water.epa.gov/drink/guide/upload/book_waterontap_full.pdf Accessed: March 15, 2014.

40. International Bottled Water Association: *U.S. consumption of bottled water shows continued growth, increasing 6.2 percent in 2012; Sales up 6.7 percent.* 2013. http://www.bottledwater.org/us-consumption-bottled-water-shows-continued-growth-increasing-62-percent-2012-sales-67-percent Accessed: March 15, 2014.

41. U.S. Environmental Protection Agency: *Water health series: Bottled water basics.* 2005. http://water.epa.gov/drink/info/upload/2005_09_14_faq_fs_healthseries_bottledwater.pdf Accessed: March 15, 2014.

42. International Bottled Water Association: *Recycling.* 2014. http://www .bottledwater.org/education/recycling Accessed: March 15, 2014.

43. Centers for Disease Control and Prevention: *Traveler's health: Water disinfection.* Updated April 2013. http://wwwnc.cdc.gov/travel/page/water-disinfection Accessed: March 15, 2014.

20 Global Nutrition

Infant undernutrition in a developing country

MONIQUE, A HAITIAN MOTHER, BRINGS HER 10-month-old son, Louis, to a free local health clinic because she is worried about the baby's health. Louis is weak and has chronic diarrhea. The physician who weighs and observes the baby determines Louis is undernourished and suffering from a water-borne infection. When asked about Louis's diet, Monique reports that she is still feeding the child a ready-to-use infant formula and gives him cooked rice. Monique admits that she dilutes the formula with an equal amount of water that comes from a local stream before feeding the formula to the baby.

The physician gives an antibiotic to the baby and tells Monique to avoid diluting the formula. The doctor also provides her with a supply of a peanut-based supplement to mix into the cooked rice. A clinic worker tells the mother to boil and cool the water before using it.

After 3 months, Monique returns to the clinic with her son. She is pleased that the child no longer has diarrhea and his growth rate has increased dramatically since she last visited the clinic.

- What are possible causes of undernutrition and diarrhea in this child?
- In this situation, why might breastfeeding have been better for the infant than formula feeding?
- Describe why the child's health has improved.

The suggested Case Study Response can be found on page 657.

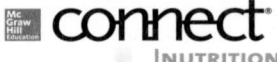

Connect | NUTRITION   Check out the Connect site at www.mcgrawhillconnect.com to further explore this case study.

The school lunch program at the Kentucky Academy in Ghana, West Africa provides a mid-day meal to children who otherwise may not have access to food or adequate amounts of food.

Throughout the world, which countries have a high prevalence of chronic undernutrition? What are the consequences of chronic undernutrition in children? Take the following quiz to test your knowledge of global nutrition, including the problem of undernutrition in the United States. The answers are found on page 660.

1. More people in the world experience undernutrition than overnutrition. ___T ___F

2. Stunting is a consequence of chronic undernutrition in infants and children. ___T ___F

3. In children, diets that are iron deficient can lead to blindness. ___T ___F

4. Individuals experiencing *marginal food security* have a reduction in both the quantity and nutritional quality of the foods they consume. ___T ___F

5. The Supplemental Nutrition Assistance Program enables low-income Americans to purchase foods as well as certain seeds for their gardens. ___T ___F

20.1 Malnutrition: A Worldwide Concern

LEARNING OUTCOMES

1 *Identify populations or groups of people that are at risk of undernutrition.*

2 *Explain factors that contribute to undernutrition.*

Malnutrition, which literally means "bad" or "ill" nutrition, was defined in Chapter 1 as a state of health that results from improper nourishment. Malnutrition can occur when diets lack nutrients (undernutrition) or contain excessive amounts of nutrients (overnutrition). Today, more people suffer from overnutrition than undernutrition. It is estimated that more than 1.4 billion people in the world are either overweight or obese.[1] Despite increasing rates of overnutrition, under-nutrition remains a serious global concern. Approximately 870 million adults and children worldwide suffer from an inadequate food intake.[2] Malnutrition can be caused by a variety of factors including poor diet, disease, and medication interactions. This chapter will focus specifically on malnutrition in the form of undernutrition resulting from inadequate food and nutrient intake.

Chronic Undernutrition

Chronic undernutrition occurs when long-term energy and nutrient intakes are insufficient to meet an individual's needs. Undernutrition can be very harmful, especially when it occurs during periods of rapid growth and elevated nutrient needs, such as pregnancy, infancy, and childhood. In addition, undernutrition is commonly seen in older adults and may partly be the result of physiological changes that occur as people age. These physiological changes include impaired digestion and absorption, diminished ability to taste, and decreased muscle mass (see Chapter 18). Because the aging process weakens the immune system, older adults have a greater risk of developing the physiological consequences of chronic undernutrition than younger adults.[3]

Undernutrition occurs in all countries; however, developing countries have much higher rates than developed countries. The prevalence of undernutrition is highest in sub-Saharan Africa and southern and eastern parts of Asia.[4] Table 20.1 compares the prevalence of undernutrition across all developed and developing countries, as well as in various developing countries from across the globe.

Factors That Contribute to Undernutrition

Throughout the world, social, environmental, economic, political, and other factors contribute to undernutrition (Fig. 20.1). Poverty, however, is the leading risk factor for undernutrition in both developed and developing countries. More than a billion people live on the equivalent of less than $1.25 per day, and those living in chronic poverty unquestionably struggle to obtain enough food to meet their nutrition needs.[5] Furthermore, many developing nations owe large sums of money to wealthy countries. High national debts often cause government leaders to cut or eliminate

chronic undernutrition state of under-nutrition occurring when energy and nutrient intakes are insufficient to meet an individual's needs over an extended period of time

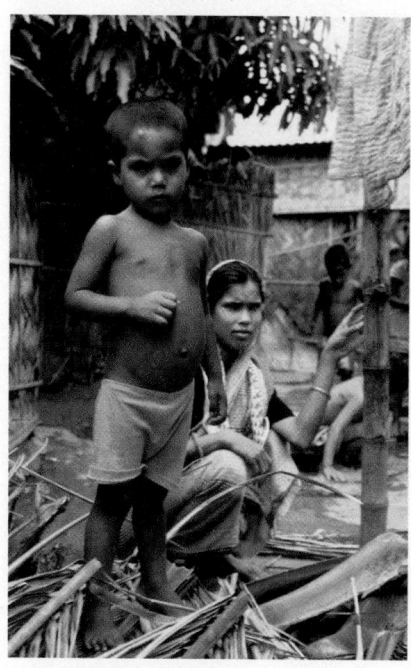

The child and young woman live in Bangladesh, located in Southern Asia. Bangladesh is a developing country where poverty and undernutrition rates are widespread.

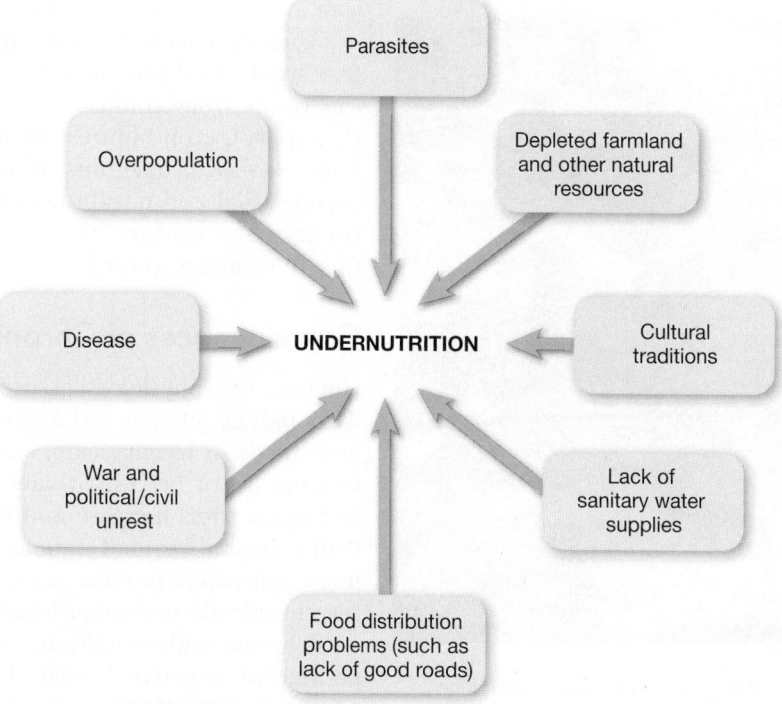

FIGURE 20.1 Factors that contribute to undernutrition. Many factors, including war, disease, and overpopulation, contribute to undernutrition in developing countries.

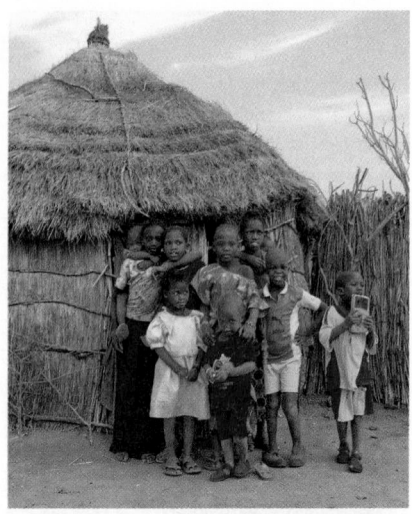

Many families in developing countries do not have access to electricity, sewage systems, and running water. These African children are in front of a grass hut home.

stunting reduced adult size as a consequence of chronic undernutrition in infancy and childhood

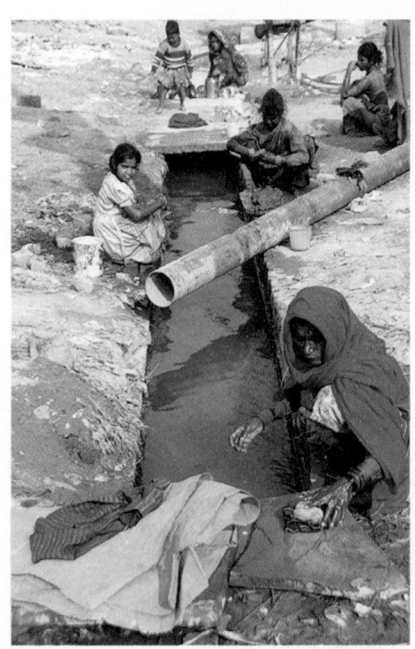

In developing countries, poor sanitation practices and lack of clean cooking and drinking water contribute to the spread of diseases.

TABLE 20.1 Prevalence of Undernutrition Among Selected Countries, 2010–2012

Region or Country	People Undernourished (in millions)	Population Undernourished (as a percent of total)
World	868	12.5
All developed countries	16	1.4
All developing countries	852	14.9
Selected developing regions		
Africa (all countries)	239	22.9
Northern	4	2.7
Sub-Saharan	37.8	26.8
Asia	563	13.9
Central	6	7.4
Eastern	167	11.5
Southern	304	17.6
Southeastern	65	10.9
Western	21	10.9
Caribbean	7	17.8
Latin American	42	7.7
Oceania	1	12.1

Adapted from: Table 1.1 in Food and Agriculture Organization of the United Nations: *The state of food insecurity in the world.* 2012. http://www.fao.org/docrep/016/i3027e/i3027e.pdf.

basic services that would reduce undernutrition and poverty, including health care and education programs.

Undernutrition is common among impoverished people in developing countries where food production and supplies are inadequate. Regional food shortages can result from traditional dietary practices (e.g., consuming a diet with little variety), crop failures, local warfare, and political instability and corruption. Impoverished people must also cope with infectious diseases, parasitic infections, overcrowded and unsafe housing conditions, and polluted water supplies. In the twenty–first century, over one–third of the world's population still lacks access to safe drinking water.[6]

Consequences of Chronic Undernutrition

Hunger, the physiological need for food, usually accompanies undernutrition. Although significant reductions in the rates of chronically undernourished have been made in recent years, one in eight people is not able to access enough food to meet his or her nutritional needs.[7] Studies show that diet diversity improves as income rates increase and families are able to purchase more nutrient–dense fruits, vegetables, and animal sources of food.[8] These foods, which are typically more expensive, provide many of the micronutrients that are lacking in diets of the chronically undernourished.

Chronic undernutrition, especially when it occurs early in life, can result in permanent negative health effects such as decreased cognitive ability, reduced adult size **(stunting)**, and compromised reproductive functioning.[9] Furthermore, chronic undernutrition depresses the body's immune system, increasing the risk of infectious diseases, such as measles. These costs of childhood undernutrition contribute to decreased productivity (ability to work and earn an income) in adulthood, which continues the cycle of poverty and undernutrition for generations. Each year, undernutrition may account for over $1 trillion in lost revenue and health care costs throughout the world.[8]

Undernutrition During Pregnancy

A mother's nutritional status before and during pregnancy has a significant impact on both her health and her baby's health. Having a healthy weight is usually necessary for a woman's fertility. Undernourished women with poor nutrient intakes are less likely to become pregnant, yet pregnancies still occur. Worldwide, between 10 and 20% of pregnant women are underweight. This rate is even higher in highly populated parts of the world, such as India, where nearly 40% of pregnant women have BMIs below 18.5 kg/m^2.[10]

Maternal undernutrition increases the likelihood of delivering a low−birth−weight infant. Babies born at less than ideal birth weights are more likely to die before reaching the age of 1 year than babies born at normal weights.[11] In developing countries, as many as 16% of newborns are low birth weight compared to 8% of infants born in the United States.[10,12] Because many newborns in developing countries are not weighed at birth, the percentage of low−birth−weight babies may be much higher.[11] Additionally, studies conducted in countries that have frequent food shortages indicate that poor nutrition during pregnancy may increase the risk for such diseases as high blood pressure, obesity, and even *schizophrenia*, a severe form of mental illness, later in life.[13]

Iron deficiency anemia and stunting in pregnant women who have a history of chronic undernutrition account for one−fifth of maternal deaths worldwide.[10] Stunting in a pregnant woman can increase the need for a caesarian delivery ("C−section") because the fetus's head may be too large to pass through the mother's pelvis. In many developing countries, access to safe operating rooms may be limited, and women who have stunting may be more likely to die while giving birth than pregnant women who are adequately nourished.

Undernutrition During Infancy

According to various international health agencies, the first 2 years of an infant's life are the critical time period for avoiding undernutrition.[14] Efforts to reduce undernutrition include providing adequate amounts of vitamins and minerals through diet and supplements, increasing access to safe water, using special therapeutic foods, and improving breastfeeding rates. As described in Chapter 16, breastfeeding has many benefits. In developing countries, however, many new mothers do not exclusively breastfeed their babies for more than a few weeks.[10] Infant formulas are nutritious substitutes for breast milk, but they are generally more expensive, and parents may add excessive amounts of water in order to extend the formula. This practice dilutes the nutritional value of the formula and increases the likelihood of contaminating it with disease−causing microbes. In infants, the diarrhea that results from drinking formula made with unsanitary water can cause dehydration, serious illness, and even death.

Undernutrition During Childhood Years

Each year, 35% of deaths in children under 5 years of age, or 3.5 million children, are related to maternal or child undernutrition.[10] The **under−5 mortality rate** is frequently used to evaluate the health of infants and young children from a global perspective. The under−5 mortality rate is expressed as the number of newborns in a population, per 1000 live births, who are likely to die before they reach 5 years of age. Table 20.2 identifies the under−5 mortality rates in several countries. The United Nations (UN) has made reducing child mortality rates one of its main goals.[7]

under-5 mortality rate number of newborns in a population, per 1000 live births, who are likely to die before they reach 5 years of age

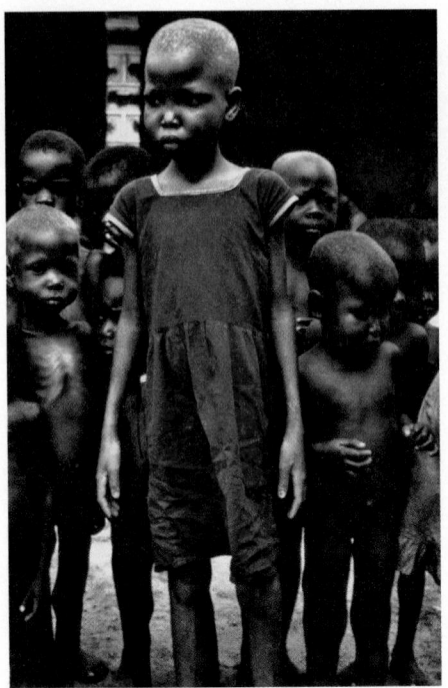

FIGURE 20.2 Chronic undernutrition. This photograph shows a group of undernourished children outside a Nigerian orphanage during the late 1960s.

TABLE 20.2 Under-5 Mortality Rates for Selected Countries, 2012

Country	Rate per 1000 Live Births
Afghanistan	99
Ethiopia	68
Guinea	101
Mali	128
Niger	114
Sierra Leone	182
China	14
Denmark	4
Germany	4
Haiti	76
Iceland	2
India	56
Japan	3
Mexico	16
United States	7

Adapted from: The World Bank: *Data: Mortality rate, under-5 (per 1000 live births).* http://data.worldbank.org/indicator/SH.DYN .MORT Accessed: March 18, 2014.

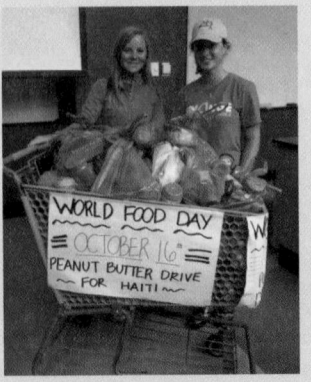

When undernourished children are able to survive, they often have stunted growth, blindness, and/or impaired intellectual development as a result of having experienced severe nutrient deficiencies (Fig. 20.2). Worldwide, one in every four children is stunted and about one in every five children is underweight as a result of undernutrition.[2] Children who are chronically undernourished often perform poorly in school, particularly if they are iron deficient.[15] Regular breakfast consumption in children who are undernourished is positively associated with academic performance.[16]

Undernutrition Among Older Adults

Worldwide, the number of older persons who are undernourished is unknown, but as many as half of the older adults in some countries experience undernutrition.[3] As mentioned previously, a weakened immune system due to advanced age can increase the negative effects that undernutrition has on older adults. Undernutrition among older adults increases the risk for acute illness, longer hospitalizations, and death.[3]

By 2025, the world's population of people who are 60 years of age and older is expected to be at least 1 billion, with about three-fourths of these older persons living in low-income countries.[17] Ways to reduce undernutrition among older adults include improving nutrition education that targets older adults and their caregivers, enhancing government assistance programs, and providing nutrition supplementation.

ASSESS YOUR PROGRESS

1. Name at least two groups of people at risk for undernutrition.
2. List at least three factors that contribute to undernutrition.

20.2 Undernutrition: Common Micronutrient Deficiencies

LEARNING OUTCOMES

1. *Identify the four leading micronutrient deficiencies worldwide.*
2. *Describe major health concerns that can result from micronutrient deficiencies.*

Over 2 million people in the world suffer from micronutrient deficiencies.[18] Globally, four micronutrients are identified as top public health concerns: vitamin A, iron, iodine, and zinc. Worldwide, lack of nutrient–dense foods and variety in the diet are the leading causes of micronutrient deficiencies. Eliminating both vitamin A and zinc deficiencies may be the single most effective intervention for reducing complications of undernutrition on a global scale. One report estimates that every $1 spent on vitamin A and zinc supplementation in developing countries could generate $17 in benefits from reduced health care costs and improved income.[19] This section of the chapter will review the effects of vitamin A, iron, iodine, and zinc deficiencies throughout the world.

Vitamin A

As described in Chapter 9, vitamin A is important for immunity, vision, reproduction, and cellular growth. Lack of vitamin A is the leading cause of childhood blindness, or xerophthalmia. Approximately 250 million children around the world do not consume enough vitamin A, and as many as 500,000 children develop blindness each year as a result of this deficiency.[20] Additionally, a vitamin A deficiency contributes to a weakened immune system that cannot effectively combat infectious diseases, such as measles, which is common in developing countries that do not have programs to immunize children against the virus.[21]

Providing dietary supplements that contain preformed vitamin A or the provitamin A carotenoids, such as beta–carotene, is vital for regions that lack adequate access to foods that contain the vitamin or its precursors. By giving the supplements twice a year to children who live in areas with high rates of vitamin A deficiency, mortality can be reduced by 23% and childhood blindness by 70%.[18] Section 20.4 provides information on *Golden Rice*, a breakthrough in biotechnology that provides a locally grown food source of beta–carotene to those living in areas most prone to vitamin A deficiency.

Iron

Iron deficiency is the most prevalent micronutrient deficiency worldwide and one of the only micronutrient deficiencies that is common in developed countries. Iron is critical for hemoglobin development and sufficient oxygen delivery to the brain and muscles. Pregnancy increases a woman's requirement for iron; the additional iron is necessary to supply the placenta and developing fetus with adequate amounts of the mineral. Iron–rich foods such as red meats; dark, leafy greens; and iron–fortified cereals are typically consumed on a limited basis by many individuals living in poverty.

Regardless of one's age, having a diet that lacks iron can interrupt normal cognitive functioning and reduce physical activity levels. Therefore, widespread iron deficiency in a country contributes to decreased overall productivity among the population. Studies suggest that productivity rates would significantly increase

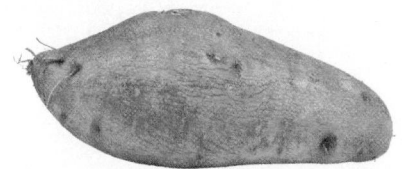

One medium sweet potato, baked with the skin on, provides the Recommended Daily Allowance of vitamin A (adult) in the form of beta-carotene.

on a global scale if iron deficiency anemia were eliminated. As a result of the increased productivity, the number of people living in poverty would be reduced.[22]

Women with iron–deficiency anemia are at greater risk for serious complications during childbirth, including hemorrhage, or uncontrolled bleeding, which can be deadly. According to health experts, maternal mortality rates could be decreased by 20% with appropriate iron supplementation during pregnancy.[18]

Iodine

Recall from Chapter 12 that iodine is essential for normal metabolism and thyroid functioning. The most common result of iodine deficiency is a goiter. In addition, iodine deficiency during pregnancy can result in intellectual disability in the developing fetus (cretinism). High rates of intellectual disability can negatively influence the average intelligence level of a population. The average intelligence quotient, or IQ score, is as much as 13 points higher in countries with populations that have adequate dietary iodine status versus countries with populations that experience widespread deficiencies of the mineral.[18]

Iodine is present in seawater and the soil, especially soil near coastal waters. Natural food sources of iodine include dairy foods and seafood products, both of which are often not accessible in adequate amounts on a global scale. Fortification of salt with iodine is a simple and relatively inexpensive method to prevent the trace mineral's deficiency, but not all countries fortify salt at this time. Reasons for not fortifying salt include increased cost to producers, lack of technology for adding iodine to salt in developing countries, and negative perceptions among the population regarding the safety of the iodized salt.

Zinc

Adequate dietary zinc stimulates immunity, which increases a person's resistance to infection, prevents stunting in children, and contributes to normal sexual maturation in adolescents. During prenatal development, the fetus has a high demand for zinc. Therefore, women who have low zinc status prior to becoming pregnant will further deplete their zinc stores during pregnancy, unless they obtain zinc supplementation.[23] Babies born to mothers who are deficient in zinc are highly likely to be deficient as well. In malnourished children, zinc supplements appear to lessen the severity of diarrhea, indicating a relationship between low zinc levels and diarrhea. Annually, nearly half a million deaths of children throughout the world who are under 5 years of age are associated with zinc deficiency.[18]

Sources of zinc typically include more expensive animal foods, including red meats, poultry, and seafood. Although zinc is found in many grains, a food group that forms the basis of diets in the majority of developing countries, grains also contain phytic acid. This compound inhibits the absorption of zinc from the gastrointestinal tract.[23] Chapter 12 provides more details on the effects of phytic acid on the absorption of minerals.

ASSESS YOUR PROGRESS

3 Identify the four leading micronutrient deficiencies worldwide.

4 Describe at least one health concern for each of the four leading micronutrient deficiencies listed in question 3.

20.3 Food Insecurity in the United States

LEARNING OUTCOMES

1 *Summarize the categories of food security.*

2 *Describe characteristics of individuals living in the United States who are likely to be food insecure.*

3 *Identify nutrition assistance programs available to Americans who experience food insecurity, and describe persons who are eligible for such assistance.*

4 *Identify resources within communities that help alleviate hunger in the United States.*

Although undernutrition is common in adults and children who live in poverty–stricken developing countries, undernutrition also occurs in wealthy, developed nations such as the United States. Many people living in the United States experience **food insecurity**. A person who is food insecure does not have access to enough nourishing food at all times to lead a healthy, active life. Conversely, when a person experiences **food security**, he or she is able to include a variety of nutritious foods in his or her diet and obtain these foods without depending on the assistance of others or the government.

There are four categories for classifying people as being food secure or food insecure:[24]

- *High food security* includes individuals who experience no concerns or problems with purchasing enough food.

- *Marginal food security* includes individuals who may experience some anxiety or worry regarding their ability to purchase enough food; however, they make little to no changes in the quality or quantity of their food intake.

- *Low food security* includes individuals who experience reduced nutritional quality of their diet due to a limited ability to purchase enough nutrient–dense food.

- *Very low food security* includes individuals who experience reductions in both the quality and quantity of their diet due to an inability to purchase enough food.

Hunger in the United States

In the United States, the rate of food insecurity has reached its highest level within the last 20 years.[25] Causes of food insecurity and hunger in the United States are similar to those in developing countries. In the United States, however, the negative effects that poor sanitation, wars, and civil unrest have on food availability are not the concerns they are in less developed nations.

Americans who are unemployed, work in low–paying jobs, or have excessive medical and housing expenses often experience food insecurity. Food insecurity may also affect older adults who live on fixed incomes, especially if they are forced to choose between purchasing nutritious food and buying life–extending medications. Research conducted by the U.S. Department of Agriculture (USDA) identified individuals who are more likely to be food insecure than other members of the population. Americans who are more likely to be food insecure include:[25]

- Households with children, especially if a single woman is the head of the household;

- Households that live at 185% of the poverty threshold;

- Hispanic families and black, non–Hispanic families;

food insecurity state in which individuals are concerned about running out of food or not having enough money to buy more food

food security state in which individuals have access to enough food at all times to lead healthy, active lives

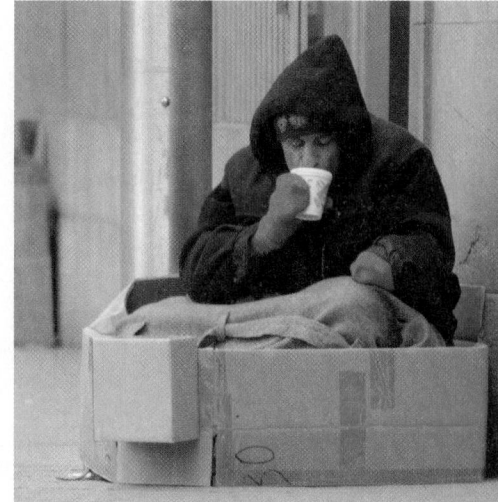

In the United States, members of the homeless population typically experience food insecurity.

- Households living in metropolitan areas; and

- Households in the southern and western regions of the country, including the states of Alabama, Arkansas, California, Georgia, Mississippi, North Carolina, and Texas.

Currently, 15% of Americans are food insecure, with approximately 9% living in low food security and 6% living in very low food security.[25] Individuals who experience very low food security frequently report that they do not always eat when they are hungry; they eat less than they feel they should; they skip meals more than three times a month or even go an entire day without eating; and they have lost weight because of not eating.

DID **YOU** KNOW?

Many Americans think that "eating healthy" has to be expensive. However, a study published by the USDA revealed that for less than $2.50 per day, Americans can consume their recommended number of fruits and vegetables. That amount is about 50 cents per serving! Results from the study indicate that watermelon (17 cents per serving) and dried pinto beans (13 cents per serving) are the least expensive fruit and vegetable, respectively, while fresh raspberries ($2.06 per serving) and frozen asparagus tips ($2.07 per serving) are the most expensive. To read more about this study. visit http://www.ers .usda.gov/media/133274/eib71_ reportsummary.pdf .

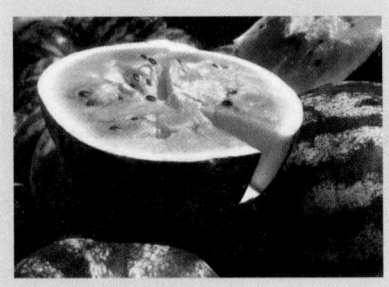

FRESH TIPS

Dried legumes, such as pinto beans, are an inexpensive yet nutritious food that contains both carbohydrates and proteins. The dried beans can often be purchased in bulk. To prepare the beans for use, the beans need to be soaked by one of three methods: hot soak, traditional soak, and quick soak. To quick soak beans:

- Place a premeasured amount of beans in a large pot.

- Add 10 cups of water for every 2 cups of beans.

- Bring the water to a boil for 2 to 3 minutes.

- Drain the beans, discarding the soak water.

- Rinse the beans in cold water.

Visit the U.S. Dry Bean Council's website at http://www.usdrybeans.com/ for information on the varieties of dried beans available, how to properly cook dry beans, and recipe ideas.

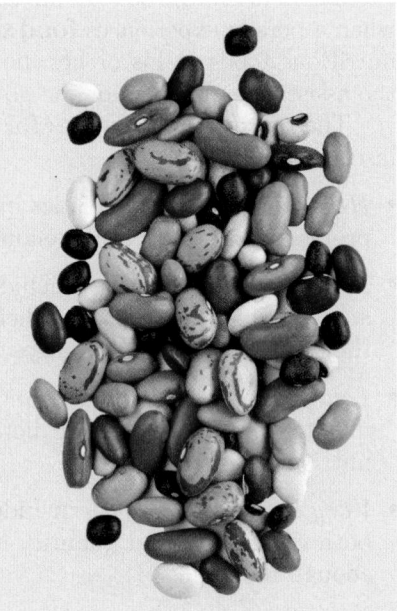

Eliminating Food Deserts

Many Americans simply do not have enough money to purchase nutrient–dense foods. However, a considerable number of Americans live in places that have few supermarkets and the people lack transportation to access grocery stores that are beyond their neighborhood. *Food deserts* are areas in which a large proportion of residents experience difficulty in obtaining nutritious foods. The USDA defines **food deserts** as areas with numerous low–income people living farther than 1 mile away from grocery stores in urban areas or farther than 10 miles away from grocery stores in rural areas.[26] To find food deserts in the United States, visit the USDA's Food Access Research Atlas at http://www.ers.usda.gov/ data–products/food–access–research–atlas/go–to–the–atlas.aspx.

Food deserts can negatively influence the health of individuals living in them, because a person's diet reflects the nutritional quality and variety of foods avail– able to purchase. When grocery stores or supermarkets are scarce in an area of town that has fast–food restaurants or convenience stores, individuals are more likely to get their food from the most convenient places. Fast–food restaurants and convenience stores typically have limited selections of healthy foods such as fruits and vegetables.

food deserts regions or areas in which a large proportion of those living there experience difficulty in obtaining nutritious food

In 2010, First Lady Michelle Obama launched *Let's Move*, a comprehensive program that aims to eliminate childhood obesity in America. One effort within this program included the *Healthy Food Financing Initiative* (*HFFI*), a cooperative initiative designed to increase the accessibility of healthy foods and employment rates in areas that have been identified as food deserts.[27] HFFI provides financial incentives such as tax credits, grants, and low–cost loans to retailers that offer nutritious foods in these areas. Since the initiative's start, funding has been provided for numerous programs that enhance the quality of food available in food deserts.

HFFI also offers financial aid to grocery stores, farmers' markets, and similar food sources that experience difficulty obtaining and marketing nutritious items in food deserts. In many of Philadelphia's low–income neighborhoods, locally owned ("mom and pop") convenience stores are selling fresh produce, because of assistance from the Healthy Corner Stores Network, supported by the HFFI. The network helps small grocery store owners provide and promote fruits and vegetables for their customers.

A creative example of how HFFI helps communities is the Casa Azafram Community Center in Nashville, Tennessee. The community center received a grant to open a commercial kitchen that can be rented (for a low cost) by community members, especially women, who want to start a business that involves making healthy foods and selling them to the public. The people who use the kitchen for this purpose also receive professional support and guidance for food– and business–related concerns, including food safety, product marketing, and financial management. An estimated 50 new jobs were created in Nashville as a result of the development of the commercial kitchen.[28]

Providing Free Food to Low-Income Americans

Many local churches and charitable organizations provide free food to members of the community who are in need. Individuals, however, must be able to get to and from such food distribution locations to receive this help. Mobile food pantries are an innovative way for these programs to distribute food to those in need who do not have transportation or who live in areas that lack food distribution centers. Mobile food pantries are simply large vehicles that carry food to low–income neighborhoods and rural counties where food distribution programs may be limited (Fig. 20.3). According to Feeding America, the nation's largest food distribution program, one mobile food pantry vehicle distributes an average of 900,000 pounds of food per year.[29]

Major U.S. Food Assistance Programs

Low–income individuals, especially children, may be able to obtain food aid from several different food assistance programs in the United States. Many of these programs are operated by the Food and Nutrition Service (FNS) within the USDA (Table 20.3). The Department of Health and Human Services (DHHS) and nonprofit agencies also provide support to those who are hungry. Each program differs in the population it serves and type of assistance provided, but most programs use income to determine eligibility for obtaining the assistance.

Supplemental Nutrition Assistance Program

The **Supplemental Nutrition Assistance Program (SNAP)**, formerly known as the Food Stamp Program, is the largest food assistance program in the United States. The program aids an estimated 28 million people each month.[31] SNAP enables qualified low–income participants to use monthly cash allotments and a special debit card to purchase foods from authorized stores. Participants are not allowed to buy any nonfood items, vitamins, medicines, alcohol, or ready–to–eat hot foods with their benefits, but they can use them to purchase most other foods,

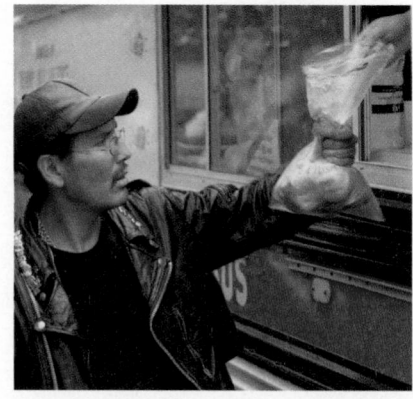

FIGURE 20.3 Mobile food pantries.
Mobile food pantries are an innovative way to get nutritious foods to areas that lack healthy food options.

DID **YOU** KNOW?

As of January 2014, the U.S. Department of Education Office of Postsecondary Education defines "low income" as an income less than $17,505 for an individual, less than $23,595 for a two-person family unit, and less than $35,775 for a four-person family unit.[30]

Supplemental Nutrition Assistance Program (SNAP) assistance program that enables qualified low-income participants to use monthly cash allotments and a special debit card to purchase foods from authorized stores

TABLE 20.3 Major Federally Subsidized Food Assistance Programs in the United States

Program	Agency	General Eligibility Requirements	Description
Supplemental Nutrition Assistance Program (SNAP)	FNS	Low-income individuals and families	Participants are provided with an electronic benefit transfer card and monthly cash allotments to purchase approved food items.
Special Supplemental Nutrition Assistance Program for Women, Infants, and Children (WIC)	FNS	Low-income pregnant, breastfeeding or postpartum women, infants, and children up to 5 years of age who are at nutritional risk	Participants receive checks or vouchers to purchase approved food items. Additionally, nutrition education, health referrals, and breastfeeding support are provided.
WIC Farmers' Market Nutrition Program	FNS	Same eligibility as WIC, except infants must be above the age of 4 months	Participants receive coupons to purchase fresh, unprepared fruits and vegetables that are locally grown and sold at farmers' markets and approved roadside stands.
National School Lunch Program (NSLP) and School Breakfast Program (SBP)	FNS	Low-income children of school age	Public and nonprofit schools receive cash subsidies in order to provide free or reduced-fee meals to students. Meals must meet specific nutrition standards.
Summer Food Service Program (SFSP)	FNS	Children enrolled at nonprofit sites providing summer meals in areas with a high number of low-income children	Facilities that serve free meals and snacks to low-income children during summer months or extended school vacations receive cash reimbursements. Sites can be schools, churches, camps, community centers, and other nonprofit programs.
Special Milk Program (SMP)	FNS	Children enrolled in schools, child care institutions, and eligible camps that do not participate in other federal nutrition programs	Programs that provide free or reduced-price milk to children receive cash reimbursements and subsidies to facilities. Milk provided must be pasteurized and meet specific nutrition guidelines.
Child and Adult Care Food Program	FNS	Children enrolled in organized child care programs and older adults in adult care programs	Programs receive cash reimbursement for nutritious meals and snacks supplied to participants.
Food Distribution Program on Indian Reservations	FNS	Low-income American Indian or non-Indian households on reservations; members of federally recognized Native American tribes	Participants receive monthly food packages. This program is an alternative to SNAP and includes a nutrition education program.
Commodity Supplemental Food (CSFP)	FNS	Low-income pregnant, breastfeeding, and postpartum women, infants, and children up to 6 years of age who are at nutritional risk; low-income adults age 60 or older who are at nutritional risk	Participants receive distributed foods from the USDA. This program is an alternative to WIC, and participants may not be eligible for both.
Food Distribution Disaster Assistance	FNS	Individuals and families in financial need that have recently experienced a disaster	Provides individuals, families, and relief agencies assistance in areas affected by a disaster, including natural disasters such as a flood, hurricane, or tornado; assistance can include food provided at mass feeding sites and distributed to households, as well as emergency SNAP benefits.
The Emergency Food Assistance Program (TEFAP)	FNS	States and programs set income standards for those eligible to receive distributed foods.	The USDA provides foods to state distribution agencies or food banks that will, in turn, distribute to other food-distributing programs.
Elderly Nutrition Program	DHHS	Adults age 60 or older; while income is not evaluated, priority is given to low-income areas	Gives programs and facilities cash grants in order to provide congregate and home-delivered meals to eligible adults; meals must meet specific nutrition standards.
Senior Farmers' Market Nutrition Program	FNS	Low-income adults age 60 or older	Provides participants with coupons to purchase fresh, unprepared fruits and vegetables that are locally grown and sold at farmers' markets and approved roadside stands

Source: U.S. Department of Agriculture Food and Nutrition Service: *Programs and services.* http://www.fns.usda.gov/programs-and-services Accessed: August 5, 2013.

as well as garden seeds and plants that produce food. SNAP operates in all 50 states as well as the District of Columbia, Puerto Rico, and the Virgin Islands.

In addition to increasing participants' capability of purchasing nutrient–dense foods, SNAP also offers nutrition education to those who qualify. The nutrition education component of the program, or "SNAP–ed," focuses on providing dietary recommendations, low–cost healthy recipes, and tips for eating well on a limited budget.

Although it may seem contradictory, obesity and food insecurity can occur within the same family or even affect the same individual. This situation happens when families must sacrifice food quality for quantity because they have a limited food budget or when food–insecure individuals overeat just because extra food is available. Skipping meals and/or experiencing stress that is related to financial concerns can lead to overeating and other unhealthy food practices among the food insecure. To address the increasing rates of obesity among SNAP participants, obesity prevention education is now included in SNAP–ed. For more information about the SNAP program, visit http://www.fns.usda .gov/snap/supplemental–nutrition–assistance–program–snap .

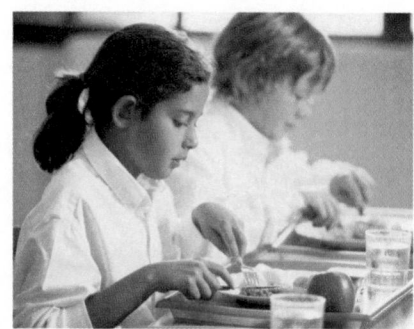

FIGURE 20.4 National School Lunch Program. Every day, 31 million children receive a nutritious reduced-price or free lunch through the National School Lunch Program.

Special Supplemental Nutrition Assistance Program for Women, Infants, and Children

The Special Supplemental Nutrition Assistance Program for Women, Infants, and Children (WIC) provides nutrition education including breastfeeding support, referrals for health and social services, and checks or vouchers to purchase specific foods. For more information about WIC, see Chapter 16.

School Food Programs

Some food assistance programs support schools and other child care institutions that provide nourishing foods to children. The National School Lunch Program (Fig. 20.4) provides reimbursements to schools that offer free or reduced–cost nutritious lunches for eligible low–income students and after–school snacks at sites that meet certain eligibility requirements. The **School Breakfast Program** reimburses schools and other nonprofit agencies for the cost of providing a nutritious morning meal to eligible low–income children. Additional programs that deliver food support to children include the **Special Milk Program**, which enables students to receive free or reduced–cost milk with meals, and the **Summer Food Service Program**, which provides financial support to qualifying facilities that serve free meals and snacks to students during the summer, when schools in low–income neighborhoods are not in session.

Programs for Older Adults

As mentioned in Chapter 18, loss of appetite, low income, and even the inability to drive to the grocery store can negatively affect an older adult's intake of nutritious food. The **Elderly Nutrition Program** provides financial assistance for nonprofit programs that provide free meals to adults 60 years of age and older, regardless of their income. Meals can be either **congregate meals**, that is, a group meal served 5 days a week in a community location such as a senior center, or delivered to participants' homes. Congregate meals enable older adults to enjoy the company of other people who are their age. Many communities also have **Meals on Wheels** programs in which volunteers deliver meals that have been prepared at the community site to home–bound individuals who might not be able to obtain nutrient–dense meals without such assistance.

Taking Action Against Food Insecurity

Food banks are nonprofit organizations that act as distribution centers for surplus foods. By receiving donations from the government as well as private

School Breakfast Program program through which schools and other nonprofit agencies are reimbursed for the cost of providing a nutritious morning meal to eligible low-income children

Special Milk Program program that enables eligible students to receive free or reduced-cost milk with meals

Summer Food Service Program program that provides financial support to qualifying facilities that serve free meals and snacks to students during the summer

Elderly Nutrition Program program that provides financial assistance for nonprofit programs that provide free meals to adults 60 years of age and older, regardless of their income

congregate meals meals served in a community location so people can socialize while they eat

Meals on Wheels program in which volunteers deliver meals that have been prepared at a community site to home-bound individuals

food banks nonprofit organizations that act as distribution centers for surplus food

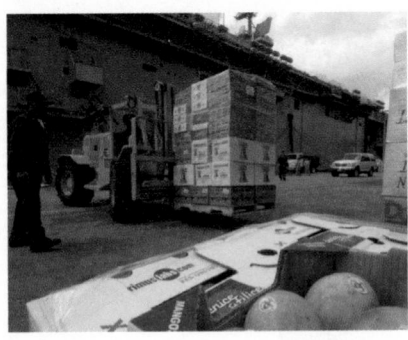

Feeding America, the nation's largest food bank, serves over 3 billion pounds of food and other essential products annually.

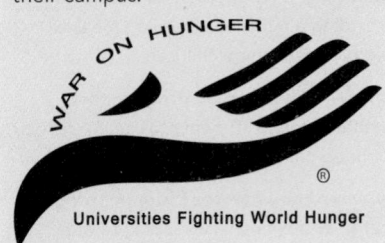
food pantry nonprofit service that provides food to people in need

soup kitchens establishments where prepared meals are provided to those who are hungry, typically for free

organizations and individuals, food banks may charge a small fee to redistribute foods to people who use the resources to help feed persons who are food insecure. Sites and groups that are eligible to obtain the food include homeless shelters, **food pantries**, **soup kitchens**, and other nonprofit hunger—relief charities.

Feeding America is the nation's largest network of food banks with over 200 facilities across the country.[29] In addition to being a food bank, Feeding America sponsors other nutrition—related programs. The Backpack Program, for example, provides packaged nutritious foods for low—income children to take home with them over the weekend, when they do not have access to free school breakfasts or lunches.

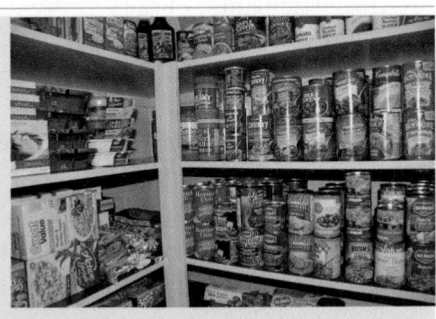
ASSESS YOUR PROGRESS

5 List the four categories of food security.

6 Identify at least three groups of people who are most likely to experience food insecurity.

7 Explain how food deserts can affect the health of those living there.

8 Identify at least three nutrition assistance programs available to Americans who experience food insecurity, and explain how they help reduce hunger.

9 Name at least two resources in communities from which people can obtain food.

20.4 Preventing and Treating Undernutrition

LEARNING OUTCOMES

1 *Identify prevention and treatment opportunities for worldwide undernutrition.*

2 *Describe how sustainable living and agriculture practices affect undernutrition and world hunger.*

The causes of undernutrition and hunger are complex and, therefore, difficult to eliminate. This section discusses biotechnology and the fortification of food as effective measures for the prevention and treatment of undernutrition.

TABLE 20.4 Major Global Food Aid Programs and Their Efforts to Reduce Undernutrition

Global Food Aid Program	Program's Methods to Eliminate Undernutrition
Catholic Relief Agencies www.crs.org	Assists impoverished persons outside of the United States; efforts include providing relief aid in response to major emergencies and support for measures that reduce poverty and the spread of infectious diseases
Global Alliance for Improved Nutrition www.gainhealth.org	Reduces malnutrition through sustainable strategies designed to improve the health and nutrition of populations at risk
Micronutrient Initiative www.micronutrient.org	Strives to eliminate micronutrient deficiencies worldwide by offering knowledge and technology concerning the nutrient fortification of food to the food industry
The World Bank www.worldbank.org	Strives to eliminate extreme poverty by providing low-interest loans, interest-free credits, and grants to developing countries; investments can be for efforts to improve people's health and agricultural production
United Nations Children's Fund (UNICEF) www.unicef.org	Strives to save and improve children's lives by providing health care and immunizations, clean water, nutrition education, and emergency relief
UN's Food and Agriculture Organization www.fao.org	Develops worldwide strategies to meet the following objectives: • Eliminate hunger and malnutrition • Improve production and sustainability of agriculture • Decrease rural poverty • Ensure efficiency of agriculture and food systems
UN's World Food Programme www.wfp.org	Strives to reduce worldwide hunger by distributing emergency food aid to needy populations across the globe. The World Food Programme is the world's largest agency that promotes efforts to reduce undernutrition.
UN's World Health Organization www.who.int	Directs and coordinates efforts to manage health concerns within the UN's system by providing leadership on global health matters, developing the health research agenda, setting standards, developing evidence-based policies, and monitoring and assessing international health trends

Table 20.4 identifies a few of the major global food aid agencies striving to eliminate undernutrition, along with the efforts being made by each of them to reach this goal.

In the short run, wealthy countries can provide food aid to keep impoverished people in less developed nations from starving to death. In the long run, families and small farmers in underdeveloped nations need to learn new and more efficient methods of growing, processing, preserving, and distributing nutritious regional food products. In addition, governments can support programs that encourage breastfeeding and fortify locally grown or commonly consumed foods with vitamins and minerals that are often deficient in local diets.

Population control is critical for preserving the Earth's resources for future generations. Impoverished parents in poor countries typically have many children, because they expect only a few to survive and reach adulthood. As they grow older, the impoverished parents expect to receive care and financial support from their surviving adult children. When people are financially secure, adequately nourished, and well educated, they tend to have fewer, healthier children, in part, because financially secure persons do not need to rely on their adult children for support later in life. Thus, ways to slow population growth include providing well-paying jobs, improving public education, and increasing access to health care services in developing countries.

Biotechnology

Biotechnology involves the use of living things—plants, animals, and microbes—to manufacture new products. Biotechnology in agriculture can include the use of

biotechnology use of living things to produce new products

genetic modification (GM) altering an organism's genetic material in effort to create a new organism with different traits; also called genetic engineering

genetically modified organisms (GMOs) organisms that have been genetically modified

both traditional practices, such as cross−breeding of plants and animals, and pro−gressive practices, such as the alteration of genes. **Genetic modification (GM)**, also called genetic engineering, involves altering a plant or animal's genetic material in an effort to create a new plant or animal with different traits. For example, genes that produce a desirable trait in one organism, such as requir−ing less water to grow, can be transferred into the DNA of another organism so the second organism displays that same desirable trait. Plant and animal prod−ucts that have been genetically altered are referred to as **genetically modified organisms (GMOs)**.

Biotechnology has led to the development of crops that supply higher yields, resist pests and diseases, are tolerant of drought conditions and temperature extremes, and are nutritionally enhanced. Many of the major GM crops that are grown worldwide are modified to be tolerant to *herbicides*, which are pesticides specifically designed to kill unwanted plants such as weeds, and to require fewer pesticides in general. Examples of these crops include corn, soybeans, canola, and sugar beets.

Golden Rice is a plant that has been developed specifically to provide greater amounts of nutrients essential for human health (Fig. 20.5). Rice is a staple in the diets of millions of people in developing countries. By altering certain genes of rice plants, researchers were able to develop a kind of rice that is rich in beta−carotene, a vitamin A precursor. Golden Rice can be grown in countries experiencing high levels of vitamin A deficiency to provide an inexpensive source of this nutrient for the population.[32] The beta−carotene in Golden Rice has been found to be as effective as pure beta−carotene in oil and more effective than beta−carotene in spinach in providing vitamin A to young children.[33] At this time, no GM foods of animal origin have been approved for human consumption, although scientists have developed a type of salmon that has been genetically engineered to grow faster.

By increasing food production or modifying the nutritional content of foods, biotechnology offers another way of alleviating the world food crisis, but GM is controversial. Although foods produced from GM organisms appear to be safe for humans, some individuals are concerned about the potential for negative effects of such genetic manipulations on individual and environmental health, particularly after long−term consumption of GMOs.[34] The development of herbicide−resistant weeds and the presence of undeclared food allergens in GM foods are just a few of the concerns that are being investigated by scientists.[35,36]

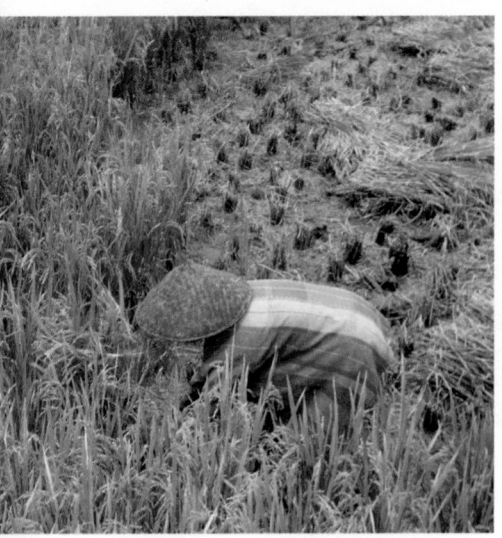

FIGURE 20.5 Growing Golden Rice. Golden Rice is a genetically modified organism that contains more beta-carotene than traditional rice.

Fortification of Foods

As defined in Chapter 3, fortification is the addition of any nutrient to food, generally at a level that exceeds what is naturally in the food. In developing countries where micronutrient deficiencies are common, widespread commercial fortification of staple foods can be a cost−efficient way to improve the con−sumption of the much−needed nutrients.

For fortification to be successful for preventing and treating undernutri−tion, foods selected to be fortified should be those that are commonly con−sumed and relatively inexpensive so that low−income individuals can afford them.[37] Examples of foods that are frequently fortified include wheat and maize flours, cereals, vegetable oils, milk, sugar, salt, and condiments such as soy sauce. Americans regularly consume iodized salt, milk fortified with vitamins A and D, and enriched grain products.

ready-to-use therapeutic foods (RUTFs) shelf-stable foods fortified with calories, protein, and micronutrients that are used for the treatment of undernutrition

Ready-to-Use Therapeutic Foods and Micronutrient Powders

Ready−to−use therapeutic foods (RUTFs) are energy−dense pastes that are enriched with micronutrients. RUTFs are often distributed to families by clinic workers and doctors. Their use has shown to be effective in treating under—nutrition, especially among young children in developing countries.[38] RUTFs are typically packaged in single doses for easy use and to reduce waste. Most RUTFs do not require refrigeration or dilution with water, which makes them very safe to use in areas where sanitation problems exist. The most common RUTFs are pastes made from peanuts, skimmed milk powder, vegetable fats, and micronutrients, such as *Mother Administered Nutritive Aid* (*MANA*) and *Plumpy'nut®* (Fig. 20.6).

Micronutrient powders are single—dose packages of powdered micronutri—ents, such as iron, vitamin A, and zinc.[39] Similarly to RUTFs, these powders are designed to prevent micronutrient deficiencies; however, they must be added to foods to be consumed. The majority of micronutrient powders are used for infants who are being weaned from breast milk, a time when undernutrition is prevalent in susceptible populations. One example of a micronutrient powder is *Sprinkles*, which contains iron, zinc, and vitamins folic acid, A, and C. Studies show that when Sprinkles is used as recommended for 60 to 120 days, rates of iron deficiency anemia can be drastically reduced in devel—oping countries.[40]

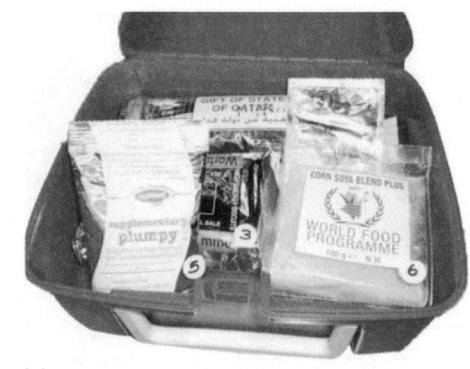
(a)

Sustainable Living Practices

Our current system of food production relies primarily on conventional agricul—tural methods. In general, conventional farming requires considerable amounts of water and pesticides that can harm the environment. Irrigation systems often remove fresh water from rivers and other natural sources at a faster rate than it is restored. This activity reduces water flow to many communities. The water that runs off conventional farms can carry precious topsoil with it, along with pesticides that pollute waterways. Such farming methods also release green—house gases, especially carbon dioxide and methane, which contribute to global warming. Furthermore, the need for new farmland often requires cutting down trees so that forests can be converted to croplands. The loss of forests eliminates native wild animal and plant habitats. About 40% of the Earth's land (excluding Greenland and Antarctica) is used for food production; very little suitable land remains to be farmed.[41] What can be done to feed the world's population without destroying the Earth's natural resources?

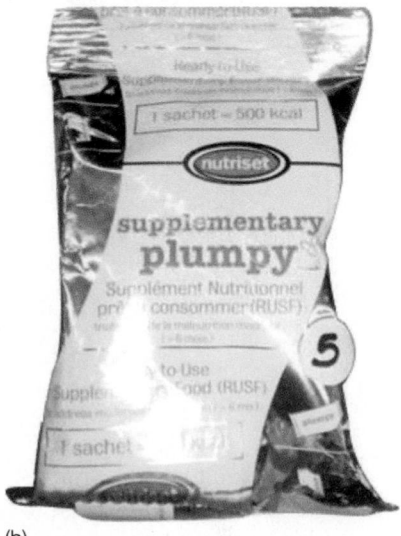
(b)

FIGURE 20.6 Ready-to-use therapeutic foods (RUTFs). (a) Hunger relief organizations pack lunch boxes with a variety of RUTFs. (b) *Plumpy'nut.*

What's Sustainable Agriculture?

Sustainable agriculture involves farming methods that meet the demand for more food without depleting natural resources and harming the environment. The challenge is finding ways for farmers and ranchers to move from primarily conventional farming techniques to sustainable agriculture. Farming needs to be profitable for farmers and ranchers, so any switch from conventional to sustain—able agricultural methods must not reduce their profit margins.

To solve the problems created by conventional agricultural methods, an international team developed the following five points for establishing a universal policy:[41]

1. Stop expanding agricultural activity, especially into tropical forests and grasslands.

2. Find ways to improve crop yields on existing farms.
   - Biotechnology in agriculture has led to the development of crops that supply higher yields, resist pests, or tolerate drought conditions.
   - By increasing food production or modifying the nutritional content of foods, biotechnology offers a way of reducing the world food crisis.

sustainable agriculture farming methods that do not deplete natural resources or harm the environment while meeting the demand for food

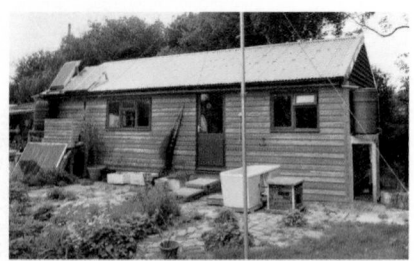

Rain barrels can capture fresh water that can then be used in a variety of ways, including watering of a garden. Rain barrels can be purchased from garden centers and hardware stores, or they can be made out of large plastic barrels or trash containers.

3. Find ways to use natural resources and pesticides more efficiently.
   - Use irrigation systems that apply water directly to a plant's base instead of spraying it into the air, where much of the water evaporates.
   - Rely more on nonchemical methods of pest management (see Chapter 19).

4. Eat less meat. Sixty percent of the world's crops (primarily grains) are grown for human consumption. Most of the remaining crops are used to feed cattle and other farm animals. It takes about 30 pounds of grains to produce 1 pound of hamburger. By eating less meat, especially beef, more grains could be produced to feed people. Grass—fed beef also spares grains for human consumption, because grass is not eaten by people.

5. Reduce food waste. About 30% of food is wasted. In many instances, the food spoils before it is eaten or it is thrown out as garbage. Cutting portion sizes and better menu planning can reduce the amount of food that people waste each day.[42]

DID YOU KNOW?

Food service establishments, including university dining facilities, produce significant amounts of edible food waste. Plate waste is food that is served to an individual but not consumed. A plate waste study at an all-you-can-eat university dining facility found that 57 g of edible food was disposed of per individual tray, amounting to over 1.5 tons of food waste over a 6-week period.[43] Plate waste awareness education programs and trayless dining appear to reduce plate waste on college campuses.[43,44]

ASSESS YOUR PROGRESS

10. List at least two international agencies that sponsor programs to reduce undernutrition worldwide.
11. What is a GMO?
12. Identify at least two examples of foods that are often fortified with micronutrients to reduce malnutrition in developing countries.
13. What is sustainable agriculture?

SUMMARY

SECTION 20.1 **Malnutrition: A Worldwide Concern**

- Malnutrition is a state of health that results from improper nourishment and can occur when diets are either lacking or exceeding in nutrients.
- Although more people suffer from overnutrition, chronic undernutrition is still a serious global concern and results from an inadequate food and nutrient intake. Poverty is the leading risk factor for undernutrition.

SECTION 20.2 **Undernutrition: Common Micronutrient Deficiencies**

- Vitamin A, iron, iodine, and zinc deficiencies are top public health concerns throughout the world. Complications from these deficiencies can include fatigue, diarrhea, cognitive impairment, blindness, and even death. Lack of nutrient-dense foods and variety in the diet are the leading causes of micronutrient deficiencies.

SECTION 20.3 Food Insecurity in the United States

- Undernutrition also occurs in developed nations such as the United States, especially among those individuals living in food insecurity. Causes of food insecurity include being unemployed, having a low-paying job and excessive expenses, and living in a food desert.
- Several different food assistance programs are available in the United States to help low-income individuals obtain food.
- Food banks, food pantries, and soup kitchens are community resources available for hungry, low-income individuals.

SECTION 20.4 Preventing and Treating Undernutrition

- Food aid, government support, widespread fortification of foods, biotechnology, and population control are all methods that can reduce undernutrition.

Get the most out of your study of nutrition with McGraw-Hill's innovative suite of adaptive learning products including McGraw-Hill LearnSmart®, SmartBook®, McGraw-Hill LearnSmart Achieve®, and McGraw-Hill LearnSmart Prep®. Visit www.learnsmartadvantage.com.

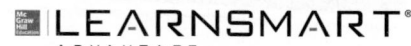

CASE STUDY RESPONSE

INFANT UNDERNUTRITION IN A DEVELOPING COUNTRY

THIS HAITIAN INFANT'S UNDERNUTRITION CAN most likely be attributed to his mother's diluting the formula and using only half of the amount necessary to meet the infant's nutritional needs. The diarrhea experienced by Louis could be caused by Monique's use of water from a stream that was contaminated with diarrhea-causing pathogens. The child's malnutrition may have also contributed to his diarrhea.

Breastfeeding could have offered a number of advantages over formula feeding for Monique and Louis. Breast milk is inexpensive compared to infant formula. Additionally, there is no need to add water to breast milk, and this could have eliminated a potential cause of the diarrhea.

The clinic worker provided Monique with a ready-to-use therapeutic food that added energy, protein, and micronutrients to the infant's diet. By being provided with adequate nutrition for a few months, Louis was able to gain weight and grow in length. In addition, the clinic worker educated Monique on how to make the potentially contaminated water safer for her and her son to consume.

Critical Thinking

1. Explain the relationship between a country's maternal mortality rate and poverty rate.

2. You are working at a county health department clinic in a major city. A 19-year-old woman with a 2-year-old daughter come into the clinic seeking help so she can obtain food for herself and her child. Which federal nutrition assistance programs would you recommend for this mother? What kinds of information would you need to obtain to be able to recommend a particular nutrition assistance program for the woman and/or her child?

3. In the United States, certain food assistance programs provide garden seeds. Which garden seeds would you recommend for a person living in a low-income urban area who has access to a small plot of land with rich soil?

4. A friend is afraid to eat corn because it contains GMOs. What would you tell your friend concerning the safety of GMOs?

5. Have you considered volunteering at a food bank or soup kitchen in your community? Explain why you would or would not volunteer for such local food aid efforts.

Modifying Recipes for Healthy Living

Tim plans to attend a football tailgate party, and the party's host asked him to bring a chili to share with about eight people. After searching online, Tim found a recipe for a chili that is made with a large amount of lean ground beef. He is unable to afford the lean ground beef in the amount called for in the recipe, and he is unsure of how to make the recipe more affordable. Review this recipe and offer suggestions to modify the recipe to make it a vegetarian, bean-based chili that is nutritious and more affordable.

HEARTY CHILI WITH BEEF

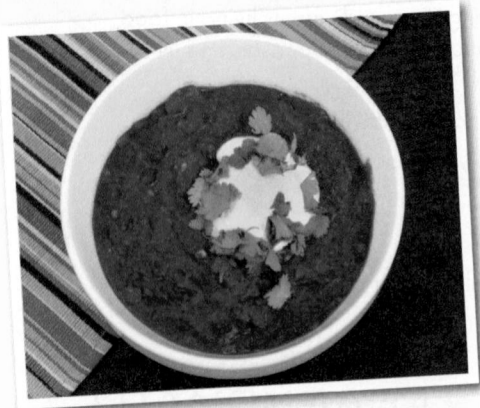

INGREDIENTS

4 lb lean ground sirloin beef

1 medium white or yellow onion, chopped

2 cloves garlic, minced

2 tsp ground cumin

2 Tbsp chili powder

1 tsp salt

½ tsp black pepper

1 Tbsp apple cider vinegar

2 cups water

1 28-oz can whole, peeled tomatoes (with juice)

2 Tbsp yellow cornmeal

Garnishes for serving: low-fat sour cream and sliced green onions (optional)

PREPARATION STEPS

1. Heat a large pot over medium heat and add ground beef. Using the side of a spoon, break up the ground beef while it is cooking. Cook, stirring occasionally, until ground beef is completely browned.

2. Transfer cooked beef to a large bowl, leaving behind the beef drippings in the pot. Set beef aside. Add onions to pot and sauté until soft, about 5 minutes.

3. Return cooked beef to the pot and stir in garlic, spices, vinegar, water, tomatoes with juice, and cornmeal.

4. Bring chili to a boil, and then reduce to a simmer. Cook, stirring occasionally, until chili thickens, about 20 minutes.

5. Serve hot. Garnish with low-fat sour cream and sliced green onions, if desired. Serves eight. (Chili can also be made the day before and reheated. Be sure to transfer hot chili into smaller containers before placing in the fridge to cool, and reheat chili to 165°F before serving.)

STEP 1 Brainstorm

Examine this recipe and other chili recipes found either online or in cookbooks. What less costly ingredients are in other chili recipes that could be substituted for part of the lean ground beef that is in this recipe?

STEP 2 Develop a modified version of this recipe

After reviewing other recipes and considering ingredients, modify this recipe to be more affordable. List the ingredients, amounts of ingredients needed, and the preparation steps for the new recipe.

STEP 3 Find the cost difference

Go to a grocery store to determine the cost of 4 pounds of lean ground beef, preferably ground sirloin. Calculate the cost of a single serving of the chili that is made with the ground sirloin and the cost of a serving of the chili that is made by following the modified recipe. Was your modified recipe more affordable? If so, by what percentage?

OPTIONAL ACTIVITIES

STEP 4 Analyze nutrient contents of the original and modified recipes by using a computer software program

Develop a table that compares the number of calories and amounts of total fat, saturated fat, protein, and fiber in each chili recipe. How did your modifications change the nutrient composition of the chili?

STEP 5 Test your new recipe

Keep notes on any changes that you make to amounts of the ingredients as you prepare the chili.

STEP 6 Reflect on your findings

How did the modified chili appear and taste?

Practice Test

Select the best answer.

1. Which of the following groups of individuals is least likely to experience harmful consequences from chronic undernutrition?

   a. infants
   b. pregnant women
   c. older adults
   d. young adults

2. Which of the following health effects is least likely to occur as a result of chronic undernutrition in childhood?

   a. reduced height and weight
   b. increased cognitive abilities
   c. reduced effectiveness of the immune system
   d. increased susceptibility to infectious diseases

3. Which of the following countries has the highest under-5 mortality rate?

   a. United States
   b. Iceland
   c. Germany
   d. Denmark

4. Lack of _____ in the diet is the leading cause of childhood blindness worldwide.

   a. vitamin C
   b. iron
   c. vitamin A
   d. zinc

5. _____ deficiency during pregnancy can significantly impair the intelligence level of the developing fetus.

   a. Vitamin A
   b. Iodine
   c. Zinc
   d. Vitamin C

6. A family with members who worry each month about having enough money to purchase food, even though their diet quality and quantity is adequate, is most likely experiencing

   a. high food security.
   b. marginal food security.
   c. low food security.
   d. very low food security.

7. Which of the following situations is an example of food security?

   a. A family is able to obtain enough food each month through the use of food assistance programs.
   b. A family is able to purchase enough food for the majority of the month but usually must decrease food intake during the last week.
   c. A family must follow a budget but is able to provide enough nutritious food for each member to live a healthy and active life.
   d. A family relies on weekly food donations from community charities to obtain enough to eat.

8. An example of a GMO is a

   a. form of bacteria that does not require oxygen to survive.
   b. kind of corn that tolerates heat better than other kinds of corn.
   c. chemically coated variety of pumpkin seeds that grow in compost.
   d. type of lettuce that needs water to mature and develop leaves.

9. A food _____ is an area in which a large proportion of people who live there experience difficulty accessing nutritious food.

   a. wasteland
   b. famine
   c. shortage
   d. desert

10. Which of the following federal food assistance programs offers monthly financial assistance to low-income participants for purchasing eligible foods?

    a. Supplemental Nutrition Assistance Program
    b. The Emergency Food Assistance Program
    c. Food Distribution Disaster Assistance
    d. Commodity Supplemental Food Program

11. Which of the following federal food assistance programs offers food assistance to Americans who have been affected by a tornado or flood?

    a. Supplemental Food Assistance Program
    b. The Emergency Food Assistance Program
    c. Food Distribution Disaster Assistance
    d. Commodity Supplemental Food Program

12. Which of the following federal food assistance programs provides low-income children with meals and snacks when school is not in session?

    a. Special Milk Program
    b. National School Lunch Program
    c. Summer Food Service Program
    d. School Breakfast Program

13. The Healthy Food Financing Initiative

    a. distributes food vouchers to older adult Americans who have low incomes and are nutritionally at risk.
    b. grants money to public and private schools that offer nutrition education classes.
    c. provides funding for programs that improve the accessibility of nutritious food in food deserts.
    d. prepares financially sound budgets for families in major metropolitan areas that are not food secure.

14. A _____ is a nonprofit organization that distributes commodity foods to groups that prepare free or low-cost meals for people who are hungry.

    a. food pantry
    b. food bank
    c. soup kitchen
    d. congregate meal center

15. Which of the following shelf-stable, nutrient-fortified foods has been developed to treat undernutrition among young children in developing countries?

    a. whey powders
    b. GMO peanuts
    c. Golden Rice
    d. ready-to-use therapeutic foods

ANSWERS TO PRACTICE TEST

1-d; 2-b; 3-a; 4-c; 5-b; 6-b; 7-c; 8-b; 9-d; 10-a; 11-c; 12-c; 13-c; 14-b; 15-d

ANSWERS TO CHAPTER 20 QUIZ Yourself

1. More people in the world experience undernutrition than overnutrition. **False** (p. 641)
2. Stunting is a consequence of chronic undernutrition in infants and children. **True** (p. 642)
3. In children, diets that are iron deficient can lead to blindness. **False** (p. 645)
4. Individuals experiencing *marginal food security* have a reduction in both the quantity and nutritional quality of the foods they consume. **False** (p. 647)
5. The Supplemental Nutrition Assistance Program enables low-income Americans to purchase foods as well as certain seeds for their gardens. **True** (p. 651)

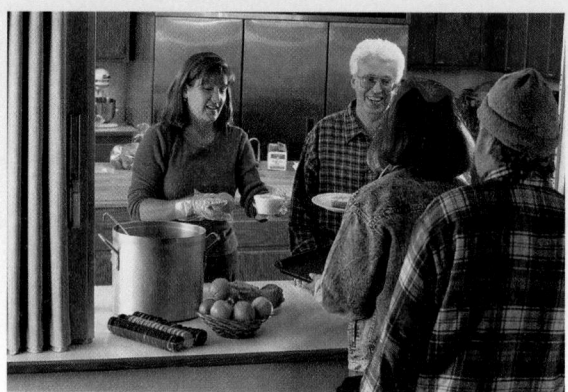

References

1. World Health Organization: *Obesity and overweight: Fact sheet no. 311.* Updated March 2013. http://www.who.int/mediacentre/factsheets/fs311/en/ Accessed: March 18, 2014.

2. Academy of Nutrition and Dietetics: Position of the Academy of Nutrition and Dietetics: Nutrition security in developing nations: Sustainable food, water, and health. *Journal of the Academy of Nutrition and Dietetics* 113(4): 581, 2013.

3. Underweight, undernutrition, and the aging: Population Reference Bureau's *Today's Research on Aging,* Issue 8, October 2007. http://www.prb.org/pdf07/TodaysResearchAging8.pdf Accessed: March 18, 2014.

4. Food and Agriculture Organization of the United Nations: *The state of food insecurity in the world.* 2012. http://www.fao.org/docrep/016/i3027e/i3027e.pdf Accessed: March 18, 2014.

5. The World Bank: *Poverty and Equity Data.* ND. http://povertydata.worldbank.org/poverty/home/ Accessed March 18, 2014.

6. Centers for Disease Control and Prevention: *Global water, sanitation, & hygiene: Global WASH fast facts: Information on water, sanitation, and hygiene.* Updated November 2013. http://www.cdc.gov/healthywater/global/wash_statistics.html Accessed: March 18, 2014.

7. United Nations: *The millennium development goals report.* 2013. http://www.un.org/millenniumgoals/pdf/report-2013/mdg-report-2013-english.pdf Accessed: March 18, 2014.

8. Food and Agriculture Organization of the United Nations: *The state of food and agriculture: Food systems for better nutrition.* 2013. http://www.fao.org/docrep/018/i3300e/i3300e.pdf Accessed: March 18, 2014.

9. Neufield LM, Osendarp SJ: Global, regional and country trends in underweight and stunting as indicators of nutrition and health of populations. *Nestle Nutrition Institute Workshop Series* 78:11, 2014.

10. Black RE and others: Maternal and child undernutrition: Global and regional exposures and health consequences. *Lancet* 371:243, 2008.

11. United Nations Children's Fund: *Tracking progress on child and maternal nutrition: A survival and development priority.* November 2009. http://www.unicef.org/publications/files/Tracking_Progress_on_Child_and_Maternal_Nutrition_EN_110309.pdf Accessed: March 18, 2014.

12. Centers for Disease Control and Prevention: *FastStats: Birthweight and gestation.* Updated February 2014. http://www.cdc.gov/nchs/fastats/birthwt.htm Accessed: March 18, 2014.

13. World Health Organization: *Mental health and psychological well-being among children in severe food shortage situations.* 2006. http://www.who.int/nmh/publications/msd_MHChildFSS9.pdf Accessed: March 18, 2014.

14. World Food Programme: Hunger. *What is malnutrition?* ND. http://www.wfp.org/hunger/malnutrition Accessed: March 18, 2014.

15. Taras H: Nutrition and student performance at school. *Journal of School Health* 75(6):199, 2005.

16. Adolphus K and others: The effects of breakfast on behavior and academic performance in children and adolescents. *Frontiers in Human Neuroscience* 7:425, 2013.

17. World Health Organization: *Nutrition for older persons: Aging and nutrition: A growing global challenge.* ND. http://www.who.int/nutrition/topics/ageing/en/index.html Accessed: March 18, 2014.

18. Stang B: *Investing in the future: A united call to action on vitamin and mineral deficiencies: Global report 2009.* http://www.unitedcalltoaction.org/documents/Investing_in_the_future.pdf Accessed: March 18, 2014.

19. Copenhagen Consensus Center: *Press release: The world's best investment: Vitamins for undernourished children, according to top economists, including 5 Nobel Laureates.* May 30, 2008. http://www.copenhagenconsensus.com/sites/default/files/Copenhagen_Consensus_2008_Results_Press_Release.pdf Accessed: March 18, 2014.

20. World Health Organization: *Nutrition: Micronutrient deficiencies: Vitamin A deficiency.* ND. http://www.who.int/nutrition/topics/vad/en/ Accessed: March 18, 2014.

21. National Institutes of Health: *Dietary supplement fact sheet: Vitamin A.* Updated June 2013. http://ods.od.nih.gov/factsheets/VitaminA-HealthProfessional/ Accessed: March 18, 2014.

22. World Health Organization: *Nutrition: Micronutrient deficiencies: Iron deficiency anaemia.* ND. http://www.who.int/nutrition/topics/ida/en/ Accessed: March 18, 2014.

23. National Institutes of Health: *Dietary supplement fact sheet: Zinc.* Updated June 2013. http://ods.od.nih.gov/factsheets/Zinc-HealthProfessional/ Accessed: March 18, 2014.

24. U.S. Department of Agriculture Economic Research Service: *Definitions of food security.* Updated September 2013. http://www.ers.usda.gov/topics/food-nutrition-assistance/food-security-in-the-us/definitions-of-food-security.aspx Accessed: March 18, 2014.

25. U.S. Department of Agriculture Economic Research Service: *Key statistics and graphics.* Updated September 2013. http://www.ers.usda.gov/topics/food-nutrition-assistance/food-security-in-the-us/key-statistics-graphics.aspx Accessed: March 18, 2014.

26. U.S. Department of Agriculture Economic Research Service: *Food access research atlas: About the atlas.* Updated March 2013. http://www.ers.usda.gov/data-products/food-access-research-atlas/about-the-atlas.aspx Accessed: March 18, 2014.

27. Let's Move: *Eat healthy: Healthy communities.* ND. http://www.letsmove.gov/healthy-communities Accessed: March 18, 2014.

28. U.S. Department of Health and Human Services, Administration for Children and Families: *CED grants.* ND. http://www.acf.hhs.gov/programs/ocs/programs/ced/ced-grantees Accessed March 18, 2014.

29. Feeding America: *Hunger & poverty statistics.* ND. http://feedingamerica.org/hunger-in-america/hunger-facts/hunger-and-poverty-statistics.aspx Accessed: March 18, 2014.

30. U.S. Department of Education, Office of Postsecondary Education: *Federal TRIO programs current-year low-income levels.* Updated January 2014. http://www2.ed.gov/about/offices/list/ope/trio/incomelevels.html Accessed March 18, 2014.

31. U.S. Department of Agriculture Food and Nutrition Service: *Programs and services.* Updated December 2013. http://www.fns.usda.gov/programs-and-services Accessed: March 18, 2014.

32. Golden Rice Project: *Golden rice will reach those who need it at no additional cost.* ND. http://www.goldenrice.org/ Accessed: March 18, 2014.

33. Tang G and others: β-carotene in Golden Rice is as good as β-carotene in oil at providing vitamin A to children. *American Journal of Clinical Nutrition* 96:1185S, 2012.

34. Union of Concerned Scientists: *Genetic engineering in agriculture.* Updated November 2012. http://www.ucsusa.org/food_and_agriculture/our-failing-food-system/genetic-engineering/ Accessed: March 18, 2014.

35. Winter CK, Gallegos LK. *Safety of genetically engineered food.* Agricultural Biotechnology in California Series, Publication 8180, 2006. http://anrcatalog.ucdavis.edu/pdf/8180.pdf Accessed March 18, 2014.

36. Center for Science in the Public Interest: *Straight talk on genetically engineered foods: Answers to frequently asked questions.* Washington, DC: 2012. http://cspinet.org/new/pdf/biotech-faq.pdf Accessed March 18, 2014.

37. Project Healthy Children: *FAQ: What foods can be fortified?* ND. http://projecthealthychildren.org/why-food-fortification/faq/ Accessed: March 18, 2014.

38. World Health Organization: Maternal, newborn, child, and adolescent health. *Malnutrition.* ND. http://www.who.int/maternal_child_adolescent/topics/child/malnutrition/en/ Accessed: March 18, 2014.

39. World Health Organization: e-Library of Evidence for Nutrition Actions. *Multiple micronutrient powders for home fortification of foods consumed by children 6–23 months of age.* ND. http://www.who.int/elena/titles/micronutrientpowder_infants/en/ Accessed: March 18, 2014.

40. Sprinkles Global Health Initiative: *Proof of efficacy, safety and effectiveness: Community-based studies on Sprinkles involving both anemic and non-anemic children have been completed in Northern Canada, China, Bangladesh, India and Pakistan, Ghana, Bolivia and Haiti.* ND. http://www.sghi.org/about_sprinkles/proof_safety.html Accessed: March 18, 2014.

41. Foley JA: Can we feed the world and sustain the planet? *Scientific American* 305(5):60, 2011.

42. Sarjahani A and others: Food and non-edible, compostable waste in a university dining facility. *Journal of Hunger and Environmental Nutrition* 4(1):95–102, 2009.

43. Whitehair KJ and others: Written messages improve edible food waste behaviors in a university dining facility. *Journal of the Academy of Nutrition and Dietetics* 113(1):63, 2013.

44. Thiagarajah K, Getty VM: Impact on plate waste of switching from a tray to a trayless delivery system in a university dining hall and employee response to the switch. *Journal of the Academy of Nutrition and Dietetics* 113(1):141, 2013.

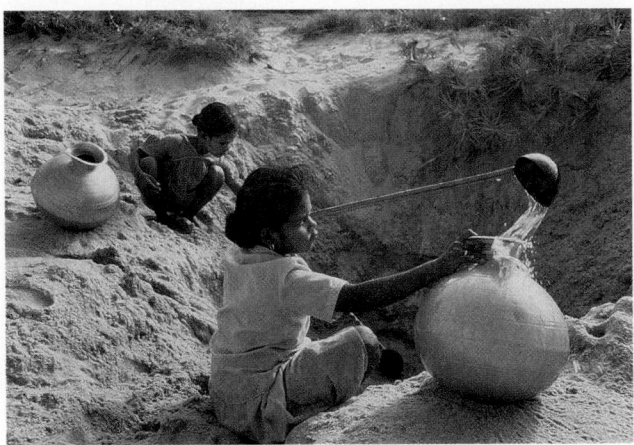

Appendixes

Appendixes

English-Metric Conversions

LENGTH

English (USA)	Metric
inch (in)	= 2.54 cm, 25.4 mm
foot (ft)	= 0.30 m, 30.48 cm
yard (yd)	= 0.91 m, 91.4 cm
mile (statute) (5280 ft)	= 1.61 km, 1609 m
mile (nautical) (6077 ft, 1.15 statute mi)	= 1.85 km, 1850 m

Metric	English (USA)
millimeter (mm)	= 0.039 in (thickness of a dime)
centimeter (cm)	= 0.39 in
meter (m)	= 3.28 ft, 39.4 in
kilometer (km)	= 0.62 mi, 1091 yd, 3273 ft

WEIGHT

English (USA)	Metric
grain	= 64.80 mg
ounce (oz)	= 28.35 g
pound (lb)	= 453.60 g, 0.45 kg
ton (short—2000 lb)	= 0.91 metric ton (907 kg)

Metric	English (USA)
milligram (mg)	= 0.002 grain (0.000035 oz)
gram (g)	= 0.04 oz (1/28 of an oz)
kilogram (kg)	= 35.27 oz, 2.20 lb
metric ton (1000 kg)	= 1.10 tons

VOLUME

English (USA)	Metric
cubic inch	= 16.39 cc
cubic foot	= 0.03 m³
cubic yard	= 0.765 m³
teaspoon (tsp)	= 5 mL
tablespoon (Tbsp)	= 15 mL
fluid ounce	= 0.03 liter (30 mL)*
cup (c)	= 237 mL
pint (pt)	= 0.47 liter
quart (qt)	= 0.95 liter
gallon (gal)	= 3.79 liters

Metric	English (USA)
milliliter (mL)	= 0.03 oz
liter (L)	= 2.12 pt
liter	= 1.06 qt
liter	= 0.27 gal

1 liter ÷ 1000 = 1 milliliter or 1 cubic centimeter (10^{-3} liter)*
1 liter ÷ 1,000,000 = 1 microliter (10^{-6} liter)
*1 mL = 1 cc

Metric and Other Common Units

Unit/Abbreviation	Other Equivalent Measure
milligram/mg	1/1000 of a gram
microgram/μg	1/1,00,000 of a gram
deciliter/dL	1/10 of a liter (about 1/2 cup)
milliliter/mL	1/1000 of a liter (5 mL is about 1 tsp)
International Unit/IU	Crude measure of vitamin activity generally based on growth rate seen in animals

Fahrenheit-Celsius Conversion Scale

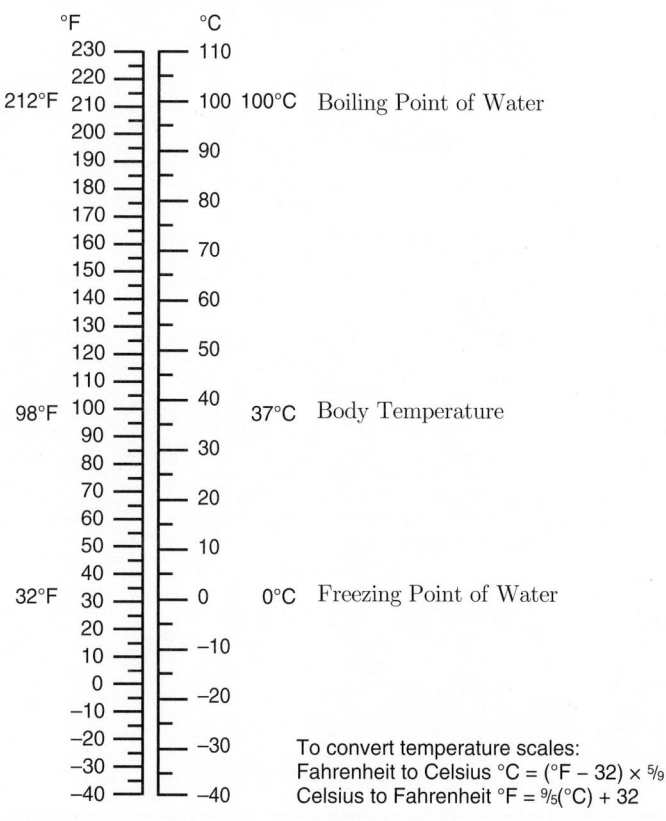

To convert temperature scales:
Fahrenheit to Celsius $°C = (°F - 32) \times 5/9$
Celsius to Fahrenheit $°F = 9/5(°C) + 32$

Household Units

3 teaspoons	= 1 tablespoon
4 tablespoons	= 1/4 cup
5 1/3 tablespoons	= 1/3 cup
8 tablespoons	= 1/2 cup
10 2/3 tablespoons	= 2/3 cup
16 tablespoons	= 1 cup
1 tablespoon	= 1/2 fluid ounce

1 cup	= 8 fluid ounces
1 cup	= 1/2 pint
2 cups	= 1 pint
4 cups	= 1 quart
2 pints	= 1 quart
4 quarts	= 1 gallon

Appendix B
Basic Chemistry Concepts

From Atoms to Molecules

Matter is comprised of atoms that contain certain particles, including protons and electrons (Fig. B.1). Protons are positively charged particles in the nucleus, the central region of an atom. Electrons are small, negatively charged particles that are located in a "cloud" surrounding the nucleus. The number of electrons surrounding the nucleus equals the number of protons within the nucleus. Thus, the negative and positive charges cancel out each other, making an atom neutral, which means it has no electrical charge.

More than 100 different types of atoms exist, and each type is an *element*, a substance that cannot be separated into simpler substances by ordinary chemical or physical means. Elements are the building blocks of matter. Chemists use letters as symbols to represent elements. For example, the symbols for carbon, nitrogen, and sodium are C, N, and Na, respectively. Table B.1 lists several elements, most of which are essential for human nutrition.

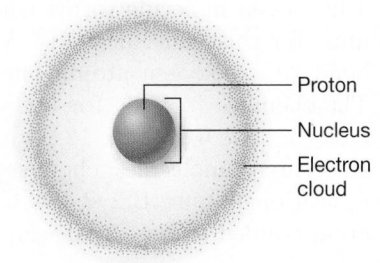

FIGURE B.1

IONS

An atom has no electrical charge (*neutral*) if it has the same number of protons and electrons. When an atom (or group of atoms) gains or loses one or more electrons, it has an electrical charge and is called an *ion*. If an atom gains one electron, it becomes an ion with a negative charge (*anion*), because electrons are negatively charged. A negative charge is indicated with a minus sign ($-$) after the chemical symbol or formula, such as OH^-, which is the *hydroxide* ion. If an atom loses an electron, it becomes an ion with a positive charge (*cation*), because it has an extra proton, and protons are positively charged. A positive charge is indicated with a plus sign ($+$) after the chemical symbol or formula. The formula for the positively charged hydrogen ion is simply H^+, which means it is a proton.

MOLECULES AND COMPOUNDS

When atoms interact, they may share or transfer electrons, which results in a *chemical bond* (attraction) between the atoms. A covalent chemical bond forms when the atoms share electrons, forming a *molecule*. Molecules can contain the same element or different elements. Although a molecule is comprised of atoms, as a structural unit, a molecule acts independently and has different characteristics than the atoms of the elements that form it.

A *compound* forms when two or more different atoms are attracted to each other. A hydrogen molecule (H_2) is not a compound, because it is comprised of the same element. Glucose is a molecule as well as a compound because it is comprised of three different elements: carbon, hydrogen, and oxygen.

TABLE B.1 Elements in the Body

Element	Symbol
Hydrogen	H
Oxygen	O
Carbon	C
Nitrogen	N
Calcium	Ca
Phosphorus	P
Potassium	K
Sulfur	S
Sodium	Na
Chloride	Cl
Magnesium	Mg
Iron	Fe
Iodine	I
Copper	Cu
Zinc	Zn
Manganese	Mn
Cobalt	Co
Chromium	Cr
Selenium	Se
Molybdenum	Mo
Fluoride*	F
Tin	Sn
Silicon†	Si
Vanadium†	V
Nickel†	Ni
Boron†	B
Arsenic†	As

*Although fluoride is not essential, the mineral helps strengthen teeth and bones.

†When experimental animals are fed diets that are deficient in these mineral elements, they eventually develop deficiency symptoms. However, there have been no reports of widespread deficiencies of these minerals in human populations. Therefore, scientists have not established human requirements for them.

Ionic Bonds   Positively charged ions are attracted to negatively charged ions. This kind of attraction forms *ionic bonds*. Common table salt, for example, is comprised of sodium (Na^+) and chloride (Cl^-) ions that are held together by ionic bonds. When an ionic molecule, such as table salt (NaCl), is dissolved in water, the sodium and chloride atoms separate (*dissociate*), forming a solution that can conduct electricity. Thus, sodium and chloride ions are called *electrolytes*. Electrolytes have many important functions in the body, including helping to maintain proper fluid balance.

Chemical Formulas

Chemists use a chemical formula to identify a particular molecule. For example, a hydrogen molecule forms when two hydrogen atoms bind together. The formula for this molecule is H_2. A water molecule forms when two hydrogen atoms bond to an oxygen atom. The chemical formula for a water molecule is H_2O. The chemical formula for the simple sugar glucose is $C_6H_{12}O_6$, which means the molecule has 6 carbon, 12 hydrogen, and 6 oxygen atoms. When illustrating the structure of molecules, chemists may use straight lines to show the bonding configuration. Figure B.2 shows CH_4 (*methane*), which is comprised of one carbon atom bonded to four hydrogen atoms.

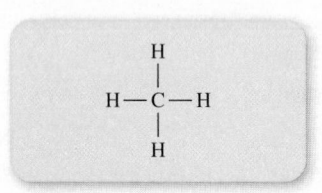

FIGURE B.2 Methane (CH_4).

MULTIPLE BONDS

Some atoms that share electrons form single bonds, but a few atoms, including carbon, can form multiple bonds. Each carbon atom (C) has four bonding sites, and as a result, carbon atoms can covalently bond to each other by single, double (Fig. B.3a), and even triple bonds (Fig. B3b). Carbon's ability to bond to other carbon atoms as well as form multiple bonds with a neighboring carbon atom contributes to the formation of a vast array of organic (carbon−containing) compounds.

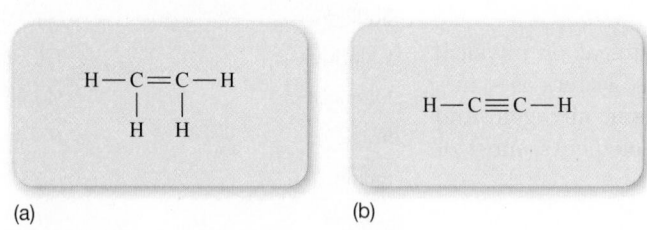

(a)   (b)

FIGURE B.3 Covalent bonding. Double bond (*a*) and triple bond (*b*).

What Is a Chemical Reaction?

Most molecules can undergo chemical reactions, processes that change the arrangement of atoms in the molecules. Chemical equations are used to depict the substances involved in reactions (Fig. B.4). In general, a reaction shows *reactants* to the left of the arrow and *products* to the right side of the arrow. If the reaction is not easy to reverse, the arrow points only toward the product. Some reactions are reversible, so the arrow is depicted as in Figure B.5.

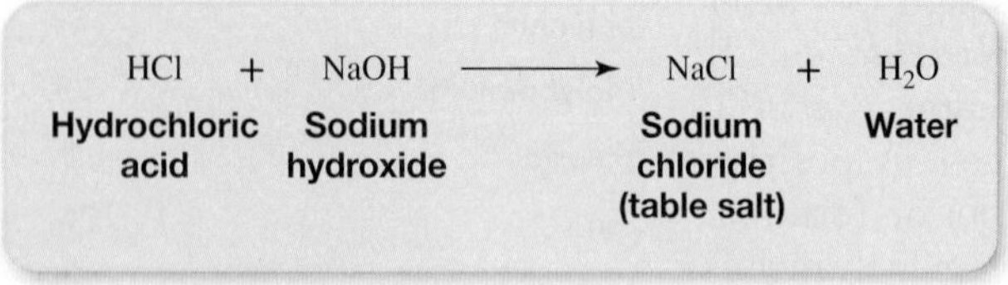

The elements that comprise the molecules that react are never destroyed, but they combine with other elements to form new molecules or compounds. *Synthesis* reactions involve the combination of smaller chemical units to form larger ones. Cells, for example, synthesize large protein molecules by combining smaller units (amino acids). *Decomposition* reactions involve the breaking down of molecules. Digestion, the process by which large molecules in food are broken down into smaller ones, requires decomposition reactions. When elements or compounds combine or decompose, the new substances that form as a result often have physical and chemical characteristics (*properties*) that are different from those of the reactants.

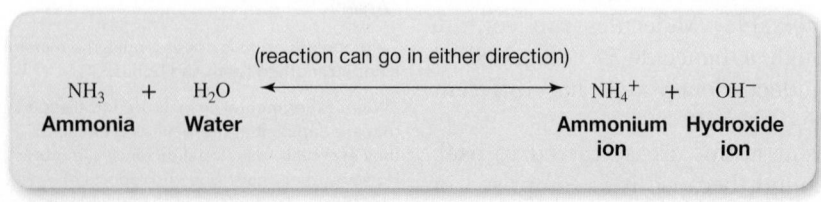

FIGURE B.4 Example chemical equation.

FIGURE B.5 Reversible reaction. Some reactions can go in either direction, as indicated by the reversible arrow in this example.

OXIDATION-REDUCTION REACTIONS

In living systems, chemical reactions often involve the loss and gain of electrons and energy. Oxidation occurs when a molecule loses an electron to another molecule and releases energy as a result. When this occurs, the molecule that loses the electron has been oxidized, and the molecule that accepts or gains the electron is the *oxidizing agent*. The oxidizing agent has undergone reduction, because it has gained an electron (a negative charge). Therefore, the oxidizing agent has been reduced, and the molecule that was oxidized when it gave up the electron is the *reducing agent*. Such reactions are referred to as oxidation–reduction or redox reactions. To help recall which molecule has been oxidized and which has been reduced, use the memory aid "OIL RIG," for **O**xidation **I**s **L**osing; **R**eduction **I**s **G**aining."

ENZYMES

Life depends upon chemical reactions; however, many of these reactions occur slowly or do not occur spontaneously. Living cells produce enzymes, proteins that facilitate (catalyze) chemical reactions, enabling them to occur quickly. In general, the names of enzymes end with *–ase*, such as sucrase and alcohol dehydrogenase. A few enzymes have retained their classic names, including pepsin and rennin, enzymes involved in digestion. Many enzymes are secreted in an inactive form, and they must be activated to catalyze reactions. *Pepsinogen*, for example, is the inactive form of pepsin. *Cofactors* are ions or small molecules that regulate enzyme activity. A *coenzyme* is a type of cofactor (see Chapters 8 and 10).

Solutions

A solution is an evenly distributed mixture of two or more compounds. In living things, water is the *solvent*, the primary component of solutions. The human body, for example, is about 60% water. A substance that dissolves in the solvent is a *water–soluble solute*. Many beverages and foods are solutions that have water as the solvent (Fig. B.6). A sports drink, for example, is a solution that is mostly water, the solvent. The drink has relatively small amounts of sugar, minerals, colorings, and flavorings (solutes) dissolved in the water.

In living systems, the solubility of a substance describes how easily it dissolves, that is, forms a solution, in a liquid solvent. Many naturally occurring substances, including simple carbohydrates such as sugar and all mineral elements, are water soluble because they dissolve in water. Other substances, such as fat, are insoluble in water, so they will not dissolve in water (Fig. B.7). Blood has a high water content, a characteristic that makes it easier for the body to transport and eliminate watersoluble substances than water–insoluble materials.

WHAT ARE ACIDS AND BASES?

Acids are substances that dissociate when dissolved in water and release H^+. Bases are substances that accept H^+ when dissolved in water. Many bases, such as sodium hydroxide (NaOH), release hydroxide ions (OH^-), which accept H^+. Many of the chemicals people encounter daily are either acidic or basic (*alkaline*). As one can tell by their names, phosphoric acid in soft drinks and ascorbic acid (better known as vitamin C) are acids. Ammonia, baking soda, and sodium hydroxide, an ingredient of many hair removal products, are bases.

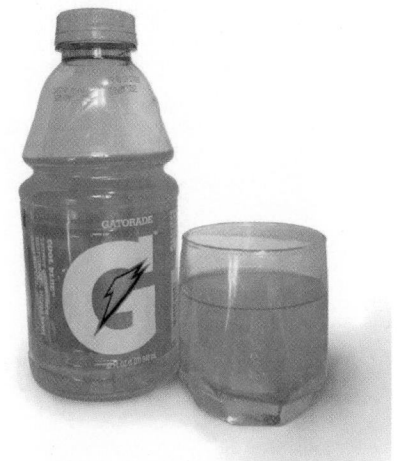

FIGURE B.6 Solutions. Sports drinks are an example of a solution, a mixture of water, sugar, minerals, colorings, and flavorings.

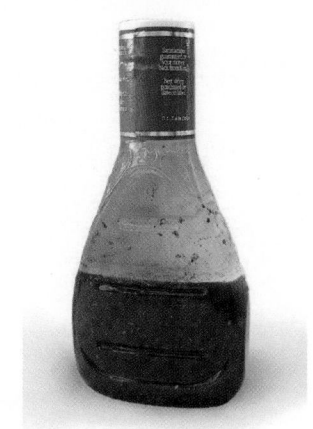

FIGURE B.7 Solubility. In this bottle of salad dressing, the fat is insoluble in water, resulting in separation of the two substances.

Anatomy and Physiology for the Study of Nutrition

Anatomy is the scientific study of cells and other body structures; physiology is the scientific study of how cells and body structures function. This appendix reviews some basic information about human anatomy and physiology, including the organization of the body into organ systems.

THE CELL

A cell is the smallest living functional unit in an organism. The human body has about 100 trillion cells. Most human cells contain several different types of *organelles*, structures that have specific functions. Figure C.1 shows a cell with various organelles. Table C.1 summarizes major functions of these organelles.

The organelles are surrounded by a watery fluid called cytoplasm. Many chemical reactions occur in the cytoplasm. Each human cell has a plasma membrane that defines the boundaries of the cell and holds the cytoplasm in place. The plasma membrane also controls the passage of materials into and out of the cell.

FROM CELLS TO SYSTEMS

Cells that have similar characteristics and functions are usually joined together into larger masses called tissues. There are four major types of tissues:

- *Epithelial tissue* lines or covers surfaces, forming a barrier that protects structures but allows certain

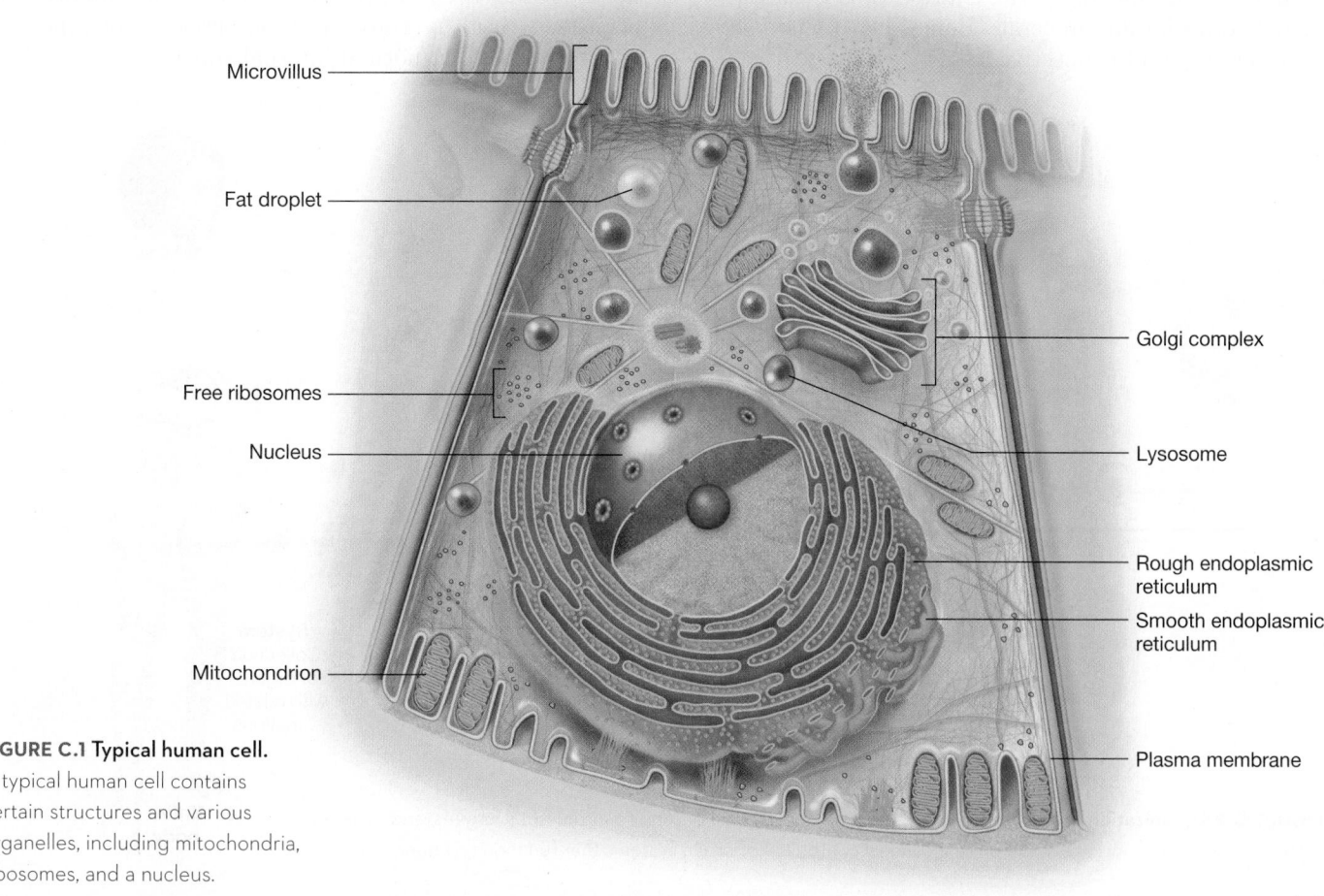

FIGURE C.1 Typical human cell.
A typical human cell contains certain structures and various organelles, including mitochondria, ribosomes, and a nucleus.

Microvillus

Fat droplet

Free ribosomes

Nucleus

Mitochondrion

Golgi complex

Lysosome

Rough endoplasmic reticulum

Smooth endoplasmic reticulum

Plasma membrane

TABLE C.1 Summary of Selected Organelles and Their Functions

Organelle	Function
Nucleus	Contains DNA that controls cellular activities
Ribosome	Forms proteins from amino acids
Rough Endoplasmic Reticulum	Synthesizes proteins (has ribosomes attached to it)
Smooth Endoplasmic Reticulum	Synthesizes carbohydrates and lipids, stores calcium
Golgi Apparatus	Prepares and distributes newly synthesized proteins and lipids for secretion or use within the cell
Lysosome	Stores digestive enzymes
Mitochondrion	Major site of ATP production (aerobic conditions)
Microvillus	Increases surface area of plasma membrane, which enhances ability to absorb and secrete substances

materials to enter. The outermost layer of skin and mucous membranes of the mouth are examples of epithelial tissue.

- *Connective tissue* holds structures together, supports and cushions moving parts, transports substances, and stores fat and minerals. Bones, blood, and body fat are types of connective tissue.

- *Muscle tissue* is necessary for movement.

- *Nervous tissue* conducts electrical signals that transmit information to cells throughout the body.

An *organ* is composed of various tissues that function in a related fashion. The brain, for example, is an organ because it contains different types of nervous tissue. An *organ system* is a group of organs that work together for a similar purpose. The urinary system, for example, includes the kidneys and the bladder. Two major functions of the urinary system are filtering blood and excreting wastes in urine. A living organism is comprised of organ systems that function together to support the needs of the organism. Figure C.2 illustrates how cells in the body are organized into tissues, organs, and organ systems. Table C.2 lists each system's major organs or tissues and summarizes their primary functions.

All organ systems must work together in a coordinated manner to maintain good health. When one system fails to function correctly, the functioning of the other systems is soon affected. The body's ability to maintain *homeostasis*, an internal chemical and physical environment that supports life and good health, is critical. Internal conditions such as body temperature and blood pressure normally fluctuate throughout the day, but the body strives to maintain such factors within fairly specific limits. Changes in the cell's internal and external environment can disrupt homeostasis, and sickness and even death can result if the abnormality persists. A healthy body, however, uses various mechanisms to regain its normal internal status.

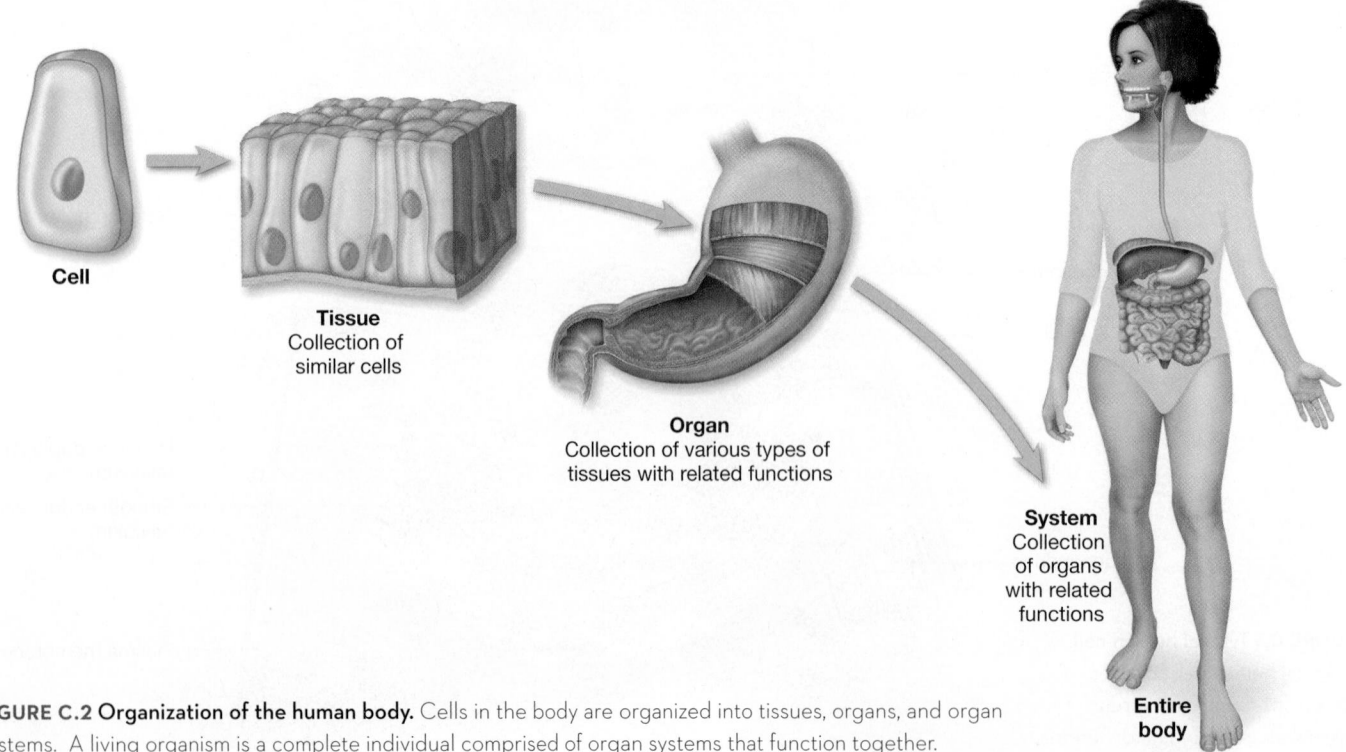

Cell

Tissue
Collection of similar cells

Organ
Collection of various types of tissues with related functions

System
Collection of organs with related functions

Entire body

FIGURE C.2 Organization of the human body. Cells in the body are organized into tissues, organs, and organ systems. A living organism is a complete individual comprised of organ systems that function together.

TABLE C.2 The Organ Systems and Their Primary Functions

System	Major Organs or Tissues	Primary Functions
Digestive	Mouth, salivary glands, esophagus, stomach, intestines, pancreas, liver, gallbladder	Digestion and absorption of nutrients
Cardiovascular	Heart, blood vessels, blood	Circulation of blood throughout the body
Respiratory	Nose, pharynx, larynx, trachea, bronchi, lungs	Exchange of oxygen and carbon dioxide
Lymphatic and Immune	Lymphatic fluid, white blood cells, lymph vessels and nodes, spleen, thymus	Defense and immunity against infectious agents, fluid balance, white blood cell production, absorption of fat-soluble nutrients from intestinal tract
Urinary	Kidneys, bladder	Elimination of salts, water, and wastes; maintenance of fluid balance
Muscular	Muscles	Movement and stability of the body
Skeletal	Bones, tendons, ligaments	Support, movement, protection, and production of blood cells
Nervous	Brain, spinal cord, nerves, sensory receptors	Thought processes, regulation and coordination of many body activities, detection of changes in external and internal environments
Endocrine	Glands or organs that secrete hormones (chemical messengers)	Regulation and coordination of many body activities, including growth, nutrient balance, and reproduction
Integumentary	Skin, hair, nails	Protection and immunity, regulation of body temperature, vitamin D synthesis
Reproductive	Gonads and genitals	Procreation (creating children)

Adapted from: Widmaier EP, and others: *Vander's human physiology,* 12th ed. Boston: McGraw-Hill Publishing Company, 2011.

Appendix D

Major Monosaccharides, Amino Acids, and Vitamins

Major Monosaccharides

```
        H
        |
        C═O
        |
   H ── C ── OH
        |
  HO ── C ── H
        |
   H ── C ── OH
        |
   H ── C ── OH
        |
   H ── C ── OH
        |
        H
```
Glucose

```
        H
        |
   H ── C ── OH
        |
        C═O
        |
  HO ── C ── H
        |
   H ── C ── OH
        |
   H ── C ── OH
        |
   H ── C ── OH
        |
        H
```
Fructose

```
        H
        |
        C═O
        |
   H ── C ── OH
        |
  HO ── C ── H
        |
  HO ── C ── H
        |
   H ── C ── OH
        |
   H ── C ── OH
        |
        H
```
Galactose

Amino Acids

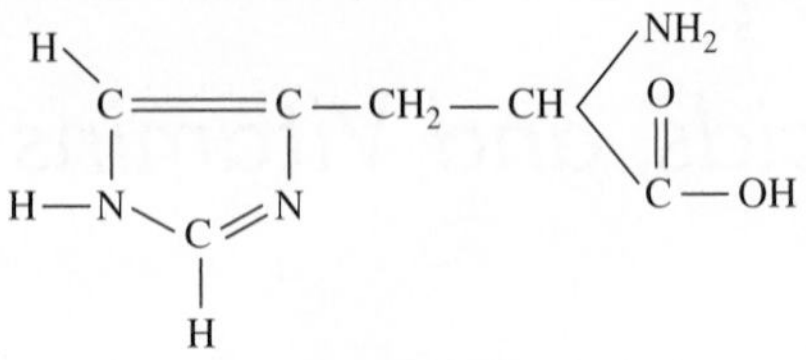

Histidine (His)
(essential)

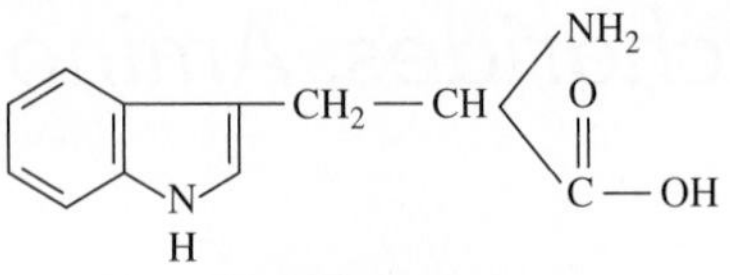

Tryptophan (Trp)
(essential)

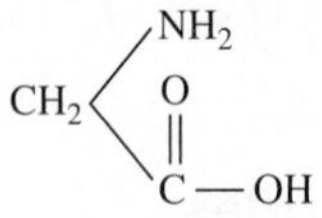

Glycine (Gly)

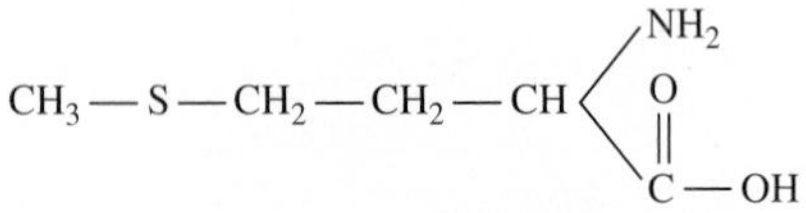

Methionine (Met)
(essential)

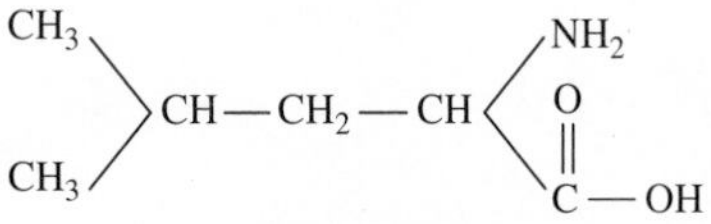

Leucine (Leu)
(essential)

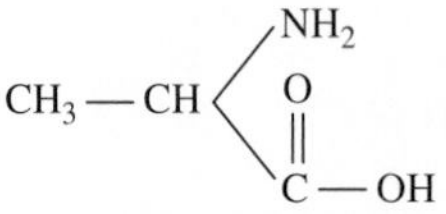

Alanine (Ala)

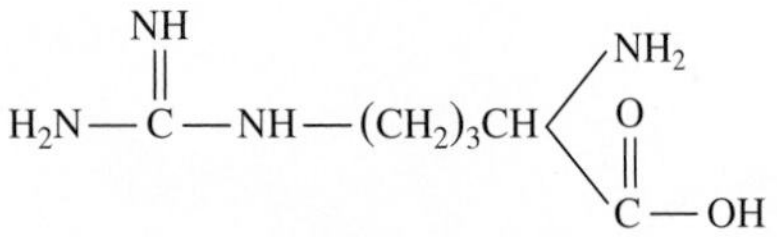

Arginine (Arg)
(essential in infancy)

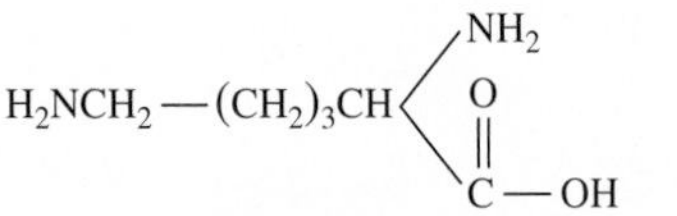

Lysine (Lys)
(essential)

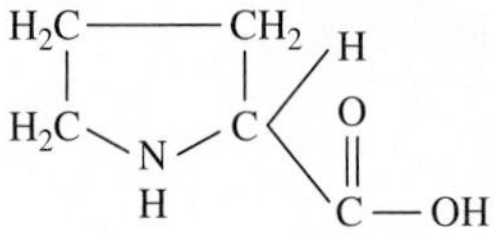

Proline (Pro)

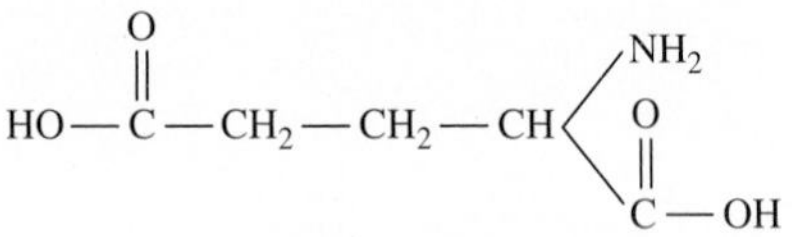

Glutamic Acid (Glu)

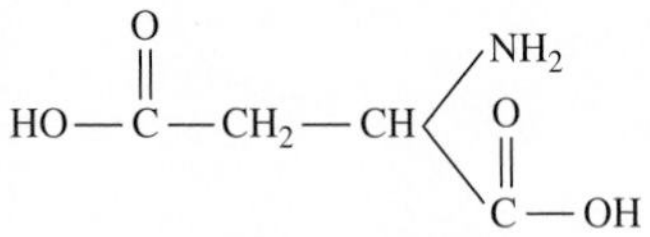

Aspartic Acid (Asp)

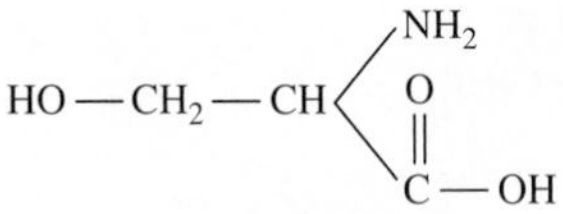

Serine (Ser)

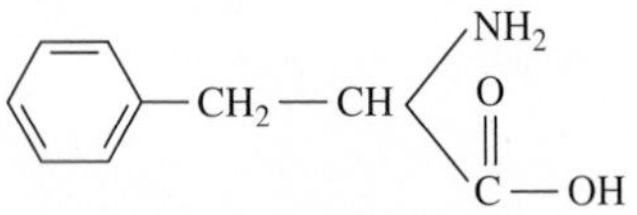

Phenylalanine (Phe)
(essential)

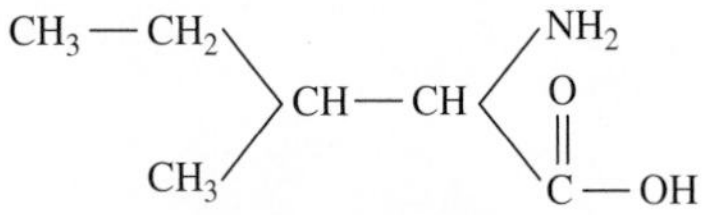

Isoleucine (Ile)
(essential)

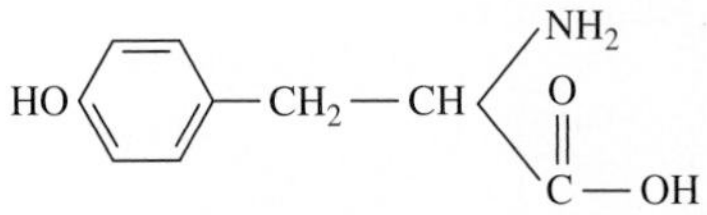

Tyrosine (Tyr)

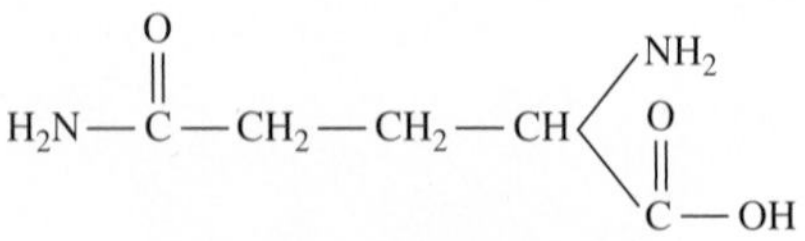

Glutamine (Gln)

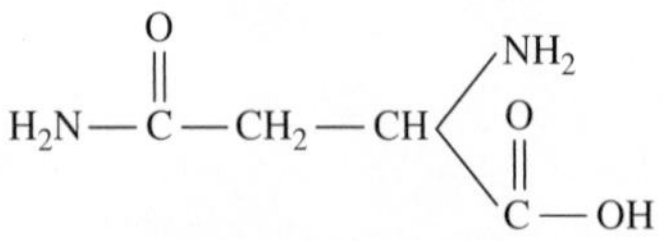

Asparagine (Asn)

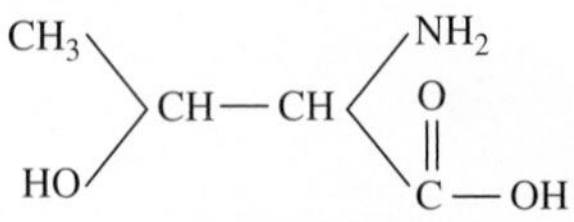

Threonine (Thr)
(essential)

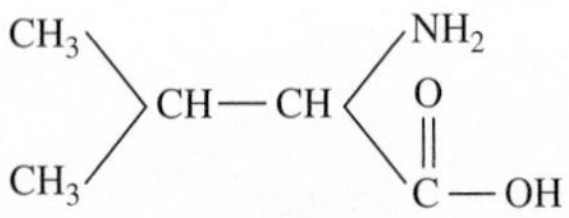

Valine (Val)
(essential)

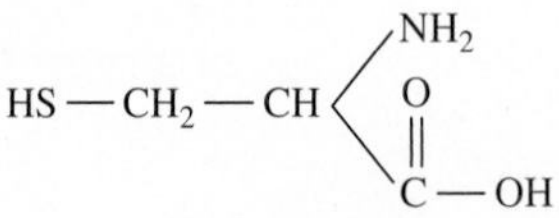

Cysteine (Cys)

Vitamins

Provitamin A

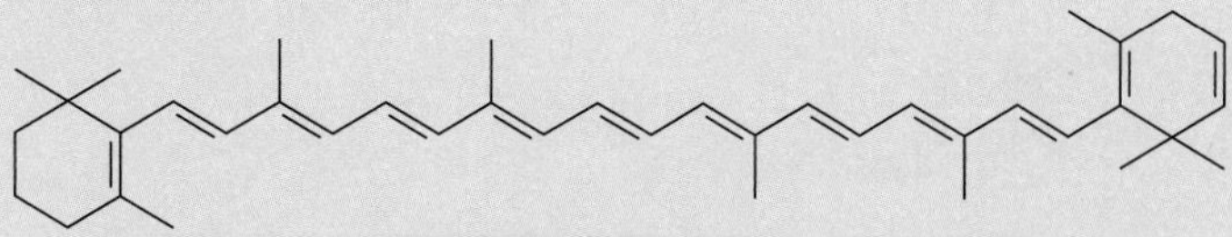

Beta-carotene

Preformed Vitamin A

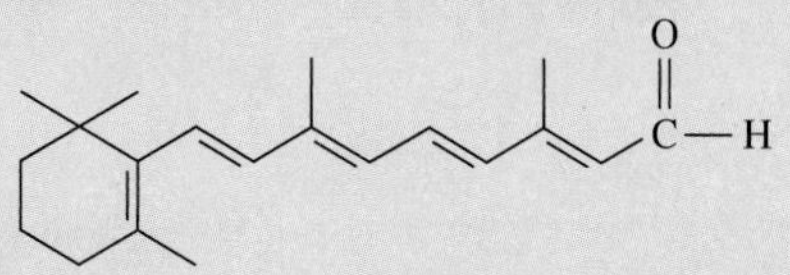

Retinal

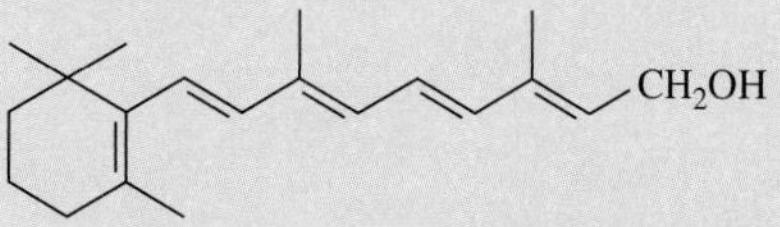

Retinol

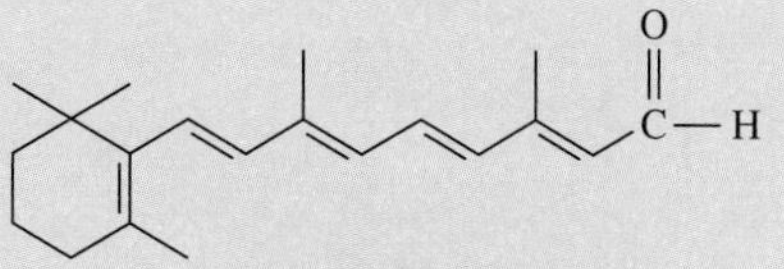

Retinoic acid

Vitamin A family

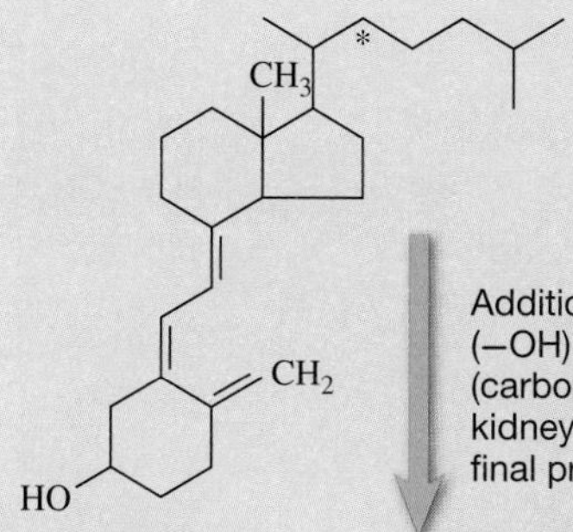

CH_3

Addition of hydroxyl groups
(—OH) by the liver
(carbon #25) and then by the
kidney (carbon #1) yields the
final product.

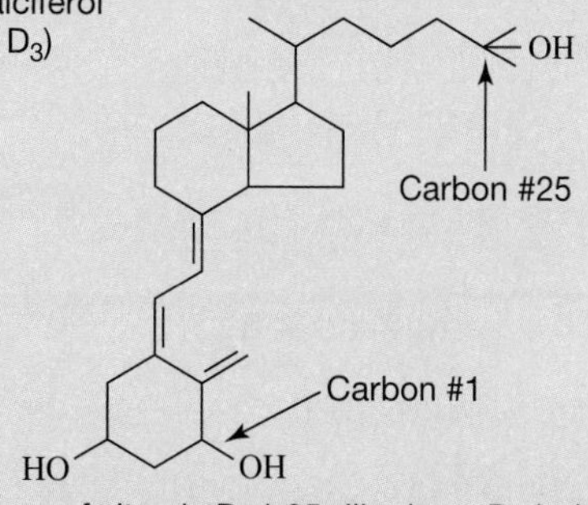

HO

Cholecalciferol
(vitamin D_3)

CH_2

OH

Carbon #25

Carbon #1

HO   OH

Active form of vitamin D: 1,25 dihydroxy D_3 (calcitriol)

The form produced by the body is called cholecalciferol
(vitamin D_3). A form typically found in or added to foods is
ergocalciferol (vitamin D_2). It has a double bond in the
starred position in the top structure.

Vitamin D family

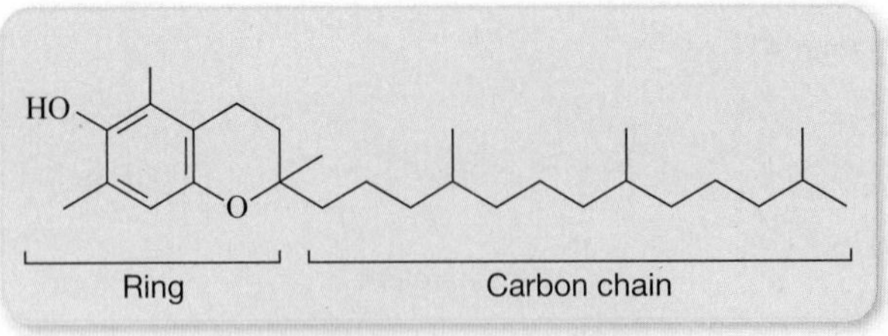
Ring
Carbon chain

Vitamin E (alpha-tocopherol)

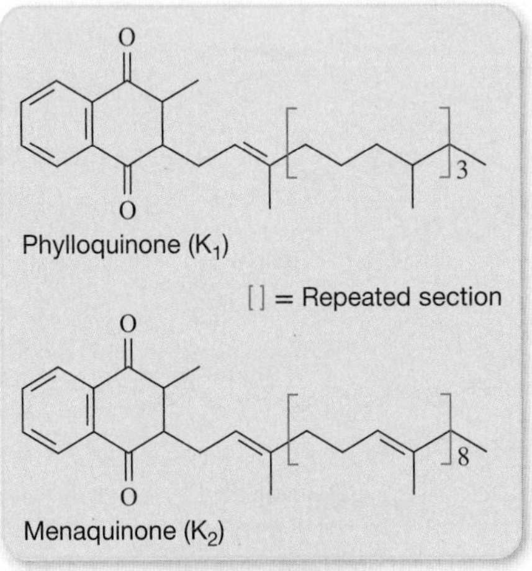
Phylloquinone (K_1)
[ ] = Repeated section
Menaquinone (K_2)

Vitamin K family

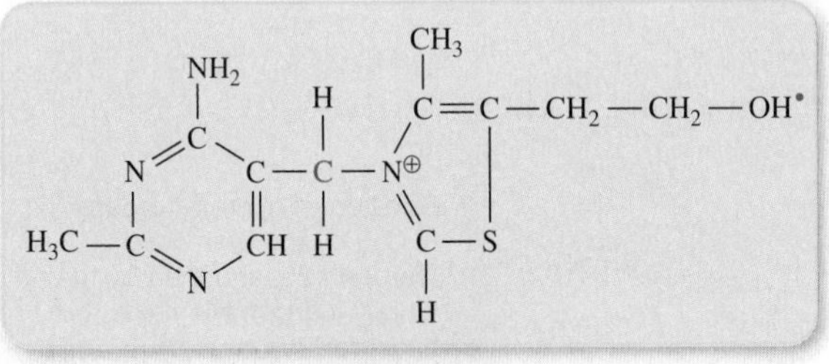

Thiamin

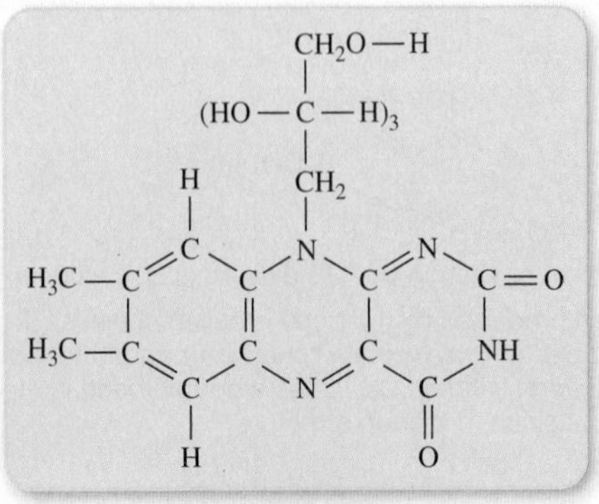

Riboflavin

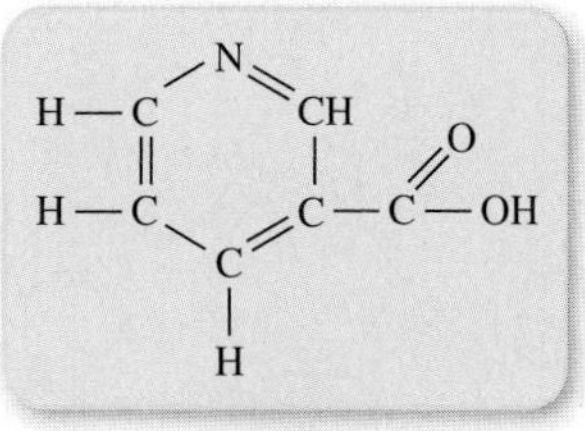

Niacin

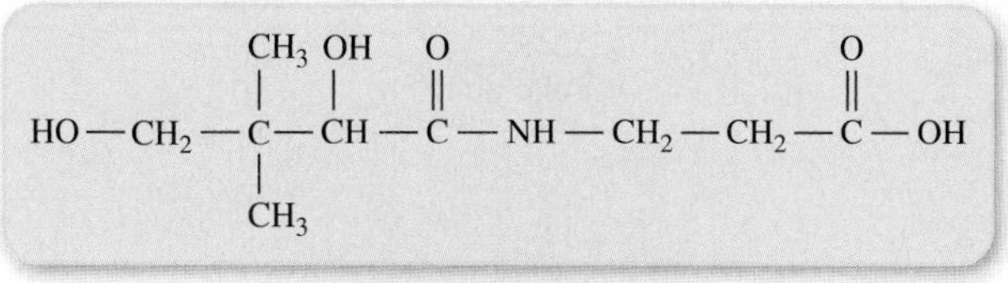

Pantothenic acid

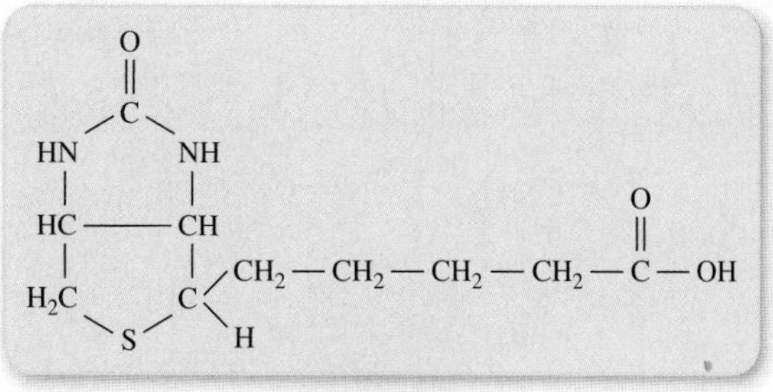

Biotin

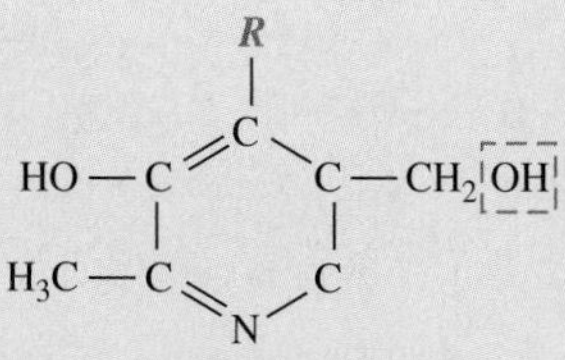

Vitamin B-6

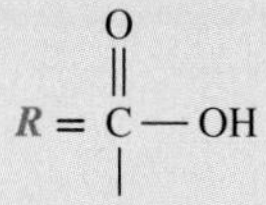

$$R = \overset{O}{\overset{\|}{C}} - OH \quad \text{pyridoxal}$$

$$R = CH_2OH \quad \text{pyridoxine}$$

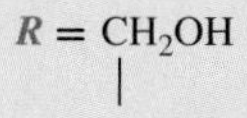

$$R = CH_2NH_2 \quad \text{pyridoxamine}$$

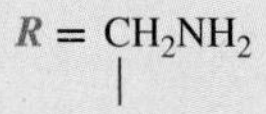

Boxed area = Hydroxyl group where
phosphate is added

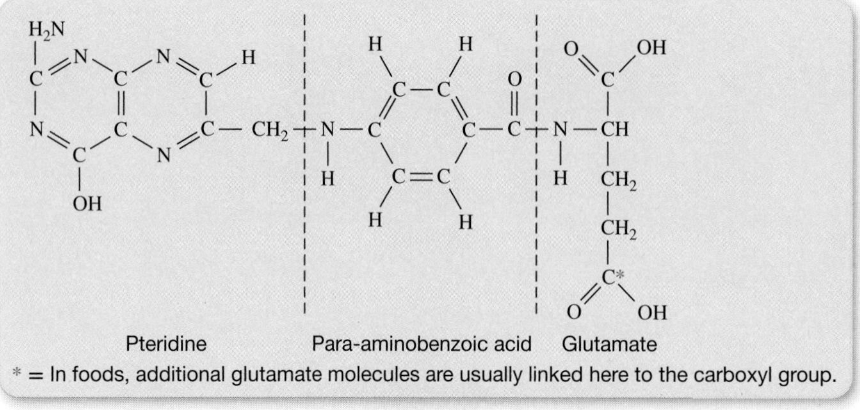

Pteridine   Para-aminobenzoic acid   Glutamate

* = In foods, additional glutamate molecules are usually linked here to the carboxyl group.

Folic acid

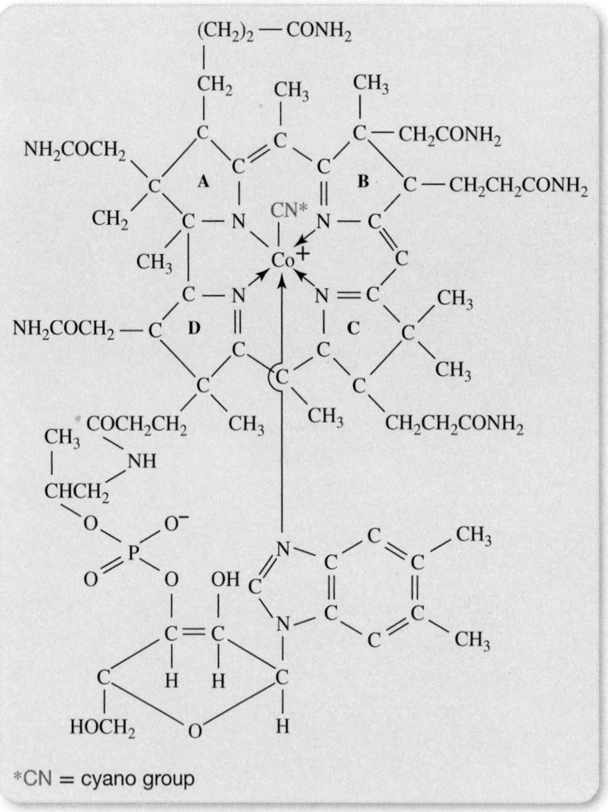

*CN = cyano group

Vitamin B-12 (cyanocobalamin)

Boxed area = Ascorbic acid (vitamin C) undergoes reversible oxidation and reduction by loss of 2 hydrogens (red) and 2 electrons (not shown).

Ascorbic acid (reduced)

Dehydroascorbic acid (oxidized)

Appendix E
Vitamins Involved in Energy Metabolism

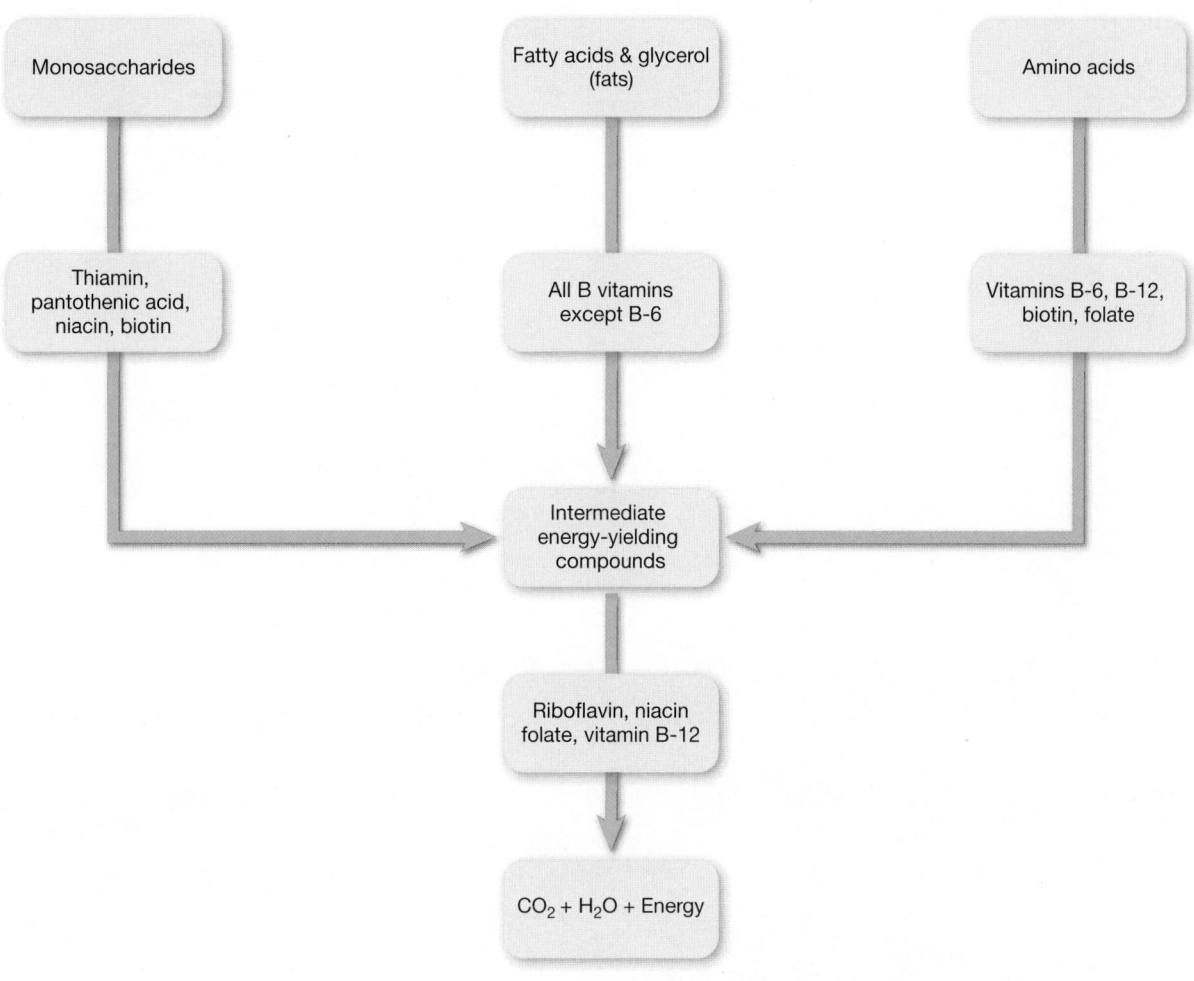

Monosaccharides

Fatty acids & glycerol (fats)

Amino acids

Thiamin, pantothenic acid, niacin, biotin

All B vitamins except B-6

Vitamins B-6, B-12, biotin, folate

Intermediate energy-yielding compounds

Riboflavin, niacin folate, vitamin B-12

$CO_2 + H_2O$ + Energy

Appendix F
Nutrition Assessment

Nutrition Assessment

In early 1970s, physician Charles E. Butterworth, Jr. determined that the majority of patients who had long-term hospital stays were malnourished and starving. In some cases, the patient's malnourished condition complicated the existing disease state and increased the individual's risk for dying. In 1974, Dr. Butterworth's article "The Skeleton in the Hospital Closet" exposed *hospital malnutrition* as a serious problem.[1] Today, trained professionals who work in hospital settings are required to screen every patient within 24 hours of admittance to assess the individual's risk for malnutrition.

Nutrition assessment is the process in which specific patient data are collected, evaluated, and interpreted to determine the nutritional status of an individual or population.[2] During the assessment process, clinicians evaluate the patient for weight; history of poor dietary intake and/or signs of starvation, such as loss of muscle mass and/or subcutaneous fat; and key laboratory values. Assessment data are used to develop nutrition interventions that will improve nutritional status, often resulting in better patient outcomes, fewer days in the hospital, and reduced health care costs.[3]

THE FIRST STEP: NUTRITION SCREENING

Nutrition assessment is a highly involved process that requires a RD/RDN or other trained health care professional. Because full nutrition assessments can be time consuming and expensive, health care practitioners conduct an initial *nutrition screening* to determine whether an individual needs a more in-depth nutrition assessment. **Nutrition screening** is the process of identifying characteristics, such as low body weight, that are known to be associated with chronic nutrition problems, and identifying individuals who are malnourished or at nutritional risk.[2] Table F.1 lists the key health-related criteria assessed by conducting nutrition screening.

Data obtained from the screening are recorded on a special screening form. The criteria used to develop the form are based on several factors, including the life stages of the population being screened (e.g., children, young adults, older adults) and the type of facility (e.g., hospital or long-term care facility).

Health care professionals may offer health screenings in community settings, such as at shopping malls or churches. The goal of such screenings is to identify individuals at risk for common chronic diseases, including hypertension and cardiovascular disease. For example, blood pressure testing can be used in screening for hypertension. In comparison to community screenings, dietitians working in hospitals or long-term care facilities typically screen patients for changes in appetite or body weight. This information is then used along with key laboratory measurements to evaluate patients' state of nutritional health.

Following the initial screening, the health care provider can make one of the following decisions:

- No further follow-up is needed.

- The patient should be rescreened after a period of time.

- A full nutrition assessment is necessary.

TABLE F.1 Nutrition Screening: Key Criteria

Change in appetite
Diarrhea or constipation
Dietary intake
Disease diagnosis
Food allergies
Height
Weight
Laboratory measurements: blood and/or urine samples
Lifestyle factors
Nausea or vomiting
Unintentional weight gain or weight loss

Full Nutrition Assessment

The four main techniques used to assess nutritional status are historical assessment, anthropometric assessment, laboratory (biochemical) assessment, and clinical assessment. Each of these is described in the following sections.

HISTORICAL ASSESSMENT

The **historical assessment** obtains personal health−related information that is gathered by interviewing the patient. A detailed personal and social history, personal and family medical history, use of medications and complementary medicine, and dietary data including dietary intake and supplement use are often collected as part of the historical assessment. The historical assessment provides clues to the patient's current health status and risk for future health problems. Health care professionals use this information to determine follow−up questions to ask the patient about his or her health status, so they can make an appropriate diagnosis and prescribe the best treatment. The information gathered from the history can help the health care professional consider all aspects of the patient that may contribute to impaired nutritional status. This section focuses on methods of collecting dietary data.

DIETARY ASSESSMENT

Dietary assessment is the process of gathering information about a person's eating habits, food and dietary supplement intake, and motivations for his or her food selections to identify possible nutrient imbalances. A variety of dietary assessment methods are available to assess a person's usual food and supplement intake. Dietitians select the appropriate dietary assessment method by evaluating the type of dietary information that is needed, how it will be utilized, and the interest and motivation of the individual who is providing the dietary information.

Advances in technology have introduced new methods for collecting dietary intake information. These technologies empower the client or patient to enter his or her own food choices into specialized dietary software. The person can immediately see the results and share them with the dietetics professional. This section will discuss both traditional methods and new technology available to collect dietary intake data for dietary assessment.

24−hour Dietary Recall. A **24−hour dietary recall** documents food, beverage and supplement intake over the previous 24 hours. The recall is typically used to gather data for population studies or to provide the dietitian with a general idea of an individual's dietary habits. To obtain the most accurate dietary intake data, trained interviewers should establish trust with their client, ask nonjudgmental questions, and use the *multiple−pass method* of interviewing subjects.

The multiple−pass method involves having the interviewer ask the client to freely recall everything he or she has consumed in the past 24 hours. After the first "pass" of data collection, the assessor reviews the list and asks the client to provide more details, such as portion size, preparation method, and clarification on the food type (e.g., regular, reduced fat, or fat−free salad dressing). In the third and final pass, the reviewer reads the foods and beverages that are on the list to the client and asks him or her to include information that may have been omitted.

When collecting a 24−hour dietary recall, interviewers should ask respondents about activities they participated in during the previous day to help them remember food and beverage intake associated with those activities. For example, remembering that it was a coworker's birthday may remind the woman being interviewed that she had a piece of cake at lunchtime.

A 24−hour dietary recall is useful because it takes very little time to administer, is inexpensive, and respondents can usually provide details about the foods and beverages they consumed. However, respondents may not accurately report their food intake. Most respondents tend to un−derreport consumption of foods and beverages that may be perceived as "unhealthy." Conversely, intake of foods considered "healthy," such as fruits and vegetables, are often overreported. Because of the short time frame, the information gathered should not be generalized to characterize a person's usual food intake. The previous day's intake may not be typical for the individual, or the person may forget foods that were eaten. Using the multiple−pass method and obtaining 24−hour dietary recalls on several nonconsecutive days can minimize these limitations.

Food Frequency Questionnaire. The **food frequency questionnaire** asks the respondent to recall how frequently he or she eats specified foods during a given time frame, which can range from several weeks to 1 year. Food frequency questionnaires can be tailored to target specific food groups, ethnic foods, and foods that are rich in specific nutrients, such as calcium or iron. Comprehensive food frequency questionnaires will list between 100 to 150 foods, whereas food frequency questionnaires targeting a particular food group or set of nutrients may list only 20 to 30 foods. Respondents are asked to recall the serving size, number of servings consumed, and frequency of consumption over a period of time (several months to 1 year). Results from the questionnaire provide information about dietary patterns and intake of specific nutrients over time.

Food frequency questionnaires are useful because they take little time to administer, are inexpensive, and do not require a trained professional to administer them. These questionnaires are the most commonly used dietary assessment tool in large epidemiological studies of diet and health. However, because the questionnaire is self−reported, respondents may misclassify foods and report incorrect portion sizes. In addition, the foods listed on the questionnaire may not reflect the foods the person typically eats. Combining the results of the food frequency questionnaire with the results of a 24–hour dietary recall can improve the accuracy of the data.

Food Record. A **food record**, also called a **food diary**, gives the responsibility for recording food intake to the client, rather than the interviewer. To complete a food record, the client is asked to record everything he or she eats and drinks over a specified period of time, typically for 3 days. Records are kept for as little as 1 day and as many as 7 days, if the individual is highly motivated. Details on the time of consumption, location of consumption, type of food or beverage, method of preparation, and portion size are recorded.

For the best accuracy, clients should be encouraged to record their food intake on both weekday and weekend days and when the food or beverage is consumed. Many individuals consume more high–calorie and high–fat foods on weekends, particularly if they eat meals away from home.

Food records are an effective method of obtaining dietary information when the health care professional is working with highly cooperative individuals who are motivated to keep detailed records of their intake. By keeping detailed food records, clients often become more aware of their personal eating habits and are more likely to assume responsibility for negative eating habits and be receptive to dietary advice. Food records should not be used with individuals who have poor reading skills, are unmotivated, and/or lack the time to keep detailed intake records.

Technological Advances in Collecting Diet Information. Advances in digital technology created a variety of new tools to collect dietary intake data. Computer programs and mobile electronic device "apps" are designed to reduce errors and costs commonly associated with traditional dietary collection methods and improve accessibility. People who are comfortable using mobile electronic devices can record their food intake anytime and anyplace,

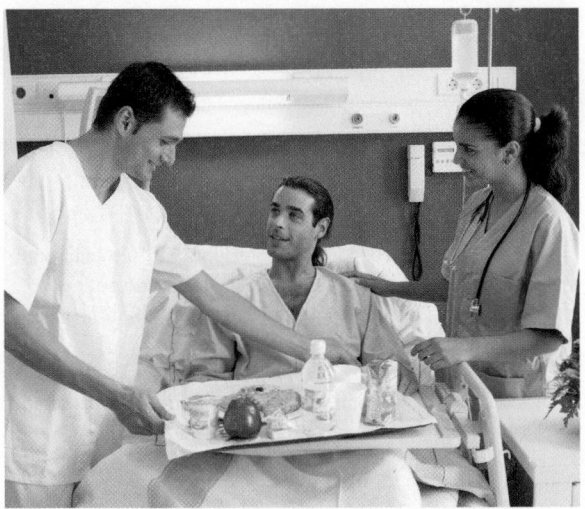

which often leads to a more accurate food record and increased patient compliance.

Computerized Weighing and Recording Systems. Computerized weighing and recording of food systems are used to reduce error in reporting and to expedite collection and analysis of dietary intake. A food recording electronic device is an example of a computerized weighing and recording system that allows the users to identify the food they are eating in a database and weigh the food item on a scale. The scale then sends the data directly to a standardized database on the computer. A variety of intake reports can then be created for a specified period of time.[4]

Automated Self–Administered 24–Hour Dietary Recalls. The automated self–administered 24–hour dietary recall (ASA24™) is an example of an online software application that is designed for research studies, such as those conducted by the U.S. Department of Health and Human Services. ASA24 allows research participants to log in from their home computer. The software program presents images of the foods and an avatar that offers instructions for selecting the correct food and portion eaten. The information entered by the participant is sent directly to the researcher. A drawback of using this system is the limited database of foods currently available and typically consumed in the United States.[5]

Mobile Applications. In recent years, a variety of applications (apps) have become available to electronic mobile device users who want to track and analyze their diet. Options include free apps, apps that are available for a fee, and a free app that has an incomplete database that can be expanded by paying a fee.

The majority of apps require the individual to enter food intake data directly into the system. A variety of input methods are available, including entering specific foods and the quantity consumed, entering food groups and the quantity consumed, entering the calorie and/or carbohydrate quantity of the foods consumed, or entering intake information into a food frequency questionnaire format. Systems known as "semiautomatic" apps allow the user to scan the barcode off of a food item. The nutritional information from the food item is directly entered into the software.[6]

While there are several benefits to using nutrition apps, electronic mobile device technology is still in its infancy and there are several limitations. The databases often have limited food options and may not offer information on micronutrients and subcategories of macronutrients (e.g., omega–3 fatty acids). Most apps, particularly the free apps, do not provide a standard serving–size reference to help the user accurately assess the size of the portion eaten. This limitation presents a problem, because most people are not trained to estimate portion sizes accurately. Nevertheless, the future of nutrition apps as a means of collecting reliable food data is promising because the technology continues to improve.

Strengths and Weaknesses of Dietary Assessment Tools.

Each of the tools described in the previous sections has both strengths and weaknesses in its ability to record, monitor, and evaluate dietary intake. Table F.2 provides a summary of these strengths and weaknesses.

ANTHROPOMETRIC ASSESSMENT

Anthropometric assessment uses physical measurements of weight, height (also known as *stature*) or length, body composition, and distribution of fat on the body to determine health and nutrition status. Health care professionals compare the values of physical measurements against population standards that are sex—and age-specific to determine the patient's risk for certain chronic diseases, such as cardiovascular disease and type 2 diabetes. Collecting and comparing measurements over time alerts the health care professional to changes in an individual's nutritional and health status.

As with all categories of nutritional assessment, it is important to include a variety of appropriate anthropometric measurements to ensure the correct diagnosis is

TABLE F.2 Dietary Assessment Tools: Pros and Cons

Dietary Assessment Tool	Strengths	Limitations
24-hour dietary recall	• Administered by a trained professional • Requires little time to administer • Little respondent burden • Respondent can provide details on foods consumed. • Inexpensive	• A single day is often not reflective of one's habitual food intake. • Relies on memory of the respondent, which may be less than accurate • Respondent may over- or underreport intake. • Entry of intake into computerized system for evaluation is time-consuming.
Food frequency questionnaire	• Many questionnaires are self-administered. • Computer-readable questionnaires minimize labor and time required. • Inexpensive • Shows trends in food intake over time and seasons • Little respondent burden	• Respondent may not properly classify foods. • Some foods can fit into multiple categories, which can reduce reliability of data. • Foods listed may not be representative of what the respondent normally consumes. • Relies on the memory of the respondent
Food record (diary)	• Respondent lists food immediately, instead of relying on memory. • Respondent can provide details on food consumed. • Food intake can be recorded for multiple days. • Provides more information about variety in the diet and habitual food intake • Inexpensive	• Respondent burden is high. • Quality of diary is dependent on the motivation and training of respondent. • Respondent must be able to read and write. • Food intake may change through record keeping. • Respondent may over- or underreport intake. • Entry of intake into computerized system for evaluation is time-consuming.
Computerized recording systems	• Respondent lists food immediately and does not rely on memory. • Respondent can provide details about food consumed. • Food intake can be recorded for multiple days. • Interactive and engaging recording systems can enhance the enjoyment of the respondent. • Analysis of diet immediate through computerized system	• Equipment can be expensive. • Respondent must be trained and comfortable with using technology. • Equipment can malfunction.
Mobile applications	• Respondent lists food immediately and does not rely on memory. • Food intake can be entered anytime and anyplace. • Analysis of diet is immediate. • Energy expenditure and energy intake can be assessed. • Macronutrient intake can be assessed. • Bar code of manufactured foods can be scanned into the mobile device.	• Limited food databases • Nutrient profiles for macronutrients and sub-macronutrients (e.g., omega-3 fatty acids) are limited or do not exist. • Individuals recording the data may not be trained to accurately determine portion sizes. • Standard serving sizes may not be available as references. • Access may be limited if the respondent is in an area that has poor mobile device service. • Cost of mobile device and apps

made about an individual's health and nutrition status. For example, recall from Chapter 13 that body mass index (BMI) does not account for body composition (e.g., body fat), which is an important measure for evaluating health and risk for chronic disease. Therefore, measures of body composition or distribution of body fat should also be included in the anthropometric assessment.

Weight and Height   Weight and height are the most commonly collected anthropometric measurements. These measurements are relatively easy to obtain and provide useful information throughout the entire life cycle. As shown in Figure F.1, electronic and balance beam scales are used to measure weight. Electronic scales are porta- ble, have displays that are easy to read, and provide the results faster than a balance beam scale. All scales should be calibrated on a regular basis and immediately after they are moved to ensure the measurements are accurate. It is important to consider variations between scales when comparing measured values to previous values from two different scales. Ideally, an individual should be measured at the same time of day, wear similar clothing, and obtain his or her weight from the same scale over a period of time to reduce variables that could influence the accuracy of the measurement.

Infants are weighed on a balance beam scale (Fig. F.2). To obtain the most accurate measurement, infants should be weighed either unclothed or in only a dry diaper. In- fants may be fussy during the measurement, making it a challenge to obtain an accurate measurement; multiple measurements may be required to obtain an average and, therefore, valid reading. An alternative method of ob- taining an infant's weight is to have the caregiver hold the infant while standing on a platform scale and then subtracting the adult's weight from the scale.

Height in older children and adults is measured with the individual standing erect against a flat wall. As seen in Figure F.3, the person's shoulders are relaxed and arms are at the sides. The individual's feet should be shoeless

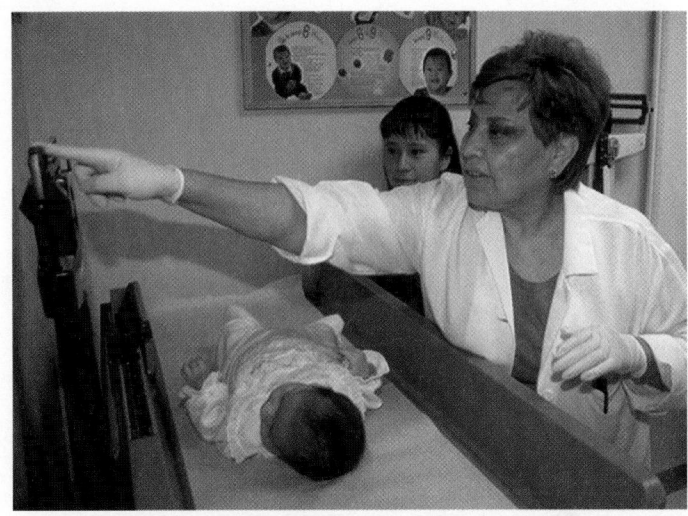

FIGURE F.2 Balance beam scale for weighing infants.

and flat on the floor. The person should be looking straight so the top of the head is parallel to the floor. Because infants and toddlers may be unable to stand on their own, their length is measured while they are lying on a table (*supine*) with a measuring board (Fig. F.4). The infant's head is placed against one end of the mea- suring board, and his or her legs are straightened and placed flush against the base of the measuring board that is at the infant's feet. This measurement may be uncom- fortable for the child and often requires two clinicians to ensure an accurate measurement is taken.

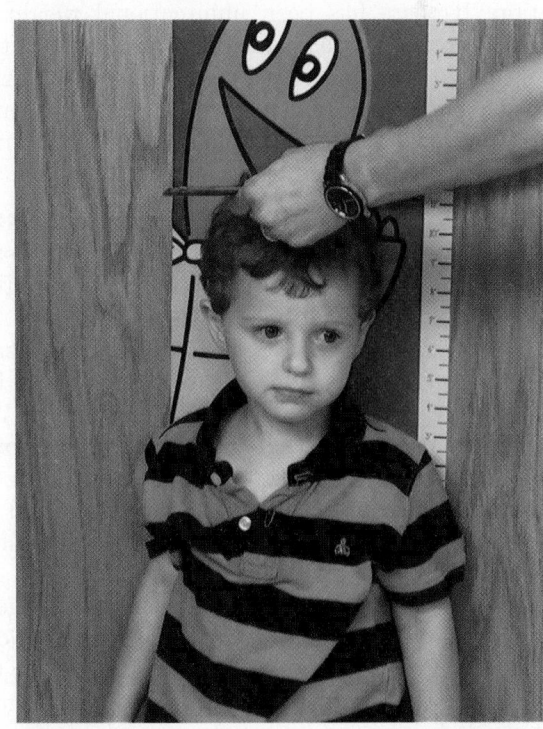

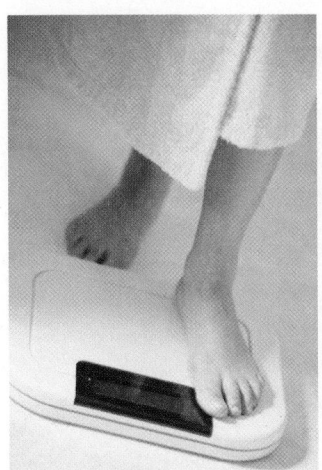 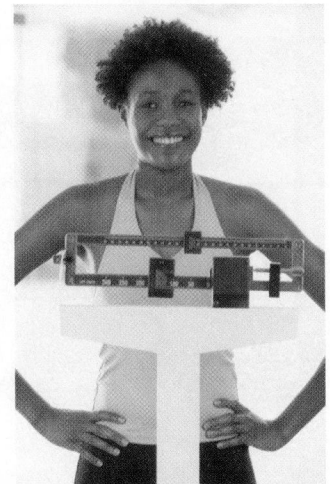

FIGURE F.1 Electronic and balance beam scales for measuring weight.

FIGURE F.3 Measuring height in older children.

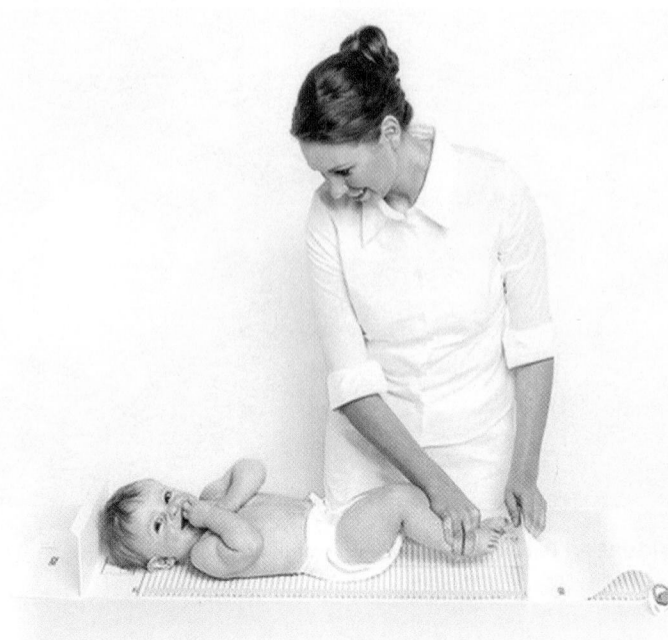

FIGURE F.4 Measuring height in infants and toddlers.

Body weight in adults is interpreted by comparing the measured weight to weight−for−height standards and evaluating changes in weight that occur over time. BMI is the preferred standard used by health care profession−als to assess weight status and subsequent risk for chronic disease. See Chapter 13 for detailed instructions on how to calculate BMI and how to interpret the results in the adult population. If there has been unintentional weight loss, calculating percent weight change is a useful indicator to determine whether an individual is at risk for malnutrition. Weight changes of greater than 10% within a 6−month period of time generally indicate the need for further med−ical assessment by a trained health care professional.[7]

***Using Growth Charts: Children*.** **Growth charts** are used to evaluate weight and height (or length) status of adolescents, children, toddlers, and infants. Growth charts for infants from birth to 2 years of age have been developed by the World Health Organization (WHO) and the Centers for Disease Control and Pre−vention (CDC). The CDC recommends using the WHO growth charts to assess the growth and development of infants. These charts provide a standard for how an infant should grow in optimal conditions, and they were developed using high−quality studies designed to develop growth charts.[8]

Growth charts for infants include weight−for−age and length−for−age. Growth charts for children and adoles−cents ages 2 to 20 years have been developed by the CDC and include stature−for−age and BMI−for−age.[8–10] Weight and height are plotted on weight−for−age, stature−for−age (or length−for−age), and BMI−for−age growth charts to determine a percentile ranking when compared to population data. To plot the measurements on the growth chart, first find the child's age on the hor−izontal axis. Use a straightedge to draw a vertical line up from that point. Second, find the appropriate mea−sure for stature (or length), weight, or BMI on the ver−tical axis and use a straightedge to draw a horizontal line from that point. Draw a small dot where the two lines meet. Weight−for−age, length−for−age, and weight−for−length growth charts for infants birth to 2 years and height−for−age, stature−for−age, and BMI−for−age growth charts for children and adolescents 2 to 20 years are available at http://www.cdc.gov/growthcharts.

Weight status in adolescents and children is interpreted by calculating the BMI and comparing it against popula−tion standards. BMI is plotted on age− and sex−specific BMI charts developed by the CDC to determine a percentile ranking against population data of adolescents and children. Clinicians should look for a consistent pattern of growth over a period of time on the percentile chart to ensure the child or teen is growing properly, rather than looking at an individual point on the chart. As long as a child is growing along the curve, there are generally no concerns about the youngster's health. Adolescents and children who are below the 5th percentile or above the 95th percentile should have a further assessment conducted by a pediatric medical spe−cialist.[9,10] Figure F.5, which is on page A−29, provides an example growth chart for a 2−year−old female child.

Weight and height for infants are plotted on weight−for−age and length−for−age growth charts to deter−mine a percentile ranking against population data. Infants who are less than the 2nd or higher than the 98th percen−tile ranges should have a further assessment conducted by a pediatric medical specialist.

HEAD CIRCUMFERENCE

Head circumference is used to evaluate growth and brain development during the first 2 years of life. As shown in Figure F.6, head circumference is measured with a

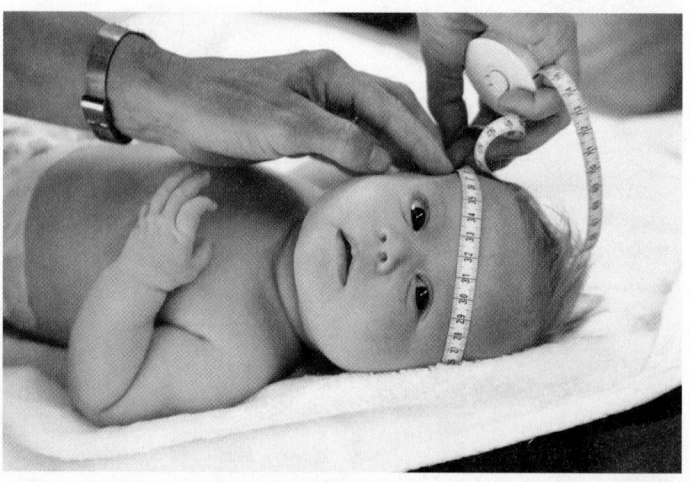

FIGURE F.6 Measuring head circumference.

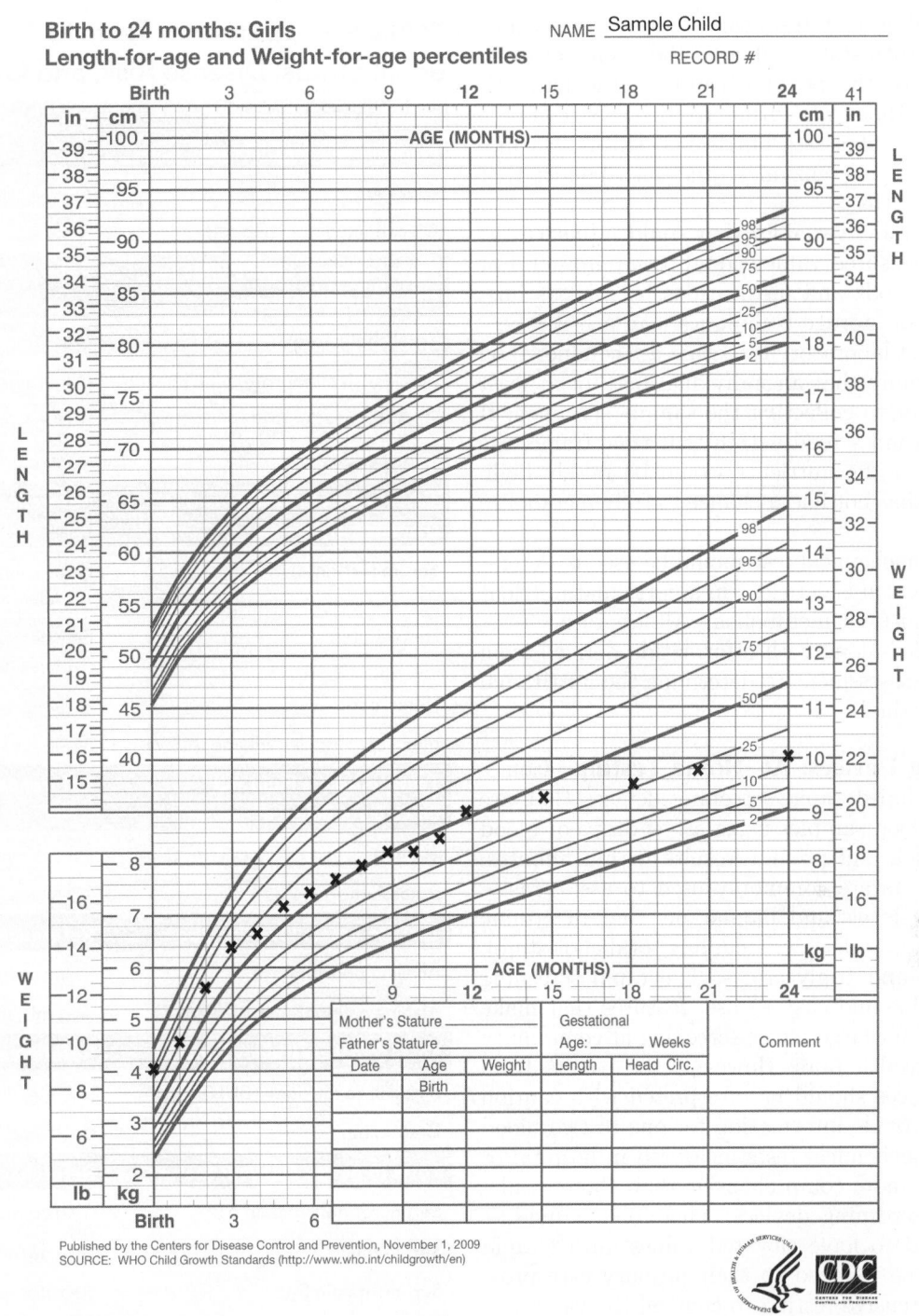

Birth to 24 months: Girls
Length-for-age and Weight-for-age percentiles

NAME Sample Child

RECORD #

Published by the Centers for Disease Control and Prevention, November 1, 2009
SOURCE: WHO Child Growth Standards (http://www.who.int/childgrowth/en)

FIGURE F.5 Sample growth chart: length-for-age and weight-for-age.

nonstretchable measuring tape. The clinician places the tape around the largest region of the infant's or toddler's head, which is just above the eyebrows and where the top of the ears attach to the head. The tape should extend from the front of the head to around the widest part of the back of the child's head. To ensure an accurate value, the measurement should be taken three times and an average value derived from the measurements. Once measured, the value is plotted on a gender–specific growth chart. Head–circumference–for–age growth charts developed by the WHO are used to assess head circumference among children ages birth to 2 years (available at http://www.cdc.gov/growthcharts).

LABORATORY (BIOCHEMICAL) ASSESSMENT

Laboratory (or biochemical) assessment is an objective and quantitative evaluation of nutritional markers obtained from blood, urine, feces, and tissues. The results of some laboratory tests can accurately determine an individual's health status, whereas the results of other tests offer clues to the possible cause of the patient's health problem.[11] Blood and urine are the most common specimens collected to assess nutritional status, because they contain nutrients, enzymes, and metabolites that reflect nutrition status.

To ensure accuracy, variables that could influence the outcome of the measured value should be minimized. For example, certain foods and medications, as well as improper collection or storage techniques, can affect laboratory values. Most laboratory tests that are conducted on blood samples require that an individual fast for at least 8 to 12 hours prior to collecting the sample specimen. If an individual consumes food within that time frame, the measured values of the nutrients would be falsely high, because the body has not had a chance to fully metabolize the nutrient.

No one single biochemical test should be used to determine whether a person is deficient in a particular nutrient or has impaired nutrient metabolism. All laboratory tests should be evaluated along with information derived from other methods of assessment to determine the nutritional status of an individual.

Rapid Screening Devices: At–Home Testing Companies have developed rapid screening devices that are able to analyze blood samples using a few drops of blood from a finger prick and provide results within minutes. These types of tests are commonly used to assess fasting blood glucose levels and biomarkers that determine risk for cardiovascular disease, including total cholesterol, HDL cholesterol, and triglycerides. The rapid screening devices are portable and easy to use, features that make the devices useful for large–scale screening at community events, such as health fairs. However, the results from the screening devices should be interpreted with caution since they only provide information for one to two blood measurements. Biochemical tests measured in hospital or clinic settings are more comprehensive than those available with rapid screening devices. Therefore, individuals who are found to have elevated values during rapid screening should be referred to their primary care provider for more extensive testing to confirm the values.

Biochemical Tests Used in the Hospital or Clinical Setting Results of biochemical tests provide objective and quantitative values related to risk for disease, disease management, organ or tissue function, and nutritional status. Most medical facilities run a *comprehensive metabolic panel* that gives results for a standard set of biochemical measurements. Table F.3 lists tests commonly included in a comprehensive metabolic panel, as well as tests used to measure nutritional status, the normal range for the test, and what the test indicates if the values are outside of the reference range. In many instances, the health care professional orders more specialized tests than

TABLE F.3 Laboratory Tests to Assess Nutritional Status, Disease Risk, and Organ Function

Tests to Assess Glucose Management for Diabetes	Reference Range
Glucose	65–100 mg/dL
Glycohemoglobin (Hb A$_{1c}$)	< 6.5 %
Tests to Assess Lipid Profile for Cardiovascular Disease	**Reference Range**
Total cholesterol	< 200 mg/dL
Low-density lipoprotein (LDL)	< 100 mg/dL
High-density lipoprotein (HDL)	≥ 60 mg/dL
Triglycerides	< 150 mg/dL
Tests to Assess Risk for and Diagnosis of Anemia	**Reference Range**
Serum ferritin	Females: 12–150 ng/mL; Males: 30–320 ng/mL*
Hemoglobin	Females: 12–16 g/dL; Males: 14–18 g/dL
Hematocrit	37–54%
Mean corpuscular volume (MCV)	82–98 fL†
Tests to Assess Fluid and Electrolyte Balance	**Reference Range**
Sodium	135–145 mmol/L
Potassium	3.3–5.1 mmol/L
Tests to Assess Liver Function	**Reference Range**
Alkaline phosphatase	39–117 mU/mL
Alanine amino transferase (ALT)	5–57 mU/mL
Tests to Assess Kidney Function	**Reference Range**
Blood urea nitrogen (BUN)	6–19 mg/dL
Creatinine	0.4–1.2 mg/dL
Tests to Assess Nutrient Status	**Reference Range**
Serum retinol (vitamin A)	0.3–1.20 mg/L
Serum folate	1.8–9 ng/mL
Serum vitamin B-12	200–1100 pg/mL‡
Serum vitamin C	0.6–2 mg/dL
Serum vitamin D	15–75 pg/mL
Serum vitamin E	≤ 6.0 mg/L
Urinary calcium (24-hr specimen)	< 40 mg/dL
Serum phosphate (phosphorus)	2.8–4.1 mg/dL
Serum zinc	60–150 µg/dL

*ng/mL = nanograms per milliliter

†fL = femtoliter

‡pg/mL = picograms per milliliter

Sources: Chernecky C, Berger B: *Laboratory tests and diagnostic procedures* 6th ed. St. Louis: Elsevier, 2013; Lee R, Nieman D: *Nutritional assessment*, 6th ed. New York: McGraw-Hill, 2013.

TABLE F.4 Physical Signs in Nutritional Assessment

	Clinical Findings	What This Finding Might Indicate
Hair	Falls out, corkscrew, dry, brittle "flag-sign" (striped)	Deficiency of protein or vitamin C Excess of vitamin A
Nails	Brittle, pale, spoon-shaped	Deficiency of iron or protein
Skin	Scaly, flaky, dry, cracked, rough, spotty, off-color (red or yellow)	Deficiency of protein, essential fatty acids, vitamin A, or vitamin C Excess of niacin (red) or beta carotene (yellow)
Mouth	Missing, discolored, or decayed teeth, swollen gums, gums that bleed easily, swollen tongue, cracked skin around the corners	Deficiency of vitamin C, B vitamins, or minerals (fluoride)
Glands	Swollen glands in neck	Deficiency of iodine or protein
Eyes	Redness, foamy spots; vision adjusts slowly or poorly to darkness	Deficiency of vitamin A, B vitamins, zinc, or iron
Bones and Joints	Bowlegs or knock knees, bumps on skull or ends of bones, beading or bumps on ribs	Deficiency of vitamin D or calcium
Muscles	Loss of muscle tone, "wasting" of muscles	Deficiency of protein
Other	Swelling, edema	Deficiency of protein

Source: Lee R. and Nieman D. Nutritional assessment, 6th ed. New York: McGraw-Hill, 2013.

those that are included in the metabolic panel to confirm a diagnosis or monitor a patient's progress.

CLINICAL ASSESSMENT (PHYSICAL EXAMINATION)

The physical examination is the process in which a medical professional examines the physical characteristics of a patient for signs of disease and malnutrition. During the physical exam, the health care professional asks the patient specific questions seeking answers that will help him or her determine the correct diagnosis. Signs are clinical observations that go unnoticed by a patient but are clear to a trained professional. Symptoms are reported directly by the patient. Vital signs such as blood pressure, temperature, heart rate, and respiratory rate are taken as part of the physical exam. In addition to the vital signs, the clinician evaluates the patient's hair, skin, eyes, mouth, throat, and major organ systems.

Nutritional deficiencies are usually apparent in areas of the body where the cellular turnover rate is the highest, including the skin, nails, hair, and digestive tract. Clinicians are trained to evaluate these structures or tissues to detect signs and symptoms of malnutrition. Table F.4 identifies key physical signs used in nutritional assessment. Chapters 7, 9, 10, 11, and 12 provide additional information regarding the clinical signs associated with protein, vitamin, and mineral malnutrition.[12]

References

1. Butterworth, C: The skeleton in the hospital closet. *Nutrition Today* March/April:436,1974.
2. Academy of Nutrition and Dietetics: *International dietetics & nutrition terminology (IDNT) reference manual.* 4th ed. Chicago: Academy of Nutrition and Dietetics, 2012.
3. Philipson TJ and others: Impact of oral nutritional supplementation on hospital outcomes. *American Journal of Management Care* 19(2):121, 2013.
4. Thompson F and others: Need for technological innovation in dietary assessment. *Journal of the Academy of Nutrition and Dietetics* 110:48, 2010.
5. Stumbo P: New technology in dietary assessment: A review of digital methods in improving food record accuracy. *Proceedings of the Nutrition Society* 72:70, 2013.
6. Rusin M and others: Functionalities and input methods for recording food intake: A systemic review. *International Journal of Medical Informatics* 82:653, 2013.
7. Charney P, Marian M: *Pocket guide to nutrition screening and nutrition assessment.* 2nd ed. Chicago: Academy of Nutrition and Dietetics, 2008.
8. Centers for Disease Control: *WHO growth standards are recommended for use in the U.S. for infants and children 0 to 2 years of age.* 2013. http://www.cdc.gov/growthcharts/who_charts.htm Accessed December 14, 2013.
9. Centers for Disease Control and Prevention: Frequently asked questions about the 2000 CDC growth charts. 2013. http://www.cdc.gov/growthcharts/growthchart_faq.htm Accessed December 14, 2013.
10. Centers for Disease Control and Prevention: *Other growth chart resources.* 2013. http://www.cdc.gov/nccdphp/dnpao/growthcharts/resources/index.htm#interpretation Accessed December 14, 2013.
11. U.S. Food and Drug Administration: *Medical devices.* 2013. http://www.fda.gov/MedicalDevices/default.htm Accessed December 14, 2013.
12. Lee R, Nieman D: *Nutritional assessment.* 6th ed. New York: McGraw−Hill, 2013.

Key Terms

anthropometric assessment
physical measurements of height, weight, body composition, and distribution of body fat

clinical assessment
physical examination, including measurement of blood pressure, temperature, heart rate, and/or bowel sounds in addition to observations of the patient's physical status from skin, eyes, hair, nails, and other parts of the body

dietary assessment
process of gathering information about a person's eating habits, food and supplement intake, and motivations for their food selections

food frequency questionnaire
dietary assessment tool that asks respondents to recall how frequently they eat specified foods during a given time frame

food record (food diary)
dietary assessment tool in which an individual records everything he or she eats and drinks over a specified period of time, typically for 3 days

growth charts
specialized charts used to evaluate weight and height (or length) status in adolescents, children, toddlers, and infants. Charts are developed by the World Health Organization (WHO) and Centers for Disease Control and Prevention (CDC).

historical assessment
assessment of an individual's personal history, family medical history, socioeconomic status, use of medications and complementary medicine, and lifestyle habits

laboratory (biochemical) assessment
data obtained from blood, plasma, urinary, or fecal samples

nutrition assessment
process in which patient data are collected, evaluated, and interpreted to determine the nutritional status of an individual or population

nutrition screening
process of identifying characteristics known to be associated with nutrition problems and identifying individuals who are malnourished or at nutritional risk

24–hour dietary recall
dietary assessment tool that includes documentation of food, beverage, and supplement intake over the previous 24–hour period

Appendix G
Daily Values Table

Dietary Constituent	Unit of Measure	Daily Values for People Over 4 Years of Age (as of January 2016)	Proposed Nutrient Standards for Daily Value*
Total fat	g	65	65
Saturated fatty acids	"	20	20
Protein	"	50	50
Cholesterol	mg	300	300
Total carbohydrate	g	300	300
Fiber	"	25	28
Vitamin A	μg (RAEs)	1500	900
Vitamin D	μg	10	20
Vitamin E	mg	14–20	15
Vitamin K	μg	80	120
Vitamin C	mg	60	90
Folate	μg	400	400
Thiamin	mg	1.5	1.2
Riboflavin	"	1.7	1.3
Niacin	"	20	16
Vitamin B-6	"	2	1.7
Vitamin B-12	μg	6	2.4
Biotin	mg	0.03	30
Pantothenic acid	"	10	5
Calcium	"	1000	1300
Phosphorus	"	1000	1250
Iodine	μg	150	150
Iron	mg	18	18
Magnesium	"	400	420
Copper	"	2	0.9
Zinc	"	15	11
Sodium	"	2400	2300
Potassium	"	3500	4700
Chloride	"	3400	2300
Manganese	"	2	2.3
Selenium	μg	70	55
Chromium	"	120	35
Molybdenum	"	75	45

Abbreviations: g = gram, mg = milligram, μg = microgram, RAEs = retinol activity equivalents, ATE = alpha tocopherol equivalent

*Proposed standards from: U.S. Department of Health and Human Services, Food and Drug Administration: Food labeling: Revision of the Nutrition and Supplement Facts labels. 21 CFR Part 101 [Docket No. FDA-2012-N-1210] RIN 0910-AF22. *Federal Register* 79(41), March 3, 2014.

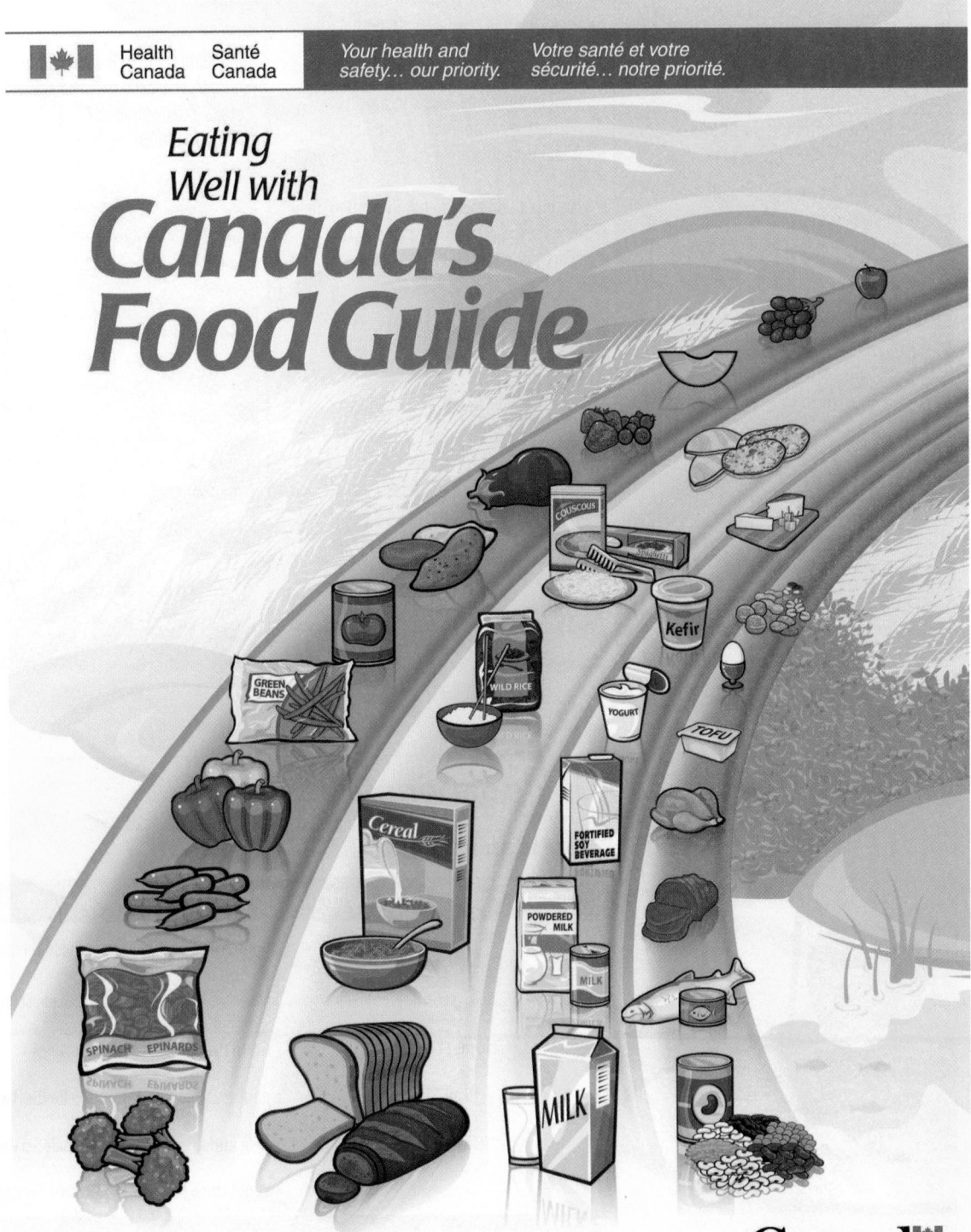

Advice for different ages and stages...

Children

Following *Canada's Food Guide* helps children grow and thrive.

Young children have small appetites and need calories for growth and development.

- Serve small nutritious meals and snacks each day.
- Do not restrict nutritious foods because of their fat content. Offer a variety of foods from the four food groups.
- Most of all... be a good role model.

Women of childbearing age

All women who could become pregnant and those who are pregnant or breastfeeding need a multivitamin containing **folic acid** every day. Pregnant women need to ensure that their multivitamin also contains **iron**. A health care professional can help you find the multivitamin that's right for you.

Pregnant and breastfeeding women need more calories. Include an extra 2 to 3 Food Guide Servings each day.

Here are two examples:
- Have fruit and yogurt for a snack, or
- Have an extra slice of toast at breakfast and an extra glass of milk at supper.

Men and women over 50

The need for **vitamin D** increases after the age of 50.

In addition to following *Canada's Food Guide*, everyone over the age of 50 should take a daily vitamin D supplement of 10 µg (400 IU).

How do I count Food Guide Servings in a meal?

Here is an example:

Vegetable and beef stir-fry with rice, a glass of milk and an apple for dessert		
250 mL (1 cup) mixed broccoli, carrot and sweet red pepper	=	2 **Vegetables and Fruit** Food Guide Servings
75 g (2 ½ oz.) lean beef	=	1 **Meat and Alternatives** Food Guide Serving
250 mL (1 cup) brown rice	=	2 **Grain Products** Food Guide Servings
5 mL (1 tsp) canola oil	=	part of your **Oils and Fats** intake for the day
250 mL (1 cup) 1% milk	=	1 **Milk and Alternatives** Food Guide Serving
1 apple	=	1 **Vegetables and Fruit** Food Guide Serving

Recommended Number of *Food Guide Servings* per Day

	Children			Teens		Adults			
Age in Years	2-3	4-8	9-13	14-18		19-50		51+	
Sex	Girls and Boys			Females	Males	Females	Males	Females	Males
Vegetables and Fruit	4	5	6	7	8	7-8	8-10	7	7
Grain Products	3	4	6	6	7	6-7	8	6	7
Milk and Alternatives	2	2	3-4	3-4	3-4	2	2	3	3
Meat and Alternatives	1	1	1-2	2	3	2	3	2	3

The chart above shows how many Food Guide Servings you need from each of the four food groups every day.

Having the amount and type of food recommended and following the tips in *Canada's Food Guide* will help:

• Meet your needs for vitamins, minerals and other nutrients.

• Reduce your risk of obesity, type 2 diabetes, heart disease, certain types of cancer and osteoporosis.

• Contribute to your overall health and vitality.

What is One Food Guide Serving?
Look at the examples below.

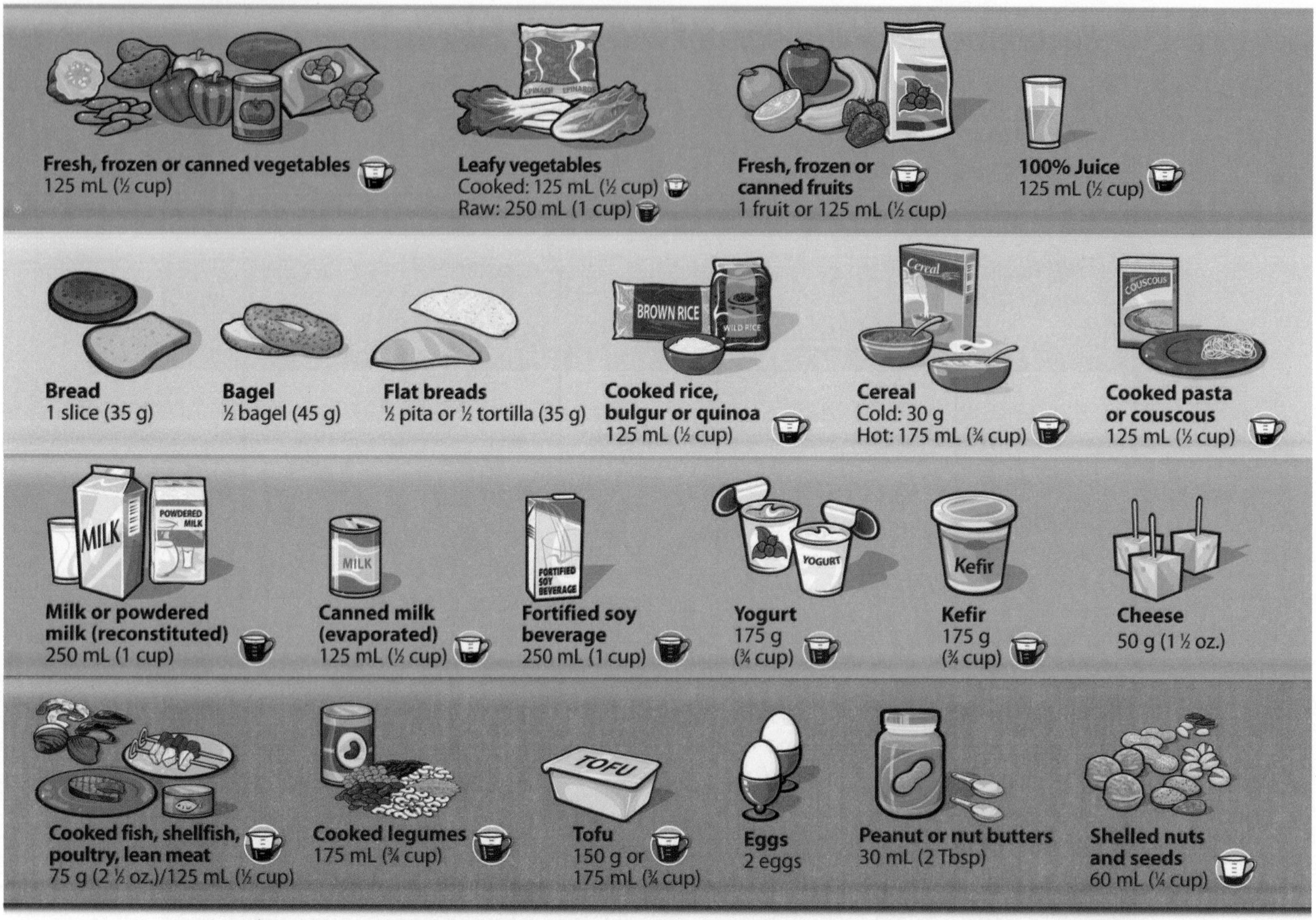

Fresh, frozen or canned vegetables
125 mL (½ cup)

Leafy vegetables
Cooked: 125 mL (½ cup)
Raw: 250 mL (1 cup)

Fresh, frozen or canned fruits
1 fruit or 125 mL (½ cup)

100% Juice
125 mL (½ cup)

Bread
1 slice (35 g)

Bagel
½ bagel (45 g)

Flat breads
½ pita or ½ tortilla (35 g)

Cooked rice, bulgur or quinoa
125 mL (½ cup)

Cereal
Cold: 30 g
Hot: 175 mL (¾ cup)

Cooked pasta or couscous
125 mL (½ cup)

Milk or powdered milk (reconstituted)
250 mL (1 cup)

Canned milk (evaporated)
125 mL (½ cup)

Fortified soy beverage
250 mL (1 cup)

Yogurt
175 g
(¾ cup)

Kefir
175 g
(¾ cup)

Cheese
50 g (1 ½ oz.)

Cooked fish, shellfish, poultry, lean meat
75 g (2 ½ oz.)/125 mL (½ cup)

Cooked legumes
175 mL (¾ cup)

Tofu
150 g or
175 mL (¾ cup)

Eggs
2 eggs

Peanut or nut butters
30 mL (2 Tbsp)

Shelled nuts and seeds
60 mL (¼ cup)

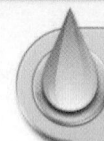

Oils and Fats

- Include a small amount – 30 to 45 mL (2 to 3 Tbsp) – of unsaturated fat each day. This includes oil used for cooking, salad dressings, margarine and mayonnaise.
- Use vegetable oils such as canola, olive and soybean.
- Choose soft margarines that are low in saturated and trans fats.
- Limit butter, hard margarine, lard and shortening.

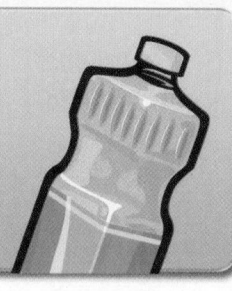

Make each Food Guide Serving count...
wherever you are – at home, at school, at work or when eating out!

▶ **Eat at least one dark green and one orange vegetable each day.**
- Go for dark green vegetables such as broccoli, romaine lettuce and spinach.
- Go for orange vegetables such as carrots, sweet potatoes and winter squash.

▶ **Choose vegetables and fruit prepared with little or no added fat, sugar or salt.**
- Enjoy vegetables steamed, baked or stir-fried instead of deep-fried.

▶ **Have vegetables and fruit more often than juice.**

▶ **Make at least half of your grain products whole grain each day.**
- Eat a variety of whole grains such as barley, brown rice, oats, quinoa and wild rice.
- Enjoy whole grain breads, oatmeal or whole wheat pasta.

▶ **Choose grain products that are lower in fat, sugar or salt.**
- Compare the Nutrition Facts table on labels to make wise choices.
- Enjoy the true taste of grain products. When adding sauces or spreads, use small amounts.

▶ **Drink skim, 1%, or 2% milk each day.**
- Have 500 mL (2 cups) of milk every day for adequate vitamin D.
- Drink fortified soy beverages if you do not drink milk.

▶ **Select lower fat milk alternatives.**
- Compare the Nutrition Facts table on yogurts or cheeses to make wise choices.

▶ **Have meat alternatives such as beans, lentils and tofu often.**

▶ **Eat at least two Food Guide Servings of fish each week.***
- Choose fish such as char, herring, mackerel, salmon, sardines and trout.

▶ **Select lean meat and alternatives prepared with little or no added fat or salt.**
- Trim the visible fat from meats. Remove the skin on poultry.
- Use cooking methods such as roasting, baking or poaching that require little or no added fat.
- If you eat luncheon meats, sausages or prepackaged meats, choose those lower in salt (sodium) and fat.

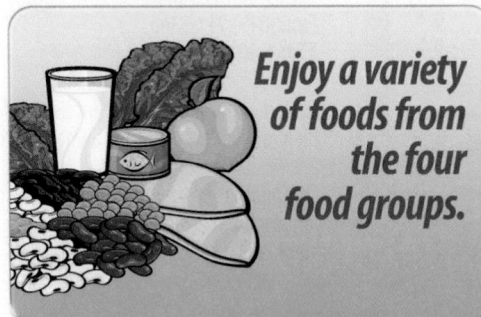

Enjoy a variety of foods from the four food groups.

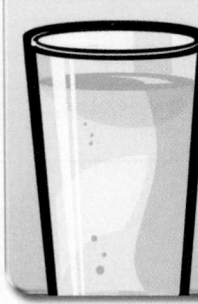

Satisfy your thirst with water!

Drink water regularly. It's a calorie-free way to quench your thirst. Drink more water in hot weather or when you are very active.

* Health Canada provides advice for limiting exposure to mercury from certain types of fish. Refer to www.healthcanada.gc.ca for the latest information.

Eat well and be active today and every day!

The benefits of eating well and being active include:

- Better overall health.
- Lower risk of disease.
- A healthy body weight.
- Feeling and looking better.
- More energy.
- Stronger muscles and bones.

Be active

To be active every day is a step towards better health and a healthy body weight.

Canada's Physical Activity Guide recommends building 30 to 60 minutes of moderate physical activity into daily life for adults and at least 90 minutes a day for children and youth. You don't have to do it all at once. Add it up in periods of at least 10 minutes at a time for adults and five minutes at a time for children and youth.

Start slowly and build up.

Eat well

Another important step towards better health and a healthy body weight is to follow *Canada's Food Guide* by:

- Eating the recommended amount and type of food each day.
- Limiting foods and beverages high in calories, fat, sugar or salt (sodium) such as cakes and pastries, chocolate and candies, cookies and granola bars, doughnuts and muffins, ice cream and frozen desserts, french fries, potato chips, nachos and other salty snacks, alcohol, fruit flavoured drinks, soft drinks, sports and energy drinks, and sweetened hot or cold drinks.

Read the label

- Compare the Nutrition Facts table on food labels to choose products that contain less fat, saturated fat, trans fat, sugar and sodium.
- Keep in mind that the calories and nutrients listed are for the amount of food found at the top of the Nutrition Facts table.

Limit trans fat

When a Nutrition Facts table is not available, ask for nutrition information to choose foods lower in trans and saturated fats.

Nutrition Facts
Per 0 mL (0 g)

Amount	% Daily Value
Calories 0	
Fat 0 g	0 %
Saturates 0 g	0 %
+ Trans 0 g	
Cholesterol 0 mg	
Sodium 0 mg	0 %
Carbohydrate 0 g	0 %
Fibre 0 g	0 %
Sugars 0 g	
Protein 0 g	

Vitamin A	0 %	Vitamin C	0 %
Calcium	0 %	Iron	0 %

Take a step today...

✓ Have breakfast every day. It may help control your hunger later in the day.

✓ Walk wherever you can – get off the bus early, use the stairs.

✓ Benefit from eating vegetables and fruit at all meals and as snacks.

✓ Spend less time being inactive such as watching TV or playing computer games.

✓ Request nutrition information about menu items when eating out to help you make healthier choices.

✓ Enjoy eating with family and friends!

✓ Take time to eat and savour every bite!

For more information, interactive tools, or additional copies visit Canada's Food Guide on-line at: **www.healthcanada.gc.ca/foodguide**

or contact:

Publications
Health Canada
Ottawa, Ontario K1A 0K9
E-Mail: publications@hc-sc.gc.ca
Tel.: 1-866-225-0709
Fax: (613) 941-5366
TTY: 1-800-267-1245

Également disponible en français sous le titre : Bien manger avec le Guide alimentaire canadien

This publication can be made available on request on diskette, large print, audio-cassette and braille.

Appendix I
Food Composition Table

The following is a list of abbreviations used in the Food Composition Table:

Abbreviation Key

Unit/Amt = Unit/Amount
Wt (g) = Weight in grams
Energy (kcal) = Kilocalories
Prot (g) = Protein
Carb (g) = Carbohydrate
Fiber (g) = Dietary fiber
Fat (g) = Total fat
Sat (g) = Saturated fat
Mono (g) = Monounsaturated fat
Poly (g) = Polyunsaturated fat
Chol (mg) = Cholesterol
Vit A (RE) = Vitamin A
Thia (mg) = Thiamin
Ribo (mg) = Riboflavin
Niac (mg NE) = Niacin
Vit B6 (mg) = Vitamin B–6
Vit B12 (µg) = Vitamin B–12
Fol (µg) = Folate
Vit C (mg) = Vitamin C
Vit D (IU) = Vitamin D
Vit E (mg AT) = Vitamin E

Cal (mg) = Calcium
Iron (mg) = Iron
Magn (mg) = Magnesium
Phos (mg) = Phosphorus
Pota (mg) = Potassium
Sodi (mg) = Sodium
Zinc (mg) = Zinc
Wat (%) = Water
Alco (g) = Alcohol
Caff (g) = Caffeine

g = gram
mg = milligram
µg = microgram
mg AT = milligrams of alpha–tocopheral
mg NE = milligrams of Niacin Equivalents
oz = ounce
lb = pound
Tbs = tablespoon
tsp = teaspoon

► Note: Some nutrient or food component values are not included in the database because of the lack of accuate information. These are indicated by a — (dash) in the particular nutrient or food component column.

PAGE KEY: A-42 Beverages and Beverage Mixes A-44 Candies A-46 Cereals A-48 Cheeses and Substitutes A-50 Dairy Products and Substitutes A-52 Desserts A-56 Eggs and Egg Substitutes
A-56 Fats, Oils, Margarines, and Shortenings A-58 Fruits A-60 Grain Products and Baked Goods A-62 Grains and Flours A-64 Meats and Meat Substitutes A-68 Nuts, Seeds, and Products

Code	Food Name	Unit/ Amt	Wt (g)	Energy (kcal)	Prot (g)	Carb (g)	Fiber (g)	Fat (g)	Sat (g)	Mono (g)	Poly (g)	Chol (mg)	Vit A (RE)
BEVERAGES AND BEVERAGE MIXES													
Alcoholic Beverages and Mixes													
22515	Alcohol, tequila, 80 proof	1 fl oz	28	64	0	0	0	0	0.0	0.0	0.0	0	0
22594	Alcohol, vodka, 80 proof	1 fl oz	28	64	0	0	0	0	0.0	0.0	0.0	0	0
22670	Alcohol, whiskey, 80 proof	1 fl oz	28	64	0	0	0	0	0.0	0.0	0.0	0	0
34066	Beer, amber ale	12 fl oz	356	169	2	14	0	0	0.0	0.0	0.0	0	
22500	Beer, can/btl, 12 fl oz	12 fl oz	356	153	2	13	0	0	0.0	0.0	0.0	0	0
34053	Beer, Light	12 fl oz	353	105	1	5	0	0	0.0	0.0	0.0	0	
34052	Malt Beverage	12 fl oz	353	185	0	21	0	0	0.0	0.0	0.0	0	
22557	Mixed Drink, margarita	1 ea	77	170	0	11	0	0	0.0	0.0	0.0	0	0
22539	Mixed Drink, tequila sunrise, 6.8 fl oz can	1 ea	211	232	1	24	0	0	0.0			0	20
22577	Wine, all table types	5 fl oz	148	123	0	4	0	0	0.0	0.0	0.0	0	0
Carbonated Drinks													
20055	Soda, 7 Up	8 fl oz	246	103	0	27	0	0	0.0	0.0	0.0	0	0
20207	Soda, 7 Up, diet	1 cup	246	0	0	0	0	0	0.0	0.0	0.0	0	0
20006	Soda, club	8 fl oz	237	0	0	0	0	0	0.0	0.0	0.0	0	0
20148	Soda, Coca-Cola	1 btl	430	170	0	46	0	0	0.0	0.0	0.0	0	0
20166	Soda, cola	8 fl oz	249	100	0	28	0	0	0.0	0.0	0.0	0	0
443	Soda, cola, caff free	1 can	368	151	0	39	0	0	0.0	0.0	0.0	0	0
20167	Soda, cola, diet, w/asp	8 fl oz	240	0	0	0	0	0	0.0	0.0	0.0	0	0
4796	Soda, Dr. Pepper	1 cup	246	100	0	27	0	0	0.0	0.0	0.0		0
4800	Soda, fruit punch, juicy red, Hawaiian Punch, cnd	1 cup	248	130	0	33	0	0	0.0	0.0	0.0		0
20009	Soda, root beer	1 cup	246	101	0	26	0	0	0.0	0.0	0.0	0	0
20032	Soda, Sprite	8 fl oz	264	106	0	27	0	0				0	0
Coffee and Tea													
20439	Coffee, espresso, restaurant prep	8 fl oz	240	5	0	0	0	0	0.2	0.0	0.2	0	0
20023	Coffee, reg, inst, prep w/water	8 fl oz	238	5	0	1	0	0	0.0	0.0	0.0	0	0
20014	Tea, brewed w/tap water	1 cup	237	2	0	1	0	0	0.0	0.0	0.0	0	0
20681	Tea, green	0.5 btl	252	100	0	25	0	0	0.0	0.0	0.0	0	0
20853	Tea, herbal, Echinacea Complete Care, brewed	1 cup	237	0	0	0	0	0	0.0	0.0	0.0	0	0
20857	Tea, herbal, Ginseng Energy, brewed	1 cup	237	0	0	0	0	0	0.0	0.0	0.0	0	0
20036	Tea, herbal, not chamomile, brewed	1 cup	237	2	0	0	0	0	0.0	0.0	0.0	0	0
20542	Tea, iced, black, lemon	1 can	368	120	0	33	0	0	0.0	0.0	0.0	0	0
30451	Tea, iced, inst	2 tsp	1	0	0	0	0	0	0.0	0.0	0.0	0	0
Fruit Flavored Drinks													
20004	Drink, breakfast, orange, prep f/pwd	8 fl oz	271	133	0	34	0	0	0.0	0.0	0.0	0	209
20737	Drink, fruit punch	0.5 btl	252	110	0	29	0	0	0.0	0.0	0.0		
20176	Drink, fruit punch, noncarbonated	8 fl oz	240	133	0	33	0	0	0.0	0.0	0.0	0	
20761	Drink, Island Punch	0.4 btl	252	110	0	27	0	0	0.0	0.0	0.0	0	0
4794	Drink, lemonade, Country Time, cnd	1 cup	247	90	0	23	0	0	0.0	0.0	0.0		0
20746	Drink, pink lemonade	0.5 btl	252	110	0	26	0	0	0.0	0.0	0.0	0	

PAGE KEY: A-70 Prepared Foods A-78 Restaurants A-90 Salad Dressings and Dips A-92 Sauces and Gravies A-94 Snack Foods A-94 Spices, Flavors, and Seasonings A-96 Sports Bars and Drinks A-96 Supplemental Foods and Formulas A-96 Sweeteners and Sweet Substitutes A-98 Vegetables and Legumes A-108 Miscellaneous

Thia (mg)	Ribo (mg)	Niac (mg NE)	Vit B6 (mg)	Vit B12 (µg)	Fol (µg)	Vit C (mg)	Vit D (IU)	Vit E (mg AT)	Cal (mg)	Iron (mg)	Magn (mg)	Phos (mg)	Pota (mg)	Sodi (mg)	Zinc (mg)	Wat (%)	Alco (g)	Caff (g)
0.00	0.00	0.00	0.00	0.00	0.0	0.0	0.0	0.0	0	0.00	0.0	1	1	0	0.0	67	9.28	0.00
												1				67	9.28	
												1	1			67	9.28	
														44			18.65	0.00
0.01	0.09	1.83	0.15	0.07	21.4	0.0	0.0	0.0	14	0.07	21.4	50	96	14	0.0	92	13.88	0.00
0.03	0.03	1.40							11				59	11		333	14.11	0.00
0.03	0.03	0.87							38				51	20			16.94	0.00
0.00	0.00	0.03	0.00	0.00	1.2	1.0	0.0	0.0	2	0.05	1.4	4	15	4	0.0	37	18.50	0.00
0.07	0.02	0.40	0.10	0.00	23.2	40.7			0	0.03	14.8	21	21	120	1.3	79	19.82	0.00
0.00	0.02	0.25	0.07	0.00	1.5	0.0	0.0	0.0	12	0.55	16.3	30	147	7	0.2	87	15.39	0.00
			0.00			0.0						46		51			0.00	0.00
0.00	0.00		0.00	0.00		0.0								36			0.00	0.00
0.00	0.00	0.00	0.00	0.00	0.0	0.0	0.0	0.0	12	0.01	2.4	0	5	50	0.2	100	0.00	0.00
						0.0			0	0.00				55			0.00	40.00
						0.0			0	0.00		36	10	20			0.00	25.00
0.00	0.00	0.00	0.00	0.00		0.0	0.0	0.0	7	0.07	0.0	40	11	15	0.0	90	0.00	0.00
						0.0			0	0.00		27	20	25			0.00	24.00
						0.0								35			0.00	27.20
																		27.20
						0.0								90			0.00	0.00
																		27.20
0.00	0.00	0.00	0.00	0.00	0.0	0.0	0.0	0.0	12	0.11	2.5	0	2	32	0.2	89	0.00	0.00
0.00	0.00	0.03	0.00	0.00	0.0	0.0	0.0	0.0	5	0.28	2.6	0	3	24	0.1	90	0.00	0.00
0.00	0.41	12.50	0.00	0.00	2.4	0.5	0.0	0.0	5	0.31	192.0	17	276	34	0.1	98	0.00	508.79
0.00	0.00	0.56	0.00	0.00	0.0	0.0		0.0	10	0.10	9.5	7	72	10	0.0	99	0.00	61.97
0.00	0.02	0.00	0.00	0.00	11.8	0.0	0.0	0.0	0	0.05	7.1	2	88	7	0.0	100	0.00	47.40
0.00	0.00	0.00	0.00	0.00	0.0	0.0	0.0	0.0	6	0.00	2.1	0	2	10	0.0		0.00	18.00
						35.0			0	0.00				0	7.5		0.00	0.00
			0.50	1.50		0.0			0	0.00				0			0.00	0.00
0.01	0.00	0.00	0.00	0.00	2.4	0.0	0.0	0.0	5	0.18	2.4	0	21	2	0.1	100	0.00	0.00
						0.0			0	0.00				45			0.00	
						0.0			0	0.00				0		1	0.00	25.00
0.00	0.23	2.76	0.28	0.00	0.0	80.0		0.0	141	0.00	2.7	52	68	14	0.0	87	0.00	0.00
0.00	0.00	0.00	0.00	0.00	0.0	0.0	0.0	0.0	6	0.00	2.2	1	23	10	0.0		0.00	0.00
		0.00				43.3						0	0	30			0.00	0.00
0.00	0.00	0.00	0.00	0.00	0.0	0.0	0.0	0.0	6	0.00	2.0	0	2	10	0.0		0.00	0.00
						0.0								90			0.00	0.00
0.00	0.00	0.00	0.00	0.00	0.4	0.0	0.0	0.0	7	0.01	2.4	0	8	10	0.0		0.00	0.00

Code	Food Name	Unit/Amt	Wt (g)	Energy (kcal)	Prot (g)	Carb (g)	Fiber (g)	Fat (g)	Sat (g)	Mono (g)	Poly (g)	Chol (mg)	Vit A (RE)
Juices													
3008	Juice, apple, unswtnd, cnd/btl	1 cup	248	114	0	28	0	0	0.1	0.0	0.1	0	0
1853	Juice, grape	8 fl oz	236	150	0	38	0	0	0.0	0.0	0.0	0	
794	Juice, grapefruit	8 fl oz	236	120	0	29	0	0	0.0	0.0	0.0	0	
1854	Juice, orange	1 cup	236	120	0	29	0	0	0.0	0.0	0.0	0	
3090	Juice, orange, fresh	1 cup	248	112	2	26	0	0	0.1	0.1	0.1	0	50
3094	Juice, orange, unswtnd, fzn conc, 6 fl oz can	1 fl oz	36	56	1	14	0	0	0.0	0.0	0.0	0	13
6507	Juice, vegetable, cnd	1 cup	243	50	2	10	2	0	0.0	0.0	0.0	0	400
Other Beverages													
14	Drink, chocolate, dry mix	2.5 tsp	22	89	1	20	1	1	0.4	0.2	0.0	0	0
38362	Drink, horchata de arroz, rice beverage, Mexican	1 cup	245	100	0	25	0	0	0.0	0.0	0.0	0	0
62057	Drink, Instant Breakfast, classic French vanilla, dry mix	1 indv pkt	36	130	5	27	0	0	0.0	0.0	0.0	3	
101	Drink, Instant Breakfast, prep w/1% milk	1 cup	281	233	15	36	0	3	1.8			14	469
20589	Drink, sugar cane, Puerto Rican	1 cup	240	164	0	42	0	0	0.0	0.0	0.0	0	0
12	Hot Cocoa, dry mix	3 tsp	28	111	2	23	1	1	0.7	0.4	0.0	0	0
20051	Water, bottled, Poland Spring	1 cup	237	0	0	0	0	0	0.0	0.0	0.0	0	0
20041	Water, tap, municipal	1 cup	237	0	0	0	0	0	0.0	0.0	0.0	0	0
CANDIES													
23076	Candy Bar, 3 Musketeers, fun size	2 ea	28	122	1	22	0	4	2.4	0.7	0.1	1	6
23125	Candy Bar, 5th Avenue, 2 oz	1 ea	56	270	5	35	2	13	3.7	5.9	1.9	3	8
23049	Candy Bar, Almond Joy, 1.7 oz	1 ea	49	235	2	29	2	13	8.6	2.6	0.6	2	4
23110	Candy Bar, Baby Ruth, 2.1-oz bar	1 ea	60	275	3	39	1	13	7.3	3.3	1.6	0	0
23066	Candy Bar, Butterfinger, 2.16-oz bar	1 ea	60	275	3	44	1	11	5.7	3.1	1.9	0	0
23116	Candy Bar, Caramello, 1.6 oz	1 ea	45	208	3	29	1	10	5.7	2.4	0.3	12	27
23118	Candy Bar, carob, unswtnd, 3-oz bar	1 ea	87	470	7	49	3	27	25.2	0.4	0.3	1	1
23060	Candy Bar, Kit Kat, 1.5-oz bar	1 ea	42	218	3	27	0	11	7.5	2.5	0.4	5	10
23037	Candy Bar, Mars almond, 1.76-oz bar	1 ea	50	234	4	31	1	12	3.6	5.3	2.0	8	8
23146	Candy Bar, milk chocolate, 1.5-oz bar	1 ea	42	223	4	24	1	13	7.7	3.3	0.3	10	19
23038	Candy Bar, Milky Way, 2.05-oz bar	1 ea	58	264	2	41	1	10	7.0	1.3	0.2	5	18
23035	Candy Bar, Mounds, 1.9 oz	1 ea	53	258	2	31	2	14	10.9	0.2	0.1	1	0
23040	Candy Bar, Snickers, 2-oz bar	1 ea	57	280	4	35	1	14	5.2	4.5	1.7	7	27
23149	Candy Bar, Twix, caramel cookie, 2.06-oz pkg	1 pkg	58	291	3	38	1	14	11.0	1.7	0.4	4	12
17410	Candy Bar, Twix, chocolate fudge cookie	2 ea	51	280	4	29	2	17	2.5	7.3	6.4	3	5
23506	Candy, California Gold, peanuts, yogurt cvrd, natural	22 pce	40	220	5	17	2	15	2.0			0	1
23015	Candy, caramels	1 ea	10	39	0	8	0	1	0.3	0.2	0.4	1	1
92647	Candy, Good N Plenty, snack	1 ea	17	60	0	14	0	0	0.0	0.0	0.0	0	0
23412	Candy, gummy worms	10 ea	74	293	0	73	0	0	0.0	0.0	0.0	0	0
92653	Candy, hard, lollipop	1 ea	17	60	0	16	0	0	0.0	0.0	0.0	0	0
23033	Candy, jellybeans, sml	10 ea	11	41	0	10	0	0				0	0
52154	Candy, licorice, twists, black, tray	4 ea	40	140	1	36	0	0	0.0	0.0	0.0	0	0
52155	Candy, licorice, twists, original red, tray	4 ea	40	140	1	34	0	0	0.0	0.0	0.0	0	
92644	Candy, malt choc, Whoppers	9 ea	20	90	1	15	0	4	3.0			0	0
23047	Candy, milk chocolate peanut, M&M	0.25 cup	42	219	4	26	2	11	4.3	3.4	1.5	3	9
92642	Candy, Milk Duds	7 ea	21	90	1	15	0	4	1.0			0	
23424	Candy, peanut butter cups, Reese's, mini	1 ea	7	36	1	4	0	2	0.8	0.9	0.4	0	1
23021	Candy, peanuts, milk chocolate cvrd	10 ea	40	208	5	20	2	13	5.8	5.2	1.7	4	16

PAGE KEY: A-70 Prepared Foods   A-78 Restaurants   A-90 Salad Dressings and Dips   A-92 Sauces and Gravies   A-94 Snack Foods   A-94 Spices, Flavors, and Seasonings   A-96 Sports Bars and Drinks
A-96 Supplemental Foods and Formulas   A-96 Sweeteners and Sweet Substitutes   A-98 Vegetables and Legumes   A-108 Miscellaneous

Thia (mg)	Ribo (mg)	Niac (mg NE)	Vit B6 (mg)	Vit B12 (µg)	Fol (µg)	Vit C (mg)	Vit D (IU)	Vit E (mg AT)	Cal (mg)	Iron (mg)	Magn (mg)	Phos (mg)	Pota (mg)	Sodi (mg)	Zinc (mg)	Wat (%)	Alco (g)	Caff (g)
0.05	0.03	0.18	0.03	0.00	0.0	2.2	0.0	0.0	20	0.30	12.4	17	250	10	0.0	88	0.00	0.00
														10			0.00	0.00
														0			0.00	0.00
														0			0.00	0.00
0.21	0.07	0.99	0.10	0.00	74.4	124.0	0.0	0.1	27	0.50	27.3	42	496	2	0.1	88	0.00	0.00
0.10	0.01	0.25	0.05	0.00	55.0	49.0	0.0	0.3	11	0.11	12.1	20	239	1	0.1	58	0.00	0.00
						60.0			40	0.72			520	620			0.00	0.00
0.00	0.02	0.10	0.00	0.00	1.1	0.2	0.0	0.1	8	0.68	21.6	28	130	46	0.3	1	0.00	7.92
0.00	0.00	0.14	0.00	0.00	0.4	0.1		0.0	12	0.34	3.5	5	6	7	0.1	89	0.00	0.00
0.30	0.14	5.00	0.40	0.60	80.0	27.0	0.0		250	4.50	80.0	250	240	100	3.0		0.00	0.00
0.40	0.47	5.48	0.52	1.53	117.7	30.9	100.0	5.4	406	4.86	118.5	392	731	267	4.1		0.00	0.00
0.07	0.03	0.05	0.00	0.00	0.0	0.0		0.0	12	2.25	8.0	5	39	42	0.2	81	0.00	0.00
0.02	0.15	0.15	0.02	0.10	1.7	0.1	0.0	0.1	37	0.33	23.2	88	199	141	0.4	2	0.00	5.03
0.00	0.00	0.00	0.00	0.00	0.0	0.0	0.0	0.0	2	0.01	2.4	0	0	2	0.0	100	0.00	0.00
0.00	0.00	0.00	0.00	0.00	0.0	0.0	0.0	0.0	7	0.00	2.4	0	2	7	0.0	100	0.00	0.00
0.00	0.01	0.05	0.00	0.03	1.1	0.1	0.0	0.3	15	0.18	8.1	19	37	54	0.2	6	0.00	1.96
0.07	0.05	2.18	0.05	0.10	20.2	0.2	0.0	1.5	41	0.67	34.7	79	194	126	0.6	2	0.00	2.79
						0.3			31	0.62		55	124	70		8	0.00	
0.02	0.07	0.75	0.02	0.03	7.2	0.0	0.0	0.6	28	0.37	25.8	56	149	138	0.4	7	0.00	2.40
0.07	0.03	1.59	0.03	0.01	16.8	0.0	0.0	1.0	22	0.46	28.8	58	132	138	0.6	1	0.00	0.60
						0.8			96	0.49		68	153	55		7	0.00	
0.05	0.09	0.20	0.00	0.23	5.9	0.0	0.0	0.1	52	0.41	15.5	57	97	23	0.0	2	0.00	5.88
0.01	0.15	0.46	0.02	0.18	4.5	0.3	0.0	3.9	84	0.55	36.0	117	162	85	0.6	4	0.00	2.00
						0.9			105	0.37		87	184	42		1	0.00	
0.02	0.05	0.09	0.00	0.10	2.3	0.4	9.3	0.5	67	0.28	11.6	39	72	97	0.4	6	0.00	3.48
0.02	0.02	0.15	0.05	0.00	3.2	0.2	0.0	0.1	11	1.11	29.1	48	170	77	0.6	9	0.00	9.01
0.02	0.07	2.04	0.05	0.09	15.4	0.3	0.0	0.9	53	0.40	41.0	108	184	136	1.4	6	0.00	4.55
0.09	0.11	0.63	0.00	0.18	15.1	0.3	0.0	0.4	61	0.46	15.7	61	108	115	0.6	4	0.00	4.05
0.07	0.10	0.56	0.01	0.17	4.6	0.5	0.0	1.4	66	0.67	23.5	75	158	136	0.5	2	0.00	5.09
						0.0			31	0.00				10		2	0.00	0.00
0.00	0.02	0.00	0.00	0.02	0.4	0.0	0.0	0.0	14	0.00	1.7	12	22	25	0.0	8	0.00	0.00
						0.0			0	0.11				40			0.00	0.00
0.00	0.00	0.00	0.00	0.00	0.0	0.0	0.0	0.0	2	0.30	0.7	1	4	33	0.0	1	0.00	0.00
						0.0			0	0.00				10		1	0.00	0.00
0.00	0.00	0.00	0.00	0.00	0.0	0.0	0.0	0.0	0	0.00	0.2	0	4	6	0.0	6	0.00	0.00
						0.0			0	0.00				60			0.00	0.00
						0.0			0					20			0.00	
						0.0			40	0.18				65			0.00	
0.02	0.05	1.42	0.03	0.14	23.4	0.0	0.0	1.2	43	0.49	29.3	81	147	21	0.7	2	0.00	4.25
														40		1	0.00	
0.00	0.00	0.31	0.00	0.01	3.5	0.0	0.0	0.0	5	0.07	4.3	11	24	25	0.1	1	0.00	0.49
0.05	0.07	1.70	0.03	0.20	20.4	0.0	0.0	1.0	42	0.51	38.4	85	201	16	1.0	2	0.00	5.59

Code	Food Name	Unit/ Amt	Wt (g)	Energy (kcal)	Prot (g)	Carb (g)	Fiber (g)	Fat (g)	Sat (g)	Mono (g)	Poly (g)	Chol (mg)	Vit A (RE)
23517	Candy, raisins, Crystal Dark, chocolate cvrd	35 pce	40	160	1	27	2	7	4.0			0	2
23485	Candy, Skittles, original, bite size, 2.17-oz pkg	1 pkg	62	251	0	56	0	3	2.6	0.0	0.0	0	0
23144	Candy, Starburst, fruit chews, original	8 ea	40	163	0	33	0	3	3.1	0.0	0.0	0	0
4149	Candy, SweeTarts	8 ea	15	50	0	13	0	0	0.0	0.0	0.0	0	0
92769	Candy, Tootsie Roll	6 pce	40	155	1	35	0	1	0.4	0.8	0.1	1	0
23082	Chewing Gum, stick	1 stk	3	11	0	3	0	0	0.0	0.0	0.0	0	0
91256	Fudge, plain	1 svg	43	188	0	27	0	9	6.0			11	10
23007	Marshmallows	1 ea	7	23	0	6	0	0	0.0	0.0	0.0	0	0

CEREALS

Hot Cereals

Code	Food Name	Unit/ Amt	Wt (g)	Energy (kcal)	Prot (g)	Carb (g)	Fiber (g)	Fat (g)	Sat (g)	Mono (g)	Poly (g)	Chol (mg)	Vit A (RE)
40190	Cereal, hot, multigrain, plain, ckd w/water & salt	0.5 cup	120	74	3	17	4	0	0.1			0	0
40239	Cereal, hot, oatmeal, maple, ckd w/water & salt	0.5 cup	120	85	3	16	2	1	0.2	0.3	0.3	0	350
40072	Cereal, hot, oatmeal, plain, fort, inst, prep w/water	1 cup	234	159	6	27	4	3	0.6	0.9	1.0	0	435
40186	Cereal, hot, wheat, ckd w/water & salt	0.5 cup	124	95	3	20	1	1	0.1	0.1	0.2	0	0
40089	Grits, corn, plain, inst, prep w/water	1 cup	219	166	3	35	2	1	0.2	0.2	0.4		
38571	Grits, hominy, yellow, quick, dry	0.25 cup	37	125	3	29	2	1	0.2	0.2	0.3	0	42

Ready to Eat Cereals

Code	Food Name	Unit/ Amt	Wt (g)	Energy (kcal)	Prot (g)	Carb (g)	Fiber (g)	Fat (g)	Sat (g)	Mono (g)	Poly (g)	Chol (mg)	Vit A (RE)
40095	Cereal, All-Bran	0.5 cup	31	81	4	23	9	2	0.2	0.2	0.7	0	163
40258	Cereal, Alpha-Bits, svg	1 svg	32	130	3	27	1	2	0.0			0	150
40098	Cereal, Apple Jacks	1 cup	28	102	1	25	3	1	0.1	0.1	0.2	0	146
61233	Cereal, Banana Nut Crunch	1 cup	59	249	5	44	4	6	0.8	2.2	2.6	0	225
40394	Cereal, Basic 4	1 cup	55	197	4	43	3	2	0.8	0.7	0.5	0	142
61203	Cereal, bran flakes	0.75 cup	30	96	3	24	5	1	0.1	0.1	0.3	0	225
40297	Cereal, Cheerios	1 cup	28	103	3	21	3	2	0.3	0.5	0.6	0	243
40325	Cereal, Chex, corn	1 cup	31	114	2	26	1	1	0.1	0.1	0.2	0	144
40335	Cereal, Chex, wheat	0.75 cup	47	169	5	38	5	1	0.2	0.1	0.4	0	140
40126	Cereal, Cinnamon Toast Crunch	0.75 cup	31	128	2	25	1	3	0.4	1.0	0.9	0	308
61272	Cereal, Coco Roos, chocolate	0.75 cup	30	119	1	27	1	1	0.1	0.5	0.1	0	180
40102	Cereal, Cocoa Krispies	0.75 cup	31	118	2	27	1	1	0.6	0.1	0.1	0	153
40425	Cereal, Cocoa Puffs	0.75 cup	27	104	1	23	2	1	0.0	0.9	0.0	0	150
40103	Cereal, Complete Oat Bran Flakes	0.75 cup	30	105	3	23	4	1	0.2	0.5	0.3	0	235
40324	Cereal, Cookie Crisp	1 cup	26	98	1	22	1	1	0.2	0.3	0.4	0	148
40206	Cereal, Corn Pops	1 cup	32	124	1	29	3	0	0.1	0.1	0.2	0	144
4354	Cereal, Cranberry Almond Crunch	0.75 cup	51	197	4	40	3	3	0.0	1.5	0.9	0	202
40017	Cereal, crispy rice	1 cup	28	102	2	24	0	0	0.1	0.1	0.1	0	197
61179	Cereal, Familia	1 cup	122	473	12	90	10	8	0.9	3.9	2.0	0	1
40130	Cereal, Fiber One	0.5 cup	30	60	2	25	14	1	0.1	0.1	0.4	0	1
40218	Cereal, Froot Loops	1 cup	29	108	1	25	3	1	0.6	0.1	0.1	0	136
61306	Cereal, frosted flakes	0.75 cup	30	116	2	27	1	0	0.0	0.0	0.1	0	356
40043	Cereal, Frosted Mini Wheats	5 ea	51	175	5	42	5	1	0.2	0.1	0.5	0	0
61204	Cereal, Fruity Pebbles	0.75 cup	30	120	1	26	0	1	0.3	0.5	0.4	0	225
60964	Cereal, Go Lean	1 cup	52	148	14	30	10	1	0.2	0.2	0.6	0	5
40299	Cereal, Golden Grahams	0.75 cup	30	113	2	25	1	1	0.1	0.5	0.3	0	142
40197	Cereal, granola, w/raisins, low fat	0.66 cup	60	226	5	47	4	3	0.8	1.2	1.0	0	196
40265	Cereal, Grape Nuts Flakes	0.75 cup	29	106	3	24	3	1	0.2			0	150

Thia (mg)	Ribo (mg)	Niac (mg NE)	Vit B6 (mg)	Vit B12 (µg)	Fol (µg)	Vit C (mg)	Vit D (IU)	Vit E (mg AT)	Cal (mg)	Iron (mg)	Magn (mg)	Phos (mg)	Pota (mg)	Sodi (mg)	Zinc (mg)	Wat (%)	Alco (g)	Caff (g)
					1.0				16	3.00				40		4	0.00	
0.00	0.00	0.00	0.00	0.00	0.0	41.4	0.0	0.1	0	0.00	0.6	1	7	9	0.0	4	0.00	0.00
0.00	0.00	0.00	0.00	0.00	0.4	23.5	0.0	0.1	0	0.00	0.4	2	1	1	0.0	9	0.00	0.00
0.00	0.00	0.00	0.00	0.00	0.0	0.0	0.0	0.0	0	0.00	0.1	0	0	0	0.0		0.00	0.00
0.01	0.02	0.07	0.00	0.00	3.6	0.0		0.3	14	0.31	8.8	23	46	18	0.2	7	0.00	2.79
0.00	0.00	0.00	0.00	0.00	0.0	0.0	0.0	0.0	0	0.00	0.0	0	0	0	0.0	3	0.00	0.00
						0.0			0	0.18				42			0.00	0.00
0.00	0.00	0.00	0.00	0.00	0.1	0.0	0.0	0.0	0	0.01	0.1	1	0	6	0.0	16	0.00	0.00
0.11	0.05	1.53	0.05	0.00	12.1	0.0			14	1.05	54.2	107	151	99	0.9	83	0.00	0.00
0.34	0.40	4.67	0.46	1.38	6.0	14.2		0.1	65	4.19	26.4	124	106	130	0.7	83	0.00	0.00
0.61	0.50	7.07	0.68	0.00	103.0	0.0	0.0	0.2	187	13.94	60.8	180	143	115	1.5	84	0.00	0.00
0.12	0.05	1.19	0.03	0.00	14.9	0.0		0.6	11	0.89	28.6	88	133	95	0.9	81	0.00	0.00
0.31	0.30	3.66	0.10		59.1	0.0		0.0	140	14.68	19.7	55	74	412	0.4	81	0.00	0.00
0.18	0.14	1.59	0.09	0.00	57.0	0.0			1	1.51	14.8	46	62	1	0.3	12	0.00	0.00
0.69	0.83	4.59	3.72	5.82	406.1	6.2	40.0	0.4	121	5.46	112.2	356	316	81	3.8	2	0.00	0.00
						0.0			100	2.70				210			0.00	0.00
0.47	0.62	7.57	0.70	1.67	110.9	16.6	40.0	0.0	3	4.51	9.8	22	34	124	2.1	3	0.00	0.00
0.37	0.41	5.00	0.50	1.50	99.7	0.1	40.1	0.7	21	16.20	48.4	183	171	230	1.5	4	0.00	0.00
0.37	0.41	5.00	0.50	1.50	100.1	0.0	40.2	0.6	250	4.50	31.9	100	157	322	3.8	6	0.00	0.00
0.37	0.43	5.00	0.50	1.50	99.9	0.0	39.9	0.3	17	8.10	64.2	152	185	220	1.5	4	0.00	0.00
0.54	0.44	5.34	0.50	1.74	273.0	6.8	40.0	0.2	114	8.89	40.0	100	171	160	4.4	4	0.00	0.00
0.38	0.43	5.17	0.51	1.54	206.8	6.2	41.2	0.1	103	9.30	15.5	22	46	236	3.9	2	0.00	0.00
0.34	0.40	4.69	0.46	1.40	376.0	5.6	37.6	0.4	94	13.53	37.6	150	173	298	3.5	2	0.00	0.00
0.62	0.62	7.38	0.56	1.62	116.6	7.3	41.2	0.6	140	5.65	13.0	50	47	217	5.3	3	0.00	0.00
0.36	0.58	5.84	0.75	1.86	200.1	6.2	54.6	0.1	122	5.84	6.9	42	59	135	5.2	2	0.00	1.20
0.46	0.69	4.96	1.01	2.15	197.5	15.0	40.3	0.1	40	6.88	11.8	32	59	131	1.5	3	0.00	0.93
0.34	0.37	4.50	0.44	1.35	89.9	5.4	40.0	0.2	90	4.05	7.3	18	72	147	3.4	2	0.00	0.54
1.64	1.79	21.00	2.09	6.03	403.5	63.0	42.0	12.6	16	18.89	45.0	105	120	210	15.6	3	0.00	0.00
0.31	0.37	4.32	0.43	1.29	86.6	5.2	40.0	0.2	100	3.90	7.0	40	48	144	3.2	2	0.00	0.51
0.37	0.43	4.98	0.50	1.50	100.2	6.1	51.2	0.0	4	1.78	8.0	17	47	124	1.5	2	0.00	0.00
0.34	0.37	4.46	0.44	0.00	89.2	13.4	35.7	1.0	15	1.61	28.6	89	116	115	1.3	6	0.00	0.00
0.56	0.79	8.10	0.54	1.52	169.7	18.1	33.9	0.0	1	9.15	6.4	27	31	214	0.4	4	0.00	0.00
0.38	0.67	2.20	0.11	0.34	19.5	0.7	0.0	1.4	211	3.39	386.7	411	603	61	2.3	2	0.00	0.00
0.37	0.43	5.00	0.50	1.50	99.9	6.0	0.0	0.3	100	4.50	39.9	150	180	106	3.8	3	0.00	0.00
0.37	0.43	4.98	0.49	1.50	100.0	13.3	40.0	0.0	3	4.61	10.1	23	41	132	1.5	3	0.00	0.00
0.64	0.95	11.94	1.20	1.66	144.6	18.5	51.6	0.0	0	4.30	2.4	10	20	172	0.1	2	0.00	0.00
0.50	0.50	5.09	0.50	1.52	102.5	0.0	0.0	0.3	17	16.31	47.4	153	180	5	1.5	6	0.00	0.00
0.37	0.41	5.01	0.56	1.66	99.9	0.0	39.9	0.4	2	1.79	5.7	17	33	190	1.7	3	0.00	0.00
0.25	0.10	0.20	0.28	0.00	22.4	0.0	0.0	0.3	73	2.59	84.2	247	482	86	1.8	2	0.00	0.00
0.37	0.43	5.00	0.50	1.50	99.9	6.0	39.9	0.2	97	4.50	8.1	39	57	256	3.6	2	0.00	0.00
0.36	0.41	4.98	1.98	6.00	400.2	1.2	40.2	1.4	19	2.51	44.4	140	120	144	3.8	4	0.00	0.00
0.37	0.43	5.00	0.50	1.50	100.0	0.0	40.0		11	8.10	29.9	88	99	125	1.2	3	0.00	0.00

PAGE KEY: A-42 Beverages and Beverage Mixes A-44 Candies A-46 Cereals A-48 Cheeses and Substitutes A-50 Dairy Products and Substitutes A-52 Desserts A-56 Eggs and Egg Substitutes A-56 Fats, Oils, Margarines, and Shortenings A-58 Fruits A-60 Grain Products and Baked Goods A-62 Grains and Flours A-64 Meats and Meat Substitutes A-68 Nuts, Seeds, and Products

Code	Food Name	Unit/ Amt	Wt (g)	Energy (kcal)	Prot (g)	Carb (g)	Fiber (g)	Fat (g)	Sat (g)	Mono (g)	Poly (g)	Chol (mg)	Vit A (RE)
60969	Cereal, Harmony	1.25 cup	55	201	6	43	2	1	0.3	0.4	0.3	0	150
61344	Cereal, Healthy Fiber, multigrain flakes	0.75 cup	28	100	3	23	4	0	0.0	0.0	0.0	0	20
60958	Cereal, Heart to Heart, honey tstd oat	0.75 cup	33	118	4	25	4	2	0.3	0.4	0.4	0	125
61259	Cereal, Honey Bunches of Oats, w/almond	0.75 cup	31	126	2	24	1	3	0.3	1.3	0.8	0	225
40427	Cereal, Honey Graham Oh!s	0.75 cup	27	111	1	23	1	2	1.6	0.2	0.2	0	199
40068	Cereal, Honey Smacks	0.75 cup	27	105	2	24	1	1	0.1	0.2	0.2	0	153
40055	Cereal, hot, pilaf, 7 whole grain, ckd	0.5 cup	140	170	6	30	6	3	0.0			0	0
61340	Cereal, Just Flakes, oats	0.75 cup	28	100	4	19	3	2	0.0			0	0
40010	Cereal, Kix	1.25 cup	30	110	2	25	3	1	0.1	0.2	0.3	0	265
40300	Cereal, Lucky Charms	0.75 cup	27	110	2	22	1	1	0.2	0.3	0.3	0	151
40418	Cereal, Mueslix, w/raisins dates & almonds	0.67 cup	55	196	5	40	4	3	0.4	1.6	1.0	0	90
61217	Cereal, Oreo O's	0.75 cup	27	112	1	22	1	2	0.4	0.9	0.9	0	225
40216	Cereal, Product 19	1 cup	30	100	2	25	1	0	0.1	0.1	0.2	0	216
40209	Cereal, Raisin Bran	1 cup	59	190	5	46	7	1	0.2	0.2	0.4	0	261
40210	Cereal, Rice Krispies	1.25 cup	33	128	2	28	0	0	0.1	0.1	0.1	0	379
40018	Cereal, rice, puffed	1 cup	14	54	1	12	0	0	0.0	0.0	0.0	0	0
61558	Cereal, Shredded Wheat, biscuits	2 ea	47	160	5	37	6	1	0.0			0	0
40211	Cereal, Special K	1 cup	31	117	6	23	3	1	0.1	0.1	0.2	0	225
61214	Cereal, Toasties, corn flakes	1 cup	28	101	2	24	1	0	0.0	0.0	0.0	0	216
40021	Cereal, Total, wheat	0.75 cup	30	96	3	22	3	1	0.2	0.1	0.2	0	150
38026	Cereal, wheat germ, tstd	0.25 cup	28	108	8	14	4	3	0.5	0.4	1.9	0	3
40307	Cereal, Wheaties	0.75 cup	27	94	3	22	3	0	0.1	0.1	0.3	0	150
40040	Cereal, Wheaties, raisin bran	1 cup	55	183	4	45	5	1	0.2	0.1	0.4	0	150

CHEESES AND SUBSTITUTES

Natural Cheeses

Code	Food Name	Unit/ Amt	Wt (g)	Energy (kcal)	Prot (g)	Carb (g)	Fiber (g)	Fat (g)	Sat (g)	Mono (g)	Poly (g)	Chol (mg)	Vit A (RE)
47855	Cheese, blue	1 oz	28	100	6	1	0	8	5.3	2.2	0.2	21	58
47859	Cheese, brie, 1" cube	1 oz	28	95	6	0	0	8	4.9	2.3	0.2	28	50
47863	Cheese, cheddar, 1" cube	1 slc	28	113	7	0	0	9	5.9	2.6	0.3	29	76
1551	Cheese, cheddar, fat free, 1" cube	1 oz	28	40	8	1	0	0	0.0	0.0	0.0	3	60
1008	Cheese, cheddar, shredded	0.25 cup	28	114	7	0	0	9	6.0	2.7	0.3	30	77
47864	Cheese, cheddar, slice	1 slc	28	113	7	0	0	9	5.9	2.6	0.3	29	76
47865	Cheese, colby, 1" cube	1 slc	28	110	7	1	0	9	5.7	2.6	0.3	27	76
1010	Cheese, colby, shredded	0.25 cup	28	111	7	1	0	9	5.7	2.6	0.3	27	77
47866	Cheese, colby, slice	1 slc	28	110	7	1	0	9	5.7	2.6	0.3	27	76
47871	Cheese, feta, 1" cube	1 oz	28	75	4	1	0	6	4.2	1.3	0.2	25	36
1080	Cheese, goat, soft	1 oz	28	76	5	0	0	6	4.1	1.4	0.1	13	83
1054	Cheese, gouda	1 oz	28	101	7	1	0	8	5.0	2.2	0.2	32	47
1017	Cheese, monterey jack, shredded	0.25 cup	28	105	7	0	0	9	5.4	2.5	0.3	25	58
47885	Cheese, monterey jack, slice	1 slc	28	104	7	0	0	8	5.3	2.5	0.3	25	57
1553	Cheese, mozzarella, fat free, 1" cube	1 oz	28	40	8	1	0	0	0.0	0.0	0.0	3	60
13348	Cheese, mozzarella, string, sticks	1 ea	28	50	8	1	0	2	1.0			5	40
47891	Cheese, muenster	1 slc	28	103	7	0	0	8	5.4	2.4	0.2	27	84
1075	Cheese, parmesan, grated	1 Tbs	5	22	2	0	0	1	0.9	0.4	0.1	4	12
1510	Cheese, pepper jack, 1" cube	1 cubic inch	28	110	7	1	0	9	5.0			30	60
47900	Cheese, provolone, slice	1 slc	28	98	7	1	0	7	4.8	2.1	0.2	19	68
1064	Cheese, ricotta, whole milk	0.25 cup	62	108	7	2	0	8	5.1	2.2	0.2	32	76

PAGE KEY: A-70 Prepared Foods   A-78 Restaurants   A-90 Salad Dressings and Dips   A-92 Sauces and Gravies   A-94 Snack Foods   A-94 Spices, Flavors, and Seasonings   A-96 Sports Bars and Drinks
A-96 Supplemental Foods and Formulas   A-96 Sweeteners and Sweet Substitutes   A-98 Vegetables and Legumes   A-108 Miscellaneous

Thia (mg)	Ribo (mg)	Niac (mg NE)	Vit B6 (mg)	Vit B12 (µg)	Fol (µg)	Vit C (mg)	Vit D (IU)	Vit E (mg AT)	Cal (mg)	Iron (mg)	Magn (mg)	Phos (mg)	Pota (mg)	Sodi (mg)	Zinc (mg)	Wat (%)	Alco (g)	Caff (g)
1.50	0.85	10.01	1.00	4.17	399.9	30.2	40.2	13.5	600	9.02	24.2	100	91	355	7.5	3	0.00	0.00
0.15	0.17	2.00	0.20	0.60	40.0	0.0			0	0.72			100	15		1	0.00	0.00
0.15	0.05	0.60	2.00	6.01	400.0	30.0	0.0	13.5	14	1.82	8.6	31	96	82	1.5	3	0.00	0.00
0.37	0.41	5.00	0.50	1.50	100.1	0.0	40.0	0.5	11	8.10	21.4	60	70	136	0.3	3	0.00	0.00
0.50	0.56	6.61	0.66	0.00	400.1	7.9	0.0	0.2	3	5.94	12.2	39	44	165	5.0	3	0.00	0.00
0.37	0.43	5.00	0.50	1.50	101.3	6.1	40.0	0.1	6	0.34	15.9	46	40	51	0.4	2	0.00	0.00
						0.0			20	1.44				15			0.00	0.00
						0.0			20	1.08			80	190			0.00	0.00
0.58	0.60	7.28	0.68	1.71	236.1	7.6	39.9	0.1	171	9.60	15.3	57	56	189	5.2	3	0.00	0.00
0.46	0.51	6.01	0.51	1.60	201.2	6.3	40.0	0.1	108	4.96	15.9	64	49	195	4.4	3	0.00	0.00
0.43	0.43	5.50	2.03	6.05	405.9	0.2	16.0	4.0	32	4.51	49.0	100	240	170	3.7	9	0.00	0.00
0.37	0.41	5.00	0.50	1.50	99.9	0.0	0.0	0.4	5	1.79	14.9	32	49	128	1.5	2	0.00	0.81
1.50	1.71	20.01	2.06	6.00	399.9	61.2	39.3	13.5	5	18.09	15.9	40	50	207	15.3	3	0.00	0.00
0.66	0.93	8.64	1.04	3.01	150.4		40.1	0.4	28	7.53	74.3	215	335	251	2.1	9	0.00	0.00
0.60	0.73	7.03	0.99	3.13	177.9	15.5	40.9	0.0	2	11.35	8.6	42	29	185	0.4	4	0.00	0.00
0.05	0.03	0.49	0.00	0.00	21.6	0.0	0.0	0.0	1	0.40	4.2	17	16	1	0.2	4	0.00	0.00
						0.0			20	1.08				0		3	0.00	0.00
0.52	0.58	7.13	1.98	6.05	399.9	21.0	0.0	4.7	8	8.68	19.2	68	20	204	0.9	3	0.00	0.00
0.37	0.43	5.00	0.50	1.50	100.0	0.0	40.0	0.1	1	5.40	4.5	15	33	200	0.1	4	0.00	0.00
1.50	1.70	20.00	2.00	6.00	399.9	60.0	99.9	13.5	1000	18.00	24.0	80	92	197	15.0	3	0.00	0.00
0.46	0.23	1.58	0.28	0.00	99.4	1.7	0.0	4.5	13	2.56	90.4	324	268	1	4.7	6	0.00	0.00
0.68	0.75	9.00	0.89	2.70	180.1	5.4	35.9	0.3	18	7.55	28.9	90	94	199	6.8	3	0.00	0.00
0.75	0.85	10.01	1.00	3.02	200.2	0.0	40.2	0.3	0	7.48	42.4	140	227	251	7.5	7	0.00	0.00
0.00	0.10	0.28	0.05	0.34	10.2	0.0	6.0	0.1	150	0.09	6.5	110	73	395	0.8	42	0.00	0.00
0.01	0.15	0.10	0.07	0.46	18.4	0.0	5.7	0.1	52	0.14	5.7	53	43	178	0.7	48	0.00	0.00
0.00	0.10	0.01	0.01	0.23	5.0	0.0	6.7	0.1	202	0.18	7.8	143	27	174	0.9	37	0.00	0.00
									400					220		18	0.00	0.00
0.00	0.10	0.01	0.01	0.23	5.1	0.0	6.8	0.1	204	0.18	7.9	145	28	175	0.9	37	0.00	0.00
0.00	0.10	0.01	0.01	0.23	5.0	0.0	6.7	0.1	202	0.18	7.8	143	27	174	0.9	37	0.00	0.00
0.00	0.10	0.02	0.01	0.23	5.0	0.0	6.7	0.1	192	0.20	7.3	128	36	169	0.9	38	0.00	0.00
0.00	0.10	0.02	0.01	0.23	5.1	30.0	6.8	0.1	194	0.20	7.3	129	36	171	0.9	38	0.00	0.00
0.00	0.10	0.02	0.01	0.23	5.0	0.0	6.7	0.1	192	0.20	7.3	128	36	169	0.9	38	0.00	0.00
0.03	0.23	0.28	0.11	0.47	9.1	0.0	4.5	0.1	140	0.18	5.4	96	18	316	0.8	55	0.00	0.00
0.01	0.10	0.11	0.07	0.05	3.4	0.0	4.3	0.1	40	0.54	4.5	73	7	104	0.3	61	0.00	0.00
0.00	0.09	0.01	0.01	0.43	6.0	0.0	5.7	0.1	198	0.07	8.2	155	34	232	1.1	41	0.00	0.00
0.00	0.10	0.02	0.01	0.23	5.1	0.0	6.2	0.1	211	0.20	7.6	125	23	151	0.8	41	0.00	0.00
0.00	0.10	0.02	0.01	0.23	5.0	0.0	6.2	0.1	209	0.20	7.6	124	23	150	0.8	41	0.00	0.00
									400					220		18	0.00	0.00
						0.0			200	0.00				220			0.00	0.00
0.00	0.09	0.02	0.01	0.40	3.4	0.0	6.2	0.1	201	0.10	7.6	131	38	176	0.8	42	0.00	0.00
0.00	0.01	0.00	0.00	0.10	0.5	0.0	1.1	0.0	55	0.03	1.9	36	6	76	0.2	21	0.00	0.00
						0.0			200	0.00				170		10	0.00	0.00
0.00	0.09	0.03	0.01	0.40	2.8	0.0	5.6	0.1	212	0.15	7.8	139	39	245	0.9	41	0.00	0.00
0.00	0.11	0.05	0.02	0.20	7.4	0.0	6.2	0.1	128	0.23	6.8	98	65	52	0.7	72	0.00	0.00

PAGE KEY: A-42 Beverages and Beverage Mixes   A-44 Candies   A-46 Cereals   A-48 Cheeses and Substitutes   A-50 Dairy Products and Substitutes   A-52 Desserts   A-56 Eggs and Egg Substitutes
A-56 Fats, Oils, Margarines, and Shortenings   A-58 Fruits   A-60 Grain Products and Baked Goods   A-62 Grains and Flours   A-64 Meats and Meat Substitutes   A-68 Nuts, Seeds, and Products

Code	Food Name	Unit/ Amt	Wt (g)	Energy (kcal)	Prot (g)	Carb (g)	Fiber (g)	Fat (g)	Sat (g)	Mono (g)	Poly (g)	Chol (mg)	Vit A (RE)
47908	Cheese, Swiss, 1" cube	1 oz	28	108	8	2	0	8	5.0	2.1	0.3	26	64
47912	Cheese, Swiss, slice	1 slc	28	106	8	2	0	8	5.0	2.0	0.3	26	63
1047	Cottage Cheese, 1% fat	0.5 cup	113	81	14	3	0	1	0.7	0.3	0.0	5	13
1014	Cottage Cheese, 2% fat	0.5 cup	113	97	13	4	0	3	1.1	0.5	0.1	11	24
47848	Cottage Cheese, fat free, sml curd	0.5 cup	126	90	12	8	0	0	0.0	0.0	0.0	10	40
1015	Cream Cheese	1 Tbs	14	50	1	1	0	5	2.8	1.2	0.2	16	54
1452	Cream Cheese, fat free	1 oz	28	30	4	2	0	0	0.2	0.1	0.0	3	3
Processed Cheeses and Substitutes													
1001	Cheese Product, American, cold pack	1 oz	28	94	6	2	0	7	4.4	2.0	0.2	18	48
48332	Cheese, American, past, proc, fat free, 1" cube	1 oz	28	42	6	4	0	0	0.1	0.1	0.0	3	125
48314	Cheese, American, past, proc, low fat, 1" cube	1 oz	28	51	7	1	0	2	1.3	0.6	0.1	10	17
1096	Cheese, American, past, proc, low fat, shredded	0.25 cup	28	51	7	1	0	2	1.2	0.6	0.1	10	17
47918	Cheese, pimento, past, proc, 1" cube	1 oz	28	106	6	0	0	9	5.6	2.5	0.3	27	73
48311	Cottage Cheese Substitute, soy	0.5 cup	112	170	14	8	0	9	1.3	2.0	5.1	0	5
DAIRY PRODUCTS AND SUBSTITUTES													
Creams and Substitutes													
506	Cream Substitute, pwd	1 tsp	2	11	0	1	0	1	0.7	0.0	0.0	0	0
54315	Cream Substitute, soy milk, plain	1 Tbs	15	15	0	1	0	1	0.0			0	0
500	Cream, half & half	1 indv pkt	15	20	0	1	0	2	1.1	0.5	0.1	6	15
501	Cream, light	1 Tbs	15	29	0	1	0	3	1.8	0.8	0.1	10	28
503	Cream, whipping, heavy, whipped	1 Tbs	8	26	0	0	0	3	1.7	0.8	0.1	10	31
504	Sour Cream, cultured	1 Tbs	12	23	0	0	0	2	1.4	0.6	0.1	6	21
54383	Sour Cream, fat free	2 Tbs	32	24	1	5	0	0	0.0	0.0	0.0	3	24
Milks and Non-Dairy Milks													
7	Buttermilk, low fat, cultured	1 cup	245	98	8	12	0	2	1.3	0.6	0.1	10	37
17	Eggnog	1 cup	254	224	12	20	0	11	6.6	3.3	0.5	150	152
4	Milk, 1%, w/add vit A & D	1 cup	244	102	8	12	0	2	1.5	0.7	0.1	12	142
2	Milk, 2%, w/add vit A & D	1 cup	244	122	8	12	0	5	3.1	1.4	0.2	20	136
18	Milk, chocolate, 2%, w/add vit A & D	1 cup	250	190	7	30	2	5	2.9	1.1	0.2	20	162
21109	Milk, chocolate, rducd fat, w/add calc	1 cup	250	195	7	30	2	5	2.9	1.1	0.2	20	162
173	Milk, evaporated, Carnation, w/add vit D	30 ml	32	40	2	3	0	2	1.5			10	0
23	Milk, goat, w/add vit D	1 cup	244	168	9	11	0	10	6.5	2.7	0.4	27	142
1	Milk, whole, 3.25%, w/add vit D	1 cup	244	149	8	12	0	8	4.6	2.0	0.5	24	115
66	Milk, whole, dry pwd, w/add vit D	0.25 cup	32	159	8	12	0	9	5.4	2.5	0.2	31	84
24043	Rice Milk, w/add calc vit A & D	8 fl oz	240	113	1	22	1	2	0.0	1.5	0.8	0	151
20033	Soy Milk	1 cup	243	131	8	15	1	4	0.5	1.0	2.3	0	1
20920	Soy Milk, chocolate	1 cup	250	145	5	24	2	4	0.5			0	103
Yogurt													
2836	Yogurt, cherry, fruit on the bottom	1 indv cup	227	220	9	42	1	2	1.0			10	0
15408	Yogurt, fruit, nonfat, 8-oz cntr	1 cup	245	233	11	47	0	0	0.3	0.1	0.0	5	7
2000	Yogurt, plain, low fat, 12g prot, 8-oz cntr	1 cup	245	154	13	17	0	4	2.5	1.0	0.1	15	35
11979	Yogurt, plain, nonfat	1 cup	226	120	12	17	0	0	0.0	0.0	0.0	5	100
71587	Yogurt, soy, vanilla	1 ea	170	150	5	25	1	3	0.0			0	0
2015	Yogurt, vanilla, low fat, 11g prot, 8-oz cntr	1 cup	245	208	12	34	0	3	2.0	0.8	0.1	12	30

Thia (mg)	Ribo (mg)	Niac (mg NE)	Vit B6 (mg)	Vit B12 (µg)	Fol (µg)	Vit C (mg)	Vit D (IU)	Vit E (mg AT)	Cal (mg)	Iron (mg)	Magn (mg)	Phos (mg)	Pota (mg)	Sodi (mg)	Zinc (mg)	Wat (%)	Alco (g)	Caff (g)
0.01	0.07	0.02	0.01	0.94	1.7	0.0	5.7	0.1	224	0.05	10.8	161	22	54	1.2	37	0.00	0.00
0.01	0.07	0.02	0.01	0.93	1.7	0.0	5.6	0.1	221	0.05	10.6	159	22	54	1.2	37	0.00	0.00
0.01	0.18	0.14	0.07	0.70	13.6	0.0	0.0	0.0	69	0.15	5.7	151	97	459	0.4	82	0.00	0.00
0.05	0.21	0.11	0.01	0.50	11.3	0.0	0.0	0.0	103	0.17	7.9	184	95	373	0.5	81	0.00	0.00
						0.0			80	0.00				450			0.00	0.00
0.00	0.01	0.01	0.00	0.03	1.6	0.0	3.6	0.0	14	0.05	1.3	15	20	47	0.1	54	0.00	0.00
0.00	0.07	0.07	0.00	0.27	9.9	0.0	0.0	0.0	100	0.05	6.2	148	79	199	0.4	72	0.00	0.00
0.00	0.12	0.01	0.03	0.36	1.4	0.0			141	0.23	8.5	113	103	274	0.9	43	0.00	0.00
0.01	0.14	0.05	0.02	0.31	7.7	0.0	0.0	0.1	195	0.07	10.2	265	82	433	1.0	57	0.00	0.00
0.00	0.10	0.01	0.01	0.21	2.6	0.0	1.4	0.1	194	0.11	6.8	234	51	405	0.9	59	0.00	0.00
0.00	0.10	0.01	0.01	0.21	2.5	0.0	1.4	0.1	193	0.11	6.8	234	51	404	0.9	59	0.00	0.00
0.00	0.10	0.01	0.01	0.20	2.3	0.7	6.2	0.1	174	0.11	6.2	211	46	405	0.8	39	0.00	0.00
0.00	0.15	0.56	0.07	0.00	24.8	0.0	0.0	0.7	212	6.30	256.5	250	224	22	1.9	71	0.00	0.00
0.00	0.00	0.00	0.00	0.00	0.0	0.0	0.0	0.0	0	0.01	0.1	8	16	4	0.0	2	0.00	0.00
						0.0			0	0.00				10		86	0.00	0.00
0.00	0.01	0.00	0.00	0.05	0.5	0.1	1.2	0.0	16	0.00	1.5	14	20	6	0.1	81	0.00	0.00
0.00	0.01	0.00	0.00	0.02	0.3	0.1	2.1	0.1	14	0.00	1.4	12	18	6	0.0	74	0.00	0.00
0.00	0.00	0.00	0.00	0.00	0.3	0.0	2.0	0.1	5	0.00	0.5	5	6	3	0.0	58	0.00	0.00
0.00	0.01	0.00	0.00	0.02	0.8	0.1	1.7	0.1	13	0.01	1.2	14	17	10	0.0	74	0.00	0.00
0.00	0.05	0.01	0.00	0.10	3.5	0.0	0.0	0.0	40	0.00	3.2	30	41	45	0.2	81	0.00	0.00
0.07	0.37	0.14	0.07	0.54	12.2	2.5	2.5	0.1	284	0.11	27.0	218	370	257	1.0	90	0.00	0.00
0.09	0.47	0.27	0.12	1.13	2.5	3.8	124.5	0.5	330	0.50	48.3	277	419	137	1.2	83	0.00	0.00
0.05	0.44	0.23	0.09	1.14	12.2	0.0	117.1	0.0	305	0.07	26.8	232	366	107	1.0	90	0.00	0.00
0.10	0.44	0.21	0.09	1.28	12.2	0.5	119.6	0.1	293	0.05	26.8	224	342	115	1.2	89	0.00	0.00
0.10	0.46	0.40	0.05	0.82	5.0	0.0	122.5	0.1	272	0.60	35.0	255	422	165	1.0	82	0.00	2.50
0.10	1.40	0.40	0.05	0.82	5.0	0.0		0.1	485	0.60	35.0	190	308	165	1.0	82	0.00	2.50
	0.10					0.0	24.0		80	0.00		60	90	30		24		0.00
0.11	0.34	0.68	0.10	0.17	2.4	3.2	124.4	0.2	327	0.11	34.2	271	498	122	0.7	87	0.00	0.00
0.10	0.40	0.21	0.09	1.10	12.2	0.0	124.4	0.2	276	0.07	24.4	205	322	105	0.9	88	0.00	0.00
0.09	0.38	0.20	0.10	1.03	11.8	2.8	134.4	0.2	292	0.15	27.2	248	426	119	1.1	2	0.00	0.00
0.05	0.34	0.93	0.09	1.50	4.8	0.0	100.8	1.1	283	0.47	26.4	134	65	94	0.3	89	0.00	0.00
0.15	0.17	1.25	0.18	0.00	43.7	0.0	0.0	0.3	61	1.55	60.8	126	287	124	0.3	88	0.00	0.00
	0.51			3.07	25.0	0.0	122.5		308	1.47	40.0		360	102	0.6	86	0.00	
						0.0			300	0.00			480	150			0.00	0.00
0.10	0.43	0.25	0.10	1.14	22.1	1.7	0.0	0.1	372	0.17	36.8	292	475	142	1.8	75	0.00	0.00
0.10	0.51	0.28	0.11	1.37	27.0	2.0	2.5	0.1	448	0.20	41.7	353	573	172	2.2	85	0.00	0.00
					2.4				450	0.00				180			0.00	0.00
					29.9				299	1.45				20		79	0.00	0.00
0.10	0.49	0.25	0.10	1.29	27.0	2.0	2.5	0.0	419	0.17	39.2	331	537	162	2.0	79	0.00	0.00

Code	Food Name	Unit/ Amt	Wt (g)	Energy (kcal)	Prot (g)	Carb (g)	Fiber (g)	Fat (g)	Sat (g)	Mono (g)	Poly (g)	Chol (mg)	Vit A (RE)
DESSERTS													
Brownies and Dessert Squares													
47019	Brownie, prep f/recipe, 2" square	1 ea	24	112	1	12		7	1.8	2.6	2.3	18	46
Cakes													
46004	Cake, angel food, 1/12 of 9"	1 pce	28	72	2	16	0	0	0.0	0.0	0.1	0	0
46098	Cake, applesauce, w/o icing	1 pce	87	313	3	52	2	12	2.4	5.0	3.5	22	10
46103	Cake, banana, w/o icing	1 pce	87	262	3	46	1	8	1.6	3.6	2.1	32	83
46262	Cake, carrot, buttercream frosted	1 pce	71	280	2	36	1	15	3.5			35	100
46120	Cake, chocolate, w/fluffy white icing, prep f/recipe, slice	1 pce	91	280	3	43	1	11	2.7			23	50
46005	Cake, coffee, cinnamon, w/crumb topping prep f/mix 1/8 of 8"	1 pce	56	178	3	30	1	5	1.0	2.2	1.8	27	20
46205	Cake, fruit	1 pce	43	139	1	26	2	4	0.5	1.8	1.4	2	3
46000	Cake, gingerbread, prep f/rec, 1/9 of 8" square	1 pce	74	263	3	36		12	3.1	5.3	3.1	24	10
71650	Cake, lemon, layer, 9", FS	1 pce	88	290	2	43	0	12	3.5			35	
46016	Cake, pound, w/butter, 12 oz	1 pce	28	109	2	14	0	6	3.2	1.7	0.3	62	44
46077	Cake, shortcake, biscuit type, prep f/recipe	1 svg	55	190	3	27	1	8	2.1	3.3	2.0	2	10
12722	Cake, snack, chocolate, w/cream	3 ea	85	280	3	54	0	6	2.0			75	20
46078	Cake, sponge, prep f/recipe, 1/12 of 10"	1 pce	63	187	5	36	1	3	0.8	1.0	0.4	107	49
46012	Cake, yellow, w/chocolate icing, 1/8 of 18 oz	1 pce	64	243	2	35	1	11	3.0	6.1	1.4	35	21
49001	Cheesecake, no bake, prep f/dry mix, 1/12 of 9"	1 pce	99	271	5	35	2	13	6.6	4.5	0.8	29	99
46426	Cupcake, chocolate, w/frosting, low fat	1 ea	43	131	2	29	2	2	0.5	0.8	0.2	0	(RE)
Cookies													
91664	Cookie, almond	2 ea	29	170	2	19	0	10	3.0			0	0
93285	Cookie, animal, vanilla	9 ea	28	120	2	20	1	4	1.5			0	0
90637	Cookie, chocolate chip bar, prep f/recipe w/marg, 2" square	1 ea	32	156	2	19	1	9	2.6	3.3	2.7	10	50
47031	Cookie, chocolate chip, enrich, higher fat, med 2.25"	1 ea	10	47	1	6	0	2	1.0	0.7	0.3	0	0
42726	Cookie, chocolate chip, refrig dough, svg	1 svg	28	135	1	17	1	7	2.0	2.5	0.5	5	
47041	Cookie, chocolate wafer	1 ea	6	26	0	4	0	1	0.3	0.3	0.2	0	0
92323	Cookie, chocolate, biscotti style, low fat	2 ea	30	120	3	23	3	3	0.0			0	0
47012	Cookie, fig bar	1 ea	16	56	1	11	1	1	0.2	0.5	0.4	0	1
47043	Cookie, fortune	1 ea	8	30	0	7	0	0	0.1	0.1	0.0	0	0
50962	Cookie, Fudge Stripes	3 ea	31	160	2	21	1	7	4.0			0	0
47077	Cookie, granola	1 ea	13	60	1	9	1	2	1.6	0.2	0.2	0	0
47737	Cookie, lemon drop	3 ea	33	160	1	20	0	8	2.0			0	0
47161	Cookie, newton, fig	2 ea	31	116	2	19	2	3	1.0	1.0	0.0	0	
47496	Cookie, oatmeal raisin, home style, svg	1 ea	26	106	1	18	1	3	0.7	1.3	0.3	2	1
49102	Cookie, peanut butter	1 ea	15	72	1	9	0	4	0.7	1.9	0.8	0	0
47061	Cookie, raisin, soft type	1 ea	15	60	1	10	0	2	0.5	1.1	0.3	0	1
92328	Cookie, sandwich, Cookie Cremes, chocolate, w/cream	1 indv pkt	80	385	3	59	0	15	3.0			0	0
50973	Cookie, sandwich, lemon creme, sugar free	3 ea	28	130	1	19	0	7	1.5			0	0
47071	Cookie, sandwich, vanilla, w/creme, 1 3/4"	1 ea	10	48	0	7	0	2	0.3	0.8	0.8	0	0
50960	Cookie, shortbread, pecan	1 ea	16	80	1	9	0	5	1.0			5	0
47045	Cookie, snap, ginger	1 ea	7	29	0	5	0	1	0.2	0.4	0.1	0	0
47011	Cookie, snickerdoodle, prep f/recipe	1 ea	20	80	1	12	0	3	2.1			9	25
47064	Cookie, sugar	1 ea	15	72	1	10	0	3	0.8	1.8	0.4	8	4
47738	Cookie, Tagalongs	2 ea	28	150	3	13	2	10	4.0			0	0

PAGE KEY: A-70 Prepared Foods   A-78 Restaurants   A-90 Salad Dressings and Dips   A-92 Sauces and Gravies   A-94 Snack Foods   A-94 Spices, Flavors, and Seasonings   A-96 Sports Bars and Drinks   A-96 Supplemental Foods and Formulas   A-96 Sweeteners and Sweet Substitutes   A-98 Vegetables and Legumes   A-108 Miscellaneous

Thia (mg)	Ribo (mg)	Niac (mg NE)	Vit B6 (mg)	Vit B12 (µg)	Fol (µg)	Vit C (mg)	Vit D (IU)	Vit E (mg AT)	Cal (mg)	Iron (mg)	Magn (mg)	Phos (mg)	Pota (mg)	Sodi (mg)	Zinc (mg)	Wat (%)	Alco (g)	Caff (g)
0.02	0.05	0.23	0.01	0.03	7.0	0.1			14	0.43	12.7	32	42	82	0.2	13	0.00	
0.02	0.14	0.25	0.00	0.01	9.8	0.0			39	0.15	3.4	91	26	210	0.0	33	0.00	0.00
0.12	0.12	1.09	0.05	0.03	5.6	0.9	2.8	1.6	17	1.39	10.6	45	145	141	0.2	23	0.00	0.00
0.14	0.17	1.16	0.20	0.07	11.5	2.9	3.1	1.2	26	1.11	15.5	50	168	181	0.3	33	0.10	0.00
0.05	0.07	0.40			8.0	0.0			20	0.72				230			0.00	0.00
0.10	0.12	0.82	0.01	0.07	29.3	0.1	2.9	0.9	18	0.93	10.8	41	64	207	0.3	51	0.00	
0.09	0.10	0.85	0.02	0.07	26.9	0.1	10.6	0.1	76	0.80	10.1	120	63	236	0.3	30	0.00	0.00
0.01	0.03	0.34	0.01	0.00	8.6	0.2	0.0	0.4	14	0.88	6.9	22	66	138	0.1	25	0.00	0.00
0.14	0.11	1.28	0.14	0.03	24.4	0.1			53	2.13	51.8	40	325	242	0.3	28	0.00	0.00
														250			0.00	0.00
0.03	0.05	0.37	0.00	0.07	11.5	0.0			10	0.38	3.1	38	33	111	0.1	25	0.00	0.00
0.17	0.15	1.41	0.01	0.03	29.2	0.1			113	1.39	8.8	79	58	278	0.3	28	0.00	0.00
						0.0			20	0.36				230			0.00	
0.10	0.18	0.75	0.03	0.23	24.6	0.0			26	1.00	5.7	63	89	144	0.4	29	0.00	0.00
0.07	0.10	0.80	0.01	0.10	14.1	0.0			24	1.33	19.2	103	114	216	0.4	22	0.00	
0.11	0.25	0.49	0.05	0.31	29.7	0.5			170	0.46	18.8	232	209	376	0.5	44	0.00	0.00
0.01	0.05	0.31	0.00	0.00	6.5	0.0			15	0.66	10.8	79	96	178	0.2	23	0.00	0.86
						0.0			0	0.00				75			0.00	0.00
						0.0			0	0.00				80		2	0.00	0.00
0.05	0.05	0.43	0.02	0.02	10.6	0.1			12	0.79	17.6	32	72	116	0.3	6	0.00	5.11
0.01	0.01	0.18	0.00	0.00	4.9	0.0	0.0	0.2	3	0.31	3.9	8	15	34	0.1	6	0.00	1.10
										0.72				85		9	0.00	
0.00	0.01	0.17	0.00	0.00	3.7				2	0.23	3.2	8	13	41	0.1	4	0.00	0.41
						0.0			0	0.72				50	0		0.00	
0.02	0.02	0.30	0.00	0.00	5.6	0.0	0.0	0.1	10	0.46	4.3	10	33	56	0.1	16	0.00	0.00
0.00	0.00	0.15	0.00	0.00	5.3	0.0	0.0	0.0	1	0.11	0.6	3	3	22	0.0	8	0.00	0.00
						0.0			0	0.72				110			0.00	
0.07	0.02	0.23	0.05	0.00	10.5	0.1		0.0	9	0.37	13.1	46	47	43	0.2	3	0.00	0.00
0.14	0.10	1.04	0.00	0.01	32.4	0.0	1.3	0.2	0	0.72	5.1	33	34	150	0.1	2	0.00	0.00
										0.69		78		116			0.00	
0.07	0.03	0.43			12.2				10	0.62			74	88		12	0.00	0.00
0.02	0.02	0.63	0.00	0.00	10.8	0.0	0.0	0.3	5	0.37	6.8	13	25	62	0.1	6	0.00	0.00
0.02	0.02	0.30	0.00	0.00	4.8	0.1	0.0	0.3	7	0.34	3.2	12	21	51	0.0	13	0.00	0.00
						0.0			0	4.26				296		0	0.00	
						0.0			0	0.36				50		1	0.00	0.00
0.02	0.01	0.27	0.00	0.00	5.0	0.0	0.0	0.2	3	0.21	1.4	8	9	35	0.0	2	0.00	0.00
						0.0			0	0.00				50		1	0.00	
0.00	0.01	0.23	0.00	0.00	6.1	0.0	0.0	0.1	5	0.44	3.4	6	24	39	0.0	5	0.00	0.00
0.05	0.03	0.40	0.00	0.00	13.6	0.1	2.7	0.1	8	0.46	2.1	10	23	75	0.1	5	0.00	0.00
0.02	0.02	0.40	0.00	0.02	8.0	0.0	0.9	0.0	3	0.31	1.8	12	9	54	0.1	5	0.00	0.00
0.10	0.03	1.37	0.02	0.00	30.5	0.0	0.0	0.8	0	0.72	17.1	40	71	85	0.3		0.00	0.00

PAGE KEY: A-42 Beverages and Beverage Mixes   A-44 Candies   A-46 Cereals   A-48 Cheeses and Substitutes   A-50 Dairy Products and Substitutes   A-52 Desserts   A-56 Eggs and Egg Substitutes   A-56 Fats, Oils, Margarines, and Shortenings   A-58 Fruits   A-60 Grain Products and Baked Goods   A-62 Grains and Flours   A-64 Meats and Meat Substitutes   A-68 Nuts, Seeds, and Products

Code	Food Name	Unit/ Amt	Wt (g)	Energy (kcal)	Prot (g)	Carb (g)	Fiber (g)	Fat (g)	Sat (g)	Mono (g)	Poly (g)	Chol (mg)	Vit A (RE)
47739	Cookie, Thin Mints	4 ea	28	140	1	18	1	8	2.0			0	0
47740	Cookie, Trefoils	5 ea	32	160	2	20	0	8	1.0			0	0
47044	Cookies, fudge, cake type	1 ea	21	73	1	16	1	1	0.2	0.4	0.1	0	0
47183	Cracker, graham, cinnamon	24 ea	30	130	2	23	1	4	1.0	1.0	2.0	0	0
Doughnuts, Pastries, and Sweet Rolls													
45523	Croissant, cheese, med	1 ea	57	236	5	27	1	12	6.1	3.7	1.4	32	120
45572	Danish, cheese	1 ea	71	266	6	26	1	16	4.8	8.0	1.8	16	26
45630	Doughnut, buttermilk, glazed	1 ea	64	270	3	35	0	13	3.0			15	0
45518	Doughnut, cake, chocolate, glazed/sugared, med, 3"	1 ea	42	175	2	24	1	8	2.2	4.7	1.0	24	5
71335	Doughnut, cake, holes	1 ea	14	59	1	6	0	3	1.0	1.8	0.4	1	0
45507	Doughnut, filled, jelly, 3 1/2" oval	1 ea	85	289	5	33	1	16	4.1	8.7	2.0	22	15
71343	Doughnut, glazed, enrich, lrg, 4 1/4"	1 ea	75	299	5	38	2	14	4.1	7.5	2.1	22	4
70161	Fritter, apple, fzn	1 pce	62	130	2	18	1	6	1.8			2	2
45593	Pastry, toaster, apple cinnamon	1 ea	52	205	2	37	1	5	0.9	3.1	1.4	0	100
45594	Pastry, toaster, brown sugar cinnamon	1 ea	50	219	3	32	1	9	1.0	3.6	4.6	0	100
45595	Pastry, toaster, cherry	1 ea	52	204	2	37	1	5	0.9	3.0	1.6	0	100
45601	Pastry, toaster, chocolate fudge, frosted	1 ea	52	201	3	37	1	5	1.0	2.7	1.1	0	100
45782	Pastry, toaster, s'mores	1 ea	52	204	3	36	1	5	1.5	3.1	0.9	0	100
42746	Pastry, toaster, strawberry swirl Danish	1 ea	62	254	3	37	1	11	3.0	3.6	4.4	0	0
42266	Turnover, apple, w/icing, kit, refrig	1 ea	57	180	2	24	0	8	2.0			0	0
Frozen Desserts													
46110	Cake, ice cream, chocolate roll, 12 oz	1 pce	34	101	1	14	0	5	2.1	1.8	0.8	15	22
90721	Frozen Dessert Pop, 1.75 fl oz bar	1 ea	52	41	0	10	0	0	0.0	0.0	0.0	0	0
23051	Frozen Dessert, slushy	1 cup	193	247	1	63	0	0	0.0	0.0	0.0	0	0
2045	Frozen Yogurt Cone, chocolate, sml	1 ea	78	168	4	24	1	7	4.2	2.3	0.4	1	37
2044	Frozen Yogurt Sandwich	1 ea	85	181	4	32	0	4	2.3	1.3	0.4	1	37
72125	Frozen Yogurt, chocolate	0.5 cup	87	110	3	19	2	3	2.0	0.8	0.1	11	35
625	Frozen Yogurt, vanilla, low fat	0.5 cup	106	200	9	31	0	4	2.5			65	40
72188	Ice Cream Bar, Fudgsicle	1 ea	61	90	3	16	1	2	1.0			5	0
25537	Ice Cream Cone, sundae, chocolate, classic	1 ea	94	310	5	34	2	17	9.0			15	20
71778	Ice Cream Sandwich	1 ea	70	190	3	28	0	8	4.0			20	40
71814	Ice Cream, neapolitan	0.5 cup	65	130	2	16	0	7	4.0			25	40
71810	Ice Cream, rocky road	0.5 cup	65	160	3	19	1	8	4.5			25	40
2008	Ice Cream, soft serve, French vanilla	0.5 cup	86	191	4	19	1	11	6.4	3.0	0.4	78	142
2018	Ice Cream, strawberry	0.5 cup	68	130	2	15	0	7	4.0			20	40
2004	Ice Cream, vanilla	0.5 cup	66	137	2	16	0	7	4.5	2.0	0.3	29	79
72119	Ice Cream, vanilla, fat free	0.5 cup	68	94	3	20	1	0	0.0	0.0	0.0	0	137
2011	Sherbet, orange	0.5 cup	74	107	1	22	1	1	0.9	0.4	0.1	1	9
Pies and Fruit Desserts													
62352	Cheesecake, cherry, FS	1 cntr	113	330	6	27	1	22	13.0			100	300
49064	Cobbler, berry, ckd f/fzn	0.25 ea	120	370	3	41	1	21	5.0			5	0
49023	Crisp, cherry	0.5 cup	123	352	3	56	1	14	2.4	6.2	4.3	1	125
45535	Crust, pie, enrich, rtb, fzn, 9"	1 ea	173	791	11	84	4	45	14.1	21.0	5.5	0	0
45500	Crust, pie, graham cracker, prep f/recipe, bkd, 9"	1 ea	239	1181	10	156	4	60	12.4	27.2	16.5	0	488
48004	Pie, apple, w/enrich flour, 1/6 of 8"	1 pce	117	277	2	40	2	13	4.4	5.1	2.6	0	39
48023	Pie, banana cream, no bake, prep f/mix, 1/8 of 9"	1 slc	92	231	3	29	1	12	6.4	4.2	0.7	27	92

PAGE KEY: A-70 Prepared Foods   A-78 Restaurants   A-90 Salad Dressings and Dips   A-92 Sauces and Gravies   A-94 Snack Foods   A-94 Spices, Flavors, and Seasonings   A-96 Sports Bars and Drinks   A-96 Supplemental Foods and Formulas   A-96 Sweeteners and Sweet Substitutes   A-98 Vegetables and Legumes   A-108 Miscellaneous

Thia (mg)	Ribo (mg)	Niac (mg NE)	Vit B6 (mg)	Vit B12 (µg)	Fol (µg)	Vit C (mg)	Vit D (IU)	Vit E (mg AT)	Cal (mg)	Iron (mg)	Magn (mg)	Phos (mg)	Pota (mg)	Sodi (mg)	Zinc (mg)	Wat (%)	Alco (g)	Caff (g)
0.05	0.05	0.49	0.00	0.00	14.9	0.0	0.0	0.1	200	0.44	4.6	14	19	80	0.1		0.00	0.00
0.14	0.09	1.08	0.00	0.00	33.4	0.0	0.1	0.1	0	0.36	4.1	20	20	90	0.1		0.00	0.00
0.05	0.03	0.25	0.00	0.01	9.0	0.0			7	0.51	6.7	17	29	40	0.1	12	0.00	0.00
						0.0			100	1.08				150		0	0.00	0.00
0.30	0.18	1.23	0.03	0.18	42.2	0.1	0.0	0.8	30	1.23	13.7	74	75	206	0.5	21	0.00	0.00
0.12	0.18	1.41	0.02	0.14	42.6	0.1	1.4	0.2	25	1.13	10.6	77	70	229	0.5	31	0.00	0.00
						0.0			60	1.08				290		12	0.00	0.00
0.01	0.02	0.20	0.00	0.03	18.9	0.0	0.0	0.1	89	0.94	14.3	68	45	167	0.2	16	0.00	0.41
0.02	0.01	0.28	0.00	0.00	11.2	0.2	0.0	0.3	4	0.41	2.2	37	16	78	0.1	23	0.00	0.00
0.27	0.11	1.82	0.09	0.18	57.8	0.0	0.0	0.4	21	1.50	17.0	72	67	204	0.6	36	0.00	0.00
0.23	0.14	1.96	0.02	0.07	81.0	0.9	0.0	1.1	34	2.80	13.5	104	75	237	0.9	23	0.00	0.00
0.05	0.05	0.60				3.0			20	0.54			22	285		75	0.00	0.00
0.15	0.17	1.98	0.20	0.00	41.6	0.0			12	1.82	5.7	28	47	174	0.3	12	0.00	0.00
0.15	0.17	2.00	0.20	0.00	40.0	0.0			16	1.79	8.0	32	68	190	0.6	10	0.00	0.00
0.15	0.17	1.98	0.20	0.00	41.6	0.0			15	1.82	8.3	44	59	220	0.6	12	0.00	0.00
0.15	0.15	1.98	0.20	0.00	52.0	0.0			20	1.82	15.1	44	82	229	0.3	12	0.00	
0.15	0.15	1.98	0.20	0.00	52.0	0.0			15	1.82	10.9	39	65	213	0.2	12	0.00	
						0.0			20	1.08				170		16	0.00	0.00
						0.0			0	0.72				260			0.00	0.00
0.03	0.07	0.30	0.00	0.07	2.3	0.1	3.5	0.3	42	0.50	9.1	40	57	45	0.2	39	0.02	
0.00	0.00	0.00	0.00	0.00	0.0	0.4	0.0	0.0	0	0.28	0.5	0	8	4	0.1	80	0.00	0.00
0.00	0.00	0.00	0.00	0.00	0.0	1.9		0.0	4	0.31	1.9	2	6	42	0.0	67	0.00	0.00
0.07	0.18	0.68	0.05	0.18	4.7	0.5		0.2	99	0.97	30.8	116	197	84	0.6	53	0.00	
0.03	0.15	0.34	0.05	0.18	7.3	0.5		0.1	95	0.34	12.0	98	151	57	0.4	52	0.00	0.00
0.02	0.15	0.11	0.02	0.05	10.4	0.0	2.6	0.1	87	0.40	21.8	77	204	55	0.2	71	0.00	2.60
						0.0			250	0.00				55			0.00	
						0.0			80	0.36				65		40	0.00	
						0.0			60	0.36				115			0.00	
						0.0	0.0		40	0.72				170			0.00	
						2.0	0.0		60	0.00				55		40	0.00	
						0.0	0.0		60	0.36				65			0.00	
0.03	0.15	0.07	0.03	0.43	7.7	0.7	24.9	0.5	113	0.18	10.3	100	152	52	0.4	60	0.00	0.00
						6.0			60	0.00				25			0.00	0.00
0.02	0.15	0.07	0.02	0.25	3.3	0.4	5.3	0.2	84	0.05	9.2	69	131	53	0.5	61	0.00	
0.02	0.17	0.10	0.02	0.31	4.8	0.0	0.0	0.0	101	0.00	14.3	102	205	66	0.7	64	0.00	
0.01	0.07	0.05	0.01	0.10	3.0	1.7	0.0	0.0	40	0.10	5.9	30	71	34	0.4	66	0.00	0.00
						1.2			60	1.08				250			0.00	0.00
						3.6			20	1.08				220			0.00	0.00
0.10	0.12	0.99	0.07	0.07	8.1	1.4		2.2	76	1.75	9.9	161	110	418	0.2	40	0.00	0.00
0.47	0.28	4.67	0.09	0.00	121.1	0.0		0.8	33	4.50	26.0	125	168	708	0.8	18	0.00	0.00
0.25	0.41	5.09	0.09	0.05	57.4	0.0	38.2	5.5	50	5.19	43.0	155	210	1365	1.1	4	0.00	0.00
0.02	0.02	0.31	0.03	0.00	31.6	3.7	0.0	1.8	13	0.52	8.2	28	76	235	0.2	52	0.00	0.00
0.09	0.12	0.64	0.02	0.18	19.3	0.5			67	0.41	11.0	154	104	267	0.3	51	0.00	0.00

Code	Food Name	Unit/ Amt	Wt (g)	Energy (kcal)	Prot (g)	Carb (g)	Fiber (g)	Fat (g)	Sat (g)	Mono (g)	Poly (g)	Chol (mg)	Vit A (RE)
48025	Pie, blueberry, 1/6 of 8"	1 slc	117	271	2	41	1	12	2.0	5.0	4.1	0	55
48005	Pie, cherry, 1/6 of 8"	1 slc	117	304	2	47	1	13	3.0	6.8	2.4	0	68
48031	Pie, chocolate cream, 1/6 of 8"	1 pce	113	344	3	38	2	22	5.6	12.6	2.7	6	0
71646	Pie, key lime, w/o topping, 10", FS	1 pce	113	420	6	55		20	12.0			20	40
48040	Pie, peach, 1/6 of 8"	1 pce	117	261	2	38	1	12	1.8	5.0	4.4	0	19
48012	Pie, pecan	1 pce	133	541	6	79	3	22	3.5	11.1	4.7	56	69
48000	Pie, pumpkin	1 pce	133	323	5	46	2	13	2.6	6.1	2.4	35	747
49015	Strudel, apple	1 pce	71	195	2	29	2	8	1.5	2.3	3.8	4	5
Puddings and Gelatins													
92977	Gelatin, cherry, sugar free, snack cup	1 svg	92	10	1	0	0	0	0.0	0.0	0.0	0	0
23337	Gelatin, grape, dry mix, svg	1 svg	22	80	2	19	0	0	0.0	0.0	0.0	0	0
23052	Gelatin, prep f/dry mix w/water	0.5 cup	135	84	2	19	0	0	0.0	0.0	0.0	0	0
48001	Pie Filling, apple, 21-oz can	1 oz	28	28	0	7	0	0				0	1
48015	Pie Filling, cherry, 21-oz can	1 oz	28	33	0	8	0	0		0.0	0.0	0	6
48044	Pie Filling, pumpkin, cnd	0.5 cup	135	140	1	36	11	0	0.1	0.0	0.0	0	1120
58203	Pudding, all flvrs, not choc, low cal, inst	1 svg	8	28	0	7	0	0	0.0	0.0	0.0	0	0
2649	Pudding, rice, prep f/dry mix w/2% milk	0.5 cup	140	155	5	29	0	2	1.4	0.6	0.1	8	66
57995	Pudding, Snack Pack, vanilla, fat free, FS	1 indv cup	99	90	2	20	0	0	0.0	0.0	0.0	0	0
Toppings													
46037	Frosting, chocolate, creamy, rte	2 Tbs	41	163	0	26	0	7	2.3	3.7	0.9	0	0
46039	Frosting, cream cheese, creamy, rte	2 Tbs	33	137	0	22	0	6	1.5	1.2	2.0	0	0
46330	Frosting, lemon	2 Tbs	33	140	0	23	0	5	1.0			0	0
54308	Syrup, caramel	2 Tbs	39	100	1	25	0	0	0.0	0.0	0.0	0	0
23437	Syrup, chocolate	2 Tbs	39	100	1	24		0	0.0	0.0	0.0	0	0
23069	Topping, butterscotch	2 Tbs	41	103	1	27	0	0	0.0	0.0	0.0	0	11
23070	Topping, caramel	2 Tbs	41	103	1	27	0	0	0.0	0.0	0.0	0	11
23014	Topping, chocolate fudge	2 Tbs	38	133	2	24	1	3	1.5	1.5	0.1	0	0
92528	Topping, hot fudge	1 Tbs	19	70	1	10		2	1.0			5	
23071	Topping, marshmallow cream, 7-oz jar	1 jar	198	638	2	156	0	1	0.1	0.2	0.1	0	0
23164	Topping, strawberry	2 Tbs	42	107	0	28	0	0	0.0	0.0	0.0	0	1
510	Topping, whipped cream, pressurized	1 Tbs	4	9	0	0	0	1	0.5	0.2	0.0	3	7
565	Topping, whipped, lite	2 Tbs	9	20	0	3		1	1.0			0	0
EGGS AND EGG SUBSTITUTES													
19581	Egg Substitute, new	0.25 cup	61	30	6	1	0	0	0.0	0.0	0.0	0	60
19507	Egg Whites, raw	0.25 cup	61	32	7	0	0	0				0	0
19510	Eggs, hard bld, lrg	1 ea	50	78	6	1	0	5	1.6	2.0	0.7	186	75
19509	Eggs, whole, lrg, fried	1 ea	46	90	6	0	0	7	2.0	2.8	1.5	184	102
19501	Eggs, whole, raw, lrg	1 ea	50	72	6	0	0	5	1.6	1.8	1.0	186	80
FATS, OILS, MARGARINES, AND SHORTENINGS													
8000	Butter, salted	1 Tbs	14	102	0	0	0	12	7.3	3.0	0.4	31	99
8003	Fat, bacon grease	1 Tbs	13	116	0	0	0	13	5.0	5.8	1.4	12	0
8084	Oil, canola	1 Tbs	14	124	0	0	0	14	1.0	8.9	3.9	0	0
8009	Oil, corn, salad or cooking	1 Tbs	14	120	0	0	0	14	1.8	3.8	7.4	0	0
8008	Oil, olive, salad or cooking	1 Tbs	14	119	0	0	0	14	1.9	9.8	1.4	0	0
90965	Oil, veg, pure	1 Tbs	14	120	0	0	0	14	1.5	6.0	6.0	0	0

Thia (mg)	Ribo (mg)	Niac (mg NE)	Vit B6 (mg)	Vit B12 (µg)	Fol (µg)	Vit C (mg)	Vit D (IU)	Vit E (mg AT)	Cal (mg)	Iron (mg)	Magn (mg)	Phos (mg)	Pota (mg)	Sodi (mg)	Zinc (mg)	Wat (%)	Alco (g)	Caff (g)
0.00	0.03	0.34	0.03	0.00	31.6	3.2	0.0	1.2	9	0.34	5.8	27	58	256	0.2	52	0.00	0.00
0.02	0.02	0.23	0.05	0.00	31.6	1.1	0.0	0.9	14	0.56	9.4	34	95	288	0.2	46	0.00	0.00
0.03	0.11	0.76	0.01	0.00	14.7	0.0			41	1.21	23.7	77	144	154	0.3	44	0.00	0.00
						0.0			150	0.72				200			0.00	0.00
0.07	0.03	0.23	0.02	0.00	33.9	1.1	0.0	1.1	9	0.57	7.0	26	146	227	0.1	54	0.00	0.00
0.27	0.10	1.74	0.05	0.15	42.6	0.0	6.7	1.1	29	1.24	29.3	110	132	210	1.2	18	0.00	0.00
0.23	0.15	1.47	0.07	0.46	34.6	0.0	4.0	1.0	85	1.20	18.6	108	222	450	0.5	50	0.00	0.00
0.02	0.01	0.23	0.02	0.15	19.9	1.2	0.0	1.0	11	0.30	6.4	23	106	111	0.1	44	0.00	0.00
						0.0			0	0.00				45			0.00	0.00
						0.0			0	0.00				80	1		0.00	0.00
0.00	0.00	0.00	0.00	0.00	1.4	0.0	0.0	0.0	4	0.02	1.4	30	1	101	0.0	84	0.00	0.00
0.00	0.00	0.00	0.00	0.00	0.0	0.5	0.0	0.0	1	0.07	0.6	2	13	13	0.0	73	0.00	0.00
0.00	0.00	0.03	0.00	0.00	1.1	1.0	0.0		3	0.07	2.0	4	30	5	0.0	71	0.00	0.00
0.01	0.15	0.50	0.20	0.00	47.2	4.7	0.0		50	1.42	21.6	61	186	281	0.4	71	0.00	0.00
0.00	0.00	0.00	0.00	0.00	0.1	0.0	0.0	0.0	11	0.02	0.4	189	2	340	0.0	7	0.00	0.00
0.10	0.20	0.62	0.05	0.34	5.6	1.0	47.6		147	0.51	18.2	122	182	153	0.5	73	0.00	0.00
						0.0			60	0.00				160			0.00	0.00
0.00	0.00	0.05	0.00	0.00	0.4	0.0	0.0	0.6	3	0.57	8.6	32	80	75	0.1	17	0.00	0.81
0.00	0.00	0.00	0.00	0.00	0.0	0.0			1	0.05	0.7	1	12	63	0.0	15	0.00	0.00
						0.0			0	0.00			15	70		5	0.00	0.00
						0.0			20	0.00				105		13	0.00	0.00
						0.0			0	0.36				25		14	0.00	7.00
0.00	0.03	0.01	0.00	0.03	0.8	0.1	0.0		22	0.07	2.9	19	34	143	0.1	32	0.00	0.00
0.00	0.03	0.01	0.00	0.03	0.8	0.1	0.0		22	0.07	2.9	19	34	143	0.1	32	0.00	0.00
0.00	0.02	0.09	0.00	0.01	1.5	0.1	0.0	1.0	19	0.49	18.2	37	108	131	0.3	22	0.00	2.66
														80	0.00	5		
0.00	0.00	0.15	0.00	0.00	2.0	0.0	0.0	0.0	6	0.43	4.0	16	10	158	0.1	20	0.00	0.00
0.00	0.00	0.07	0.00	0.00	2.5	5.8	0.0	0.0	3	0.11	1.7	2	21	9	0.0	33	0.00	0.00
0.00	0.00	0.00	0.00	0.00	0.1	0.0	0.6	0.0	4	0.00	0.4	3	5	5	0.0	61	0.00	0.00
						0.0			0	0.00				0		5	0.00	0.00
	0.85		0.07	0.60	32.0	0.0	16.0	0.8	20	1.08			85	125	0.6		0.00	0.00
0.00	0.27	0.05	0.00	0.05	2.4	0.0	0.0	0.0	4	0.05	6.7	9	99	101	0.0	88	0.00	0.00
0.02	0.25	0.02	0.05	0.56	22.0	0.0	43.5	0.5	25	0.60	5.0	86	63	62	0.5	75	0.00	0.00
0.01	0.23	0.03	0.07	0.44	23.5	0.0	40.5	0.6	29	0.87	6.0	99	70	95	0.6	69	0.00	0.00
0.01	0.23	0.03	0.09	0.43	23.5	0.0	41.0	0.5	28	0.87	6.0	99	69	71	0.6	76	0.00	0.00
0.00	0.00	0.00	0.00	0.01	0.4	0.0	8.5	0.3	3	0.00	0.3	3	3	101	0.0	16	0.00	0.00
0.00	0.00	0.00	0.00	0.00	0.0	0.0	13.0	0.1	0	0.00	0.0	0	0	19	0.0	0	0.00	0.00
0.00	0.00	0.00	0.00	0.00	0.0	0.0	0.0	2.4	0	0.00	0.0	0	0	0	0.0	0	0.00	0.00
0.00	0.00	0.00	0.00	0.00	0.0	0.0	0.0	1.9	0	0.00	0.0	0	0	0	0.0	0	0.00	0.00
0.00	0.00	0.00	0.00	0.00	0.0	0.0	0.0	1.9	0	0.07	0.0	0	0	0	0.0	0	0.00	0.00
						0.0	3.0		0	0.00				0		0	0.00	0.00

PAGE KEY: A-42 Beverages and Beverage Mixes   A-44 Candies   A-46 Cereals   A-48 Cheeses and Substitutes   A-50 Dairy Products and Substitutes   A-52 Desserts   A-56 Eggs and Egg Substitutes   A-56 Fats, Oils, Margarines, and Shortenings   A-58 Fruits   A-60 Grain Products and Baked Goods   A-62 Grains and Flours   A-64 Meats and Meat Substitutes   A-68 Nuts, Seeds, and Products

Code	Food Name	Unit/ Amt	Wt (g)	Energy (kcal)	Prot (g)	Carb (g)	Fiber (g)	Fat (g)	Sat (g)	Mono (g)	Poly (g)	Chol (mg)	Vit A (RE)
8135	Margarine & Butter, blend, w/soybean oil	1 Tbs	14	101	0	0	0	11	2.0	4.3	3.4	2	123
8490	Margarine, soft, safflower oil	1 Tbs	14	100	0	0	0	11	1.4	6.7	1.9	0	50
8007	Shortening, household, part hydrog, soybean & cttnsd oil	1 Tbs	13	113	0	0	0	13	3.2	5.7	3.3	0	0
90963	Shortening, veg	1 Tbs	12	110	0	0	0	12	3.0	4.0	3.0	0	0
250	Spread, Benecol	1 Tbs	14	70	0	0	0	8	1.0	4.5	2.0	0	100
44437	Spread, light, tub	1 Tbs	14	50	0	0	0	5	1.0	1.5	2.5	0	100
FRUITS													
Dried Fruits													
23404	Fruit Leather, roll, lrg	1 ea	21	78	0	18	0	1	0.1	0.3	0.1	0	1
3202	Raisins, golden, seedless, packed cup	0.25 cup	41	125	1	33	2	0	0.1	0.0	0.1	0	0
Canned Fruits													
3147	Applesauce, swtnd, cnd	1 cup	246	167	0	43	3	0	0.1	0.0	0.1	0	1
71774	Mandarin Oranges, cnd, w/light syrup	0.5 cup	126	77	1	20	1	0	0.0	0.0	0.0	0	106
27169	Olives, black, jumbo, cnd	1 ea	8	7	0	0	0	1	0.1	0.4	0.0	0	3
9539	Olives, green, pickled, cnd	1 ea	3	4	0	0	0	0	0.1	0.3	0.0	0	1
71114	Pineapple, chunks, cnd, w/juice	0.5 cup	124	75	1	20	1	0	0.0	0.0	0.0	0	5
Fresh and Frozen Fruits													
3001	Apples, fresh, med 3", USDA	1 ea	182	95	0	25	4	0	0.1	0.0	0.1	0	10
3157	Apricots, whole, fresh, USDA	1 ea	35	17	0	4	1	0	0.0	0.1	0.0	0	67
3016	Avocado, avg, fresh	1 ea	201	322	4	17	13	29	4.3	19.7	3.7	0	29
3020	Banana, fresh, med, 7" to 7 7/8" long	1 ea	118	105	1	27	3	0	0.1	0.0	0.1	0	8
3029	Blueberries, fresh	0.5 cup	74	42	1	11	2	0	0.0	0.0	0.1	0	4
3036	Cherries, sweet, fresh	0.5 cup	77	49	1	12	2	0	0.0	0.0	0.0	0	5
3770	Chicle, fresh, pulp	0.5 cup	120	100	1	24	6	1	0.2	0.6	0.0	0	7
3191	Currants, red, fresh	0.25 cup	28	16	0	4	1	0	0.0	0.0	0.0	0	1
3676	Figs, fresh, lrg, 2 1/2"	1 ea	64	47	0	12	2	0	0.0	0.0	0.1	0	9
3818	Grapefruit, pink, fresh, 3 3/4"	0.5 ea	123	52	1	13	2	0	0.0	0.0	0.0	0	141
3820	Grapefruit, red, fresh, 3 3/4"	0.5 ea	123	52	1	13	2	0	0.0	0.0	0.0	0	141
3055	Grapes, Thompson seedless, fresh	0.5 cup	76	52	1	14	1	0	0.0	0.0	0.0	0	5
3634	Guava, fresh	0.5 cup	82	56	2	12	4	1	0.2	0.1	0.3	0	51
3249	Java Plum, fresh	1 ea	3	2	0	0		0				0	0
3065	Kiwi, fresh, 2"	1 ea	69	42	1	10	2	0	0.0	0.05	0.2	0	6
3071	Limes, peeled, fresh, 2"	1 ea	67	20	0	7	2	0	0.0	0.0	0.0	0	3
71769	Mandarin Oranges, fresh, med, 2 1/2"	1 ea	88	47	1	12	2	0	0.0	0.1	0.1	0	60
3221	Mango, fresh, whole	1 ea	336	202	3	50	5	1	0.3	0.5	0.2	0	364
3076	Melon, cantaloupe, fresh, med, 5"	0.25 ea	138	47	1	11	1	0	0.1	0.0	0.1	0	467
71102	Melon, honeydew, fresh, 5 1/4"	1 ea	1000	360	5	91	8	1	0.4	0.0	0.6	0	50
3215	Nectarines, fresh, medium 2 1/2"	1 ea	142	62	2	15	2	0	0.0	0.1	0.2	0	47
3082	Oranges, all types, fresh, med, 2 5/8"	1 ea	131	62	1	15	3	0	0.0	0.0	0.0	0	29
3720	Papaya, fresh, lrg	0.25 ea	195	84	1	21	3	1	0.2	0.1	0.1	0	185
3199	Passion Fruit, purple, fresh	0.5 cup	118	114	3	28	12	1	0.1	0.1	0.5	0	150
3096	Peaches, fresh, med, w/o skin, 2.66"	1 ea	150	58	1	14	2	0	0.0	0.1	0.1	0	49
3103	Pears, fresh, med	1 ea	178	103	1	28	6	0	0.0	0.0	0.1	0	4
3112	Pineapple, fresh	1 ea	905	452	5	119	13	1	0.1	0.1	0.4	0	52
3745	Plantain, fresh, med	1 ea	179	218	2	57	4	1	0.3	0.1	0.1	0	202
3121	Plums, fresh, 2 1/8"	1 ea	66	30	0	8	1	0	0.0	0.1	0.0	0	23

PAGE KEY: A-70 Prepared Foods A-78 Restaurants A-90 Salad Dressings and Dips A-92 Sauces and Gravies A-94 Snack Foods A-94 Spices, Flavors, and Seasonings A-96 Sports Bars and Drinks A-96 Supplemental Foods and Formulas A-96 Sweeteners and Sweet Substitutes A-98 Vegetables and Legumes A-108 Miscellaneous

Thia (mg)	Ribo (mg)	Niac (mg NE)	Vit B6 (mg)	Vit B12 (µg)	Fol (µg)	Vit C (mg)	Vit D (IU)	Vit E (mg AT)	Cal (mg)	Iron (mg)	Magn (mg)	Phos (mg)	Pota (mg)	Sodi (mg)	Zinc (mg)	Wat (%)	Alco (g)	Caff (g)
0.00	0.00	0.00	0.00	0.00	0.3	0.0	0.1	0.5	1	0.00	0.1	1	3	89	0.0	17	0.00	0.00
						0.0		3.0	0	0.00				90		3	0.00	0.00
0.00	0.00	0.00	0.00	0.00	0.0	0.0	0.0	0.8	0	0.00	0.0	0	0	0	0.0	0	0.00	0.00
						0.0		3.0	0	0.00				0		0	0.00	0.00
						0.0		2.7	0	0.00				110		6	0.00	0.00
						0.0			0	0.00				90		9	0.00	0.00
0.01	0.00	0.01	0.05	0.00	0.4	25.2	0.0	0.1	7	0.20	4.2	7	62	67	0.0	10	0.00	0.00
0.00	0.07	0.46	0.12	0.00	1.2	1.3	0.0	0.0	22	0.74	14.4	47	308	5	0.1	15	0.00	0.00
0.03	0.05	0.18	0.07	0.00	2.5	4.2	0.0	0.4	7	0.30	7.4	15	184	5	0.1	82	0.00	0.00
0.07	0.05	0.56	0.05	0.00	6.3	24.9	0.0	0.1	9	0.46	10.1	13	98	8	0.3	83	0.00	0.00
0.00	0.00	0.00	0.00	0.00	0.0	0.1	0.0	0.1	8	0.28	0.3	0	1	61	0.0	84	0.00	0.00
0.00	0.00	0.00	0.00	0.00	0.1	0.0	0.0	0.1	1	0.00	0.3	0	1	42	0.0	75	0.00	0.00
0.11	0.01	0.34	0.09	0.00	6.2	11.8	0.0	0.0	17	0.34	17.4	7	152	1	0.1	84	0.00	0.00
0.02	0.05	0.17	0.07	0.00	5.5	8.4	0.0	0.3	11	0.21	9.1	20	195	2	0.1	86	0.00	0.00
0.00	0.00	0.20	0.01	0.00	3.1	3.5	0.0	0.3	5	0.14	3.5	8	91	0	0.1	86	0.00	0.00
0.12	0.25	3.49	0.51	0.00	162.8	20.1	0.0	4.2	24	1.11	58.3	105	975	14	1.3	73	0.00	0.00
0.03	0.09	0.77	0.43	0.00	23.6	10.3	0.0	0.1	6	0.31	31.9	26	422	1	0.2	75	0.00	0.00
0.02	0.02	0.31	0.03	0.00	4.4	7.2	0.0	0.4	4	0.20	4.4	9	57	1	0.1	84	0.00	0.00
0.01	0.02	0.11	0.03	0.00	3.1	5.4	0.0	0.1	10	0.28	8.5	16	171	0	0.1	82	0.00	0.00
0.00	0.01	0.23	0.03	0.00	16.9	17.7			25	0.95	14.5	14	233	14	0.1	78	0.00	0.00
0.00	0.00	0.02	0.01	0.00	2.2	11.5	0.0	0.0	9	0.28	3.6	12	77	0	0.1	84	0.00	0.00
0.03	0.02	0.25	0.07	0.00	3.8	1.3	0.0	0.1	22	0.23	10.9	9	148	1	0.1	79	0.00	0.00
0.05	0.03	0.25	0.07	0.00	16.0	38.4	0.0	0.2	27	0.10	11.1	22	166	0	0.1	88	0.00	0.00
0.05	0.03	0.25	0.07	0.00	16.0	38.4	0.0	0.2	27	0.10	11.1	22	166	0	0.1	88	0.00	0.00
0.05	0.05	0.14	0.05	0.00	1.5	8.2	0.0	0.1	8	0.27	5.3	15	144	2	0.1	81	0.00	0.00
0.05	0.02	0.88	0.09	0.00	40.4	188.3	0.0	0.6	15	0.20	18.1	33	344	2	0.2	81	0.00	0.00
0.00	0.00	0.00	0.00	0.00		0.4			1	0.00	0.4	1	2	0		83	0.00	0.00
0.01	0.01	0.23	0.03	0.00	17.2	64.0	0.0	1.0	23	0.20	11.7	23	215	2	0.1	83	0.00	0.00
0.01	0.00	0.12	0.02	0.00	5.4	19.5	0.0	0.1	22	0.40	4.0	12	68	1	0.1	88	0.00	0.00
0.05	0.02	0.33	0.07	0.00	14.1	23.5	0.0	0.2	33	0.12	10.6	18	146	2	0.1	85	0.00	0.00
0.09	0.12	2.25	0.40	0.00	144.5	122.3	0.0	3.0	37	0.54	33.6	47	564	3	0.3	83	0.00	0.00
0.05	0.02	1.00	0.10	0.00	29.0	50.6	0.0	0.1	12	0.28	16.6	21	368	22	0.2	90	0.00	0.00
0.37	0.11	4.17	0.87	0.00	190.0	180.0	0.0	0.2	60	1.70	100.0	110	2280	180	0.9	90	0.00	0.00
0.05	0.03	1.60	0.03	0.00	7.1	7.7	0.0	1.1	9	0.40	12.8	37	285	0	0.2	88	0.00	0.00
0.10	0.05	0.37	0.07	0.00	39.3	69.7	0.0	0.2	52	0.12	13.1	18	237	0	0.1	87	0.00	0.00
0.03	0.05	0.69	0.07	0.00	72.2	118.9	0.0	0.6	39	0.49	41.0	20	355	16	0.2	88	0.00	0.00
0.00	0.15	1.76	0.11	0.00	16.5	35.4	0.0	0.0	14	1.88	34.2	80	411	33	0.1	73	0.00	0.00
0.03	0.05	1.21	0.03	0.00	6.0	9.9	0.0	1.1	9	0.37	13.5	30	285	0	0.3	89	0.00	0.00
0.01	0.03	0.28	0.05	0.00	12.5	7.5	0.0	0.2	16	0.30	12.5	20	212	2	0.2	84	0.00	0.00
0.70	0.28	4.53	1.00	0.00	162.9	432.6	0.0	0.2	118	2.61	108.6	72	986	9	1.1	86	0.00	0.00
0.09	0.10	1.23	0.54	0.00	39.4	32.9	0.0	0.3	5	1.07	66.2	61	893	7	0.3	65	0.00	0.00
0.01	0.01	0.28	0.01	0.00	3.3	6.3	0.0	0.2	4	0.10	4.6	11	104	0	0.1	87	0.00	0.00

PAGE KEY: A-42 Beverages and Beverage Mixes   A-44 Candies   A-46 Cereals   A-48 Cheeses and Substitutes   A-50 Dairy Products and Substitutes   A-52 Desserts   A-56 Eggs and Egg Substitutes   A-56 Fats, Oils, Margarines, and Shortenings   A-58 Fruits   A-60 Grain Products and Baked Goods   A-62 Grains and Flours   A-64 Meats and Meat Substitutes   A-68 Nuts, Seeds, and Products

Code	Food Name	Unit/ Amt	Wt (g)	Energy (kcal)	Prot (g)	Carb (g)	Fiber (g)	Fat (g)	Sat (g)	Mono (g)	Poly (g)	Chol (mg)	Vit A (RE)
3197	Pomegranate, fresh, 4"	1 ea	282	234	5	53	11	3	0.3	0.3	0.2	0	0
3648	Raspberries, fresh	0.5 cup	62	32	1	7	4	0	0.0	0.0	0.2	0	2
3209	Rhubarb, fresh, diced	0.5 cup	61	13	1	3	1	0	0.0	0.0	0.1	0	6
3134	Strawberries, fresh, whole	0.5 cup	72	23	0	6	1	0	0.0	0.0	0.1	0	1
71991	Tangelo, fresh, med	1 ea	109	50	1	15	3	0	0.0			0	0
3717	Tangerines, fresh, lrg, 2 3/4"	1 ea	120	64	1	16	2	0	0.0	0.1	0.1	0	82
3143	Watermelon, fresh, 1/16 melon	1 pce	286	86	2	22	1	0	0.0	0.1	0.1	0	163

GRAIN PRODUCTS AND BAKED GOODS

Bars

Code	Food Name	Unit/ Amt	Wt (g)	Energy (kcal)	Prot (g)	Carb (g)	Fiber (g)	Fat (g)	Sat (g)	Mono (g)	Poly (g)	Chol (mg)	Vit A (RE)
53227	Bar, cereal, mixed berry	1 ea	37	137	2	27	1	3	0.6	1.9	0.4	0	150
23100	Bar, granola, almond, hard	1 ea	24	119	2	15	1	6	3.0	1.9	0.9	0	1
47591	Bar, granola, cinnamon	1 ea	21	90	2	14	1	3	0.2			0	0
63342	Bar, granola, oat, fruit & nut	1 ea	28	111	2	22	1	2	0.2	0.0	1.4	0	8
47592	Bar, granola, oats 'n honey	1 ea	21	90	2	14	1	3	0.2			0	0
23059	Bar, granola, plain, hard	1 ea	25	118	3	16	1	5	0.6	1.1	3.0	0	8

Breads and Rolls

Code	Food Name	Unit/ Amt	Wt (g)	Energy (kcal)	Prot (g)	Carb (g)	Fiber (g)	Fat (g)	Sat (g)	Mono (g)	Poly (g)	Chol (mg)	Vit A (RE)
71165	Bagel, egg, 3"	1 ea	69	192	7	37	2	1	0.3	0.3	0.4	17	23
42001	Biscuit, buttermilk, prep f/recipe, 2.5"	1 ea	60	212	4	27	1	10	2.6	4.2	2.5	2	10
71195	Biscuit, plain, prep f/recipe, 2.5"	1 ea	60	212	4	27	1	10	2.6	4.2	2.5	2	10
42205	Biscuit, whole wheat	1 ea	63	199	6	30	5	7	1.7	3.0	2.2	2	14
42004	Bread Crumbs, plain, grated, dry	0.25 cup	27	107	4	19	1	1	0.3	0.3	0.6	0	0
42042	Bread, cracked wheat, reg slice	1 slc	25	65	2	12	1	1	0.2	0.5	0.2	0	0
42530	Bread, French, hot & crusty twin, 4" slice	4	50	150	5	29	1	2	0.5			0	0
71207	Bread, French, lrg slice	1 slc	96	277	11	54	2	2	0.5	0.3	0.8	0	0
42047	Bread, multigrain, slice	1 slc	26	69	3	11	2	1	0.2	0.2	0.5	0	0
42049	Bread, oatmeal, slice	1 slc	27	73	2	13	1	1	0.2	0.4	0.5	0	1
42007	Bread, pita, white, enrich, lrg, 6 1/2"	1 ea	60	165	5	33	1	1	0.1	0.1	0.3	0	0
42051	Bread, raisin, enrich, slice	1 slc	26	71	2	14	1	1	0.3	0.6	0.2	0	0
57235	Bread, rye, mild	1 pce	32	70	3	13	4	0	0.0			0	0
42012	Bread, wheat, slice	1 slc	25	66	3	12	1	1	0.2	0.2	0.4	0	0
42138	Bread, white, prep f/recipe w/2% milk, slice	1 slc	42	120	3	21	1	2	0.5	0.5	1.2	1	10
71020	Bread, whole grain, slice	1 slc	26	69	3	11	2	1	0.2	0.2	0.5	0	0
71939	Bread, wraps, thin thin	1 ea	35	109	4	21	0	1	0.0			0	0
42036	Breadsticks, plain, 7 5/8" x 5/8"	1 ea	10	41	1	7	0	1	0.1	0.4	0.4	0	0
42020	Bun, hamburger	1 ea	43	120	4	21	1	2	0.5	0.5	0.8	0	0
42021	Bun, hot dog/frankfurter	1 ea	43	120	4	21	1	2	0.5	0.5	0.8	0	0
42504	Bun, sandwich	1 ea	46	130	5	22	1	3	1.0			0	0
42115	Cornbread, prep f/dry mix, pce	1 pce	60	188	4	29	1	6	1.6	3.1	0.7	37	28
42016	Croutons, plain, dry	0.25 cup	8	31	1	6	0	0	0.1	0.2	0.1	0	0
42015	Croissant, butter, med	1 ea	57	231	5	26	1	12	6.6	3.1	0.6	38	120
42394	English Muffin	1 ea	57	130	5	25	1	1	0.0			0	0
44515	Muffin, plain, prep f/recipe w/2% milk	1 ea	57	169	4	24	2	6	1.2	1.6	3.3	22	23
42018	Roll, dinner, brown & serve	1 ea	28	87	3	15	1	2	0.4	0.5	0.7	1	0
42022	Roll, hard, 3 1/2"	1 ea	57	167	6	30	1	2	0.3	0.6	1.0	0	0
71358	Roll, hoagie, whole wheat, med	1 ea	94	250	8	48	7	4	0.8	1.1	2.0	0	0

PAGE KEY: A-70 Prepared Foods   A-78 Restaurants   A-90 Salad Dressings and Dips   A-92 Sauces and Gravies   A-94 Snack Foods   A-94 Spices, Flavors, and Seasonings   A-96 Sports Bars and Drinks   A-96 Supplemental Foods and Formulas   A-96 Sweeteners and Sweet Substitutes   A-98 Vegetables and Legumes   A-108 Miscellaneous

Thia (mg)	Ribo (mg)	Niac (mg NE)	Vit B6 (mg)	Vit B12 (μg)	Fol (μg)	Vit C (mg)	Vit D (IU)	Vit E (mg AT)	Cal (mg)	Iron (mg)	Magn (mg)	Phos (mg)	Pota (mg)	Sodi (mg)	Zinc (mg)	Wat (%)	Alco (g)	Caff (g)
0.18	0.15	0.82	0.20	0.00	107.2	28.8	0.0	1.7	28	0.85	33.8	102	666	8	1.0	78	0.00	0.00
0.01	0.01	0.37	0.02	0.00	12.9	16.1	0.0	0.5	15	0.41	13.5	18	93	1	0.3	86	0.00	0.00
0.00	0.01	0.18	0.00	0.00	4.3	4.9	0.0	0.2	52	0.12	7.3	9	176	2	0.1	94	0.00	0.00
0.01	0.01	0.28	0.02	0.00	17.3	42.3	0.0	0.2	12	0.30	9.4	17	110	1	0.1	91	0.00	0.00
				0.00		30.0			40	0.00				0		92	0.00	0.00
0.07	0.03	0.44	0.09	0.00	19.2	32.0	0.0	0.2	44	0.18	14.4	24	199	2	0.1	85	0.00	0.00
0.09	0.05	0.50	0.12	0.00	8.6	23.2	0.0	0.1	20	0.68	28.6	31	320	3	0.3	91	0.00	0.00
0.37	0.40	4.98	0.51	0.00	40.0	0.0			14	1.80	9.6	36	70	105	1.5	14	0.00	0.00
0.07	0.01	0.15	0.00	0.00	2.9	0.0			8	0.60	19.4	55	66	61	0.4	3	0.00	0.00
						0.0			0	0.54				80		2	0.00	0.00
0.14	0.11	1.42	0.21	0.00	44.8	0.0	0.0	0.3	10	1.48	23.8	68	67	70	0.5	7	0.00	0.00
						0.0			0	0.54				80		2	0.00	0.00
0.07	0.02	0.40	0.01	0.00	5.8	0.2			15	0.74	24.2	69	84	74	0.5	4	0.00	0.00
0.37	0.15	2.38	0.05	0.10	60.7	0.4			9	2.75	17.2	58	47	348	0.5	33	0.00	0.00
0.20	0.18	1.76	0.01	0.05	36.6	0.1			141	1.74	10.8	98	73	348	0.3	29	0.00	0.00
0.20	0.18	1.76	0.01	0.05	36.6	0.1			141	1.74	10.8	98	73	348	0.3	29	0.00	0.00
0.15	0.11	2.20	0.12	0.07	13.0	0.2	10.1	1.3	155	1.69	56.9	199	200	210	1.2	28	0.00	0.00
0.25	0.10	1.78	0.02	0.09	28.9	0.0	0.0	0.0	49	1.29	11.6	45	53	198	0.4	7	0.00	0.00
0.09	0.05	0.92	0.07	0.00	15.2	0.0			11	0.69	13.0	38	44	134	0.3	36	0.00	0.00
0.23	0.17	2.00			40.0	0.0			60	1.44				300		14	0.00	0.00
0.41	0.28	4.57	0.10	0.00	142.1	0.2	0.0	0.2	42	3.48	26.9	109	123	492	0.9	28	0.00	0.00
0.07	0.02	1.04	0.07	0.00	19.5	0.0	0.0	0.1	27	0.64	20.3	59	60	109	0.4	37	0.00	0.00
0.10	0.05	0.85	0.01	0.00	16.7	0.0	0.0	0.1	18	0.73	10.0	34	38	127	0.3	37	0.00	0.00
0.36	0.20	2.77	0.01	0.00	64.2	0.0	0.0	0.2	52	1.57	15.6	58	72	322	0.5	32	0.00	0.00
0.09	0.10	0.89	0.01	0.00	27.6	0.0	0.0	0.1	17	0.75	6.8	28	59	81	0.2	34	0.00	0.00
0.15	0.14	3.00	0.30	0.89	80.0	0.0			100	1.79	60.0			70	2.2	15	0.00	0.00
0.09	0.07	1.29	0.02	0.00	21.2	0.1	0.0	0.0	36	0.87	12.0	39	46	130	0.3	36	0.00	0.00
0.17	0.15	1.50	0.01	0.02	38.2	0.1			24	1.25	8.0	48	61	151	0.3	35	0.00	0.00
0.07	0.02	1.04	0.07	0.00	19.5	0.0		0.1	27	0.64	20.3	59	60	109	0.4	37	0.00	0.00
						0.0			40	1.41				188			0.00	0.00
0.05	0.05	0.52	0.00	0.00	16.2	0.0	0.0	0.1	2	0.43	3.2	12	12	66	0.1	6	0.00	0.00
0.17	0.14	1.78	0.02	0.09	47.7	0.0	0.0	0.0	59	1.42	9.0	27	40	206	0.3	35	0.00	0.00
0.17	0.14	1.78	0.02	0.09	47.7	0.0	0.0	0.0	59	1.42	9.0	27	40	206	0.3	35	0.00	0.00
0.23	0.14	1.20			32.0	0.0			40	1.08				220		15	0.00	0.00
0.15	0.15	1.23	0.05	0.10	33.0	0.1			44	1.13	12.0	226	77	467	0.4	32	0.00	0.00
0.05	0.01	0.40	0.00	0.00	9.9	0.0			6	0.31	2.3	9	9	52	0.1	6	0.00	0.00
0.21	0.14	1.25	0.02	0.00	50.2	0.1	0.0	0.5	21	1.15	9.1	60	67	198	0.4	23	0.00	0.00
0.21	0.17	2.00			40.0	0.0			0	1.79				170		25	0.00	0.00
0.15	0.17	1.32	0.01	0.09	29.1	0.2			114	1.36	9.7	87	69	266	0.3	38	0.00	0.00
0.15	0.10	1.50	0.02	0.03	28.3	0.1	0.0	0.1	50	1.03	7.3	34	39	150	0.3	28	0.00	0.00
0.27	0.18	2.42	0.01	0.00	54.1	0.0	0.0	0.2	54	1.87	15.4	57	62	310	0.5	31	0.00	0.00
0.23	0.14	3.46	0.18	0.00	28.2	0.0	0.0	0.8	100	2.26	79.9	211	256	377	1.9	33	0.00	0.00

PAGE KEY: A-42 Beverages and Beverage Mixes   A-44 Candies   A-46 Cereals   A-48 Cheeses and Substitutes   A-50 Dairy Products and Substitutes   A-52 Desserts   A-56 Eggs and Egg Substitutes   A-56 Fats, Oils, Margarines, and Shortenings   A-58 Fruits   A-60 Grain Products and Baked Goods   A-62 Grains and Flours   A-64 Meats and Meat Substitutes   A-68 Nuts, Seeds, and Products

Code	Food Name	Unit/ Amt	Wt (g)	Energy (kcal)	Prot (g)	Carb (g)	Fiber (g)	Fat (g)	Sat (g)	Mono (g)	Poly (g)	Chol (mg)	Vit A (RE)
42185	Roll, Mexican, bolillo	1 ea	117	307	10	61	2	2	0.5	0.2	0.6	1	4
71359	Roll, submarine, whole wheat, med	1 ea	94	250	8	48	7	4	0.8	1.1	2.0	0	0
42037	Stuffing, bread, prep f/dry mix	0.5 cup	100	177	3	22	3	9	1.7	3.8	2.6	0	125
Crackers													
90163	Cookies, biscuit, arrowroot	1 ea	5	22	0	4	0	1	0.2	0.4	0.1	0	0
43503	Cracker Crumbs, graham, plain	1 cup	84	355	6	65	2	8	1.3	3.4	3.2	0	0
47026	Crackers, animal	6 ea	15	67	1	11	0	2	0.5	1.1	0.3	0	0
70963	Crackers, butter, Ritz, original	5 ea	16	79	1	10	0	4	0.9	1.0	1.7		
71273	Crackers, cheese, 1" square	15 ea	15	75	2	9	0	4	1.4	1.8	0.4	2	4
11717	Crackers, Club, original	4 ea	14	70	1	9	0	3	1.0	1.0	1.0	0	0
47378	Crackers, graham, honey	8 ea	31	140	2	23	1	4	1.0	1.5	1.0	0	0
43535	Crackers, matzoh, egg	1 ea	28	109	3	22	1	1	0.2	0.2	0.1	23	4
43509	Crackers, melba toast, plain, pce, 3 3/4" x 1 3/4" x 1/8"	3 ea	15	59	2	11	1	0	0.1	0.1	0.2	0	0
43506	Crackers, saltine	5 ea	15	63	1	11	0	1	0.3	0.3	0.6	0	0
43581	Crackers, wheat, original	16 ea	31	150	3	21	1	6	1.0			0	0
Pancakes, French Toast, and Waffles													
42156	French Toast, prep f/recipe w/2% milk	1 pce	65	149	5	16		7	1.8	2.9	1.7	75	84
45192	Pancakes, buttermilk, fzn	1 ea	39	90	2	15	0	3	0.6	1.1	0.8	4	67
45072	Waffles, buttermilk, fzn	2 ea	71	179	4	29	1	6	1.4	1.9	0.5	6	0
Pastas													
38048	Chow Mein Noodles, dry	0.5 cup	22	119	2	13	1	7	1.0	1.7	3.9	0	0
91205	Pasta, acini di pepe, enrich, dry	1 svg	57	207	8	42	2	1	0.2			0	0
38365	Pasta, egg, FS	0.75 cup	68	200	8	33	1	4	1.0			40	0
91211	Pasta, lasagna, enrich, dry	1 svg	55	200	7	41	2	1	0.2			0	0
38102	Pasta, macaroni, enrich, ckd	1 cup	140	221	8	43	3	1	0.2	0.2	0.4	0	0
38551	Pasta, rice, ckd	1 cup	176	192	2	44	2	0	0.0	0.0	0.0	0	0
38580	Pasta, semolina, elbow, twists, dry	0.75 cup	56	201	7	41	2	1	0.3	0.2	0.8	0	0
38105	Pasta, shells, sml, enrich, ckd	1 cup	115	182	7	35	2	1	0.2	0.2	0.4	0	0
38118	Pasta, spaghetti, enrich, ckd	1 cup	140	221	8	43	3	1	0.2	0.2	0.4	0	0
49116	Wrappers, egg roll, 7" square	1 ea	32	93	3	19	1	0	0.1	0.1	0.2	3	1
Tortillas and Taco Shells													
42359	Taco Shells, corn, yellow	2 ea	28	120	2	19	2	5	1.0	2.0	0.5	0	0
42023	Tortilla, corn, rtb	1 ea	24	52	1	11	2	1	0.1	0.2	0.3	0	0
90646	Tortilla, flour, rtb, 6"	1 ea	30	94	2	15	1	2	0.6	1.2	0.5	0	0
GRAINS AND FLOURS													
38030	Flour, all purpose, white, bleached, enriched	0.25 cup	31	114	3	24	1	0	0.0	0.0	0.1	0	0
46086	Flour, cake, white, enriched, unsifted	0.25 cup	34	124	3	27	1	0	0.0	0.0	0.1	0	0
38032	Flour, whole wheat	0.25 cup	30	102	4	22	3	1	0.1	0.1	0.4	0	0
38017	Oats, rolled, old fashioned, dry	0.5 cup	40	150	5	27	4	3	0.5	1.0	1.0	0	0
38010	Rice, brown, long grain, ckd	0.5 cup	98	108	3	22	2	1	0.2	0.3	0.3	0	0
38082	Rice, brown, med grain, ckd	0.5 cup	98	109	2	23	2	1	0.2	0.3	0.3	0	0
38013	Rice, white, long grain, ckd	0.5 cup	79	103	2	22	0	0	0.1	0.1	0.1	0	0
38021	Rice, wild, ckd	0.5 cup	82	83	3	17	1	0	0.0	0.0	0.2	0	0
2730	Tapioca, quick cooking, dry	1.5 tsp	6	20	0	5	0	0	0.0	0.0	0.0	0	0
38027	Wheat, bulgur, dry	0.25 cup	35	120	4	27	6	0	0.1	0.1	0.2	0	0
38068	Wheat, sprouted	0.25 cup	27	53	2	11	0	0	0.1	0.0	0.2	0	0

PAGE KEY: A-70 Prepared Foods   A-78 Restaurants   A-90 Salad Dressings and Dips   A-92 Sauces and Gravies   A-94 Snack Foods   A-94 Spices, Flavors, and Seasonings   A-96 Sports Bars and Drinks   A-96 Supplemental Foods and Formulas   A-96 Sweeteners and Sweet Substitutes   A-98 Vegetables and Legumes   A-108 Miscellaneous

Thia (mg)	Ribo (mg)	Niac (mg NE)	Vit B6 (mg)	Vit B12 (µg)	Fol (µg)	Vit C (mg)	Vit D (IU)	Vit E (mg AT)	Cal (mg)	Iron (mg)	Magn (mg)	Phos (mg)	Pota (mg)	Sodi (mg)	Zinc (mg)	Wat (%)	Alco (g)	Caff (g)
0.69	0.46	6.59	0.03	0.00	41.1	0.0	0.3	0.1	14	3.80	22.1	90	98	7	0.8	37	0.00	0.00
0.23	0.14	3.46	0.18	0.00	28.2	0.0	0.0	0.8	100	2.26	79.9	211	256	377	1.9	33	0.00	0.00
0.14	0.10	1.48	0.03	0.00	39.0	0.0	0.0	1.4	32	1.09	12.0	42	74	524	0.3	65	0.00	0.00
0.01	0.01	0.17	0.00	0.00	5.0	0.0	0.0	0.0	2	0.12	0.9	6	5	24	0.0	4	0.00	0.00
0.18	0.25	3.46	0.05	0.00	38.6	0.0	0.0	0.3	20	3.13	25.2	87	113	401	0.7	4	0.00	0.00
0.05	0.05	0.51	0.00	0.00	15.5	0.0	0.0	0.0	6	0.40	2.7	17	15	72	0.1	4	0.00	0.00
0.07	0.03	0.77	0.00		11.5			0.6	25	0.72	3.0	44	19	141	0.1	3	0.00	0.00
0.09	0.05	0.69	0.07	0.07	22.8	0.0	0.0	0.0	23	0.72	5.4	33	22	149	0.2	3	0.00	0.00
						0.0			0	0.36				150			0.00	0.00
						0.0			100	1.08				150		1	0.00	0.00
0.21	0.17	1.41	0.01	0.05	6.7	0.0			11	0.75	6.7	41	42	6	0.2	6	0.00	0.00
0.05	0.03	0.62	0.00	0.00	18.6	0.0	0.0	0.1	14	0.56	8.9	29	30	90	0.3	5	0.00	0.00
0.09	0.05	0.79	0.00	0.00	21.0	0.0	0.0	0.2	3	0.76	3.8	17	24	167	0.1	4	0.00	0.00
						0.0			20	1.08				280		0	0.00	0.00
0.12	0.20	1.05	0.05	0.20	27.9	0.2			65	1.09	11.0	76	87	311	0.4	55	0.00	0.00
0.10	0.10	1.33	0.14	0.40	20.1	0.5			14	1.20	7.0	132	40	196	0.2	47	0.00	0.00
						0.0		0.5	154	4.21	14.0	248	88	615	0.3	30	0.00	0.00
0.12	0.09	1.34	0.01	0.00	20.2	0.0	0.0	0.8	4	1.05	11.7	36	27	99	0.3	1	0.00	0.00
0.46	0.25	3.05			122.0	0.0			10	1.83	30.6	80	82	3	0.7	10	0.00	0.00
						0.0			0	1.79				140			0.00	0.00
0.43	0.25	2.95			117.7	0.0			10	1.76	29.6	77	79	3	0.6	10	0.00	0.00
0.37	0.18	2.35	0.07	0.00	102.2	0.0	0.0	0.1	10	1.78	25.2	81	62	1	0.7	62	0.00	0.00
0.02	0.00	0.12	0.00	0.00	5.3	0.0	0.0		7	0.25	5.3	35	7	33	0.4	74	0.00	0.00
0.49	0.20	3.33	0.07	0.00	10.3	0.0		0.1	12	1.61		105		3	0.7	6	0.00	0.00
0.31	0.15	1.94	0.05	0.00	83.9	0.0	0.0	0.1	8	1.47	20.7	67	51	1	0.6	62	0.00	0.00
0.37	0.18	2.35	0.07	0.00	102.2	0.0	0.0	0.1	10	1.78	25.2	81	62	1	0.7	62	0.00	0.00
0.17	0.11	1.74	0.00	0.00	27.5	0.0			15	1.08	6.4	26	26	183	0.2	29	0.00	0.00
						0.0			40	0.36				190		1	0.00	0.00
0.01	0.01	0.36	0.05	0.00	1.2	0.0	0.0	0.1	19	0.30	17.3	75	45	11	0.3	46	0.00	0.00
0.15	0.07	1.07	0.01	0.00	31.2	0.0	0.0	0.1	39	1.00	6.6	37	46	191	0.2	30	0.00	0.00
0.25	0.15	1.84	0.00	0.00	57.2	0.0	0.0	0.0	5	1.45	6.9	34	33	1	0.2	12	0.00	0.00
0.31	0.15	2.32	0.00	0.00	63.7	0.0	0.0	0.0	5	2.50	5.5	29	36	1	0.2	13	0.00	0.00
0.15	0.05	1.49	0.11	0.00	13.2	0.0	0.0	0.2	10	1.08	41.1	107	109	1	0.8	11	0.00	0.00
						0.0			0	1.79				0			0.00	0.00
0.09	0.01	1.49	0.14	0.00	3.9	0.0	0.0	0.0	10	0.40	41.9	81	42	5	0.6	73	0.00	0.00
0.10	0.00	1.29	0.15	0.00	3.9	0.0	0.0		10	0.51	42.9	75	77	1	0.6	73	0.00	0.00
0.12	0.00	1.16	0.07	0.00	45.8	0.0	0.0	0.0	8	0.94	9.5	34	28	1	0.4	68	0.00	0.00
0.03	0.07	1.05	0.10	0.00	21.3	0.0	0.0	0.2	2	0.49	26.2	67	83	2	1.1	74	0.00	0.00
						0.0			0	0.00				0		1	0.00	0.00
0.07	0.03	1.78	0.11	0.00	9.4	0.0	0.0	0.0	12	0.86	57.4	105	144	6	0.7	9	0.00	0.00
0.05	0.03	0.82	0.07	0.00	10.3	0.7	0.0		8	0.57	22.1	54	46	4	0.4	48	0.00	0.00

PAGE KEY: A-42 Beverages and Beverage Mixes   A-44 Candies   A-46 Cereals   A-48 Cheeses and Substitutes   A-50 Dairy Products and Substitutes   A-52 Desserts   A-56 Eggs and Egg Substitutes   A-56 Fats, Oils, Margarines, and Shortenings   A-58 Fruits   A-60 Grain Products and Baked Goods   A-62 Grains and Flours   A-64 Meats and Meat Substitutes   A-68 Nuts, Seeds, and Products

Code	Food Name	Unit/ Amt	Wt (g)	Energy (kcal)	Prot (g)	Carb (g)	Fiber (g)	Fat (g)	Sat (g)	Mono (g)	Poly (g)	Chol (mg)	Vit A (RE)
MEATS AND MEAT SUBSTITUTES													
Beef and Veal													
10740	Beef, cubed patty, FS	1 ea	91	251	15	2	0	20	8.1			64	11
58115	Beef, ground, hamburger, bkd, 10% fat	3 oz	85	182	23	0	0	9	3.7	4.0	0.3	73	0
58120	Beef, ground, hamburger, bkd, 15% fat	3 oz	85	204	22	0	0	12	4.6	5.3	0.4	77	0
58125	Beef, ground, hamburger, bkd, 20% fat	3 oz	85	216	21	0	0	14	5.2	6.1	0.4	77	0
58110	Beef, ground, hamburger, bkd, 5% fat	3 oz	85	148	23	0	0	5	2.5	2.2	0.3	62	0
10051	Beef, jerky, lrg pce	1 pce	20	82	7	2	0	5	2.2	2.3	0.2	10	0
10472	Beef, liver, brsd	3 oz	85	162	25	4	0	4	1.4	0.6	0.5	337	8042
11487	Beef, porterhouse steak, brld, 1/8" trim	3 oz	85	253	20	0	0	19	7.2	8.2	0.7	60	0
11407	Beef, prime rib, brld, 1/8" trim	3 oz	85	301	21	0	0	24	9.8	10.3	0.8	71	0
11228	Beef, rib pot roast, lean, rstd, 0" trim	3 oz	85	202	23	0	0	11	4.6	4.8	0.3	69	0
10806	Beef, T-bone steak, brld, 0" trim	3 oz	85	210	21	0	0	14	5.2	6.1	0.5	51	0
11491	Beef, T-bone steak, brld, 1/8" trim	3 oz	85	238	21	0	0	17	6.4	7.3	0.6	53	0
10933	Beef, tenderloin, filet mignon, rstd, 1/8" trim	3 oz	85	276	20	0	0	21	8.3	8.7	0.9	72	0
10908	Beef, top round steak, brsd, 1/8" trim	3 oz	85	202	29	0	0	9	3.2	3.5	0.4	77	0
11292	Beef, top sirloin steak, lean, brld, 0" trim	3 oz	85	156	26	0	0	5	1.9	2.0	0.2	70	0
10846	Beef, whole rib, brld, 1/8" trim	3 oz	85	287	19	0	0	23	9.2	9.7	0.8	70	0
11531	Veal, avg of all cuts, ckd	3 oz	85	196	26	0	0	10	3.6	3.7	0.7	97	0
Chicken													
81202	Chicken, breast, fillet, grilled	1 ea	85	100	20	1	0	2				45	0
81186	Chicken, breast, oven rstd, fat free, sliced	2 pce	42	33	7	1	0	0	0.1	0.1	0.0	15	0
15004	Chicken, broiler/fryer, breast, w/o skin, rstd	1 ea	86	142	27	0	0	3	0.9	1.1	0.7	73	5
15001	Chicken, broiler/fryer, breast, w/skin, rstd	1 ea	98	193	29	0	0	8	2.1	3.0	1.6	82	27
15080	Chicken, broiler/fryer, dark meat, w/skin, rstd	3 oz	85	215	22	0	0	13	3.7	5.3	3.0	77	51
15057	Fried Chicken, broiler/fryer, breast, w/o skin	3 oz	85	159	28	0	0	4	1.1	1.5	0.9	77	6
14725	Nuggets, chicken, ckd f/fzn	4 pce	80	237	12	11	2	16	3.2	7.1	3.5	34	0
Fish, Seafood, and Shellfish													
19000	Clams, mixed species, stmd, sml	3 oz	85	126	22	4	0	2	0.2	0.1	0.5	57	145
19037	Crab, Alaska king, imit f/surimi	3 oz	85	81	6	13	0	0	0.1	0.1	0.1	17	0
17179	Fish, catfish, channel, farmed, fillet, bkd/brld	3 oz	85	122	16	0	0	6	1.3	2.6	1.2	56	1
17090	Fish, haddock, fillet, bkd/brld	3 oz	85	77	17	0	0	0	0.1	0.1	0.2	56	18
17049	Fish, mackerel, Atlantic, fillet, bkd/brld	3 oz	85	223	20	0	0	15	3.6	6.0	3.7	64	46
17121	Fish, orange roughy, fillet, bkd/brld	3 oz	85	89	19	0	0	1	0.0	0.4	0.2	68	20
17093	Fish, perch, ocean, Atlantic, fillet, bkd/brld	3 oz	85	82	16	0	0	2	0.3	0.5	0.3	54	13
17171	Fish, salmon, pink, fillet, bkd/brld	3 oz	85	130	21	0	0	4	0.8	1.4	0.8	47	36
17068	Fish, sole, fillet, bkd/brld	3 oz	85	73	13	0	0	2	0.5	0.6	0.4	48	10
71139	Fish, sturgeon, mixed species, bkd/brld, 4.5 x 2 1/8 x 7/8	3 oz	85	115	18	0	0	4	1.0	2.1	0.8	65	224
17101	Fish, tuna, bluefin, fillet, bkd/brld	3 oz	85	156	25	0	0	5	1.4	1.7	1.6	42	644
19006	Lobster, northern, stmd	3 oz	85	76	16	0	0	1	0.2	0.2	0.3	124	1
19142	Scallops, ckd, lrg	6 lrg	84	140	27	5	0	1	0.0			65	30
19012	Shrimp, mixed species, stmd, lrg	4 ea	22	26	5	0	0	0	0.0	0.0	0.0	46	20
Game Meats													
14009	Bison, rstd	3 oz	85	122	24	0	0	2	0.8	0.8	0.2	70	0
40551	Deer, rstd	3 oz	85	134	26	0	0	3	1.1	0.7	0.5	95	0
14014	Elk, rstd	3 oz	85	124	26	0	0	2	0.6	0.4	0.3	62	0

PAGE KEY: A-70 Prepared Foods   A-78 Restaurants   A-90 Salad Dressings and Dips   A-92 Sauces and Gravies   A-94 Snack Foods   A-94 Spices, Flavors, and Seasonings   A-96 Sports Bars and Drinks   A-96 Supplemental Foods and Formulas   A-96 Sweeteners and Sweet Substitutes   A-98 Vegetables and Legumes   A-108 Miscellaneous

Thia (mg)	Ribo (mg)	Niac (mg NE)	Vit B6 (mg)	Vit B12 (µg)	Fol (µg)	Vit C (mg)	Vit D (IU)	Vit E (mg AT)	Cal (mg)	Iron (mg)	Magn (mg)	Phos (mg)	Pota (mg)	Sodi (mg)	Zinc (mg)	Wat (%)	Alco (g)	Caff (g)
0.10						8.0			17	1.89				53			0.00	0.00
0.02	0.15	4.44	0.30	2.13	5.1	0.0		0.3	11	2.46	17.9	164	255	52	5.7	61	0.00	0.00
0.02	0.15	4.19	0.28	2.11	5.1	0.0	6.0	0.4	15	2.32	17.0	158	243	54	5.5	59	0.00	0.00
0.03	0.14	3.94	0.28	2.10	6.0	0.0	6.8	0.4	20	2.19	16.2	152	230	57	5.3	58	0.00	0.00
0.02	0.15	4.69	0.30	2.13	5.1	0.0		0.3	7	2.58	18.7	169	268	49	5.8	65	0.00	0.00
0.02	0.02	0.34	0.03	0.20	26.8	0.0	2.2	0.1	4	1.08	10.2	81	119	416	1.6	23	0.00	0.00
0.15	2.91	14.90	0.86	60.02	215.2	1.6	41.7	0.4	5	5.55	17.9	423	299	67	4.5	59	0.00	0.00
0.09	0.18	3.46	0.30	1.83	6.0	0.0			7	2.32	19.6	159	273	54	3.9	53	0.00	0.00
0.07	0.15	3.46	0.28	2.50	6.0	0.0			11	1.89	18.7	151	282	54	4.9	47	0.00	0.00
0.07	0.18	3.77	0.21	2.22	7.7	0.0	7.7	0.1	7	2.40	21.3	178	304	62	6.3	58	0.00	0.00
0.09	0.20	3.63	0.31	1.86	6.0	0.0		0.2	4	2.84	20.4	169	257	57	4.0	58	0.00	0.00
0.09	0.18	3.51	0.30	1.85	6.0	0.0			7	2.41	20.4	164	286	56	4.0	55	0.00	0.00
0.07	0.21	2.54	0.20	2.08	6.8	0.0			8	2.65	18.7	173	282	48	3.4	48	0.00	0.00
0.05	0.20	3.09	0.23	2.23	7.7	0.0	6.0	0.1	4	2.69	20.4	183	271	38	3.7	55	0.00	0.00
0.07	0.12	7.42	0.56	1.45	8.5	0.0	3.4	0.3	17	1.66	22.1	208	334	54	4.9	63	0.00	0.00
0.07	0.14	2.77	0.23	2.46	5.1	0.0			9	1.86	17.0	152	268	54	4.5	48	0.00	0.00
0.05	0.27	6.78	0.25	1.34	12.8	0.0	0.0	0.3	19	0.98	22.1	203	276	74	4.0	57	0.00	0.00
						0.0			0	1.08				410			0.00	0.00
0.00	0.00	1.44	0.05	0.03	0.4	0.0			3	0.12	3.8	25	28	457	0.1	77	0.00	0.00
0.05	0.10	11.78	0.51	0.28	3.4	0.0	4.3	0.2	13	0.88	24.9	196	220	64	0.9	65	0.00	0.00
0.05	0.11	12.46	0.55	0.31	3.9	0.0	4.9	0.3	14	1.04	26.5	210	240	70	1.0	62	0.00	0.00
0.05	0.18	5.40	0.25	0.25	6.0	0.0			13	1.15	18.7	143	187	74	2.1	59	0.00	0.00
0.07	0.10	12.56	0.54	0.31	3.4	0.0	4.3	0.4	14	0.97	26.4	209	235	67	0.9	60	0.00	0.00
0.07	0.05	3.56	0.14	0.10	2.4	0.0	8.8	1.0	25	0.93	20.8	158	212	446	1.0	49	0.00	0.00
0.12	0.36	2.84	0.09	84.11	24.7	18.8			78	23.78	15.3	287	534	95	2.3	64	0.00	0.00
0.02	0.07	0.52	0.10	0.47	0.0	0.0	0.0	0.1	11	0.33	36.6	240	77	715	0.3	75	0.00	0.00
0.01	0.09	2.17	0.15	2.35	10.2	0.0	8.5	0.8	8	0.23	19.6	210	311	101	0.5	75	0.00	0.00
0.01	0.05	3.50	0.28	1.80	11.1	0.0	19.6	0.5	12	0.18	22.1	236	299	222	0.3	80	0.00	0.00
0.14	0.34	5.82	0.38	16.15	1.7	0.3			13	1.34	82.5	236	341	71	0.8	53	0.00	0.00
0.03	0.05	1.54	0.05	0.40	4.3	0.0		1.6	9	0.95	15.3	87	154	59	0.3	67	0.00	0.00
0.03	0.05	1.02	0.07	1.46	8.5	0.0	49.3	0.8	29	0.23	23.0	255	192	295	0.3	74	0.00	0.00
0.07	0.10	8.14	0.58	4.01	4.3	0.0	444.0	0.4	7	0.37	27.2	266	373	77	0.4	71	0.00	0.00
0.01	0.01	1.09	0.10	1.11	5.1	0.0	118.2	0.7	21	0.20	18.7	263	168	309	0.3	81	0.00	0.00
0.07	0.07	8.59	0.20	2.13	14.5	0.0	438.0	0.5	14	0.76	38.3	230	310	59	0.5	70	0.00	0.00
0.23	0.25	8.96	0.44	9.25	1.7	0.0			9	1.11	54.4	277	275	43	0.7	59	0.00	0.00
0.01	0.00	1.55	0.10	1.22	9.4	0.0	0.9	0.9	82	0.25	36.6	157	196	413	3.4	78	0.00	0.00
						0.0			40	2.51			430	310			0.00	0.00
0.00	0.00	0.58	0.05	0.37	5.3	0.0	0.9	0.5	20	0.07	8.1	67	37	208	0.4	72	0.00	0.00
0.09	0.23	3.16	0.34	2.43	6.8	0.0	0.0	0.3	7	2.91	22.1	178	307	48	3.1	67	0.00	0.00
0.15	0.50	5.71				0.0			6	3.79	20.4	192	285	46	2.3	65	0.00	0.00
					7.7	0.0			4	3.08	20.4	153	279	52	2.7	66	0.00	0.00

PAGE KEY: A-42 Beverages and Beverage Mixes   A-44 Candies   A-46 Cereals   A-48 Cheeses and Substitutes   A-50 Dairy Products and Substitutes   A-52 Desserts   A-56 Eggs and Egg Substitutes   A-56 Fats, Oils, Margarines, and Shortenings   A-58 Fruits   A-60 Grain Products and Baked Goods   A-62 Grains and Flours   A-64 Meats and Meat Substitutes   A-68 Nuts, Seeds, and Products

Code	Food Name	Unit/Amt	Wt (g)	Energy (kcal)	Prot (g)	Carb (g)	Fiber (g)	Fat (g)	Sat (g)	Mono (g)	Poly (g)	Chol (mg)	Vit A (RE)
Lamb													
40354	Lamb, Austl, average of all cuts, ckd, 1/8" trim	3 oz	85	218	21	0	0	14	6.8	5.7	0.6	74	
13628	Lamb, average of all cuts, ckd, choice, 1/8" trim	3 oz	85	230	22	0	0	15	6.3	6.5	1.1	82	0
13524	Lamb, ground, brld, 20% fat	3 oz	85	241	21	0	0	17	6.9	7.1	1.2	82	0
Lunchmeat													
11815	Beef, roast, Italian, deli	2 oz	57	60	11	1	0	1	0.5			20	0
57966	Frank, beef, 97% fat free	1 ea	49	45	6	3	0	2	1.0			15	0
57967	Frank, beef, rducd fat	1 ea	49	120	6	0	0	10	4.5			25	0
13010	Frankfurter, beef & pork	1 ea	45	137	5	1	0	12	4.8	6.2	1.2	22	8
58220	Frankfurter, beef pork & turkey, fat free	1 ea	57	62	7	6	0	1	0.3	0.4	0.2	23	0
13008	Frankfurter, beef, 5" x 7/8"	1 ea	57	188	6	2	0	17	6.7	8.2	0.7	30	0
13274	Frankfurter, low sod	1 ea	57	178	7	1	0	16	6.9	7.8	0.8	35	0
13012	Frankfurter, turkey	1 ea	45	100	6	2	0	8	1.8	2.6	1.8	35	0
13038	Lunchmeat Loaf, beef & pork, w/bbq, 1/16" slice	1 pce	23	40	4	1	0	2	0.7	1.0	0.2	9	2
13000	Lunchmeat, beef, thin slice, oval	1 pce	9	11	2	0	0	0	0.1	0.1	0.0	4	0
58284	Lunchmeat, bologna, beef, low fat	1 oz	28	58	3	1	0	4	1.5	1.8	0.1	12	0
10439	Lunchmeat, bologna, beef, slice	1 pce	38	100	5	1	0	8	3.5			20	0
11829	Lunchmeat, bologna, chicken, slice	1 pce	38	100	4	1	0	9	2.5			45	20
16996	Lunchmeat, bologna, fat free	1 svg	28	22	4	2	0	0	0.1	0.1	0.0	7	0
58184	Lunchmeat, chicken breast, oven roast, deli sliced	3 pce	52	50	10	1	0	0	0.0			20	0
58149	Lunchmeat, chicken breast, oven rstd, slice	1 slc	28	20	5	0	0	0	0.0	0.0	0.0	10	
58167	Lunchmeat, ham, brown sugar, slice	2 pce	45	60	8	4	0	1	0.0			10	0
13261	Lunchmeat, ham, extra lean, 5% fat, sliced, oval	1 slc	24	26	5	0	0	1	0.2	0.2	0.1	11	0
11819	Lunchmeat, ham, smkd, deli	2 oz	57	60	9	2	0	2	0.5			30	0
58199	Lunchmeat, roast beef, choice, deli sliced	2 pce	45	50	9	0	0	2	0.5			25	0
13112	Lunchmeat, turkey breast, hickory smkd, 98% fat free, svg	1 svg	28	30	5	1		0	0.0			10	0
13114	Lunchmeat, turkey breast, oven rstd, fat free	1 oz	28	24	4	1	0	0	0.1	0.1	0.0	9	0
13020	Pastrami, turkey, slices	1 pce	28	38	5	1	0	2	0.5	0.6	0.5	19	1
13201	Salami, hard, slice	3 pce	27	99	7	0	0	8	3.0	4.0	0.8	26	2
13025	Salami, turkey, ckd, svg	1 oz	28	49	5	0	0	3	0.8	0.9	0.7	22	1
13182	Sausage, beef, Smokies	1 ea	43	127	5	1	0	11	4.8	5.5	0.4	27	0
13021	Sausage, pepperoni, beef & pork, slice	1 pce	2	10	0	0	0	1	0.3	0.3	0.1	2	0
58353	Sausage, pork, link, ckd f/fzn, USDA	1 ea	48	128	9	0	0	10	2.7	4.2	1.1	47	7
13184	Sausage, Smokies, link	1 ea	43	130	5	1	0	12	4.0	5.7	1.2	27	0
58232	Sausage, turkey, ckd f/fresh	1 svg	57	112	14	0	0	6	1.3	1.7	1.5	52	9
Meat Substitutes													
7564	Tempeh	0.5 cup	83	160	15	8		9	1.8	2.5	3.2	0	0
90040	Tofu, fermented & salted, w/calc sulfate, block	1 ea	11	13	1	1		1	0.1	0.2	0.5	0	0
27044	Vegetarian Meat, bacon bits	1 Tbs	7	33	2	2	1	2	0.3	0.4	0.9	0	0
7509	Vegetarian Meat, bacon, strips	1 ea	15	46	2	1	0	4	0.7	1.1	2.3	0	1
7558	Vegetarian Meat, beef, fillet	1 ea	85	246	20	8	5	15	2.4	3.7	7.9	0	0
7561	Vegetarian Meat, beef, patty	1 ea	56	110	12	4	3	5	0.8	1.2	2.6	0	0
7547	Vegetarian Meat, chicken	0.5 cup	84	188	20	3	3	11	1.5	2.3	6.1	0	0
7549	Vegetarian Meat, fish sticks	1 ea	28	81	6	3	2	5	0.8	1.2	2.6	0	0
92148	Vegetarian Meat, hot dog	1 ea	70	163	14	5	3	10	1.4	2.7	5.5	0	0

PAGE KEY: A-70 Prepared Foods   A-78 Restaurants   A-90 Salad Dressings and Dips   A-92 Sauces and Gravies   A-94 Snack Foods   A-94 Spices, Flavors, and Seasonings   A-96 Sports Bars and Drinks   A-96 Supplemental Foods and Formulas   A-96 Sweeteners and Sweet Substitutes   A-98 Vegetables and Legumes   A-108 Miscellaneous

Thia (mg)	Ribo (mg)	Niac (mg NE)	Vit B6 (mg)	Vit B12 (µg)	Fol (µg)	Vit C (mg)	Vit D (IU)	Vit E (mg AT)	Cal (mg)	Iron (mg)	Magn (mg)	Phos (mg)	Pota (mg)	Sodi (mg)	Zinc (mg)	Wat (%)	Alco (g)	Caff (g)
0.10	0.28	4.63	0.31	2.44					14	1.63	18.7	166	256	65	4.0	59	0.00	0.00
0.09	0.21	5.57	0.11	2.19	16.2	0.0			14	1.63	20.4	164	270	61	4.0	56	0.00	0.00
0.09	0.20	5.69	0.11	2.22	16.2	0.0	1.7	0.1	19	1.51	20.4	171	288	69	4.0	55	0.00	0.00
						0.0			0	1.08				360			0.00	0.00
						0.0			0	1.08				400		37	0.00	0.00
						0.0			0	0.72				360		31	0.00	0.00
0.09	0.05	1.19	0.05	0.57	1.8	0.0	16.2	0.1	5	0.51	4.5	39	75	504	0.8	56	0.00	0.00
0.09	0.09	1.98	0.10	0.60	3.4	13.7	1.1	0.0	31	1.00	8.0	75	125	455	1.7	72	0.00	0.00
0.01	0.07	1.35	0.05	0.98	2.8	0.0	20.5	0.1	8	0.86	8.0	91	89	650	1.4	52	0.00	0.00
0.02	0.05	1.37	0.07	0.87	2.3	0.0	21.1	0.1	11	0.81	1.7	50	95	177	1.2	57	0.00	0.00
0.01	0.07	1.65	0.05	0.37	4.0	0.0	10.3	0.3	67	0.66	6.3	77	176	485	0.8	63	0.00	0.00
0.07	0.05	0.51	0.05	0.38	2.1	0.0	8.3		13	0.27	3.9	30	76	307	0.6	65	0.00	0.00
0.00	0.02	0.43	0.03	0.18	0.3	0.0	0.2	0.0	1	0.18	1.8	24	29	104	0.3	73	0.00	0.00
0.00	0.02	0.70	0.03	0.40	1.4	0.3	4.3	0.1	3	0.28	3.4	50	42	335	0.5	65	0.00	0.00
						0.0			0	0.36				340		23	0.00	0.00
						1.2			40	0.72				350		23	0.00	0.00
						0.0			4	0.25	6.2	43	44	274	0.3	78	0.00	0.00
						0.0			0	0.36				430		38	0.00	0.00
														240		22	0.00	0.00
						0.0			0	0.36				490			0.00	0.00
0.07	0.05	1.37	0.09	0.09	0.0	0.0	6.7	0.1	1	0.17	5.0	69	156	254	0.4	74	0.00	0.00
						0.0			0	0.36				430		42	0.00	0.00
						0.0			0	1.08				250			0.00	0.00
						0.0			0	0.00				260		21	0.00	0.00
						0.0			3	0.31	7.7	66	58	338	0.2	76	0.00	0.00
0.01	0.07	1.00	0.07	0.07	1.4	2.3	2.8	0.1	3	1.20	4.0	57	98	280	0.6	72	0.00	0.00
0.15	0.07	1.36	0.11	0.50	0.8	0.0	16.7		3	0.49	5.7	49	96	534	0.9	38	0.00	0.00
0.11	0.09	1.12	0.11	0.28	2.8	0.0	6.8	0.1	11	0.34	6.2	75	61	285	0.7	69	0.00	0.00
					4.7	0.0			5	0.75	6.5	99	74	416	1.3	56	0.00	0.00
0.00	0.00	0.09	0.00	0.02	0.1	0.0	0.2		0	0.02	0.4	4	6	33	0.0	31	0.00	0.00
0.34	0.11	1.34	0.12	0.43	0.5	0.0			4	0.55	9.1	91	115	259	1.4	59	0.00	0.00
						0.0			4	0.50	7.3	103	77	433	0.9	56	0.00	0.00
0.05	0.15	3.25	0.18	0.69	3.4	0.4	3.4	0.1	13	0.85	12.0	115	170	379	2.2	65	0.00	0.00
0.05	0.30	2.19	0.18	0.07	19.9	0.0	0.0		92	2.24	67.2	221	342	7	0.9	60	0.00	0.00
0.01	0.00	0.03	0.00	0.00	3.2	0.0	0.0		135	0.21	6.4	8	8	316	0.2	70	0.00	0.00
0.03	0.00	0.10	0.00	0.07	8.9	0.1	0.0	0.5	7	0.05	6.7	15	10	124	0.1	8	0.00	0.00
0.66	0.07	1.12	0.07	0.00	6.3	0.0	0.0	1.0	3	0.36	2.9	10	26	220	0.1	49	0.00	0.00
0.93	0.75	10.19	1.27	3.56	86.7	0.0	0.0	2.9	81	1.70	19.6	382	510	416	1.2	45	0.00	0.00
0.50	0.34	5.59	0.67	1.34	43.7	0.0	0.0	1.0	16	1.17	10.1	193	101	308	1.0	58	0.00	0.00
0.05	0.20	1.22	0.58	1.83	63.8	0.0	0.0	2.3	29	2.75	14.3	281	45	596	0.6	59	0.00	0.00
0.31	0.25	3.35	0.41	1.17	28.6	0.0	0.0	1.1	27	0.56	6.4	126	168	137	0.4	45	0.00	0.00
0.31	0.57	2.20	0.05	1.63	54.6	0.0	0.0	1.3	23	0.99	12.6	241	69	330	0.8	58	0.00	0.00

Code	Food Name	Unit/ Amt	Wt (g)	Energy (kcal)	Prot (g)	Carb (g)	Fiber (g)	Fat (g)	Sat (g)	Mono (g)	Poly (g)	Chol (mg)	Vit A (RE)
7551	Vegetarian Meat, lunchmeat, slices	1 pce	14	26	2	1	0	2	0.2	0.3	0.6	0	0
90626	Vegetarian Meat, sausage, slices	1 slc	28	72	5	3	1	5	0.8	1.3	2.6	0	0
Pork and Ham													
27096	Bacon Bits, real, svg	1 svg	7	25	3	0	0	2	0.5			5	0
92207	Bacon, cured, microwaved	1 pce	5	25	2	0	0	2	0.6	0.8	0.2	6	1
92208	Bacon, cured, pan fried	1 pce	8	42	3	0	0	3	1.0	1.4	0.4	9	1
28143	Canadian Bacon, svg	1 svg	56	68	9	1		3	1.0	1.4	0.3	27	0
12184	Pork, chop, blade loin, w/bone, brld	1 ea	219	506	52	0	0	31	9.5	10.7	4.1	171	9
12192	Pork, chop, center loin, w/bone, brld	3 oz	85	178	22	0	0	9	3.0	3.6	1.2	71	2
93445	Pork, cured ham & wtr product, pan brld	3 oz	85	105	13	4	0	4	1.3	1.8	0.6	38	11
12307	Pork, cured ham, lean, 8% fat, rstd	0.5 cup	70	116	15	0	0	5	1.8	2.6	0.7	40	0
12099	Pork, ground, ckd	3 oz	85	253	22	0	0	18	6.6	7.9	1.6	80	2
12296	Pork, patty, chopette, fzn, 3.2 oz, FS	1 ea	91	240	14	1	1	20	7.2	8.7	1.9	56	15
12010	Pork, ribs, spareribs, brsd	3 oz	85	338	25	0	0	26	9.5	11.5	2.3	103	3
12060	Pork, roast, top loin, rstd	3 oz	85	163	22	0	0	8	2.4	3.0	0.8	68	1
12237	Pork, tenderloin, chop, brld	3 oz	85	171	25	0	0	7	2.5	2.8	0.6	80	2
Turkey													
51101	Turkey, avg, dark meat, w/o skin, rstd	3 oz	85	160	24	0	0	6	1.9	1.5	2.0	72	0
16028	Turkey, avg, dark meat, w/skin, rstd	3 oz	85	188	23	0	0	10	3.0	3.1	2.6	76	0
16158	Turkey, avg, light meat, w/o skin, rstd	3 oz	85	134	25	0	0	3	0.9	0.5	0.7	59	0
16027	Turkey, avg, light meat, w/skin, rstd	3 oz	85	168	24	0	0	7	2.0	2.4	1.7	65	0
16204	Turkey, ground, raw, svg	4 oz	113	192	20	0	0	12	3.5			91	0
16351	Turkey, jerky, original	1 pce	30	86	15	3	0	1	0.0			32	64
NUTS, SEEDS, AND PRODUCTS													
4507	Coconut, fresh, shredded	2 Tbs	10	35	0	2	1	3	3.0	0.1	0.0	0	0
4559	Coconut, milk, cnd	2 Tbs	28	56	1	1		6	5.3	0.3	0.1	0	0
4575	Coconut, tstd f/dried	3 Tbs	15	89	1	7	1	7	6.3	0.3	0.1	0	0
4572	Nut Butter, almond	2 Tbs	32	196	7	6	3	18	1.3	10.4	4.4	0	0
4571	Nuts, almonds, dry rstd, salted, whole	22 ea	28	169	6	6	3	15	1.1	9.2	3.7	0	0
4505	Nuts, almonds, oil rstd, unsalted	0.25 cup	39	238	8	7	4	22	1.7	13.7	5.3	0	0
4549	Nuts, almonds, whole, dry rstd, unsalted	22 ea	28	169	6	6	3	15	1.1	9.2	3.7	0	0
4642	Nuts, beechnuts, dried	1 oz	28	163	2	9		14	1.6	6.2	5.7	0	0
4536	Nuts, Brazil, dried, lrg	6 ea	28	186	4	3	2	19	4.3	7.0	5.8	0	0
4750	Nuts, Brazil, dried, unblanched, shelled	0.25 cup	33	218	5	4	2	22	5.0	8.2	6.8	0	0
4519	Nuts, cashews, dry rstd, salted, whole	0.25 cup	34	197	5	11	1	16	3.1	9.4	2.7	0	0
4596	Nuts, cashews, oil rstd, salted, whole	0.25 cup	32	187	5	10	1	15	2.7	8.4	2.8	0	0
4622	Nuts, cashews, oil rstd, unsalted, whole	0.25 cup	32	187	5	10	1	15	2.7	8.4	2.8	0	0
4516	Nuts, macadamia, dried, whole	0.25 cup	34	241	3	5	3	25	4.0	19.7	0.5	0	0
4594	Nuts, mixed, w/o peanuts, oil rstd, unsalted	0.25 cup	36	221	6	8	2	20	3.3	11.9	4.1	0	1
4592	Nuts, mixed, w/peanuts, dry rstd, salted	0.25 cup	34	203	6	9	3	18	2.4	10.8	3.7	0	0
4533	Nuts, mixed, w/peanuts, oil rstd, unsalted	0.25 cup	36	219	6	8	4	20	3.1	11.3	4.7	0	1
4541	Nuts, peanuts, dry rstd, salted	30 ea	30	176	7	6	2	15	2.1	7.4	4.7	0	0
4756	Nuts, peanuts, dry rstd, unsalted	0.25 cup	36	214	9	8	3	18	2.5	9.0	5.7	0	0
4763	Nuts, peanuts, oil rstd, salted	0.25 cup	36	216	10	5	3	19	3.1	9.4	5.5	0	0
4755	Nuts, peanuts, oil rstd, unsalted	32 ea	28	163	7	5	2	14	1.9	6.8	4.4	0	0

PAGE KEY: A-70 Prepared Foods   A-78 Restaurants   A-90 Salad Dressings and Dips   A-92 Sauces and Gravies   A-94 Snack Foods   A-94 Spices, Flavors, and Seasonings   A-96 Sports Bars and Drinks   A-96 Supplemental Foods and Formulas   A-96 Sweeteners and Sweet Substitutes   A-98 Vegetables and Legumes   A-108 Miscellaneous

Thia (mg)	Ribo (mg)	Niac (mg NE)	Vit B6 (mg)	Vit B12 (µg)	Fol (µg)	Vit C (mg)	Vit D (IU)	Vit E (mg AT)	Cal (mg)	Iron (mg)	Magn (mg)	Phos (mg)	Pota (mg)	Sodi (mg)	Zinc (mg)	Wat (%)	Alco (g)	Caff (g)
0.56	0.03	1.55	0.11	0.56	14.0	0.0	0.0	0.4	6	0.25	3.2	62	28	100	0.2	65	0.00	0.00
0.66	0.10	3.13	0.23	0.00	7.3	0.0	0.0	0.6	18	1.03	10.1	63	65	249	0.4	50	0.00	0.00
						0.0			0	0.00				220			0.00	0.00
0.02	0.00	0.50	0.01	0.07	0.1	0.0		0.0	1	0.05	1.6	24	25	104	0.2	16	0.00	0.00
0.03	0.01	0.91	0.02	0.10	0.2	0.0	3.4	0.0	1	0.10	2.8	44	47	192	0.3	12	0.00	0.00
						0.8			3	0.50	10.6		156	569	1.0	73	0.00	0.00
1.07	0.68	17.36	1.07	1.45	0.0	0.0	87.6	0.5	123	1.90	43.8	528	690	162	6.9	61	0.00	0.00
0.50	0.20	6.92	0.56	0.50	0.0	0.0	25.5	0.1	20	0.67	21.3	187	293	47	1.8	62	0.00	0.00
0.25	0.11	3.64	0.28	0.37	1.7	0.0	28.9	0.1	7	0.62	14.5	204	231	1181	1.4	71	0.00	0.00
0.51	0.20	3.73	0.23	0.47	2.1	0.0	22.4	0.2	6	0.98	13.3	174	253	970	1.8	66	0.00	0.00
0.60	0.18	3.57	0.33	0.46	5.1	0.6	17.9	0.2	19	1.10	20.4	192	308	62	2.7	53	0.00	0.00
0.58	0.20	3.93				0.6			27	0.18		157	292	163	3.1		0.00	0.00
0.34	0.31	4.65	0.30	0.92	3.4	0.0	88.5	0.3	40	1.57	20.4	222	272	79	3.9	40	0.00	0.00
0.46	0.20	6.03	0.58	0.49	0.0	0.0	17.0	0.1	6	0.54	21.3	190	297	39	1.8	64	0.00	0.00
0.81	0.31	4.30	0.43	0.82	5.1	0.9			4	1.17	29.8	247	378	54	2.5	61	0.00	0.00
0.05	0.20	3.09	0.31	0.31	7.7	0.0	6.8	0.5	27	1.98	20.4	174	247	67	3.8	63	0.00	0.00
0.05	0.20	3.00	0.27	0.31	7.7	0.0	3.4	0.5	28	1.92	19.6	167	233	65	3.5	60	0.00	0.00
0.05	0.10	5.82	0.46	0.31	5.1	0.0	6.8	0.1	16	1.14	23.8	186	259	54	1.7	66	0.00	0.00
0.05	0.10	5.34	0.40	0.30	5.1	0.0	4.3	0.1	18	1.20	22.1	177	242	54	1.7	63	0.00	0.00
						0.0			0	0.00				142		79	0.00	0.00
						0.0			21	1.15				589		9	0.00	0.00
0.00	0.00	0.05	0.00	0.00	2.6	0.3	0.0	0.0	1	0.23	3.2	11	36	2	0.1	47	0.00	0.00
0.00	0.00	0.18	0.00	0.00	4.0	0.3	0.0		5	0.93	13.0	27	62	4	0.2	73	0.00	0.00
0.00	0.01	0.09	0.05	0.00	1.4	0.2	0.0		4	0.50	13.8	32	83	6	0.3	1	0.00	0.00
0.00	0.30	1.00	0.02	0.00	17.0	0.0	0.0	7.7	111	1.12	89.3	163	239	69	1.1	2	0.00	0.00
0.01	0.27	1.00	0.03	0.00	15.0	0.0	0.0	6.7	76	1.09	79.7	133	202	96	0.9	3	0.00	0.00
0.03	0.31	1.44	0.05	0.00	10.6	0.0	0.0	10.2	114	1.44	107.5	183	274	0	1.2	3	0.00	0.00
0.01	0.27	1.00	0.03	0.00	15.0	0.0	0.0	6.7	76	1.09	79.7	133	202	1	0.9	3	0.00	0.00
0.09	0.10	0.25	0.18	0.00	32.0	4.4			0	0.69	0.0	0	288	11	0.1	7	0.00	0.00
0.17	0.00	0.07	0.02	0.00	6.2	0.2	0.0	1.6	45	0.68	106.6	206	187	1	1.2	3	0.00	0.00
0.20	0.00	0.10	0.02	0.00	7.3	0.2	0.0	1.9	53	0.81	125.0	241	219	1	1.3	3	0.00	0.00
0.07	0.07	0.47	0.09	0.00	23.6	0.0	0.0	0.3	15	2.05	89.1	168	194	219	1.9	2	0.00	0.00
0.11	0.07	0.56	0.10	0.00	8.1	0.1	0.0	0.3	14	1.95	88.0	171	204	99	1.7	3	0.00	0.00
0.11	0.07	0.56	0.10	0.00	8.1	0.1	0.0	0.3	14	1.95	88.0	171	204	4	1.7	3	0.00	0.00
0.40	0.05	0.82	0.09	0.00	3.7	0.4	0.0	0.2	28	1.24	43.5	63	123	2	0.4	1	0.00	0.00
0.18	0.17	0.70	0.05	0.00	20.2	0.2	0.0		38	0.93	90.4	162	196	4	1.7	3	0.00	0.00
0.07	0.07	1.61	0.10	0.00	17.1	0.1	0.0	3.7	24	1.26	77.1	149	204	229	1.3	2	0.00	0.00
0.18	0.07	1.79	0.09	0.00	29.5	0.2	0.0		38	1.13	83.4	165	206	4	1.8	2	0.00	0.00
0.12	0.02	4.05	0.07	0.00	43.5	0.0	0.0	2.3	16	0.68	52.8	107	197	244	1.0	2	0.00	0.00
0.15	0.03	4.94	0.09	0.00	52.9	0.0	0.0	2.5	20	0.81	64.2	131	240	2	1.2	2	0.00	0.00
0.02	0.02	4.98	0.17	0.00	43.2	0.3	0.0	2.5	22	0.55	63.4	143	261	115	1.2	1	0.00	0.00
0.07	0.02	4.00	0.07	0.00	35.3	0.0	0.0	1.9	25	0.50	51.8	145	191	2	1.9	2	0.00	0.00

Code	Food Name	Unit/ Amt	Wt (g)	Energy (kcal)	Prot (g)	Carb (g)	Fiber (g)	Fat (g)	Sat (g)	Mono (g)	Poly (g)	Chol (mg)	Vit A (RE)
4665	Nuts, peanuts, Spanish, oil rstd, unsalted	0.25 cup	37	213	10	6	3	18	2.8	8.1	6.3	0	0
4517	Nuts, peanuts, Spanish, raw	0.25 cup	36	208	10	6	3	18	2.8	8.1	6.3	0	0
4578	Nuts, pecans, halves	0.25 cup	25	171	2	3	2	18	1.5	10.1	5.3	0	1
4624	Nuts, pine	10 ea	1	7	0	0	0	1	0.1	0.2	0.3	0	0
4525	Nuts, walnuts, black, dried, chpd	0.25 cup	31	193	8	3	2	18	1.1	4.7	11.0	0	1
4626	Peanut Butter, chunky	2 Tbs	32	188	8	7	3	16	2.6	7.9	4.7	0	0
4627	Peanut Butter, creamy	2 Tbs	32	188	8	6	2	16	3.4	7.7	4.5	0	0
63338	Peanut Butter, creamy, rducd fat	2 Tbs	36	187	9	13	2	12	2.1	5.8	3.3	0	0
4636	Peanut Butter, creamy, unsalted	2 Tbs	32	188	8	6	2	16	3.3	7.6	4.4	0	0
62939	Peanut Butter, crunchy, rducd fat	2 Tbs	36	190	8	15	2	12	2.5			0	0
4747	Peanut Butter, rducd fat	1 Tbs	16	81	4	5	1	5	1.0	2.8	1.6	0	
4777	Seeds, flax/linseed, whole	0.25 cup	42	224	8	12	11	18	1.5	3.2	12.1	0	
4545	Seeds, sunflower, kernels, dried	0.25 cup	35	204	7	7	3	18	1.6	6.5	8.1	0	2
4597	Seeds, sunflower, kernels, dry rstd, salted	0.25 cup	32	186	6	8	3	16	1.7	3.0	10.5	0	0
4551	Seeds, sunflower, kernels, dry rstd, unsalted	0.25 cup	32	186	6	8	4	16	1.7	3.0	10.5	0	0
4552	Seeds, sunflower, oil rstd, salted	0.25 cup	34	200	7	8	4	17	2.4	2.7	11.6	0	0
63261	Soy Nuts, wheat free	0.33 cup	30	144	12	9	4	7	1.0			1	3

PREPARED FOODS

Canned Foods

Code	Food Name	Unit/ Amt	Wt (g)	Energy (kcal)	Prot (g)	Carb (g)	Fiber (g)	Fat (g)	Sat (g)	Mono (g)	Poly (g)	Chol (mg)	Vit A (RE)
50595	Broth, beef, clear, cnd	1 cup	198	15	2	0	0	0	0.0			0	0
50596	Broth, chicken, clear, cnd, rts	1 cup	198	15	1	1	0	0	0.0			5	0
57701	Chili, turkey, w/beans, cnd	1 svg	247	210	17	28	6	3	1.0			45	100
7760	Chili, vegetarian, cnd	1 svg	38	30	3	4	2	0	0.1	0.1	0.1	0	25
56001	Chili, w/beans, cnd	1 cup	256	287	15	30	11	14	6.0	6.0	0.9	44	86
50901	Chili, w/beef, cnd, rts	1 cup	245	190	16	34	8	2	0.5			5	100
28167	Chili, w/o beans, cnd	1 cup	240	283	18	15		17	5.4	5.9	1.1	50	
14804	Chowder, clam, New England, chunky, microwv	1 cup	245	201	6	17	3	12	2.5			10	0
17535	Dish, rice bowl, cheddar broccoli, microwv	1 bowl	74	290	8	51	2	7	2.5			10	0
57655	Macaroni & Cheese, can	1 svg	244	200	8	28	1	6	2.1	1.5	0.7	15	44
92620	Ravioli, beef, w/meat sauce, cnd	1 cup	212	260	11	39	5	7	3.0			10	100
90856	Refried Beans, fat free, cnd	0.5 cup	130	110	7	21	6	0	0.0	0.0	0.0	0	0
9096	Refried Beans, original, cnd, FS	0.5 cup	128	100	6	18	5	2	1.0			0	0
9095	Refried Beans, spicy, cnd, FS	0.5 cup	128	100	6	18	6	2	1.0			0	0
50061	Soup, bean & pork, cond, 11.5-oz can	0.5 cup	130	168	8	22	8	6	1.5	2.1	1.8	3	87
50003	Soup, beef noodle, prep f/cnd w/water	1 cup	244	83	5	9	1	3	1.1	1.2	0.5	5	25
50080	Soup, chicken mushroom, prep f/cnd w/water	1 cup	244	132	4	9	0	9	2.4	4.0	2.3	10	113
50569	Soup, chicken noodle, rts, cnd	1 cup	259	90	6	13	1	1	0.5			10	500
50020	Soup, chicken rice, prep f/cnd w/water	1 cup	243	58	4	7	1	2	0.4	0.9	0.4	7	41
50091	Soup, chicken vegetable, prep f/cnd w/water	1 cup	248	77	4	9	1	3	0.9	1.3	0.6	10	198
50654	Soup, cream of chicken, cond, cnd	1 cup	252	227	6	18	0	15	4.3	5.2	2.7	20	113
50666	Soup, cream of mushroom, cond, cnd	0.5 cup	121	103	2	8	0	7	1.7	1.3	1.7	0	10
50049	Soup, cream of mushroom, prep f/cnd w/water	1 cup	248	104	2	8	0	7	1.7	1.3	1.7	0	10
50999	Soup, gumbo, zesty, rts, cnd	1 cup	244	100	6	15	3	2	1.0			10	40
91617	Soup, lentil, cnd	1 cup	206	130	8	19	9	4	0.5			0	300
50009	Soup, minestrone, prep f/cnd w/water	1 cup	241	82	4	11	1	3	0.6	0.7	1.1	2	234

PAGE KEY: A-70 Prepared Foods   A-78 Restaurants   A-90 Salad Dressings and Dips   A-92 Sauces and Gravies   A-94 Snack Foods   A-94 Spices, Flavors, and Seasonings   A-96 Sports Bars and Drinks
A-96 Supplemental Foods and Formulas   A-96 Sweeteners and Sweet Substitutes   A-98 Vegetables and Legumes   A-108 Miscellaneous

Thia (mg)	Ribo (mg)	Niac (mg NE)	Vit B6 (mg)	Vit B12 (µg)	Fol (µg)	Vit C (mg)	Vit D (IU)	Vit E (mg AT)	Cal (mg)	Iron (mg)	Magn (mg)	Phos (mg)	Pota (mg)	Sodi (mg)	Zinc (mg)	Wat (%)	Alco (g)	Caff (g)
0.11	0.02	5.48	0.09	0.00	46.3	0.0	0.0		37	0.83	61.7	142	285	2	0.7	2	0.00	0.00
0.25	0.05	5.80	0.12	0.00	87.6	0.0	0.0		39	1.42	68.6	142	272	8	0.8	6	0.00	0.00
0.15	0.02	0.28	0.05	0.00	5.4	0.3	0.0	0.3	17	0.62	29.9	69	101	0	1.1	4	0.00	0.00
				0.00		0.0			0	0.05				0		2	0.00	0.00
0.01	0.03	0.15	0.18	0.00	9.7	0.5	0.0	0.6	19	0.97	62.8	160	163	1	1.1	5	0.00	0.00
0.02	0.03	4.38	0.12	0.00	29.4	0.0	0.0	2.0	14	0.61	51.2	102	238	156	0.9	1	0.00	0.00
0.01	0.02	4.28	0.17	0.00	23.7	0.0	0.0	2.9	14	0.60	49.3	115	208	147	0.9	2	0.00	0.00
0.10	0.01	5.26	0.10	0.00	21.6	0.0	0.0	3.3	13	0.68	61.2	133	241	194	1.0	1	0.00	0.00
0.01	0.02	4.28	0.17	0.00	23.7	0.0	0.0	2.9	14	0.60	49.3	115	208	5	0.9	2	0.00	0.00
		5.00	0.11	0.00	24.0	0.0			0	0.72	60.0			220	0.9		0.00	0.00
		2.07		0.00					6	0.31		59	115	89		3	0.00	0.00
0.68	0.07	1.28	0.20	0.00	36.5	0.3	0.0	0.1	107	2.41	164.6	270	341	13	1.8	7	0.00	0.00
0.51	0.11	2.92	0.46	0.00	79.4	0.5	0.0	12.3	27	1.84	113.8	231	226	3	1.8	5	0.00	0.00
0.02	0.07	2.25	0.25	0.00	75.8	0.4	0.0	8.4	22	1.22	41.3	370	272	131	1.7	1	0.00	0.00
0.02	0.07	2.25	0.25	0.00	75.8	0.4	0.0	8.4	22	1.22	41.3	370	272	1	1.7	1	0.00	0.00
0.10	0.09	1.38	0.27	0.00	79.0	0.4	0.0	12.3	29	1.44	42.9	384	163	138	1.8	2	0.00	0.00
				0.00		0.0			63	1.91						2	0.00	0.00
						0.0			0	0.00				890			0.00	0.00
						0.0			0	0.00				960			0.00	0.00
						0.0			80	2.70				1250			0.00	0.00
						0.0			7	0.58			109	149			0.00	0.00
0.11	0.27	0.92	0.34	0.00	58.9	4.4	0.0	1.3	120	8.77	115.2	394	934	1336	5.1	76	0.00	0.00
						2.4			100	4.50				480			0.00	0.00
0.07	0.27	2.99	0.31	2.45		4.3			72	4.82	48.0	185	444	934	2.7	78	0.00	0.00
						0.0			81	1.78				870		84	0.00	0.00
0.23	0.25	1.60			60.0	0.0			150	1.44			350	950			0.00	0.00
0.25	0.28	2.89	0.09	0.37	31.7	0.0	0.0	0.1	85	2.20	22.0	115	205	737	1.1	81	0.00	0.00
0.15	0.17	4.00			60.0	0.0			40	1.79				1070			0.00	0.00
						0.0			0	0.00				460		100	0.00	0.00
						0.0			40	1.98				510		100	0.00	0.00
						0.0			40	1.98				630		100	0.00	0.00
0.07	0.02	0.55	0.03	0.03	31.2	1.6	0.0	1.1	78	1.99	42.9	127	390	922	1.0	70	0.00	0.00
0.07	0.05	1.03	0.03	0.20	19.5	0.5	0.0	1.2	20	1.07	7.3	46	98	930	1.5	92	0.00	0.00
0.01	0.10	1.62	0.05	0.05	0.0	0.0			29	0.87	9.8	27	154	798	1.0	90	0.00	0.00
						0.0			20	0.36				870			0.00	0.00
0.01	0.01	1.12	0.01	0.17	0.0	0.2	0.0	0.1	22	0.75	0.0	22	100	578	0.3	94	0.00	0.00
0.03	0.05	1.25	0.05	0.11	5.0	1.0	0.0	0.4	17	0.88	7.4	42	159	972	0.4	93	0.00	0.00
0.02	0.11	0.99	0.00	0.00	5.0	0.3	0.0	1.4	35	2.67	10.1	78	123	1769	0.7	83	0.00	0.00
0.05	0.05	0.50	0.00	0.00	2.4	0.0	0.0	1.0	15	1.34	4.8	31	75	849	0.2	84	0.00	0.00
0.05	0.05	0.51	0.00	0.00	2.5	0.0	0.0	1.0	17	1.34	5.0	32	74	789	0.2	92	0.00	0.00
						3.6			40	0.72				480			0.00	0.00
0.15	0.07	1.01	0.20	0.00	151.7	6.0	0.0	0.7	20	2.70	35.1	156	416	590	1.1		0.00	0.00
0.05	0.03	0.93	0.10	0.00	36.2	1.2			34	0.92	7.2	55	313	612	0.7	91	0.00	0.00

PAGE KEY: A-42 Beverages and Beverage Mixes   A-44 Candies   A-46 Cereals   A-48 Cheeses and Substitutes   A-50 Dairy Products and Substitutes   A-52 Desserts   A-56 Eggs and Egg Substitutes
A-56 Fats, Oils, Margarines, and Shortenings   A-58 Fruits   A-60 Grain Products and Baked Goods   A-62 Grains and Flours   A-64 Meats and Meat Substitutes   A-68 Nuts, Seeds, and Products

Code	Food Name	Unit/ Amt	Wt (g)	Energy (kcal)	Prot (g)	Carb (g)	Fiber (g)	Fat (g)	Sat (g)	Mono (g)	Poly (g)	Chol (mg)	Vit A (RE)
50486	Soup, onion, French, cond, cnd	0.5 cup	126	45	2	6	1	1	1.0	0.0	0.5	5	0
50050	Soup, pea, green, prep f/cnd w/water	1 cup	259	158	8	26	5	3	1.4	1.0	0.4	0	8
50407	Soup, split pea, rducd sod, cnd	1 cup	253	180	10	30	5	2	0.8	0.9	0.4	5	140
50504	Soup, tomato, cond, cnd	0.5 cup	74	54	1	12	1	0	0.0	0.0	0.0	0	
40699	Soup, vegetable, rts, cnd	1 cup	264	100	3	21	3	0	0.0			0	700
50181	Soup, won ton	1 cup	241	182	14	14	1	7	2.3	3.0	1.0	53	99
57659	Stew, beef, cnd, svg	1 svg	196	194	9	15	2	11	4.3	5.0	0.5	25	44
Dry and Prepared from Dry Foods													
50192	Broth, beef, dry cube	1 cube	4	6	1	1	0	0	0.1	0.1	0.0	0	0
50193	Broth, chicken, dehyd, cube	1 cube	5	10	1	1	0	0	0.1	0.1	0.1	1	0
66106	Casserole, potato, scalloped, prep, f/dry, FS	0.5 cup	140	120	2	24	2	3	1.0			0	0
38650	Pilaf, wheat, dry	0.25 cup	56	170	7	40	8	1	0.0			0	0
5138	Mashed Potatoes, flakes, prep f/dry w/whl milk & marg	0.5 cup	105	119	2	16	2	6	1.5	2.4	1.6	4	52
91856	Soup, beef vegetable, in a cup, dry	1 svg	35	150	5	27	1	2	1.0			0	80
50037	Soup, chicken noodle, prep f/dehyd w/water	1 cup	245	56	2	9	0	1	0.3	0.5	0.4	10	3
50036	Soup, cream of chicken, prep f/dehyd w/water	1 cup	261	107	2	13	0	5	3.4	1.2	0.4	3	41
50039	Soup, mushroom, prep f/dehyd w/water, pkt	1 cup	253	83	2	11	1	5	0.8	2.3	1.5	0	20
50040	Soup, onion, prep f/dehyd w/water	1 cup	230	28	1	6	1	0	0.0	0.0	0.0	0	0
92163	Soup, ramen noodle, any flvr, dry	1 svg	43	187	5	27	1	7	3.2	2.8	0.6	0	1
15773	Soup, tomato, prep f/dry w/water	1 cup	265	101	2	19	1	2	0.8	0.6	0.2	5	93
50044	Soup, vegetable beef, prep f/dry w/water	1 cup	253	53	3	8	1	1	0.6	0.5	0.1	0	24
Frozen and Refrigerated Foods													
83063	Bowl, fried rice	1 svg	340	450	18	77	6	8	0.5			0	700
82019	Burrito, bean & cheese, ckd	1 ea	142	300	9	46	4	9	4.5			15	40
49171	Chicken Tenders, breast, ckd f/fzn	3 ea	85	240	11	16	1	14	4.0			25	0
7762	Corn Dog, vegetarian, fzn	1 ea	71	150	7	22	3	4	0.5	1.0	2.5	0	0
81223	Dish, chicken breast, patty, brd, ckd f/fzn	1 ea	90	210	13	10	0	13	3.0			45	0
16260	Dish, chicken, alfredo, w/broccoli, fzn	1 ea	326	300	25	34	2	7	3.0			50	20
56958	Dish, creamed corn, low fat, fzn	0.5 cup	118	110	2	24	2	1	0.0			0	0
70749	Dish, fish & chips	1 svg	156	350	16	38	4	15	4.5			30	40
57290	Dish, green beans, w/almonds, fzn	0.75 cup	116	80	3	8	3	4	0.0			0	20
11055	Dish, meatballs, Swedish, w/pasta, fzn	1 ea	326	560	32	47	3	27	12.0			100	300
83107	Dish, pasta, chicken cacciatore	1.25 cup	295	330	23	44	3	6				40	450
70605	Dish, potatoes O'Brien, fzn	0.75 cup	85	60	1	13	2	0	0.0	0.0	0.0	0	0
1729	Dish, potatoes, rstd, w/ham, bowl, fzn	1 ea	241	210	17	26	6	4	2.0			30	20
17373	Dish, rice bowl w/ chicken, sweet & sour, fzn, prep	1 ea	340	428	19	76	2	5	1.1	1.7	1.4	54	211
70702	Dish, shrimp, popcorn, breaded, fzn	20 ea	112	270	11	28	1	13	2.0	5.0	2.0	35	0
18139	Dish, skillet, Easy Espress, chicken & dumplings, fzn	1 svg	340	370	23	41	5	13	3.5			60	900
16918	Dish, turkey, mostly white meat, w/gravy & stuffing	1 ea	255	240	13	30	2	9	2.0			20	40
6571	Dish, twice baked potatoes, cheddar, fzn, FS	1 ea	141	180	4	24	2	7	2.5			5	0
14069	Dish, veal & beef patty, brd, fzn, 3.2 oz, FS	1 ea	91	202	11	12	2	12	5.5	5.1	0.6	33	20
6592	Dish, vegetables, broccoli carrot cauliflower, teriyaki, fzn	1.25 cup	110	70	2	7	2	4	1.0			0	350
83009	Egg Roll, pork, restaurant style, ckd	1 ea	170	220	5	24	2	11	2.5			10	60
70830	Eggs, scrambled, low fat	1 svg	170	240	12	18	2	13	3.0			40	225
83154	Fajita, chicken, w/vegetables, fzn	2.25 cup	205	131	9	11	3	5	0.9			22	174

PAGE KEY: A-70 Prepared Foods   A-78 Restaurants   A-90 Salad Dressings and Dips   A-92 Sauces and Gravies   A-94 Snack Foods   A-94 Spices, Flavors, and Seasonings   A-96 Sports Bars and Drinks   A-96 Supplemental Foods and Formulas   A-96 Sweeteners and Sweet Substitutes   A-98 Vegetables and Legumes   A-108 Miscellaneous

Thia (mg)	Ribo (mg)	Niac (mg NE)	Vit B6 (mg)	Vit B12 (µg)	Fol (µg)	Vit C (mg)	Vit D (IU)	Vit E (mg AT)	Cal (mg)	Iron (mg)	Magn (mg)	Phos (mg)	Pota (mg)	Sodi (mg)	Zinc (mg)	Wat (%)	Alco (g)	Caff (g)
						0.0			20	0.00			559	650		91	0.00	0.00
0.10	0.05	1.20	0.05	0.00	2.6	1.6	0.0	0.2	31	1.88	38.8	122	184	870	1.7	85	0.00	0.00
0.18	0.07	1.15	0.18	0.02	50.6	0.0	0.0	0.5	43	1.95	35.4	137	463	420	1.0	82	0.00	0.00
						3.6			0	0.43			411	286		80	0.00	
						0.0			40	0.72				900			0.00	0.00
0.40	0.25	4.59	0.20	0.40	18.8	3.4		0.4	31	1.75	20.6	153	316	543	1.1	84	0.00	0.00
0.14	0.10	2.15	0.17	0.98	27.4	1.4	0.0	0.5	24	4.86	15.7	82	319	760	2.0	81	0.00	0.00
0.00	0.00	0.11	0.00	0.03	1.2	0.0	0.0	0.0	2	0.07	1.8	8	15	864	0.0	3	0.00	0.00
0.00	0.01	0.18	0.00	0.00	1.5	0.0	0.0	0.0	9	0.09	2.7	9	18	1152	0.0	2		0.00
						6.0			40	0.36			240	480			0.00	0.00
						0.0			20	1.08				640			0.00	0.00
0.11	0.05	0.69	0.00	0.00	7.3	10.2	0.0		51	0.23	18.9	59	245	349	0.2	76	0.00	0.00
						3.6			0	0.36				990			0.00	0.00
0.20	0.07	1.05	0.01	0.05	17.1	0.0	0.0	0.1	5	0.49	7.4	29	32	561	0.2	94	0.00	0.00
0.10	0.20	2.60	0.05	0.25	5.2	0.5	0.0	0.6	76	0.25	5.2	97	214	1185	1.6	91	0.00	0.00
0.01	0.02	0.60	0.01	0.05	5.1	1.0	0.0	0.6	13	0.46	7.6	23	96	1020	0.1	92	0.00	0.00
0.02	0.02	0.14	0.05	0.00	0.0	0.2	0.0	0.0	21	0.11	9.2	21	71	796	0.1	96	0.00	0.00
0.43	0.10	1.75	0.03	0.10	48.6	0.1	0.0	0.6	12	1.72	9.9	51	77	875	0.4	5	0.00	0.00
0.28	0.46	2.45	0.15	0.15	29.2	5.3	0.0	0.6	77	0.47	26.5	87	294	943	0.3	90	0.00	0.00
0.15	0.20	1.85	0.10	0.07	20.2	2.0	0.0	0.2	15	0.52	12.6	35	182	789	0.3	94	0.00	0.00
0.58	0.21	5.86	0.55	0.00	222.6	3.6	0.0	0.6	150	6.30	75.1	283	481	1090	1.6		0.00	0.00
						0.0			40	0.72				690			0.00	0.00
						0.0			20	0.72				450			0.00	0.00
						0.0			0	1.08			60	500			0.00	0.00
						0.0			0	0.72				400			0.00	0.00
						12.0			100	1.79				530			0.00	0.00
						3.6			0	0.00				320		90	0.00	0.00
						1.2			150	1.44				930			0.00	0.00
						3.6			60	0.72				410			0.00	0.00
						2.4			100	3.59				1250			0.00	0.00
						12.0			40	3.59				890			0.00	0.00
						0.0			0	0.00			160	20		70	0.00	0.00
						24.0			100	1.08				600			0.00	0.00
0.25	0.18	7.71	0.54	1.09	61.2	10.2	3.4	0.8	44	1.19	47.6	320	418	1132	1.3	69	0.00	0.00
						0.0			40	1.44				610			0.00	0.00
						2.4			80	1.44				1120			0.00	0.00
						6.0			40	1.08				830			0.00	0.00
						24.0			60	1.79				320			0.00	0.00
0.15	0.14	3.61				0.0			30	1.62		115	241	368	3.5		0.00	0.00
						21.0			20	0.36				490			0.00	0.00
						0.0			20	1.08				390			0.00	0.00
						4.8			40	0.72				620			0.00	0.00
						36.6			17	0.62				637				

PAGE KEY: A-42 Beverages and Beverage Mixes A-44 Candies A-46 Cereals A-48 Cheeses and Substitutes A-50 Dairy Products and Substitutes A-52 Desserts A-56 Eggs and Egg Substitutes A-56 Fats, Oils, Margarines, and Shortenings A-58 Fruits A-60 Grain Products and Baked Goods A-62 Grains and Flours A-64 Meats and Meat Substitutes A-68 Nuts, Seeds, and Products

Code	Food Name	Unit/ Amt	Wt (g)	Energy (kcal)	Prot (g)	Carb (g)	Fiber (g)	Fat (g)	Sat (g)	Mono (g)	Poly (g)	Chol (mg)	Vit A (RE)
5791	French Fries, cottage cut, par fried, fzn	10 ea	65	99	2	16	2	4	1.8	1.5	0.3	0	0
749	French Fries, crinkle, 1/2" x 17/32", 80% ckd, fzn, FS	3 oz	85	120	2	20	1	4	1.0			0	0
5691	French Fries, shoestring, battered, fzn, FS	1 svg	85	170	4	17	1	10	3.0			0	0
5592	French Fries, w/salt, ckd f/fzn	10 ea	50	82	1	14	1	3	0.5	1.6	0.2	0	0
5790	French Fries, w/salt, fzn	10 ea	89	131	2	22	2	4	0.9	2.8	0.3	0	0
56800	French Toast, cinnamon swirl	1 svg	156	440	14	35	2	28	12.0			150	60
70611	Hash Browns, breakfast, diced, extra crispy, microwv, fzn	0.75 cup	77	160	1	20	2	8	1.5			0	0
6578	Hash Browns, shreds, fzn, FS	1 svg	85	60	1	13	1	0	0.0	0.0	0.0	0	0
11118	Meal, beef, pot roast, fzn	1 ea	312	300	20	41	8	6	2.0			40	250
70150	Meal, burrito, beef & bean, w/salsa, fzn	1 ea	305	540	24	62	8	22	9.2	8.8	1.8	49	81
15957	Meal, chicken & noodles, homestyle, ckd f/fzn	1 cup	340	390	12	44	7	19	7.0			50	700
17888	Meal, chicken fajita, supreme, w/veg rice & beans, fzn	1 ea	262	260	17	32	4	7	3.0	2.0	1.5	40	200
446	Meal, egg roll, w/fried rice & chicken, ckd f/fzn	1 ea	241	330	12	51	5	9	3.0			60	200
1753	Meal, enchilada & tamale, beef, combination ckd f/fzn	1 ea	312	450	10	56	9	20	8.0			30	150
1756	Meal, fish sticks, ckd f/fzn	1 ea	187	290	11	33	4	13	4.5			30	100
70766	Meal, meatloaf	1 ea	468	640	24	65	6	31	14.0			45	60
11071	Meal, steak, salisbury	1 ea	461	610	34	46	10	33	17.0			80	150
16912	Meal, turkey, breast, traditional, fzn	1 ea	298	290	22	40	5	4	2.0			45	80
58543	Meatballs, chicken & turkey, chipotle	3 ea	64	110	10	2	1	7	2.0			60	
70623	Onion Rings, fzn	5 ea	81	180	2	21	2	10	2.0			0	0
56995	Pizza, bagel, cheese & pepperoni, fzn	4 ea	88	220	9	30	2	7	3.0			15	40
45082	Pizza, Canadian bacon, fzn, 1/4 ea	1 pce	135	329	17	28	1	17	4.8	8.0	2.9	12	180
56782	Pizza, cheese, fzn, for one	1 ea	184	497	21	48	4	24				40	
56781	Pizza, deluxe, fzn, for one	1 ea	234	582	23	51	4	32	10.0	9.0	3.0	20	245
70898	Pizza, pepperoni, ckd/fzn, svg	1 pce	146	432	16	42	3	22	7.0	10.0	3.4	22	0
56779	Pizza, pepperoni, fzn, for one	1 ea	191	546	20	50	4	30	9.0	7.0	2.0	20	263
56778	Pizza, sausage, fzn, for one	1 ea	213	571	23	49	4	32	10.0	7.0	3.0	20	272
57178	Pizza, supreme, fzn, 1/5 of 12"	1 pce	130	300	14	30	3	14	6.0			30	60
16163	Pot Pie, chicken	1 ea	198	410	10	43	2	22	9.0			25	200
16915	Pot Pie, turkey	1 ea	198	400	10	42	3	21	8.0			25	100
7906	Potato Wedges, fzn, USDA	3 oz	85	105	2	22	2	2	0.5	1.2	0.1	0	0
23834	Quesadilla, chicken & cheese, fzn	1 ea	85	190	9	22	1	7	3.0			15	60
56868	Ravioli, cheese, w/tomato sauce, fzn	1 ea	340	380	19	47	5	13	8.0			80	200
70826	Sandwich, breakfast, sausage egg cheese, w/biscuit	1 ea	156	460	16	37	3	28	11.0			115	0
17002	Sticks, fish, ckd f/fzn, 4" x 1" x 1/2"	1 ea	28	70	3	6	0	4	0.8	1.2	1.6	8	7
1717	Stir Fry, chicken & veg, fzn	1 ea	337	360	19	57	5	6	2.0			25	350
6602	Stir Fry, teriyaki, fzn	1.5 cup	170	50	3	11	3	0	0.0	0.0	0.0	0	40
11050	Stroganoff, beef, fzn	1 ea	276	380	22	34	2	17	5.0			70	40
70598	Tater Tots, fzn	9 ea	86	160	2	20	2	8	1.5			0	0
57140	Tortellini, three cheese, fzn	81 g	81	250	11	37	2	7	3.5			35	0

Prepared and Generic Foods

Code	Food Name	Unit/ Amt	Wt (g)	Energy (kcal)	Prot (g)	Carb (g)	Fiber (g)	Fat (g)	Sat (g)	Mono (g)	Poly (g)	Chol (mg)	Vit A (RE)
7084	Bean Cakes, Japanese style	1 ea	32	130	2	16	1	7	1.0	2.9	2.6	0	0
7165	Beans, bbq, FS	0.5 cup	100	160	6	32	6	2	0.5				
56234	Chop Suey, pork, w/noodles	1 cup	220	448	22	31	4	27	4.8	7.7	12.8	48	19
57618	Chow Mein, pork, w/noodles	1 cup	220	448	22	31	4	27	4.8	7.7	12.8	48	19
56238	Chow Mein, shrimp, w/noodles	1 cup	220	272	17	24	3	13	1.9	3.1	6.9	82	15

PAGE KEY: A-70 Prepared Foods   A-78 Restaurants   A-90 Salad Dressings and Dips   A-92 Sauces and Gravies   A-94 Snack Foods   A-94 Spices, Flavors, and Seasonings   A-96 Sports Bars and Drinks   A-96 Supplemental Foods and Formulas   A-96 Sweeteners and Sweet Substitutes   A-98 Vegetables and Legumes   A-108 Miscellaneous

Thia (mg)	Ribo (mg)	Niac (mg NE)	Vit B6 (mg)	Vit B12 (μg)	Fol (μg)	Vit C (mg)	Vit D (IU)	Vit E (mg AT)	Cal (mg)	Iron (mg)	Magn (mg)	Phos (mg)	Pota (mg)	Sodi (mg)	Zinc (mg)	Wat (%)	Alco (g)	Caff (g)
0.05	0.00	1.15	0.11	0.00	9.8	5.5	0.0		5	0.68	10.4	30	220	21	0.2	67	0.00	0.00
						4.8			20	0.72		1		15			0.00	0.00
						3.6			0	0.36				330			0.00	0.00
0.05	0.01	1.11	0.09	0.00	14.0	6.7	0.0	0.1	6	0.37	13.0	48	226	194	0.2	62	0.00	0.00
0.09	0.03	1.80	0.15	0.00	31.1	15.4	0.0	0.1	8	0.55	18.7	74	363	295	0.3	67	0.00	0.00
0.34	0.37	3.00				0.0			80	1.79			184	580			0.00	0.00
						2.4			0	0.36				290		47	0.00	0.00
						9.0			0	0.72		1		10			0.00	0.00
						18.0			20	1.79				600			0.00	0.00
0.49	0.44	5.69	0.31	1.08	134.4	20.1		1.6	144	5.53	70.7	350	685	881	3.6	63	0.00	0.00
0.27	0.28	5.69				0.0			60	1.79			374	1080			0.00	0.00
						15.0			100	1.08				600			0.00	0.00
						0.0			40	1.08				1270			0.00	0.00
						0.0			150	1.79				1530			0.00	0.00
						3.6			60	1.79				820			0.00	0.00
						18.0			150	5.40				1870			0.00	0.00
						4.8			200	5.40				1620			0.00	0.00
0.44	0.25	6.00				36.0			20	1.44		270	540	460			0.00	0.00
														540			0.00	0.00
						0.0			40	0.72			85	160			0.00	0.00
						0.0			60	0.72			160	480		40	0.00	0.00
					100.0	0.0		3.0	301	1.21	35.0	418	290	976	3.0	70	0.00	0.00
								2.0			48.0	386	342		4.0	85	0.00	0.00
0.30	0.81	3.52	0.25	2.00	80.0	0.0		2.0	332	2.56	61.0	480	498	1367	5.0		0.00	0.00
0.33	0.34	3.60	0.14	0.82	68.6	2.8			220	3.51	35.0	302	289	902	2.2	42	0.00	0.00
0.25	0.70	2.57	0.20	2.00	97.0	0.0		4.0	336	2.03	53.0	443	416	1353	4.0	86	0.00	0.00
0.30	0.76	2.84	0.23	2.00	109.0	0.0		4.0	371	2.27	60.0	505	456	1363	0.0		0.00	0.00
						0.0			150	1.44				690			0.00	0.00
						1.2			20	1.79				780			0.00	0.00
						2.4			20	1.79				700			0.00	0.00
0.09	0.02	1.30	0.30	0.00		9.5	0.0		13	0.60	16.2	74	335	42	0.3	68	0.00	0.00
						6.0			100	1.44				460			0.00	0.00
						9.0			300	1.79				1000			0.00	0.00
						0.0			150	1.79				1060		71	0.00	0.00
0.03	0.02	0.44	0.00	0.36	9.0	0.0	3.9	0.3	7	0.28	7.8	51	60	118	0.1	53	0.00	0.00
						4.8			40	2.70				600			0.00	0.00
						42.0			40	1.08				650			0.00	0.00
						0.0			80	2.70				990			0.00	0.00
						0.0			0	0.36			250	420		54	0.00	0.00
						0.0			0	0.00				300		25	0.00	0.00
0.07	0.05	0.55	0.01	0.00	9.1	0.0	0.0	1.2	3	0.67	6.1	21	58	1	0.2	23	0.00	0.00
														640			0.00	0.00
0.77	0.43	6.23	0.41	0.41	41.8	20.2		2.7	45	3.29	52.8	249	489	848	2.6	62	0.00	0.00
0.77	0.43	6.23	0.41	0.41	41.8	20.2		2.7	45	3.29	52.8	249	489	848	2.6	62	0.00	0.00
0.23	0.23	4.46	0.18	0.58	45.1	9.4		1.3	58	3.42	51.2	220	391	710	1.3	74	0.00	0.00

PAGE KEY: A-42 Beverages and Beverage Mixes   A-44 Candies   A-46 Cereals   A-48 Cheeses and Substitutes   A-50 Dairy Products and Substitutes   A-52 Desserts   A-56 Eggs and Egg Substitutes   A-56 Fats, Oils, Margarines, and Shortenings   A-58 Fruits   A-60 Grain Products and Baked Goods   A-62 Grains and Flours   A-64 Meats and Meat Substitutes   A-68 Nuts, Seeds, and Products

Code	Food Name	Unit/ Amt	Wt (g)	Energy (kcal)	Prot (g)	Carb (g)	Fiber (g)	Fat (g)	Sat (g)	Mono (g)	Poly (g)	Chol (mg)	Vit A (RE)
11016	Dish, beef, w/sweet & sour	1 cup	252	336	16	28	2	18	6.1	7.2	2.6	54	33
56200	Dish, chicken & noodles, w/tomato sauce	1 cup	224	291	20	31	2	9	2.1	3.8	2.5	74	143
15921	Dish, chicken breast, sweet & sour	1 svg	131	118	8	15	1	3	0.5	0.9	1.4	23	22
15915	Dish, chicken breast, teriyaki	3 oz	85	118	18	4	0	2	0.6	0.7	0.6	55	11
56193	Dish, chicken, w/noodles & mushroom soup sauce	1 cup	224	311	22	30	1	11	3.1	2.9	3.8	81	28
5514	Dish, mushrooms, batter dipped, fried	5 ea	70	156	2	11	1	12	1.5	3.6	6.0	2	6
5643	Dish, mushrooms, stuffed	2 ea	48	138	5	13	1	7	2.2	3.1	1.6	6	50
5644	Dish, okra, batter dipped, fried	0.5 cup	46	88	1	7	1	6	0.8	1.6	3.5	1	19
12081	Dish, pork chop, breaded, brld/bkd	1 ea	100	259	25	6	0	14	5.1	6.2	1.5	72	2
12900	Dish, pork, sweet & sour	1 cup	226	231	15	25	2	8	2.1	3.2	2.3	39	31
58383	Dish, shredded beef, w/original bbq sauce, ckd	1 cup	224	360	28	44	0	8	2.0			60	160
92798	Dish, shredded pork, w/original bbq sauce, ckd	1 cup	224	360	24	44	0	8	2.0			60	160
56287	Egg Foo Yung, chicken	1 ea	86	121	8	4	1	8	1.9	2.8	2.3	167	87
56110	Egg Roll, w/o meat	1 ea	64	101	3	10	1	6	1.2	2.9	1.3	30	16
19516	Eggs, scrambled	1 ea	61	91	6	1	0	7	2.0	2.7	1.5	169	99
15013	Fried Chicken, breast, broiler/fryer, w/skin, batter fried	1 ea	140	364	35	13	0	18	4.9	7.6	4.3	119	28
15003	Fried Chicken, breast, broiler/fryer, w/skin, flour fried	1 ea	98	218	31	2	0	9	2.4	3.4	1.9	87	15
15113	Fried Chicken, drk meat, broiler/fryer, w/skin, batter fried	3 oz	85	253	19	8		16	4.2	6.4	3.8	76	26
56242	Gumbo, New Orleans style, w/rice	1 cup	244	193	14	17	2	8	1.6	2.6	2.7	40	63
56150	Hash, beef	1 cup	190	312	21	21	2	16	4.9	5.7	3.3	57	0
56239	Jambalaya, shrimp, w/rice, Creole	1 cup	243	310	27	28	1	9	1.8	3.8	2.8	181	133
5272	Mashed Potatoes, prep f/rec w/whole milk & margarine	1 cup	210	233	4	36	3	9	2.0	3.9	2.4	2	99
5137	Mashed Potatoes, prep f/recipe w/whole milk	0.5 cup	105	87	2	18	2	1	0.3	0.1	0.1	2	8
57411	Ravioli, beef, square, preckd, FS	9 pce	146	300	14	40	1	8	3.8			77	
56231	Shepherds Pie, beef	1 cup	243	278	17	32	3	9	2.6	4.0	1.7	37	78
56100	Spaghetti, w/meatballs, prep f/recipe	1 svg	248	362	18	28	3	18	4.8			65	164
7559	Stew, vegetarian	1 cup	247	304	42	17	3	7	1.2	1.8	3.8	0	232
91818	Sushi, California roll	1 ea	198	292	8	49	3	3	1.0			3	90
91814	Sushi, Maki, roll, cucumber	6 pce	85	120	3	25	2	1	0.0			0	50
91464	Tamales, w/beef & sauce, FS	2 ea	190	310	6	26	4	23	10.0			20	200
57407	Tortellini, beef filled, preckd, FS	1 cup	128	250	11	38	2	6	3.5			40	20
5989	Vegetables, succotash, ckd w/salt, drnd	0.5 cup	96	107	5	23	5	1	0.1	0.1	0.4	0	28
Salads													
52061	Salad, chicken, FS	0.5 cup	100	250	10	9	2	20	4.0			55	20
52066	Salad, egg, FS	0.5 cup	100	230	9	8	0	18	4.0			240	0
69197	Salad, Field Greens	1 cup	57	10	1	3	1	0	0.0	0.0	0.0	0	200
52010	Salad, fruit, chilled, FS	0.66 cup	110	60	1	14	2	0	0.0	0.0	0.0	0	0
3312	Salad, fruit, w/citrus, fresh	1 cup	175	99	1	25	3	1	0.1	0.0	0.1	0	14
52029	Salad, macaroni, elbow, classic, FS	0.5 cup	106	197	3	25	2	9	1.5			8	
4839	Salad, pasta, Greek, w/feta cheese, FS	0.66 cup	140	200	6	27	3	8	2.0			5	
56005	Salad, potato, prep f/recipe	1 cup	250	358	7	28	3	20	3.6	6.2	9.3	170	88
52065	Salad, seafood, FS	0.5 cup	100	230	6	14	8	17	2.5			20	0
5537	Salad, spinach, w/o dressing	1 cup	74	108	5	11	2	5	1.4	2.2	0.7	77	176
52060	Salad, tuna, FS	0.5 cup	100	260	12	9	2	19	3.0			30	20

Thia (mg)	Ribo (mg)	Niac (mg NE)	Vit B6 (mg)	Vit B12 (µg)	Fol (µg)	Vit C (mg)	Vit D (IU)	Vit E (mg AT)	Cal (mg)	Iron (mg)	Magn (mg)	Phos (mg)	Pota (mg)	Sodi (mg)	Zinc (mg)	Wat (%)	Alco (g)	Caff (g)
0.11	0.18	2.61	0.31	1.59	12.7	21.6		1.2	27	2.69	33.7	151	336	930	3.9	74	0.00	0.00
0.27	0.23	5.73	0.31	0.20	16.5	11.8		2.1	34	2.90	47.2	177	478	658	1.9	72	0.00	0.00
0.05	0.07	3.08	0.18	0.07	5.8	12.1		0.7	15	0.83	20.8	75	185	506	0.7	79	0.00	0.00
0.05	0.12	5.82	0.31	0.18	8.1	2.1		0.2	18	1.13	23.4	132	205	1118	1.3	67	0.56	0.00
0.21	0.25	5.34	0.18	0.33	13.0	0.8		1.0	72	2.45	36.2	201	220	550	2.2	71	0.00	0.00
0.10	0.25	2.25	0.03	0.02	8.3	1.2		2.3	15	1.22	6.8	119	154	112	0.4	63	0.00	0.00
0.15	0.25	2.64	0.07	0.10	11.0	2.8	25.0	0.8	100	1.49	14.3	107	209	298	0.7	43	0.07	0.00
0.09	0.07	0.72	0.05	0.01	19.0	5.2	5.5	1.5	30	0.62	17.9	61	95	61	0.2	67	0.00	0.00
0.81	0.30	4.75	0.41	0.62	5.8	0.5	12.0	0.4	24	1.00	26.8	240	400	415	2.2	52	0.00	0.00
0.55	0.20	3.63	0.40	0.34	10.3	19.6	27.1	1.1	28	1.44	34.4	149	386	839	1.5	77	0.00	0.00
						0.0			0	2.88				1480			0.00	0.00
						0.0			0	2.88				1520			0.00	0.00
0.05	0.23	0.88	0.11	0.34	22.3	3.1		1.1	27	0.81	11.4	96	136	132	0.8	76	0.00	0.00
0.07	0.10	0.80	0.05	0.05	13.4	2.9		0.9	14	0.81	9.1	38	97	274	0.3	70	0.00	0.00
0.01	0.23	0.05	0.07	0.46	22.0	0.0	43.9	0.7	40	0.80	6.7	101	81	88	0.6	76	0.00	0.00
0.15	0.20	14.72	0.60	0.41	21.0	0.0	8.4	1.5	28	1.75	33.6	259	281	385	1.3	52	0.00	0.00
0.07	0.12	13.47	0.56	0.33	5.9	0.0			16	1.16	29.4	228	254	74	1.1	57	0.00	0.00
0.10	0.18	4.76	0.20	0.23	15.3	0.0			18	1.22	17.0	123	157	251	1.8	49	0.00	0.00
0.20	0.15	4.51	0.20	2.41	45.6	13.5		1.4	71	2.60	40.1	152	446	542	15.2	83	0.00	0.00
0.15	0.20	3.74	0.49	1.79	16.5	7.1		1.2	19	2.46	36.4	204	587	470	5.0	69	0.00	0.00
0.28	0.10	4.76	0.21	1.17	12.2	16.9		2.3	104	4.38	63.6	300	439	370	1.7	72	0.00	0.00
0.18	0.09	2.47	0.51	0.15	18.9	22.0	14.7	0.9	44	0.55	39.9	101	685	699	0.6	75	0.00	0.00
0.09	0.03	1.16	0.23	0.07	8.4	6.5	8.4	0.0	25	0.28	18.9	48	311	317	0.3	78	0.00	0.00
									119	2.10				400			0.00	0.00
0.20	0.18	3.90	0.58	1.25	21.1	16.4		1.3	40	2.18	46.9	193	764	312	3.9	75	0.00	0.00
0.25	0.30	4.38	0.28	0.94	67.7	16.3	16.9	2.5	92	3.32	43.7	173	479	1133	3.4		0.00	0.00
1.73	1.48	29.63	2.72	5.42	254.4	0.0	0.0	1.2	77	3.21	313.7	543	296	988	2.7	70	0.00	0.00
						4.8			20	1.08				952			0.00	0.00
						0.0			0	0.36				90			0.00	0.00
						1.8			40	1.08				870			0.00	0.00
						1.2			60	1.79				490			0.00	0.00
0.15	0.09	1.26	0.10	0.00	31.7	7.9	0.0		16	1.46	50.9	112	394	243	0.6	68	0.00	0.00
						1.2			40	0.36				600			0.00	0.00
						0.0			40	1.44				570			0.00	0.00
										0.47				20			0.00	0.00
					54.0				0	18.00				10		95	0.00	0.00
0.07	0.05	0.41	0.23	0.00	14.1	29.2	0.0	0.6	16	0.31	17.4	18	309	1	0.1	84	0.00	0.00
														560			0.00	0.00
														780			0.00	0.00
0.18	0.15	2.22	0.34	0.00	17.5	25.0	0.0		48	1.62	37.5	130	635	1322	0.8	76	0.00	0.00
						0.0			20	0.36				770			0.00	0.00
0.12	0.28	1.66	0.10	0.20	59.9	6.7	0.0	0.9	46	1.46	27.1	83	242	227	0.6	70	0.00	0.00
						0.0			20	0.36				580			0.00	0.00

PAGE KEY: A-42 Beverages and Beverage Mixes   A-44 Candies   A-46 Cereals   A-48 Cheeses and Substitutes   A-50 Dairy Products and Substitutes   A-52 Desserts   A-56 Eggs and Egg Substitutes
A-56 Fats, Oils, Margarines, and Shortenings   A-58 Fruits   A-60 Grain Products and Baked Goods   A-62 Grains and Flours   A-64 Meats and Meat Substitutes   A-68 Nuts, Seeds, and Products

Code	Food Name	Unit/ Amt	Wt (g)	Energy (kcal)	Prot (g)	Carb (g)	Fiber (g)	Fat (g)	Sat (g)	Mono (g)	Poly (g)	Chol (mg)	Vit A (RE)
Sandwiches													
56009	Sandwich, BLT, w/white	1 ea	124	318	10	29	2	18	4.1			20	49
56281	Sandwich, bologna	1 ea	83	256	7	26	1	13	4.1	6.3	2.1	16	37
70755	Sandwich, egg cheese	1 ea	119	350	12	30	1	20	8.0			110	0
56013	Sandwich, grilled cheese, w/white	1 ea	119	399	17	30	1	23	11.9			53	167
56014	Sandwich, grilled cheese, w/whole wheat	1 ea	132	431	20	30	4	27	13.8			60	192
56030	Sandwich, ham, w/whole wheat	1 ea	169	379	27	29	4	18	3.9			59	7
56267	Sandwich, pastrami	1 ea	134	331	14	27	2	18	6.2	8.7	1.0	51	3
56041	Sandwich, peanut butter & jam, w/whole wheat	1 ea	114	398	13	51	5	17	3.6			0	1
56286	Sandwich, salami	1 ea	82	234	8	25	1	11	3.4	5.2	1.9	19	35
56048	Sandwich, tuna salad, w/white	1 ea	122	326	13	35	1	14	1.9			13	15
56052	Sandwich, turkey, w/white	1 ea	156	346	24	29	1	14	1.9			43	8
56053	Sandwich, turkey, w/whole wheat	1 ea	169	360	27	29	4	16	2.3			47	8
RESTAURANTS													
Arby's													
9011	Chicken Tenders, crispy	1 reg	131	359	23	28	2	17	2.7			42	0
8986	French Fries, curly, med	1 svg	128	408	5	48	4	22	3.2			0	0
37627	Hash Browns, cake	1 sml	100	255	2	16	2	14	2.0			0	0
37621	Salad, Market Fresh, farmhouse chicken, crispy, w/o dressing	1 ea	349	460	32	29	4	25	9.0			65	600
81476	Sandwich, Arby's melt, roast beef	1 ea	146	320	18	38	2	11	3.5			30	0
69056	Sandwich, beef 'n cheddar	1 reg	195	430	23	42	2	19	6.0			45	20
56341	Sandwich, chicken, rstd	1 ea	189	400	24	40	3	16	2.5			50	20
56342	Sandwich, ham & Swiss melt	1 ea	131	300	18	37	2	8	3.5			35	20
8992	Sandwich, Market Fresh, roast beef & Swiss	1 ea	345	820	40	84	6	37	11.0			80	250
81477	Sandwich, Market Fresh, roast beef gyro, w/flatbread	1 ea	220	420	20	32	2	23	6.0			50	100
81504	Sandwich, reuben, Market Fresh, corned beef & Swiss, w/rye	1 ea	295	690	36	65	4	32	9.0			80	40
56336	Sandwich, roast beef	1 reg	154	350	23	37	2	13	4.5			45	0
9025	Sauce, dipping, honey dijon	1 indv pkt	28	130	0	5	0	12	2.0			10	0
9008	Sticks, mozzarella, brd, fried, reg	8 pce	137	432	20	36	1	23	8.6			50	100
A&W Restaurant													
81303	Cheeseburger	1 ea	191	500	28	43	3	24	9.0			90	200
81305	Cheeseburger, deluxe, w/bacon	1 ea	278	600	32	44	4	33	12.0			110	250
81319	French Fries, cheese, svg	1 svg	170	390	4	50	4	19	5.0			5	0
81343	French Fries, sml	1 svg	113	313	4	45	4	13	3.3			0	0
81352	Frozen Dessert, Polar Swirl, Oreo, med	1 ea	397	833	16	125	2	30	11.7			54	350
81330	Frozen Dessert, sundae, hot fudge	1 ea	189	350	8	54	1	11	6.0			30	150
81311	Hamburger	1 ea	177	460	26	39	3	22	8.0			75	40
81341	Ice Cream Float, root beer, med	1 ea	467	330	4	70	0	4	2.5			15	100
81358	Milk Shake, vanilla, med	1 ea	475	719	12	97	0	31	18.8			134	250
81310	Sandwich, chicken, grilled	1 ea	262	430	37	37	4	15	3.5			90	40
81315	Sandwich, hot dog, chili & cheese	1 ea	154	350	13	27	2	21	8.0			45	40
Burger King													
56352	Cheeseburger	1 ea	133	380	19	32	4	20	9.1	7.6	2.0	60	
57001	Cheeseburger, double	1 ea	197	570	35	32	2	34	17.0			110	100
56355	Cheeseburger, Whopper	1 ea	316	790	35	53	3	48	18.3	16.0	12.0	114	
57000	Cheeseburger, Whopper Jr	1 ea	180	460	21	33	2	27	10.0			60	80
9087	Chicken Tenders, 4 pce svg	4 pce	62	179	11	11	1	10				32	

PAGE KEY: A-70 Prepared Foods   A-78 Restaurants   A-90 Salad Dressings and Dips   A-92 Sauces and Gravies   A-94 Snack Foods   A-94 Spices, Flavors, and Seasonings   A-96 Sports Bars and Drinks   A-96 Supplemental Foods and Formulas   A-96 Sweeteners and Sweet Substitutes   A-98 Vegetables and Legumes   A-108 Miscellaneous

Thia (mg)	Ribo (mg)	Niac (mg NE)	Vit B6 (mg)	Vit B12 (µg)	Fol (µg)	Vit C (mg)	Vit D (IU)	Vit E (mg AT)	Cal (mg)	Iron (mg)	Magn (mg)	Phos (mg)	Pota (mg)	Sodi (mg)	Zinc (mg)	Wat (%)	Alco (g)	Caff (g)
0.40	0.25	3.69	0.15	0.34	66.3	6.0	6.8	2.3	68	2.20	22.0	123	239	631	1.0	69	0.00	0.00
0.28	0.20	2.73	0.07	0.37	18.7	0.0		0.8	60	1.96	15.4	74	112	598	0.9	41	0.00	0.00
						1.2			150	1.79				890			0.00	0.00
0.28	0.40	2.36	0.07	0.40	60.4	0.0	9.7	1.0	407	2.00	26.5	470	162	1155	2.0	45	0.00	0.00
0.23	0.36	2.46	0.15	0.46	36.6	0.0	10.8	1.4	439	2.31	68.2	619	264	1291	3.1	44	0.00	0.00
0.89	0.38	7.30	0.50	0.66	34.6	0.2	27.5	3.1	58	3.47	72.4	378	502	1339	3.7	83	0.00	0.00
0.28	0.27	4.76	0.12	0.97	21.2	2.0		0.3	68	2.64	23.1	135	243	1335	2.7	53	0.00	0.00
0.28	0.20	6.42	0.20	0.00	76.3	2.1	0.0	3.2	80	2.66	75.2	201	336	465	1.5	25	0.00	0.00
0.30	0.28	2.96	0.09	1.07	17.2	0.0		0.7	58	2.25	16.1	80	117	612	0.9	44	0.00	0.00
0.30	0.23	5.88	0.12	0.66	62.5	1.1	72.0	2.8	76	2.40	24.5	152	168	588	0.7	56	0.00	0.00
0.31	0.28	9.27	0.41	1.74	60.3	0.0	15.0	3.3	72	2.18	30.9	250	306	1586	1.3	85	0.00	0.00
0.25	0.21	10.06	0.52	1.91	35.4	0.0	16.4	3.9	53	2.46	71.2	356	417	1734	2.2	84	0.00	0.00
						0.0			12	0.86				730			0.00	0.00
						2.3			25	1.72				930			0.00	0.00
						1.8			10	0.72				435			0.00	0.00
						12.0			250	1.79				1090			0.00	0.00
						0.0			80	3.59				900			0.00	0.00
						1.2			100	4.50				1220			0.00	0.00
						1.2			80	1.79				950			0.00	0.00
						0.0			150	2.70				1070			0.00	0.00
						9.0			450	7.19				1760			0.00	0.00
						9.0			80	3.59				1040			0.00	0.00
						9.0			350	6.30				1970			0.00	0.00
						0.0			60	3.59				960			0.00	0.00
						0.0			0	0.00				160			0.00	0.00
						0.0			399	0.72				1476			0.00	0.00
1.04	0.56	7.78	0.31	1.12	225.7	2.4	4.8	0.9	150	4.50	41.3	272	341	870	4.0		0.00	0.00
1.07	0.64	10.57	0.50	1.77	227.3	6.0	10.5	1.7	200	5.40	52.2	415	601	1390	5.9		0.00	0.00
0.18	0.05	2.16	0.33	0.01	16.3	18.0	0.6	0.2	40	0.00	19.4	68	433	880	0.5		0.00	0.00
0.10	0.01	1.20	0.18	0.00	7.7	19.6	0.0	0.1	0	0.00	12.1	31	203	465	0.3		0.00	0.00
0.30	0.93	1.46	0.20	1.54	61.0	0.0	138.2	1.8	467	4.19	132.8	541	946	646	2.6		0.00	25.64
						0.0			200	0.36				140			0.00	
0.89	0.50	8.38	0.36	1.48	194.8	2.4	3.9	1.1	100	4.50	37.2	279	395	690	4.7		0.00	0.00
						0.0			150	0.36				120			0.00	0.00
0.20	0.66	0.31	0.14	1.46	15.5	0.0	150.9	0.8	438	1.69	40.9	332	538	212	1.6		0.00	0.00
0.79	0.46	16.78	0.73	0.33	168.0	6.0	4.1	1.1	100	3.59	50.6	339	494	1080	1.8		0.00	0.00
0.73	0.37	5.00	0.18	0.91	138.6	1.2	21.2	0.6	80	1.79	19.2	152	235	1080	2.0		0.00	0.00
0.40	0.31	4.51	0.11			0.3		0.1	124	3.32	31.9	190	237	801	3.2	45	0.00	0.00
						0.0			250	4.50				1020			0.00	0.00
0.67	0.62	8.09	0.23		161.2	0.6		0.3	259	6.32	56.9	357	534	1431	5.1	55	0.00	0.00
						4.8			150	3.59				740			0.00	0.00
0.07	0.07	4.63	0.21		4.3	0.4		0.5	9	0.37	15.5	141	163	447	0.4	46	0.00	0.00

PAGE KEY: A-42 Beverages and Beverage Mixes   A-44 Candies   A-46 Cereals   A-48 Cheeses and Substitutes   A-50 Dairy Products and Substitutes   A-52 Desserts   A-56 Eggs and Egg Substitutes   A-56 Fats, Oils, Margarines, and Shortenings   A-58 Fruits   A-60 Grain Products and Baked Goods   A-62 Grains and Flours   A-64 Meats and Meat Substitutes   A-68 Nuts, Seeds, and Products

Code	Food Name	Unit/ Amt	Wt (g)	Energy (kcal)	Prot (g)	Carb (g)	Fiber (g)	Fat (g)	Sat (g)	Mono (g)	Poly (g)	Chol (mg)	Vit A (RE)
42429	French Toast, sticks	5 ea	107	373	6	44	1	19	4.3	10.2	2.7	0	
56351	Hamburger	1 ea	121	333	17	33	2	15	6.1	6.4	1.5	42	
56354	Hamburger, Whopper	1 ea	291	678	31	54	5	37	12.4	13.6	9.9	87	
56999	Hamburger, Whopper Jr	1 ea	167	410	18	32	2	23	7.0			50	40
9040	Onion Rings	1 sml	51	176	3	22	2	9	2.2			0	0
56362	Sandwich, BK Big Fish	1 ea	263	710	24	67	4	38	14.0			50	20
56360	Sandwich, chicken	1 ea	224	660	25	53	3	39	8.0			70	20
Carl's Junior													
91421	Baked Potato, Great Stuff, w/bacon & cheese	1 ea	411	630	20	76	6	29	7.0			35	150
91433	Burrito, breakfast	1 ea	185	480	27	26	2	30	13.0			465	150
91404	Cheeseburger, Western Bacon	1 ea	225	650	32	63	2	30	12.0			80	40
91414	French Fries, svg	1 svg	92	290	5	37	3	14	3.0			0	0
91406	Hamburger, Jr	1 ea	134	330	18	34	1	13	5.0			45	0
91403	Hamburger, Super Star	1 ea	345	790	42	49	2	46	14.0			130	100
91419	Nuggets, chicken, Chicken Stars, svg	1 ea	90	280	12	15	0	19	4.5			40	0
91425	Salad, garden	1 ea	137	50	3	4	2	2	1.5			10	600
91407	Sandwich, chicken, bbq flvr, charbroiled	1 ea	199	280	25	37	2	3	1.0			60	60
91411	Sandwich, chicken, crispy, bacon Swiss	1 ea	291	720	32	66	3	36	10.0			75	80
91413	Sandwich, fish, Carl's Catch	1 ea	201	510	18	50	1	27	7.0			80	60
Chick-fil-A													
69188	Fried Chicken, breast, fillet, brd	1 ea	105	230	23	10	0	11	2.5			60	40
52139	Salad, carrot raisin, sml	1 sml	91	130	1	22	2	5	1.0			0	1700
52135	Salad, Chick-N-Strips	1 ea	315	340	30	19	3	16	5.0			85	600
69152	Sandwich, chicken	1 ea	170	410	28	38	1	16	3.5			60	40
69183	Wrap, Cool, chicken Caesar	1 ea	227	460	38	51	3	11	6.0			85	150
69184	Wrap, Cool, chicken, chargrilled	1 ea	240	390	31	53	3	7	3.0			70	450
69182	Wrap, Cool, chicken, spicy	1 ea	225	390	31	51	3	7	3.5			70	40
Chili's													
4823	Dish, pasta, veggie	1 svg	632	680	34	102	6	13	4.0			125	619
4824	Dish, pasta, veggie, w/chicken	1 svg	717	786	53	106	6	15	5.0			167	631
4822	Meal, chicken, platter	1 svg	652	563	38	83	4	9	3.0			58	736
4826	Salad, chicken, w/dressing	1 ea	445	272	29	27	6	5	1.0			47	416
4825	Sandwich, chicken	1 ea	553	527	44	70	11	8	2.0			43	620
Dairy Queen													
2352	Blended Drink, Arctic Rush Freeze, blue raspberry, med	1 med	518	560	12	89	0	14	9.0			50	200
56372	Cheeseburger, double, homestyle	1 ea	226	640	34	34	1	34	18.0			125	150
2131	Frozen Dessert, banana split	1 ea	374	520	9	94	3	13	10.0			30	150
72141	Frozen Dessert, Blizzard, banana split, med	1 med	382	570	13	93	1	16	10.0			55	250
2368	Frozen Dessert, Blizzard, Oreo cookies, med	1 med	334	680	14	100	1	25	12.0			50	200
56368	Hamburger, homestyle	1 ea	142	350	17	33	1	14	7.0			50	60
72131	Ice Cream Cone, soft serve, vanilla, choc dipped, lrg	1 lrg	312	670	13	83	0	32	21.0			45	200
2142	Ice Cream Cone, soft serve, vanilla, lrg	1 lrg	284	470	12	74	0	14	9.0			45	200
2143	Ice Cream Cone, soft serve, vanilla, med	1 med	199	330	9	53	0	10	6.0			30	150
2134	Ice Cream Sandwich, DQ	1 ea	85	190	4	31	1	5	3.0			10	40
2348	Ice Cream, soft serve, chocolate	1 sml	135	215	6	32	0	7	5.0			22	150
16287	Meal, chicken strip, w/gravy toast & fries, 4 pce basket	1 meal	432	1360	39	103	8	63	11.0			100	40

PAGE KEY: A-70 Prepared Foods   A-78 Restaurants   A-90 Salad Dressings and Dips   A-92 Sauces and Gravies   A-94 Snack Foods   A-94 Spices, Flavors, and Seasonings   A-96 Sports Bars and Drinks
A-96 Supplemental Foods and Formulas   A-96 Sweeteners and Sweet Substitutes   A-98 Vegetables and Legumes   A-108 Miscellaneous

Thia (mg)	Ribo (mg)	Niac (mg NE)	Vit B6 (mg)	Vit B12 (µg)	Fol (µg)	Vit C (mg)	Vit D (IU)	Vit E (mg AT)	Cal (mg)	Iron (mg)	Magn (mg)	Phos (mg)	Pota (mg)	Sodi (mg)	Zinc (mg)	Wat (%)	Alco (g)	Caff (g)
0.30	0.18	2.75	0.05	0.00		0.0		0.9	57	2.04	20.3	93	119	458	0.5	34	0.00	0.00
0.40	0.27	4.78	0.11		77.4	0.2		0.0	62	3.04	29.0	144	220	551	2.6	45	0.00	0.00
0.62	0.50	8.35	0.25		136.8	0.6		0.4	113	12.72	52.4	262	492	911	8.2	56	0.00	0.00
						4.8			80	3.59				520		91	0.00	0.00
						0.0			64	0.00				257			0.00	0.00
						0.0			80	3.59				1200			0.00	0.00
						0.0			80	2.70				1330			0.00	0.00
						36.0			150	4.50				1700			0.00	0.00
						0.0			350	2.70				750			0.00	0.00
						1.2			200	4.50				1430			0.00	0.00
						21.0			0	1.08				170		34	0.00	0.00
						2.4			60	3.59				480			0.00	0.00
						9.0			100	5.40				910			0.00	0.00
						0.0			20	1.08				330		42	0.00	0.00
						15.0			80	0.72				60			0.00	0.00
						4.8			80	2.70				830			0.00	0.00
						6.0			250	3.59				1610			0.00	0.00
						2.4			150	1.79				1030			0.00	0.00
						0.0			40	1.08				990			0.00	0.00
						3.6			20	0.36				90			0.00	0.00
						6.0			150	1.08				680			0.00	0.00
						0.0			100	2.70				1300			0.00	0.00
						0.0			400	3.59				1540			0.00	0.00
						4.8			200	3.59				1120			0.00	0.00
						4.8			200	3.59				1150			0.00	0.00
						7.0			245	7.00				760			0.00	0.00
						7.0			249	8.00				1195			0.00	0.00
						33.0			172	8.00				3284			0.00	0.00
						16.0			36	4.00				1475			0.00	0.00
						26.0			306	9.00				2923			0.00	0.00
						0.0			400	2.70				190			0.00	0.00
						0.0			200	4.50				1230			0.00	0.00
						18.0			250	2.70				160			0.00	
						9.0			450	3.59				230			0.00	
						0.0			400	3.59				530			0.00	
						0.0			40	2.70				680			0.00	0.00
						0.0			400	2.70				220			0.00	
						0.0			400	2.70				200			0.00	0.00
						0.0			250	1.79				140			0.00	0.00
						0.0			100	1.08				135			0.00	
						0.0			150	0.89				110			0.00	
						1.2			100	6.30				2910			0.00	0.00

PAGE KEY: A-42 Beverages and Beverage Mixes   A-44 Candies   A-46 Cereals   A-48 Cheeses and Substitutes   A-50 Dairy Products and Substitutes   A-52 Desserts   A-56 Eggs and Egg Substitutes   A-56 Fats, Oils, Margarines, and Shortenings   A-58 Fruits   A-60 Grain Products and Baked Goods   A-62 Grains and Flours   A-64 Meats and Meat Substitutes   A-68 Nuts, Seeds, and Products

Code	Food Name	Unit/ Amt	Wt (g)	Energy (kcal)	Prot (g)	Carb (g)	Fiber (g)	Fat (g)	Sat (g)	Mono (g)	Poly (g)	Chol (mg)	Vit A (RE)
2224	Milk Shake, chocolate, med	1 med	550	790	18	130	0	21	13.0			70	250
56383	Onion Rings	1 side	113	360	6	47	2	16	2.0			0	0
71690	Sandwich, bbq beef	1 ea	142	270	16	43	1	4	1.0			30	60
56374	Sandwich, hot dog, beef	1 ea	110	290	11	22	1	17	7.0			35	40
Domino's Pizza													
91365	Breadsticks	1 svg	37	116	3	18	1	4	0.8			0	4
91366	Breadsticks, cheesy	1 svg	43	142	4	18	1	6	2.0			6	18
91369	Fried Chicken, Buffalo wings	1 ea	25	50	6	2	0	2	0.6			26	8
91370	Fried Chicken, Buffalo wings, hot	1 ea	25	45	5	0	0	2	0.6			26	27
93265	Pizza, deep dish, ultimate, cheese, 14"	1 pce	121	332	14	41	3	13	4.9	3.6	2.3	17	99
93259	Pizza, deep dish, ultimate, pepperoni, 14"	1 pce	127	366	15	41	3	16	6.2	5.1	2.6	22	94
93263	Pizza, ExtravaganZZa Feast, 14"	1 pce	151	368	16	39	3	17	6.6	5.5	2.2	30	82
56386	Pizza, hand tossed, cheese, 12"	2 pce	159	375	15	55	3	11	4.8			23	131
91360	Pizza, hand tossed, Hawaiian feast, 12"	2 pce	204	450	21	58	3	16	7.2			41	173
91361	Pizza, hand tossed, pepperoni feast, 12"	2 pce	196	534	24	56	3	25	10.9			57	175
91357	Pizza, hand tossed, veggie feast, 12"	2 pce	203	439	19	57	4	16	7.1			34	181
93267	Pizza, thin crust, cheese, 14"	1 pce	39	123	5	11	1	7	2.6	1.6	1.4	8	39
Dunkin' Donuts													
45702	Doughnut, cake, choc glazed	1 ea	73	290	3	33	1	16	3.5			0	0
45716	Doughnut, raised, Bavarian kreme	1 ea	67	210	3	30	1	9	2.0			0	0
45708	Doughnut, raised, glazed	1 ea	35	140	2	19	1	6	1.2			0	0
42636	Fritter, apple	1 ea	164	600	8	82	2	28	6.0			0	0
14119	Salad, Mediterranean	1 ea	425	220	10	23	5	11	3.5			15	1600
14120	Salad, Oriental	1 ea	397	580	30	39	4	35	5.0			45	1500
El Pollo Loco													
4012	Guacamole	1 svg	48	51	0	5	0	3	0.0			0	
1656	Salad, tostada	1 ea	476	740	34	83	11	33	9.0			65	
28104	Salsa, avocado	1 svg	28	18	0	1	0	1	0.0			0	
7204	Taco, chicken, soft	1 ea	108	237	17	18	1	11	5.0			45	
49112	Tortilla, corn, 6"	1 ea	28	70	1	14	1	1	0.0			0	
Hardee's													
9280	Cheeseburger	1 ea	124	313	16	26	1	14	7.0			40	
9284	Chicken Strips, brd, fried, 5-pce svg	5 pce	92	201	18	13	0	8	1.7			25	
9286	French Fries, Crispy Curls, reg	1 svg	96	340	5	41	0	18	4.0			0	
6146	French Fries, reg	1 svg	113	340	4	45	0	16	2.0			0	
56412	Hamburger	1 ea	110	265	14	26	1	10	4.0			35	
56418	Sandwich, roast beef, regular	1 ea	123	310	17	26	2	16	6.0			43	
56404	Sandwich, sausage egg, w/biscuit	1 ea	156	617	19	44		41	12.9			224	
56403	Sandwich, sausage, w/biscuit	1 ea	114	553	13	44		36	11.0			30	
In-N-Out Burger													
81118	Cheeseburger, Double Double, w/lettuce bun	1 ea	362	520	33	11	3	39	17.0			120	250
81117	Cheeseburger, Double Double, w/mustard & ketchup	1 ea	330	590	37	41	3	32	17.0			115	250
81115	Cheeseburger, w/lettuce bun	1 ea	300	330	18	11	3	25	9.0			60	200
81114	Cheeseburger, w/mustard & ketchup	1 ea	268	400	22	41	3	18	9.0			60	200
81119	French Fries	1 svg	125	400	7	54	2	18	5.0			0	0

Thia (mg)	Ribo (mg)	Niac (mg NE)	Vit B6 (mg)	Vit B12 (µg)	Fol (µg)	Vit C (mg)	Vit D (IU)	Vit E (mg AT)	Cal (mg)	Iron (mg)	Magn (mg)	Phos (mg)	Pota (mg)	Sodi (mg)	Zinc (mg)	Wat (%)	Alco (g)	Caff (g)
						0.0			600	4.50				350			0.00	
						2.4			20	1.08				840			0.00	0.00
						0.0			60	2.70				830			0.00	0.00
						0.0			60	1.79				900			0.00	0.00
						0.1			6	0.87				152			0.00	0.00
						0.1			47	0.92				183		14	0.00	0.00
						0.1			6	0.31				175			0.00	0.00
						1.1			5	0.30				354			0.00	0.00
0.28	0.30	5.13		0.56		0.0		1.1	179	3.57	30.2	244	198	679	1.7	42	0.00	0.00
0.20	0.31	5.05		0.70		0.0		1.1	142	3.29	31.8	257	224	668	1.9	41	0.00	0.00
0.20	0.33	4.90		0.82		0.0		1.2	171	3.50	33.2	278	263	689	1.9	51	0.00	0.00
						0.0			187	2.99				776			0.00	0.00
						1.9			274	3.29				1102			0.00	0.00
						0.1			279	3.40				1349		87	0.00	0.00
						1.3			279	3.44				987			0.00	0.00
0.02	0.03	0.40		0.31		0.0		0.6	87	0.28	10.1	117	72	194	0.6	40	0.00	0.00
						0.0			0	0.00				370			0.00	
0.25	0.15	1.64	0.01	0.00	58.6	0.0	0.0	0.7	0	0.72	9.3	40	58	270	0.2		0.00	0.00
						0.0			0	0.56				194			0.00	0.00
						0.0			0	2.16				720			0.00	0.00
						42.0			200	5.40				760			0.00	0.00
						36.0			100	3.59				1510			0.00	0.00
														272				
														1823				
														226				
														526				
														35		36		
														895			0.00	0.00
														736			0.00	0.00
														950			0.00	0.00
														390		46	0.00	0.00
														663			0.00	0.00
														804			0.00	0.00
														1359			0.00	0.00
														1305			0.00	0.00
						12.0			350	4.50				1160			0.00	0.00
						12.0			350	5.40				1520			0.00	0.00
						12.0			200	2.70				720			0.00	0.00
						12.0			200	3.59				1080			0.00	0.00
						0.0			20	1.79				245			0.00	0.00

PAGE KEY: A-42 Beverages and Beverage Mixes   A-44 Candies   A-46 Cereals   A-48 Cheeses and Substitutes   A-50 Dairy Products and Substitutes   A-52 Desserts   A-56 Eggs and Egg Substitutes
A-56 Fats, Oils, Margarines, and Shortenings   A-58 Fruits   A-60 Grain Products and Baked Goods   A-62 Grains and Flours   A-64 Meats and Meat Substitutes   A-68 Nuts, Seeds, and Products

Code	Food Name	Unit/ Amt	Wt (g)	Energy (kcal)	Prot (g)	Carb (g)	Fiber (g)	Fat (g)	Sat (g)	Mono (g)	Poly (g)	Chol (mg)	Vit A (RE)
81112	Hamburger, w/lettuce bun	1 ea	275	240	13	11	3	17	4.0			40	150
81111	Hamburger, w/mustard & ketchup	1 ea	243	310	16	41	3	10	4.0			35	150
24329	Milk Shake, vanilla	15 fl oz	312	680	9	78	0	37	25.0			90	150
Jack in the Box													
56434	Cheeseburger	1 ea	131	350	18	31	1	17	8.0			50	
15162	Chicken Strips, breast, brd, fried, 4-pce svg	4 pce	201	500	35	36	3	25	6.0			80	
62548	Dish, fish & chips, svg	1 svg	252	680	18	60	4	41	10.0			35	
56433	Hamburger	1 ea	118	310	16	30	1	14	6.0			40	
2163	Milk Shake, chocolate, medium	1 ea	413	859	15	117	1	37	23.6			148	
2165	Milk Shake, vanilla, medium	1 ea	373	746	14	84	1	38	23.6			151	
56446	Onion Rings, svg	1 svg	119	500	6	51	3	30	6.0			0	
56448	Salad, side, w/o dressing	1 ea	137	60	3	5	2	3	1.5			10	
69035	Sandwich, chicken	1 ea	145	400	15	38	2	21	4.5			35	
56378	Taco, beef, monster	1 ea	112	240	8	20	3	14	5.0			20	
56377	Taco, beef, regular	1 ea	76	160	5	15	2	8	3.0			15	
Jamba Juice													
81280	Breadsticks, pizza, w/add prot	1 svg	76	230	9	33	2	6	1.5			5	60
81227	Smoothie, Banana Berry, 16 fl oz	16 fl oz	475	270	2	66	3	2	0.0			0	20
81245	Smoothie, Coldbuster, 16 fl oz	16 fl oz	476	280	3	65	3	2	0.0			5	700
81266	Smoothie, Orange Dream Machine, 16 fl oz	16 fl oz	504	410	15	84	1	2	1.0			5	80
81253	Smoothie, PowerBoost, 16 fl oz	16 fl oz	519	280	4	67	6	1	0.0			0	600
81283	Smoothie, Razzmatazz, 16 fl oz	16 fl oz	490	300	2	72	3	1	0.0			0	20
Kentucky Fried Chicken													
42331	Biscuit	1 ea	52	185	4	22	1	9	2.2	6.1	0.6	1	
56451	Cole Slaw, svg	0.5 cup	96	138	1	15	2	8	1.2	1.9	4.7	2	1
6152	Corn, cob, large	1 ea	162	150	5	26	7	3	1.0			0	0
15163	Fried Chicken, breast, original rec	1 ea	201	444	45	11		24	5.5	8.6	7.6	165	38
56453	Mashed Potatoes, w/gravy, svg	1 svg	136	130	2	18	1	4	1.0			0	20
6188	Potato Wedges, svg	10 pce	123	348	5	41	4	18	3.7	10.9	2.2	0	
Long John Silver's													
56477	Cornbread, hush puppies, svg	1 svg	23	60	1	9	1	2	0.5			0	0
56461	Dish, fish, batter dipped, reg	1 pce	92	230	11	16	0	13	4.0			30	
19108	Dish, shrimp, battered	1 ea	14	45	2	3	0	3	1.0			15	0
69030	Sandwich, fish, batter dipped	1 ea	177	440	17	47	3	21	5.0			40	60
91388	Sticks, cheese, brd, fried	3 ea	45	140	4	12	1	8	2.0			10	40
McDonald's													
69009	Cheeseburger	1 ea	119	313	15	33	1	14	5.3	4.3	0.4	42	58
69010	Cheeseburger, Big Mac	1 ea	219	563	26	44	4	33	8.3	7.6	0.7	79	82
69012	Cheeseburger, Quarter Pounder	1 ea	199	513	29	40	3	28	11.2	9.2	0.9	94	111
47147	Cookie, McDonaldland, pkg	1 pkg	57	255	4	41	1	9	1.8	4.6	1.2		0
19579	Eggs, scrambled, svg	1 svg	102	197	15	2		15	4.1	5.3	2.2	436	186
81438	French Fries, sml	1 svg	71	224	3	28	3	11	1.5	5.5	3.3	0	0
2171	Frozen Dessert, sundae, hot fudge	1 ea	179	333	7	54	1	11	6.4	1.9	0.4	23	145
69008	Hamburger	1 ea	105	265	13	32	1	10	3.1	3.3	0.2	28	12
69011	Hamburger, Quarter Pounder	1 ea	171	417	24	38	3	20	6.9	7.2	0.5	67	19
2169	Milk Shake, vanilla, triple thick, sml, 16 fl oz	1 ea	354	552	12	94	0	16	8.0	3.9	0.8	50	323

PAGE KEY: A-70 Prepared Foods   A-78 Restaurants   A-90 Salad Dressings and Dips   A-92 Sauces and Gravies   A-94 Snack Foods   A-94 Spices, Flavors, and Seasonings   A-96 Sports Bars and Drinks   A-96 Supplemental Foods and Formulas   A-96 Sweeteners and Sweet Substitutes   A-98 Vegetables and Legumes   A-108 Miscellaneous

Thia (mg)	Ribo (mg)	Niac (mg NE)	Vit B6 (mg)	Vit B12 (µg)	Fol (µg)	Vit C (mg)	Vit D (IU)	Vit E (mg AT)	Cal (mg)	Iron (mg)	Magn (mg)	Phos (mg)	Pota (mg)	Sodi (mg)	Zinc (mg)	Wat (%)	Alco (g)	Caff (g)
						12.0			40	2.70				370			0.00	0.00
						12.0			40	3.59				730			0.00	0.00
						12.0			300	0.00				390			0.00	0.00
													270	790			0.00	0.00
													530	1260			0.00	0.00
													960	1100			0.00	0.00
													250	600			0.00	0.00
													944	354				0.00
													825	288			0.00	0.00
													140	420			0.00	0.00
													200	65			0.00	0.00
													240	730			0.00	0.00
													220	390			0.00	0.00
													190	270			0.00	0.00
0.37	0.25	3.00	0.03	0.00	80.0	4.8	0.0	0.8	80	2.70	8.0	20	130	450	0.3		0.00	0.00
0.05	0.10	0.80	0.60	0.11	16.0	9.0	0.0	0.4	80	0.72	24.0	40	540	35	0.3		0.00	0.00
0.23	0.14	2.00	0.30	0.00	100.0	684.0	0.0	10.1	60	0.72	40.0	60	800	15	7.5		0.00	0.00
0.23	0.25	0.80	0.11	0.47	60.0	78.0	100.0	0.0	400	0.72	32.0	300	540	230	0.6		0.00	0.00
2.70	2.89	34.00	3.59	4.80	360.0	198.0	240.0	12.1	600	1.44	240.0	80	810	30	7.5		0.00	0.00
0.05	0.17	4.00	0.69	0.11	100.0	36.0	0.0	0.0	80	1.08	24.0	60	570	45	0.3		0.00	0.00
0.23	0.10	1.65	0.01	0.07	50.2	0.2	1.2	0.7	31	1.47	7.8	305	60	548	0.3	29	0.00	0.00
0.03	0.00	0.20	0.11	0.02	19.9	13.9	0.2	0.5	27	0.20	8.6	19	134	180	0.1	74	0.00	0.00
						6.0			60	1.08				10			0.00	0.00
0.09	0.23	17.85	0.68	0.62					62	1.19	52.3	458	547	1184	1.6	57		
						2.4			0	0.36				380			0.00	0.00
0.18	0.01	2.63	0.25	0.00	36.3	4.5	0.0	1.0	32	1.29	36.9	130	642	931	0.5	44	0.00	0.00
						0.0			20	0.36				200		10	0.00	0.00
0.11	0.07	1.46	0.07	1.59	25.7	4.8	0.0	1.4	20	1.79	34.4	207	170	700	0.4	50	0.00	0.00
0.02	0.01	0.38	0.01	0.07	5.6	1.2	10.8	0.4	0	0.00	3.8	22	22	125	0.1	6	0.00	0.00
0.28	0.18	2.92	0.12	1.84	66.6	9.0	0.0	1.8	60	3.59	46.9	267	224	1120	0.6	88	0.00	0.00
0.02	0.03	0.28	0.01	0.25	6.3	0.0	0.0	0.5	100	0.72	6.3	74	27	320	0.4	20	0.00	0.00
0.27	0.31	4.78		1.01	70.2	0.7			199	2.79	23.8	167	238	745	2.3	45	0.00	0.00
0.38	0.46	7.40		1.92	100.7	0.9			254	4.38	43.8	267	396	1007	4.2	51	0.00	0.00
0.33	0.69	7.65		2.50	101.5	1.6			287	4.17	43.8	320	436	1152	5.2	49	0.00	0.00
0.20	0.17	2.05	0.07		58.1			1.1	10	1.91	9.7	63	56	275	0.3	4	0.00	
0.10	0.62	0.07	0.18	1.10	71.4			1.5	67	2.11	12.2	266	142	196	1.5	67	0.00	
0.23	0.02	1.96	0.37		42.6	5.2			12	0.61	22.7	94	398	161	0.3	40	0.00	0.00
0.07	0.40	0.27	0.09	0.98	0.0			0.3	249	1.49	34.0	229	440	168	1.0	59	0.00	
0.25	0.25	4.76		0.87	67.2	0.6			127	2.76	21.0	112	213	532	2.0	46	0.00	0.00
0.31	0.58	7.61		2.19	95.8	1.5			144	4.11	37.6	212	388	730	4.6	50	0.00	0.00
0.12	0.74	0.38	0.17	1.95	0.0			0.0	428	0.25	42.5	354	623	188	1.5	65	0.00	0.00

Code	Food Name	Unit/ Amt	Wt (g)	Energy (kcal)	Prot (g)	Carb (g)	Fiber (g)	Fat (g)	Sat (g)	Mono (g)	Poly (g)	Chol (mg)	Vit A (RE)
27070	Mustard, hot, pkt	1 indv pkt	28	53	1	8	1	2	0.3	0.5	1.0		0
15174	Nuggets, chicken, McNuggets, 4 pce svg	4 pce	64	186	10	11	1	12	2.0	5.2	3.8	28	0
48136	Pie, snack, apple	1 ea	77	249	2	34	2	12	3.1	7.1	0.8		
34745	Sandwich, breakfast, bacon egg cheese, w/biscuit, lrg	1 ea	154	480	15	43	3	27	12.0			235	150
69006	Sandwich, breakfast, McMuffin, sausage cheese	1 ea	115	383	15	28	2	24	8.3	8.9	3.7	45	60
69007	Sandwich, breakfast, McMuffin, sausage egg cheese	1 ea	165	452	21	29	1	29	9.9	10.9	4.6	254	111
69004	Sandwich, breakfast, sausage egg, w/biscuit	1 ea	163	507	18	31	1	36	14.1	12.6	5.2	248	104
81475	Sandwich, chicken, club, premium grilled	1 ea	269	594	46	53	3	22	7.8	6.7	5.8	124	191
69013	Sandwich, Filet O Fish	1 ea	142	390	16	39	1	19	3.7	5.5	8.0	40	25
53254	Sauce, dipping, honey mustard, tangy	1 indv pkt	43	72	1	12	1	2	0.4	0.6	1.2		0
42747	Sweet Roll, cinnamon	1 ea	105	418	8	56	2	19	4.7	9.5	3.0	61	132
Pizza Hut													
92495	Chicken, wings, mild, 2 pce svg	2 pce	53	110	11	1	0	7	2.0			70	60
56489	Pizza, hand tossed, cheese, 12" med	1 pce	96	260	11	30	2	10	4.8	2.8	1.8	23	88
57372	Pizza, hand tossed, ham, 12" med	1 pce	98	220	12	29	2	6	3.0			20	60
57377	Pizza, hand tossed, Italian sausage, 12" med	1 pce	111	290	13	30	2	12	6.0			30	60
57376	Pizza, hand tossed, pork, 12" med	1 pce	111	270	13	30	3	11	5.0			25	60
57787	Pizza, pan, cheese, 6" personal	1 pce	63	160	7	18	1	7	3.0			15	40
57383	Pizza, pan, Meat Lover's, 12" med	1 pce	123	340	15	29	2	19	7.0			35	60
56482	Pizza, pan, pepperoni, 12" med	1 pce	96	286	11	29	2	14	5.1	4.2	3.3	24	46
57382	Pizza, pan, Veggie Lover's, 12" med	1 pce	119	260	10	30	2	12	4.0			15	80
Starbucks													
20592	Coffee, cappuccino, w/2% milk, tall	1 ea	169	90	6	9	0	4	2.0			15	60
20639	Coffee, cappuccino, w/whole milk, tall	1 ea	169	110	6	9	0	6	3.0			15	40
20659	Coffee, iced, latte, Caffe, w/2% milk, tall	1 ea	289	100	6	10	0	4	2.5			15	60
Subway													
91790	Chili, con carne	1 cup	240	310	17	28	9	14	5.0			35	150
91784	Chowder, clam, New England	1 cup	240	140	5	19	7	4	1.0			15	150
91786	Chowder, potato cheese	1 cup	240	210	7	22	2	10	7.0			25	300
91801	Mustard, honey, fat free	1.5 Tbs	21	30	0	7	0	0	0.0	0.0	0.0	0	0
52119	Salad, chicken, breast, rstd	1 ea	303	140	16	12	3	3	1.0			45	150
52115	Salad, club	1 ea	322	150	17	12	3	4	1.5			35	150
69119	Sandwich, beef steak cheese, w/white, 6"	1 ea	256	390	24	48	5	14	5.0			35	100
69125	Sandwich, chicken breast, rstd, w/white, 6"	1 ea	236	320	23	47	5	5	2.0			45	60
69115	Sandwich, ham, w/white, 6"	1 ea	232	290	18	46	4	5	1.5			25	60
69129	Sandwich, meatball, w/white, 6"	1 ea	287	530	24	53	6	26	10.0			55	150
69121	Sandwich, roast beef, w/white, 6"	1 ea	222	290	19	45	4	5	2.0			20	60
69137	Sandwich, turkey breast, w/ham, w/white, 6"	1 ea	232	290	20	46	4	5	1.5			25	60
69111	Sandwich, turkey, w/white, 6"	1 ea	222	280	18	46	4	4	1.5			20	60
69109	Sandwich, veggie delite, w/white, 6"	1 ea	166	230	9	44	4	3	1.0			0	60
Taco Bell													
56519	Burrito, bean	1 ea	198	404	16	55	8	14	4.8	5.9	1.7	18	13
57678	Burrito, chicken, grilled, Stuft	1 ea	325	680	35	76	7	26	7.0			70	100
57677	Burrito, chili cheese	1 ea	156	390	16	40	3	18	9.0			40	150
45585	Dessert, cinnamon twists, svg	1 svg	35	160	1	28	0	5	1.0			0	0
57665	Gordita, beef, supreme	1 ea	153	310	14	30	3	16	7.0			35	100

PAGE KEY: A-70 Prepared Foods   A-78 Restaurants   A-90 Salad Dressings and Dips   A-92 Sauces and Gravies   A-94 Snack Foods   A-94 Spices, Flavors, and Seasonings   A-96 Sports Bars and Drinks   A-96 Supplemental Foods and Formulas   A-96 Sweeteners and Sweet Substitutes   A-98 Vegetables and Legumes   A-108 Miscellaneous

Thia (mg)	Ribo (mg)	Niac (mg NE)	Vit B6 (mg)	Vit B12 (µg)	Fol (µg)	Vit C (mg)	Vit D (IU)	Vit E (mg AT)	Cal (mg)	Iron (mg)	Magn (mg)	Phos (mg)	Pota (mg)	Sodi (mg)	Zinc (mg)	Wat (%)	Alco (g)	Caff (g)
0.00	0.01	0.10	0.01	0.05	0.0	0.0		0.2	9	0.23	6.7	16	23	253	0.1	59	0.00	0.00
0.10	0.07	4.73	0.25	0.20	17.9	0.8			9	0.57	14.1	212	161	404	0.4	47	0.00	0.00
0.23	0.15	2.02	0.03		87.0	24.9		1.5	15	1.52	5.4	28	49	153	0.2	37	0.00	0.00
						0.0			150	3.59				1270			0.00	0.00
0.40	0.33	4.80	0.18	0.51	79.3	0.0		0.3	258	2.34	24.1	187	216	797	1.5	39	0.00	0.00
0.43	0.56	4.82	0.25	1.14		0.0		0.8	284	3.25	29.7	282	282	944	2.0	50	0.00	0.00
0.50	0.62	4.84	0.23	0.98	138.6	0.0		1.6	95	3.30	21.2	494	269	1082	1.7	45	0.00	0.00
0.46	0.50	15.00				11.8			256	3.69				1695		53	0.00	0.00
0.36	0.25	3.41		1.04	69.6	0.1			163	2.09	28.4	168	248	689	0.7	46	0.00	0.00
0.00	0.01	0.09	0.01	0.07	0.0	0.0		0.3	10	0.18	5.2	15	21	165	0.1	63	0.00	0.00
0.31	0.28	2.52	0.10		108.1	0.0		1.9	60	1.80	19.9	109	147	397	0.9	20	0.00	0.00
						0.0			0	0.72				320			0.00	0.00
0.25	0.25	3.16	0.10	0.67		0.0		0.7	201	1.87	21.1	239	166	658	1.6	43	0.00	0.00
						6.0			150	1.79				550			0.00	0.00
						3.6			150	1.79				660			0.00	0.00
						3.6			150	1.79				640			0.00	0.00
						0.0			100	1.44				310			0.00	0.00
						6.0			150	2.70				750			0.00	0.00
0.28	0.23	3.69	0.12	0.61		0.0		0.7	140	2.04	21.1	197	191	664	1.5	41	0.00	0.00
						9.0			150	2.70				470			0.00	0.00
						0.0			200	0.00				70			0.00	75.00
						0.0			200	0.00				70			0.00	75.00
						0.0			200	0.00				80			0.00	75.00
						12.0			60					900			0.00	0.00
						0.0			60	1.79				900			0.00	0.00
						0.0			200	0.00				1010			0.00	0.00
						0.0			0	0.00				140			0.00	0.00
						30.0			40	1.08				800			0.00	0.00
						30.0			40	18.00				1110			0.00	0.00
						24.0			150	8.10				1210			0.00	0.00
						21.0			60	5.40				1000			0.00	0.00
						21.0			60	3.59				1270			0.00	0.00
						27.0			150	5.40				1360			0.00	0.00
						21.0			60	6.30				910			0.00	0.00
						21.0			60	3.59				1220			0.00	0.00
						21.0			60	3.59				1010			0.00	0.00
						21.0			60	3.59				510			0.00	0.00
0.40	0.30	3.39	0.23	0.00	99.0			1.0	232	4.57	61.4	337	533	1216	1.7	55	0.00	0.00
						6.0			300	3.59				1950			0.00	0.00
						0.0			300	1.79				1080			0.00	0.00
						0.0			0	0.36				150			0.00	0.00
						4.8			150	2.70				590			0.00	0.00

PAGE KEY: A-42 Beverages and Beverage Mixes   A-44 Candies   A-46 Cereals   A-48 Cheeses and Substitutes   A-50 Dairy Products and Substitutes   A-52 Desserts   A-56 Eggs and Egg Substitutes   A-56 Fats, Oils, Margarines, and Shortenings   A-58 Fruits   A-60 Grain Products and Baked Goods   A-62 Grains and Flours   A-64 Meats and Meat Substitutes   A-68 Nuts, Seeds, and Products

Code	Food Name	Unit/ Amt	Wt (g)	Energy (kcal)	Prot (g)	Carb (g)	Fiber (g)	Fat (g)	Sat (g)	Mono (g)	Poly (g)	Chol (mg)	Vit A (RE)
56533	Nachos, svg	1 svg	99	362	5	36	4	22	4.7	12.6	2.6	4	2
56531	Pizza, Mexican	1 ea	216	550	21	46	7	31	11.0			45	150
57685	Quesadilla, cheese	1 ea	142	490	19	39	3	28	13.0			55	100
57689	Quesadilla, chicken	1 ea	184	540	28	40	3	30	13.0			80	150
56537	Salad, taco, w/salsa	1 ea	533	906	36	80	16	49	15.9	21.2	4.0	101	33
53604	Sauce, border, mild, svg	1 indv pkt	28	5	0	1	0	0	0.0	0.0	0.0	0	60
56524	Taco, beef	1 ea	78	184	8	14	3	11	3.6	4.2	1.6	24	6
56525	Taco, soft, beef	1 ea	99	217	12	20	3	10	4.2	4.3	1.0	28	8
56689	Taco, soft, chicken	1 ea	99	200	14	19	2	7	2.6	2.8	1.0	37	2
56528	Tostada	1 ea	170	250	11	29	7	10	4.0			15	100
Taco John's													
57576	Burrito, bean, w/cheese	1 ea	187	380	15	53	10	12	5.0			15	
57577	Burrito, beefy	1 ea	187	430	22	41	8	20	9.0			55	
57585	Chimichanga, beef & bean, platter	1 ea	422	760	27	88	9	34	11.0			50	
49127	Dessert, churros	1 ea	55	230	2	31	1	11	2.0			10	
57586	Enchilada, double	1 ea	422	720	37	54	11	40	18.0			105	
2479	Frozen Dessert, Choco Taco	1 ea	113	300	4	38	1	15	7.0			15	
57589	Mexi Rolls	1 svg	213	480	20	33	3	30	10.0			50	
57593	Nachos, svg	1 svg	142	380	6	38	1	23	6.0			10	
57600	Taco	1 ea	94	180	9	13	3	10	4.0			25	
57596	Taco Burger, w/cheese	1 ea	142	280	14	28	3	12	5.0			35	
57601	Taco, soft shell	1 ea	113	220	11	21	4	10	5.0			25	
Taco Time													
56540	Burrito, bean, crisp	1 ea	149	427	15	53	9	18	5.0			12	
56542	Burrito, bean, soft	1 ea	191	380	16	58	13	10	4.0			15	
56621	Burrito, chicken, crisp	1 ea	135	422	17	32	2	25	8.0			54	
56541	Burrito, meat, crisp	1 ea	149	552	34	39	7	30	10.0			58	
56543	Burrito, meat, soft	1 ea	191	491	31	48	12	21	8.0			56	
56620	Burrito, veggie	1 ea	312	491	21	70	10	16	6.0			24	
56550	Cheeseburger, taco	1 ea	213	633	31	48	7	36	10.0			66	
7141	Dish, refritos beans, w/cheese sauce & chips, svg	1 svg	198	326	18	44	13	10	5.0			22	
45586	Empanada, fruit filled	1 ea	113	250	5	37		9				0	
56554	Nachos, svg	1 svg	298	680	26	61	11	38	19.0			78	
50979	Quesadilla, cheddar melt	1 ea	92	205	11	17	1	11	6.0			30	
56556	Salad, taco	1 ea	213	479	30	30	7	28	11.0			63	
56545	Taco	1 ea	113	295	22	16	5	17	7.0			48	
56655	Taco, soft, super	1 ea	298	510	29	50	11	23	12.0			60	
Wendy's													
56579	Baked Potato, bacon & cheese	1 ea	366	460	19	67	7	13	5.0			30	0
56580	Baked Potato, broccoli & cheese	1 ea	396	340	10	70	8	2	1.5			5	150
56574	Cheeseburger, deluxe, w/bacon	1 ea	275	640	37	46	2	35	14.0			125	150
56570	Cheeseburger, jr	1 ea	129	330	17	32	2	15	6.7	5.7	1.5	46	
56571	Cheeseburger, jr, w/bacon	1 ea	137	310	17	25	1	16	6.0			50	100
50311	Chili, sml	1 sml	227	190	14	19	5	6	2.5			40	40
71831	French Fries, med	1 svg	142	453	6	56	5	23	4.5	12.1	5.3		
71834	Frozen Dessert, Frosty, jr	1 ea	113	149	4	27	4	3	1.8	0.8	0.1	18	

PAGE KEY: A-70 Prepared Foods A-78 Restaurants A-90 Salad Dressings and Dips A-92 Sauces and Gravies A-94 Snack Foods A-94 Spices, Flavors, and Seasonings A-96 Sports Bars and Drinks A-96 Supplemental Foods and Formulas A-96 Sweeteners and Sweet Substitutes A-98 Vegetables and Legumes A-108 Miscellaneous

Thia (mg)	Ribo (mg)	Niac (mg NE)	Vit B6 (mg)	Vit B12 (µg)	Fol (µg)	Vit C (mg)	Vit D (IU)	Vit E (mg AT)	Cal (mg)	Iron (mg)	Magn (mg)	Phos (mg)	Pota (mg)	Sodi (mg)	Zinc (mg)	Wat (%)	Alco (g)	Caff (g)
0.11	0.12	0.89	0.18	0.00	12.9			1.0	88	1.11	51.5	280	180	509	1.1	34	0.00	0.00
						6.0			350	3.59				1030			0.00	0.00
						0.0			500	1.44				1150			0.00	0.00
						2.4			500	1.79				1380			0.00	0.00
0.80	0.56	8.02	0.55	2.13	229.2			2.9	506	9.43	143.9	549	1221	1935	6.2	67	0.00	0.00
						0.0			0	0.00				210			0.00	0.00
0.07	0.15	1.50	0.10	0.75	14.8			0.5	62	1.47	25.7	139	168	349	1.7	56	0.00	0.00
0.15	0.20	2.56	0.09	0.76	51.5			0.4	115	2.41	19.8	161	179	626	1.6	56	0.00	0.00
0.20	0.15	6.30	0.15	0.37	47.5			0.3	104	1.70	21.8	222	235	600	0.8	56	0.00	0.00
						4.8			150	1.44				710			0.00	0.00
														830			0.00	0.00
														870			0.00	0.00
														1930			0.00	0.00
														120			0.00	0.00
														2090			0.00	0.00
														110			0.00	
														1270			0.00	0.00
														970			0.00	0.00
														270			0.00	0.00
														600			0.00	0.00
														470			0.00	0.00
														453			0.00	0.00
														715			0.00	0.00
														795			0.00	0.00
														1000			0.00	0.00
														1197			0.00	0.00
														643			0.00	0.00
														1291			0.00	0.00
														525			0.00	0.00
														46			0.00	0.00
														1250			0.00	0.00
														255			0.00	0.00
														895			0.00	0.00
														609			0.00	0.00
														590			0.00	0.00
						42.0			150	3.59				990			0.00	0.00
						66.0			200	3.59				490			0.00	0.00
						12.0			200	5.40				1620			0.00	0.00
0.46	0.21	3.97	1.23	1.67		0.8	5.7		119	3.58	28.4	173	230	851	2.8	48	0.00	0.00
						3.6			100	2.70				670			0.00	0.00
						2.4			60	1.79				830			0.00	0.00
0.25	0.09	3.51	0.56		24.1	7.2			21	2.74	48.3	195	816	244	0.8	39	0.00	0.00
0.07	0.81	0.38	0.00	0.67	5.4	0.0	35.6		145	1.17	22.6	127	209	111	0.5	69	0.00	5.63

PAGE KEY: A-42 Beverages and Beverage Mixes   A-44 Candies   A-46 Cereals   A-48 Cheeses and Substitutes   A-50 Dairy Products and Substitutes   A-52 Desserts   A-56 Eggs and Egg Substitutes   A-56 Fats, Oils, Margarines, and Shortenings   A-58 Fruits   A-60 Grain Products and Baked Goods   A-62 Grains and Flours   A-64 Meats and Meat Substitutes   A-68 Nuts, Seeds, and Products

Code	Food Name	Unit/ Amt	Wt (g)	Energy (kcal)	Prot (g)	Carb (g)	Fiber (g)	Fat (g)	Sat (g)	Mono (g)	Poly (g)	Chol (mg)	Vit A (RE)
2177	Frozen Dessert, Frosty, med	1 ea	298	393	10	70	10	8	4.9	2.1	0.3	48	
15176	Nuggets, chicken, 5-pce svg	5 pce	75	250	12	12	1	17	3.7	8.5	4.3	38	
52083	Salad, side, w/o dressing	1 ea	168	35	1	8	2	0	0.0	0.0	0.0	0	550
56588	Salad, taco, Southwest, w/o dressing & toppings	1 ea	438	400	27	26	7	22	11.0			85	600
81443	Sandwich, chicken, Ultimate Grill	1 ea	225	403	33	42	2	11	2.3	3.3	4.1	90	

White Castle

Code	Food Name	Unit/ Amt	Wt (g)	Energy (kcal)	Prot (g)	Carb (g)	Fiber (g)	Fat (g)	Sat (g)	Mono (g)	Poly (g)	Chol (mg)	Vit A (RE)
13497	Cheeseburger	1 ea	66	160	7	13	0	9	4.5			20	0
13499	Cheeseburger, bacon	1 ea	73	200	10	13	0	12	5.0			30	0
13700	Cheeseburger, double	1 ea	119	290	14	19	1	18	9.0			45	1
13498	Cheeseburger, jalapeno	1 ea	68	170	8	13	0	10	5.0			25	0
13774	Chicken Rings, 6-pce svg	6 pce	110	340	18	15	0	23	4.5			80	0
13782	Dish, Fish Nibblers, 14-pce svg	14 pce	117	280	19	24	5	16	3.5			30	0
13496	Hamburger, Slyder	1 ea	59	140	6	13	0	7	3.0			15	0
13705	Sandwich, chicken breast, w/cheese	1 ea	82	210	13	21	0	8	2.5			25	0
13708	Sandwich, fish, w/cheese	1 ea	77	180	10	18	0	8	2.5			25	0

SALAD DRESSINGS AND DIPS

Dips

Code	Food Name	Unit/ Amt	Wt (g)	Energy (kcal)	Prot (g)	Carb (g)	Fiber (g)	Fat (g)	Sat (g)	Mono (g)	Poly (g)	Chol (mg)	Vit A (RE)
8824	Dip, bean, black, mild	2 Tbs	30	30	2	5	1	0	0.0	0.0	0.0	0	0
53685	Dip, bean, original	2 Tbs	35	40	2	5	1	1	0.0			0	0
27138	Dip, creamy ranch	2 Tbs	31	60	1	3	0	4	3.0			0	0
44805	Dip, French onion	2 Tbs	28	50	1	4	0	3	1.5			10	20
27136	Dip, green onion	2 Tbs	31	60	1	3	0	4	3.0			0	0
27132	Dip, guacamole	2 Tbs	32	50	1	3	0	4	2.5			0	0
90861	Dip, salsa con queso, medium	2 Tbs	32	40	1	2	0	3	1.0			5	20
44950	Dip, salsa con queso, mild	2 Tbs	32	40	1	3	0	3	1.5			5	0
44415	Dip, salsa, grande	2 Tbs	28	50	1	1	0	5	3.0			15	40
27143	Dip, spinach parmesan	2 Tbs	29	90	2	2	0	9	3.0			15	80
44414	Dip, Veggie	2 Tbs	28	50	1	2	0	5	3.0			15	60
44425	Guacamole, med	2 Tbs	28	57	1	3	2	5	1.0			0	10
7957	Hummus	1 Tbs	15	25	1	2	1	1	0.2	0.6	0.5	0	0

Lower Calorie Salad Dressings

Code	Food Name	Unit/ Amt	Wt (g)	Energy (kcal)	Prot (g)	Carb (g)	Fiber (g)	Fat (g)	Sat (g)	Mono (g)	Poly (g)	Chol (mg)	Vit A (RE)
44722	Salad Dressing, blue cheese, rducd cal	1 Tbs	16	14	0	2	0	0	0.1	0.2	0.1	2	11
44465	Salad Dressing, buttermilk, light	1 Tbs	15	30	0	3	0	2	0.2	0.4	0.6	2	3
8138	Salad Dressing, Caesar, low cal	1 Tbs	15	16	0	3	0	1	0.1	0.2	0.4	0	0
44467	Salad Dressing, French, fat free	1 Tbs	16	21	0	5	0	0	0.0	0.0	0.0	0	1
44729	Salad Dressing, French, rducd cal	1 Tbs	16	32	0	4	0	2	0.3	0.5	1.2	0	3
44498	Salad Dressing, Italian, fat free	1 Tbs	14	7	0	1	0	0	0.0	0.0	0.0	0	1
44720	Salad Dressing, Italian, rducd cal	1 Tbs	14	28	0	1	0	3	0.4	0.7	1.6	0	0
8493	Salad Dressing, ranch, fat free	2 Tbs	34	50	0	11	0	0	0.0	0.0	0.0	0	0
44497	Salad Dressing, thousand island, fat free	1 Tbs	16	21	0	5	1	0	0.0	0.1	0.1	1	0
20263	Salad Dressing, vinaigrette, red wine, fat free	2 Tbs	32	15	0	3	0	0	0.0	0.0	0.0	0	0

Regular Salad Dressings

Code	Food Name	Unit/ Amt	Wt (g)	Energy (kcal)	Prot (g)	Carb (g)	Fiber (g)	Fat (g)	Sat (g)	Mono (g)	Poly (g)	Chol (mg)	Vit A (RE)
44705	Salad Dressing, Caesar	1 Tbs	15	80	0	0	0	9	1.3	2.0	4.8	6	1
90838	Salad Dressing, Caesar Italian, w/oregano	2 Tbs	31	100	1	2	0	10	1.5			0	0
8015	Salad Dressing, French	1 Tbs	16	73	0	2	0	7	0.9	1.3	3.4	0	7
8569	Salad Dressing, French, creamy	1 Tbs	16	80	0	2	0	8	1.2			0	0

PAGE KEY: A-70 Prepared Foods   A-78 Restaurants   A-90 Salad Dressings and Dips   A-92 Sauces and Gravies   A-94 Snack Foods   A-94 Spices, Flavors, and Seasonings   A-96 Sports Bars and Drinks   A-96 Supplemental Foods and Formulas   A-96 Sweeteners and Sweet Substitutes   A-98 Vegetables and Legumes   A-108 Miscellaneous

Thia (mg)	Ribo (mg)	Niac (mg NE)	Vit B6 (mg)	Vit B12 (µg)	Fol (µg)	Vit C (mg)	Vit D (IU)	Vit E (mg AT)	Cal (mg)	Iron (mg)	Magn (mg)	Phos (mg)	Pota (mg)	Sodi (mg)	Zinc (mg)	Wat (%)	Alco (g)	Caff (g)
0.18	2.15	1.03	0.00	1.75	14.2	0.0	94.0		381	3.09	59.6	334	551	292	1.3	69	0.00	14.85
0.05	0.09	4.53	0.18	0.25	25.9	1.0	6.1		18	0.56	18.0	215	177	509	0.5	43	0.00	0.00
						15.0			40	0.72				25			0.00	0.00
						15.0			450	2.70				1140			0.00	0.00
0.87	0.57	9.35	0.31	0.74	75.8	2.5	4.6		56	3.49	54.0	378	497	961	1.3	60	0.00	0.00
						0.0			60	0.72				360		35	0.00	0.00
						0.0			60	0.72				500			0.00	0.00
						0.0			100	1.08				650			0.00	0.00
						0.0			40	0.72				410		35	0.00	0.00
						0.0			20	1.79				670			0.00	0.00
						0.0			250	1.08				870			0.00	0.00
						0.0			0	0.72				240		32	0.00	0.00
						0.0			40	0.36				710			0.00	0.00
						0.0			40	0.00				420			0.00	0.00
						1.2			20	0.36				100			0.00	0.00
						0.0			0	0.36				170			0.00	0.00
						0.0			0	0.00				190			0.00	0.00
						0.0			40	0.00				150			0.00	0.00
						0.0			0	0.00				170			0.00	0.00
						0.0			0	0.00				240			0.00	0.00
						0.0			20	0.00				300			0.00	0.00
						0.0			0	0.00				330			0.00	0.00
						1.2			20	0.00				130			0.00	0.00
0.00	0.03	0.05	0.02	0.09	7.6	0.0	3.3	0.6	40	0.00	5.9	48	49	200	0.2		0.00	0.00
						0.0			20	0.00				125			0.00	0.00
						1.8			10	0.18				147		19	0.00	0.00
0.02	0.00	0.09	0.02	0.00	12.5	0.0	0.0		6	0.37	10.7	26	34	57	0.3	67	0.00	0.00
0.00	0.00	0.00	0.00	0.01	4.5	0.0	0.0	0.1	11	0.01	0.6	8	8	150	0.0	78	0.00	0.00
0.00	0.00	0.00	0.00	0.00	0.6	0.1	0.0	0.2	6	0.10	0.9	29	20	168	0.1	62	0.00	0.00
0.00	0.00	0.00	0.00	0.00	0.3	0.0	0.0	0.1	4	0.02	0.3	3	4	172	0.0	73	0.00	0.00
0.00	0.00	0.01	0.00	0.00	2.2	0.0	0.0	0.0	1	0.09	0.5	0	13	136	0.0	65	0.00	0.00
0.00	0.00	0.00	0.00	0.00	0.3	0.0	0.0	0.5	2	0.05	0.0	2	13	134	0.0	59	0.00	0.00
0.00	0.00	0.01	0.00	0.03	1.7	0.1	0.0	0.1	4	0.05	0.7	15	14	158	0.1	86	0.00	0.00
0.00	0.00	0.00	0.00	0.00	0.4	0.1	0.0	0.1	1	0.01	0.3	1	5	150	0.0	70	0.00	0.00
						0.0			0	0.00				330			0.00	0.00
0.03	0.00	0.03	0.00	0.00	1.9	0.0	0.0	0.1	2	0.03	0.6	0	20	126	0.0	66	0.00	0.00
						0.0			0	0.00				400			0.00	0.00
0.00	0.00	0.00	0.00	0.00	0.3	0.0	0.7	0.7	7	0.15	0.3	3	4	178	0.0	34	0.00	0.00
						0.0			20	0.00				470			0.00	0.00
0.00	0.00	0.02	0.00	0.01	0.0	0.6	0.0	0.8	4	0.12	0.8	3	11	134	0.0	37	0.00	0.00
						0.0			0	0.00				135			0.00	0.00

PAGE KEY: A-42 Beverages and Beverage Mixes A-44 Candies A-46 Cereals A-48 Cheeses and Substitutes A-50 Dairy Products and Substitutes A-52 Desserts A-56 Eggs and Egg Substitutes
A-56 Fats, Oils, Margarines, and Shortenings A-58 Fruits A-60 Grain Products and Baked Goods A-62 Grains and Flours A-64 Meats and Meat Substitutes A-68 Nuts, Seeds, and Products

Code	Food Name	Unit/ Amt	Wt (g)	Energy (kcal)	Prot (g)	Carb (g)	Fiber (g)	Fat (g)	Sat (g)	Mono (g)	Poly (g)	Chol (mg)	Vit A (RE)
8579	Salad Dressing, honey dijon	1 Tbs	16	55	0	3	0	5	0.8			0	0
44699	Salad Dressing, Italian	2 Tbs	31	70	0	0	0	8	1.0			0	0
44590	Salad Dressing, ranch	1 Tbs	15	73	0	1	0	8	1.2	1.7	4.2	5	2
8024	Salad Dressing, thousand island	1 Tbs	16	59	0	2	0	6	0.8	1.3	2.9	4	4
SAUCES AND GRAVIES													
Gravies													
53564	Gravy, beef, fat free, cnd	0.25 cup	59	15	1	3	0	0	0.0	0.0	0.0	0	
53022	Gravy, chicken, cnd	0.25 cup	60	47	1	3	0	3	0.8	1.5	0.9	1	1
53038	Gravy, mushroom, dry pkt, svg	1 svg	21	69	2	14	1	1	0.5	0.3	0.0	1	0
53040	Gravy, onion, dehyd pkt, svg	1 svg	24	77	2	16	1	1	0.4	0.2	0.0	0	0
53044	Gravy, turkey, dry pkt, svg	1 svg	7	26	1	5		1	0.1	0.2	0.2	1	1
Salsas													
53676	Salsa	2 Tbs	30	10	0	2	0	0	0.0	0.0	0.0	0	0
93340	Salsa, garden style, med	2 Tbs	31	10	1	2	1	0	0.0	0.0	0.0	0	40
91457	Salsa, green chili tomato, chunky, FS	2 Tbs	31	7	0	3	0	0	0.0			0	
53584	Salsa, hot, cnd	2 Tbs	32	5	0	2	0	0	0.0	0.0	0.0	0	20
92617	Salsa, lime & garlic	2 Tbs	32	12	0	3	1	0	0.0	0.0	0.0	0	20
91458	Salsa, picante, chunky, FS	2 Tbs	31	7	0	1		0	0.0			0	
53207	Salsa, restaurant, chunky, med	2 Tbs	31	10	0	2	0	0	0.0	0.0	0.0	0	0
92618	Salsa, rstd peppers & garlic	2 Tbs	32	10	0	2	1	0	0.0	0.0	0.0	0	40
53466	Salsa, rts	1 Tbs	16	4	0	1	0	0	0.0	0.0	0.0	0	5
93342	Salsa, thick & chunky, med	2 Tbs	31	10	1	2	0	0	0.0	0.0	0.0	0	
90864	Salsa, thick 'n chunky, medium	2 Tbs	31	15	0	2	1	0	0.0	0.0	0.0	0	0
16818	Salsa, verde	2 Tbs	32	15	0	2	0	0	0.0			0	20
Sauces													
9559	Sauce, alfredo	0.25 cup	61	110	1	2	0	10	3.5			30	40
53000	Sauce, barbecue	1 fl oz	31	47	0	11	0	0	0.0	0.0	0.1	0	7
53320	Sauce, barbecue, sweet & sour	2 Tbs	34	45	0	10	0	0	0.0	0.0	0.0	0	0
53420	Sauce, barbecue, teriyaki	2 Tbs	36	60	0	12	0	0	0.0	0.0	0.0	0	0
9558	Sauce, cheese, cheddar, rts	0.25 cup	61	90	2	2	0	8	2.5			25	20
9054	Sauce, enchilada, FS	0.25 cup	61	20	0	3	0	1	0.0			0	75
53233	Sauce, enchilada, green chile, mild	0.25 cup	61	20	0	3	0	1	0.0			0	0
9466	Sauce, hollandaise, prep w/water f/dry mix	2 Tbs	32	10	0	2	0	0	0.0	0.0	0.0	0	0
53432	Sauce, marinara, FS	0.5 cup	127	120	2	20	2	4	1.0			0	50
53627	Sauce, pasta, garlic & herb, cnd	0.5 cup	126	50	2	10	2	0	0.0	0.0	0.0	0	40
53629	Sauce, pasta, traditional, cnd	0.5 cup	126	50	2	11	2	0	0.0	0.0	0.0	0	30
53471	Sauce, pepper, Tabasco, rts	1 tsp	5	1	0	0	0	0	0.0	0.0	0.0	0	8
7479	Sauce, picante	2 Tbs	32	8	0	2	1	0	0.0	0.0	0.0	0	10
53363	Sauce, pizza, deluxe, rts	0.25 cup	63	34	1	5	1	1	0.3	0.3	0.1	2	42
53461	Sauce, plum, rts	1 Tbs	19	35	0	8	0	0	0.0	0.0	0.1	0	1
53714	Sauce, sloppy joe, original recipe, cnd	0.25 cup	67	70	1	16	0	0	0.0	0.0	0.0	0	250
9486	Sauce, spaghetti, Italian style, dry mix	1 Tbs	8	25	0	5		0	0.0	0.0	0.0	0	
51016	Sauce, spaghetti, traditional, cnd	0.5 cup	125	60	2	15	3	1	0.0			0	75
53718	Sauce, spaghetti, w/meat, cnd	0.5 cup	125	60	3	14	3	1	0.0			0	150
92310	Sauce, steak	1 Tbs	16	5	0	1	0	0	0.0	0.0	0.0	0	0

PAGE KEY: A-70 Prepared Foods   A-78 Restaurants   A-90 Salad Dressings and Dips   A-92 Sauces and Gravies   A-94 Snack Foods   A-94 Spices, Flavors, and Seasonings   A-96 Sports Bars and Drinks   A-96 Supplemental Foods and Formulas   A-96 Sweeteners and Sweet Substitutes   A-98 Vegetables and Legumes   A-108 Miscellaneous

Thia (mg)	Ribo (mg)	Niac (mg NE)	Vit B6 (mg)	Vit B12 (µg)	Fol (µg)	Vit C (mg)	Vit D (IU)	Vit E (mg AT)	Cal (mg)	Iron (mg)	Magn (mg)	Phos (mg)	Pota (mg)	Sodi (mg)	Zinc (mg)	Wat (%)	Alco (g)	Caff (g)
						0.0			0	0.00				105			0.00	0.00
						0.0			0	0.00				350		22	0.00	0.00
0.00	0.00	0.00	0.00	0.05	0.6	0.5	0.6	0.6	5	0.09	0.8	24	9	164	0.1	38	0.00	0.00
0.23	0.00	0.07	0.00	0.00	0.0	0.0	0.5	0.6	3	0.18	1.3	4	17	138	0.0	47	0.00	0.00
														300		91	0.00	0.00
0.00	0.02	0.25	0.00	0.05	1.2	0.0	0.0	0.1	12	0.28	1.2	17	65	252	0.5	85	0.00	0.00
0.03	0.07	0.77	0.01	0.15	6.5	1.5	0.0	0.0	48	0.20	7.1	43	55	1382	0.3	3	0.00	0.00
0.05	0.10	0.88	0.01	0.17	7.4	1.7			67	0.23	8.2	49	63	1005	0.2	4	0.00	0.00
0.00	0.02	0.18	0.00	0.03	5.7	0.0			10	0.23	3.1	18	30	307	0.1	5	0.00	0.00
						2.4			0	0.00			55	115		28	0.00	0.00
						3.6			0	0.00				220		27	0.00	0.00
														167			0.00	0.00
						2.4			0	0.00			95	170		30	0.00	0.00
						1.8			0	0.00				210		87	0.00	0.00
														247		29	0.00	0.00
						2.4			0	0.00				230		28	0.00	0.00
						0.0			0	0.00				230		30	0.00	0.00
0.00	0.00	0.00	0.02	0.00	0.6	0.3	0.0	0.2	4	0.07	2.4	5	48	96	0.1	90	0.00	0.00
						4.8			0	0.00				180		27	0.00	0.00
						0.0			0	0.00				240		28	0.00	0.00
						1.2			0	0.00			65	230		88	0.00	0.00
						0.0			40	0.00				390			0.00	0.00
0.00	0.00	0.15	0.00	0.00	0.6	0.2	0.0	0.2	4	0.07	3.8	5	65	265	0.0	60	0.00	0.00
						0.0			0	0.00				420			0.00	0.00
						0.0			0	0.36				440		23	0.00	0.00
						0.0			60	0.00				480		47	0.00	0.00
						1.2			0	0.00				380			0.00	0.00
						1.2			0	0.00				340			0.00	0.00
						0.0			0	0.00				105			0.00	0.00
				0.00		1.2			0	0.72				480			0.00	0.00
						6.0			40	1.08				390			0.00	0.00
						6.0			40	1.08				390			0.00	0.00
0.00	0.00	0.00	0.00	0.00	0.0	0.2	0.0	0.0	1	0.05	0.6	1	6	30	0.0	95	0.00	0.00
														250		90	0.00	0.00
0.03	0.02	0.89	0.09	0.00	6.3	7.1		1.6	34	0.56	13.2	32	223	117	0.2	87	0.00	0.00
0.00	0.01	0.18	0.00	0.00	1.1	0.1			2	0.27	2.3	4	49	102	0.0	54	0.00	0.00
						1.2			0	1.08				680			0.00	0.00
														490			0.00	0.00
						9.0			40	1.44				590			0.00	0.00
						9.0			40	1.44				720			0.00	0.00
						0.0			0	0.00				200		15	0.00	0.00

PAGE KEY: A-42 Beverages and Beverage Mixes   A-44 Candies   A-46 Cereals   A-48 Cheeses and Substitutes   A-50 Dairy Products and Substitutes   A-52 Desserts   A-56 Eggs and Egg Substitutes
A-56 Fats, Oils, Margarines, and Shortenings   A-58 Fruits   A-60 Grain Products and Baked Goods   A-62 Grains and Flours   A-64 Meats and Meat Substitutes   A-68 Nuts, Seeds, and Products

Code	Food Name	Unit/ Amt	Wt (g)	Energy (kcal)	Prot (g)	Carb (g)	Fiber (g)	Fat (g)	Sat (g)	Mono (g)	Poly (g)	Chol (mg)	Vit A (RE)
53620	Sauce, stir fry	1 Tbs	18	20	1	4	0	0	0.0	0.0	0.0	0	0
53264	Sauce, sweet & sour	1 oz	28	48	0	12	0	0	0.0			0	0
9720	Sauce, taco, medium	2 Tbs	32	10	0	2	1	0	0.0	0.0	0.0	0	0
8983	Sauce, tartar	2 Tbs	28	139	0	1	0	15	2.7	0.7	2.3	11	6
53004	Sauce, teriyaki, rts	1 Tbs	18	16	1	3	0	0				0	0
33768	Sauce, Thai peanut	1 Tbs	17	60	2	5	0	4	0.5			0	0
SNACK FOODS													
44278	Chips, corn, original	32 ea	28	160	2	15	1	10	1.5			0	0
44256	Chips, multigrain, Sun Chips, original	16 pce	28	139	2	19	2	6	0.6	3.3	1.8	0	0
61236	Chips, potato, bkd	10 ea	12	56	1	9	1	2	0.3	1.2	0.5	0	0
43703	Chips, potato, classic, svg	1 ea	28	150	2	15	1	10	1.0	6.0	3.0	0	0
44241	Chips, potato, rducd fat, svg	1 svg	28	140	2	18	1	7	1.0	4.0	2.0	0	0
12947	Chips, potato, unsalted	1 oz	28	140	2	16	1	8	0.7			0	0
44301	Chips, tortilla, blue corn	18 pce	28	110	3	22	2	2	0.0			0	0
44224	Chips, tortilla, cool ranch, svg	1 svg	28	140	2	18	1	7	1.0			0	0
61156	Chips, tortilla, light, bkd	10 ea	16	74	1	12	1	2	0.5	1.0	0.8	0	1
44225	Chips, tortilla, nacho cheese, svg	1 svg	28	140	2	17	1	8	1.5			0	0
4039	Chips, tortilla, salsa verde, svg	1 svg	28	140	2	19	1	7	1.0			0	40
44223	Chips, tortilla, tstd corn, svg	1 svg	28	140	2	18	1	7	1.0			0	0
44298	Chips, tortilla, yellow corn	18 pce	28	110	3	22	2	2	0.0			0	0
44022	Popcorn Cake	1 ea	10	38	1	8	0	0	0.0	0.1	0.1	0	1
43701	Popcorn, caramel coated, original	0.5 cup	28	120	2	23	1	2	0.0			0	0
44014	Popcorn, caramel coated, w/o peanuts	1 oz	28	122	1	22	1	4	1.0	0.8	1.3	1	1
44038	Popcorn, cheese flvrd	1 cup	11	58	1	6	1	4	0.7	1.1	1.7	1	5
44066	Popcorn, low fat, low sod, microwv	1 cup	8	34	1	6	1	1	0.1	0.3	0.3	0	1
44013	Popcorn, oil popped, microwv	1 cup	11	64	1	5	1	5	0.8	1.1	2.6	0	2
44072	Popcorn, white, air popped	1 cup	8	31	1	6	1	0	0.0	0.1	0.2	0	0
44015	Pretzels, hard	5 ea	30	114	3	24	1	1	0.1	0.3	0.3	0	0
61182	Pretzels, soft, med	1 ea	115	389	9	80	2	4	0.8	1.2	1.1	3	0
60899	Rice Cake, brown	1 ea	20	74	1	16	0	0	0.1	0.2	0.2		0
14262	Rice Cake, butter popped corn	1 ea	9	35	1	8	0	0	0.0	0.0	0.0	0	0
14248	Rice Cake, caramel corn	1 ea	13	50	1	11	0	0	0.0	0.0	0.0	0	0
44312	Rice Cake, caramel corn, mini	7 ea	15	60	1	13	0	0	0.0	0.0	0.0	0	0
44016	Rice Cake, plain	1 ea	9	35	1	7	0	0	0.1	0.1	0.1	0	0
61768	Snack, bagel, crisps, plain, bkd	6 ea	28	130	3	18	0	6	2.5			0	0
44032	Snack, mix, Chex	0.67 cup	30	127	3	22	1	3	0.4	0.9	1.3	0	0
44248	Snack, puffs, cheese, svg	1 svg	28	160	2	15	1	10	1.5			0	0
44058	Trail Mix, regular	0.25 cup	38	173	5	17		11	2.1	4.7	3.6	0	1
44059	Trail Mix, w/chocolate chips salted nuts & seeds	0.25 cup	36	177	5	16		12	2.2	4.9	4.1	1	2
SPICES, FLAVORS, AND SEASONINGS													
26001	Herb, basil, dried, ground	1 tsp	1	3	0	1	1	0	0.0	0.0	0.0	0	1
5359	Herb, chives, fresh	1 Tbs	3	1	0	0	0	0	0.0	0.0	0.0	0	13
26501	Herb, cilantro, ground	1 tsp	1	2	0	0	0	0					4
26009	Herb, oregano, ground	1 tsp	2	5	0	1	1	0	0.0	0.0	0.0	0	3
26012	Herb, parsley, fresh, chpd	1 Tbs	4	1	0	0	0	0	0.0	0.0	0.0	0	32

PAGE KEY: A-70 Prepared Foods   A-78 Restaurants   A-90 Salad Dressings and Dips   A-92 Sauces and Gravies   A-94 Snack Foods   A-94 Spices, Flavors, and Seasonings   A-96 Sports Bars and Drinks   A-96 Supplemental Foods and Formulas   A-96 Sweeteners and Sweet Substitutes   A-98 Vegetables and Legumes   A-108 Miscellaneous

Thia (mg)	Ribo (mg)	Niac (mg NE)	Vit B6 (mg)	Vit B12 (µg)	Fol (µg)	Vit C (mg)	Vit D (IU)	Vit E (mg AT)	Cal (mg)	Iron (mg)	Magn (mg)	Phos (mg)	Pota (mg)	Sodi (mg)	Zinc (mg)	Wat (%)	Alco (g)	Caff (g)
						0.0			0	0.00				520				0.00
						0.0			2	0.02				101			0.00	0.00
						0.0			0	0.00				170			0.00	0.00
						0.7			6	0.14			38	153		39	0.00	0.00
0.00	0.00	0.23	0.01	0.00	1.4	0.0	0.0	0.0	4	0.31	11.0	28	40	690	0.0	68	0.07	0.00
						0.0			0	0.00				135				0.00
		0.03				0.0			20	0.00		40		170		0	0.00	0.00
0.03	0.00	0.60	0.05	0.00	7.1	0.0		2.0	6	0.49	21.5	63	66	93	0.5	2	0.00	0.00
0.03	0.00	0.49	0.05	0.0	0.0	0.0	0.0	0.3	15	0.10	5.2	33	87	76	0.1	1	0.00	0.00
0.02		1.20	0.07			6.0			0	0.36	16.0	40		180		0	0.00	0.00
0.02	0.02	1.20	0.07			6.0			0	0.36		40	310	180			0.00	0.00
						4.8			0	0.36				5	1	1		0.00
						0.0			60	0.36				140		0		0.00
0.02	0.02	0.23	0.07	0.03	6.9	0.0		0.9	20	0.36	16.0	60	52	170	0.2	1	0.00	0.00
0.03	0.03	0.07	0.02	0.00	2.6	0.0	0.0	0.6	25	0.25	15.5	51	44	137	0.2	1	0.00	0.00
0.05			0.07			0.0			20	0.36		60		180		1	0.00	0.00
			0.03			0.0			20	0.36	16.0	40		210			0.00	0.00
		0.40	0.07			0.0			40	0.00		60		120			0.00	0.00
						0.0			60	0.36				160		0		0.00
0.00	0.01	0.60	0.01	0.00	1.8	0.0	0.0	0.0	1	0.18	15.9	28	33	29	0.4	5		0.00
						0.0			0	0.72				70		0	0.00	0.00
0.01	0.01	0.62	0.00	0.00	1.4	0.0	0.0	0.3	12	0.49	9.9	24	31	58	0.2	3	0.00	0.00
0.00	0.02	0.15	0.02	0.05	1.2	0.1	0.0		12	0.25	10.0	40	29	98	0.2	2	0.00	0.00
0.02	0.00	0.17	0.00	0.00	1.4	0.0	0.0	0.4	1	0.18	12.1	21	19	39	0.3	3	0.00	0.00
0.00	0.00	0.12	0.00	0.00	2.8	0.0	0.0	0.3	0	0.21	8.7	22	20	116	0.3	1	0.00	0.00
0.01	0.01	0.15	0.01	0.00	1.8	0.0			1	0.20	10.5	24	24	0	0.3	4	0.00	0.00
0.15	0.10	1.53	0.00	0.00	55.8	0.0	0.0	0.1	5	1.55	8.7	34	41	407	0.4	3	0.00	0.00
0.46	0.33	4.90	0.01	0.00	27.6	0.0	0.0	0.6	26	4.51	24.1	91	101	926	1.1	15	0.00	0.00
						0.0			5	0.15			67	57		5	0.00	0.00
						0.0			0	0.00				45			0.00	0.00
						0.0			0	0.00				30			0.00	0.00
						0.0			0	0.00				150			0.00	0.00
0.03	0.00	0.58	0.05	0.00	1.8	0.0	0.0	0.0	1	0.12	14.2	33	25	14	2.0	0	0.00	0.00
						0.0			0	1.08				70			0.00	0.00
0.10	0.05	1.30	0.02		15.0				10	0.89	12.3	46	59	361	0.3	3	0.00	0.00
0.09	0.07	0.80				0.0			0	0.72		40		370		1	0.00	0.00
0.17	0.07	1.76	0.10	0.00	26.6	0.5			29	1.13	59.2	129	257	86	1.2	9	0.00	0.00
0.15	0.07	1.61	0.09	0.00	23.7	0.5			40	1.24	58.8	141	237	44	1.1	7	0.00	
0.00	0.01	0.07	0.01	0.00	4.3	0.0	0.0	0.1	31	1.25	10.0	4	37	1	0.1	10	0.00	0.00
0.00	0.00	0.01	0.00	0.00	3.1	1.7	0.0	0.0	3	0.05	1.3	2	9	0	0.0	91	0.00	0.00
		0.00				0.2			6	0.31		4				5	0.00	0.00
0.00	0.00	0.07	0.01	0.00	4.3	0.0	0.0	0.3	29	0.66	4.9	3	23	0	0.0	10	0.00	0.00
0.00	0.00	0.05	0.00	0.00	5.8	5.1	0.0	0.3	5	0.23	1.9	2	21	2	0.0	88	0.00	0.00

PAGE KEY: A-42 Beverages and Beverage Mixes   A-44 Candies   A-46 Cereals   A-48 Cheeses and Substitutes   A-50 Dairy Products and Substitutes   A-52 Desserts   A-56 Eggs and Egg Substitutes
A-56 Fats, Oils, Margarines, and Shortenings   A-58 Fruits   A-60 Grain Products and Baked Goods   A-62 Grains and Flours   A-64 Meats and Meat Substitutes   A-68 Nuts, Seeds, and Products

Code	Food Name	Unit/ Amt	Wt (g)	Energy (kcal)	Prot (g)	Carb (g)	Fiber (g)	Fat (g)	Sat (g)	Mono (g)	Poly (g)	Chol (mg)	Vit A (RE)
26033	Herb, thyme, ground	1 tsp	1	4	0	1	1	0	0.0	0.0	0.0	0	5
7503	Miso	0.5 cup	138	274	16	36	7	8	1.6	1.7	4.4	0	12
90931	Mustard, deli	1 tsp	5	6	0	0	0	0	0.0			0	0
26632	Salt Substitute, no sod, pkt	1 indv pkt	1	0	0	0	0	0	0.0	0.0	0.0	0	0
26014	Salt, table	0.25 tsp	2	0	0	0	0	0	0.0	0.0	0.0	0	0
669	Seasoning, garlic salt	0.25 tsp	1	0	0	0	0	0	0.0	0.0	0.0		
26604	Seasoning, lemon pepper	1 tsp	2	2	0	0	0	0	0.0	0.0	0.0	0	0
26028	Seasoning, poultry	1 tsp	2	5	0	1	0	0	0.0	0.0	0.0	0	4
26004	Spice Blend, curry, pwd	1 tsp	2	6	0	1	1	0	0.0	0.1	0.1	0	2
26002	Spice, chili pepper, pwd	1 tsp	3	8	0	1	1	0	0.1	0.1	0.2	0	80
26003	Spice, cinnamon, ground	1 tsp	3	6	0	2	1	0	0.0	0.0	0.0	0	1
26019	Spice, clove, ground	1 tsp	2	7	0	1	1	0	0.1	0.0	0.1	0	1
26065	Spice, garlic, pwd	1 tsp	3	8	0	2	1	0				0	0
26008	Spice, onion, pwd	1 tsp	2	8	0	2	0	0	0.0	0.0	0.0	0	0
26010	Spice, paprika	1 tsp	2	6	0	1	1	0	0.0	0.0	0.2	0	113
26522	Spice, pepper, black, ground	1 tsp	2	8	0	2	1	0					2

SPORTS BARS AND DRINKS

Code	Food Name	Unit/ Amt	Wt (g)	Energy (kcal)	Prot (g)	Carb (g)	Fiber (g)	Fat (g)	Sat (g)	Mono (g)	Poly (g)	Chol (mg)	Vit A (RE)
62714	Bar, energy, carrot cake	1 ea	68	234	10	41	5	4	1.8			0	884
62278	Bar, energy, chocolate	1 ea	68	247	10	47	4	2	0.9	0.7	0.4	0	0
62715	Bar, energy, chocolate almond fudge	1 ea	68	231	10	38	5	5	0.9			0	276
62709	Bar, energy, chocolate chip	1 ea	68	238	10	42	5	4	0.9			0	278
62716	Bar, energy, cookies & cream	1 ea	68	225	10	39	5	4	1.5			0	277
62710	Bar, energy, peanut butter	1 ea	68	240	12	38	5	5	0.8			0	277
62275	Bar, energy, Performance, apple cinnamon	1 ea	65	230	8	45	2	4	0.5			0	0
62561	Bar, energy, Performance, chocolate peanut butter	1 ea	65	240	9	44	1	4	1.0			0	150
62821	Bar, energy, Performance, vanilla crisp	1 ea	65	240	8	45	1	4	0.5			0	0
63031	Drink, protein, Max Whey, all flvrs, pwd, scoop	1 scp	27	88	20	3	0	1				25	0
20650	Drink, sports, berry	8 fl oz	244	63	0	16	0	0	0.0	0.0	0.0	0	0
20559	Drink, sports, Powerade, lemon lime, rtd, svg	8 fl oz	244	78	0	19	0	0	0.0	0.0	0.1	0	0

SUPPLEMENTAL FOODS AND FORMULAS

Code	Food Name	Unit/ Amt	Wt (g)	Energy (kcal)	Prot (g)	Carb (g)	Fiber (g)	Fat (g)	Sat (g)	Mono (g)	Poly (g)	Chol (mg)	Vit A (RE)
62833	Carbohydrate Gel, chocolate	1 ea	41	120	0	28		2	1.0				
62795	Drink, Boost High Protein, vanilla, rtu, SD	8 fl oz	256	240	15	33	0	6	0.5			10	200
62796	Drink, Boost Plus, vanilla, rtu, SD	8 fl oz	256	360	14	45	0	14	1.5			10	200
62162	Drink, Boost, vanilla, rtu, SD	8 fl oz	256	240	10	41	0	4	0.5			5	250
63156	Drink, breakfast, chocolate, inst, SD	0.25 cup	34	130	8	24	0	1	0.5	0.2	0.1	5	300
4055	Drink, Instant Breakfast, straw, prep w/whole milk, SD	8 fl oz	279	290	15	37		9				40	350
4054	Drink, Instant Breakfast, van, prep w/whole milk, SD	8 fl oz	279	290	15	37		9				40	350
34577	Drink, protein, soy, chocolate	1 cntr	341	230	15	37	3	3	0.5	1.5	1.0	0	125
4340	Formula, Ensure Plus, vanilla, rtu	1 cup	252	355	13	50	0	11	1.5	2.9	7.0	5	375
62136	Pudding, Boost, vanilla, rtu, indv, SD	1 ea	142	240	7	33	0	9	1.0			5	150
29341	Shake, nutrition, Myoplex Lite, chocolate fudge, rtd	1 cntr	346	170	20	20	5	2	0.0			10	500

SWEETENERS AND SWEET SUBSTITUTES

Jams, Jellies, and Glazes

Code	Food Name	Unit/ Amt	Wt (g)	Energy (kcal)	Prot (g)	Carb (g)	Fiber (g)	Fat (g)	Sat (g)	Mono (g)	Poly (g)	Chol (mg)	Vit A (RE)
90974	Fruit Spread, apricot, 100% fruit	1 Tbs	19	40	0	10	0	0	0.0	0.0	0.0	0	0
90976	Fruit Spread, blueberry, 100% fruit	1 Tbs	19	40	0	10	0	0	0.0	0.0	0.0	0	0
90984	Fruit Spread, concord grape, 100% fruit	1 Tbs	19	40	0	10	0	0	0.0	0.0	0.0	0	0

PAGE KEY: A-70 Prepared Foods   A-78 Restaurants   A-90 Salad Dressings and Dips   A-92 Sauces and Gravies   A-94 Snack Foods   A-94 Spices, Flavors, and Seasonings   A-96 Sports Bars and Drinks   A-96 Supplemental Foods and Formulas   A-96 Sweeteners and Sweet Substitutes   A-98 Vegetables and Legumes   A-108 Miscellaneous

Thia (mg)	Ribo (mg)	Niac (mg NE)	Vit B6 (mg)	Vit B12 (µg)	Fol (µg)	Vit C (mg)	Vit D (IU)	Vit E (mg AT)	Cal (mg)	Iron (mg)	Magn (mg)	Phos (mg)	Pota (mg)	Sodi (mg)	Zinc (mg)	Wat (%)	Alco (g)	Caff (g)
0.00	0.00	0.07	0.00	0.00	3.8	0.7	0.0	0.1	26	1.73	3.1	3	11	1	0.1	8	0.00	0.00
0.12	0.31	1.25	0.27	0.10	26.1	0.0	0.0	0.0	78	3.42	66.0	219	289	5126	3.5	43	0.00	0.00
						0.0			6	0.10				78		74	0.00	0.00
						0.0			0		0.0		530	0			0.00	0.00
0.00	0.00	0.00	0.00	0.00	0.0	0.0	0.0	0.0	0	0.00	0.0	0	0	581	0.0	0	0.00	0.00
						0.00								240		0	0.00	0.00
0.00	0.00	0.00	0.00	0.00	0.0	0.0	0.0	0.0	3	0.10	0.8	1	6	461	0.0	2	0.00	0.00
0.00	0.00	0.03	0.01	0.00	2.1	0.2	0.0	0.0	15	0.52	3.4	3	10	0		9	0.00	0.00
0.00	0.00	0.07	0.01	0.00	3.1	0.2	0.0	0.4	10	0.58	5.1	7	31	1	0.1	10	0.00	0.00
0.00	0.02	0.31	0.05	0.00	0.8	0.0	0.0	1.0	9	0.46	4.0	8	53	44	0.1	11	0.00	0.00
0.00	0.00	0.02	0.00	0.00	0.2	0.1	0.0	0.1	26	0.21	1.6	2	11	0		11	0.00	0.00
0.00	0.00	0.02	0.00	0.00	2.0	1.7	0.0	0.2	14	0.18	5.5	2	23	5	0.0	7	0.00	0.00
0.00	0.00	0.01		0.00		0.1			3	0.01			38	1		6	0.00	0.00
0.00	0.00	0.00	0.01	0.00	1.5	0.6	0.0	0.0	9	0.09	2.7	8	24	2	0.1	5	0.00	0.00
0.00	0.02	0.23	0.05	0.00	1.1	0.0	0.0	0.7	5	0.49	4.1	7	52	2	0.1	11	0.00	0.00
						0.00			9	0.18				0		12	0.00	0.00
0.37	0.28	3.54	0.41	0.98	87.0	67.1		20.2	275	5.32	103.2	298	246	170	3.2	11	0.00	0.00
5.48	1.30	22.17	1.50	3.80	418.2	62.8		5.6	343	7.96	168.6	418	246	99	6.8	10	0.00	0.00
0.38	0.31	3.63	0.43	0.98	84.6	65.7		20.8	278	5.73	128.3	304	232	139	3.7	13	0.00	0.00
0.34	0.28	3.49	0.38	0.98	85.6	66.1		20.3	265	5.21	95.5	286	206	76	3.5	10	0.00	0.00
0.34	0.27	3.45	0.43	0.98	85.1	66.2		20.3	279	5.23	102.6	266	212	179	3.2	13	0.00	0.00
0.40	0.30	6.25	0.41	0.98	96.2	65.8		20.4	268	5.30	113.7	305	301	289	3.6	10	0.00	0.00
0.23	0.17					42.0			250	4.50			105	200			0.00	0.00
0.44	0.50	6.00	0.60	3.59	240.0	36.0			300	3.59	60.0	150	105	200	2.2		0.00	
0.23	0.17		0.50			42.0			150	2.70		150	105	200			0.00	
						0.0			0	0.00				35			0.00	
0.02	0.00	0.54	0.05	0.00	0.0	1.0	0.0	0.0	2	0.11	0.0	24	37	95	0.0	93	0.00	0.00
0.02	0.00	3.81	0.37	3.33	0.0	0.0	0.0	0.0	2	0.21	0.0	2	44	54	0.0	92	0.00	0.00
						9.0							40	200			0.00	25.00
0.37	0.43	5.00	0.69	2.09	140.0	60.0	80.0		350	4.50	100.0	300	380	170	4.5		0.00	0.00
0.37	0.43	5.00	0.69	2.09	140.0	60.0	80.0		350	4.50	100.0	300	380	170	4.5		0.00	0.00
0.37	0.43	5.00	0.69	2.09	140.0	60.0	160.0		300	4.50	100.0	300	400	130	4.5		0.00	0.00
0.44	0.25	7.00	0.60	1.50	140.0	21.0			200	6.30	28.0	150	350	110	4.5		0.00	1.00
0.52	0.68	7.00	0.69	2.09	140.0	21.0	140.0	4.8	450	6.30	140.0	400	620	210	5.3		0.00	0.00
0.52	0.68	7.00	0.69	2.09	140.0	21.0	140.0	4.8	450	6.30	140.0	400	620	210	5.3		0.00	0.00
0.37	0.43	5.00	0.50	1.50	100.0	30.0	100.0		250	4.50	100.0	250	360	220	3.8		0.00	0.00
0.37	0.43	5.00	0.50	1.50	100.8	30.0	100.8	3.4	199	4.51	100.8	199	441	239	3.8	70	0.00	0.00
0.23	0.25	3.00	0.40	1.20	80.0	36.0	80.0		250	2.70	60.0	200	250	125	3.0	93	0.00	0.00
0.75	0.85	10.00	1.00	3.00	360.0	60.0	200.0		200	2.70	100.0	400	450	380	7.5		0.00	
						0.0			0	0.00				0		9	0.00	0.00
						0.0			0	0.00				0		9	0.00	0.00
						0.0			0	0.00				0		9	0.00	0.00

PAGE KEY: A-42 Beverages and Beverage Mixes   A-44 Candies   A-46 Cereals   A-48 Cheeses and Substitutes   A-50 Dairy Products and Substitutes   A-52 Desserts   A-56 Eggs and Egg Substitutes   A-56 Fats, Oils, Margarines, and Shortenings   A-58 Fruits   A-60 Grain Products and Baked Goods   A-62 Grains and Flours   A-64 Meats and Meat Substitutes   A-68 Nuts, Seeds, and Products

Code	Food Name	Unit/ Amt	Wt (g)	Energy (kcal)	Prot (g)	Carb (g)	Fiber (g)	Fat (g)	Sat (g)	Mono (g)	Poly (g)	Chol (mg)	Vit A (RE)
90979	Fruit Spread, strawberry, 100% fruit	1 Tbs	19	40	0	10	0	0	0.0	0.0	0.0	0	0
23054	Jam	1 Tbs	20	56	0	14	0	0	0.0	0.0	0.0	0	0
23003	Jelly	1 Tbs	21	56	0	15	0	0	0.0	0.0	0.0	0	0
23005	Marmalade, orange	1 Tbs	20	49	0	13	0	0	0.0	0.0	0.0	0	1
92229	Preserves	1 Tbs	20	56	0	14	0	0	0.0	0.0	0.0	0	0
Sugars and Syrups													
25309	Honey, light	1 Tbs	21	64	0	17	0	0	0.0	0.0	0.0	0	0
25003	Molasses	1 Tbs	20	58	0	15	0	0	0.0	0.0	0.0	0	0
25201	Sugar, brown, unpacked	1 tsp	3	11	0	3	0	0	0.0	0.0	0.0	0	0
63415	Sugar, powdered	0.25 cup	37	140	0	37	0	0	0.0	0.0	0.0		
25006	Sugar, white, granulated	1 tsp	4	16	0	4	0	0	0.0	0.0	0.0	0	0
25010	Syrup, corn, dark	1 Tbs	20	57	0	16	0	0	0.0	0.0	0.0	0	0
25000	Syrup, corn, light	1 Tbs	22	62	0	17	0	0				0	0
63334	Syrup, dietetic	1 Tbs	15	6	0	7	0	0	0.0	0.0	0.0	0	0
23042	Syrup, pancake	1 Tbs	20	47	0	12	0	0	0.0	0.0	0.0	0	0
VEGETABLES AND LEGUMES													
Canned Vegetables and Legumes													
7867	Artichokes, hearts, cnd, pieces	0.5 cup	100	38	2	6	0	0	0.0	0.0	0.0	0	12
6262	Asparagus, spears, cut, cnd	0.5 cup	119	20	2	3	1	0	0.0	0.0	0.0	0	30
5199	Carrots, cnd, drnd, slices	0.5 cup	73	18	0	4	1	0	0.0	0.0	0.1	0	815
7933	Chili Peppers, green, cnd	0.25 cup	35	7	0	2	1	0	0.0	0.0	0.1	0	4
6268	Corn, sweet, whl kernel, cnd	0.33 cup	77	80	2	16	1	0	0.0			0	0
9520	Greens, turnip, cnd, unsalted	0.5 cup	72	14	1	2	1	0	0.1	0.0	0.1	0	429
38077	Hominy, white, cnd	0.5 cup	82	59	1	12	2	1	0.1	0.2	0.3	0	0
5094	Mushrooms, cnd, drnd, pces/slices	0.5 cup	78	20	1	4	2	0	0.0	0.0	0.1	0	0
7275	Peas, garbanzo, cnd	0.5 cup	126	100	5	17	4	2	0.0			0	0
93303	Pickles, bread & butter, slices	1 ea	8	7	0	2	0	0	0.0	0.0	0.0	0	6
27013	Pickles, dill, slices	1 ea	7	1	0	0	0	0	0.0	0.0	0.0	0	1
90585	Pickles, sweet, slices	1 ea	8	7	0	2	0	0	0.0	0.0	0.0	0	6
5227	Pimentos, cnd	1 Tbs	12	3	0	1	0	0	0.0	0.0	0.0	0	32
5964	Pumpkin, cnd, w/salt	0.5 cup	122	42	1	10	4	0	0.2	0.0	0.0	0	1906
6393	Sauerkraut, crisp	30 g	30	5	0	1	1	0	0.0	0.0	0.0	0	0
5595	Spinach, cnd, w/liquid	0.5 cup	117	22	2	3	2	0	0.1	0.0	0.2	0	753
6459	Sprouts, bean, cnd, svg	1 svg	83	12	1	2	1	0	0.0			0	0
5162	Sweet Potatoes, dark orange, mashed f/cnd	0.5 cup	128	129	3	30	2	0	0.1	0.0	0.1	0	1109
5181	Tomato Paste, unsalted, 6-oz can	0.25 cup	66	54	3	12	3	0	0.1	0.0	0.1	0	100
5180	Tomato Sauce, cnd	0.5 cup	122	29	2	7	2	0	0.0	0.0	0.1	0	53
51000	Tomatoes, chunky, chili style, cnd	0.5 cup	128	30	1	8	2	0	0.0	0.0	0.0	0	50
51001	Tomatoes, chunky, pasta style, cnd	0.5 cup	128	45	1	11	2	0	0.0	0.0	0.0	0	50
6927	Tomatoes, crushed, cnd	0.5 cup	128	41	2	9	2	0	0.1	0.1	0.1	0	89
51005	Tomatoes, dices, w/liquid, cnd	0.5 cup	126	25	1	6	2	0	0.0	0.0	0.0	0	50
5630	Tomatoes, green, pickled	0.5 cup	71	26	1	6	1	0	0.0	0.1	0.1	0	59
6293	Tomatoes, puree, cnd	0.25 cup	63	20	1	4	0	0	0.0	0.0	0.0	0	50
9169	Tomatoes, stewed, cnd	0.5 cup	121	45	1	10	2	0	0.0	0.0	0.0	0	30
51022	Tomatoes, stwd, original recipe, cnd	0.5 cup	126	35	1	9	2	0	0.0	0.0	0.0	0	50

PAGE KEY: A-70 Prepared Foods   A-78 Restaurants   A-90 Salad Dressings and Dips   A-92 Sauces and Gravies   A-94 Snack Foods   A-94 Spices, Flavors, and Seasonings   A-96 Sports Bars and Drinks
A-96 Supplemental Foods and Formulas   A-96 Sweeteners and Sweet Substitutes   A-98 Vegetables and Legumes   A-108 Miscellaneous

Thia (mg)	Ribo (mg)	Niac (mg NE)	Vit B6 (mg)	Vit B12 (µg)	Fol (µg)	Vit C (mg)	Vit D (IU)	Vit E (mg AT)	Cal (mg)	Iron (mg)	Magn (mg)	Phos (mg)	Pota (mg)	Sodi (mg)	Zinc (mg)	Wat (%)	Alco (g)	Caff (g)
						0.0			0	0.00				0		9	0.00	0.00
0.00	0.01	0.00	0.00	0.00	2.2	1.8	0.0	0.0	4	0.10	0.8	4	15	6	0.0	30	0.00	0.00
0.00	0.00	0.00	0.00	0.00	0.4	0.2	0.0	0.0	1	0.03	1.3	1	11	6	0.0	30	0.00	0.00
0.00	0.00	0.00	0.00	0.00	1.8	1.0	0.0	0.0	8	0.02	0.4	1	7	11	0.0	33	0.00	0.00
0.00	0.01	0.00	0.00	0.00	2.2	1.8	0.0	0.0	4	0.10	0.8	4	15	6	0.0	30	0.00	0.00
0.00	0.05	0.05	0.00	0.00	2.1	0.1	0.0	0.0	1	0.05	0.4	1	10	1	0.0	17	0.00	0.00
0.00	0.00	0.18	0.12	0.00	0.0	0.0	0.0	0.0	41	0.93	48.4	6	293	7	0.1	22	0.00	0.00
0.00	0.00	0.00	0.00	0.00	0.0	0.0	0.0	0.0	2	0.01	0.3	0	4	1	0.0	1	0.00	0.00
														0		0	0.00	0.00
0.00	0.00	0.00	0.00	0.00	0.0	0.0	0.0	0.0	0	0.00	0.0	0	0	0	0.0	0	0.00	0.00
0.00	0.00	0.00	0.00	0.00	0.0	0.0	0.0	0.0	4	0.07	1.6	2	9	31	0.0	22	0.00	0.00
0.00	0.00	0.00	0.00	0.00	0.0	0.0	0.0	0.0	3	0.00	0.2	0	0	14	0.1	23	0.00	0.00
0.00	0.00	0.00	0.00	0.00	0.0	0.0	0.0	0.0	0	0.00	0.0	0	0	3	0.0	50	0.00	0.00
0.00	0.00	0.00	0.00	0.00	0.0	0.0	0.0	0.0	1	0.00	0.4	2	3	16	0.0	38	0.00	0.00
			0.00			4.5			0	1.35			0	250		72	0.00	0.00
						6.0			0	0.36				420			0.00	0.00
0.00	0.01	0.40	0.07	0.00	6.6	2.0	0.0	0.5	18	0.46	5.8	18	131	177	0.2	93	0.00	0.00
0.00	0.00	0.21	0.03	0.00	18.8	11.9	0.0		13	0.46	1.4	4	39	138	0.0	93	0.00	0.00
						1.2			0	0.00				230		58	0.00	0.00
0.00	0.03	0.25	0.02	0.00	66.2	11.2	0.0	1.1	85	1.09	14.4	15	102	21	0.2	95	0.00	0.00
0.00	0.00	0.02	0.00	0.00	0.8	0.0	0.0	0.0	8	0.50	13.2	29	7	173	0.9	83	0.00	0.00
0.07	0.01	1.24	0.05	0.00	9.4	0.0	6.2	0.0	9	0.62	11.7	51	101	332	0.6	91	0.00	0.00
						0.0			20	1.08				280			0.00	0.00
0.00	0.00	0.00	0.00	0.00	0.1	0.1	0.0	0.0	5	0.01	0.5	1	8	34	0.0	76	0.00	0.00
0.00	0.00	0.00	0.00	0.00	0.1	0.1	0.0	0.0	3	0.02	0.5	1	6	61	0.0	94	0.00	0.00
0.00	0.00	0.00	0.00	0.00	0.1	0.1	0.0	0.0	5	0.01	0.5	1	8	34	0.0	76	0.00	0.00
0.00	0.00	0.07	0.02	0.00	0.7	10.2	0.0	0.1	1	0.20	0.7	2	19	2	0.0	93	0.00	0.00
0.02	0.07	0.44	0.07	0.00	14.7	5.1	0.0	1.3	32	1.70	28.2	43	252	295	0.2	90	0.00	0.00
						3.6			0	0.00				220		28	0.00	0.00
0.01	0.11	0.31	0.09	0.00	67.9	15.8	0.0		97	1.85	65.5	37	269	373	0.5	93	0.00	0.00
						14.2			10	0.25				20		96	0.00	0.00
0.02	0.10	1.22	0.30	0.00	14.0	6.6	0.0	1.4	38	1.70	30.6	66	268	96	0.3	74	0.00	0.00
0.03	0.10	2.00	0.14	0.00	7.9	14.3	0.0	2.8	24	1.95	27.5	54	664	64	0.4	74	0.00	0.00
0.02	0.07	1.19	0.11	0.00	13.5	8.6	0.0	1.7	16	1.25	19.6	32	405	642	0.2	91	0.00	0.00
						9.0			20	0.36				670			0.00	0.00
						9.0			20	0.36				560			0.00	0.00
0.10	0.07	1.55	0.18	0.00	16.6	11.7	0.0		43	1.65	25.5	41	374	168	0.3	89	0.00	0.00
						9.0			20	1.44			280	200			0.00	0.00
0.03	0.01	0.28	0.05	0.00	5.3	20.0	0.0	0.2	11	0.36	7.5	19	128	89	0.1	90	0.00	0.00
						9.0			0	0.36				15		57	0.00	0.00
						12.0			40	0.36			280	330			0.00	0.00
						12.0			20	1.08			300	360			0.00	0.00

PAGE KEY: A-42 Beverages and Beverage Mixes   A-44 Candies   A-46 Cereals   A-48 Cheeses and Substitutes   A-50 Dairy Products and Substitutes   A-52 Desserts   A-56 Eggs and Egg Substitutes   A-56 Fats, Oils, Margarines, and Shortenings   A-58 Fruits   A-60 Grain Products and Baked Goods   A-62 Grains and Flours   A-64 Meats and Meat Substitutes   A-68 Nuts, Seeds, and Products

Code	Food Name	Unit/ Amt	Wt (g)	Energy (kcal)	Prot (g)	Carb (g)	Fiber (g)	Fat (g)	Sat (g)	Mono (g)	Poly (g)	Chol (mg)	Vit A (RE)
7885	Tomatoes, stwd, unsalted, cnd	0.5 cup	123	35	1	7	2	0	0.0	0.0	0.0	0	50
7896	Tomatoes, whole, peeled, cnd	0.5 cup	121	25	1	4	1	0	0.0	0.0	0.0	0	50
7873	Vegetables, peas & carrots, cnd	0.5 cup	123	50	4	10	3	0	0.0	0.0	0.0	0	500
6460	Waterchestnuts, slices, cnd	1 svg	130	65	1	16	6	0	0.0			0	0
Cooked Vegetables and Legumes													
5000	Artichokes, globe, ckd, drnd, med	1 ea	120	64	3	14	10	0	0.1	0.0	0.2	0	2
5003	Asparagus, ckd, drnd	0.5 cup	90	20	2	4	2	0	0.0	0.0	0.1	0	91
5249	Bamboo Shoots, slices, ckd, drnd	0.5 cup	60	7	1	1	1	0	0.0	0.0	0.1	0	0
7012	Beans, black, mature, ckd	0.5 cup	86	114	8	20	7	0	0.1	0.0	0.2	0	1
4450	Beans, blackeyed, mature, ckd	0.5 cup	86	99	7	18	6	0	0.1	0.0	0.2	0	1
7027	Beans, broad, mature, ckd	0.5 cup	85	94	6	17	5	0	0.1	0.1	0.1	0	1
4444	Beans, fava, mature, ckd	0.5 cup	85	94	6	17	5	0	0.1	0.1	0.1	0	1
7045	Beans, French, mature, ckd	0.5 cup	88	114	6	21	8	1	0.1	0.0	0.4	0	0
7031	Beans, goa, mature, ckd	0.5 cup	86	126	9	13		5	0.7	1.9	1.3	0	0
7021	Beans, great northern, mature, ckd	0.5 cup	88	104	7	19	6	0	0.1	0.0	0.2	0	0
7008	Beans, kidney, all types, mature, ckd	0.5 cup	88	112	8	20	6	0	0.1	0.0	0.2	0	0
7006	Beans, lentils, mature, ckd	0.5 cup	99	115	9	20	8	0	0.1	0.1	0.2	0	1
90019	Beans, lentils, mature, ckd w/salt	0.5 cup	99	113	9	19	8	0	0.1	0.1	0.2	0	1
7058	Beans, lima, baby, mature, ckd	0.5 cup	91	115	7	21	7	0	0.1	0.0	0.2	0	0
7059	Beans, mung, mature, ckd	0.5 cup	101	106	7	19	8	0	0.1	0.1	0.1	0	2
7022	Beans, navy, mature, ckd	0.5 cup	91	127	7	24	10	1	0.1	0.1	0.4	0	0
7050	Beans, pink, mature, ckd	0.5 cup	84	126	8	24	4	0	0.1	0.0	0.2	0	0
7013	Beans, pinto, mature, ckd	0.5 cup	86	122	8	22	8	1	0.1	0.1	0.2	0	0
7053	Beans, white, mature, ckd	0.5 cup	90	124	9	22	6	0	0.1	0.0	0.1	0	0
5022	Beets, ckd, drnd, sliced	0.5 cup	85	37	1	8	2	0	0.0	0.0	0.1	0	3
5407	Borage, ckd, drnd	4 oz	113	28	2	4		1	0.2	0.3	0.1	0	497
90415	Broccoli, spear, 5" long, ckd, drnd	1 ea	37	13	1	3	1	0	0.0	0.0	0.1	0	57
5234	Broccoli, spears, ckd f/fzn, drnd	0.5 cup	92	26	3	5	3	0	0.0	0.0	0.1	0	93
5033	Brussels Sprouts, ckd, drnd	0.5 cup	78	28	2	6	2	0	0.1	0.0	0.2	0	60
5038	Cabbage, ckd, drnd, shredded	0.5 cup	75	17	1	4	1	0	0.0	0.0	0.0	0	6
5075	Cabbage, kale, ckd, drnd	0.5 cup	65	18	1	4	1	0	0.0	0.0	0.1	0	885
5238	Cabbage, red, ckd, drnd, shredded	0.5 cup	75	22	1	5	2	0	0.0	0.0	0.0	0	2
5358	Carrots, ckd f/fzn, drnd, slices	0.5 cup	73	27	0	6	2	0	0.1	0.0	0.2	0	1236
5047	Carrots, ckd, drnd, slices	0.5 cup	78	27	1	6	2	0	0.0	0.0	0.1	0	1329
5052	Cauliflower, florets, ckd, drnd	3 ea	54	12	1	2	1	0	0.0	0.0	0.1	0	1
7266	Cauliflower, green, ckd, head	0.125 ea	56	18	2	4	2	0	0.0	0.0	0.1	0	8
5894	Celery, w/salt, diced, drnd, ckd	0.5 cup	75	14	1	3	1	0	0.0	0.0	0.1	0	39
5567	Corn, white, sweet, cob, ckd f/fzn, drnd	1 ea	63	59	2	14	1	0	0.1	0.1	0.2	0	0
5560	Corn, white, sweet, kernels f/one ear, ckd, drnd	0.5 cup	78	76	3	17	2	1	0.2	0.3	0.5	0	0
6019	Corn, white, sweet, kernels, ckd f/fzn w/salt, drnd	0.5 cup	82	66	2	16	2	0	0.1	0.1	0.2	0	0
5393	Corn, white, sweet, kernels, ckd f/fzn, drnd	0.5 cup	82	66	2	16	2	0	0.1	0.1	0.2	0	0
5365	Corn, yellow, sweet, cob, kernels, ckd f/fzn, drnd	0.5 cup	82	78	3	18	2	1	0.1	0.2	0.3	0	19
5379	Corn, yellow, sweet, kernels, ckd, drnd	0.5 cup	74	72	3	16	2	1	0.1	0.3	0.4	0	20
5639	Cucumber, ckd	0.5 cup	90	14	1	3	1	0	0.0	0.0	0.1	0	21
5072	Eggplant, ckd, drnd, 1" cubes	0.5 cup	50	17	0	4	1	0	0.0	0.0	0.0	0	2

PAGE KEY: A-70 Prepared Foods   A-78 Restaurants   A-90 Salad Dressings and Dips   A-92 Sauces and Gravies   A-94 Snack Foods   A-94 Spices, Flavors, and Seasonings   A-96 Sports Bars and Drinks   A-96 Supplemental Foods and Formulas   A-96 Sweeteners and Sweet Substitutes   A-98 Vegetables and Legumes   A-108 Miscellaneous

Thia (mg)	Ribo (mg)	Niac (mg NE)	Vit B6 (mg)	Vit B12 (µg)	Fol (µg)	Vit C (mg)	Vit D (IU)	Vit E (mg AT)	Cal (mg)	Iron (mg)	Magn (mg)	Phos (mg)	Pota (mg)	Sodi (mg)	Zinc (mg)	Wat (%)	Alco (g)	Caff (g)
				0.00		12.0			40	1.44			150	15			0.00	0.00
				0.00		12.0			20	0.72			200	220			0.00	0.00
				0.00		9.0			20	1.08			0	330			0.00	0.00
				0.00		0.0			4	0.34				16		86	0.00	0.00
0.05	0.10	1.33	0.10	0.00	106.8	8.9	0.0	0.2	25	0.73	50.4	88	343	72	0.5	84	0.00	0.00
0.15	0.12	0.98	0.07	0.00	134.1	6.9	0.0	1.3	21	0.81	12.6	49	202	13	0.5	93	0.00	0.00
0.00	0.02	0.18	0.05	0.00	1.2	0.0	0.0		7	0.14	1.8	12	320	2	0.3	96	0.00	0.00
0.20	0.05	0.43	0.05	0.00	128.1	0.0	0.0		23	1.80	60.2	120	305	1	1.0	66	0.00	0.00
0.17	0.05	0.41	0.09	0.00	177.8	0.3	0.0	0.2	21	2.15	45.3	133	238	3	1.1	70	0.00	0.00
0.07	0.07	0.60	0.05	0.00	88.4	0.3	0.0	0.0	31	1.27	36.5	106	228	4	0.9	72	0.00	0.00
0.07	0.07	0.60	0.05	0.00	88.4	0.3	0.0	0.0	31	1.27	36.5	106	228	4	0.9	72	0.00	0.00
0.11	0.05	0.47	0.09	0.00	66.4	1.1	0.0		56	0.95	49.6	90	327	5	0.6	67	0.00	0.00
0.25	0.10	0.70	0.03	0.00	8.6	0.0	0.0		122	3.72	46.4	132	241	11	1.2	67	0.00	0.00
0.14	0.05	0.60	0.10	0.00	90.3	1.2	0.0		60	1.88	44.2	146	346	2	0.8	69	0.00	0.00
0.14	0.05	0.50	0.10	0.00	115.0	1.1	0.0	0.0	31	1.96	37.2	122	358	1	0.9	67	0.00	0.00
0.17	0.07	1.04	0.18	0.00	179.2	1.5	0.0	0.1	19	3.29	35.6	178	365	2	1.3	70	0.00	0.00
0.17	0.07	1.04	0.18	0.00	179.2	1.5	0.0	0.1	19	3.29	35.6	178	365	236	1.3	70	0.00	0.00
0.15	0.05	0.60	0.07	0.00	136.5	0.0	0.0		26	2.18	48.2	116	365	3	0.9	67	0.00	0.00
0.17	0.05	0.57	0.07	0.00	160.6	1.0	0.0	0.2	27	1.40	48.5	100	269	2	0.8	73	0.00	0.00
0.21	0.05	0.58	0.12	0.00	127.4	0.8	0.0	0.0	63	2.15	48.2	131	354	0	0.9	64	0.00	0.00
0.21	0.05	0.47	0.15	0.00	142.0	0.0	0.0	0.8	44	1.94	54.9	139	429	2	0.8	61	0.00	0.00
0.17	0.05	0.27	0.20	0.00	147.1	0.7	0.0	0.8	39	1.78	42.8	126	373	1	0.8	63	0.00	0.00
0.10	0.03	0.12	0.07	0.00	72.5	0.0	0.0	0.8	81	3.30	56.4	101	502	5	1.2	63	0.00	0.00
0.01	0.02	0.28	0.05	0.00	68.0	3.1	0.0	0.0	14	0.67	19.6	32	259	65	0.3	87	0.00	0.00
0.07	0.18	1.07	0.10	0.00	11.3	36.9	0.0		116	4.13	64.6	62	557	100	0.2	92	0.00	0.00
0.01	0.05	0.20	0.07	0.00	40.0	24.0	0.0	0.5	15	0.25	7.8	25	108	15	0.2	89	0.00	0.00
0.05	0.07	0.41	0.11	0.00	27.6	36.9	0.0	1.2	47	0.56	18.4	51	166	22	0.3	91	0.00	0.00
0.07	0.05	0.46	0.14	0.00	46.8	48.4	0.0	0.3	28	0.93	15.6	44	247	16	0.3	89	0.00	0.00
0.05	0.02	0.18	0.07	0.00	22.5	28.1	0.0	0.1	36	0.12	11.2	25	147	6	0.2	93	0.00	0.00
0.02	0.05	0.31	0.09	0.00	8.4	26.6	0.0	0.6	47	0.57	11.7	18	148	15	0.2	91	Alco	Caff
0.05	0.03	0.28	0.17	0.00	18.0	25.8	0.0	0.1	32	0.50	12.8	25	196	21	0.2	91	0.00	0.00
0.01	0.02	0.30	0.05	0.00	8.0	1.7	0.0	0.7	26	0.38	8.0	23	140	43	0.3	90	0.00	0.00
0.05	0.02	0.50	0.11	0.00	10.9	2.8	0.0	0.8	23	0.27	7.8	23	183	45	0.2	90	0.00	0.00
0.01	0.02	0.21	0.09	0.00	23.8	23.9	0.0	0.0	9	0.17	4.9	17	77	8	0.1	93	0.00	0.00
0.03	0.05	0.37	0.11	0.00	23.1	40.8	0.0		18	0.40	10.7	32	156	13	0.4	89	0.00	0.00
0.02	0.03	0.23	0.05	0.00	16.5	4.6	0.0	0.3	32	0.31	9.0	19	213	245	0.1	94	0.00	0.00
0.10	0.03	0.95	0.14	0.00	19.5	3.0	0.0		2	0.37	18.3	47	158	3	0.4	73	0.00	0.00
0.07	0.03	1.30	0.10	0.00	15.7	4.9	0.0	0.1	2	0.43	24.3	72	198	2	0.4	73	0.00	0.00
0.07	0.05	1.07	0.10	0.00	25.6	2.6	0.0	0.1	3	0.28	15.7	47	121	202	0.3	77	0.00	0.00
0.07	0.05	1.07	0.10	0.00	25.6	2.6	0.0	0.1	3	0.28	15.7	47	121	4	0.3	77	0.00	0.00
0.14	0.05	1.25	0.18	0.00	25.6	4.0	0.0	0.1	2	0.50	23.9	62	207	3	0.5	73	0.00	0.00
0.07	0.03	1.25	0.10	0.00	17.1	4.1	0.0	0.1	2	0.34	19.4	57	162	1	0.5	73	0.00	0.00
0.01	0.01	0.21	0.03	0.00	10.1	4.7	0.0	0.1	15	0.27	11.6	20	144	2	0.2	95	0.00	0.00
0.03	0.00	0.30	0.03	0.00	6.9	0.6	0.0	0.2	3	0.11	5.4	7	61	0	0.1	90	0.00	0.00

PAGE KEY: A-42 Beverages and Beverage Mixes   A-44 Candies   A-46 Cereals   A-48 Cheeses and Substitutes   A-50 Dairy Products and Substitutes   A-52 Desserts   A-56 Eggs and Egg Substitutes   A-56 Fats, Oils, Margarines, and Shortenings   A-58 Fruits   A-60 Grain Products and Baked Goods   A-62 Grains and Flours   A-64 Meats and Meat Substitutes   A-68 Nuts, Seeds, and Products

Code	Food Name	Unit/ Amt	Wt (g)	Energy (kcal)	Prot (g)	Carb (g)	Fiber (g)	Fat (g)	Sat (g)	Mono (g)	Poly (g)	Chol (mg)	Vit A (RE)
5025	Greens, beet, ckd, drnd	0.5 cup	72	19	2	4	2	0	0.0	0.0	0.1	0	551
5061	Greens, collard, chpd, ckd, drnd	0.5 cup	95	25	2	5	3	0	0.0	0.0	0.2	0	771
5096	Greens, mustard, ckd, drnd	0.5 cup	70	10	2	1	1	0	0.0	0.1	0.0	0	443
5426	Greens, purslane, ckd, drnd	0.5 cup	58	10	1	2		0				0	106
24128	Greens, Swiss chard, bld, drnd, chpd	0.5 cup	88	18	2	4	2	0	0.0	0.0	0.0	0	536
5185	Greens, turnip, chpd, ckd, drnd	0.5 cup	72	14	1	3	3	0	0.0	0.0	0.1	0	549
5640	Hominy, ckd	0.5 cup	82	59	1	12	2	1	0.1	0.2	0.3	0	0
5092	Mushrooms, ckd, drnd	0.5 cup	78	22	2	4	2	0	0.0	0.0	0.1	0	0
5384	Mushrooms, shiitake, ckd, whole	4 ea	72	40	1	10	2	0	0.0	0.1	0.0	0	0
7508	Natto, fermented soybeans	0.5 cup	88	186	16	13	5	10	1.4	2.1	5.4	0	0
5099	Okra, ckd, drnd, slices	0.5 cup	80	18	1	4	2	0	0.0	0.0	0.1	0	23
7811	Onion, red, ckd, drnd, chpd	0.5 cup	105	46	1	11	1	0	0.0	0.0	0.1	0	0
5108	Onion, white, ckd, drnd, chpd	0.5 cup	105	46	1	11	1	0	0.0	0.0	0.1	0	0
7812	Onion, yellow, ckd, drnd, chpd	0.5 cup	105	46	1	11	1	0	0.0	0.0	0.1	0	0
5212	Parsnips, ckd, drnd	0.5 cup	78	55	1	13	3	0	0.0	0.1	0.0	0	0
5213	Peas, black eyed, immature, ckd, drnd	0.5 cup	82	80	3	17	4	0	0.1	0.0	0.1	0	65
7056	Peas, catjang cowpeas, ckd	0.5 cup	86	100	7	17	3	1	0.2	0.1	0.3	0	1
4441	Peas, chickpea, mature, ckd	0.5 cup	82	134	7	22	6	2	0.2	0.5	0.9	0	2
7001	Peas, garbanzo, mature, ckd	0.5 cup	82	134	7	22	6	2	0.2	0.5	0.9	0	2
5939	Peas, green, ckd f/fzn w/salt, drnd	0.5 cup	80	62	4	11	4	0	0.0	0.0	0.1	0	168
7020	Peas, green, split, ckd	0.5 cup	98	116	8	21	8	0	0.1	0.1	0.2	0	1
5126	Peppers, bell, green, sweet, ckd, drnd, chpd	1 cup	135	38	1	9	2	0	0.0	0.0	0.1	0	63
9549	Peppers, bell, green, sweet, sauteed	1 svg	85	108	1	4	2	10	1.4	2.0	5.0	0	23
5278	Peppers, bell, red, sweet, ckd, drnd, chpd	0.5 cup	68	19	1	5	1	0	0.0	0.0	0.1	0	200
5334	Potatoes, baked, med, 2 1/4" to 3 1/4"	1 ea	173	161	4	37	4	0	0.1	0.0	0.1	0	2
5130	Potatoes, baked, peeled		61	57	1	13	1	0	0.0	0.0	0.0	0	0
5948	Potatoes, baked, peeled, salted	0.5 cup	61	57	1	13	1	0	0.0	0.0	0.0	0	0
6996	Potatoes, baked, salted	0.5 cup	61	57	2	13	1	0	0.0	0.0	0.0	0	1
9250	Potatoes, red, w/skin, baked, med, 2 1/4" to 3 1/4"	1 ea	173	154	4	34	3	0	0.0	0.0	0.1	0	2
5512	Potatoes, rstd	1 ea	93	132	3	30	3	0	0.0	0.0	0.1	0	0
9247	Potatoes, w/skin, baked, med, 2 1/4"-3 1/4"	1 ea	173	163	4	36	4	0	0.0	0.0	0.1	0	2
9366	Potatoes, white, baby, ckd	0.5 cup	85	70	2	15	1	0	0.0	0.0	0.0	0	0
9368	Potatoes, yukon gold, ckd	0.5 cup	85	70	2	15	1	0	0.0	0.0	0.0	0	0
7226	Rutabaga, ckd, drnd, mashed	0.5 cup	120	47	2	10	2	0	0.0	0.0	0.1	0	0
5013	Snap Beans, green, ckd f/fzn, drnd	0.5 cup	68	19	1	4	2	0	0.0	0.0	0.1	0	38
7015	Soybeans, mature, ckd	0.5 cup	86	149	14	9	5	8	1.1	1.7	4.4	0	1
90028	Soybeans, mature, ckd w/salt	0.5 cup	86	149	14	9	5	8	1.1	1.7	4.4	0	1
5147	Spinach, ckd, drnd	0.5 cup	90	21	3	3	2	0	0.0	0.0	0.1	0	943
5459	Sprouts, soybean, mature, stmd	0.5 cup	47	38	4	3	0	2	0.3	0.5	1.2	0	2
5316	Squash, acorn, ckd, mashed	0.5 cup	122	42	1	11	3	0	0.0	0.0	0.0	0	100
5317	Squash, butternut, bkd, cubes	0.5 cup	102	41	1	11	3	0	0.0	0.0	0.0	0	1143
5455	Squash, spaghetti, bkd/ckd, drnd	0.5 cup	78	21	1	5	1	0	0.0	0.0	0.1	0	9
6922	Squash, spaghetti, ckd w/salt, drnd	0.5 cup	78	21	1	5	1	0	0.0	0.0	0.1	0	9
5152	Squash, summer, all types, ckd, drnd, slices	0.5 cup	90	18	1	4	1	0	0.1	0.0	0.1	0	19
5981	Squash, winter, all types, bkd w/salt, cubes	0.5 cup	102	40	1	9	3	1	0.1	0.0	0.3	0	535
5667	Squash, zucchini, slices, stmd	0.5 cup	90	13	1	3	1	0	0.0	0.0	0.1	0	29

PAGE KEY: A-70 Prepared Foods   A-78 Restaurants   A-90 Salad Dressings and Dips   A-92 Sauces and Gravies   A-94 Snack Foods   A-94 Spices, Flavors, and Seasonings   A-96 Sports Bars and Drinks
A-96 Supplemental Foods and Formulas   A-96 Sweeteners and Sweet Substitutes   A-98 Vegetables and Legumes   A-108 Miscellaneous

Thia (mg)	Ribo (mg)	Niac (mg NE)	Vit B6 (mg)	Vit B12 (µg)	Fol (µg)	Vit C (mg)	Vit D (IU)	Vit E (mg AT)	Cal (mg)	Iron (mg)	Magn (mg)	Phos (mg)	Pota (mg)	Sodi (mg)	Zinc (mg)	Wat (%)	Alco (g)	Caff (g)
0.07	0.20	0.36	0.10	0.00	10.1	17.9	0.0	1.3	82	1.37	49.0	30	654	174	0.4	89	0.00	0.00
0.03	0.10	0.55	0.11	0.00	88.3	17.3	0.0	0.8	133	1.10	19.0	28	110	15	0.2	92	0.00	0.00
0.02	0.03	0.30	0.07	0.00	51.1	17.7	0.0	0.8	52	0.49	10.5	29	141	11	0.1	94	0.00	0.00
0.01	0.05	0.25	0.03	0.00	5.2	6.0	0.0		45	0.43	38.5	21	281	25	0.1	94	0.00	0.00
0.02	0.07	0.31	0.07	0.00	7.9	15.8	0.0	1.7	51	1.98	75.2	29	480	157	0.3	93	0.00	0.00
0.02	0.05	0.30	0.12	0.00	85.0	19.7	0.0	1.4	99	0.57	15.8	21	146	21	0.1	93	0.00	0.00
0.00	0.00	0.02	0.00	0.00	0.8	0.0	0.0	0.0	8	0.50	13.2	29	7	173	0.9	83	0.00	0.00
0.05	0.23	3.48	0.07	0.00	14.0	3.1	6.2	0.0	5	1.36	9.4	68	278	2	0.7	91	0.00	0.00
0.02	0.11	1.08	0.10	0.00	15.1	0.2	20.2	0.0	2	0.31	10.1	21	84	3	1.0	83	0.00	0.00
0.14	0.17	0.00	0.10	0.00	7.0	11.4	0.0	0.0	190	7.53	100.6	152	638	6	2.7	55	0.00	0.00
0.10	0.03	0.69	0.15	0.00	36.8	13.0	0.0	0.2	62	0.21	28.8	26	108	5	0.3	93	0.00	0.00
0.03	0.01	0.17	0.14	0.00	15.7	5.5	0.0	0.0	23	0.25	11.5	37	174	3	0.2	88	0.00	0.00
0.03	0.01	0.17	0.14	0.00	15.7	5.5	0.0	0.0	23	0.25	11.5	37	174	3	0.2	88	0.00	0.00
0.03	0.01	0.17	0.14	0.00	15.7	5.5	0.0	0.0	23	0.25	11.5	37	174	3	0.2	88	0.00	0.00
0.05	0.03	0.56	0.07	0.00	45.2	10.1	0.0	0.8	29	0.44	22.6	54	286	8	0.2	80	0.00	0.00
0.07	0.11	1.15	0.05	0.00	104.8	1.8	0.0	0.2	106	0.92	42.9	42	345	3	0.8	75	0.00	0.00
0.14	0.03	0.61	0.07	0.00	121.4	0.3	0.0		22	2.60	82.1	121	321	16	1.6	70	0.00	0.00
0.10	0.05	0.43	0.10	0.00	141.0	1.1	0.0	0.3	40	2.36	39.4	138	239	6	1.3	60	0.00	0.00
0.10	0.05	0.43	0.10	0.00	141.0	1.1	0.0	0.3	40	2.36	39.4	138	239	6	1.3	60	0.00	0.00
0.23	0.07	1.17	0.09	0.00	47.2	7.9	0.0	0.0	19	1.22	17.6	62	88	258	0.5	80	0.00	0.00
0.18	0.05	0.87	0.05	0.00	63.7	0.4	0.0	0.0	14	1.25	35.3	97	355	2	1.0	69	0.00	0.00
0.07	0.03	0.63	0.31	0.00	21.6	100.4	0.0	0.7	12	0.62	13.5	24	224	3	0.2	92	0.00	0.00
0.03	0.03	0.49	0.17	0.00	1.7	150.4	0.0	1.2	7	0.25	6.8	13	114	14	0.1	83	0.00	0.00
0.03	0.01	0.31	0.15	0.00	10.9	116.3	0.0	1.1	6	0.31	6.8	12	113	1	0.1	92	0.00	0.00
0.10	0.07	2.44	0.54	0.00	48.4	16.6	0.0	0.1	26	1.87	48.4	121	926	17	0.6	75	0.00	0.00
0.05	0.00	0.85	0.18	0.00	5.5	7.8	0.0	0.0	3	0.20	15.2	30	239	3	0.2	75	0.00	0.00
0.05	0.00	0.85	0.18	0.00	5.5	7.8	0.0	0.0	3	0.20	15.2	30	239	147	0.2	75	0.00	0.00
0.03	0.02	0.86	0.18	0.00	17.1	5.9	0.0	0.0	9	0.66	17.1	43	326	6	0.2	75	0.00	0.00
0.11	0.09	2.75	0.37	0.00	46.7	21.8	0.0	0.1	16	1.21	48.4	125	943	21	0.7	77	0.00	0.00
0.11	0.05	2.34	0.40	0.00	19.2	26.3	0.0	0.1	12	1.26	35.0	77	905	10	0.7	62	0.00	0.00
0.07	0.07	2.64	0.37	0.00	65.7	21.8	0.0	0.1	17	1.11	46.7	130	941	12	0.6	75	0.00	0.00
						18.0			0	0.72				5		67	0.00	0.00
						18.0			0	0.72				5		67	0.00	0.00
0.10	0.05	0.86	0.11	0.00	18.0	22.6	0.0	0.4	58	0.63	27.6	67	391	24	0.4	89	0.00	0.00
0.01	0.05	0.25	0.03	0.00	15.5	2.8	0.0	0.0	28	0.44	12.8	20	107	1	0.2	91	0.00	0.00
0.12	0.25	0.34	0.20	0.00	46.4	1.5	0.0	0.3	88	4.42	74.0	211	443	1	1.0	63	0.00	0.00
0.12	0.25	0.34	0.20	0.00	46.4	1.5	0.0	0.3	88	4.42	74.0	211	443	204	1.0	63	0.00	0.00
0.09	0.20	0.43	0.21	0.00	131.4	8.8	0.0	1.9	122	3.21	78.3	50	419	63	0.7	91	0.00	0.00
0.10	0.01	0.50	0.05	0.00	37.6	3.9	0.0	0.1	28	0.62	28.2	63	167	5	0.5	79	0.00	0.00
0.11	0.00	0.64	0.14	0.00	13.5	8.0	0.0		32	0.68	31.9	33	322	4	0.1	90	0.00	0.00
0.07	0.01	0.99	0.12	0.00	19.5	15.5	0.0	1.3	42	0.62	29.7	28	291	4	0.1	88	0.00	0.00
0.02	0.01	0.62	0.07	0.00	6.2	2.7	0.0	0.1	16	0.25	8.5	11	91	14	0.2	92	0.00	0.00
0.02	0.01	0.62	0.07	0.00	6.2	2.7	0.0	0.1	16	0.25	8.5		91	197	0.2	92	0.00	0.00
0.03	0.03	0.46	0.05	0.00	18.0	4.9	0.0	0.1	24	0.31	21.6	35	173	1	0.4	94	0.00	0.00
0.09	0.01	0.72	0.07	0.00	28.7	9.8	0.0	0.1	14	0.34	8.2	20	448	243	0.3	89	0.00	0.00
0.05	0.02	0.34	0.07	0.00	16.9	6.9	0.0	0.1	14	0.37	19.8	29	223	3	0.2	95	0.00	0.00

PAGE KEY: A-42 Beverages and Beverage Mixes   A-44 Candies   A-46 Cereals   A-48 Cheeses and Substitutes   A-50 Dairy Products and Substitutes   A-52 Desserts   A-56 Eggs and Egg Substitutes   A-56 Fats, Oils, Margarines, and Shortenings   A-58 Fruits   A-60 Grain Products and Baked Goods   A-62 Grains and Flours   A-64 Meats and Meat Substitutes   A-68 Nuts, Seeds, and Products

Code	Food Name	Unit/Amt	Wt (g)	Energy (kcal)	Prot (g)	Carb (g)	Fiber (g)	Fat (g)	Sat (g)	Mono (g)	Poly (g)	Chol (mg)	Vit A (RE)
5327	Squash, zucchini, w/skin, ckd, drnd, slices	0.5 cup	90	14	1	2	1	0	0.1	0.0	0.1	0	101
5544	Taro, ckd, slices, Tahitian	0.5 cup	68	30	3	5		0	0.1	0.0	0.2	0	121
5229	Taro, poi	0.5 cup	120	134	0	33	0	0	0.0	0.0	0.1	0	8
5536	Tomatoes, green, ckd, fried	1 ea	144	284	5	19	1	22	4.6	9.4	6.4	41	82
5178	Tomatoes, red, ckd f/fresh	0.5 cup	120	22	1	5	1	0	0.0	0.0	0.1	0	59
5177	Tomatoes, red, ckd f/fresh, med	1 ea	123	22	1	5	1	0	0.0	0.0	0.1	0	60
5628	Tomatoes, red, fried	1 ea	101	168	3	12	1	13	2.7	5.5	3.8	24	57
5183	Turnips, ckd, drnd, cubes	0.5 cup	78	17	1	4	2	0	0.0	0.0	0.0	0	0
5187	Vegetables, ckd f/fzn, drnd, 10-oz pkg	0.5 cup	91	59	3	12	4	0	0.0	0.0	0.1	0	389
5123	Vegetables, peas & carrots, ckd f/fzn, drnd	0.5 cup	80	38	2	8	2	0	0.1	0.0	0.2	0	761
5168	Yams, tropical, ckd/bkd, cubes	0.5 cup	68	79	1	19	3	0	0.0	0.0	0.0	0	8

Dried Vegetables and Legumes

Code	Food Name	Unit/Amt	Wt (g)	Energy (kcal)	Prot (g)	Carb (g)	Fiber (g)	Fat (g)	Sat (g)	Mono (g)	Poly (g)	Chol (mg)	Vit A (RE)
9918	Onion, green, freeze dried, Just Green Onions, svg	1 svg	43	150	9	28	4	1	0.0			0	1200
7259	Potatoes, dehyd	1 oz	28	104	2	23	1	0					0
5446	Tomatoes, sun dried	0.5 cup	27	70	4	15	3	1	0.1	0.1	0.3	0	24

Fresh Vegetables and Legumes

Code	Food Name	Unit/Amt	Wt (g)	Energy (kcal)	Prot (g)	Carb (g)	Fiber (g)	Fat (g)	Sat (g)	Mono (g)	Poly (g)	Chol (mg)	Vit A (RE)
7440	Artichokes, Calif, fresh	1 ea	340	85	7	20	10	0	0.0	0.0	0.0	0	0
5001	Asparagus, fresh	0.5 cup	67	13	1	3	1	0	0.0	0.0	0.0	0	51
6757	Broccoli, fresh	0.5 cup	46	15	1	3	1	0	0.0	0.0	0.0	0	28
5032	Brussels Sprouts, fresh	0.5 cup	44	19	1	4	2	0	0.0	0.0	0.1	0	33
5036	Cabbage, fresh, shredded	1 cup	70	18	1	4	2	0	0.0	0.0	0.0	0	7
5208	Cabbage, kale, fresh, chpd	1 cup	67	34	2	7	1	0	0.1	0.0	0.2	0	1030
5042	Cabbage, red, fresh, shredded	1 cup	70	22	1	5	1	0	0.0	0.0	0.1	0	78
9329	Carrots, baby, fresh	0.75 cup	85	40	1	9	2	0	0.0	0.0	0.0	0	1250
5049	Cauliflower, fresh	0.5 cup	54	13	1	3	1	0	0.0	0.0	0.0	0	0
90436	Celery, stalk, sml, 5" long, fresh	1 ea	17	3	0	1	0	0	0.0	0.0	0.0	0	8
7927	Chili Peppers, banana, fresh	0.25 cup	31	8	1	2	1	0	0.0	0.0	0.1	0	11
7931	Chili Peppers, jalapeno, fresh	1 ea	14	4	0	1	0	0	0.0	0.0	0.0	0	15
5378	Corn, yellow, sweet, kernels, fresh	0.5 cup	72	62	2	14	1	1	0.2	0.3	0.4	0	14
5071	Cucumber, w/skin, fresh, slices	0.5 cup	52	8	0	2	0	0	0.0	0.0	0.0	0	5
26005	Garlic, cloves, fresh	1 ea	3	4	0	1	0	0	0.0	0.0	0.0	0	0
7961	Greens, grape leaf, fresh	1 ea	3	3	0	1	0	0	0.0	0.0	0.0	0	83
5547	Greens, turnip, chpd, fresh	1 cup	55	18	1	4	2	0	0.0	0.0	0.1	0	637
5222	Greens, watercress, fresh, chpd	0.5 cup	17	2	0	0	0	0	0.0	0.0	0.0	0	54
9181	Jicama, fresh, chpd	0.5 cup	65	25	0	6	3	0	0.0	0.0	0.0	0	1
5083	Lettuce, iceberg, fresh, shred	1 cup	72	10	1	2	1	0	0.0	0.0	0.1	0	36
5088	Lettuce, romaine, fresh, shred	1 cup	47	8	1	2	1	0	0.0	0.0	0.1	0	409
5090	Mushrooms, fresh, pces/slices	0.5 cup	35	8	1	1	0	0	0.0	0.0	0.1	0	0
6494	Mushrooms, fresh, whole	0.5 cup	48	11	1	2	0	0	0.0	0.0	0.1	0	0
7498	Onion, red, fresh, chpd	0.5 cup	80	32	1	7	1	0	0.0	0.0	0.0	0	0
5101	Onion, white, fresh, chpd	0.5 cup	80	32	1	7	1	0	0.0	0.0	0.0	0	0
7499	Onion, yellow, fresh, chpd	0.5 cup	80	32	1	7	1	0	0.0	0.0	0.0	0	0
5120	Pea Pods, fresh, whole	0.5 cup	32	13	1	2	1	0	0.0	0.0	0.0	0	34
5116	Peas, green, fresh	0.5 cup	72	59	4	10	4	0	0.1	0.0	0.1	0	55
5124	Peppers, bell, green, sweet, fresh, chpd	0.5 cup	74	15	1	3	1	0	0.0	0.0	0.0	0	28
5128	Peppers, bell, red, sweet, fresh, chpd	0.5 cup	74	23	1	4	1	0	0.0	0.0	0.1	0	233

PAGE KEY: A-70 Prepared Foods   A-78 Restaurants   A-90 Salad Dressings and Dips   A-92 Sauces and Gravies   A-94 Snack Foods   A-94 Spices, Flavors, and Seasonings   A-96 Sports Bars and Drinks   A-96 Supplemental Foods and Formulas   A-96 Sweeteners and Sweet Substitutes   A-98 Vegetables and Legumes   A-108 Miscellaneous

Thia (mg)	Ribo (mg)	Niac (mg NE)	Vit B6 (mg)	Vit B12 (µg)	Fol (µg)	Vit C (mg)	Vit D (IU)	Vit E (mg AT)	Cal (mg)	Iron (mg)	Magn (mg)	Phos (mg)	Pota (mg)	Sodi (mg)	Zinc (mg)	Wat (%)	Alco (g)	Caff (g)
0.02	0.01	0.46	0.07	0.00	25.2	11.6	0.0	0.1	16	0.33	17.1	33	238	3	0.3	95	0.00	0.00
0.02	0.14	0.33	0.07	0.00	4.8	26.0	0.0		102	1.07	34.9	46	427	37	0.1	86	0.00	0.00
0.15	0.05	1.32	0.33	0.00	25.2	4.8	0.0	2.8	19	1.05	28.8	47	220	14	0.3	72	0.00	0.00
0.15	0.18	1.36	0.10	0.14	12.7	20.9	9.2	3.0	101	1.50	17.1	102	254	134	0.4	68	0.00	0.00
0.03	0.02	0.63	0.09	0.00	15.6	27.4	0.0	0.7	13	0.81	10.8	34	262	13	0.2	94	0.00	0.00
0.03	0.02	0.64	0.10	0.00	16.0	28.0	0.0	0.7	14	0.83	11.1	34	268	14	0.2	94	0.00	0.00
0.10	0.11	0.97	0.07	0.07	11.8	13.4	6.5	1.8	55	0.93	12.6	62	200	78	0.2	72	0.00	0.00
0.01	0.01	0.23	0.05	0.00	7.0	9.0	0.0		26	0.14	7.0	20	138	12	0.1	94	0.00	0.00
0.05	0.10	0.76	0.07	0.00	17.3	2.9	0.0	0.3	23	0.75	20.0	46	154	32	0.4	83	0.00	0.00
0.18	0.05	0.92	0.07	0.00	20.8	6.5	0.0	0.4	18	0.75	12.8	39	126	54	0.4	86	0.00	0.00
0.05	0.01	0.37	0.15	0.00	10.9	8.2	0.0	0.2	10	0.34	12.2	33	456	5	0.1	70	0.00	0.00
						54.0			300	9.00				20			0.00	0.00
0.07	0.05	1.04		0.00		3.1			8	0.79		57	261	2		6	0.00	0.00
0.14	0.12	2.44	0.09	0.00	18.4	10.6	0.0	0.0	30	2.45	52.4	96	925	566	0.5	15	0.00	0.00
0.10	0.11	2.72	0.14		136.0	20.4		1.4	68	2.45	136.0	204	578	255		91	0.00	0.00
0.10	0.09	0.66	0.05	0.00	34.8	3.8	0.0	0.8	16	1.42	9.4	35	135	1	0.4	93	0.00	0.00
0.02	0.05	0.28	0.07	0.00	28.7	40.6	0.0	0.4	21	0.33	9.6	30	144	15	0.2	89	0.00	0.00
0.05	0.03	0.33	0.10	0.00	26.8	37.4	0.0	0.4	18	0.62	10.1	30	171	11	0.2	86	0.00	0.00
0.03	0.02	0.15	0.09	0.00	30.1	25.6	0.0	0.1	28	0.33	8.4	18	119	13	0.1	92	0.00	0.00
0.07	0.09	0.67	0.18	0.00	19.4	80.4	0.0		90	1.13	22.8	38	299	29	0.3	84	0.00	0.00
0.03	0.05	0.28	0.15	0.00	12.6	39.9	0.0	0.1	32	0.56	11.2	21	170	19	0.2	90	0.00	0.00
						6.0			20	0.00				45		74	0.00	0.00
0.02	0.02	0.27	0.10	0.00	30.5	25.8	0.0	0.0	12	0.21	8.0	24	160	16	0.1	92	0.00	0.00
0.00	0.00	0.05	0.00	0.00	6.1	0.5	0.0	0.0	7	0.02	1.9	4	44	14	0.0	95	0.00	0.00
0.02	0.01	0.38	0.10	0.00	9.0	25.6	0.0	0.2	4	0.14	5.3	10	79	4	0.1	92	0.00	0.00
0.00	0.00	0.18	0.05	0.00	3.8	16.6	0.0	0.5	2	0.03	2.1	4	35	0	0.0	92	0.00	0.00
0.10	0.03	1.27	0.07	0.00	30.5	4.9	0.0	0.1	1	0.37	26.8	65	196	11	0.3	76	0.00	0.00
0.00	0.01	0.05	0.01	0.00	3.6	1.5		0.0	8	0.15	6.8	12	76	1	0.1	95	0.00	0.00
0.00	0.00	0.01	0.03	0.00	0.1	0.9	0.0	0.0	5	0.05	0.8	5	12	1	0.0	59	0.00	0.00
0.00	0.00	0.07	0.00	0.00	2.5	0.3	0.0	0.1	11	0.07	2.8	3	8	0	0.0	73	0.00	0.00
0.03	0.05	0.33	0.14	0.00	106.7	33.0	0.0	1.6	104	0.61	17.1	23	163	22	0.1	90	0.00	0.00
0.01	0.01	0.02	0.01	0.00	1.5	7.3	0.0	0.2	20	0.02	3.6	10	56	7	0.0	95	0.00	0.00
0.00	0.01	0.12	0.02	0.00	7.8	13.1	0.0	0.3	8	0.38	7.8	12	98	3	0.1	90	0.00	0.00
0.02	0.01	0.09	0.02	0.00	20.9	2.0	0.0	0.1	13	0.30	5.0	14	102	7	0.1	96	0.00	0.00
0.02	0.02	0.15	0.02	0.00	63.9	1.9	0.0	0.1	16	0.46	6.6	14	116	4	0.1	95	0.00	0.00
0.02	0.14	1.25	0.03	0.00	5.9	0.7	2.5	0.0	1	0.17	3.1	30	111	2	0.2	92	0.00	0.00
0.03	0.18	1.73	0.05	0.01	8.2	1.0	3.4	0.0	1	0.23	4.3	41	153	2	0.2	92	0.00	0.00
0.03	0.01	0.09	0.10	0.00	15.2	5.9	0.0	0.0	18	0.17	8.0	23	117	3	0.1	89	0.00	0.00
0.03	0.01	0.09	0.10	0.00	15.2	5.9	0.0	0.0	18	0.17	8.0	23	117	3	0.1	89	0.00	0.00
0.03	0.01	0.09	0.10	0.00	15.2	5.9	0.0	0.0	18	0.17	8.0	23	117	3	0.1	89	0.00	0.00
0.05	0.02	0.18	0.05	0.00	13.2	18.9	0.0	0.1	14	0.66	7.6	17	63	1	0.1	89	0.00	0.00
0.18	0.10	1.51	0.11	0.00	47.1	29.0	0.0	0.1	18	1.07	23.9	78	177	4	0.9	79	0.00	0.00
0.03	0.01	0.36	0.17	0.00	7.4	59.9	0.0	0.3	7	0.25	7.4	15	130	2	0.1	94	0.00	0.00
0.03	0.05	0.73	0.21	0.00	34.3	95.1	0.0	1.2	5	0.31	8.9	19	157	3	0.2	92	0.00	0.00

Code	Food Name	Unit/ Amt	Wt (g)	Energy (kcal)	Prot (g)	Carb (g)	Fiber (g)	Fat (g)	Sat (g)	Mono (g)	Poly (g)	Chol (mg)	Vit A (RE)
5441	Peppers, bell, yellow, sweet, fresh, lrg, 3 3/4" long	1 ea	186	50	2	12	2	0	0.1			0	37
6851	Potatoes, fresh, w/skin, med, 2 1/4" to 3 1/4"	1 ea	213	164	4	37	5	0	0.1	0.0	0.1	0	0
5143	Radishes, fresh, med, 3/4" to 1"	1 ea	4	1	0	0	0	0	0.0	0.0	0.0	0	0
7214	Rutabaga, fresh, cubes	0.5 cup	70	25	1	6	2	0	0.0	0.0	0.1	0	0
5253	Seaweed, agar, fresh	2 Tbs	10	3	0	1	0	0	0.0	0.0	0.0	0	0
5009	Snap Beans, green, fresh	0.5 cup	50	16	1	3	1	0	0.0	0.0	0.1	0	34
6863	Spinach, fresh, leaf	1 ea	10	2	0	0	0	0	0.0	0.0	0.0	0	94
5010	Sprouts, alfalfa, fresh	1 cup	33	8	1	1	1	0	0.0	0.0	0.1	0	5
6861	Sprouts, soybean, mature, fresh	0.5 cup	35	43	5	3	0	2	0.3	0.5	1.3	0	0
90538	Squash, summer, all types, fresh, sml	0.5 cup	56	9	1	2	1	0	0.0	0.0	0.1	0	11
5833	Squash, winter, all types, fresh, cubes	0.5 cup	58	20	1	5	2	0	0.0	0.0	0.0	0	79
90604	Squash, zucchini, baby, med, fresh	1 ea	11	2	0	0	0	0	0.0	0.00	0.0	0	5
6880	Sweet Potatoes, dark orange, fresh, cubes	0.5 cup	66	57	1	13	2	0	0.0	0.0	0.0	0	943
5445	Tomatillo, fresh, med	1 ea	34	11	0	2	1	0	0.0	0.1	0.1	0	4
5519	Tomatoes, green, fresh, chpd	0.5 cup	90	21	1	5	1	0	0.0	0.0	0.1	0	58
3973	Tomatoes, orange, fresh	1 ea	111	18	1	4	1	0	0.0	0.0	0.1	0	166
90530	Tomatoes, red, cherry, fresh, year round avg	1 ea	17	3	0	1	0	0	0.0	0.0	0.0	0	14
6492	Tomatoes, roma, fresh, year round avg, fresh	1 ea	62	11	1	2	1	0	0.0	0.0	0.1	0	52
9350	Vegetables, stir fry, Oriental, fresh, rtu	3 oz	85	15	1	3	1	0	0.0	0.0	0.0	0	150
5306	Yams, tropical, fresh, cubes	0.5 cup	75	88	1	21	3	0	0.0	0.0	0.1	0	10
Frozen Vegetables and Legumes													
5361	Asparagus, spears, fzn	4 ea	58	14	2	2	1	0	0.0	0.0	0.1	0	55
699	Beans, green, French cut, fzn, FS	1 svg	85	30	1	6	2	0	0.0	0.0	0.0	0	20
6222	Beans, lima, baby, fzn	0.5 cup	83	110	6	20	5	0	0.0	0.0	0.0	0	0
6372	Broccoli, cuts, fzn	0.67 cup	90	25	1	4	2	0	0.0	0.0	0.0	0	10
6551	Broccoli, florets, fzn	1.33 cup	83	20	1	4	2	0	0.0	0.0	0.0	0	10
5740	Carrots, fzn, slices	0.5 cup	64	23	0	5	2	0	0.0	0.0	0.2	0	909
6368	Corn, fzn	0.67 cup	84	80	2	17	2	0	0.0			0	0
1808	Corn, Simply Sweet, cob, fzn, 3", FS	1 ea	141	90	2	19	2	0	0.0			0	0
6018	Corn, white, sweet, kernels, fzn	0.5 cup	82	73	2	17	2	1	0.1	0.2	0.3	0	0
5821	Greens, turnip, fzn, chpd/dices, 10-oz pkg	0.5 cup	82	18	2	3	0	0	0.1	0.0	0.1	0	507
51073	Pea Pods, snow, ckd f/fzn	1 svg	85	35	2	4	2	1	0.0			0	20
6226	Peas, garden, fzn	0.67 cup	89	70	5	12	4	0	0.0	0.0	0.0	0	40
9645	Peas, sweet, fzn	0.67 cup	85	70	4	12	4	0	0.0	0.0	0.0	0	40
6219	Snap Beans, green, cut, fzn	0.67 cup	81	30	1	5	2	0	0.0	0.0	0.0	0	10
6241	Snap Beans, green, whole, fzn	1 cup	85	35	1	5	2	0	0.0	0.0	0.0	0	10
6227	Spinach, chpd, fzn	0.33 cup	83	30	2	3	1	0	0.0	0.0	0.0	0	250
1830	Spinach, leaf, fzn, FS	1 svg	85	25	2	4	2	0	0.0	0.0	0.0	0	250
6644	Vegetables, broccoli & cauliflower, fzn	0.5 cup	43	12	0	2	1	0	0.0	0.0	0.0	0	0
9821	Vegetables, broccoli cauliflower & carrots, fzn	0.75 cup	84	30	1	5	2	0	0.0	0.0	0.0	0	75
9667	Vegetables, Chinese stirfry, fzn	1 cup	85	25	2	6	2	0	0.0	0.0	0.0	0	350
6224	Vegetables, classic, fzn	0.67 cup	86	60	2	12	2	0	0.0	0.0	0.0	0	100
1844	Vegetables, homestyle stew blend, iqf, FS	1 svg	85	45	1	10	1	0	0.0	0.0	0.0	0	50
720	Vegetables, Oriental blend, fzn, FS	1 svg	85	25	1	5	2	0	0.0	0.0	0.0	0	4
9669	Vegetables, mixed, fzn	0.67 cup	85	60	2	12	2	0	0.0	0.0	0.0	0	150
6646	Vegetables, stir fry, pepper, fzn	1 cup	84	25	1	5	1	0	0.0	0.0	0.0	0	20

PAGE KEY: A-70 Prepared Foods   A-78 Restaurants   A-90 Salad Dressings and Dips   A-92 Sauces and Gravies   A-94 Snack Foods   A-94 Spices, Flavors, and Seasonings   A-96 Sports Bars and Drinks   A-96 Supplemental Foods and Formulas   A-96 Sweeteners and Sweet Substitutes   A-98 Vegetables and Legumes   A-108 Miscellaneous

Thia (mg)	Ribo (mg)	Niac (mg NE)	Vit B6 (mg)	Vit B12 (µg)	Fol (µg)	Vit C (mg)	Vit D (IU)	Vit E (mg AT)	Cal (mg)	Iron (mg)	Magn (mg)	Phos (mg)	Pota (mg)	Sodi (mg)	Zinc (mg)	Wat (%)	Alco (g)	Caff (g)
0.05	0.05	1.65	0.31	0.00	48.4	341.3	0.0		20	0.86	22.3	45	394	4	0.3	92	0.00	0.00
0.17	0.07	2.25	0.62	0.00	34.1	42.0	0.0	0.0	26	1.65	49.0	121	897	13	0.6	79	0.00	0.00
0.00	0.00	0.00	0.00	0.00	1.1	0.7	0.0	0.0	1	0.01	0.5	1	10	2	0.0	95	0.00	0.00
0.05	0.02	0.49	0.07	0.00	14.7	17.5	0.0	0.2	33	0.36	16.1	41	236	14	0.2	90	0.00	0.00
0.00	0.00	0.00	0.00	0.00	8.5	0.0	0.0	0.1	5	0.18	6.7	0	23	1	0.1	91	0.00	0.00
0.03	0.05	0.37	0.07	0.00	16.5	6.1	0.0	0.2	18	0.50	12.5	19	106	3	0.1	90	0.00	0.00
0.00	0.01	0.07	0.01	0.00	19.4	2.8	0.0	0.2	10	0.27	7.9	5	56	8	0.1	91	0.00	0.00
0.02	0.03	0.15	0.00	0.00	11.9	2.7	0.0	0.0	11	0.31	8.9	23	26	2	0.3	93	0.00	0.00
0.11	0.03	0.40	0.05	0.00	60.2	5.4	0.0		23	0.73	25.2	57	169	5	0.4	69	0.00	0.00
0.02	0.07	0.28	0.11	0.00	16.4	9.6	0.0	0.1	8	0.20	9.6	21	148	1	0.2	95	0.00	0.00
0.01	0.03	0.28	0.09	0.00	13.9	7.1	0.0	0.1	16	0.34	8.1	13	203	2	0.1	90	0.00	0.00
0.00	0.00	0.07	0.01	0.00	2.2	3.8	0.0		2	0.09	3.6	10	50	0	0.1	93	0.00	0.00
0.05	0.03	0.37	0.14	0.00	7.3	1.6	0.0	0.2	20	0.40	16.6	31	224	37	0.2	77	0.00	0.00
0.00	0.00	0.62	0.01	0.00	2.4	4.0	0.0	0.1	2	0.20	6.8	13	91	0	0.1	92	0.00	0.00
0.05	0.03	0.44	0.07	0.00	8.1	21.1	0.0	0.3	12	0.46	9.0	25	184	12	0.1	93	0.00	0.00
0.05	0.03	0.66	0.07	0.00	32.2	17.8	0.0		6	0.51	8.9	32	235	47	0.2	95	0.00	0.00
0.00	0.00	0.10	0.00	0.00	2.5	2.3	0.0	0.1	2	0.05	1.9	4	40	1	0.0	95	0.00	0.00
0.01	0.00	0.37	0.05	0.00	9.3	8.5	0.0	0.3	6	0.17	6.8	15	147	3	0.1	95	0.00	0.00
						21.0			60	0.00				35				
0.07	0.01	0.40	0.21	0.00	17.2	12.8	0.0	0.3	13	0.40	15.8	41	612	7	0.2	70	0.00	0.00
0.07	0.07	0.69	0.05	0.00	110.8	18.4	0.0		14	0.41	8.1	37	147	5	0.3	92	0.00	0.00
						9.0			40	0.72		1		0				0.00	0.00
0.18	0.07	0.52	0.10	0.00	124.8	9.0		0.2	40	1.44	59.1	115	438	240	0.8	56	0.00	0.00
						30.0			20	0.00				105			84	0.00	0.00
						30.0			20	0.36				20			77	0.00	0.00
0.02	0.01	0.30	0.05	0.00	6.4	1.6	0.0	0.4	23	0.28	7.7	21	150	44	0.2	90	0.00	0.00
						2.4			0	0.00				5			64	0.00	0.00
						4.8			0	0.36		0		0				0.00	0.00
0.07	0.05	1.41	0.15	0.00	29.7	5.3	0.0		3	0.34	14.8	57	173	2	0.3	75	0.00	0.00
0.03	0.07	0.31	0.07	0.00	60.7	22.0	0.0		97	1.24	22.1	22	151	10	0.1	93	0.00	0.00
						2.4			20	1.08				0			77	0.00	0.00
						6.0			0	1.08				0			71	0.00	0.00
						6.0			0	1.08			125	95			68	0.00	0.00
						3.6			40	0.36				0			75	0.00	0.00
						3.6			40	0.36				0			79	0.00	0.00
						1.2			80	0.72				125			77	0.00	0.00
						18.0			100	0.72		1		15				0.00	0.00
						13.5			10	0.18				12				0.00	0.00
						18.0			20	0.36				30				0.00	0.00
						18.0			20	0.36			160	15				0.00	0.00
						3.6			20	0.36				20			71	0.00	0.00
						6.0			20	0.36		0		20				0.00	0.00
						24.0			20	0.36		0		5				0.00	0.00
						4.8			20	0.36			150	20			70	0.00	0.00
						12.0			0	0.00				10				0.00	0.00

PAGE KEY: A-42 Beverages and Beverage Mixes   A-44 Candies   A-46 Cereals   A-48 Cheeses and Substitutes   A-50 Dairy Products and Substitutes   A-52 Desserts   A-56 Eggs and Egg Substitutes   A-56 Fats, Oils, Margarines, and Shortenings   A-58 Fruits   A-60 Grain Products and Baked Goods   A-62 Grains and Flours   A-64 Meats and Meat Substitutes   A-68 Nuts, Seeds, and Products

Code	Food Name	Unit/ Amt	Wt (g)	Energy (kcal)	Prot (g)	Carb (g)	Fiber (g)	Fat (g)	Sat (g)	Mono (g)	Poly (g)	Chol (mg)	Vit A (RE)
MISCELLANEOUS													
Baking Chips and Chocolates													
23519	Baking Chips, chocolate, Crystal Dark	31 pce	15	72	1	9	1	4	3.0			O	1
23012	Baking Chips, chocolate, semi sweet	1 Tbs	10	50	O	7	1	3	1.9	1.0	0.1	O	O
23200	Baking Chips, chocolate, semi sweet, w/butter	1 Tbs	11	51	O	7	1	3	1.9	1.1	0.1	2	1
23017	Baking Chips, milk chocolate	1 Tbs	10	56	1	6	O	3	1.9	0.8	0.1	2	6
23423	Baking Chips, milk chocolate, M&M, mini bits	1 Tbs	14	70	1	10	O	3	2.0			2	6
23444	Baking Chips, milk chocolate, mini Kisses	11 ea	15	80	1	9	O	4	3.0			5	O
23446	Baking Chips, peanut butter, Reese's	1 Tbs	15	80	3	7		4	4.0			O	O
28299	Baking Chips, white chocolate, chunks	0.5 oz	14	76	1	9	O	5	2.8			5	O
23401	Baking Chocolate, bar, semi sweet	1 svg	14	70	1	8	1	4	2.5			O	O
28063	Baking Chocolate, bar, unswtnd	1 svg	14	70	2	4	2	7	4.5			O	O
4355	Baking Chocolate, bar, white, premium	0.5 pce	14	80	1	8	O	4	3.0			5	O
28208	Baking Chocolate, unswntd, liquid	1 oz	28	134	3	10	5	14	7.2	2.6	3.0	O	O
28200	Cocoa Powder, unswntd	0.25 cup	22	49	4	12	7	3	1.7	1.0	0.1	O	O
Baking Ingredients													
28006	Baking Powder, low sod	0.25 tsp	1	1	O	1	O	O	0.0	0.0	0.0	O	O
28003	Baking Soda	0.25 tsp	1	O	O	O	O	O	0.0	0.0	0.0	O	O
26017	Cream of Tartar	1 tsp	3	8	O	2	O	O	0.0	0.0	0.0	O	O
28000	Yeast, baker's, dry active	1 tsp	4	13	2	2	1	O	0.0	0.2	0.0	O	O
Condiments													
9149	Catsup	1 Tbs	15	15	O	4	O	O	0.0	0.0	0.0	O	14
27032	Catsup, low sod	1 Tbs	15	15	O	4	O	O	0.0	0.0	0.0	O	14
8069	Dressing, mayonnaise, fat free	1 Tbs	16	11	O	2	O	O	0.1			2	3
93294	Dressing, mayonnaise, light, omega plus	1 Tbs	14	47	O	1	O	5	0.5	2.3	1.6	5	O
44719	Dressing, mayonnaise, rducd cal, cholest free	1 Tbs	15	49	O	1	O	5	0.7	1.1	2.8	O	O
8503	Dressing, mayonnaise, real	1 Tbs	14	100	O	O	O	11	1.5			5	O
8479	Dressing, Miracle Whip	1 Tbs	15	45	O	2	O	4	0.5			5	O
27004	Horseradish, prep	1 tsp	5	2	O	1	O	O	0.0	0.0	0.0	O	O
27000	Ketchup	1 Tbs	15	15	O	4	O	O	0.0	0.0	0.0	O	14
53591	Marinade, cooking sauce, mesquite	1 Tbs	17	10	O	3	O	O	0.0	0.0	0.0	O	O
53587	Marinade, cooking sauce, teriyaki	1 Tbs	18	25	1	5	O	O	0.0	0.0	0.0	O	O
27058	Mustard, dijon	1 tsp	5	5	O	1	O	O	0.0	0.0	0.0	O	O
435	Mustard, yellow, prep	1 tsp	5	3	O	O	O	O	0.0	0.1	0.0	O	O
27052	Relish, pickle, sweet	1 Tbs	15	20	O	5	O	O	0.0	0.0	0.0	O	18
53002	Sauce, soy, f/soy & wheat	1 Tbs	16	8	1	1	O	O	0.0	0.0	0.0	O	O
53614	Sauce, soy, less sodium	1 Tbs	16	10	1	1	O	O	0.0	0.0	0.0	O	O
53099	Sauce, worcestershire	1 Tbs	17	13	O	3	O	O	0.0	0.0	0.0	O	2
53457	Vinegar, balsamic	1 Tbs	15	10	O	2	O	O	0.0	0.0	0.0	O	
92153	Vinegar, distilled	1 Tbs	15	3	O	O	O	O	0.0	0.0	0.0	O	O

PAGE KEY: A-70 Prepared Foods   A-78 Restaurants   A-90 Salad Dressings and Dips   A-92 Sauces and Gravies   A-94 Snack Foods   A-94 Spices, Flavors, and Seasonings   A-96 Sports Bars and Drinks   A-96 Supplemental Foods and Formulas   A-96 Sweeteners and Sweet Substitutes   A-98 Vegetables and Legumes   A-108 Miscellaneous

Thia (mg)	Ribo (mg)	Niac (mg NE)	Vit B6 (mg)	Vit B12 (µg)	Fol (µg)	Vit C (mg)	Vit D (IU)	Vit E (mg AT)	Cal (mg)	Iron (mg)	Magn (mg)	Phos (mg)	Pota (mg)	Sodi (mg)	Zinc (mg)	Wat (%)	Alco (g)	Caff (g)
						0.0			5	2.00				31		1	0.00	
0.00	0.00	0.03	0.00	0.00	1.4	0.0	0.0	0.0	3	0.33	12.1	14	38	1	0.2	1	0.00	6.51
0.00	0.00	0.05	0.00	0.00	0.3	0.0			3	0.33	12.2	14	39	1	0.2	1	0.00	6.57
0.00	0.02	0.03	0.00	0.07	1.3	0.0	0.0	0.1	20	0.25	6.6	22	39	8	0.2	2	0.00	2.09
						0.1			16	0.17				10		2	0.00	2.48
						0.0			20	0.00				15		0	0.00	
						0.0			0	0.00				35			0.00	0.00
						0.0			19	0.00				14		0	0.00	
						0.0			0	0.72				0		0	0.00	
						0.0			0	1.44				0		0	0.00	
						0.0			20	0.00				15			0.00	
0.00	0.07	0.60	0.01	0.00	5.4	0.0			15	1.17	75.1	96	331	3	1.0	1	0.00	13.31
0.01	0.05	0.46	0.02	0.00	6.9	0.0	0.0	0.0	28	2.98	107.3	158	328	5	1.5	3	0.00	49.45
0.00	0.00	0.00	0.00	0.00	0.0	0.0	0.0	0.0	54	0.10	0.4	86	126	1	0.0	6	0.00	0.00
0.00	0.00	0.00	0.00	0.00	0.0	0.0	0.0	0.0	0	0.00	0.0	0	0	315	0.0	0	0.00	0.00
0.00	0.00	0.00	0.00	0.00	0.0	0.0	0.0	0.0	0	0.10	0.1	0	495	2	0.0	2	0.00	0.00
0.43	0.15	1.61	0.05	0.00	93.6	0.0	0.0	0.0	1	0.09	2.2	25	38	2	0.3	5	0.00	0.00
0.00	0.01	0.20	0.01	0.00	1.5	2.3	0.0	0.2	3	0.07	2.9	5	57	167	0.0	69	0.00	0.00
0.00	0.01	0.20	0.01	0.00	1.5	2.3	0.0	0.2	3	0.07	2.9	5	57	3	0.0	69	0.00	0.00
						0.0			1	0.01		4	8	120		82	0.00	0.00
0.00	0.00	0.00	0.00	0.01		0.0		1.5	2	0.03	0.3	4	9	119	0.0	52	0.00	0.00
0.00	0.00	0.00	0.00	0.00	0.0	0.0	0.0	0.9	0	0.00	0.0	0	10	107	0.0	56	0.00	0.00
						0.0			0	0.00				75		3	0.00	0.00
						0.0			0	0.00				125			0.00	0.00
0.00	0.00	0.01	0.00	0.00	2.9	1.2	0.0	0.0	3	0.01	1.4	2	12	16	0.0	85	0.00	0.00
0.00	0.01	0.20	0.01	0.00	1.5	2.3	0.0	0.2	3	0.07	2.9	5	57	167	0.0	69	0.00	0.00
						1.8			0	0.00			25	400			0.00	0.00
						3.0			0	0.00			40	480			0.00	0.00
						0.0			0	0.00				120			0.00	0.00
0.01	0.00	0.02	0.00	0.00	0.3	0.1	0.0	0.0	3	0.07	2.5	5	7	57	0.0	83	0.00	0.00
0.00	0.00	0.02	0.00	0.00	0.2	0.2	0.0	0.1	0	0.12	0.8	2	4	122	0.0	62	0.00	0.00
0.00	0.02	0.34	0.01	0.00	2.2	0.0	0.0	0.0	3	0.31	6.9	20	35	902	0.1	71	0.00	0.00
						0.0			0	0.00				575			0.00	0.00
0.00	0.01	0.11	0.00	0.00	1.4	2.2	0.0	0.0	18	0.89	2.2	10	136	167	0.0	79	0.00	0.00
														5				0.00
0.00	0.00	0.00	0.00	0.00	0.0	0.0	0.0	0.0	1	0.00	0.1	1	0	0	0.0	95	0.00	0.00

Glossary

absorption process of removing nutrients from the intestinal tract and enabling them to enter the circulatory or lymphatic systems

accelerometry method of measuring calorie expenditure during physical activity based on changes in speed and direction

Acceptable Macronutrient Distribution Ranges (AMDRs) ranges of carbohydrate, fat, and protein intakes that provide adequate amounts of vitamins and minerals, and may reduce the risk of diet–related chronic diseases

acetaldehyde highly toxic substance formed during the first step of the alcohol dehydrogenase pathway

acetylcholine neurotransmitter associated with attention, learning and memory, muscle control, and other nervous system functions

acetyl coenzyme A two–carbon molecule formed from pyruvate

acid–base balance maintaining the proper pH of body fluids

acidic solutions with pH values lower than 7

added sugars sugars added to foods during processing or preparation

adenosine diphosphate (ADP) molecule that forms when ATP loses its terminal phosphate group

adenosine triphosphate (ATP) high–energy phosphate compound

Adequate Intakes (AIs) dietary recommendations that assume a population's average daily nutrient intakes are adequate because no deficiency diseases are present

adiponectin hormone produced by adipose tissue that increases muscle cells' uptake of fatty acids from the bloodstream and metabolism of the fatty acids for energy

adipose (fat) cells cells that store triglycerides

adipose tissue fat cells

adjustable gastric banding surgical approach to treating obesity, also called "lap band"

adolescence period of life that begins at puberty and ends at adulthood

adulterated food food that has been intentionally or unintentionally altered and made impure

advanced glycation end products (AGEs) substances formed by glycation that cause inflammation and organ damage

aerobic capacity (VO$_2$ max) maximal oxygen uptake; a measure of the amount of the maximal amount of oxygen consumed during physical activity

aerobic exercise physical activities that involve sustained, rhythmic contractions of large muscle groups

aerobic metabolism ATP production that occurs in the presence of oxygen

aflatoxins substances produced from molds that can have toxic effects when consumed

age–related macular degeneration (AMD) eye disease resulting in changes in the macula of the eye, causing distorted vision

age–related maximum heart rate normal maximum heart rate of an individual of a given age during exercise

ageusia total loss of the ability to taste substances

air displacement method of estimating body composition by determining body volume

alcohol dehydrogenase pathway catabolic pathway that metabolizes alcohol in the liver

aldehyde dehydrogenase enzyme that helps convert acetaldehyde to acetate, a less toxic substance

aldosterone hormone secreted from adrenal glands in response to dehydration; stimulates kidneys to conserve sodium and water

alkaline solutions with pH values higher than 7

alpha–linolenic acid 18–carbon polyunsaturated fatty acid with three double bonds; an essential fatty acid

alpha–tocopherol form of vitamin E used by the body; found in most foods and vitamin E supplements

alternative sweeteners substances that sweeten foods while providing few or no kilocalories

Alzheimer's disease most common form of irreversible dementia that affects older adults

amenorrhea cessation of menstruation for 3 months or longer

amines compounds that include amino groups in their chemical structure

amino acid derivatives nitrogen–containing compounds that are not proteins but have important physiological roles

amino acids nitrogen–containing chemical units that comprise proteins

amino or **nitrogen–containing group** portion of an amino acid that contains nitrogen

amylin hormone secreted by the pancreas that slows gastric emptying and reduces hunger.

anabolic steroid drug that mimics the action of the male sex hormone testosterone

anabolism refers to metabolic pathways that build larger molecules from smaller ones

anaerobic metabolism metabolic pathways that do not require oxygen

anaphylaxis serious drop in blood pressure that occurs when sensitive people are exposed to food allergens; can be fatal

android obesity storage of excess body fat in the upper body or abdominal region, leading to an "apple shape"

anecdotes personal reports concerning a treatment's effectiveness

anencephaly type of neural tube defect in which the brain does not form properly or is missing

angiotensin II protein secreted in response to low blood volume and falling blood pressure

anorexia nervosa (AN) severe psychological disturbance characterized by self–imposed starvation

anosmia   complete inability to detect odors

antidiuretic hormone (ADH)   hormone secreted from pituitary glands in response to dehydration; stimulates kidneys to conserve water

antioxidant   substance that gives up electrons to free radicals to protect cells

apoptosis   cellular death

appetite   desire to eat appealing food

arachidonic acid (AA)   essential fatty acid; precursor to some eicosanoids

ariboflavinosis   riboflavin deficiency disease characterized by fatigue, inflammation of the mucous membranes that line the mouth and throat, and glossitis

arterial plaque   fatty buildup in the artery

arteriosclerosis   condition that results from atherosclerosis and is characterized by loss of arterial flexibility

arthritis   inflammation of a joint

atherosclerosis   long-term disease process in which plaque builds up inside arterial walls

autism spectrum disorders (ASDs, autism)   neurodevelopmental disorders characterized by deficits in social interaction, verbal and nonverbal communication, and by repetitive behaviors or interests

autonomy   independence and the ability to make decisions

avidin   protein found in raw egg whites that binds biotin, thus preventing absorption of the vitamin

B

bacteria   single-cell microorganisms

balance   refers to a level of caloric intake that enables a person to maintain a healthy weight

bariatric medicine   medical specialty that focuses on the treatment of obesity

basal metabolic rate (BMR)   measurement of basal metabolism

basal metabolism   minimum number of calories the body uses for vital physiological activities after fasting and resting for 12 hours

benign masses (tumors)   noncancerous tumors that are usually harmless

beriberi   thiamin deficiency disease characterized by weakness, poor muscular coordination, and abnormal functioning of the cardiovascular, digestive, and nervous systems

beta-carotene   carotenoid that the body can convert to vitamin A

beta-oxidation   chemical pathway that is involved in the catabolism of an activated fatty acid

bile   fluid that is produced in the liver and stored in the gallbladder until it is needed for fat digestion and absorption

bile salts   component of bile; aid in lipid digestion

binge eating   eating an amount of food that is much larger than what a normal person would eat in a brief period of time

binge-eating disorder (BED)   eating disorder featuring recurrent episodes of binge eating that are not followed by purging behaviors

bioavailability   refers to the extent to which the digestive tract absorbs a nutrient and how well the body uses it

bioelectrical impedance analysis (BIA)   technique of estimating body composition in which a device measures the conduction of a weak electrical current through body water

biological activity   describes vitamin's degree of potency or effects in the body

biological value (BV)   measure of protein quality based on how well and quickly the body converts food protein into body tissue protein

biotechnology   use of living things to produce new products

biotin   vitamin component of a coenzyme that participates in chemical reactions that add carbon dioxide to other compounds

blastocyst   mass of cells that develops after fertilization and implants in the uterine lining

blood urea nitrogen (BUN)   measure of the concentration of urea in blood

body composition   measurement of body tissues, usually expressed as percent body fat

body mass index (BMI)   numerical value of relationship between body weight and risk of chronic health problems associated with excess body fat calculated by dividing weight in kg by height in meters, squared

bolus   mass of food that has been chewed, moistened, mixed with saliva, and swallowed

bomb calorimeter   device used to measure the calories in a sample of food

bone mineralization   process by which bone tissue gains strength and rigidity

bovine spongiform encephalopathy (BSE)   neurodegenerative disease in cattle that is caused by prions; also referred to as "mad cow disease"

branched-chain amino acids (BCAAs)   amino acids with a unique branched side chain; preferentially utilized by muscle cells for energy

buffer   substance that can protect the pH of a solution

built environment   human-made resources, including buildings, roads, parks, supermarkets, and restaurants, within a community

bulimia nervosa (BN)   severe psychological condition characterized by repeated episodes of binge eating followed by unhealthy behaviors to prevent weight gain

C

cachexia   severe weight loss ("wasting")

caesarian section   surgical removal of the fetus from its mother's uterus

caffeine   drug found in many beverages and food products, including coffee, tea, and cola drinks, that stimulates the central nervous system and may enhance physical activity

calciferol   form of vitamin D found in both plant and animal foods

calcitonin   hormone secreted by the thyroid gland when blood calcium levels are too high

calcitriol (1,25-dihydroxyvitamin D)   most biologically active form of vitamin D

calcium-binding protein   protein necessary for absorption of calcium in the small intestine

calorie   amount of heat necessary to raise the temperature of 1 g (1 mL) of water 1° Celsius (C)

calorimetry   measurement of heat energy

carbohydrate counting   diabetes management tool in which an individual tracks his or her daily carbohydrate intake

carbohydrate loading   practice of manipulating physical activity and dietary intake of carbohydrates to increase muscle glycogen stores

carbohydrates   class of nutrients that is a major source of energy for the body

carbon skeleton   remains of an amino acid following deamination and removal of the nitrogen-containing component of the amino acid

carboxylic acid   organic molecule with a carboxyl (—COOH) group

carboxylic acid group carboxylic acid portion of a compound

carcinogen environmental factor, such as radiation, tobacco smoke, or a virus, that triggers cancer

cardiovascular disease (CVD) group of diseases that affect the heart and blood vessels; includes coronary artery disease, stroke, and disease of the blood vessels

carnitine molecule that helps fatty acids pass through the outer and inner mitochondrial membranes

carotenemia yellowing of the skin that results from excess beta−carotene in the body

carotenoids yellow−orange pigments in fruits and vegetables

case−control study study in which individuals with a health condition (cases) are matched to persons with similar characteristics who do not have the condition

casein high−quality protein found in milk

catabolism refers to metabolic pathways that break down larger molecules into smaller ones

cataracts condition characterized by abnormal changes in the lens of the eye that can cause blindness

causation specific practice that is responsible for an effect

cecum first segment of the large intestine

celiac disease inherited condition in which the protein gluten cannot be absorbed; results in damage to the small intestine and poor absorption of nutrients

centenarian individual who has lived for 100 years or more

cheilosis scaling and cracking of the skin around the corners of the mouth

chemical digestion refers to the breakdown of large nutrient molecules in food into smaller components, primarily by the action of enzymes

chemical pathways specific chemical reactions that occur in sequences

chief cells stomach cells that secrete some chemically inactive digestive enzymes

cholecalciferol (vitamin D₃) form of vitamin D found in animal food sources

cholecystectomy surgery to remove a diseased gallbladder

cholecystokinin (CCK) hormone secreted by the mucosa of the small intestine that stimulates the gallbladder to contract and the pancreas to release pancreatic juice into the small intestine

cholesterol lipid found in animal foods; precursor for steroid hormones, bile, and vitamin D

choline water−soluble, vitamin−like compound; component of lecithin

chronic long−term

chronic renal failure (CRF) long−term kidney failure

chronic undernutrition state of undernutrition occurring when energy and nutrient intakes are insufficient to meet an individual's needs over an extended period of time

chylomicron type of lipoprotein formed in enterocytes to transport lipids away from the GI tract

chyme semiliquid mass that forms when food mixes with gastric juice

chymotrypsin protein−splitting enzyme secreted from the pancreas

cirrhosis of the liver condition characterized by the accumulation of scar tissue in the liver, which permanently damages the organ

citric acid cycle complex series of chemical reactions that that are involved in energy metabolism

coenzyme A pantothenic acid−containing coenzyme that helps release energy from carbohydrates, fat, and protein, and is necessary for fatty acid synthesis

coenzymes group of organic cofactors that often have B vitamins in their chemical structures

cofactor ion or small molecule that an enzyme needs to function

cognitive behavioral therapy (CBT) psychological treatment approaches that address unhealthy behavior by challenging current beliefs and replacing them with more realistic thoughts

cohort study epidemiological study in which researchers collect and analyze various kinds of information about a large group of people over time

colic condition in which a young infant cries excessively for no apparent reason

collagen fibrous protein that gives strength to connective tissue such as bone, cartilage, and tendons

color additives dyes, pigments, or other substances that provide color to food

colostrum form of milk that is secreted from a woman's breast during the first few days after birth

complementary combinations mixing certain plant foods to provide all essential amino acids without adding animal protein

complex carbohydrates carbohydrates comprised of three or more monosaccharides bonded together

conception point at which a woman's egg is fertilized by a sperm; fertilization

conditionally essential amino acid amino acids that are normally nonessential but become essential under certain conditions

conditionally essential nutrients nutrients that are normally not essential but become essential under certain conditions, such as during a serious illness

congregate meals meals served in a community location so people can socialize while they eat

constipation infrequent bowel movements and feces that are difficult to eliminate

contaminated food item that is impure or unsafe for human consumption

control group in a controlled study, group that does not receive a treatment

correlation relationship between variables

cortisol catabolic hormone made in the adrenal cortex of the adrenal glands

creatine nitrogen−containing substance found in muscles; can form complex with phosphate to form phosphocreatine

creatinine nitrogen−containing waste produced by muscles

cretinism condition in infants who are born to iodine−deficient women; the infants have permanent brain damage and growth retardation

Crohn's disease type of IBD; the body's immune system cells attack normal intestinal cells, damaging parts of the intestines

cross−contamination transferring of pathogens from a contaminated food or surface to an uncontaminated food or surface.

cuproenzymes group of enzymes that require copper to function

cystic fibrosis inherited respiratory disease caused by a defective gene that leads to overproduction of thick and sticky mucus

cytochrome c component of the electron transport chain

cytochromes group of proteins necessary for certain chemical reactions involved in the release of energy from macronutrients

D

Daily Values (DVs) set of nutrient intake standards developed for labeling purposes

deamination removal of the nitrogen–containing group from an amino acid

deficiency disease state of health characterized by certain abnormal physiological changes that occur when the body lacks a nutrient

dehydration body water depletion

Delaney Clause component of the 1958 Food Additives Amendment that prevents manufacturers from adding carcinogenic compounds to foods

delayed onset of muscle soreness (DOMS) muscle soreness occurring in the 1 to 2 days following intense exercise

dementia decline in mental functioning that affects daily living

denaturation altering a protein's natural shape and function by exposing it to conditions such as heat, acids, and physical agitation

dental fluorosis abnormal change in the appearance of tooth enamel due to chronically high fluoride exposure while the teeth are developing

detraining declining physical fitness

diabetes mellitus (diabetes) group of serious chronic conditions characterized by abnormal glucose, fat, and protein metabolism

diabetic retinopathy damage to the retina caused by glycation

diabulimia term used to describe people with type I diabetes who manipulate their body weight by skipping insulin injections or using less insulin than prescribed

dialectical behavioral therapy (DBT) form of psychotherapy that strives to improve skills used to manage stress, anxiety, or feelings of inadequacy

diastolic pressure pressure in an artery that occurs when the ventricles relax between contractions

diet a person's usual pattern of food choices

dietary fiber ("fiber") nondigestible plant material; most types are polysaccharides

dietary guidance system food guide that translates the DRIs and evidence–based information concerning the effects of certain foods and food components on health into dietary recommendations

Dietary Reference Intakes (DRIs) set of energy and nutrient intake standards that can be used as references when making dietary recommendations

Dietary Supplement and Health Education Act of 1994 (DSHEA) federal legislation that allows manufacturers to classify nutrient supplements and herbal products as foods

dietary supplement product (excluding tobacco) that contains a vitamin, a mineral, an herb or other plant product, an amino acid, or a dietary substance that supplements the diet by increasing total intake

dietetics application of nutrition and food information to achieve and maintain optimal health and to treat many health–related conditions

digestion process of breaking down large food molecules into nutrients that the body can use

digestive system body system that breaks down food into its components, absorbs nutrients, and eliminates the waste

digestive tract or **gastrointestinal tract (GI tract)** alimentary canal or gut

diglyceride lipid that has two fatty acids attached to a three–carbon compound called glycerol

dipeptides compounds that consist of two amino acids

direct calorimetry measure of the amount of heat produced by someone inside a specialized chamber

direct or **positive correlation** describes the relationship that occurs when two variables increase or decrease in the same direction

disaccharide simple sugar comprised of two monosaccharides

disordered eating chaotic and abnormal food–related practices such as skipping meals, limiting food choices, following fad diets, and bingeing

diuretic substance that increases urine production

diverticula tiny pouches that form in the wall of the colon

diverticulitis condition characterized by inflamed diverticula

diverticulosis condition characterized by the presence of diverticula

DNA (deoxyribonucleic acid) hereditary material that provides instructions for making proteins

docosahexaenoic acid essential fatty acid; precursor to some eicosanoids

double–blind describes human studies in which neither the investigators nor the subjects are aware of the subjects' group assignments

dual–energy x–ray absorptiometry (DXA) technique of estimating body composition that involves scanning the body with two low–energy x–rays

dumping syndrome disorder that occurs when chyme flows too rapidly into the small intestine

duodenum first segment of the small intestine

E

eating disorders psychological disturbances that lead to certain physiological changes and serious health complications

eclampsia severe stage of preeclampsia that results in seizures

eczema skin condition characterized by tiny red blisters and itching

edema accumulation of fluid in tissues; "swelling"

edentulism condition characterized by the loss of all teeth

eicosanoids group of long–chain fatty acids with hormonelike functions

eicosapentaenoic acid essential fatty acid; precursor to some eicosanoids

Elderly Nutrition Program program that provides financial assistance for nonprofit programs that provide free meals to adults 60 years of age and older, regardless of their income

electron transport chain linked series of enzymes that synthesize water and ATP during aerobic energy metabolism

element substance that cannot be separated into simpler substances by ordinary chemical or physical means

emaciation very low body weight

embolus thrombus or part of a plaque that breaks free and travels through the bloodstream

embryo refers to the offspring from 2 to 8 weeks after conception

empty–calorie describes a food that supplies excessive calories from unhealthy types of fat, added sugar, and/or alcohol

emulsifier substance that helps water–soluble and water–insoluble compounds mix with each other

endogenous source of nitrogen from within the body

energy balance matching calorie intake to calorie output over the long term

energy density refers to the amount of energy a food provides per given weight of the food

energy drinks highly caffeinated beverages containing a variety of product–specific "energy blends"

energy intake calories from foods and beverages that contain macronutrients and alcohol

energy metabolism involves the chemical pathways that enable the human body to obtain and use energy from macronutrients and alcohol

energy output calories cells use to carry out their activities

energy the capacity to perform work.

enrichment addition of specific amounts of iron and the B vitamins thiamin, riboflavin, niacin, and folic acid to specific refined grain products

enterocytes absorptive cells that form the outer layer of a villus

enterohepatic circulation process that recycles bile salts in the body

enzyme protein that speeds up the rate of a chemical reaction without being altered in the process

epidemiology study of the occurrence, distribution, and causes of health problems in populations

epiglottis flap of tough tissue that prevents the food from entering the larynx and trachea

epinephrine (adrenaline) hormone produced by the adrenal glands; secreted in response to declining blood glucose levels

epithelial cells cells that form protective tissues that line the body

ergocalciferol (vitamin D$_2$) form of vitamin D found in plant food sources

erogenic aids foods, devices, dietary supplements, or drugs used to try to improve physical performance

esophagus muscular tube that extends about 10 inches from the pharynx to the upper portion of the stomach

essential amino acids amino acids the body cannot make or cannot make enough of to meet its needs

essential fat fat that is vital for survival; found in cell membranes, certain bones, and nervous tissue

essential fatty acids fatty acids that must be supplied by the diet; linoleic and alpha–linolenic acid are essential fatty acids

essential nutrient nutrient that must be supplied by food

Estimated Average Requirement (EAR) amount of a nutrient that should meet the needs of 50% of healthy people who are in a particular life–stage/sex group

Estimated Energy Requirement (EER) average daily energy intake that meets the needs of a healthy person who is maintaining his or her weight

ethanol simple two–carbon molecule that is more commonly called "alcohol"

Exchange System tool for estimating the energy, protein, carbohydrate, and fat contents of foods

exercise physical activities that are usually planned and structured for a purpose

exogenous source of nitrogen from outside of the body (dietary protein)

experiment systematic way of testing a hypothesis

external anal sphincter sphincter that allows feces to be expelled from the anus and is under voluntary control

extracellular water water that surrounds cells or is in blood

extrusion reflex involuntary response in which the young infant's tongue thrusts forward to remove solid or semisolid objects placed in the mouth

F

fad diet trendy practice that has widespread appeal for a period, then becomes no longer fashionable

fat–free mass weight of the body that includes body water, bones, teeth, muscles, and organs

fat malabsorption impaired fat absorption; symptoms include diarrhea, steatorrhea, and rapid weight loss

fat–soluble vitamins vitamins A, D, E, and K

fatty acid hydrocarbon chain found in lipids; one end of the chain forms a

carboxylic acid, and one end forms a methyl group

Federal Trade Commission (FTC) federal government agency that protects consumers against "unfair and deceptive acts or practices" by businesses in the United States

female athlete triad condition that occurs as a result of the interrelationships among energy availability, menstrual function, and bone mineral density in female athletes

fermentation process used to preserve or produce a variety of foods

ferritin major storage form of iron; serum concentrations are used to assess iron status

fertility ability to conceive

fetal alcohol spectrum disorders (FASDs) group of conditions that result in a child due to alcohol consumption by the mother during pregnancy

fetal alcohol syndrome (FAS) severe physical and intellectual deficits that develop in a fetus whose mother drank excessively during pregnancy

fetus refers to the offspring from 8 weeks until birth

fine motor skills control of the small muscles, particularly thumb and fingers

flavin adenine dinucleotide (FAD) riboflavin–containing coenzyme

folate B vitamin that is a component of the coenzyme tetrahydrofolic acid (THFA), includes folic acid, and is important for energy metabolism, DNA synthesis, and homocysteine metabolism

food additive any substance that becomes incorporated into food during production, packaging, transport, or storage

Food Additives Amendment U.S. legislation that requires evidence that a new food additive is safe before it can be marketed for use

Food and Nutrition Board (FNB) group of scientists who develop DRIs

food aversion intense dislike of a food that was previously enjoyed

food banks nonprofit organizations that act as distribution centers for surplus food

food–borne illness infection caused by microscopic disease–causing agents in food

food–cobalamin malabsorption malabsorption of vitamin B–12 due to the inability to release vitamin B–12 from animal protein during the digestive process; most common in those ages 50 years and older

food concocting making and eating strange food combinations

food craving sudden urge for a particular food or an unusual combination of foods

food deserts regions or areas in which a large proportion of those living there experience difficulty in obtaining nutritious food

food insecurity state in which individuals are concerned about running out of food or not having enough money to buy more food

food intolerances conditions characterized by unpleasant physical reactions following consumption of certain foods

food intoxication type of food–borne illness caused by toxins in the food or beverage

food jags periods in which a young child refuses to eat a food that he or she liked in the past or wants to eat only a particular food

food pantry nonprofit service that provides food to people in need

food rating systems variety of methods that evaluate the nutritional value of foods and display this information to consumers

food security state in which individuals have access to enough food at all times to lead healthy, active lives

fortification addition of nutrients to any food

free radical substance with an unpaired electron

fructose monosaccharide in fruits, honey, and certain vegetables; "levulose" or "fruit sugar"

full term describes an infant born between 38 and 40 weeks of gestation

fungi simple organisms that live on dead or decaying organic matter

fungicides substances used to limit the spread of fungi

G

galactose monosaccharide that is a component of lactose

gallstones hard particles that can accumulate in the gallbladder or become lodged in one of the ducts carrying bile from the gallbladder to the small intestine

gamma–tocopherol form of vitamin E that has a significantly lower biological activity than alpha–tocopherol

gastric alcohol dehydrogenase enzyme that detoxifies some alcohol while it is in the stomach

gastric banding surgical approach to treating obesity

gastric juice collection of stomach secretions that includes mucus, hydrochloric acid, intrinsic factor, and digestive enzymes

gastrin hormone that stimulates stomach motility and gastric gland secretions

gastritis inflammation of the lining of the stomach

gastroesophageal reflux disease (GERD) chronic condition characterized by frequent heartburn that can damage the esophagus

Gaucher disease most common lipid storage disease; caused by a deficiency of the enzyme glucocerebrosidase

G cells stomach cells that secrete gastrin

gene portion of DNA

Generally Recognized as Safe (GRAS) ingredients thought to be safe

genetically modified organisms (GMOs) organisms that have been genetically modified

genetic endowment inherited physical characteristics that can affect athletic performance

genetic modification (GM) altering an organism's genetic material in effort to create a new organism with different traits; also called genetic engineering

geriatrics specialty of health care that focuses on older adults

gestation pregnancy

gestational diabetes type of diabetes that develops in some pregnant women

gestational hypertension form of hypertension that occurs after 20 weeks of gestation and returns to normal by 12 weeks after the baby is delivered

ghrelin hormone secreted by the stomach and other tissues that stimulates eating

glaucoma condition characterized by increased pressure within the anterior chamber that damages the optic disk

glossitis swollen and sore tongue

glucagon hormone secreted from the alpha cells of the pancreas that helps regulate blood glucose levels

gluconeogenesis synthesis of glucose from noncarbohydrate precursors

glucose monosaccharide that is a primary fuel for muscles and other cells; "dextrose" or "blood sugar"

glutathione sulfur–containing antioxidant molecule

glutathione peroxidase family of selenoproteins that have antioxidant function

gluten type of protein found in many grains; provides texture and shape to baked products

gluten sensitivity uncomfortable symptoms develop following consumption of gluten, but the individual does not have damage to the small intestine

glycation condition that occurs when sugars bind to proteins, lipids, and nucleic acids in the body

glycemic index (GI) tool to measure the body's insulin response to a carbohydrate–containing food

glycemic load (GL) tool to measure the body's insulin response to a carbohydrate–containing food; similar to the glycemic index, but also factors in a typical serving size of the food

glycerol three–carbon alcohol that forms the "backbone" of fatty acids

glycogen highly branched storage polysaccharide in animals

glycogenesis pathway that enables certain cells to store glucose as glycogen

glycogenolysis pathway that breaks down glycogen into glucose molecules

glycolysis first phase of glucose catabolism

goblet cells intestinal cells that secrete mucus

goiter enlargement of the thyroid gland that is not the result of cancer

goitrogens compounds in food that inhibit iodide metabolism by the thyroid gland

gout form of arthritis caused by the buildup of uric acid crystals in joints

gross motors skills control of the large muscles

growth spurt period characterized by a rapid increase in growth

gynoid obesity storage of excess body fat in the buttocks and thighs, leading to a "pear shape"

H

Harris–Benedict equation formula commonly used to estimate basal metabolic rate

Hazard Analysis and Critical Control Points (HACCP) science–based, systematic approach to preventing food–borne illness by predicting which hazards are most likely to occur in a food production facility

healthy life expectancy number of years a person can expect to spend without being disabled or having serious diseases

heartburn pain generally felt in the upper chest that results from the passage of acidic contents from the stomach into the esophagus

heart failure condition in which the heart cannot pump effectively

heat cramps heat–related illness characterized by painful muscle contractions

heat exhaustion heat–related illness that can occur after intense exercise and is characterized by weakness or dizziness

heatstroke most dangerous form of heat–related illness; potentially fatal condition characterized by body temperatures of greater than 104°F

hematocrit ratio of red blood cells to total blood volume

heme iron–containing component of hemoglobin and myoglobin

heme iron form of iron found in meat that is absorbed efficiently

hemoglobin iron–containing protein in red blood cells that transports oxygen

hemoglobin A1c (HbA1c) glycosylated hemoglobin; blood test used to measure a person's average blood glucose over several months' period of time

hemorrhoids swollen veins in the anal canal

hepatic portal vein vein that transports absorbed nutrients to the liver

herbicides substances used to destroy weeds

hereditary hemochromatosis (HH) inherited genetic defect that causes people to absorb too much iron

high birth weight (HBW) infant whose birth weight is greater than 4000 g (approximately 8.8 pounds)

high–density lipoprotein (HDL) lipoprotein that transports cholesterol away from tissues and to the liver, where it can be eliminated; low HDL is linked to increased risk for cardiovascular disease

high–fructose corn syrup (HFCS) syrup obtained from the processing of corn

high–quality (complete) protein protein that contains all essential amino acids in amounts that support the deposition of protein in tissues and the growth of a young person

high–sensitivity C–reactive protein (hs–CRP) protein produced primarily by the liver in response to inflammation; a marker of CVD

homocysteine amino acid that may play a role in the development of atherosclerosis

homocysteinuria group of conditions caused by gene mutations that cause homocysteine to accumulate in the blood

hormones chemical messengers secreted by organs of the endocrine system that convey information to target cells

hormone sensitive lipase (HSL) enzyme in fat cells that removes the three fatty acids from a triglyceride

hunger uncomfortable physiological sensation that drives a person to consume food

hydration water status

hydrocarbon chain chain of carbon atoms bonded to each other and to hydrogen atoms

hydrogenation food manufacturing process that adds hydrogen atoms to liquid vegetable oil, forming trans fats

hydrolysate formulas infant formulas that contain protein that has been hydrolyzed to polypeptides or free amino acids

hydrophilic part of a molecule that attracts water

hydrophobic part of a molecule that avoids water and attracts lipids

hydroxyapatite crystalline structure that forms on the collagen protein complex as bone is made

hypercalcemia high blood calcium

hyperemesis gravidarum severe form of nausea and vomiting that occurs during pregnancy

hyperglycemia abnormally elevated blood glucose levels

hyperinsulinemia condition in which the pancreas releases an excessive amount of insulin; over time, condition may contribute to the development of type 2 diabetes

hyperkalemia high blood potassium

hypermagnesemia high blood magnesium

hyperphosphatemia high blood phos–phorus level

hypertension abnormally high blood pressure levels that persist even when the person is relaxed

hyperthyroidism abnormally high blood levels of thyroid hormone

hypochromic pale color

hypogeusia diminished ability to taste substances

hypoglycemia condition that occurs when blood glucose level is too low

hypokalemia low blood potassium

hyponatremia low blood sodium

hypothalamus structure in the brain that controls hunger and satiety

hypothesis possible explanation for an observation that guides scientific research

hypothyroidism low blood levels of thyroid hormone

I

ileocecal sphincter region of ileum that controls the rate of emptying undigested material into the large intestine

ileum last segment of the small intestine

inborn error of metabolism an inherited metabolic defect

inborn errors of metabolism conditions that occur when genes undergo mutations that disrupt metabolism of specific nutrients

incubation period length of time in which bacteria can grow and multiply in food or the digestive tract before they cause illness

indirect calorimetry determination of the amount of heat someone produces by measuring the amount of oxygen consumed and the amount of carbon dioxide produced

indirect or **unintentional food additives** substances that are accidently in foods

infancy period from birth to 12 months of age

infant formula synthetic food that simulates human milk

inflammatory bowel disease (IBD) condition that is characterized by chronic inflammation of the GI tract

inorganic refers to substances that do not contain carbon

insecticides substances used to control or kill insects

insoluble fiber forms of dietary fiber that generally do not dissolve in water; include cellulose, hemicelluloses, and lignin

insulin hormone secreted from the beta cells of the pancreas that helps regulate blood glucose levels

intensity level of exertion used to perform an activity

intentional additive food additive added purposefully by a food manufacturer to enhance the food

intracellular water water that is inside cells

intrinsic factor substance necessary for absorbing vitamin B–12

inverse or **negative correlation** describes the relationship that occurs when one variable increases and the other one decreases

in vitro describes experiments on cells or other components derived from living organisms

in vivo describes experiments that use whole living organisms

iodide form of iodine that the body absorbs and uses

ions elements or small molecules that have electrical charges

iron deficiency low iron stores in the body

iron deficiency anemia third stage of iron deficiency characterized by a lack of red blood cells or the production of red blood cells that do not contain enough hemoglobin

iron overload ingestion of toxic amounts of iron

J

jejunum middle segment of the small intestine

K

Kashin–Beck disease form of osteoarthritis caused by selenium deficiency; leads to joint deformity and dwarfism

Kayser–Fleischer rings copper deposits in the eyes that are a sign of Wilson disease

keratin tough protein found in hair, nails, and the outermost layers of skin

Keshan disease disease of the heart muscle associated with selenium deficiency

ketoacidosis condition that occurs when excess acetoacetate and beta–hydroxybutyrate in the bloodstream lower the blood's pH

ketogenesis ketone body formation

ketogenic diet high–fat diet

ketone bodies chemicals formed from the incomplete breakdown of fat

ketosis condition in which ketone bodies accumulate in the blood; can result in loss of consciousness and death in severe cases

kilocalorie (kcal) or Calorie the heat energy needed to raise the temperature of 1000 g (a liter) of water 1° Celsius (C)

kwashiorkor form of undernutrition that results from consuming adequate energy and insufficient high–quality protein

L

lactase enzyme that splits lactose molecule

lactation production of milk by mammary glands

lacteal vessel of the lymphatic system

lactic acid compound formed from pyruvate during anaerobic metabolism

lactoovovegetarian vegetarian who consumes milk products and eggs for animal protein

lactose disaccharide composed of a glucose and a galactose molecule; "milk sugar"

lactose intolerance inability to digest lactose properly because of a deficiency in the enzyme lactase

lactovegetarian vegetarian who consumes milk and milk products for animal protein

lanugo widespread, white, delicate, and dense hair

lecithin phosphatidylcholine; phospholipid found in egg yolk that acts as an emulsifier in certain foods

legumes plants that produce pods with a single row of seeds

leptin hormone secreted by the adipose tissue to signal the brain when enough energy has been stored

let–down failure condition that occurs when the let–down reflex is blocked

let–down reflex reflex that enables milk to be released from breasts

life expectancy average length of time a person born in a specific year can expect to live

life span maximum number of years an organism can live

lifestyle a routine way of living

limiting amino acid essential amino acid found in the lowest concentration in a protein source

lingual lipase enzyme secreted into saliva that begins fat digestion

linoleic acid 18–carbon polyunsaturated fatty acid with two double bonds; an essential fatty acid

lipases enzymes that break down lipids

lipids class of nutrients that do not dissolve in water; triglycerides, phospholipids, and sterols

lipogenesis synthesis of fatty acids

lipolysis process by which triglycerides (fats) are broken down and glycerol and fatty acids are released into the bloodstream

lipoprotein lipase (LPL) enzyme in capillary walls that breaks down triglycerides

lipoprotein profile series of blood tests to evaluate total cholesterol, HDL cholesterol, LDL cholesterol, and triglyceride levels

lipoproteins water–soluble structure that transports lipids through the bloodstream

listeriosis food–borne illness that results from ingesting *Listeria monocytogenes*

longevity capability of living a long life

low birth weight (LBW) infant whose birth weight is less than 2500 g (5.5 pounds)

low–density lipoprotein (LDL) lipoprotein that carries cholesterol into tissues; elevated LDL is strongly linked to increased risk of cardiovascular disease

low energy availability state of nega–tive energy balance

low–quality (incomplete) protein protein that lacks or has inadequate amounts of one or more of the essential amino acids

lower esophageal sphincter (LES) region of the lower part of the esophagus that controls flow of material into the upper part of the stomach; also known as the gastroesophageal sphincter

lumen hollow space through which food and fluids can pass (digestive tract)

lysozyme enzyme in saliva that can destroy some bacteria that are in food or the mouth

M

macronutrients nutrients that the body needs in large amounts

major minerals essential mineral elements required in amounts of 100 mg or more per day

malignant tumors masses of cancerous cells

malnutrition state of health that occurs when the body is improperly nourished

maltase enzyme that splits maltose molecule

maltose disaccharide composed of two glucose molecules; "malt sugar"

marasmic kwashiorkor form of undernutrition that results in a child with kwashiorkor who then starts to not consume enough energy; characterized by edema and wasting

marasmus form of undernutrition that results from starvation; diet lacks energy and nutrients

maternal referring to a mother

mature milk form of milk that is secreted by the breast about 2 weeks after delivery

Meals on Wheels program in which volunteers deliver meals that have been prepared at a community site to home–bound individuals

mechanical digestion refers to physical treatments that food undergoes while it is in the intestinal tract

meconium first feces passed by a newborn shortly after birth

medical nutrition therapies nutritionally modified diets for people with chronic health conditions

megadose amount of a vitamin or mineral that is very high, generally at least 10 times the recommended amount of the nutrient

megaloblastic anemia type of anemia characterized by large, immature red blood cells; deficiency of folate and/or vitamin B–12 can lead to this form of anemia

menadione synthetic form of vitamin K

menaquinone form of vitamin K in egg yolks, butter, and beef as well as synthesized by bacteria in the large intestine

menarche onset of the first menstrual cycle

metabolic syndrome condition that increases risk of type 2 diabetes and CVD

metabolic water water formed by cells as a metabolic by–product

metabolism total of all chemical processes that occur in living cells

metastasized cancer that has moved from one tissue to other parts of the body

methylmercury organic form of mercury

micelle water–soluble spherical lipid cluster; bile salts create a shell around each cluster, allowing for the structure to be suspended in watery digestive juices

microcytic small cell

microflora population of several kinds of bacteria

micronutrients nutrients that the body needs in very small amounts

microsomal ethanol–oxidizing system (MEOS) secondary pathway for processing alcohol in the liver

microvilli tiny hairlike projections that form the brush border of an enterocyte

Mifflin–St. Jeor equation method of predicting basal calorie needs of individuals who are overweight or obese

miscarriage death of an embryo or fetus that occurs before the twentieth week of gestation

mitochondria organelles that synthesize most of the ATP that cells need to function

moderation refers to eating reasonable amounts of each food

monoglyceride lipid that has one fatty acid attached to a three–carbon compound called glycerol

monosaccharide simple sugar that is the basic molecule of carbohydrates

***mono*unsaturated fatty acid (MUFA)** fatty acid that has one double bond within the carbon chains

morning sickness nausea and/or vomiting during pregnancy

mucosa innermost layer of the digestive tract wall

mucous cells cells that secrete mucus

mucus watery slippery fluid secreted by special cells

multivitamin–multimineral supplement supplement containing two or more vitamins and minerals

muscle dysmorphia unhealthy preoccupation with the body being too small or not muscular enough

mutation change to the typical sequence of a gene's DNA components

myelin sheath structure that wraps around and insulates a part of certain nerve cells

myocardial infarction heart attack

myoglobin iron–containing protein in muscle cells that controls oxygen uptake from red blood cells

MyPlate USDA's interactive Internet dietary and menu–planning guide

N

National Health and Nutrition Examination Survey (NHANES) survey that uses interviews and physical examinations to assesses the health and nutritional status of adults and children in the United States

National School Lunch Program federally assisted school meal program

negative energy balance calorie intake is less than calorie output

negative nitrogen balance state in which the body loses more nitrogen than it retains

neural tube embryonic structure that eventually develops into the brain and spinal cord

neurotransmitters chemicals produced by nerve cells that enable the cells to communicate with other nerve cells

niacin vitamin B–3; important for energy metabolism as part of nicotinamide adenine dinucleotide and nicotinamide adenine dinucleotide phosphate

nicotinamide adenine dinucleotide (NAD^+) niacin–containing coenzyme

night eating syndrome (NES) episodic food binges that are not followed by purging; binges take place after the evening meal and when the person wakens from sleep during the night

nitrogen balance (equilibrium) balancing nitrogen intake with nitrogen losses

nonalcoholic fatty liver abnormal accumulation of fat in the liver that is not caused by alcohol consumption

nonessential amino acids group of amino acids that the body can make

nonexercise activity thermogenesis (NEAT) energy expended during involuntary skeletal muscular activities such as fidgeting

nonheme iron form of iron that is not absorbed as efficiently as heme iron; found in meat, vegetables, grains, supplements, and fortified or enriched foods

nonnutritive sweeteners   group of synthetic compounds that are intensely sweet tasting compared to sugar

normal weight obesity (NWO)   normal body weight as measured by BMI but elevated percent body fat

nursing bottle caries   form of dental decay that occurs in young children who suck on a bottle that contains any sugar—containing substance for several hours at a time

nutrient—dense   describes a food that supplies more vitamins and minerals in relation to total calories

nutrient requirement   smallest amount of a nutrient that maintains a defined level of nutritional health

nutrients   life—sustaining substances in food

nutrigenetics   study of how inherited genetic variations influence the body's responses to specific nutrients and nutrient combinations

nutrigenomics   study of how nutrients affect the expression of a person's genome

nutrition   scientific study of nutrients and how the body uses them

Nutrition Facts panel   nutrition information about a food's nutrient contents that is displayed in a specific format on the food's package

nutritional genomics   study of nutrigenomics and nutrigenetics

nutritive sweeteners   substances that sweeten and contribute energy to foods

O

obesity   condition characterized by excessive and unhealthy amounts of body fat

obesogenic environment   external conditions that promote excessive weight gain

oleic acid   18—carbon monounsaturated fatty acid

oligosaccharides   carbohydrates comprised of three to 10 monosaccharides bonded together

omega—3 fatty acid   type of polyunsaturated fatty acid with the first double bond at the third carbon from the omega end of the molecule

omega—6 fatty acid   type of polyunsaturated fatty acid with the first double bond at the sixth carbon from the omega end of the molecule

omega (methyl) end   end of a fatty acid containing a methyl ($-CH_3$) group

oral cavity   mouth

oral rehydration therapy   specially prepared solutions of water and electrolytes used to prevent and treat dehydration

organic   (chemistry) refers to compounds that contain carbon

organically produced foods   foods that are produced without the use of antibiotics, hormones, synthetic fertilizers and pesticides, genetic improvements, or ionizing radiation

orthorexia nervosa (ON)   condition characterized by an extreme obsession with eating healthy foods

osmosis   movement of a solvent, usually water, through a selectively permeable membrane

osteoarthritis   condition characterized by degeneration of the bones and cartilage

osteoblasts   bone cells that add bone to where the tissue is needed

osteoclasts   bone cells that tear down bone tissue

osteomalacia   condition characterized by softening of the bones as a result of inadequate vitamin D status in adults

osteopenia   condition in which a person has weak bones that are susceptible to fracture

osteoporosis   chronic disease characterized by bones with low mass and reduced structure

"other specified" feeding or eating disorders   disordered eating behavior that does not meet the full criteria for AN, BN, or BED

overweight   having extra weight from bone, muscle, body fat, and/or body water

ovovegetarian   vegetarian who eats eggs for animal protein

ovulation   release of an ovum (egg) from an ovary

oxalic acid   substance found in spinach, collard greens, and sweet potatoes that interferes with mineral absorption

oxaloacetate   four—carbon molecule that is an important intermediate of the citric acid cycle

oxidants   free radicals that damage cell membranes, proteins, and DNA

oxidized LDL   LDL that has been damaged by free radicals

oxidizing agent or **oxidant**   substance that removes electrons from atoms or molecules

oxytocin   hormone that stimulates the release of milk from the breast

P

pancreatic amylase   enzyme secreted by pancreas that breaks down starch into maltose molecules

pancreatic lipase   digestive enzyme that removes two fatty acids from each triglyceride molecule

pantothenic acid   vitamin component of coenzyme A (CoA)

parasite   life form that lives on or in another organism and takes advantage of its host

parathyroid hormone (PTH)   hormone secreted in response to low blood calcium levels

parietal cells   stomach cells that secrete intrinsic factor and the components of hydrochloric acid into the lumen of the stomach

Parkinson's disease   neurological disorder that results from a lack of dopamine

pasteurization   process that kills the pathogens in foods and beverages as well as many microbes responsible for spoilage

pathogen   disease—causing microorganism

peak bone mass   present when bones have their maximum strength

peer review   critical analysis of an article about a study submitted to a journal that is conducted by a group of investigators who were not part of the study but are experts involved in related research

pellagra   niacin deficiency disease characterized by dermatitis, diarrhea, dementia, and death

pepsin   active enzyme that begins the enzymatic digestion of proteins

peptide bond   chemical attraction that connects two amino acids together

peptides   small chains of amino acids

peptide YY   protein hormone that signals the stomach to reduce ghrelin secretion

peripheral neuropathy   condition characterized by severe sensory nerve damage

peristalsis   waves of muscular contractions that help move material through most of the digestive tract

pernicious anemia   condition caused by the lack of intrinsic factor and characterized by vitamin B—12 deficiency, nerve damage, and megaloblastic red blood cells

personalized nutrition   making dietary choices based on one's genetic makeup

pescavegetarian   vegetarian who consumes fish, milk products, and eggs for animal protein

pesticide   substance used to kill or control unwanted insects, weeds, or other organisms

pesticide tolerances   maximum amounts of pesticide residues that can be in or on each treated food crop

pharynx   section of the alimentary canal that connects the nasal cavity with the top of the esophagus

phenylketonuria (PKU)   genetic metabolic disorder characterized by the inability to convert the amino acid phenylalanine into tyrosine, resulting in accumulation of phenylalanine

phosphocreatine (PCr)   high−energy compound used to re−form ATP under anaerobic conditions; provides energy for short bouts of high−intensity activity

phospholipid   type of lipid needed to make cell membranes and for proper functioning of nerve cells; chemically similar to a triglyceride except that one of the fatty acids is replaced by a chemical group that contains phosphorus

phosphorylation   anabolic reaction that results in the attachment of a P_i group to ADP

phototherapy   exposure to certain wavelengths of light by use of a specific lamp for prescribed amounts of time

phylloquinone   form of vitamin K in plants

physical activity   movement resulting from contraction of skeletal muscle

physical fitness   ability to perform moderate− to vigorous−intensity activities without becoming excessively fatigued

physiological dose   amount of a nutrient that is within the range of safe intake and enables the body to function optimally

phytic acid   compound found in grains, seeds, and beans that interferes with mineral absorption

phytochemicals   substances in plants that are not nutrients but may have healthful benefits

pica   eating nonfood substances

pincer grasp   use of the thumb and forefinger to pick up small objects

placebo   fake treatment

placebo effect   in studies involving human subjects, the situation that occurs when a subject reports having positive results even though he or she is taking a placebo

placenta   organ that forms on the lining of the uterus and functions to deliver nutrients and oxygen to the embryo/fetus and remove wastes

plant sterols/stanols   chemicals found in plants that are structurally similar to cholesterol

plasma   liquid portion of blood that has had the cells removed; contains clotting factors

polypeptides   proteins comprised of 50 or more amino acids

polypharmacy   condition that occurs when a person takes five or more medications each day

polysaccharides   carbohydrates comprised of 10 or more monosaccharides bonded together

polyunsaturated fatty acid (PUFA)   fatty acid that has two or more double bonds within the carbon chain

positive energy balance   calorie intake is greater than calorie output

positive nitrogen balance   state in which the body retains more nitrogen than it loses

potentially hazardous foods   foods that promote pathogen growth; these foods typically have high moisture content, neutral pH or low acidity levels, and/or high protein amounts

prebiotics   food components that beneficial bacteria in the large intestine use for fuel

preconception period   time before pregnancy

preeclampsia   condition that occurs during pregnancy; characterized by proteinuria and edema

pregravid   before pregnancy

prehypertension   persistent systolic blood pressure readings of 120 mm Hg to 139 mm Hg and diastolic readings of 80 mm Hg to 89 mm Hg

premenstrual syndrome (PMS)   condition that many women experience a few days before their menstrual period begins

prenatal   time from conception until birth

presbyopia   decline in near vision that occurs with aging

preschool−age   child who is 3 to 5 years of age

preterm   describes an infant born before the thirty−seventh week of gestation

primary structure   refers to the basic structure of protein; a linear chain of amino acids linked by peptide bonds

prions   infectious pathogens that are composed of misfolded proteins

probiotics   live microorganisms that promote good health for their human hosts

prolactin   hormone that stimulates milk production

prooxidant   substance that promotes production of free radicals

prospective cohort study   study in which a group of initially healthy people are followed over a time period and any diseases that eventually develop are recorded

prostaglandins   class of eicosanoids that produce a variety of important effects on the body

protein digestibility corrected amino acid score (PDCAAS)   measure of protein quality based on amino acid composition score and digestibility of a protein food

protein efficiency ratio (PER)   measure of protein quality based on the ability of a protein to support weight gain in a laboratory animal

protein−energy malnutrition (PEM)   occurs when the diet lacks sufficient protein and energy

proteins   large, complex organic molecules made up of amino acids

protein turnover   cellular process of breaking down proteins and recycling their amino acids

proteinuria   protein in the urine

protozoa   single−celled microorganisms that have complex cell structures

pseudoscience   presentation of information masquerading as factual and scientific

puberty   time at which a child matures physically and sexually into an adult

purging   activities that limit calorie intake or increase calorie output

pyloric sphincter   region of the stomach that regulates the flow of chyme into the small intestine

pyruvate   three−carbon molecule that results from the breakdown of glucose during glycolysis

quaternary structure   refers to the structure of protein that is comprised of two or more polypeptide chains arranged together in a unique manner

R

raffinose   nondigestible oligosaccharide made of three monosaccharides

reactive hypoglycemia (postprandial hypoglycemia)   low blood glucose that occurs within 4 hours of eating

ready–to–use therapeutic foods (RUTFs)   shelf–stable foods fortified with calories, protein, and micronutrients that are used for the treatment of undernutrition

Recommended Dietary Allowances (RDAs)   standards for recommended daily intakes of several nutrients

rectum   last section of the large intestine

reference protein   a high–quality protein against which quality of other proteins is measured

reflexes   involuntary muscular reactions that occur in response to a stimulus

registered dietitian (RD) or **registered dietitian nutritionist (RDN)**   college–trained health care professional who has extensive knowledge of foods, nutrition, and dietetics

renin   enzyme secreted in response to low blood volume and falling blood pressure

resistance exercises   physical activities, such as pull–ups and push–ups, that develop muscle strength and muscle endurance

resistant hypertension   blood pressure that remains uncontrolled while taking three medications or is controlled only through continued use of four or more medications

resistant starches   starches found in seeds, legumes, whole grains, and some fruits and vegetables that resist digestion and are not broken down in the human GI tract

resting metabolic rate (RMR)   body's rate of energy use a few hours after resting and eating

retinoids (preformed vitamin A)   family of compounds commonly called vitamin A (retinol, retinal, retinoic acid)

retinol   alcohol form of vitamin A and the most active form of vitamin A in the body

retinol–binding protein (RBP)   transports vitamin A in the blood

retinyl esters   storage form of vitamin A

retrospective cohort study   study in which researchers collect information about a group's past exposures and identify current health outcomes

R group (side chain)   part of an amino acid that determines the molecule's physical and chemical properties

rhodopsin   vitamin A–containing protein that is needed for vision in dim light

riboflavin   vitamin B–2; important for energy metabolism as part of flavin mononucleotide and flavin adenine dinucleotide

rickets   vitamin D–deficiency disorder in children resulting in improper bone growth

risk factor   personal characteristic that increases a person's chances of developing a chronic disease

rodenticides   substances used to kill mice and rats

rooting reflex   involuntary response in infants in which the child turns and opens his or her mouth as the child's cheek is stroked

Roux–en–Y gastric bypass   surgical approach to treating obesity

S

saliva   watery fluid that contains mucus and a few enzymes

salivary amylase   enzyme in saliva that begins starch digestion

salivary glands   structures that produce saliva and secrete the fluid into the oral cavity

sarcopenia   condition characterized by the loss of muscle tissue

sarcopenic obesity   type of obesity that is characterized by the loss of skeletal muscle mass combined with excessive body fat

satiety   sense that enough food or beverages have been consumed to satisfy hunger

saturated fatty acid (SFA)   fatty acid that has each carbon atom within the chain filled with hydrogen atoms

school–age   child who is 6 to 11 years of age

School Breakfast Program   program through which schools and other nonprofit agencies are reimbursed for the cost of providing a nutritious morning meal to eligible low–income children

scombrotoxin   toxin that forms as a result of bacterial breakdown of fish tissue that has been improperly stored

scurvy   vitamin C deficiency disease

secondary structure   refers to the coiling of a polypeptide chain

secretin   hormone secreted by the duodenum and first part of the jejunum that stimulates the pancreas and liver to release a bicarbonate–rich solution into the small intestine

segmentation   regular contractions of circular intestinal muscles followed by muscular relaxations that mix chyme within a short portion of the small intestine

selectively permeable membrane   barrier that allows the passage of certain substances and prevents the movement of other substances

selenoproteins   several proteins that require selenium to function; often serve as antioxidants

selenosis   selenium toxicity

semivegetarian ("flexitarian")   a person who usually avoids red meat but consumes other animal foods, including fish, poultry, eggs, and dairy products

senescence   declining organ functioning that occurs with advanced age

serum   liquid portion of blood that has had the cells and clotting factors removed

set–point theory   scientific notion that the body's fat content and body weight is genetically predetermined

7–dehydrocholesterol   precursor for vitamin D found in skin

shelf life   period of time that a food can be stored before it spoils

sickle cell anemia   inherited form of anemia

signs   physical changes associated with a disease state that are observable or measurable

simple diffusion   molecular movement from a region of higher to lower concentration

skeletal fluorosis   excess fluoride intake that changes bone structure, causing joint stiffness, bone pain, and increasing risk for bone fractures

skinfold thickness measurements   technique of estimating body composition in which calipers are used to measure the thickness of skinfolds at multiple body sites

sleeve gastrectomy   surgical approach to treating obesity

sodium sensitive   individual who may develop hypertension as a result of consuming a high–sodium diet

solid fats fats that are fairly hard at room temperature

soluble fiber forms of dietary fiber that dissolve or swell in water; include pectins, gums, mucilages, and some hemicelluloses

soup kitchens establishments where prepared meals are provided to those who are hungry, typically for free

Special Milk Program program that enables eligible students to receive free or reduced−cost milk with meals

Special Supplemental Nutrition Assistance Program for Women, Infants, and Children (WIC) federal program that provides funds to state governments so they can help specific populations obtain certain supplemental foods, basic health care services, and nutrition education

sphincters thickened regions of circular muscle that control the flow of contents at various points in the GI tract

spina bifida type of neural tube defect in which the spine does not form properly before birth and fails to enclose the spinal cord

sports anemia temporary condition that develops during the early stages of training in endurance athletes; a result of an increase in the liquid portion of blood (plasma) that results in low hemoglobin levels

sports gels carbohydrate−rich gels developed for athletes, particularly those engaged in endurance training and competition

sports nutrition practice of applying nutrition principles and research findings to improving athletic performance and recovery following a training session

stachyose nondigestible oligosaccharide made of four monosaccharides

standard drink approximately 12 ounces of beer, 5 ounces of wine, or 1 ½ ounces of liquor

starch storage polysaccharide in plants; composed of amylose and amylopectin

stearic acid 18−carbon saturated fatty acid

steatorrhea presence of lipid in the stool

sterilization process that kills or destroys all microorganisms and viruses

sterols type of lipid that has a more complex chemical structure than triglycerides and phospholipids

stomach muscular sac that stores and mixes food

stroke clot blocks an artery in the brain; brain cells that are nourished by the vessel die

stunting reduced adult size as a consequence of chronic undernutrition in infancy and childhood

subcutaneous fat accumulation of adipose cells in the tissue under the skin

suckle to draw milk

suck reflex involuntary response that enables an infant to draw milk and swallow when a nipple is put into his or her mouth

sucrase enzyme that splits sucrose molecule

sucrose disaccharide composed of a glucose and a fructose molecule; "table sugar"

sugar alcohols alternative sweeteners used to replace sucrose in some sugar−free foods; sorbitol, xylitol, and mannitol

Summer Food Service Program program that provides financial support to qualifying facilities that serve free meals and snacks to students during the summer

Supplemental Nutrition Assistance Program (SNAP) assistance program that enables qualified low−income participants to use monthly cash allotments and a special debit card to purchase foods from authorized stores

sustainable agriculture farming methods that do not deplete natural resources or harm the environment while meeting the demand for food

symptoms subjective complaints of ill health that are difficult to observe and measure

syndrome group of signs and symptoms that occur together and indicate a specific health problem

systolic pressure maximum blood pressure within an artery that occurs when the ventricles contract

T

target heart rate zone heart rate range that reflects intensity of physical exertion

teratogen an agent that causes birth defects

tertiary structure refers to the three−dimensional, twisted structure of a polypeptide chain that includes interactions between various amino acid groups on the chain

testimonial personal endorsement of a product

therapeutic lifestyle changes (TLC) actions, such as avoiding excess body fat, exercising daily, and improving the diet, that promote health and reduce risk for chronic disease

thermic effect of food (TEF) energy used to digest foods and beverages as well as absorb and further process the macronutrients

thiamin vitamin B−1; vitamin component of a coenzyme that is important for energy metabolism as part of thiamin pyrophosphate (TPP)

thrombus fixed bunch of clots that remain in place and disrupt blood flow

thyroid hormone hormones that con− trol the rate of cell metabolism and are dependent on iodine for production

tocopherols group of four structurally similar forms of vitamin E

toddler child who is 1 to 3 years of age

Tolerable Upper Intake Level (Upper Level or UL) highest average amount of a nutrient that is unlikely to harm most people when the amount is consumed daily

total body fat adipose tissue and essential fat

total body iron method of assessing iron status; the ratio of blood transferrin receptor to ferritin

total energy expenditure (TEE) amount of energy needed for all bodily functions throughout the day

total parenteral solution liquid mixture that provides nourishment to those who are unable to eat normally

total water intake water ingested by consuming beverages, including drinking water, and foods

toxins poisonous substances produced by living organisms

toxoplasmosis condition caused by infection with *Toxoplasma gondii*

trace minerals essential mineral elements required in amounts that are less than 100 mg per day

trans fats unsaturated fatty acids that have a trans double bond

transamination transfer of the nitrogen−containing group from an unneeded amino acid to a carbon skeleton to form an amino acid

transferrin transport protein for iron in the bloodstream

transferrin receptor membrane–bound receptor that attaches to iron; used to measure iron status

transitional milk combination of colostrum and mature milk

treatment (or experimental) group in a controlled study, group that receives a treatment

triglyceride lipid that has three fatty acids attached to a three–carbon compound called glycerol

trimester three–month period of pregnancy

tripeptides compounds that consist of three amino acids

trypsin protein–splitting enzyme secreted from the pancreas

25–hydroxyvitamin D inactive form of vitamin D, made in the liver from cholecalciferol

two–component model method of measuring body composition that divides the body into two compartments: fat mass and fat–free mass

type 1 diabetes autoimmune disease that results in destruction of the beta cells of the pancreas; as a result, insulin must be supplied to the affected person regularly through exogenous sources

type 2 diabetes most common type of diabetes; beta cells of the pancreas produce insulin, but the hormone's target cells are insulin–resistant, leading to elevated blood glucose levels

U

ulcerative colitis (UC) type of IBD that causes ulcers to form in the mucosa of the colon and rectum

umbilical cord structure that extends from the embryo/fetus to the placenta

under–5 mortality rate number of newborns in a population, per 1000 live births, who are likely to die before they reach 5 years of age

undernutrition lack of food

underwater weighing technique of estimating body composition that involves comparing weight on land to weight when completely submerged in a tank of water

underweight individual who has a BMI that is less than 18.5

unsaturated fatty acid fatty acid that is missing hydrogen atoms and has

one or more double bonds within the carbon chain

upper esophageal sphincter (UES) region of the upper part of the esophagus that opens to allow a mass of food to enter the esophagus

urea waste product of amino acid metabolism

uric acid derivative of purine metabolism

urinary incontinence condition in which urine leaks out of the bladder

urine urea nitrogen (UUN) measure of the concentration of urea in urine

uterus female reproductive organ that houses the embryo/fetus before birth

V

variable factor that can change and influence an outcome of a study

variety refers to a diet that contains foods from each food group

vascular dementia condition that occurs when the blood supply to the brain is reduced

vasoconstrictor substance that contributes to the constriction of blood vessels

vegan vegetarian who eats only plant foods

vegetarians people who eat plant–based diets

vermin animals that often live around sewage or garbage, such as flies, cockroaches, mice, and rats.

very–low–density lipoprotein (VLDL) lipoprotein made in the liver and that carries much of the triglycerides in the bloodstream

villi tiny, fingerlike projections of the small intestinal mucosa that are involved in digestion and nutrient absorption

virus microbe consisting of a piece of genetic material coated with protein

visceral fat accumulation of adipose cells under the abdominal muscles and over the digestive organs

vitamin complex organic molecule that regulates certain metabolic processes

vitamin B–6 B vitamin component of the coenzyme pyridoxal phosphate (PLP); important for energy metabolism, particularly protein metabolism, as a part of pyridoxal phosphate (PLP)

vitamin B–12 or cobalamin B vitamin that is a component of

coenzymes that participate in a variety of cellular processes, including transfer of CH_3 groups in the metabolism of folate

vitamin C ascorbic acid; cofactor that performs a variety of important cellular functions, primarily by donating electrons to other compounds

vitamin–like compounds substances that maintain normal metabolism; unlike with vitamins, the body synthesizes these compounds

W

water intoxication condition that occurs when too much water is consumed in a short time period or kidneys have difficulty filtering water from blood

water–soluble vitamins thiamin, riboflavin, niacin, vitamin B–6, pantothenic acid, folate, biotin, vitamin B–12, and vitamin C

weaning gradual process of shifting from breastfeeding or bottle feeding to eating solid foods and drinking from a cup

weight cycling repeated bouts of losing and gaining significant amounts of weight

Wernicke–Korsakoff syndrome degenerative brain disorder associated with a deficiency of thiamin and most commonly caused by excessive alcohol consumption.

whey protein nutrient–dense type of protein found in milk.

whey water–soluble protein in milk

whole grains intact, ground, cracked, or flaked seeds of cereal grains

Wilson disease a rare inherited disorder characterized by accumulation of toxic amounts of copper in the body

X

xerophthalmia condition affecting the eyes that results from vitamin A deficiency

xerostomia dry mouth

Z

zygote egg that has been fertilized by a sperm

Photo Credits

FRONT MATTER

Page xv: U.S. Department of Health and Human Services; p. xvi(left): © Wendy Schiff; p. xvi(right): © Ingram Publishing RF; p. xvii(top): U.S. Fish & Wildlife Service/Mary Smith; p. xvii(middle): © Rene Frederick/Digital Vision/Getty Images RF; p. xvii(bottom): © McGraw-Hill Education. Mark A. Dierker, photographer; p. xviii: © D. Hurst/Alamy RF; 7.22(Helix): © Digital Vision/Getty Images RF; 7.22(Vitamins): © McGraw-Hill Education. John Flournoy, photographer; 7.22(Wine): © FoodCollection/StockFood RF; 7.22(Bread): © Ingram Publishing RF; 12.11: © Medical-on-Line/Alamy; 6.16: © Biophoto Associates/Science Source; 6.18a: © McGraw-Hill Education. Al Telser, photographer; 6.18b: © Image Source/Getty Images RF; p. xxi(top right): © Dr. Parvinder Sethi RF.

CHAPTER 1

Opener & 1.1: © McGraw-Hill Education. Aaron Roeth Photography; 1.2: © Eric Audras/Getty Images RF: 1.3: Centers for Disease Control; Page 6: © Royalty-Free/Corbis RF; 1.5: © FoodCollection/StockFood RF; 1.5(Butter): © Comstock/Jupiter Images RF; p. 10 left: © Pixtal/PunchStock RF; p. 10(right): © Digital Vision/Getty Images RF; p. 11: U.S. Department of Health and Human Services. Office of Disease Prevention and Health Promotion. Healthy People 2020. Washington, DC.; 1.7: © Wendy Schiff; p. 12: © Purestock/SuperStock RF; p. 14: © Purestock/SuperStock RF; 1.8: © Wendy Schiff; 1.9: U.S. Department of Health and Human Services; p. 15: © McGraw-Hill Education. Mark Steinmetz, photographer; 1.10(left): © Sandy Jones/Getty Images RF; 1.10(right): © Royalty-Free/Corbis RF; p. 18(top): © Wendy Schiff; p. 18(bottom): © Lars A. Niki RF; p. 20(top): © Wendy Schiff; p. 20(bottom): © Onoky/Getty Images RF; p. 21: © Wendy Schiff; p. 23: © Tetra Images/Getty Images RF.

CHAPTER 2

Opener © McGraw-Hill Education. Aaron Roeth Photography; Page 26(top & bottom): Centers for Disease Control; p. 29(top): © Photodisc/Getty Images RF; p. 29(bottom): © Rene Frederick/Digital Vision/Getty Images RF; 2.3: Stephen Ausmus/ARS/USDA; p. 33: © Wendy Schiff; p. 34: © Pixtal/AGE fotostock RF; p. 37: © Wendy Schiff; p. 38: Courtesy of Health On the Net Foundation, www.hon.ch; p. 41: © Ingram Publishing; p. 42: © D. Hurst/Alamy RF.

CHAPTER 3

Opener: © McGraw-Hill Education. Aaron Roeth Photography; 3.1: © Ryan McVay/Getty Images RF; 3.4: © McGraw-Hill Education. Christopher Kerrigan, photographer; Page 51: © BananaStock/PunchStock RF; p. 52: © Wendy Schiff; p. 53: © C Squared Studios/Getty Images RF; p. 54(top): © Wendy Schiff; p. 54(bottom): © C Squared Studios/Getty Images RF; p. 55: © McGraw-Hill Education. Mark Dierker, photographer; 3.5, 3.6, 3.7, p. 56(bottom): U.S. Dept. of Agriculture, Center for Nutrition Policy and Promotion; p. 58(top): © Wendy Schiff; p. 58(middle): © Purestock/SuperStock RF; 3.8(Dice): © McGraw-Hill Education. Christopher Kerrigan, photographer; 3.8(Mouse): © Royalty-Free/Corbis RF; 3.8(Ball): © Radlung & Associates/Getty Images RF; 3.8(Baseball): © Ryan McVay/Getty Images RF; 3.8(Yo-yo): © Stockdisc/Getty Images RF; 3.8(Soap): © McGraw-Hill Education. Christopher Kerrigan, photographer; 3.9: Economic Research Service, U.S. Department of Agriculture; 3.11, p. 63(top): © Wendy Schiff; p. 63(bottom): © Katrina Wittkamp/Getty Images RF; 3.14, 3.15: © Wendy Schiff; p. 65(left): © Royalty-Free/Corbis RF; p. 65(right): © Wendy Schiff; 3.17, 3.18, p. 72, p. 75: © Wendy Schiff; p. 78: © Ingram Publishing/Alamy RF.

CHAPTER 4

Opener: © Science Photo Library RF/Getty Images RF; Page 84(left): © Burke/Triolo Productions/Getty Images RF; p. 84(right): © Kelly Strosnider; p. 88: © Nick Koudis/Getty Images RF; 4.12(Lemon), 4.12(Wine): © Burke/Triolo Productions/Getty Images RF; 4.12(Cola): © Royalty-Free/Corbis RF; 4.12(Tomato): © Stockdisc/PunchStock RF; 4.12(Banana): © Stockdisc/PunchStock RF; 4.12(Coffee): © Royalty-Free/Corbis RF; 4.12(Milk): © McGraw-Hill Education. Bob Coyle, photographer; 4.12(Egg): © Siede Preis/Getty Images RF; 4.12(Baking Soda): © McGraw-Hill Education. Stephen Frisch, photographer; 4.12(Ammonia): © McGraw-Hill Education. Jacques Cornell, photographer; 4.12(Oven cleaner): © McGraw-Hill Education. Ken Karp, photographer; p. 92: © Ingram Publishing RF; p. 96, p. 97: © Wendy Schiff; 4.21: © Du Cane Medical Imaging Ltd/Science Source; 4.23: © David M. Martin, M.D./Science Source; 4.24: Science Photo Library RF/Getty Images RF; p. 103: © McGraw-Hill Education. Lars A. Niki, photographer; p. 104: © Wendy Schiff; p. 107(top): © FoodCollection/StockFood RF; p. 107(bottom): © McGraw-Hill Education. Pat Watson, photographer; p. 108: © Jamie Grill/Corbis RF.

CHAPTER 5

Opener: © Ingram Publishing RF; Page 113: © Allan & Sandy Carey/Getty Images RF; p. 114(Sugar): © Wendy Schiff; p. 114(Honey): © Brand X Pictures/Getty Images RF; p. 115: © Glowimages/Getty Images RF; 5.5: © Wendy Schiff; 5.8(Wheat): © Photodisc/PunchStock RF; 5.8(Flour): © McGraw-Hill Education. Michael Scott, photographer; 5.9: © Wendy Schiff; p. 120: © FoodCollection/StockFood RF; p. 121: © PhotoLink/Getty Images RF; p. 122(top): © Lars A. Niki RF; p. 122(cola): © Royalty-Free/Corbis RF;

Publishing/SuperStock RF; 10.4: Centers for Disease Control; Page 310: © Mireille Vautier/Alamy; 10.6: Centers for Disease Control; 10.7: © Wendy Schiff; p. 312: © Royalty-Free/Corbis RF; p. 313: © Pixtal/AGE fotostock RF; p. 315: © McGraw-Hill Education. Jill Braaten, photographer; p. 316: © Burke Triolo Productions/Getty Images RF; p. 317: © FoodCollection/StockFood RF; 10.10(top): © Dr. R. King/Science Source; 10.10(bottom): © Dr. E. Walker/Science Source; p. 325: © Jupiter Images/Image–Source RF; 10.13: Centers for Disease Control; p. 327: © McGraw-Hill Education. John Flournoy, photographer; p. 329: © Brian Yarvin/Alamy RF; p. 330 © Ingram Publishing/SuperStock RF; p. 333(top): © Bjorn Heller/Getty Images RF; p. 333(bottom): © Ingram Publishing/Alamy RF; p. 334: © Daniel Koebe/Corbis RF; p. 335: © Author's Image/Glow Images RF; p. 336: © Floortje/Getty Images RF; p. 337: © Brand X Pictures/Getty Images RF; p. 338: © Rob Melnychuk/Photodisc/Getty Images RF; p. 340: Renne Comet/National Cancer Institute; p. 341: © Ingram Publishing/SuperStock RF.

CHAPTER 11

Opener: © McGraw-Hill Education. Charles D. Winters, Timeframe Photography, Inc.; Page 346(left): © Royalty-Free/Corbis RF; p. 346(right): © Brand X Pictures/ PunchStock RF; 11.4: © Stephen J. Krasemann/Science Source; p. 350: U.S. Navy photo by Seaman Aaron Shelley; 11.7: © Royalty-Free/Corbis RF; 11.8(MyPlate): U.S. Dept. of Agriculture; 11.8(Mango): © Stockdisc/PunchStock RF; 11.8(Kale): © Stockdisc/PunchStock RF; 11.8(Milk): © Ingram Publishing RF; 11.8(Cereal): © Stockbyte/Getty Images RF; 11.8(Sardines): © fStop/PunchStock RF; p. 356: © Comstock/Alamy RF; p. 358(left), 11.12(all), p. 358(right): © Wendy Schiff; 11.13(MyPlate): U.S. Dept. of Agriculture; 11.13(Orange Juice): © Stockbyte/Getty Images RF; 11.13(Broccoli): © Burke/ Triolo Productions/Getty Images RF; 11.13(Cheese): © Comstock/Jupiter Images RF; 11.13(Cereal), 11.13(Almonds): © Stockbyte/Getty Images RF; p. 359(bottom): © Wendy Schiff; p. 360(top): © Jonelle Weaver/Getty Images RF; 11.14: © Michael Klein/Photolibrary/ Getty Images; 11.15: © Sally and Richard Greenhill/Alamy; p. 361(bottom): © Dynamic Graphics/Jupiter Images RF; p. 362: © David R. Frazier Photolibrary, Inc./Alamy RF; 11.16(MyPlate): U.S.

Dept. of Agriculture; 11.16(Strawberries): © C. Squared Studios/Getty Images RF; 11.16(Carrots): © Comstock/Jupiter Images RF; 11.16(Yogurt): © Mitch Hrdlicka/ Getty Images RF; 11.16(Cereal): © Stockbyte/Getty Images RF; 11.16(Seeds): © McGraw-Hill Education. Jacques Cornell, photographer; p. 365(top): © PM Images/ Getty Images RF; p. 365(bottom): TSGT Lance Cheung, USAF/DoD Media; p. 367: © Photodisc/Getty Images RF; p. 368, p. 369: © Wendy Schiff; p. 370: © Creative Crop/Getty Images RF; 11.17(MyPlate): U.S. Dept. of Agriculture; 11.17(Pear): © Stockbyte/Getty Images RF; 11.17(Squash): © Burke/Triolo Productions/Getty Images RF; 11.17(Yogurt): © Ingram Publishing/ SuperStock RF; 11.17(Bread): © IT Stock/PunchStock RF; 11.17(Shrimp): © Comstock/Jupiter Images RF; 11.18(MyPlate): U.S. Dept. of Agriculture; 11.18(Berries): © David Cook/ blueshiftstudios/Alamy RF; 11.18(Lima Beans): © Brand Z Food/Alamy RF; 11.18(Milk): © Ingram Publishing RF; 11.18(Cereal): © McGraw-Hill Education. Jill Braaten, photographer; 11.18(Kidney Beans): © Royalty-Free/Corbis RF; p. 374: © Stockbyte/Getty Images RF; p. 375: © Pixtal/AGE fotostock RF; p. 377: © McGraw-Hill Education. Ken Karp, photographer; p. 378: © Tammy Stephenson; p. 379: © John E. Kelly/Getty Images RF.

CHAPTER 12

Opener: © Wendy Schiff; 12.2(MyPlate): U.S. Dept. of Agriculture; 12.2(Fruits): © Stockbyte/Getty Images RF; 12.2(Peas): © Ingram Publishing/SuperStock RF; 12.2(Oats): © McGraw-Hill Education. Jacques Cornell, photographer; 12.2(Beef): © Comstock/Jupiter Images RF; Page 387: © FoodCollection/StockFood RF; p. 388: © D. Hurst/Alamy RF; p. 389: © C Squared Studios/Getty Images RF; 12.6a: © Dr. R. King/Science Source; 12.6b: © McGraw-Hill Education; p. 392(top): © liquidlibrary/PictureQuest RF; p. 392(bottom): © Wendy Schiff; p. 393(left): © Hawley Almstedt; p. 393(right), p. 394: © Wendy Schiff; p. 395(all): © Burke/ Triolo Productions/Getty Images RF; p. 396: © Wendy Schiff; 12.8(MyPlate): U.S. Dept. of Agriculture; 12.8(Avocado): © Ingram Publishing/SuperStock RF; 12.8(Asparagus), 12.8(Cheese): © Burke/ Triolo Productions/Getty Images RF; 12.8(Bread) © Everyday Images/Alamy RF; 12.8(Chicken): © Comstock/Jupiter Images RF; 12.9: The National Geochemical

Survey, U.S. Geological Survey (USGS Open-File Report 2004-1001); p. 401: © Royalty-Free/Corbis RF; 12.10 © Custom Medical Stock Photo/Newscom; p. 404(Child): © Brand X Pictures/ PunchStock RF; p. 405: © Michael Lamotte/Cole Group/Getty Images RF; p. 407(Crab): © C Squared Studios/Getty Images RF; 12.11: © Medical-on-Line/ Alamy; p. 411: © Image Source/Getty Images RF; p. 412: © Jonelle Weaver/Getty Images RF.

CHAPTER 13

Opener: © Wendy Schiff; 13.1: Centers for Disease Control, Behavioral Risk Factor Surveillance System; 13.3: © McGraw-Hill Education. Dennis Strete, photographer; Page 423(top): © Caro/Alamy; 13.6: © David Madison, Photographer's Choice/ Getty Images; 13.7: © Mary Dean Coleman-Kelly; 13.8: Photo Courtesy of Hologic, Inc.; 13.9: RJL Systems; 13.10: © Danielle Good; p. 427(top): © Ingram Publishing/ SuperStock RF; 13.13: © Hawley Almstedt; p. 428: © Thinkstock/Jupiter Images RF; p. 431: © Royalty-Free/Corbis RF; 13.14: © Carolyn Harris; 13.15: © Hawley Almstedt; 13.16: © Danielle Good; p. 439: © Wendy Schiff; p. 440: © Digital Vision/ Getty Images RF; p. 441: © yellowdog/ Cultura/AGE fotostock RF; p. 442(middle): © Rob Melynchuk/Getty Images RF; p. 442(bottom): © Wendy Schiff; p. 444: © Valerie Haapala; p. 445: © Creatas/ PunchStock RF; p. 446: Federal Trade Commission; p. 449: © McGraw-Hill Education. Jill Braaten, photographer; 13.23: © Girishh/Alamy; p. 452: © fStop/ Getty Images RF; p. 455: © Royalty-Free/ Corbis RF; p. 456: © Comstock Images/ Getty Images RF.

CHAPTER 14

Opener: © Halfdark/Getty Images RF; 14.1a: Courtesy National Gallery of Art, Washington; 14.1b: © Kristy-Anne Glubish/Design Pics RF; Page 462(top); © Lars A. Niki RF; 14.3: © Image Source/ PunchStock RF; p. 463: © Radius Images/ Alamy RF; p. 464(left): © Thinkstock/ Getty Images RF; p. 464(right): Courtesy National Gallery of Art, Washington; p, 465: © Photodisc/Getty Images RF; 14.4: © John Dowland/Getty Images RF; p. 466(middle): © Wendy Schiff; p. 468: © Ingram Publishing/SuperStock RF; p. 469(top): © Plush Studios/Getty Images RF; 14.5: © Ian Hooton/Science Source RF; p. 472: © Purestock/SuperStock RF;

p. 473: © Tetra Images/Getty Images RF; p. 475: © Purestock/SuperStock RF; p. 477: © Image Source/PunchStock RF.

CHAPTER 15

Opener: © Bruce McEntire/Getty Images RF; Page 481: © Erik Isakson/Getty Images RF; 15.1: © Royalty-Free/Corbis RF; 15.2(Desk): © Stockdisc/PunchStock RF; 15.2(Yoga): © Fancy Collection/SuperStock RF; 15.2(Cyclist): © Photodisc/Getty Images RF; 15.2(Stretching): © Ingram Publishing/Alamy RF; 15.2(Bench press): © Ingram Publishing/Alamy RF; 15.2(Gardener): © Stockdisc/PunchStock RF; 15.2(Stroller): © Ingram Publishing/Fotosearch RF; p. 484: © Ingram Publishing RF; 15.3: © Wendy Schiff; p. 485(bottom): © Sam Edwards/AGE fotostock RF; p. 486(top): © Ryan McVay/Getty Images RF; 15.4: © Wendy Schiff; p. 488: © McGraw-Hill Education. Christopher Kerrigan, photographer; p. 491: © Royalty-Free/Corbis RF; p. 495: © Martin Bureau/AFP/Getty Images; p. 496: © Wendy Schiff; p. 498: © D. Fischer & P. Lyons/Cole Group/Getty Images RF; p. 499: © Wendy Schiff; p. 503(top): © Tammy Stephenson; p. 503(bottom): © Wendy Schiff; p. 504: © Wendy Schiff; p. 505: © Javier Pierini/Getty Images RF; p. 507: © Royalty-Free/Corbis RF. p. 508: © Adam C. Gregor/Alamy RF; p. 509: © Chuck Berman/Chicago Tribune/MCT via Getty Images; p. 510(middle): © Chris Hyde/Getty Images; p. 510(bottom): © Wendy Schiff; p. 512: © Comstock/Alamy RF; p. 514: © Jill Braaten RF; p. 515: © John A. Rizzo/Getty Images RF; p. 516(left & middle): © McGraw-Hill Education. Jill Braaten, photographer; p. 516(right): © McGraw-Hill Education. Mark A. Dierker, photographer; p. 520: © Thinkstock/Jupiter Images RF; p. 521: © Wendy Schiff; p. 522: © Ed Carey/Cole Group/Getty Images RF; p. 524: © Fuse/Getty Images RF.

CHAPTER 16

Opener: © Tanya Constantine/Blend Images LLC RF; Page: 526: © Rosemarie Gearhart/iStockphoto RF; 16.1: © Realistic Reflections RF; p. 530(left): © FoodCollection/StockFood RF; p. 530(right): © Wendy Schiff; p. 531: © Andersen Ross/Getty Images RF; p. 532: © Lissette Le Bon/Purestock/SuperStock RF; p. 533(top): © Wendy Schiff; p. 533(bottom): © Peter Cade/Getty Images

RF; p. 534: © Plush Studios/Blend Images LLC RF; p. 537(left): © Royalty-Free/Corbis RF; p. 537(right): © Authur S. Aubry/Getty Images RF; p. 540: © Mike Marsland/WireImage/Getty Images; 16.8: © Royalty-Free/Corbis RF; p. 543: © Getty Images RF; p. 545(top): © Jose Luis Pelaez Inc/Blend Images LLC RF; p. 545(bottom): © Jiang Jin/Purestock/SuperStock RF; 16.9: © Wendy Schiff; p. 548: © BananaStock/PunchStock RF; p. 549: © Wendy Schiff.

CHAPTER 17

Opener: © Darren Greenwood/Design Pics RF; 17.1a: © Photodisc/Getty Images RF; 17.1b: © Brand X Pictures/PunchStock RF; Page 555: © Kwame Zikomo/Purestock/SuperStock RF; p. 557(all): © Wendy Schiff; p. 558: © Creatas/PictureQuest RF; p. 559(top): © Brand X Pictures/PunchStock RF; p. 559(bottom): © Sky View/Digital Vision/Getty Images RF: 17.3: © Wendy Schiff; p. 560(bottom): © Dynamic Graphics Group/PunchStock RF; 17.4: © Royalty-Free/Corbis RF. 17.5: © Nancy Ney/Getty Images RF; p. 562(top): © BananaStock/PictureQuest RF; p. 562(middle): © Ocean/Corbis RF; p. 562(bottom): © Francisco Cruz/Purestock/SuperStock RF; p. 563: © Hero/Corbis/Glow Images RF; p. 564: © Fancy Collection/SuperStock RF; 17.6: U.S. Department of Agriculture, Center for Nutrition Policy and Promotion; p. 565(middle): © Mazer RF; p. 565(bottom): © KidStock/Getty Images RF; p. 566: © Blend Images/Gerry Images RF; p. 567(top): © Pixtal/AGE fotostock RF; 17.7: U.S. Dept. of Agriculture, Center for Nutrition Policy and Promotion; p. 568: © Purestock/Getty Images RF; p. 569: © Image Source/Getty Images RF; 17.10: © Image Source/Corbis RF; p. 573: © Rolf Bruderer/Getty Images RF; p. 576, p. 577(top): © Wendy Schiff; p. 577(bottom): © Hieng Ling Tie/AGE fotostock RF; p. 580: © Florian Franke/Purestock/SuperStock RF.

CHAPTER 18

Opener: © Don Hammond/Design Pics RF; Page 583: © Urikiri-Shashin-Kan/Alamy RF; p. 584: © Photodisc/Getty Images RF; p. 586: U.S. Dept. of Agriculture; p. 587: © S. Meltzer/PhotoLink/Photodisc/Getty Images RF; p. 588: © Photodisc/Getty Images RF; p. 589: © Brand X/Jupiter Images/Getty Images RF; p. 590:

© Wendy Schiff; p. 591: © Skip Nall/Getty Images RF; p. 592(left): © McGraw-Hill Education; p. 592(right): © Stockdisc/PunchStock RF; p. 593: © Realistic Reflections RF; p. 594(left): © Realistic Reflections RF; p. 594(right): © Ryan McVay/Getty Images RF; p. 595: © Realistic Reflections RF; p. 596: © McGraw-Hill Education. Mark Steinmetz, photographer; p. 598: © Photodisc/Getty Images RF; p. 599: © Hill Street Studios/Blend Images LLC RF; p. 600: © Wendy Schiff; p. 602: © Kristy-Anne Glubish/Design Pics RF.

CHAPTER 19

Opener: © Thinkstock/Jupiter Images RF; Page 605: © FoodCollection/StockFood RF; p. 606(top): © John A. Rizzo/Digital Vision/Getty Images RF; 19.1: © Wendy Schiff; p. 607(top): © Westend61/Alamy RF; p. 607(bottom): © Dynamic Graphics Group/IT Stock Free/Alamy RF; p. 608(left): © Tammy Stephenson; p. 608(right): © McGraw-Hill Education. Richard Hutchings, photographer; p. 608(bottom): © Brand X Pictures/PunchStock RF; p. 610(top): © Science Photo Library RF/Getty Images RF; p. 610(bottom): © FoodCollection/StockFood RF; p. 611(top): Renee Comet/National Cancer Institute (NCI); p. 611(bottom): © Eye of Science/Science Source; p. 612(middle): © Corbis/PunchStock RF; 19.3: Centers for Disease Control/Charles D. Humphrey; p. 614(top): © MedicalRF.com RF; p. 614(bottom): Centers for Disease Control/James Gatheny; 19.4: © Nick Kirk/Alamy RF; p. 616: © Royalty-Free/Corbis RF; 19.6: © Wendy Schiff; p. 618: © John A. Rizzo/Getty Images RF; 19.7, p. 620: © Wendy Schiff; 19.8: U.S. Department of Agriculture, Food Safety and Inspection Service; p. 623(top): © McGraw-Hill Education. John Thoeming, photographer; 19.9: © Lauren Petr Cromer; p. 624(middle): © Robert George Young/Getty Images RF; 19.10: Photo by Stephen Ausmus/ARS/USDA; 19.11: U.S. Department of Agriculture, Food Safety and Inspection Service; p. 625(bottom): © FoodCollection/StockFood RF; p. 627: © Charles Bowman/Alamy RF; 19.12, 19.13: © Wendy Schiff; 19.14: ARS/USDA; 19.14: ARS/USDA; p. 631: © BananaStock/Jupiter Images RF; p. 632: © vm/E+/Getty Images RF; p. 633(top): DoD/U.S. Air Force photo by Master Sgt. Mark C. Olsen; p. 633(bottom): Courtesy of

Katadyn North America; p. 636: © Stockbyte/PunchStock RF; p. 637: © Jupiter Images/Comstock Images/Alamy RF; p. 638: © Royalty-Free/Corbis RF.

CHAPTER 20

Opener: © Janet Mullins; Page 641: © 1997 IMS Communications Ltd/Capstone Design. All Rights Reserved. RF; p. 642(top): © Author's Image/PunchStock RF; p. 642(bottom): © Dr. Parvinder Sethi RF; 20.2: Centers for Disease Control/ Dr. Lyle Conrad; p. 644(bottom): © Tammy Stephenson; p. 645: © Ingram Publishing/Alamy RF; p. 647: © Ingram Publishing RF; p. 648(left): © 1997 IMS Communications Ltd/Capstone Design. All Rights Reserved. RF; p. 648(right): © Elena Elisseeva/Alamy RF; 20.3: © Don Hammond/Design Pics RF; 20.4: © Pixtal/ AGE fotostock RF; p. 652(left): U.S. Navy photo by Photographer's mate Airman Joshua T. Rodriguez; p. 652(middle): © Gina Logue; p. 652(bottom): © 2014 Universities Fighting World Hunger. All Rights Reserved.; 20.5: © MedioImages/ Getty Images RF; 20.6a-b: © Tammy Stephenson; p. 656: © John Rensten/Getty Images RF; p. 658: © Digitial Vision/ PunchStock RF; p. 660: © Getty Images RF; p. 661: Centers for Disease Control/ James Gatheny.

APPENDIX

B.6, B.7: © Wendy Schiff; Page A-23: © Custom Medical Stock Photo/Alamy RF; p. A-25: © Pixtal/AGE fotostock RF; F.1(left): © Stockbyte/Getty Images RF; F.1(right): © JGI/Blend Images LLC RF; F.2: USDA Photo by Ken Hammond; F.3: © McGraw-Hill Education; F.4: © SECA; F.6: © Pixtal/AGE fotostock RF.

Index

A

Dietary Reference Intakes (DRIs): Recommended Intakes for Individuals, Vitamins
Food and Nutrition Board, Institute of Medicine, National Academies

Life Stage Group	Vitamin A (µg/d)[a]	Vitamin C (mg/d)	Vitamin D (µg/d)[b,c]	Vitamin E (mg/d)[d]	Vitamin K (µg/d)	Thiamin (mg/d)	Riboflavin (mg/d)	Niacin (mg/d)[e]	Vitamin B-6 (mg/d)	Folate (µg/d)[f]	Vitamin B-12 (µg/d)	Pantothenic Acid (mg/d)	Biotin (µg/d)	Choline (mg/d)[g]
Infants														
0–6 mo	400*	40*	10	4*	2.0*	0.2*	0.3*	2*	0.1*	65*	0.4*	1.7*	5*	125*
7–12 mo	500*	50*	10	5*	2.5*	0.3*	0.4*	4*	0.3*	80*	0.5*	1.8*	6*	150*
Children														
1–3 y	300	15	15	6	30*	0.5	0.5	6	0.5	150	0.9	2*	8*	200*
4–8 y	400	25	15	7	55*	0.6	0.6	8	0.6	200	1.2	3*	12*	250*
Males														
9–13 y	600	45	15	11	60*	0.9	0.9	12	1.0	300	1.8	4*	20*	375*
14–18 y	900	75	15	15	75*	1.2	1.3	16	1.3	400	2.4	5*	25*	550*
19–30 y	900	90	15	15	120*	1.2	1.3	16	1.3	400	2.4	5*	30*	550*
31–50 y	900	90	15	15	120*	1.2	1.3	16	1.3	400	2.4	5*	30*	550*
51–70 y	900	90	15	15	120*	1.2	1.3	16	1.7	400	2.4[h]	5*	30*	550*
>70 y	900	90	20	15	120*	1.2	1.3	16	1.7	400	2.4[h]	5*	30*	550*
Females														
9–13 y	600	45	15	11	60*	0.9	0.9	12	1.0	300	1.8	4*	20*	375*
14–18 y	700	65	15	15	75*	1.0	1.0	14	1.2	400[i]	2.4	5*	25*	400*
19–30 y	700	75	15	15	90*	1.1	1.1	14	1.3	400[i]	2.4	5*	30*	425*
31–50 y	700	75	15	15	90*	1.1	1.1	14	1.3	400[i]	2.4	5*	30*	425*
51–70 y	700	75	15	15	90*	1.1	1.1	14	1.5	400	2.4[h]	5*	30*	425*
>70 y	700	75	20	15	90*	1.1	1.1	14	1.5	400	2.4[h]	5*	30*	425*
Pregnancy														
≤18 y	750	80	15	15	75*	1.4	1.4	18	1.9	600[j]	2.6	6*	30*	450*
19–30 y	770	85	15	15	90*	1.4	1.4	18	1.9	600[j]	2.6	6*	30*	450*
31–50 y	770	85	15	15	90*	1.4	1.4	18	1.9	600[j]	2.6	6*	30*	450*
Lactation														
≤18 y	1200	115	15	19	75*	1.4	1.6	17	2.0	500	2.8	7*	35*	550*
19–30 y	1300	120	15	19	90*	1.4	1.6	17	2.0	500	2.8	7*	35*	550*
31–50 y	1300	120	15	19	90*	1.4	1.6	17	2.0	500	2.8	7*	35*	550*

mg = milligram, µg = microgram

NOTE: This table (taken from the DRI reports; see www.nap.edu) presents Recommended Dietary Allowances (RDAs) in **bold type** and Adequate Intakes (AIs) in ordinary type followed by an asterisk (*). RDAs and AIs may both be used as goals for individual intake. RDAs are set to meet the needs of almost all (97 to 98%) individuals in a group. For healthy breastfed infants, the AI is the mean intake. The AI for other life stage and gender groups is believed to cover needs of all individuals in the group, but lack of data or uncertainty in the data prevents being able to specify with confidence the percentage of individuals covered by this intake.

[a] As retinol activity equivalents (RAEs). 1 RAE = 1 µg retinol, 12 µg β–carotene, 24 µg α–carotene, or 24 µg β–cryptoxanthin. To calculate RAEs from REs of provitamin A carotenoids in foods, divide the REs by 2. For preformed vitamin A in foods or supplements and for provitamin A carotenoids in supplements, 1 RE = 1 RAE.

[b] cholecalciferol. 1 µg cholecalciferol = 40 IU vitamin D.

[c] In the absence of adequate exposure to sunlight.

[d] As α–tocopherol. α–Tocopherol includes RRR–α–tocopherol, the only form of α–tocopherol that occurs naturally in foods, and the 2R–stereoisomeric forms of α–tocopherol (RRR–, RSR–, RRS–, and RSS–α–tocopherol) that occur in fortified foods and supplements. It does not include the 2S–stereoisomeric forms of α–tocopherol (SRR–, SSR–, SRS–, and SSS–α–tocopherol), also found in fortified foods and supplements.

[e] As niacin equivalents (NE). 1 mg of niacin = 60 mg of tryptophan; 0–6 months = preformed niacin (not NE).

[f] As dietary folate equivalents (DFE). 1 DFE = 1 µg food folate = 0.6 µg of folic acid from fortified food or as a supplement consumed with food = 0.5 µg of a supplement taken on an empty stomach.

[g] Although AIs have been set for choline, there are few data to assess whether a dietary supply of choline is needed at all stages of the life cycle, and it may be that the choline requirement can be met by endogenous synthesis at some of these stages.

[h] Because 10 to 30% of older people may malabsorb food–bound B–12, it is advisable for those older than 50 years to meet their RDA mainly by consuming foods fortified with B–12 or a supplement containing B–12.

[i] In view of evidence linking folate intake with neural tube defects in the fetus, it is recommended that all women capable of becoming pregnant consume 400 µg from supplements or fortified foods in addition to intake of food folate from a varied diet.

[j] It is assumed that women will continue consuming 400 µg from supplements or fortified food until their pregnancy is confirmed and they enter prenatal care, which ordinarily occurs after the end of the periconceptional period—the critical time for formation of the neural tube.

Dietary Reference Intakes (DRIs): Recommended Intakes for Individuals, Elements
Food and Nutrition Board, Institute of Medicine, National Academies

Life Stage Group	Calcium (mg/d)	Chromium (µg/d)	Copper (µg/d)	Fluoride (mg/d)	Iodine (µg/d)	Iron (mg/d)	Magnesium (mg/d)	Manganese (mg/d)	Molybdenum (µg/d)	Phosphorus (mg/d)	Selenium (µg/d)	Zinc (mg/d)
Infants												
0–6 mo	200*	0.2*	200*	0.01*	110*	0.27*	30*	0.003*	2*	100*	15*	2*
7–12 mo	260*	5.5*	220*	0.5*	130*	11	75*	0.6*	3*	275*	20*	3
Children												
1–3 y	700	11*	340	0.7*	90	7	80	1.2*	17	460	20	3
4–8 y	1000	15*	440	1*	90	10	130	1.5*	22	500	30	5
Males												
9–13 y	1300	25*	700	2*	120	8	240	1.9*	34	1250	40	8
14–18 y	1300	35*	890	3*	150	11	410	2.2*	43	1250	55	11
19–30 y	1000	35*	900	4*	150	8	400	2.3*	45	700	55	11
31–50 y	1000	35*	900	4*	150	8	420	2.3*	45	700	55	11
51–70 y	1000	30*	900	4*	150	8	420	2.3*	45	700	55	11
>70 y	1200	30*	900	4*	150	8	420	2.3*	45	700	55	11
Females												
9–13 y	1300	21*	700	2*	120	8	240	1.6*	34	1250	40	8
14–18 y	1300	24*	890	3*	150	15	360	1.6*	43	1250	55	9
19–30 y	1000	25*	900	3*	150	18	310	1.8*	45	700	55	8
31–50 y	1000	25*	900	3*	150	18	320	1.8*	45	700	55	8
51–70 y	1200	20*	900	3*	150	8	320	1.8*	45	700	55	8
>70 y	1200	20*	900	3*	150	8	320	1.8*	45	700	55	8
Pregnancy												
≤18 y	1300	29*	1000	3*	220	27	400	2.0*	50	1250	60	12
19–30 y	1000	30*	1000	3*	220	27	350	2.0*	50	700	60	11
31–50 y	1000	30*	1000	3*	220	27	360	2.0*	50	700	60	11
Lactation												
≤18 y	1300	44*	1300	3*	290	10	360	2.6*	50	1250	70	13
19–30 y	1000	45*	1300	3*	290	9	310	2.6*	50	700	70	12
31–50 y	1000	45*	1300	3*	290	9	320	2.6*	50	700	70	12

NOTE: This table presents Recommended Dietary Allowances (RDAs) in **bold type** and Adequate Intakes (AIs) in ordinary type followed by an asterisk (*). RDAs and AIs may both be used as goals for individual intake. RDAs are set to meet the needs of almost all (97 to 98%) individuals in a group. For healthy breastfed infants, the AI is the mean intake. The AI for other life stage and gender groups is believed to cover needs of all individuals in the group, but lack of data or uncertainty in the data prevents being able to specify with confidence the percentage of individuals covered by this intake.

Sources: Dietary Reference Intakes for Calcium, Phosphorus, Magnesium, Vitamin D, and Fluoride (1997); Dietary Reference Intakes for Thiamin, Riboflavin, Niacin, Vitamin B–6, Folate, Vitamin B–12, Pantothenic Acid, Biotin, and Choline (1998); Dietary Reference Intakes for Vitamin C, Vitamin E, Selenium, and Carotenoids (2000); Dietary Reference Intakes for Vitamin A, Vitamin K, Arsenic, Boron, Chromium, Copper, Iodine, Iron, Manganese, Molybdenum, Nickel, Silicon, Vanadium, and Zinc (2001); and Dietary Reference Intakes for Calcium and Vitamin D (2011). These reports may be accessed via www.nap.edu. The full reports are available from the National Academies Press at www.nap.edu.

Adapted from the Dietary Reference Intake series, National Academies Press. Copyright 1997, 1998, 2000, 2001, and 2011 by the National Academy of Sciences.

C

Dietary Reference Intakes (DRIs): Recommended Intakes for Individuals, Macronutrients
Food and Nutrition Board, Institute of Medicine, National Academies

Life Stage Group	Carbohydrate (g/d)	Total Fiber (g/d)	Fat (g/d)	Linoleic Acid (g/d)	α–Linolenic Acid (g/d)	Protein[a] (g/d)
Infants						
0–6 mo	60*	ND	31*	4.4*	0.5*	9.1*
7–12 mo	95*	ND	30*	4.6*	0.5*	**11.0**
Children						
1–3 y	130	19*	ND[b]	7*	0.7*	**13**
4–8 y	130	25*	ND	10*	0.9*	**19**
Males						
9–13 y	130	31*	ND	12*	1.2*	**34**
14–18 y	130	38*	ND	16*	1.6*	**52**
19–30 y	130	38*	ND	17*	1.6*	**56**
31–50 y	130	38*	ND	17*	1.6*	**56**
51–70 y	130	30*	ND	14*	1.6*	**56**
>70 y	130	30*	ND	14*	1.6*	**56**
Females						
9–13 y	130	26*	ND	10*	1.0*	**34**
14–18 y	130	26*	ND	11*	1.1*	**46**
19–30 y	130	25*	ND	12*	1.1*	**46**
31–50 y	130	25*	ND	12*	1.1*	**46**
51–70 y	130	21*	ND	11*	1.1*	**46**
>70 y	130	21*	ND	11*	1.1*	**46**
Pregnancy						
14–18 y	175	28*	ND	13*	1.4*	**71**
19–30 y	175	28*	ND	13*	1.4*	**71**
31–50 y	175	28*	ND	13*	1.4*	**71**
Lactation						
14–18 y	210	29*	ND	13*	1.3*	**71**
19–30 y	210	29*	ND	13*	1.3*	**71**
31–50 y	210	29*	ND	13*	1.3*	**71**

NOTE: This table presents Recommended Dietary Allowances (RDAs) in **bold type** and Adequate Intakes (AIs) in ordinary type followed by an asterisk (*). RDAs and AIs may both be used as goals for individual intake. RDAs are set to meet the needs of almost all (97 to 98%) individuals in a group. For healthy breastfed infants, the AI is the mean intake. The AI for other life stage and gender groups is believed to cover needs of all individuals in the group, but lack of data or uncertainty in the data prevents being able to specify with confidence the percentage of individuals covered by this intake.

[a] Based on 0.8g protein/kg body weight for reference body weight.
[b] ND = not determinable at this time.

Sources: Dietary Reference Intakes for Energy, Carbohydrate, Fiber, Fat, Fatty Acids, Cholesterol, Protein, and Amino Acids (2002). Copyright 1997, 1998, 2000, 2001, by the National Academy of Sciences. The full reports are available from the National Academies Press at www.nap.edu.
Adapted from the Dietary Reference Intakes series, National Academies Press.

D

Dietary Reference Intakes (DRIs): Recommended Intakes for Individuals, Electrolytes and Water
Food and Nutrition Board, Institute of Medicine, National Academies

Life Stage Group	Sodium (mg/d)	Potassium (mg/d)	Chloride (mg/d)	Water (L/d)
Infants				
0–6 mo	120*	400*	180*	0.7*
7–12 mo	370*	700*	570*	0.8*
Children				
1–3 y	1000*	3000*	1500*	1.3*
4–8 y	1200*	3800*	1900*	1.7*
Males				
9–13 y	1500*	4500*	2300*	2.4*
14–18 y	1500*	4700*	2300*	3.3*
19–30 y	1500*	4700*	2300*	3.7*
31–50 y	1500*	4700*	2300*	3.7*
51–70 y	1300*	4700*	2000*	3.7*
> 70 y	1200*	4700*	1800*	3.7*
Females				
9–13 y	1500*	4500*	2300*	2.1*
14–18 y	1500*	4700*	2300*	2.3*
19–30 y	1500*	4700*	2300*	2.7*
31–50 y	1500*	4700*	2300*	2.7*
51–70 y	1300*	4700*	2000*	2.7*
> 70 y	1200*	4700*	1800*	2.7*
Pregnancy				
14–18 y	1500*	4700*	2300*	3.0*
19–50 y	1500*	4700*	2300*	3.0*
Lactation				
14–18 y	1500*	5100*	2300*	3.8*
19–50 y	1500*	5100*	2300*	3.8*

NOTE: The table is adapted from the DRI reports. See www.nap.edu. Adequate Intakes (AIs) are followed by an asterisk (*). These may be used as a goal for individual intake. For healthy breastfed infants, the AI is the average intake. The AI for other life stage and gender groups is believed to cover the needs of all individuals in the group, but lack of data prevent being able to specify with confidence the percentage of individuals covered by this intake; therefore, no Recommended Dietary Allowance (RDA) was set.

Source: *Dietary Reference Intakes for Water, Potassium, Sodium, Chloride, and Sulfate* (2005). This report may be accessed via www.nap.edu.

Acceptable Macronutrient Distribution Ranges

Macronutrient	Range (percent of energy)		
	Children, 1–3 y	Children, 4–18 y	Adults
Fat	30–40	25–35	20–35
omega–6 polyunsaturated fats (linoleic acid)	5–10	5–10	5–10
omega–3 polyunsaturated fats[a] (α–linolenic acid)	0.6–1.2	0.6–1.2	0.6–1.2
Carbohydrate	45–65	45–65	45–65
Protein	5–20	10–30	10–35

[a]Approximately 10% of the total can come from longer–chain n–3 fatty acids.

SOURCE: *Dietary Reference Intakes for Energy, Carbohydrate, Fiber, Fat, Fatty Acids, Cholesterol, Protein, and Amino Acids* (2002). The report may be accessed via www.nap.edu.

Adapted from the Dietary Reference Intakes series, National Academies Press. Copyright 1997, 1998, 2000, 2001, 2011, by the National Academy of Sciences. The full reports are available from the National Academies Press at www.nap.edu.

Dietary Reference Intakes (DRIs): Tolerable Upper Intake Levels (UL[a]), Vitamins
Food and Nutrition Board, Institute of Medicine, National Academies

Life Stage Group	Vitamin A (μg/d)[b]	Vitamin C (mg/d)	Vitamin D (μg/d)	Vitamin E (mg/d)[c,d]	Vitamin K	Thiamin	Riboflavin	Niacin (mg/d)[d]	Vitamin B–6 (mg/d)	Folate (μg/d)[d]	Vitamin B–12	Pantothenic Acid	Biotin	Choline (g/d)	Carotenoids[e]
Infants															
0–6 mo	600	ND	25	ND	ND	ND	ND	ND	ND	ND	ND	ND	ND	ND	ND
7–12 mo	600	ND	38	ND	ND	ND	ND	ND	ND	ND	ND	ND	ND	ND	ND
Children															
1–3 y	600	400	63	200	ND	ND	ND	10	30	300	ND	ND	ND	1.0	ND
4–8 y	900	650	75	300	ND	ND	ND	15	40	400	ND	ND	ND	1.0	ND
Males, Females															
9–13 y	1700	1200	100	600	ND	ND	ND	20	60	600	ND	ND	ND	2.0	ND
14–18 y	2800	1800	100	800	ND	ND	ND	30	80	800	ND	ND	ND	3.0	ND
19–70 y	3000	2000	100	1000	ND	ND	ND	35	100	1000	ND	ND	ND	3.5	ND
>70 y	3000	2000	100	1000	ND	ND	ND	35	100	1000	ND	ND	ND	3.5	ND
Pregnancy															
≤18 y	2800	1800	100	800	ND	ND	ND	30	80	800	ND	ND	ND	3.0	ND
19–50 y	3000	2000	100	1000	ND	ND	ND	35	100	1000	ND	ND	ND	3.5	ND
Lactation															
≤18 y	2800	1800	100	800	ND	ND	ND	30	80	800	ND	ND	ND	3.0	ND
19–50 y	3000	2000	100	1000	ND	ND	ND	35	100	1000	ND	ND	ND	3.5	ND

[a]UL = The maximum level of daily nutrient intake likely to pose no risk of adverse effects. Unless otherwise specified, the UL represents total intake from food, water, and supplements. Due to lack of suitable data, ULs could not be established for vitamin K, thiamin, riboflavin, vitamin B–12, pantothenic acid, biotin, or carotenoids. In the absence of ULs, extra caution may be warranted in consuming levels above recommended intakes.

[b]As preformed vitamin A.

[c]As α–tocopherol; applies to any form of supplemental α–tocopherol.

[d]The ULs for vitamin E, niacin, and folate apply to synthetic forms obtained from supplements, fortified foods, or a combination of the two.

[e]β–Carotene supplements are advised only to serve as a provitamin A source for individuals at risk of vitamin A deficiency.

[f]ND = Not determinable due to lack of data of adverse effects in this age group and concern with regard to lack of ability to handle excess amounts. Source of intake should be from food only to prevent high levels of intake.

SOURCES: Dietary Reference Intakes for Calcium and Vitamin D (2011); Dietary Reference Intakes for Calcium, Phosphorus, Magnesium, Vitamin D, and Fluoride (1997); Dietary Reference Intakes for Thiamin, Riboflavin, Niacin, Vitamin B–6, Folate, Vitamin B–12, Pantothenic Acid, Biotin, and Choline (1998); Dietary Reference Intakes for Vitamin C, Vitamin E, Selenium, and Carotenoids (2000); and Dietary Reference Intakes for Vitamin A, Vitamin K, Arsenic, Boron, Chromium, Copper, Iodine, Iron, Manganese, Molybdenum, Nickel, Silicon, Vanadium, and Zinc (2001). These reports may be accessed via www.nap.edu. The full reports are available from the National Academies Press at www.nap.edu.

Adapted from the Dietary Reference Intakes series, National Academies Press. Copyright 1997, 1998, 2000, 2001, 2011, by the National Academy of Sciences.

F

Dietary Reference Intakes (DRIs): Tolerable Upper Intake Levels (UL[a]), Elements and Electrolytes[b,c]
Food and Nutrition Board, Institute of Medicine, National Academies

Life Stage Group	Arsenic[b]	Boron (mg/d)	Calcium (g/d)	Copper (µg/d)	Fluoride (mg/d)	Iodine (µg/d)	Iron (mg/d)	Magnesium (mg/d)[d]	Manganese (mg/d)	Molybdenum (µg/d)	Nickel (mg/d)	Phosphorus (g/d)	Selenium (µg/d)	Vanadium (mg/d)[e]	Zinc (mg/d)	Sodium (mg/d)	Chloride (mg/d)
Infants																	
0–6 mo	ND[f]	ND	1	ND	0.7	ND	40	ND	ND	ND	ND	ND	45	ND	4	ND	ND
7–12 mo	ND	ND	1.5	ND	0.9	ND	40	ND	ND	ND	ND	ND	60	ND	5	ND	ND
Children																	
1–3 y	ND	3	2.5	1000	1.3	200	40	65	2	300	0.2	3	90	ND	7	1500	2300
4–8 y	ND	6	2.5	3000	2.2	300	40	110	3	600	0.3	3	150	ND	12	1900	2900
Males, Females																	
9–13 y	ND	11	3	5000	10	600	40	350	6	1100	0.6	4	280	ND	23	2200	3400
14–18 y	ND	17	3	8000	10	900	45	350	9	1700	1.0	4	400	ND	34	2300	3600
19–70 y	ND	20	2.5[g]	10000	10	1100	45	350	11	2000	1.0	4	400	1.8	40	2300	3600
>70 y	ND	20	2	10000	10	1100	45	350	11	2000	1.0	3	400	1.8	40	2300	3600
Pregnancy																	
≤18 y	ND	17	3	8000	10	900	45	350	9	1700	1.0	3.5	400	ND	34	2300	3600
19–50 y	ND	20	2.5	10000	10	1100	45	350	11	2000	1.0	3.5	400	ND	40	2300	3600
Lactation																	
≤18 y	ND	17	3	8000	10	900	45	350	9	1700	1.0	4	400	ND	34	2300	3600
19–50 y	ND	20	2.5	10000	10	1100	45	350	11	2000	1.0	4	400	ND	40	2300	3600

[a]UL = The maximum level of daily nutrient intake that is likely to pose no risk of adverse effects. Unless otherwise specified, the UL represents total intake from food, water, and supplements. Due to lack of suitable data, ULs could not be established for arsenic, chromium, and silicon. In the absence of ULs, extra caution may be warranted in consuming levels above recommended intakes.

[b]Although a UL was not determined for arsenic, there is no justification for adding arsenic to food or supplements.

[c]Although silicon has not been shown to cause adverse effects in humans, there is no justification for adding silicon to supplements.

[d]The ULs for magnesium represent intake from a pharmacological agent only and do not include intake from food and water.

[e]Although vanadium in food has not been shown to cause adverse effects in humans, there is no justification for adding vanadium to food and vanadium supplements should be used with caution. The UL is based on adverse effects in laboratory animals and this data could be used to set a UL for adults but not children and adolescents.

[f]ND = Not determinable due to lack of data of adverse effects in this age group and concern with regard to lack of ability to handle excess amounts. Source of intake should be from food only to prevent high levels of intake.

[g]Upper Limit declines to 2 after age 50.

SOURCES: Dietary Reference Intakes for Calcium and Vitamin D (2011); Dietary Reference Intakes for Calcium, Phosphorus, Magnesium, Vitamin D, and Fluoride (1997); Dietary Reference Intakes for Thiamin, Riboflavin, Niacin, Vitamin B–6, Folate, Vitamin B–12, Pantothenic Acid, Biotin, and Choline (1998); Dietary Reference Intakes for Vitamin C, Vitamin E, Selenium, and Carotenoids (2000); Dietary Reference Intakes for Vitamin A, Vitamin K, Arsenic, Boron, Chromium, Copper, Iodine, Iron, Manganese, Molybdenum, Nickel, Silicon, Vanadium, and Zinc (2001); and Dietary Reference Intakes for Water, Potassium, Sodium, Chloride, and Sulfate (2004). These reports may be accessed via www.nap.edu. The full reports are available from the National Academies Press at www.nap.edu.

Adapted from the Dietary Reference Intakes series, National Academies Press. Copyright 1997, 1998, 2000, 2001, 2011, by the National Academy of Sciences.